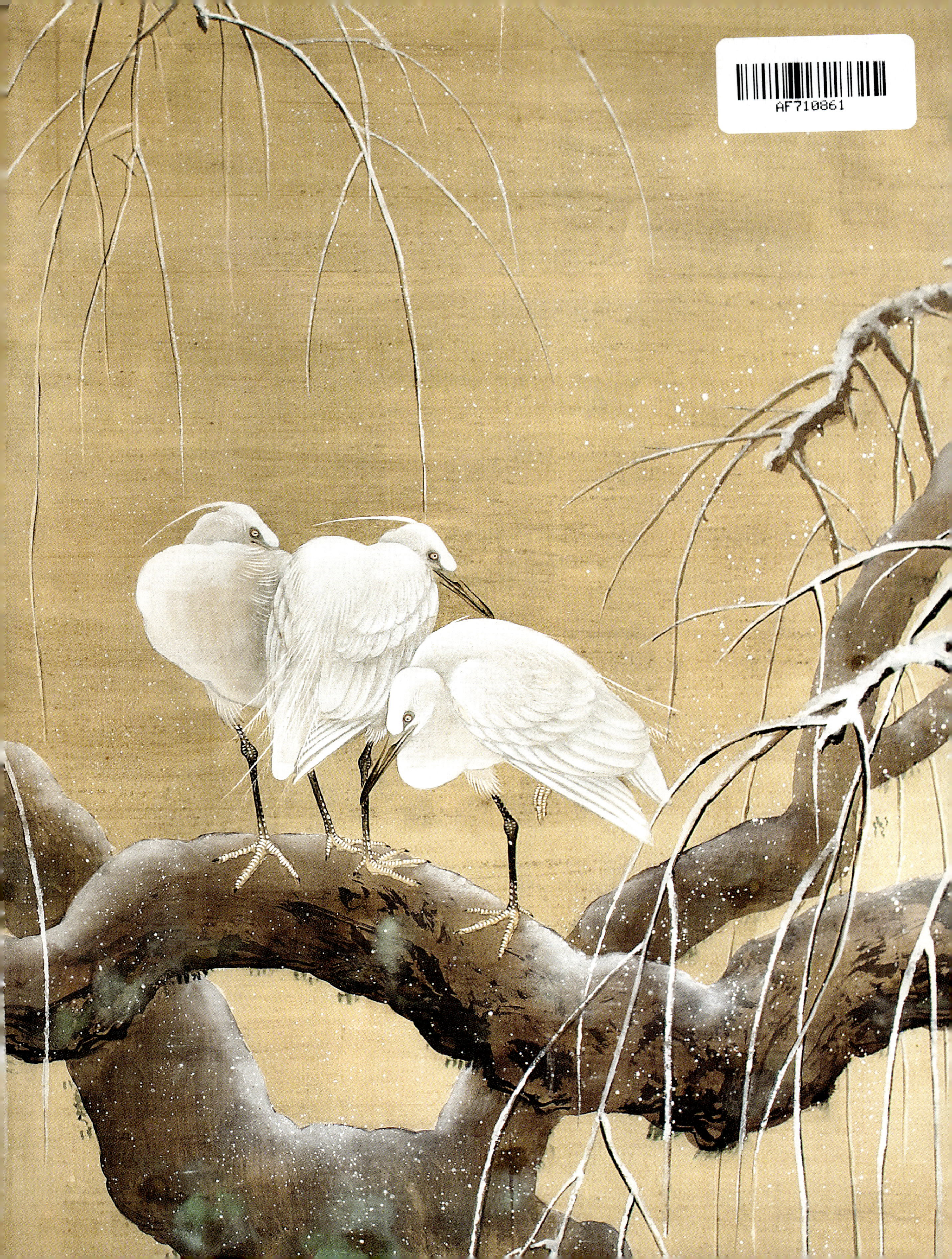

Interdisciplinary Treatment Planning, Volume II

Comprehensive Case Studies

About the Illustration on the Endsheets

In Japan and China, cranes are revered as a symbol of wisdom, longevity, and honor. Here they rest on an old and battered tree. With its snowy shoots and lichen, the gnarled tree symbolizes not only age and endurance, but also rebirth and renewal. In this masterpiece of Meiji-era painting, the snow-clad bamboo adds another layer of meaning, as it represents the flexibility and resilience of this tough plant that bends but does not break under the weight of the snow. The message for those who would seek to master treatment planning is that knowledge does not come easily, and there will be obstacles along the way. But those who study with discipline and patience will be rewarded with the ability to look beyond appearances and see the deeper meaning. This is the essence of wisdom.

Japanese Meiji Period Snow Cranes screen (detail), courtesy of Michael Ayervais Collection (www.japaneseartsite.com).

Interdisciplinary Treatment Planning, Volume II

Comprehensive Case Studies

Editor

Michael Cohen, DDS, MSD

Affiliate Assistant Professor
Department of Periodontics
University of Washington School of Dentistry
Seattle, Washington

Private practice
Seattle, Washington

quintessence books

Quintessence Publishing Co, Inc

Chicago, Berlin, Tokyo, London, Paris, Milan, Barcelona,
Istanbul, São Paulo, Mumbai, Moscow, Prague, and Warsaw

Library of Congress Cataloging-in-Publication Data

Interdisciplinary treatment planning : comprehensive case studies / [edited by] Michael Cohen.
p. ; cm.
Includes bibliographical references and index.
ISBN 978-0-86715-474-0 (hardcover)
1. Dental therapeutics--Planning. 2. Dental teams. I. Cohen, Michael, 1948-
[DNLM: 1. Tooth Diseases--surgery. 2. Comprehensive Dental Care--methods. 3. Esthetics, Dental. 4. Oral Surgical Procedures--methods. 5. Patient Care Planning. 6. Periodontal Diseases--surgery. WU 166 I606 2008]
RK318.I58 2008
617.6'01--dc22
2007047401

5 4 3 2 1

Quintessence Publishing Co, Inc
4350 Chandler Drive
Hanover Park, IL 60133
www.quintpub.com

Editor: Lisa C. Bywaters
Assistant editor: Leah Huffman
Cover and internal design: Ted Pereda
Production: Patrick Penney

Printed in China

Table of Contents

Foreword

Interdisciplinary Treatment Planning, Volume I introduced the dental profession to the Seattle Study Club community and its philosophy and focus on case planning, and it is widely anticipated that this second volume will once again achieve the same extraordinary acceptance and worldwide impact. Demonstrating the need for a detailed comprehensive treatment reference for the general practitioner and the specialist alike, and with a focus on practical case treatment, this second volume explores in further depth the essentials of interdisciplinary planning.

The unique standards set in each chapter are due not only to the astonishing quality of the clinical results displayed by all the authors but also to their strict discipline and coordination with their own respective team members. Once again in this second volume, the enthusiasm and experience of the authors permeate each chapter through their uncompromising commitment to quality dentistry and their knowledge of multiphased treatment, as well as their confidence in the vision and success of the final outcome.

The impact of this landmark text will be felt in private as well as academic settings, where I have watched postgraduate students of various specialties open the first volume in awe and read over chapters in utter amazement. To these specialty residents and general practitioners alike, the first step is to simply acquire the right mind-set and be disposed to seek collaboration with other experts from the start of their careers. The next step is to understand that this collaboration skill will develop as a lifelong endeavor and that it is a professional journey indeed.

Interdisciplinary dentistry should be given priority as early as possible because of the prime importance of diagnosis. This volume greatly elaborates on this topic and devotes considerable attention to the diagnostic phase, and the reader should appreciate the detailed lists of problems outlined in each case presentation and the organized progression that leads to a meticulous diagnosis. It is critical to note that the computation and processing of the data into each treatment sequence is multidisciplinary in nature and pooled from several other specialties, either directly or indirectly. In this fashion, the scope and quality of the diagnosis becomes considerably widened because the clinician becomes acutely aware of the nuances and fine correlations between tooth size, tooth position, gingival levels, occlusal status, implant placement, and periodontal condition.

The ability to collect and correlate the data across the specialties and sequence and coordinate multiphased treatment is a competence that is acquired over time. For many, this journey was made possible through the vision of Michael Cohen, who assembled a number of study clubs structured around one unifying principle: case planning and treatment through a practical team approach. Certainly, a consequence of this approach was the elevation of the quality of dental care in daily practice, and over the years the number of such study clubs has grown exponentially across a multitude of small and large communities nationwide. Most importantly, the foundation of this club community is based on the fact that dental practitioners cannot practice in isolation, and today more than ever, with the explosive growth of implant dentistry, esthetic dentistry, and adult orthodontics, they need to merge their own expertise with that of their team of specialists. While this is a given in an academic setting where access to specialists is within the same building, a study club approach with such a structured forum provides a tailored continuing education program within a "university without walls."

Another key foundation of the Seattle Study Club is the focus on interactive treatment planning as opposed to passive learning. The mutual interaction between the various members leads to the exploration of various treatment options and formulae and defines prognosis along with treatment expectations. In such a setting, the expertise brought by each member—

general practitioners and specialists alike—provides a very unique educational experience, and that process gets repeated on a regular basis with each session and with each new case study. I personally conducted many such seminars with a multitude of Seattle Study Clubs, and I became intimately convinced of the merit of this philosophy as I witnessed over the years the rapid progression of all the groups in their interdisciplinary planning, their comprehensive approach, and their increasing treatment standards and expectations. I can confidently say today that this interactive group learning is a mandatory component for understanding, prescribing, and practicing comprehensive interdisciplinary care.

However, as one becomes increasingly confident in interdisciplinary and multiphased treatment discussions, there is also a greater need for a systematic approach and reference as new levels of understanding and technology are reached. In this respect, this book provides the reader with the in-depth foundation for diagnosis, planning, prognosis, and sequencing that is so critical in treatment today. The clinical results emphasize the importance of a disciplined and comprehensive approach, and to my mind what makes this book so unique is that it depicts with total clarity the mental processes and the treatment philosophies of the authors and master clinicians as they contemplate their options, compute the prognosis, and weave the complex details of each treatment phase. This provides much-needed insight into decision making for tooth preservation, ridge maintenance, strategic extraction, location and number of implants with their impact on the prosthetic design and interimplant papilla levels, crown lengthening as it pertains to tooth proportion, and, conversely, gingival height as it correlates with pink porcelain design, to name a few examples.

The practicality of this textbook, with its real-life clinical situations and its didactic quality, is a reflection of what has made the Seattle Study Club journey beneficial to so many of us.

Gerard J. Chiche, DDS
Thomas P. Hinman Endowed Professor
Director, Esthetics and Implants Center
Medical College of Georgia School of Dentistry
Augusta, Georgia

Introduction & Background

Welcome, and thank you for joining me on this important second journey into interdisciplinary treatment planning. In the mid-1990s, I remember deliberating with fellow faculty members in the Graduate Periodontics Department at the University of Washington School of Dentistry on the most effective ways to synthesize diagnostic patient data into a comprehensive and consequential treatment plan. One school of thought was to work backward. This idea required one to visualize the final treatment outcome first and then use the diagnostic data to devise a plan, in step-by-step fashion, to reach the ultimate destination. Seems simple enough, right? Not so. Given that there are multiple treatment pathways, which do you choose to ensure the most predictable and successful long-term results? There are many opportunities to go astray and get "off track," even if you have the end goal in sight.

Other colleagues insisted that the most effective approach was to gather the initial data and record all that was amiss, then create a list of goals and objectives to "right the wrongs." Ultimately, one could devise a planned sequence of steps in treatment to meet each of the goals and objectives.

Following spirited discussion, it became apparent to all that an integration of the two methods was not only most ideal but indeed essential in designing an effective course of treatment. The clinician must be able to visualize the desired outcome from the outset to establish the treatment target and to set realistic patient expectations. At the same time, he or she must be able to use effective investigative skills to uncover the problems, generate ideas to resolve the problems, and then establish predictable pathways to make those ideas become a reality.

It is unfortunate that many clinicians treatment plan cases on "auto-pilot." They yield to "pre-set" thinking and solutions, reverting to what has worked well in the past in order to save time and move forward with treatment as expeditiously as possible. Although this time-saving approach may be compatible with the wishes of both the dentist and the patient, it is not always in the *best interests* of all concerned. To my way of thinking, this method of treatment planning is no more than "convenience engineering." It undermines the very essence of what makes the practice of dentistry so unique, eliminating the curiosity and intrigue associated with investigating all potential origins of the present pathology or disease. Not only does it remove the need to do more than just put the pieces of the treatment puzzle together so that they fit, but it also preempts the opportunity to move the pieces around until they actually fit better. Finally, it erodes the creativity and innovation within us as our thinking becomes more routine, resulting in monotony and the loss of passion for what we do.

Concept

I have always subscribed to the thinking that becoming skilled at anything takes not only commitment and focus, but also practice, practice, and more practice. In the best-selling book *Outliers*, by Malcolm Gladwell (Little, Brown, 2008), the author cites multiple studies substantiating that this is more than just one's personal opinion.

"The idea that excellence at performing a complex task requires a critical minimum level of practice surfaces again and again in studies of expertise. In fact, researchers have settled on what they believe is the magic number for true expertise: ten thousand hours."[1]

Gladwell quotes Dr Dan Levitin, a well-respected neurologist, as follows:

> The emerging picture from such studies is that ten thousand hours of practice is required to achieve the level of mastery associated with being a world-class expert in anything. In study after study, of composers, basketball players, fiction writers, ice skaters, concert pianists, chess players, master criminals, and what have you, this number comes up again and again . . . It seems that it takes the brain this long to assimilate all that it needs to know to achieve true mastery.[1]

In the first volume of *Interdisciplinary Treatment Planning* (2008), I maintained that for almost every case there are multiple treatment plans that will provide both clinical predictability and patient satisfaction in achieving a high level of success; this has been borne out empirically in my practice over the years. And yet I cannot emphasize more the assertion by Dr Morton Amsterdam that, although there may be multiple treatment options, there is only one correct diagnosis. The closer we come to accurately determining this diagnosis, the more successful the treatment outcome will be. Treatment planning is not magical or mystical. It is clearly a skill that can be mastered with increased knowledge, understanding, and experience.

The core and essence of Volume I was to pave the way to a higher level of proficiency in case planning by introducing and illustrating essential principles employed by master clinicians in their quest for case predictability and perfection. Each contributor's chapter concluded with a thought-provoking treatment-planning case for the reader to tackle, testing his or her true understanding of the principles introduced in that chapter.

Now comes a vital and indispensable step in improving one's treatment-planning skills: learning through repetition. The more cases one plans, the more proficient one becomes at treatment planning. This is what Volume II is all about. Although each case presents its own set of unique challenges, there are common threads between cases that stand out as primers to improving one's treatment-planning ability. These include:

· *The discipline of establishing a sound rationale for each and every step one plans to take in treatment*

This is not an easy task. It requires undivided attention and a time commitment that many clinicians are not willing to accept. However, sitting down and carefully working out even the most minute of treatment details, planning not only for success but also for potential setbacks during the course of therapy, and creating predictable strategies for recovery should anything ever fail provide the essential foundation for interdisciplinary team treatment success.

· *The understanding that every case should be approached as if the clinician has never treatment planned or treated a case before*

Each case is unique. What has worked in the past may not be successful at present or carry us predictably into the future. It is when we automatically default to what seems "tried and true" that we can be lulled into unexpected, unwanted outcomes or even failure. Once our biases and preconceived notions are eliminated from the planning process, we are more likely to focus on the unique circumstances present in a particular case and appropriately customize treatment strategies.

· *The conviction that treatment planning is optimally managed in partnership*

As I see it, when we treatment plan in isolation we are limited by our own weaknesses. No matter how skilled the clinician, imperfection is an everyday reality. The great basketball coach Pat Riley has said that "great teamwork is the only way we create the breakthroughs that define our careers." A collaborative team environment fosters unparalleled treatment outcomes.

Collaboration is the core and essence of the Seattle Study Club. It is the foundation of interdisciplinary treatment planning and brings individuals together to draw on each other's strengths. It provides a great opportunity to gain a better overall understanding of dentistry and to predictably improve one's treatment-planning skills. Ultimately, the patient is the beneficiary.

Case planning and practicing in isolation may have been possible 20 years ago, but the contemporary dentist recognizes that there is too much at stake and too much to know to go it alone.

I have always looked at the Seattle Study Club as a "university without walls"—a place where we can find all of the resources we once had in our dental school training. We are all perpetual students after graduation, and the study club is where we can most predictably grow. This is a true interdisciplinary environment where we can draw on the greatest resource that we have in our communities—each other! The idea is that everyone learns from each other to make life easier and to take the stress out of case planning and troubleshooting. If you are not taking advantage of this and working in an interdisciplinary team, you are not benefiting from the greatest asset that a club has to offer you.

Collaboration can open your horizons to many treatment options that you may never have thought of, and some of these options may fit your patients' desires better than anything you may think of presenting. Ultimately, this may be the reason that your patients accept treatment that they would otherwise have rejected. In addition, there seems to be more credibility in the eyes of patients when a team of experts is consulting and collaborating on their case. We have seen this in live treatment-planning sessions. Patients who participate in these sessions are more likely to follow through with treatment.

Interdisciplinary Treatment Planning

Volume II offers 19 new challenging treatment-planning cases. Eleven of the authors who participated in Volume I have contributed cases for this new endeavor. In addition, nineteen outstanding clinicians have been added for this project. All of the contributors were asked to follow a standardized format in developing their sections.

1. They were asked to explain why they chose their particular case for the reader to treatment plan.
2. They were asked to offer suggestions about what they thought the reader should focus on in designing his or her treatment plan.
3. They were asked to then present their case in the same format utilized in Volume I.

The treatment-planning cases are presented in two parts using the *Seattle Study Club Journal* format. Part 1 is entitled "Clinical Treatment Planning" and includes all of the diagnostic information needed by the reader to treatment plan the case. At the end of this part, there is an opportunity for the reader to pause and actually do so.

Part 2 is entitled "Active Clinical Treatment" and includes a complete narrative of all of the treatment rendered accompanied by the treatment and posttreatment images and radiographs.

In Volume II, all contributors were asked to provide an expanded "commentary" section at the end of "Active Clinical Treatment." This section includes editorial comments such as how the clinician would alter treatment if given the opportunity to begin again. What would they do differently this time around? It also contains any additional thoughts on treatment that they would like to share with the reader. Finally, it includes additional details on the philosophy, concepts, and techniques behind the treatment rendered.

Posttreatment Overlays

In Volume I, pre- and posttreatment chartings were presented on different pages within each treatment-planning exercise. This made it somewhat difficult to compare pre- and posttreatment.

In this volume, we have made the process easier by providing a posttreatment transparency for each case, which can be found in the folder included with your book. The posttreatment transparency may be superimposed over the pretreatment charting for comparison purposes.

Michael Cohen

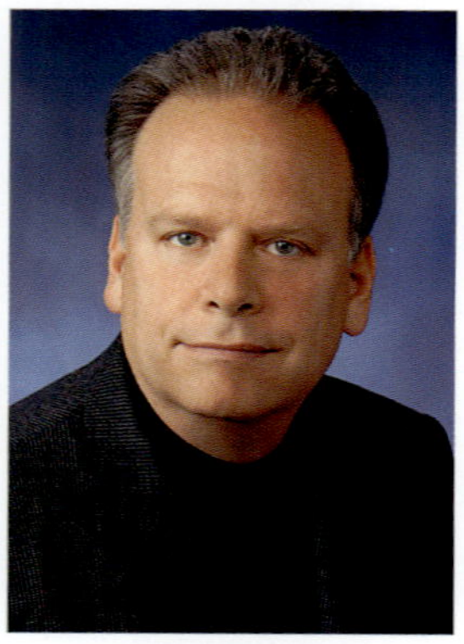

Dr Cohen received his DDS degree from McGill University in Montreal and his MS degree and certificate in periodontics from the University of Washington School of Dentistry, where he now serves as a visiting assistant clinical professor in the Department of Periodontics. He has authored numerous articles on continuing education and is the editor of *Interdisciplinary Treatment Planning: Principles, Design, Implementation* (Quintessence, 2008). For the past 25 years, Dr Cohen has lectured nationally and internationally on the topic of comprehensive treatment planning, and he maintains a private practice limited to periodontics and implants in the Seattle area.

The Seattle Study Club is the brainchild of Dr Cohen. An advanced educational organization, the Seattle Study Club consists of clinicians dedicated to raising the level of practice within their profession. This "university without walls" has more than 6,500 members in approximately 250 chapters in the United States, Canada, Australia, Germany, Spain, Taiwan, and Great Britain. Each club provides clinical treatment-planning sessions designed to increase total case management, problem-solving sessions, a faculty of specialists, and dedicated comprehensive treatment planning. National lecturers are showcased in small group settings, allowing intimate sharing of state-of-the-art treatment for the patient. The Seattle Study Club also publishes a quarterly interdisciplinary treatment-planning journal (*The Seattle Study Club Journal*) and sponsors lectures, conferences, and symposia. Guidance and assistance is also provided to each of the locally based study clubs.

The Master Clinicians

Nitzan Bichacho

Dr Bichacho is a professor of prosthodontics and head of the Ronald E. Goldstein Center for Aesthetic Dentistry and Clinical Research in the Department of Oral Rehabilitation at the Hadassah Medical Campus, Faculty of Dental Medicine, Hebrew University, Jerusalem, the institution from which he graduated in 1984. He is a past president and an active member of the European Academy of Esthetic Dentistry and serves on editorial boards of international professional publications. He is the recipient of numerous international awards for his outstanding professional achievements and contributions to oral health around the globe. Dr Bichacho conceived of and coinvented the NobelActive Implant System, and he lectures worldwide on topics in the fields of dental implant therapy, esthetic oral rehabilitation, and fixed prosthodontics, focusing on innovative treatment modalities and clinical techniques. In his private practice in Tel Aviv, he collaborates with multinational colleagues and dental technicians of world renown.

Marcelo A. Calamita

Dr Calamita received his DDS degree from the University of São Paulo, Brazil. He then obtained his certificate, MSD, and PhD in prosthodontics from the same university, where he also worked as a clinical instructor in the Department of Prosthodontics for 17 years. He has also served as an associate professor of prosthodontics at the University Braz Cubas and at the University of Guarulhos, both in São Paulo. He is currently the president of the Brazilian Academy of Aesthetic Dentistry and maintains a full-time private practice focusing on comprehensive restorative and implant dentistry. He has lectured, published articles, and coauthored book chapters on interdisciplinary treatment planning, implants, and esthetic dentistry.

Murilo Calgaro

Mr Calgaro graduated from the School of Dental Technicians, Senac São Paulo, in 2002. He also attended the Ceramic Specialization Program directed by Dr Paulo Kano at the PK Institute Training Centre, where he then became an instructor. In 2005, Mr Calgaro opened a private training center, Studio Dental, in Curitiba, Brazil. In 2007, he was invited by Dr Christian Coachman to be part of the ceramist team at Dr Eric Van Dooren's clinic in Antwerp, Belgium, where he is now the Master Ceramist. He is also the Master Ceramist for Fabio Fujiy's clinic in Campinas, Brazil, and has been working with many leading dentists around the world such as Mauro Fradeani, Nitzan Bichacho, Galip Gürel, and Sidney Kinna. He is a member of the Brazilian Academy and Society of Esthetic Dentistry.

Yen-Wei Chen

Dr Chen received his DDS degree from Taipei Medical University in Taiwan and his MSD degree and certificate in prosthodontics from the University of Washington School of Dentistry. He is an affiliate assistant professor in the Graduate Prosthodontics Program at the University of Washington and also maintains a private practice limited to prosthodontics in Seattle. Dr Chen has authored articles on the subject of esthetic dentistry and has lectured both nationally and internationally.

Stephen J. Chu

Dr Chu is an associate professor in the Department of Prosthodontics, the director of Graduate and Undergraduate Aesthetic Education, and a codirector of the Implant and Aesthetic Continuums at Columbia University School of Dentistry. He has published 23 articles and given over 100 lectures nationally and internationally on the topics of esthetic, restorative, and implant dentistry. Dr Chu is a coauthor of *Fundamentals of Color: Shade Matching and Communication in Esthetic Dentistry* (Quintessence, 2011) and *Aesthetic Restorative Dentistry: Principles and Practice* (Montage Media, 2008), and he serves on the editorial review boards of several dental journals and publications. He is the creator of Chu's Aesthetic Gauges and maintains a private practice limited to fixed prosthodontics in New York City.

Christian Coachman

Dr Coachman earned degrees in dentistry and dental technology from the University of São Paulo in 2002 and in 1995, respectively. He attended the Ceramic Specialization Program directed by Dr Dario Adolfi at the Ceramoart Training Centre, where he then became an instructor. In 1996, he opened his own laboratory and also worked as a technical consultant of Creation, Willi Geller Ceramics. In 2004, Dr Coachman was invited to become the head ceramist of the laboratory of Goldstein, Garber, and Salama, a position he held for more than 4 years. Dr Coachman currently works as a consultant and develops products for companies across the globe. He has lectured and published internationally in the fields of esthetic dentistry, oral rehabilitation, dental ceramics, and implants. He is a member of the Brazilian Academy and Society of Esthetic Dentistry.

George Duello

Dr Duello earned his dental degree from the University of Missouri–Kansas City (UMKC) School of Dentistry in 1979. He completed residency training in periodontics and received a master's degree in oral biology from the UMKC School of Dentistry in 1981. He then served in the US Air Force at MacDill Air Force Base in Tampa, Florida, as chief of Periodontics from 1981 to 1983. Dr Duello was named a diplomate of the American Board of Periodontology in 1987, and he is a member of several professional societies and associations. He is a past president of both the Missouri Society of Periodontists and the Greater St Louis Dental Society and an alumnus of the Schuster Center for Professional Development, and he currently serves as the director of the Gateway Study Club, a chapter of the Seattle Study Club in St Louis. Dr Duello has lectured nationally and internationally on contemporary periodontal and implant therapy as well as on practice management, and he has authored articles on dental implant therapy. He is also a member of the Nobel Biocare NobelKnowledge website faculty.

Stefano Gracis

Dr Gracis received his DMD degree in 1986 from the University of Pennsylvania and in 1987 from the University of Pavia in Italy. In 1990, he obtained a certificate in prosthodontics with an MSD degree from the University of Washington under the guidance of Dr Ralph Yuodelis. He then returned to Milan, Italy, where he maintains a private practice limited to prosthodontics and restorative dentistry. From 1998 to 2004, he was a guest lecturer at the University of Parma. He is an active member of both the European Academy of Esthetic Dentistry and the

Italian Academy of Prosthetic Dentistry, for which he was president from 2007 to 2008. He serves on the editorial boards of the *International Journal of Prosthodontics*, *European Journal of Esthetic Dentistry*, and *European Journal of Oral Implantology*. He has contributed several articles and two book chapters in the field of restorative dentistry and is a frequent lecturer on topics related to fixed and implant prosthodontics.

Galip Gürel

Dr Gürel earned his dental degree from the University of Istanbul Dental School in 1981. He continued his education at the University of Kentucky Department of Prosthodontics and received his MSc degree from the University of Yeditepe in Istanbul. Dr Gürel is the founder and honorary president of the Turkish Academy of Aesthetic Dentistry, president of the European Academy of Esthetic Dentistry, a member of the American Society for Dental Aesthetics, and an honorary diplomate of the American Board of Aesthetic Dentistry. He is the editor-in-chief of *Quintessence Magazine* in Turkey, is on the editorial boards of several dental publications, and is the editor of *The Science and Art of Porcelain Laminate Veneers* (Quintessence, 2003). He lectures internationally on dental esthetics and maintains a private practice limited to esthetic dentistry, with a team of specialists and laboratory technicians, in Istanbul.

Jim Janakievski

Dr Janakievski received his DDS degree from the University of Toronto, after which he completed a residency in general practice. After several years in general practice, he completed his postgraduate training at the University of Washington, where he received a certificate in periodontology with an MSD degree and a fellowship in prosthodontics. He is a diplomate of the American Board of Periodontology, serves as an affiliate assistant professor in the Department of Periodontology at the University of Washington, and maintains a private practice in Tacoma, Washington.

Greggory A. Kinzer

Dr Kinzer received his DDS degree in 1995 and an MSD and certificate in prosthodontics in 1998 from the University of Washington. Dr Kinzer currently serves as an affiliate assistant professor in the Graduate Prosthodontic Program at the University of Washington School of Dentistry. From 1998 to 2009, he taught with Dr Frank Spear at the Seattle Institute for Advanced Dental Education, prior to joining the Spear Education faculty in Scottsdale, Arizona. Dr Kinzer has written numerous articles and chapters and serves on the editorial review boards of various dental publications. He maintains a private practice in Seattle limited to comprehensive, restorative, and esthetic dentistry.

John C. Kois

Dr Kois received his DMD degree from the University of Pennsylvania School of Dental Medicine and a certificate in periodontal prosthodontics with an MSD degree from the University of Washington School of Dentistry. He maintains a private practice limited to prosthodontics in Tacoma and Seattle and is an affiliate professor in the Graduate Restorative Program at the University of Washington. Dr Kois lectures nationally and internationally, is a reviewer for many journals, and is the editor-in-chief of the *Compendium of Continuing Education in Dentistry*. He is the recipient of the 2002 Saul Schluger Memorial Award for Clinical Excellence in Diagnosis and Treatment Planning, and he received a Lifetime Achievement Award from both the World Congress of Minimally Invasive Dentistry and the American Academy of Cosmetic Dentistry. He is a past president of both the American Academy of Restorative Dentistry and the American Academy of Esthetic Dentistry and is a member of numerous other professional organizations. In addition, Dr Kois is the founder and director of the Kois Center, a didactic and clinical teaching program for restorative dentists.

Vincent O. Kokich, Jr

Dr Kokich received his dental degree from Tufts University and his master's degree in orthodontics from the University of Washington, where he teaches part-time as an affiliate assistant professor in the Department of Orthodontics. He received the Charles L. Pincus Research Award for Clinical Research from the American Academy of Esthetic Dentistry, and his current research and publications are primarily involved with esthetic interdisciplinary dentistry. He is a diplomate of the American Board of Orthodontists and a member of the Angle Society and the American Academy of Esthetic Dentistry. Dr Kokich has lectured nationally and internationally on interdisciplinary dentistry and dental esthetics, emphasizing comprehensive treatment planning and the importance of properly sequencing orthodontic, periodontal, and restorative treatment. He maintains a private practice limited to orthodontics in Tacoma, Washington.

Vincent G. Kokich, Sr

Dr Kokich is a professor in the Department of Orthodontics at the University of Washington. In 2010, he retired from his private practice limited to orthodontics in Tacoma, Washington. He has published 21 book chapters, 99 scientific articles, and 48 review articles, has given over 900 presentations worldwide, and has lectured to the orthodontic societies in over 50 different countries. Dr Kokich is the recipient of numerous distinguished awards for his contributions to dentistry, including the Saul Schluger Award in 2000 and the 2008 Charles English Community Education Award for Excellence in Teaching. He has been elected to Fellowship in the American College of Dentists, the Royal College of Surgeons of England, and the Royal College of Surgeons of Edinburgh. Dr Kokich is also the editor-in-chief of the *American Journal of Orthodontics and Dentofacial Orthopedics*.

Glenn D. Krieger

Dr Krieger graduated from dental school in 1992. Nine years later, the Academy of General Dentistry awarded him with Fellowship. He has been a member of the Seattle Study Club for over 10 years, teaching other dentists about comprehensive dental care and the latest advances in esthetic dentistry through lectures and presentations. He has twice earned a designation as one of the top 100 clinicians in continuing education by *Dentistry Today*. Dr Krieger serves as a restorative advisor to Great Blue Heron Seminars and the Renaissance Study Club, both of which are affiliates of the Seattle Study Club, and he is also the former clinical editor of *The Seattle Study Club Journal*.

Cobi J. Landsberg

Dr Landsberg graduated from the Faculty of Dental Medicine at the Hebrew University at Hadassah, Jerusalem, in 1978, and from specialized study in periodontics at Boston University in 1984. He has been a diplomate of the American Board of Periodontology since 1992. Dr Landsberg is a former chairman of the Israel Periodontal Society and is currently an instructor of periodontics in the Specialized Study Program at the Department of Periodontology, Faculty of Dental Medicine, Hebrew University. Dr Landsberg has published numerous scientific and clinical articles on periodontology and implant dentistry in the international dental literature and has lectured extensively in Israel and abroad. He is currently a member of the editorial board of *Clinical Implant Dentistry & Related Research*. Dr Landsberg maintains a private practice limited to periodontics and implant dentistry in Tel Aviv, Israel.

Sonia S. Leziy

Dr Leziy received her dental degree from McGill University in Montreal and her postgraduate degree in periodontics from the University of British Columbia, Vancouver, Canada, where she is an associate clinical professor and sessional lecturer. Dr Leziy is a fellow of both the Royal College of Dentists of Canada and the International Congress of Oral Implantologists, as well as a member of the British Columbia Society of Periodontists, the Canadian Academy of Periodontists, the American Academy of Periodontists, and the American Academy of Esthetic Dentistry. *Dentistry Today* has recognized her as one of the top 100 clinicians in continuing education in North America for the last 4 years. She has published on the topics of implant esthetics and surgical protocols and lectures internationally on implants, advanced esthetics, and periodontal plastic surgery. Dr Leziy maintains a full-time private practice in the Imperio Group Dental Health Specialists with Drs Brahm Miller (prosthodontist) and Priscilla Walsh (periodontist).

Siegfried Marquardt

Dr Marquardt graduated from the Ludwig-Maximilians-University in Munich in 1994. He has been in private practice for over 14 years in Tegernsee, Germany, specializing in periodontology, implantology, perioprosthetics, and esthetic dentistry. Dr Marquardt is the founder and CEO of the Z.a.T. Fortbildungs GmbH, which organizes and promotes international dental symposia and practical courses. In 2001, he was certified as the first specialist for esthetic dentistry in Germany by the German Association of Aesthetic Dentistry and was certified as a specialist for implantology by the European Dental Association. Dr Marquardt lectures internationally and has published articles on the topics of perioprosthetics, esthetic dentistry, and implantology. He is a member of the American Academy of Periodontology and an affiliate of the European Academy of Esthetic Dentistry, as well as a member of numerous other national and international specialist organizations. He holds professorships at the German Academy of Practice and Sciences and the Carl Zeiss Academy in Zürich. Dr Marquardt is the vice president of the German Academy of Esthetic Dentistry and the chairman of the committee for certificates and specialists. He is also the president-elect of the International Federation of Esthetic Dentistry World Meeting 2013 in Munich.

Brahm A. Miller

Dr Miller received his dental degree from McGill University in Montreal and completed his postgraduate prosthodontics certification at the Medical College of Virginia. He is a fellow and examiner of the Royal College of Dentists of Canada, a member of the Association of Prosthodontists of Canada and the British Columbia Society of Prosthodontists, and a past president and fellow of the International Congress of Oral Implantologists. Dr Miller is an associate clinical professor and sessional lecturer at the University of British Columbia. He is a member of several editorial boards, lectures extensively internationally, and has published on the topics of ceramics and advanced implant esthetics and restoration. *Dentistry Today* has recognized Dr Miller among the top 100 clinicians in continuing education in North America for the past 4 years. He maintains a full-time private practice in the Imperio Group Dental Health Specialists with periodontists Drs Sonia Leziy and Priscilla Walsh.

Ricardo Mitrani

Dr Mitrani received his DDS degree from the Unitec University of Mexico City; he then obtained a certificate in prosthodontics as well as an MSD from the University of Washington, where he served as the assistant director of the Graduate Prosthodontics Program in 2001. He currently holds academic affiliations at the University of Washington, University of Valencia in Spain, and National University of Mexico. He is a member of the International College of Dentists, American Academy of Esthetic Dentistry, American College of Prosthodontics, and American Academy of Fixed Prosthodontics. He also serves on the editorial board of the *Journal of Esthetic and Restorative Dentistry*. Dr Mitrani has authored numerous scientific publications and chapters in the fields of implant prosthodontics and esthetic dentistry and has lectured extensively internationally; he maintains a private practice limited to prosthodontics and implants in Mexico City.

Tal Morr

Dr Morr received his DMD degree from Tufts University School of Dental Medicine. He then completed a 3-year postgraduate prosthodontic program at the University of Washington School of Dentistry, where he received a certificate in prosthodontics and an MSD degree. Dr Morr currently maintains a private practice dedicated to esthetics and complex prosthetic reconstruction. He has lectured both nationally and internationally and has published articles on topics such as esthetic dentistry, complex prosthetic rehabilitation, porcelain laminate veneers, and implants. He is also a member of numerous professional organizations such as the American College of Prosthodontists, the American Academy of Esthetic Dentistry, and the American Academy of Restorative Dentistry.

Henry I. Nichols

Dr Nichols graduated from Northwestern University Dental School in 1978. Following graduation, he participated in a general practice residency program. Dr Nichols went on to complete a 3-year advanced training program in restorative dentistry at the University of Washington, which led him to focus his practice on complex restorative dentistry. Dr Nichols lectures nationally and internationally on interdisciplinary treatment planning with an emphasis on long-term efficacy. He is a contributing author of the text *Interdisciplinary Treatment Planning: Principles, Design, Implementation* (Quintessence, 2008) and also serves as a restorative advisor for the Olympic Peninsula Study Club and Great Blue Heron Seminars. Dr Nichols maintains a private practice in Port Townsend, Washington.

Robert "Tito" Norris

Dr Norris received his dental degree from the University of Texas Health Science Center (UTHSC) at San Antonio Dental School. He completed a general practice residency at the Veterans Administration Hospital in Washington, DC, followed by a residency in orthodontics at Howard University. Dr Norris then served in the US Air Force for 3 years as chief of Orthodontics at Misawa Air Base in Japan. He has lectured throughout the United States and Asia and taught as a clinical associate professor at the UTHSC. His scientific papers have been published in the *American Journal of Orthodontics and Dentofacial Orthopedics* and in *Clinical Impressions and Orthodontic Products*. He is a member of 10 different professional dental and orthodontic associations and a diplomate of the American Board of Orthodontics.

Ariel J. Raigrodski

Dr Raigrodski is a professor and director of Graduate Prosthodontics in the Department of Restorative Dentistry at the University of Washington. He is a graduate of the Hebrew University in Jerusalem and received his certificate in prosthodontics at Louisiana State University School of Dentistry, where he also completed a fellowship in implants and esthetics and earned an MS degree. Dr Raigrodski is a member of the editorial review boards of the *Journal of Esthetic and Restorative Dentistry*, the *Journal of Prosthodontics*, and the *Journal of Prosthetic Dentistry*. He is a diplomate of the American Board of Prosthodontics, a fellow of the American College of Prosthodontists and the International College of Dentists, and a member of the American Academy of Fixed Prosthodontics and other professional organizations. Dr Raigrodski's research is mainly clinical and focuses on all-ceramic restorations, dental implants, and CAD/CAM technology. He lectures both nationally and internationally and maintains a private practice in Kenmore, Washington.

J. William Robbins

Dr Robbins is a clinical professor in the Department of General Dentistry at the University of Texas Health Science Center (UTHSC) at San Antonio Dental School. He graduated from the University of Tennessee Dental School in 1973, after which he completed a rotating internship at the Veterans Administration (VA) Hospital in Leavenworth, Kansas, and a 2-year general practice residency at the VA Hospital in San Diego, California. Dr Robbins has published over 80 articles, abstracts, and chapters on a wide range of dental topics and has lectured worldwide. He also maintains a full-time private practice. He is a coeditor of the textbook *Fundamentals of Operative Dentistry – A Contemporary Approach* (Quintessence, 2006). He has won several awards, including the Presidential Teaching Award at the UTHSC, the 2002 Texas Dentist of the Year Award, and the 2003 Honorary Thaddeus V. Weclew Fellowship Award from the Academy of General Dentistry. He is a diplomate of both the Federal Services Board of General Dentistry and the American Board of General Dentistry, for which he also served as president, and a member of numerous professional organizations.

Anthony G. Sclar

Internationally considered a leader in reconstructive and esthetic dental implant surgery, Dr Sclar has been in private practice at South Florida OMS since 1989. He founded Integrated Seminars and the Sclar Center for Empowered Dental Implant Learning, where he conducts limited-attendance courses for his colleagues using unique teaching methodologies. In addition to publishing numerous journal articles and textbook chapters, Dr Sclar is the author of the textbook *Soft Tissue and Esthetic Considerations in Implant Therapy* (Quintessence, 2003). He also serves as an editor for the dental implant section of the *Journal of Oral and Maxillofacial Surgery* and as an adjunct professor and director of Clinical Research and Post Graduate Dental Implant Surgery in the Department of Oral and Maxillofacial Surgery at Nova Southeastern University College of Dental Medicine.

Ward M. Smalley

Dr Smalley is a prosthodontist and orthodontist who maintains a private practice limited to orthodontics in Seattle. He received his DDS degree in 1977, earned a certificate in fixed prosthodontics and an MSD degree in 1984, and earned a certificate in orthodontics and a second MSD in 1986, all at the University of Washington. He currently serves as an affiliate professor at the University of Washington School of Dentistry in the departments of Orthodontics, Periodontics, and Restorative Dentistry, and he also teaches part-time at the Kois Center in Seattle.

Dennis P. Tarnow

Dr Tarnow is a clinical professor of periodontology and the director of Implant Education at Columbia School of Dental Medicine. He is a former professor and chairman of the Department of Periodontology and Implant Dentistry at New York University College of Dentistry. Dr Tarnow holds certificates in periodontics and prosthodontics and is a diplomate of the American Board of Periodontology. He is a recipient of the Master Clinician Award from the American Academy of Periodontology and of the Teacher of the Year Award from New York University. Dr Tarnow maintains a private practice in New York City and has been honored with a wing named after him at New York University College of Dentistry. He has published over 100 articles on perioprosthodontics and implant dentistry, is the coauthor of three textbooks, including *Aesthetic Restorative Dentistry: Principles and Practice* (Montage Media, 2008), and lectures extensively in the United States and abroad.

Eric Van Dooren

Dr Van Dooren attended the Katholieke Universiteit Leuven in Belgium, where he received his dental degree in 1982. He maintains a private practice in Antwerp, Belgium, limited to periodontics, fixed prosthodontics, and implants. Dr Van Dooren is an active member of the European Academy of Esthetic Dentistry. In addition, he is a member of the editorial staff of both *Teamwork* (Germany) and the Belgian Dental Society. Dr Van Dooren lectures nationally and internationally, mainly on the topics of esthetics, implants, and esthetic periodontal surgery. He has published several articles in international journals and is a contributing author to *The Art of the Smile* (Quintessence, 2005).

John D. West

As founder and director of the Center for Endodontics, Dr West continues to be recognized as one of the premier educators in clinical and interdisciplinary endodontics. He received his DDS degree in 1971 from the University of Washington, where he is an affiliate associate professor. In 1975, he received his MSD in endodontics at Boston University Henry M. Goldman School of Dental Medicine, where he is a clinical instructor and recipient of the Distinguished Alumni Award. Dr West is a contributing author to several books, including *Pathways of the Pulp* (Mosby, 1998) and *Interdisciplinary Treatment Planning: Principles, Design, Implementation* (Quintessence, 2008). He is a past president of both the American Academy of Esthetic Dentistry and the Academy of Microscope Enhanced Dentistry, and he is also a member of the Northwest Network for Dental Excellence and the International College of Dentists as well as a previous consultant for the American Dental Association's prestigious Council on Dental Practice.

Acknowledgments

Editing a textbook is all-consuming. Volume I took 3 years to design, develop, and complete. Once that textbook was published, it was this author's intention to take early retirement from the literary world. In short, I wanted my life back.

Time heals; witness the birth of Volume II. This never would have happened without the encouragement and continual support of close friends, colleagues, and family:

Suzanne Cohen—The love of my life, she gave me the consideration and space to make this latest project a reality.

Carla Kimball and Janell Edwards—Seattle Study Club staff who lent their expertise in the areas of clinical case editing, compilation, and graphic design.

Dr Gerard Chiche—My close friend in life who was always there to boost my spirits whenever I contemplated quitting while I was ahead. He helped me understand the importance of leaving a legacy.

Tomoko Tsuchiya—Although I never really believed that I needed to write or edit a textbook to gain professional fulfillment, Tomoko helped me recognize the importance of making a significant contribution to dentistry and giving of myself to others.

Lisa Bywaters—Anyone who writes dental textbooks should be fortunate enough to have Lisa as a senior editor, sounding board, and coach. She was instrumental in convincing me to "pull the trigger" on Volume II and was always there to straighten me out whenever I veered off course.

The Authors—I have come to learn that most respected clinicians and academicians do not have the time to write a chapter for a textbook, especially when it isn't their own! I feel honored that so many of these esteemed individuals were willing to support me by contributing at such a high level on this project.

H.W. and Christian Haase—Why is it that when the most recognizable dentists decide to write their own textbooks, they covet the thought of being published by Quintessence? The answer is very simple. The Haases are committed to publishing the finest, highest-quality dental textbooks in the world. They do not cut corners and subscribe to the philosophy that professional excellence is a necessary precursor to financial success. I consider myself fortunate to have had the Haases both believe in and support me in the quest to realize my goals and wishes.

1

Combining Orthodontic and Restorative Therapy in Complex Cases

Stefano Gracis, DMD, MSD

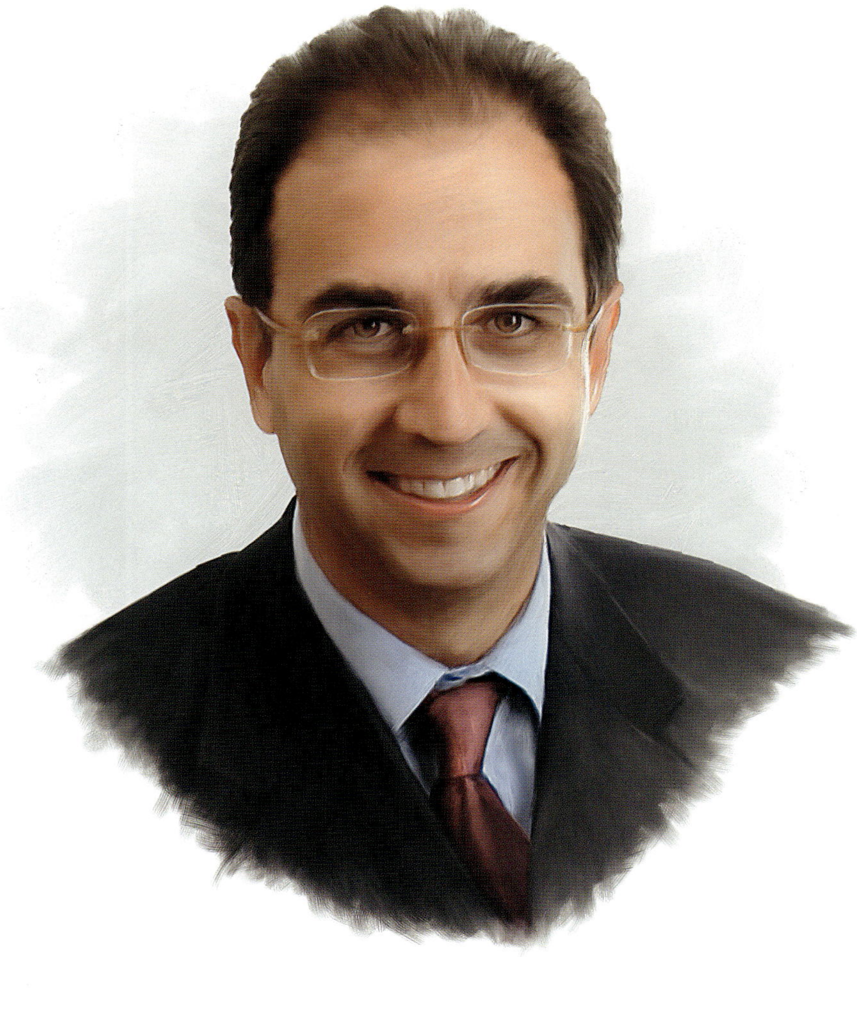

Orthodontic therapy allows the restorative dentist to be more conservative and effective and, in many cases, leads to a higher-quality treatment outcome.

Philosophy and Background

My treatment philosophy has been shaped by the outstanding teachers and mentors I encountered during my undergraduate dental education at the University of Pennsylvania and my specialty training in prosthodontics at the University of Washington. At these schools, I was exposed to what I consider many of the best minds in dentistry. These individuals not only have educated and trained me to become a caring, meticulous, and honest clinician but also have provided me with the mindset, tools, and motivation to continue to learn and improve.

One of the most important lessons learned from my university experiences is the great benefit of applying, whenever possible, a truly interdisciplinary approach to patient care. In both schools, the interaction between the restorative department and the departments of periodontics and orthodontics was more than just a formality; it was an established protocol. One of the major quests over the years since the end of my academic training and my return to Italy has been to re-create a collaborative interdisciplinary environment with like-minded specialists willing to share their thoughts and ideas, with our patients ultimately being the beneficiaries.

The reason I chose the following clinical case is that it so clearly demonstrates the philosophy and approach of our team in the treatment of complex situations. This is a very challenging case because of the damage already caused by periodontal disease, the number of teeth missing and to be removed, and the malocclusion with its edge-to-edge incisor relationship and complete lack of anterior guidance. While the first problem required the application of well-known principles and protocols for disease control and the second the relatively straightforward placement of a number of implants thanks to the generous amount of residual bone (at least in the mandible), the third aspect will likely spark discussion regarding the necessity of establishing a new anterior guidance and, if it is to be attempted, how it should be accomplished.

CASE PRESENTATION

Treating clinicians
Restorative dentistry and prosthetic rehabilitation: Stefano Gracis, DMD, MSD
Periodontal and implant surgery: Federico Gualini, MD, DDS, MSD
Orthodontic treatment: David J. De Franco, DMD, DMedSc
Endodontic treatment: Matteo Capelli, DMD
Prosthetic laboratory work: Silvano Sandrini, CDT

CLINICAL TREATMENT PLANNING

Age at initial presentation: 60 years
Initial presentation: September 1997
Active treatment completed: January 2001

Introduction and background

At the time of presentation, this 60-year-old bank officer was close to retirement. He complained that he was having great difficulty chewing because some of his teeth were painful and mobile. He had a mandibular removable partial denture (RPD) fabricated 5 years earlier that he could not wear because the teeth that were most painful, the mandibular left canine and second molar, were the teeth that anchored the RPD. He was emphatic about eliminating his RPD in favor of fixed restorations. This patient communicated his desire to address his oral health problems in a comprehensive way. He wanted to improve function but did not particularly care about esthetics or the appearance of his teeth. He seemed open to any and all recommendations related to helping him achieve his treatment goals.

Medical history

The patient was in good health with no medical contraindications to dental treatment. He was not taking any medications.

Dental history

The patient, prior to this time, had not seen a dentist for any treatment in approximately 4 years. In the past, he sought only emergency care. The mandibular RPD was fabricated about 5 years earlier, after the left first premolar was lost and the fixed prosthesis that it was supporting had to be sectioned and removed. The patient brushes his teeth twice a day with a manual toothbrush but does not floss.

Diagnostic findings

Extraoral and facial findings

- No significant facial asymmetry
- Flat to slightly concave profile with a normodivergent skeletal pattern
- Asymmetric smile
- Low smile line
- Maxillary dental midline coincident with facial midline

TMJ and mandibular range of motion

- Both TMJs within normal limits; no clicking and no pain occurring spontaneously or upon palpation
- Mouth opening and range of motion within normal limits
- No muscle discomfort or tenderness upon palpation

Pretreatment

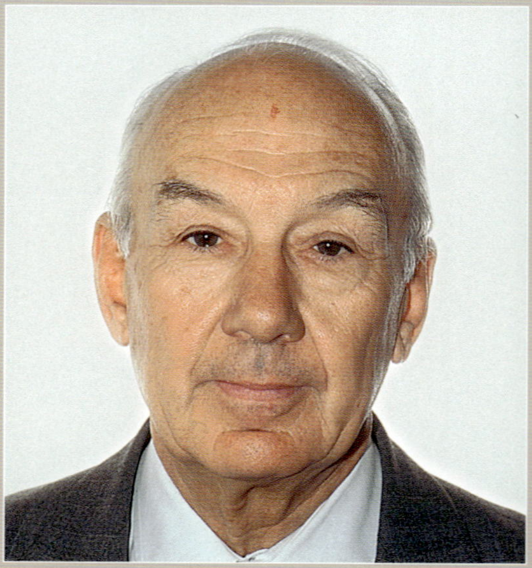

Facial view.

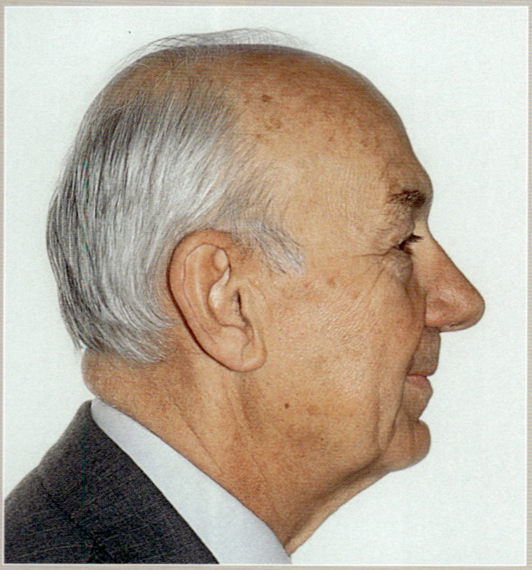

Profile view.

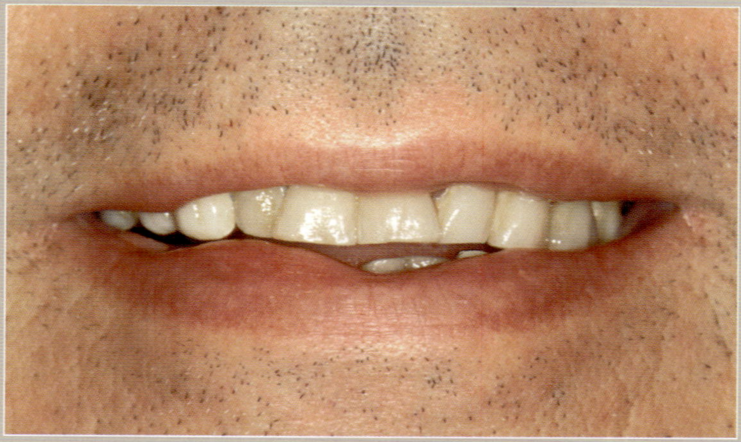

Close-up of the smile.

Intraoral findings

- Generalized bleeding upon probing with plaque and calculus deposits on all teeth
- Missing teeth nos. 1, 4, 5, 13, 16, 17, 19, 20, 21, and 32; subsequent moderate alveolar ridge resorption was evident
- Splinted teeth nos. 2 to 6, 13 to 15 with 13 cantilevered, and 30 to 31
- Defective prosthetic restorations (all)
- Class III mobility of teeth nos. 22 and 18
- Class II mobility of teeth nos. 14, 15, and 29
- Class I mobility of teeth nos. 2 to 5, 6, 7, 12, 23, 24, 28, 30, and 31
- Maxillary and mandibular dental midlines not coincident (mandibular midline shifted to the right approximately 1 mm)
- Moderate crowding of the mandibular incisors
- Incisor inclination: maxillary within norm, mandibular proclined
- Moderate tooth wear

Radiographic findings

- Horizontal slight to moderate bone loss in the maxillary and mandibular incisor regions; moderate to severe bone loss in the posterior areas with furcation involvement
- Areas of apical rarefaction around teeth nos. 3, 14, 18, 22, and 29
- Calculus deposits on several roots
- Incomplete or inadequate endodontic treatment of teeth nos. 2, 6, 18, 22, and 31

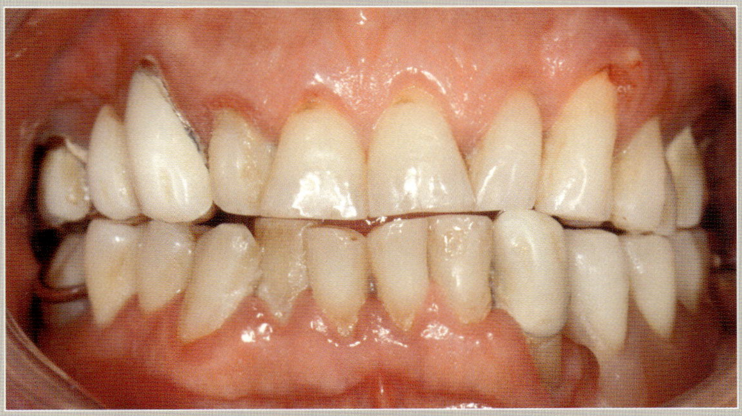

Frontal view of occlusion with the mandibular RPD in situ.

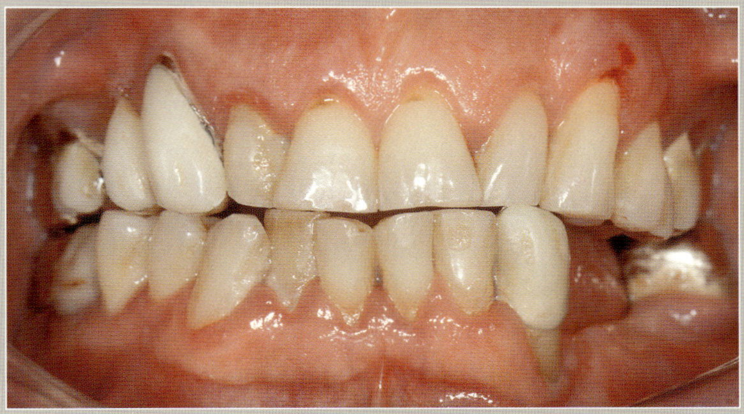

Frontal view of occlusion without the RPD.

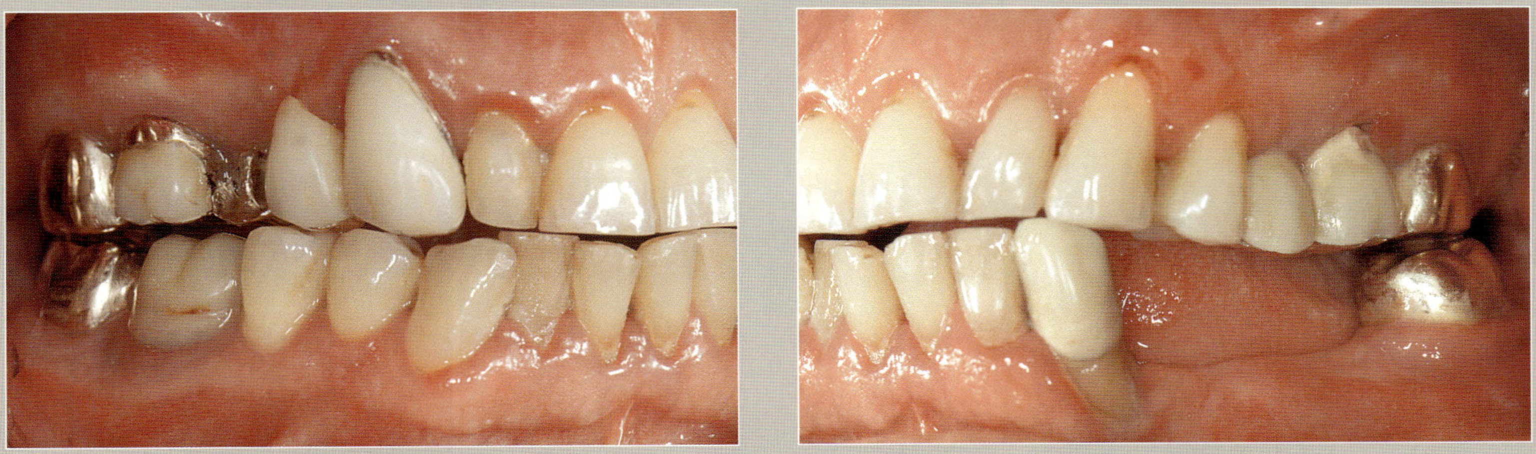

Lateral views.

Occlusal notes

- Centric relation (CR) not coincident with maximal intercuspal position (MIP) (about 1 mm anteroposterior discrepancy); initial interarch contact between teeth nos. 15 and 18
- Edge-to-edge articulation between the two arches (lack of anterior guidance)
- Canine relationship: on the right, tendency to Angle Class III; on the left, tendency to Angle Class II
- No solid occlusal contact on the right side
- Curve of Spee within normal limits

Diagnosis

- Generalized moderate to advanced periodontitis
- Multiple missing teeth
- Endodontically treated teeth
- Periapical lesions of endodontic or endodontic-periodontal origin
- Defective restorations
- Canine: Angle Class II malocclusion on the left side and Class III on the right side, with no overbite and no overjet (edge-to-edge articulation)
- Parafunctional habits

Prognosis

- General: fair; influenced by the cooperation of the patient in modifying his oral hygiene habits and the successful management of his anterior edge-to-edge articulation
- Teeth nos. 3, 14, 18, 22, and 29: hopeless
- Teeth nos. 2, 6, 12, 15, 30, and 31: questionable because of the moderate to severe attachment loss, which, in some sites, has caused furcation involvement
- Remaining dentition: good

Summary of concerns

1. Considering that the patient has neglected his oral health for many years, has his attitude and compliance changed sufficiently to allow us to carry out a complex and lengthy treatment plan?
2. What occlusal scheme can be set up and with what consequences if the patient is unwilling to undergo orthodontic therapy?

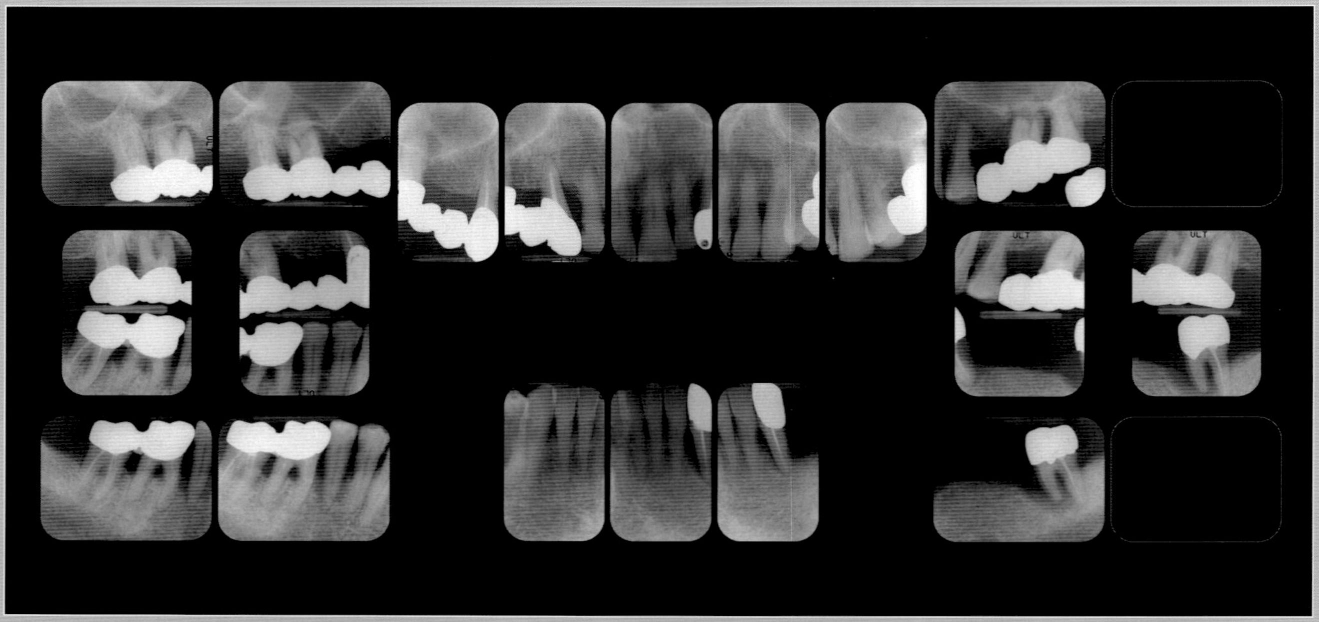

Complete-mouth radiographs at initial presentation (September 1997).

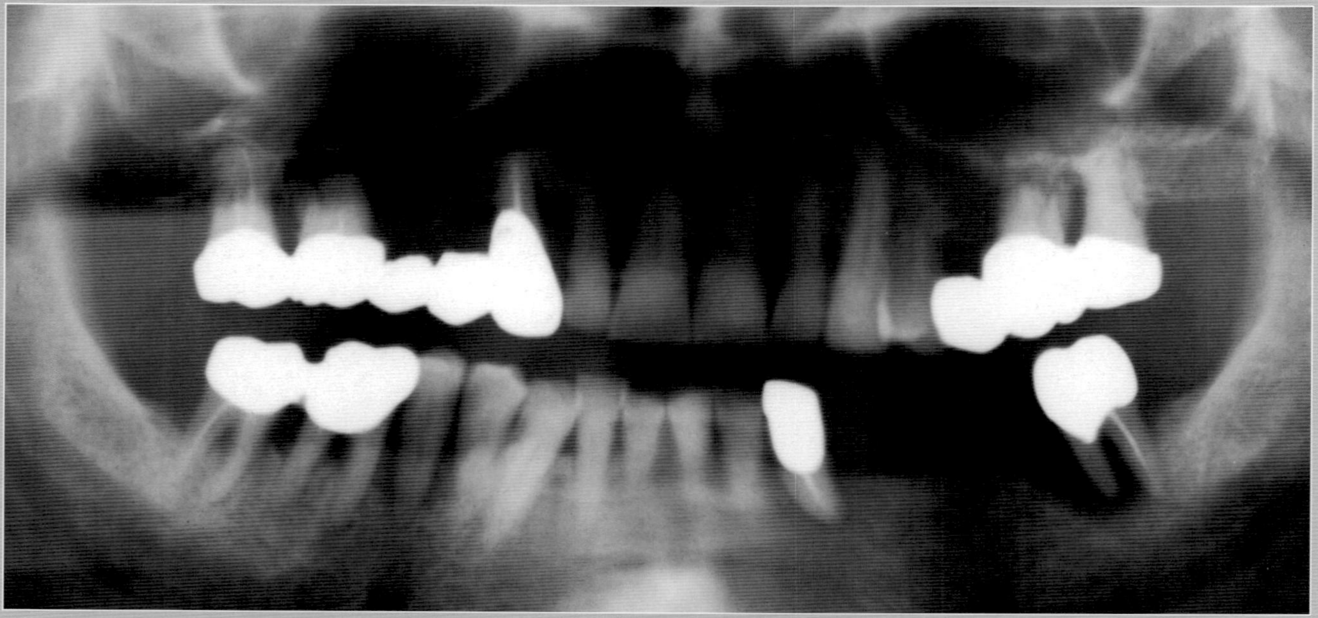

Panoramic radiograph at initial presentation (September 1997).

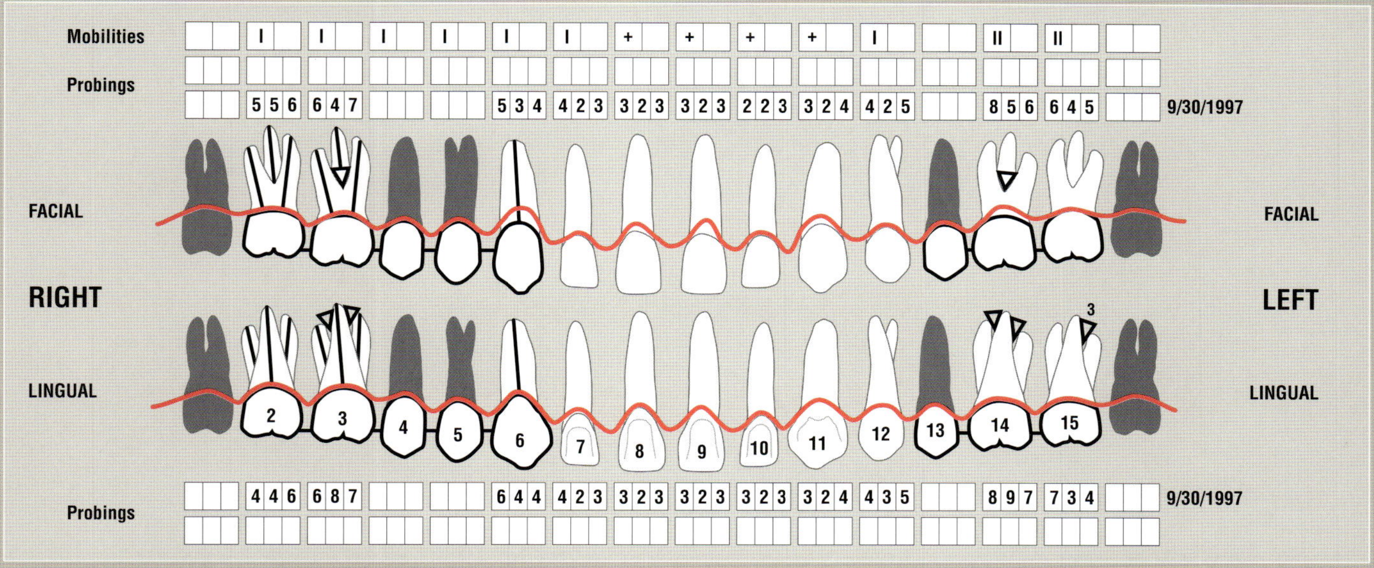

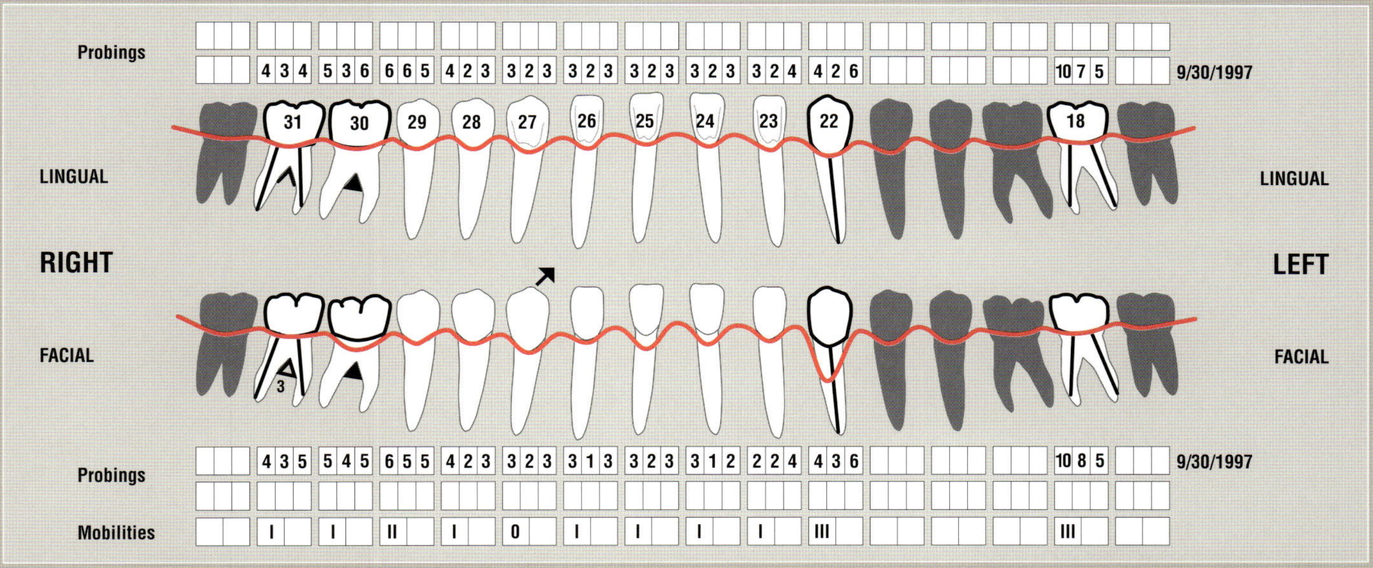

As a learning exercise, you may now outline goals/objectives of treatment and a treatment plan.

Proposed Treatment Plan

Goals/objectives of treatment

- Establish periodontal health
- Replace the missing teeth with fixed restorations
- Establish an occlusal scheme with an efficient anterior guidance and bilateral posterior support

Phase I: Initial therapy

1. Emergency care: Extraction of teeth nos.18 (abscess) and 22 (advanced bone loss with Class III mobility) and modification of the existing mandibular RPD
2. Comprehensive oral evaluation with complete-mouth and panoramic radiographs
3. Detailed periodontal assessment to determine which teeth have hopeless prognoses and require extraction in the initial stages of treatment
4. Scaling and root planing procedures, prophylaxis, and oral hygiene instruction

Phase II: Diagnostic work-up

5. Diagnostic records: Maxillary and mandibular diagnostic alginate impressions, facebow transfer, and CR record with a resin baseplate and wax occlusion rim for the mandibular arch due to the number of missing teeth on the left side
6. Diagnostic wax-up and fabrication of eggshell provisional fixed partial dentures (FPDs) in the maxillary arch for teeth nos. 2 to 6 and 12 to 15
7. Fabrication of an eggshell provisional restoration for teeth nos. 30 and 31
8. Fabrication of a provisional mandibular RPD with wire clasps to replace teeth nos. 18 to 22 and 29.

Phase III: Provisional restorative treatment and endodontic therapy

9. Maxillary arch: Removal of the existing prostheses and extraction of teeth nos. 3 and 14, followed by placement of the lab-cured provisional eggshell restorations (relined on the prepared abutments) on teeth nos. 2, 6, 12, and 15
10. Mandibular arch: Extraction of tooth no. 29, removal of the existing prosthesis on teeth nos. 30 and 31, relining of the eggshell provisional on the molars, and placement of a provisional resin RPD
11. Endodontic re-treatment of teeth nos. 2, 6, 30, and 31 and endodontic therapy on teeth nos. 12 and 15, if necessary
12. Preprosthetic reconstruction of endodontically treated teeth and relining of provisional FPDs

Phase IV: Periodontal and endodontic re-evaluation

13. New periodontal assessment of the teeth with questionable prognoses
14. Re-evaluation of the endodontically treated teeth to determine whether the canals have been fully instrumented and successfully filled and the restored abutments are structurally sound (ie, whether there is a sufficient ferrule)

Phase V: Orthodontic evaluation and planning for implant placement in the mandible

15. Referral to the orthodontist for evaluation and creation of an orthodontic setup to visualize the proposed orthodontic treatment plan
16. Fabrication of a radiographic stent to be worn during the computed tomography (CT) scan of the mandible
17. Fabrication of a surgical stent according to the information provided by the CT scan images and orthodontic setup

Phase VI: Corrective therapies in the mandible

18. Placement of three dental implants in the left posterior segment in locations compatible with planned tooth position after orthodontic treatment has been completed and relining of the provisional RPD with soft resin
19. Periodontal surgery in the mandibular right posterior segment with hemisection of teeth nos. 30 and 31 and placement of a dental implant in the position of tooth no. 29
20. Uncovering of all dental implants 3 months after initial placement, followed by seating of a provisional fixed restoration in the right and left posterior segments
21. Initiation of orthodontic treatment in the mandible to realign teeth in the anterior segment

Phase VII: Corrective therapies in the maxilla

22. Placement of dental implants in the maxillary right posterior segment (teeth nos. 3, 4, and 5) and osseous surgery around tooth no. 2 to correct the existing bony defects and to reduce periodontal pocketing
23. Tooth no. 6: If its prognosis appears to be poor during reevaluation about 8 weeks prior to implant surgery, extraction and replacement with a provisional RPD with wire clasps, and subsequent replacement with another implant
24. Teeth nos. 12 and 15: If their prognoses improve from questionable to good, osseous surgery to correct bony defects and reduce periodontal pocketing; if their prognosis worsens, placement of dental implants
25. Uncovering of dental implants in one or both maxillary posterior segments 6 months following initial placement and seating of provisional FPDs
26. Initiation of orthodontic treatment in the maxilla to slightly flare the incisors and to create space for converting the right peg lateral incisor to normal size
27. Occlusal adjustment via selective grinding of the provisional restorations to gradually decrease the vertical dimension of occlusion (VDO) and increase the overbite, implemented as overjet is created

Phase VIII: Completion of orthodontic treatment and second re-evaluation (periodontal and occlusal)

28. Evaluation of the periodontal condition of the remaining teeth to determine if any additional treatment is necessary
29. Orthodontic therapy is considered complete once the occlusal scheme allows for disocclusion of the posterior teeth in lateral and protrusive excursive movements

Phase IX: Fabrication of the definitive prosthesis

30. Clinical and laboratory phases of fabrication of the definitive tooth-supported and implant-supported prostheses
31. Delivery of an occlusal nightguard

Active Clinical Treatment

Review of the goals/objectives of treatment

- Establish a healthy and stable periodontium
- Elevate the patient's level of understanding regarding what he will need to do to ensure long-term treatment success
- Replace missing teeth and the existing RPD with fixed restorations
- Gain a stable occlusion with more ideal tooth position, bilateral posterior support, and efficient anterior guidance

Phase I: Initial therapy

At the initial examination, a full assessment of his condition was made through an extraoral and intraoral clinical examination. This included a TMJ and muscle evaluation, periodontal screening, esthetic evaluation, a full series of intraoral radiographs, and a panoramic radiograph. At that time, an antibiotic (amoxycillin 850 mg and clavulanic acid 150 mg, twice a day for 5 days) was prescribed to manage the acute infection, mainly around tooth no. 18. A few days later, the tooth was extracted along with tooth no. 22, and the existing partial denture was modified to replace them.

The patient was then scheduled for scaling and root planing under local anesthesia and oral hygiene instruction. It was important, before proceeding with any therapy, to assess his motivation and compliance. He had neglected his oral health for many years, and it wouldn't have made sense to propose sophisticated and lengthy treatment if he had not demonstrated a willingness to change his attitude. He responded positively to this initial motivational session.

At this time, I consulted with the periodontist to assess the implications of the patient's periodontally compromised posterior teeth and to help establish prognoses for their potential incorporation into a long-term treatment plan. Because of the severity of the bone loss in the premolar and molar areas and extensive furcation involvment, the prognosis for teeth nos. 3, 14, 18, 22, and 29 was hopeless. The prognosis for teeth nos. 2, 6, 12, 15, 30, and 31 was questionable, and it was determined that they should be re-evaluated following the completion of the initial phase of therapy. All other teeth were deemed to be salvageable and maintainable. An early goal was to remove the hopeless teeth as soon as possible to eliminate infection sites that would make it more difficult to effectively stabilize the periodontium.

Phase II: Diagnostic work-up

Alginate impressions were taken to obtain diagnostic casts of both arches. An arbitrary facebow transfer was recorded to mount the maxillary cast on a semi-adjustable articulator according to a horizontal reference plane.[1] Then, a maxillomandibular record was taken in CR at a slightly opened VDO to mount the mandibular cast. CR was chosen because all posterior teeth had to be restored or replaced, and, thus, a reorganizational approach had to be applied. After mounting the mandibular cast, the articulator's pin was lowered to the original VDO.

A diagnostic wax-up was made by the dental technician as part of the process of replacing the existing partial dentures in the maxillary right and left and mandibular right quadrants. From this wax-up, acrylic resin shells were manufactured to provide the patient, after relining, with provisional partial dentures for teeth nos. 2 to 6, 12 to 15, 30, and 31. These provisionals incorporated a stainless steel wire as a safety element to keep the segments together in case of breakage of the long-span provisional FPDs. A new provisional RPD was also prepared for the mandibular arch in order to replace teeth nos.18 to 22 and 29 while occluding with the new maxillary provisionals.

Phase III: Provisional restorative treatment and endodontic therapy

After removing the original partial dentures and extracting teeth nos. 3 and 14, the acrylic shells were relined on the prepared abutments using a cold-curing acrylic resin (Coldpac, Yates-Motloid). In the mandibular arch, the crowns of teeth nos. 30 and 31 were replaced by the relined provisional shell, and the provisional RPD was inserted. The new provisional restorations did not alter the patient's original VDO, resulted in significant improvement of periodontal tissues, and aided access for endodontic treatment of teeth nos. 2, 15, 30, and 31.

Phase IV: Periodontal and endodontic re-evaluation

The first re-evaluation examination was performed at approximately 4 months, and a marked improvement in gingival health demonstrated that the patient had maintained a high level of compliance with the oral hygiene regimen.

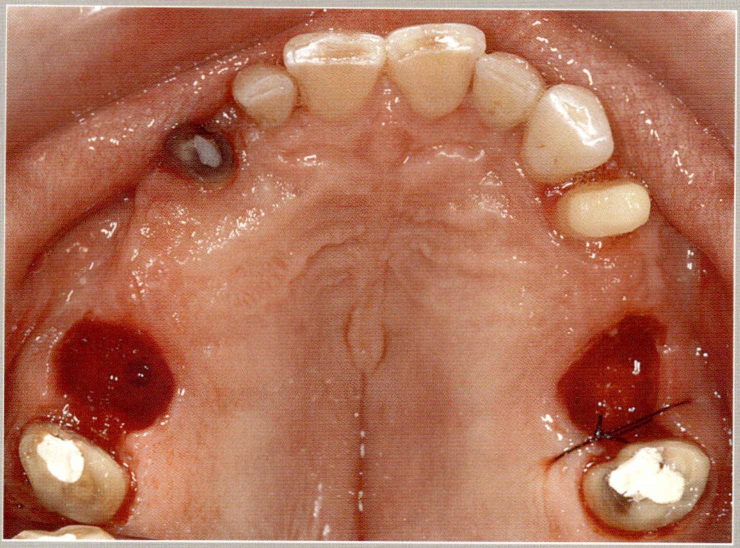

Maxillary occlusal view after removal of the existing prosthesis and extraction of teeth nos. 3 and 14.

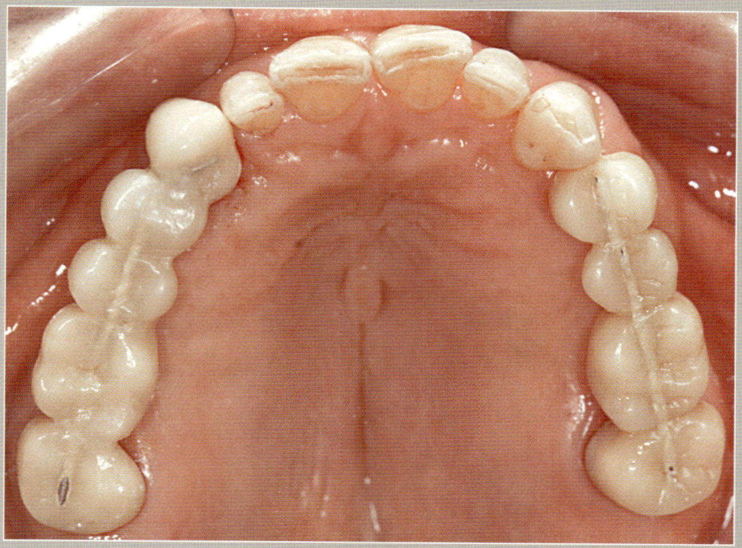

Maxillary occlusal view of lab-cured provisional shells relined on the prepared abutments.

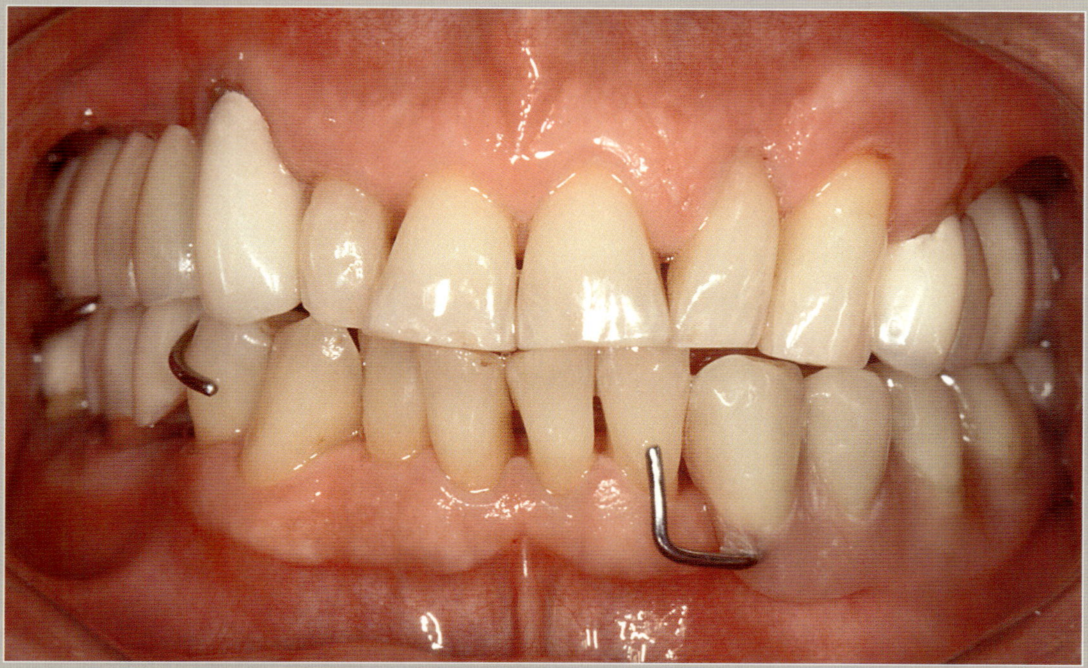

Frontal view following extraction of tooth no. 29 and delivery of mandibular provisional restorations.

In the maxillary arch, the prognosis for tooth no. 6 remained uncertain because of its compromised periodontal status, while tooth no. 12 had improved with a decrease in mobility. During this phase, tooth no. 6 was nevertheless important because a sinus elevation procedure was planned in the maxillary right posterior segment to address the lack of sufficient bone volume for implant placement in the second premolar and first molar region. By acting as a temporary abutment supporting a provisional FPD, tooth no. 6 would allow us to avoid loading the surgical area.

In the mandibular arch, endodontic treatment on teeth nos. 30 and 31 was unsuccessful because it was not possible to completely debride all canals. Nevertheless, a decision was made to proceed with surgical therapy to hemisect these teeth and modify the bony architecture in an attempt to improve their periodontal status. At the time of periodontal osseous surgery, the mesial root of tooth no. 31 was extracted, and the remaining roots were deemed too compromised to provide reliable support for a fixed prosthesis. Because the patient had ample bone volume in that area, we decided to remove the remaining roots and replace them with dental implants. First, however, an in-depth evaluation of tooth position was necessary.

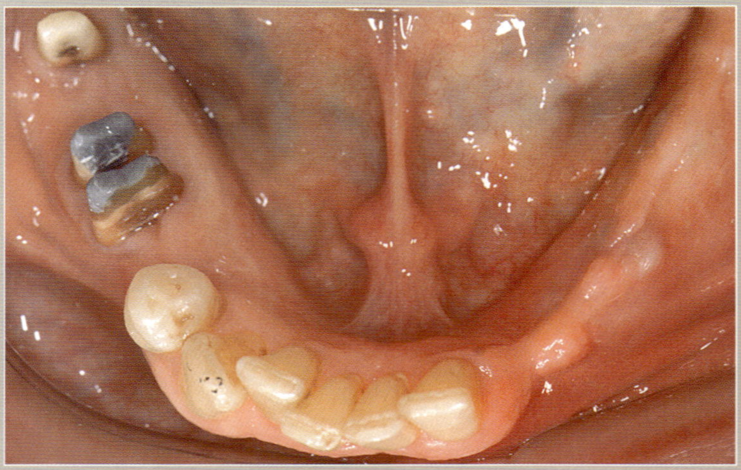

Mandibular occlusal view after the periodontal surgery performed in the right quadrant and the placement of implants in the left quadrant.

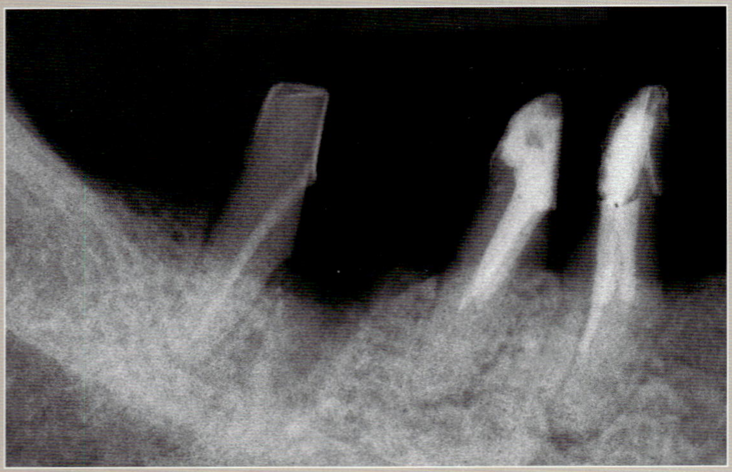

Periapical radiograph showing the periodontal and endodontic condition of the mandibular right molar roots.

Phase V: Orthodontic evaluation and planning for implant placement in the mandible

In formulating a treatment plan, the orthodontist was consulted to evaluate the possibility of gaining anterior guidance via tooth movement rather than by attempting to use restorative means. The issue of the lack of anterior guidance due to end-to-end incisal relationships (zero overbite and zero overjet) is a focal issue in devising a treatment plan that should not only resolve the pathologic conditions and replace the missing teeth but also set the stage for a predictable and stable long-term outcome. The absence of efficient canine guidance may or may not have influenced the periodontal breakdown posteriorly, but it will present a challenge in minimizing deleterious forces if dental implants are placed in posterior areas.

The orthodontic analysis focuses on six parameters: the patient's profile, skeletal scheme, maxillary and mandibular incisor inclination, degree of crowding, canine relationship, and midline alignment. Table 1 shows the initial appearance of these parameters in this patient and what they suggested in regards to therapeutic strategy.

This analysis suggests that the orthodontic treatment would result in achieving adequate overjet; however, the overbite would still be absent. There are three possible ways to restore a sufficient amount of overbite to end up with adequate anterior guidance:

1. Prosthetically restore either the maxillary or the mandibular teeth (or both) to increase their length by the amount of the desired overbite
2. Maintain the teeth as they are (do not restore them), but orthodontically extrude either the maxillary or the mandibular teeth (or both), maintaining the same VDO
3. Maintain the teeth as they are (do not restore them) and reduce the VDO

Table 2 highlights the issues that the clinician should take into consideration when attempting to choose one of the three options. From an orthodontic standpoint, all three options are equally attainable because dental implants provide sufficient anchorage for any type of tooth movement.[2-6]

The first option was ruled out due to its invasive nature and the fact that there was no true need for restorative work on most of the anterior teeth. Also, the maxillary teeth were already visible enough during smiling. Increasing the length of the mandibular teeth would have made them look unnatural because the length of the existing clinical crowns was correct.

The second option was not chosen because, when it was compared to the third, it was judged less attractive. Because there was no strong esthetic indication to increase the exposure of the maxillary and mandibular anterior teeth and all posterior units had to be prosthetically replaced, we had the opportunity to address the VDO as a variable that we could easily modify without any biologic sacrifice.

The last option requires the creation of a larger overjet because, when the VDO is decreased, the mandible rotates anteriorly and the mandibular anterior teeth approach the palatal surfaces of the maxillary anterior teeth. This made it clear from the start that orthodontic treatment would involve both arches, not just the mandible.

Once the patient had accepted orthodontic therapy, the task at hand was to obtain the necessary anchorage. The

TABLE 1 RESULTS OF ORTHODONTIC ANALYSIS		
Parameter	**Initial appearance**	**What it suggests**
Patient's profile	Flat	Do not retract the incisors.
Skeletal scheme	Normodivergent	Maintain vertical dimension.
Incisor inclination	Mandibular: within the norm Maxillary: too buccal	Retract the mandibular incisors.
Degree of crowding	Mandibular: mild to moderate	Perform interproximal stripping and alignment.
Canine relationship	Right: tendency to Class III Left: tendency to Class II	Distalize no. 27. Mesialize no. 22 (replaced by an implant).
Midline	Mandibular: to the right by 1 mm	Move mandibular teeth to the left.

TABLE 2 CONSIDERATIONS FOR CHOOSING A THERAPEUTIC OPTION		
Therapeutic option	**Questions**	**Answers**
Restore the anterior teeth.	· Do the anterior teeth need to be restored? · If so, what type of restorations do they need: conservative fillings, veneers, or full crowns? · Is clinical crown length too short?	· Maxilla: The right canine and, possibly, the right (peg-shaped) lateral incisor need to be restored. · Mandible: The left canine needs to be replaced. The patient does not mind the degree of horizontal wear of the incisal edges; on the contrary, he wants to maintain their appearance as is, unless it interferes with the treatment. · The height of all clinical crowns is acceptable.
Do not restore the teeth and, instead, use orthodontic extrusion.	· Are the maxillary anterior teeth visible when the patient smiles? · Are the mandibular anterior teeth visible when the patient smiles? · If so, is there a need to show more of either of them?	· Both the maxillary and the mandibular anterior teeth are visible when the patient speaks and smiles. · The mandibular teeth could be extruded about 1 to 2 mm without detriment, but the maxillary teeth definitely should not be repositioned more coronally.
Do not restore the teeth and, instead, orthodontically move them while decreasing the VDO.	· Is the patient's height of the lower third of the face appropriate or collapsed? · Can the patient's profile tolerate a decrease in VDO? · Is there a possibility of TMJ dysfunction if the VDO is decreased? · Can sufficient overjet be obtained orthodontically to allow an adequate overbite to be created by decreasing the VDO? · Are most or all of the posterior teeth in need of full restorations?	· The patient's face and profile appear to be in harmony, with the thirds proportioned appropriately. · If the VDO is decreased by just a couple of millimeters measured anteriorly, it would be hardly noticeable. · The possibility of TMJ dysfunction can never be ruled out, but the option of going back to the original VDO is always open. · The orthodontist has indicated that the patient can be provided with sufficient overjet even if the VDO is diminished. · All the posterior teeth need to be either restored or replaced.

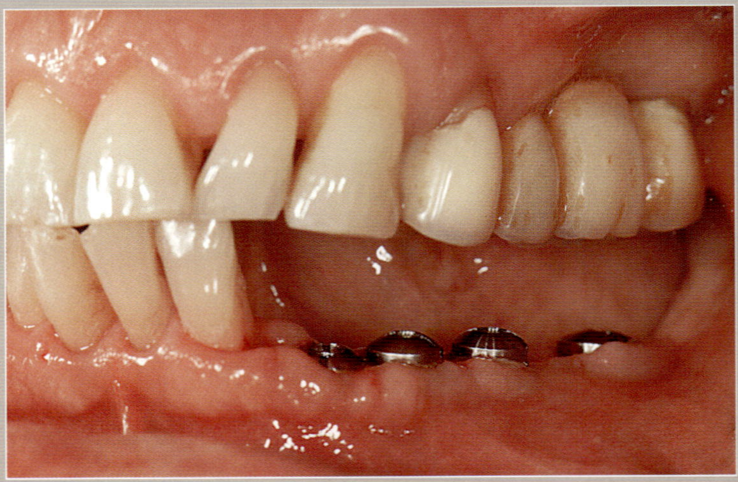

Lateral view of the four dental implants in the mandibular left posterior segment shortly after second-stage uncovering surgery.

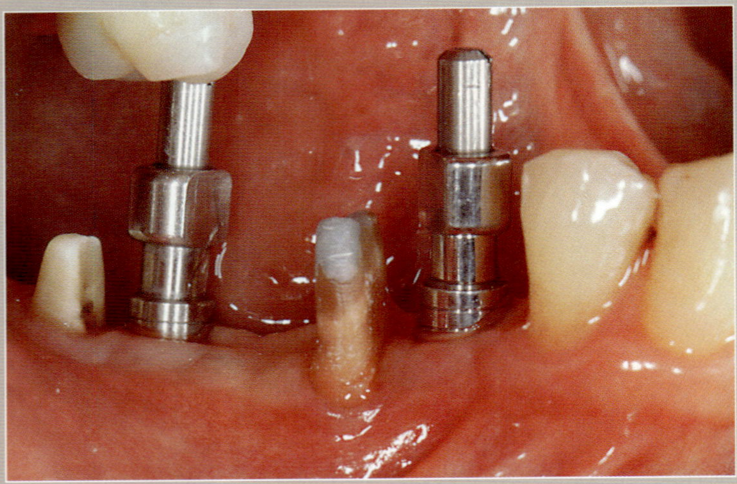

The first two implants in the mandibular right posterior area after they were uncovered. The impression copings are ready for the impression, which will allow the dental technician to fabricate an implant-supported, screw-retained provisional restoration.

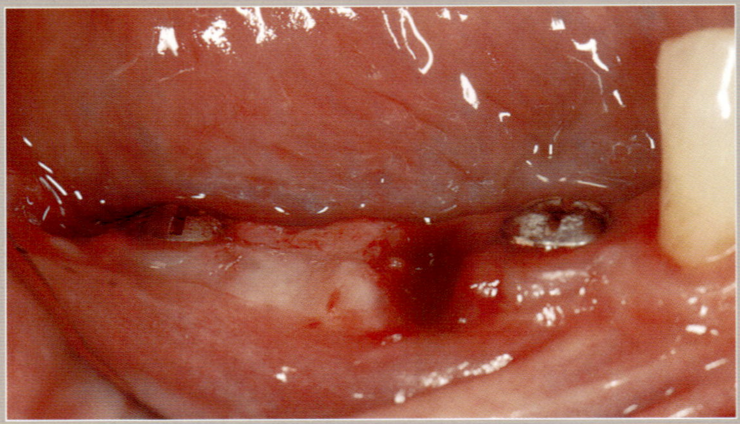

The remaining roots of the mandibular right molars were extracted on the day the implant-supported provisional was being delivered.

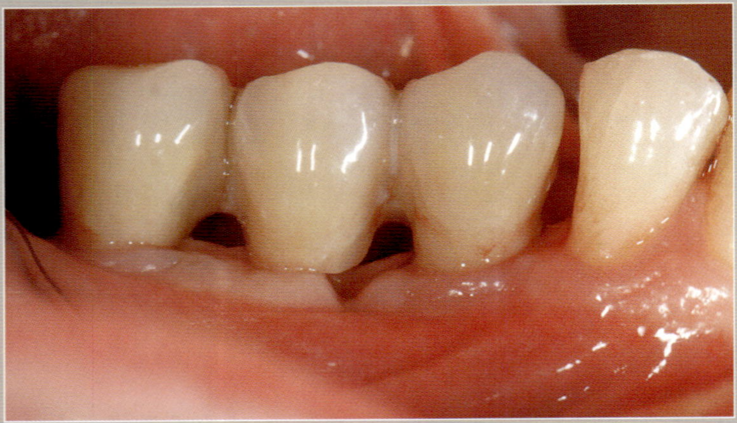

The implant-supported provisional seated on implants nos. 29 and 31. Note the diastema between the provisional restoration and tooth no. 28.

mandible was addressed first because the patient was anxious to eliminate the removable appliance.

A sinus elevation procedure was necessary in the maxillary right posterior segment to create enough bone for dental implant placement. Because the remaining mandibular teeth had to be moved lingually and slightly distally, it was of fundamental importance to locate the implants in a position that would not interfere with the orthodontic movement of the posterior teeth.

A well-established protocol[7,8] was followed to identify the most ideal sites on the edentulous ridge for implant placement. In this protocol, an orthodontic tooth setup is made under the supervision of the orthodontist. Then, the position of the implants is determined based on the mesiodistal space available and the sagittal relationship with the opposing arch. This position is subsequently transferred to the original pre-orthodontic cast, and a surgical stent is manufactured.

Phase VI: Corrective therapies in the mandible

Four screw-type dental implants (Brånemark System, Nobel Biocare) were inserted on the left side with the aid of a surgical stent, using a traditional surgical technique that requires submerging the implants. The implants in sites nos. 20, 21, and 22 were 4 mm in diameter, while the implant in site no. 19 was 5 mm in diameter. The mandibular removable appliance was kept out of the mouth for about 2 weeks and then relined with a soft resin (Visco-gel, Dentsply) to minimize the risk of placing pressure on the surgical site, which in turn minimized the risk of exposing the implants. The mesial implant was intentionally placed about 2 mm distal to tooth no. 23 in order to resolve the mandibular crowding and improve the horizontal overlap.

On the right side, in order to eliminate pressure by the appliance on the single implant site of tooth no. 29, a metal-reinforced provisional was constructed for teeth nos. 30 to 31 with tooth no. 29 as a cantilever. At the time of surgery, the distal root of tooth no. 30 was removed, two 4 × 13-mm

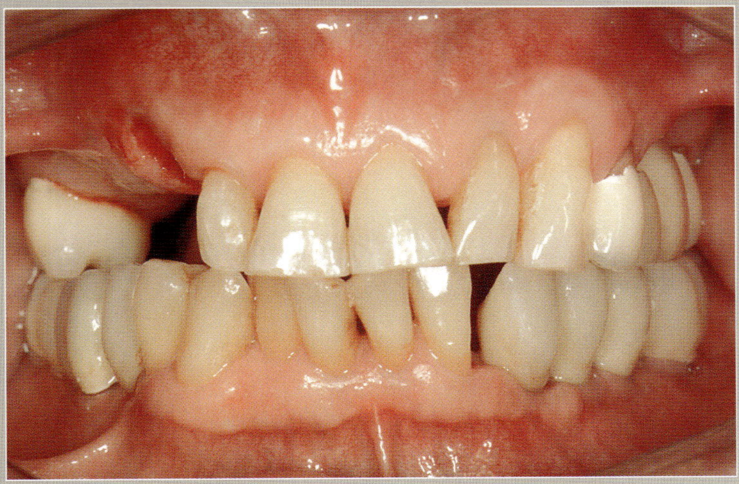

Frontal view following extraction of the maxillary right canine.

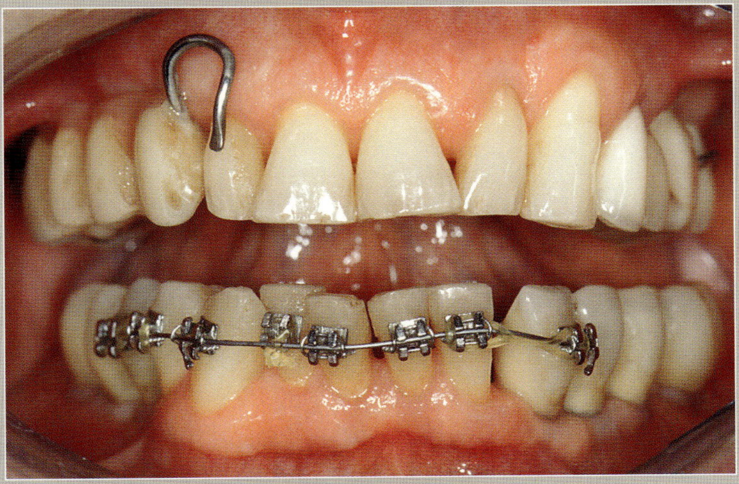

Frontal view of removable provisional appliance to replace teeth nos. 3 to 6 and initiation of orthodontic therapy in the mandible.

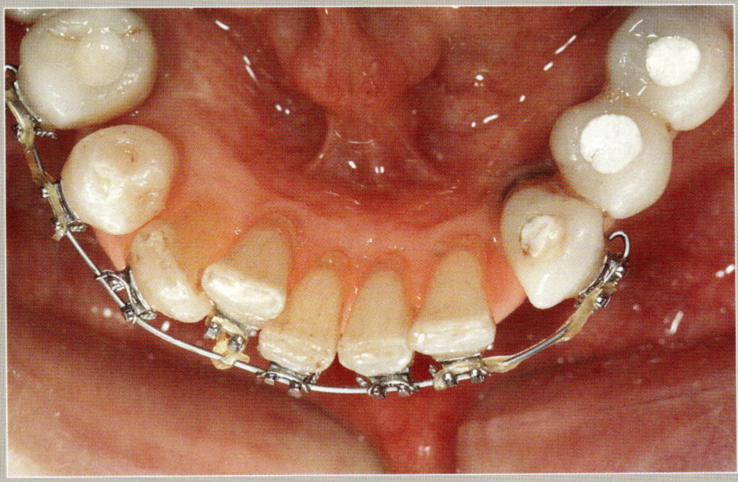

Mandibular occlusal view at the start of orthodontic therapy. Note the diastemata distal to teeth nos. 23 and 28.

regular-platform dental implants (Brånemark System, Nobel Biocare) were placed in sites nos. 29 and 31, and a new provisional was seated. Three months later, all implants were uncovered, and an impression was taken to fabricate screw-retained provisionals. At the time of the delivery of the implant-supported provisional restorations, the remaining two molar roots were extracted, and an additional 13-mm regular-platform implant (Brånemark System) was placed at site no. 30. This implant was not loaded until the end of the orthodontic phase of treatment. The mandibular screw-retained provisional restorations were constructed, maintaining a diastema between teeth nos. 22 and 23 and nos. 28 and 29 to allow for the orthodontic movement of the anterior teeth.

Orthodontic therapy was then initiated, using both provisional implant restorations as anchorage.

Phase VII: Corrective therapies in the maxilla

Tooth no. 6 was initially kept to support a provisional FPD (the first eggshell provisional was soon replaced by a metal-reinforced provisional) during the healing phases of the sinus elevation procedure. This procedure was carried out during implant placement in the mandibular left posterior segment. The bone collected from the implant sites was mixed with Bio-Oss (Geistlich) and inserted into the right sinus. Six months later, the tooth was extracted, and a provisional RPD had to be constructed to replace teeth nos. 3 to 6. Ten weeks later, four screw-type (Brånemark System) dental implants were inserted and submerged. The radiopaque stent used during the CT examination was modified and then used to identify the planned positions. The RPD was relined with a soft resin (Visco) 2 weeks later.

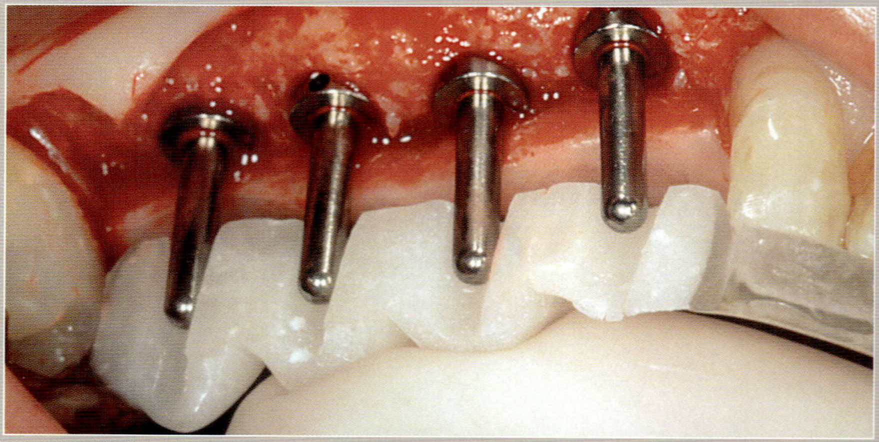

Modified radiographic stent used for identification of the mesiodistal and buccolingual position of the four maxillary implants.

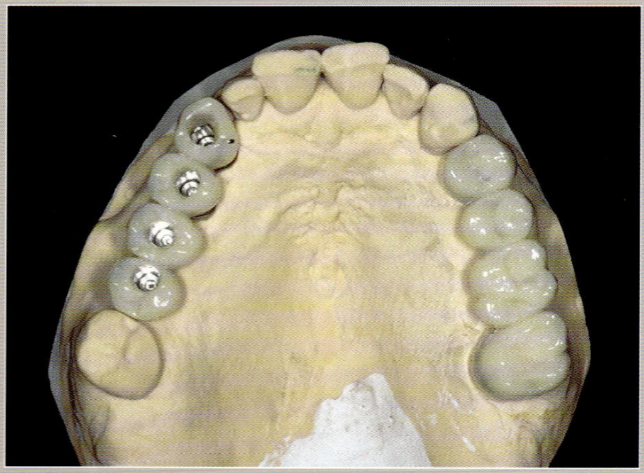

Occlusal view of maxillary provisional restorations on the cast.

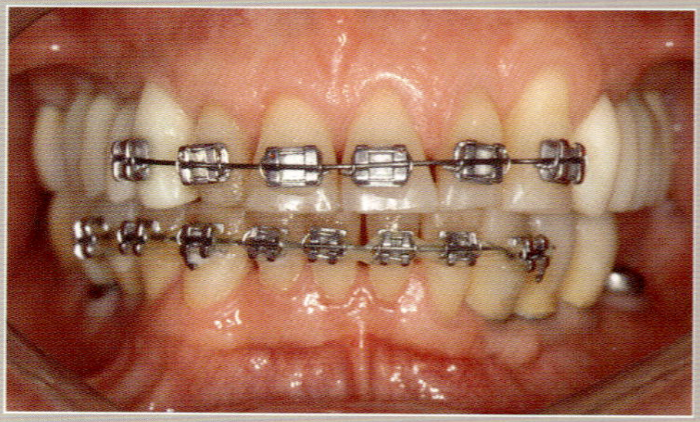

Initiation of orthodontic movement in the maxilla.

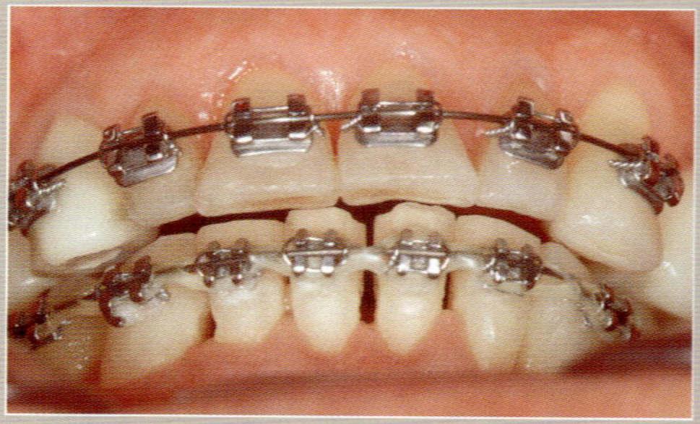

View of the overjet being created by lingual movement of the mandibular anterior teeth and buccal movement of the maxillary anterior teeth.

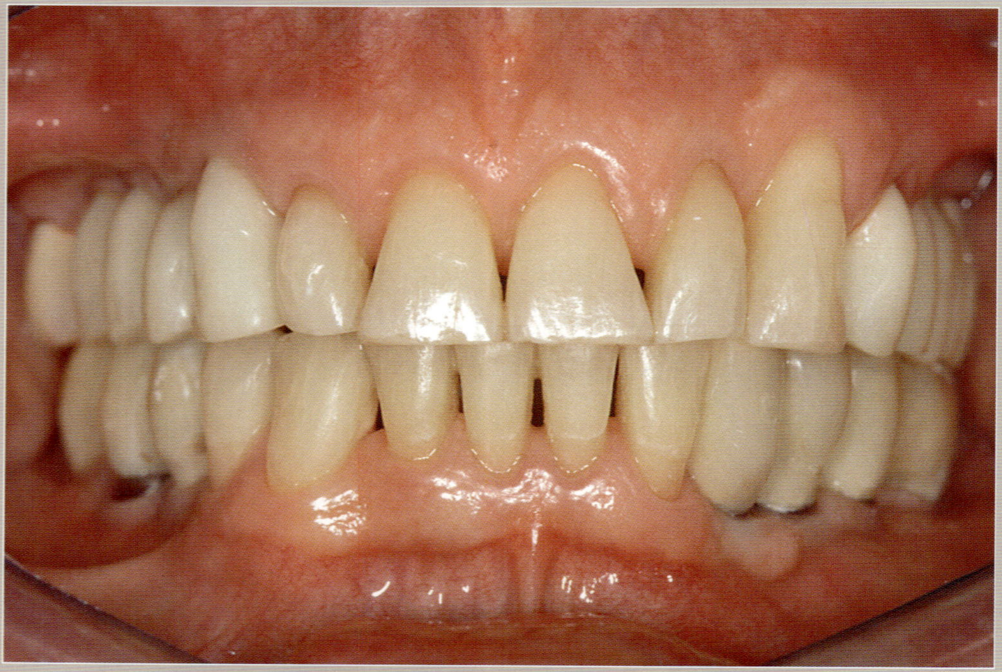

Frontal view of occlusion at the end of the orthodontic phase of treatment.

The implants were uncovered 7 months postsurgically, and a screw-retained provisional prosthesis, directly connected to the implants, was fabricated and inserted.

Ten months after the start of orthodontic movement in the mandible, it was possible to initiate orthodontic therapy in the maxilla as well. The aim of the orthodontic movement was to slightly procline the maxillary incisors to increase overjet. Also, because tooth no. 7 was smaller mesiodistally than tooth no. 10, space was allocated to properly restore it. As the orthodontist was providing the patient with overjet, repeated occlusal adjustments of the posterior provisionals were performed to decrease the VDO and, thus, obtain adequate overbite. The orthodontic phase was deemed completed once the teeth were aligned and an anterior overbite of about 2 mm was created. The efficacy of the anterior guide was checked with the provisionals before the orthodontist was asked to remove the appliance.

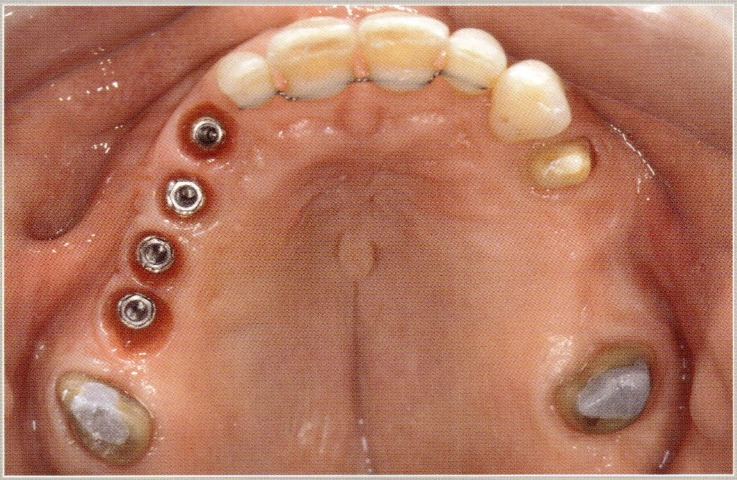 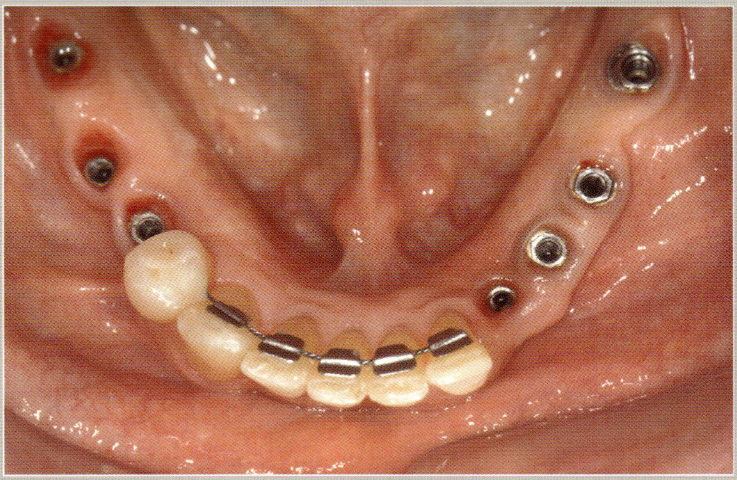

Occlusal views on the day of final impressions.

Phase VIII: Completion of orthodontic treatment and second re-evaluation (periodontal and occlusal)

Orthodontic movement of the mandibular teeth required 16 months, while orthodontic treatment in the maxilla was completed in 6 months. The movement was much slower than expected because of very dense bone as well as the compromised periodontal condition, which required the application of light forces. At the time of bracket removal, the natural teeth (nos. 7 to 11 and 23 to 28) were splinted with lingual fixed retainers.

At the time of periodontal re-evaluation, there was minimal residual periodontal pocketing. Tooth no. 12, despite being slightly mobile, was deemed suitable as an abutment for a four-unit FPD. Therefore, no additional implants were placed.

The occlusal scheme developed with the provisionals had the following features:

- CR coincident with MIP
- Bilateral contact on all posterior elements
- Light or no contact between anterior teeth
- Bilateral group function with disocclusion of the nonworking teeth
- Disocclusion of all posterior teeth in protrusion

The patient had no muscle tenderness or trismus, and the TMJ had no pathologic signs. The range of jaw movement was within normal limits. Therefore, it was decided to proceed with the definitive restorations.

Phase IX: Fabrication of the definitive prosthesis

Metal-ceramic material was chosen for the fabrication of the restorations on the remaining natural teeth (a single crown for tooth no. 2 and a four-unit FPD joining teeth nos. 12 to 15) and all implants. The material selected for all custom implant abutments was the same metal-ceramic alloy, which was applied to a prefabricated component. These materials provided the highest degree of reliability considering the parafunctional activity that the patient demonstrated at the start of therapy. For tooth no. 7, a porcelain veneer was planned in order to increase its size and match the contralateral tooth.

Much thought was given to whether adjacent implants should be restored separately or splinted. Several authors[9–13] have advocated routinely splinting adjacent implants. The reasons that have been given include sharing and distribution of the load, which decreases per-unit stress, and the possibility of adding cantilevers. Other authors[14,15] have suggested that implants may be restored separately in order to facilitate fabrication of passively fitting restorations and to increase access for adequate oral hygiene.

Certainly, in this instance, there may be a higher risk of loosening of the abutment screws or of stress concentration. Criteria that should be taken into consideration when making a decision include bone quality and quantity, crown-implant ratio, buccolingual dimension of the crowns as related to implant diameter, implant distribution, maxillomandibular relationship, and the occlusal scheme.[9,12] After an assessment of these variables was made, in this case the decision was made to restore the seven mandibular implants

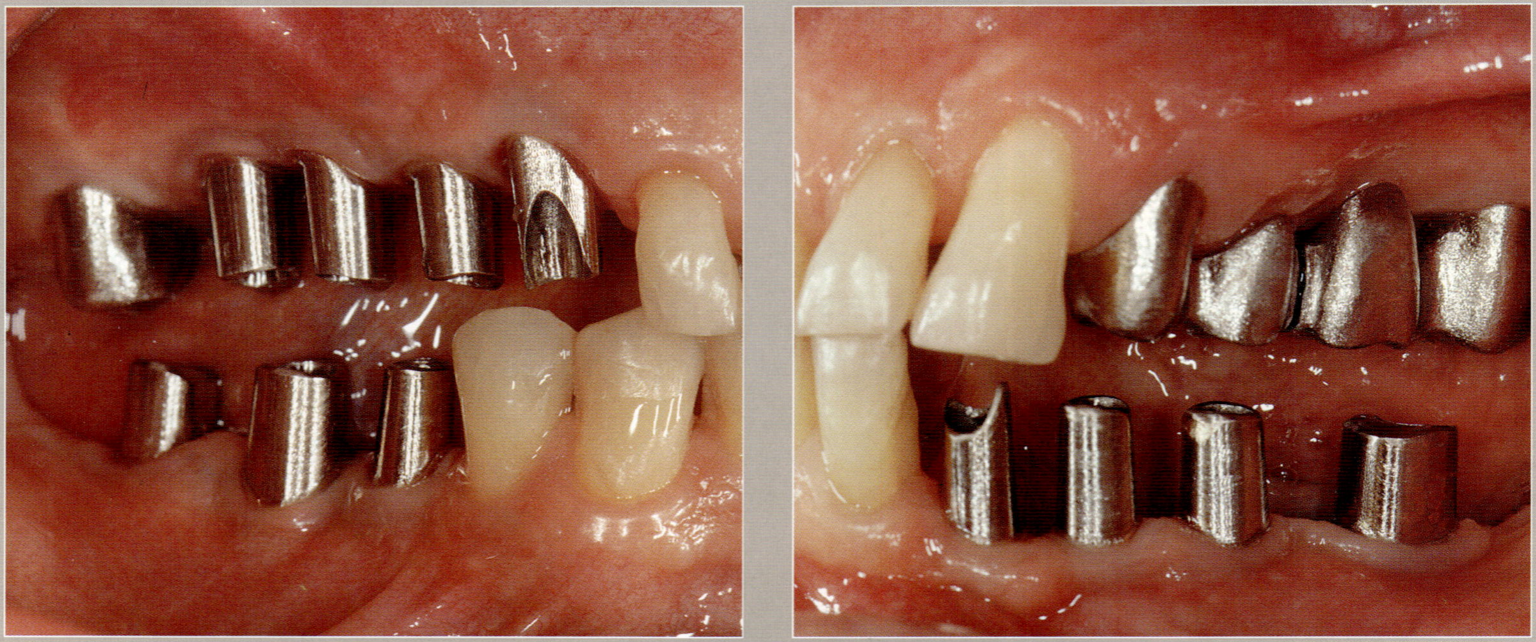

Lateral views of implant abutments and metal copings for crown of tooth no. 2 and FPD of teeth nos. 12 to 15.

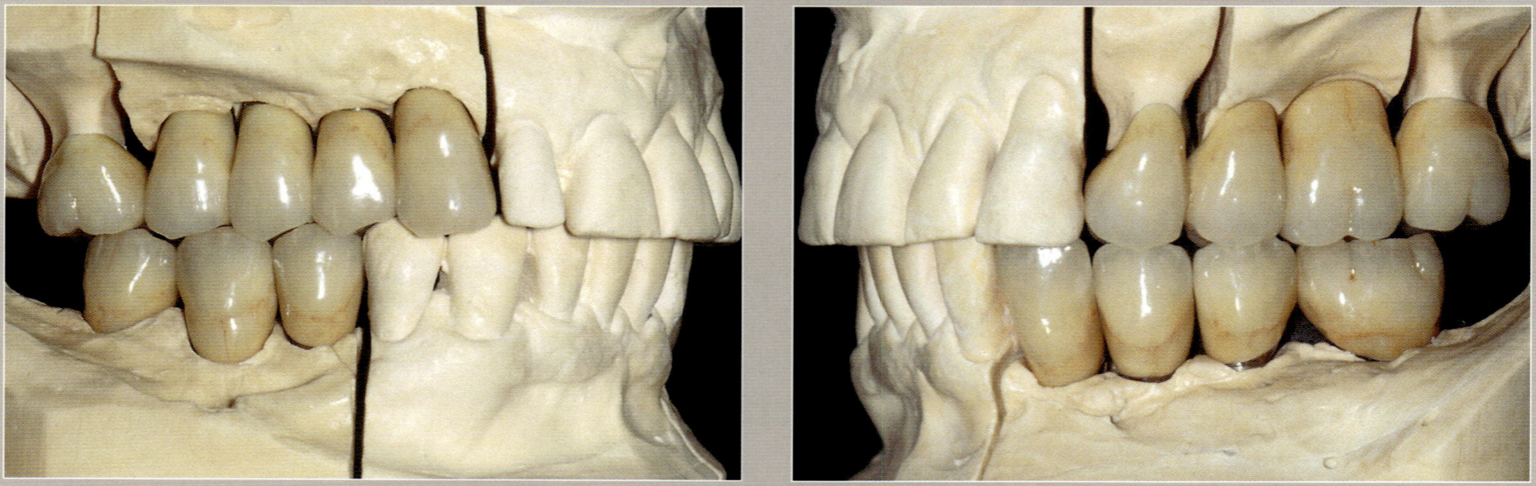

Lateral views of the finished metal-ceramic crowns in occlusion on the mounted casts.

separately and the maxillary implants splinted in twos. At the same time, attention was given to manufacturing crowns with limited buccolingual width of the occlusal table as a proven means to limit loading on the implants.[16]

Impressions were taken of the two arches using squared impression copings on the implants and a polyether material (Permadyne, 3M ESPE). The stone master casts generated were mounted on a semi-adjustable articulator (PCH, Panadent) with the aid of an earbow registration of the maxillary position and a maxillomandibular registration of CR position. The CR record was taken at the VDO dictated by the provisionals and where the definitive restorations would ultimately be constructed. Additional maxillomandibular registrations were recorded to allow cross-mounting of the stone casts with the provisional restorations. These provisionals served as a guide for developing the functional features of the definitive restorations through the modeling of a customized incisal table.[17] The articulator was set up with average settings obtained from the literature for condylar inclination (20 degrees with respect to the plane identified by the facebow), 1.5 mm of immediate mandibular lateral translation, and about 10 degrees of progressive mandibular lateral translation.[17] All crowns were constructed with metal disappearing margins on the buccal side. The implant crowns had a relatively wide lingual metal collar with a step for the tip of the rear-action hammer that could be used to remove them if necessary (eg, if the abutment screw becomes loose).

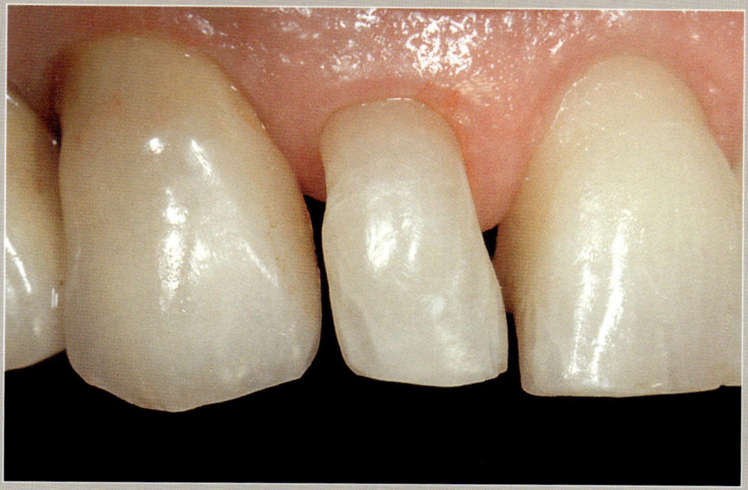

Peg lateral tooth no. 7.

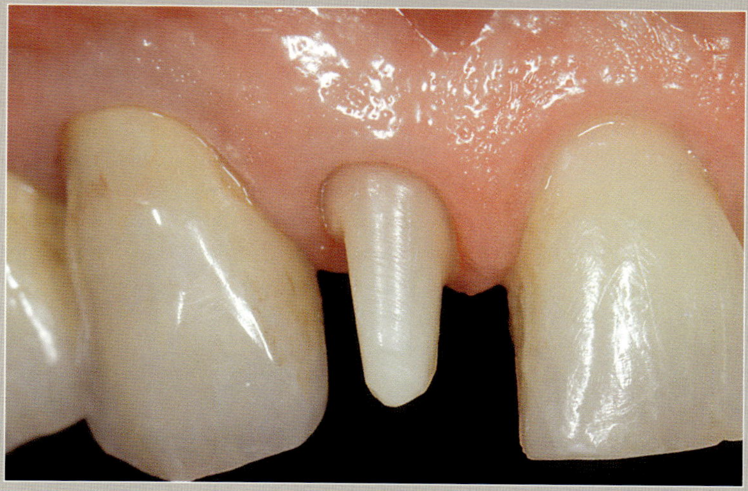

Prepared peg lateral.

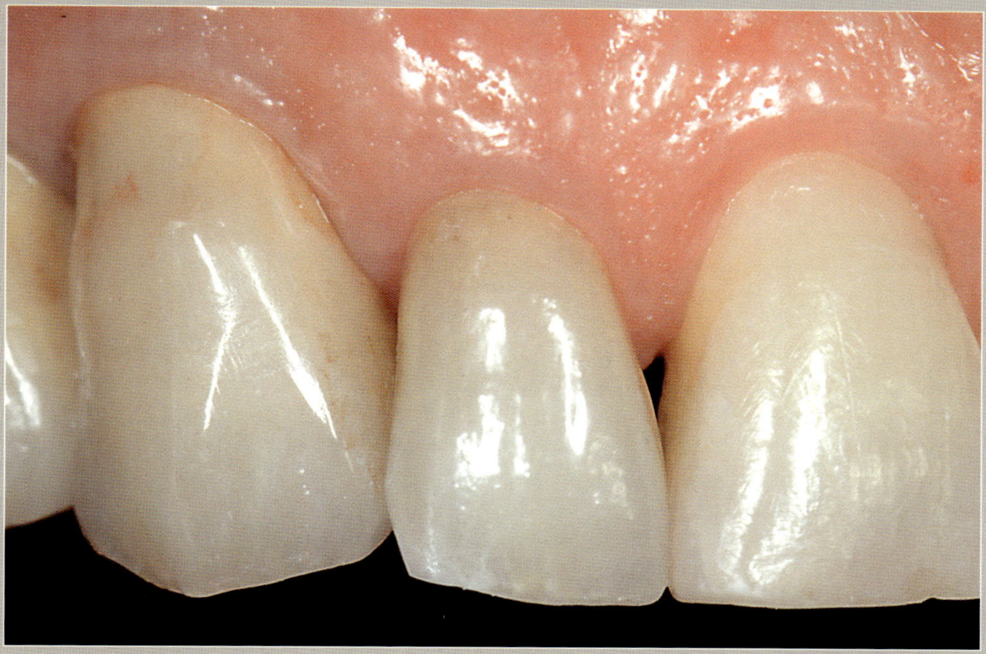

Glass-ceramic crown on tooth no. 7 cemented adhesively with a resin cement.

The titanium abutments' screws were tightened with a measured torque of 32 Ncm. All implant crowns were cemented with a temporary cement (TempBond, Kerr) and all those on natural teeth with glass-ionomer cement (Ketac-Cem, 3M ESPE).

Once restoration of the posterior teeth had been completed, the restoration of tooth no. 7 was addressed. A veneer preparation was initiated; however, in order to properly fill the interproximal spaces created by the orthodontic treatment and develop an emergence profile similar to the contralateral tooth (no. 10), it was converted to a full-crown preparation. A glass-ceramic crown (Empress II, Ivoclar Vivadent) was fabricated and cemented adhesively with a translucent resin cement (Variolink II, Ivoclar Vivadent). The tooth was left separate from tooth no. 8 and the other anterior teeth, which were connected by the orthodontic retainer.

As a final step, an occlusal appliance for the maxilla was fabricated for nighttime use and inserted during the same appointment as the delivery of the restoration for tooth no. 7. A full set of intraoral radiographs and a panoramic radiograph were taken to document the definitive periodontal and restorative status at the completion of active treatment in January 2001. Treatment took place over the course of 3 years and 4 months.

POSTTREATMENT

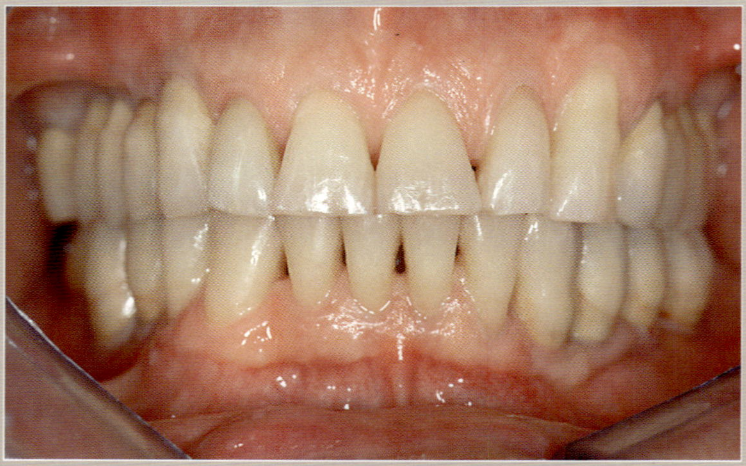

Frontal view of occlusion.

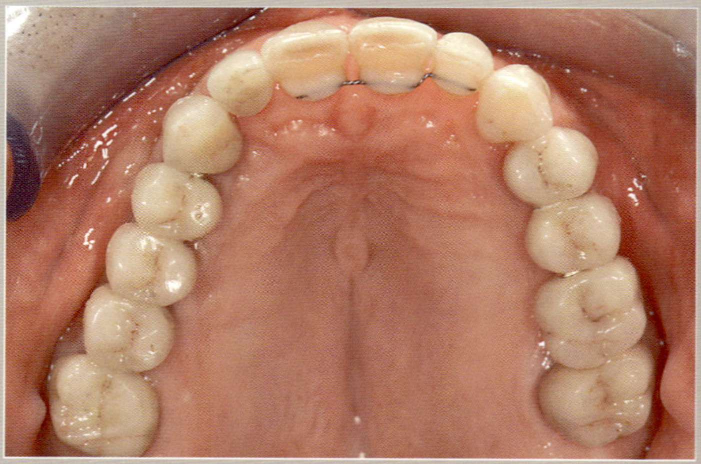

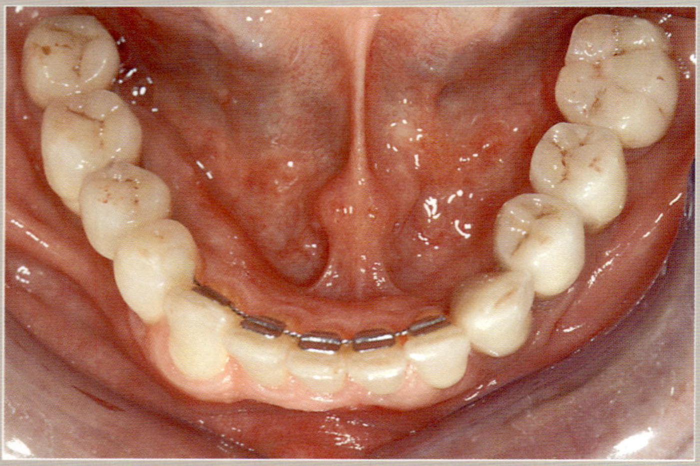

Occlusal views.

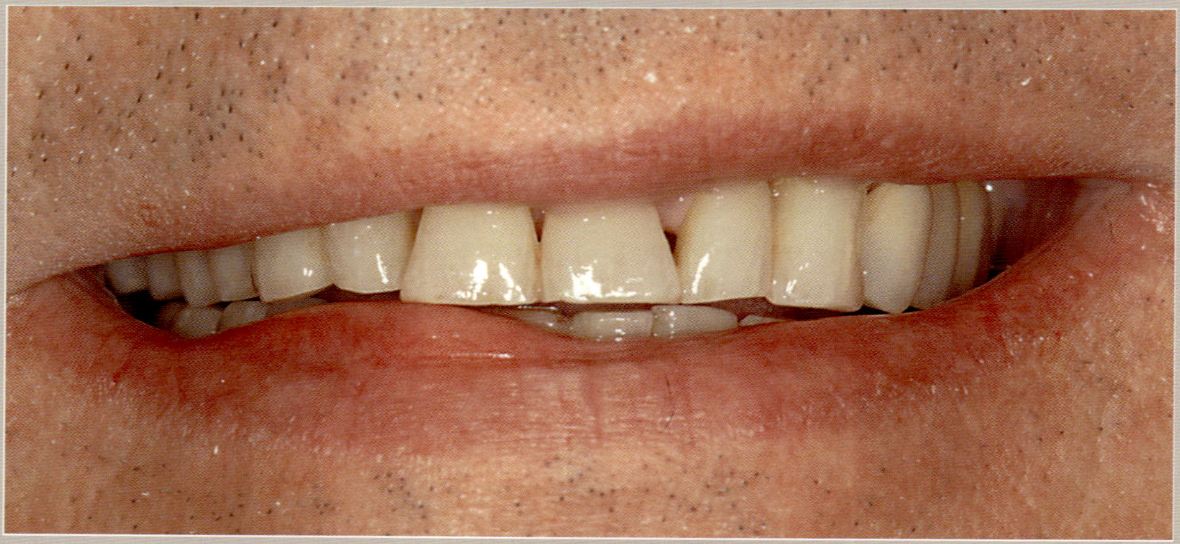

Close-up of the smile.

Phase X: Follow-up

Since the time of completion of the active treatment plan, the patient has complied with a strict 4-month maintenance schedule. During these recall sessions, the hygienist has performed scaling and root planing of all natural teeth and prophylaxis. Once a year, he has been scheduled with the restorative dentist (SG) for a complete restorative, occlusal, and periodontal examination of his rehabilitated dentition and of the nightguard. When necessary, an occlusal adjustment

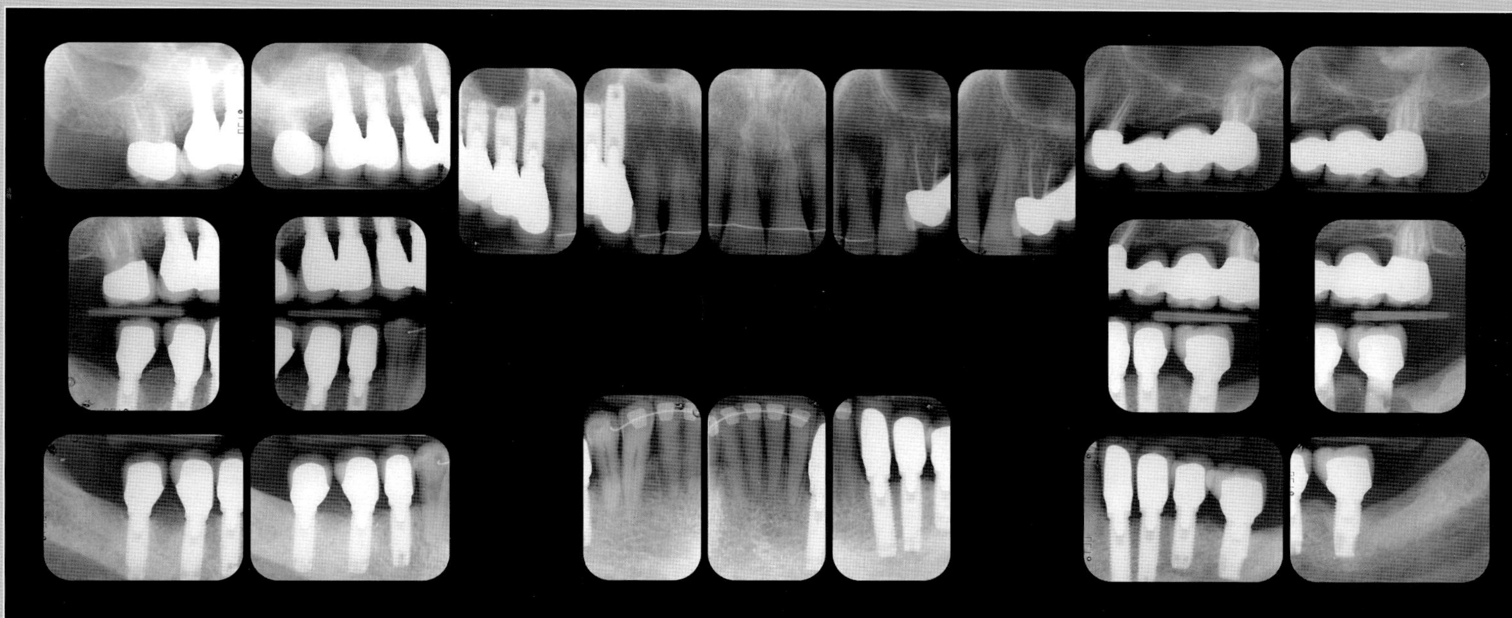

Complete-mouth radiographs at the end of treatment but before tooth no. 7 was restored (January 2001).

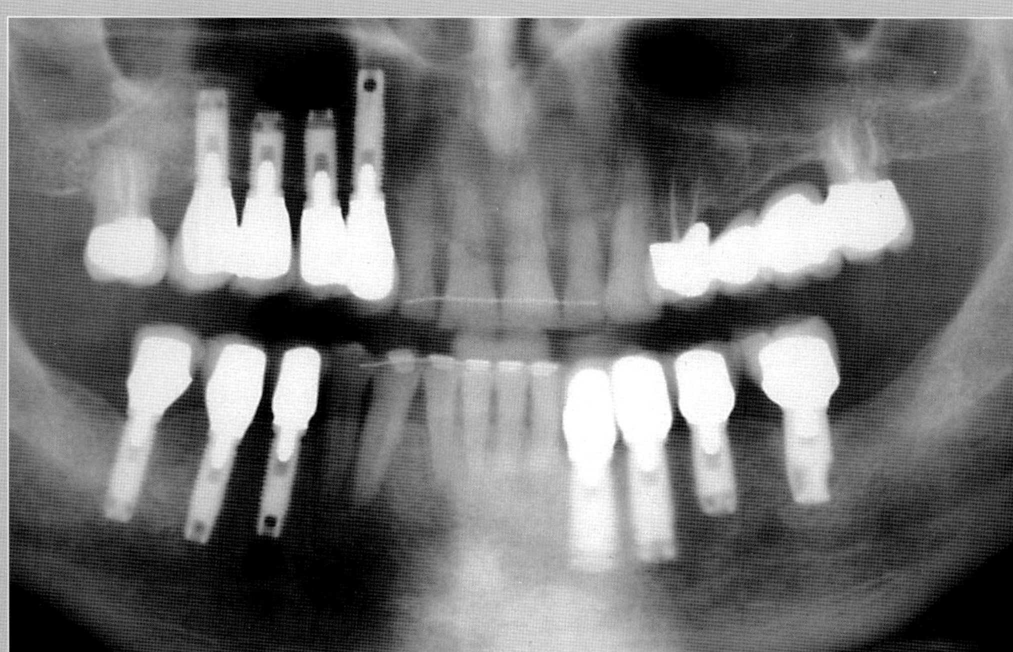

Panoramic radiograph at the end of treatment but before tooth no. 7 was restored (January 2001).

has been performed. Bitewing radiographs have been taken once a year, and periapical radiographs of the endodontically treated teeth have been taken every 2 years. A complete-mouth set of periapical radiographs and a panoramic radiograph were taken at the 9-year recall. The postorthodontic retainer applied at the end of the active orthodontic treatment is still in place.

During the past 10 years, his dentition has remained completely stable. Only minor chipping of the distolingual cusp of the implant crown at site no. 19 has been noted. This cohesive fracture was smoothed with diamond-impregnated rubber points. There has been no abutment screw loosening or fracture, and no implant crowns have been dislodged. The patient has worn the nightguard appliance regularly, and the degree of its wear has been slight. This may be taken as evidence that the initial diagnosis of parafunction, in all likelihood, was incorrect. Too often, we make the mistake of diagnosing parafunctional habits based only on the presence of occlusal or incisal wear.

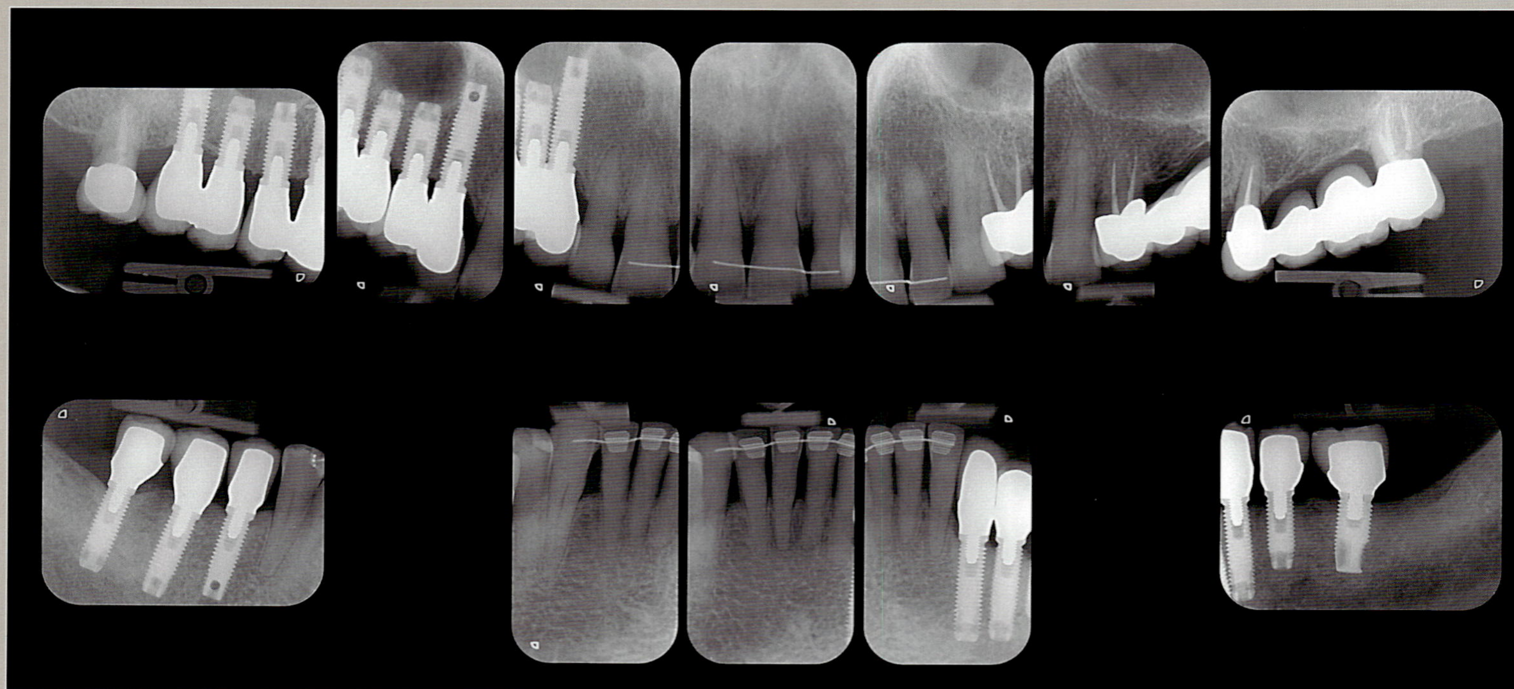

Complete-mouth radiographs at 9-year recall.

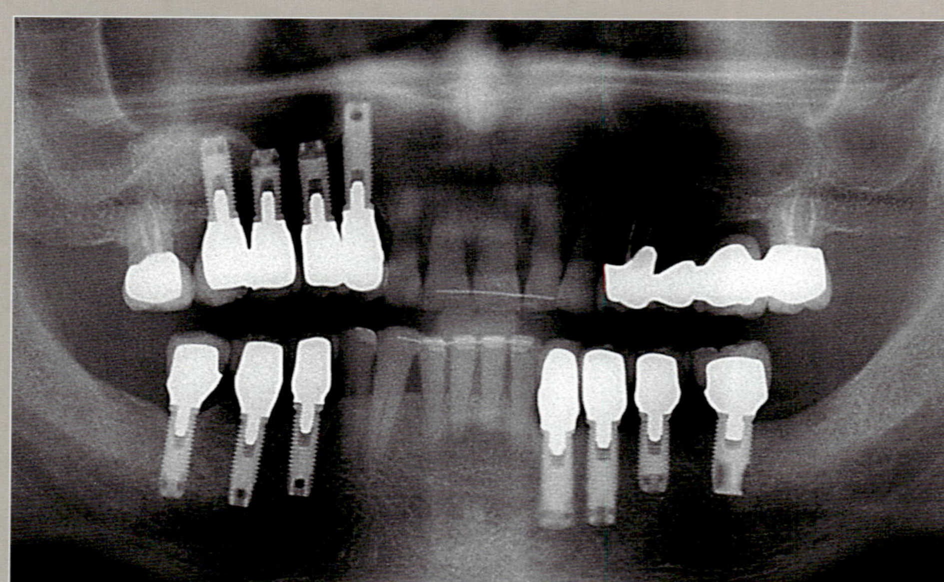

Panoramic radiograph at 9-year recall.

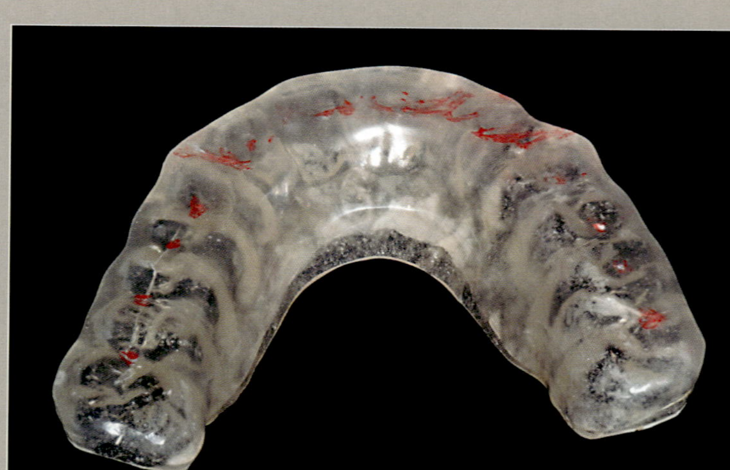

View of the occlusal surface of the nighttime appliance after 10 years of regular use. The limited amount of wear indicates that, in all likelihood, the initial diagnosis of parafunction was incorrect.

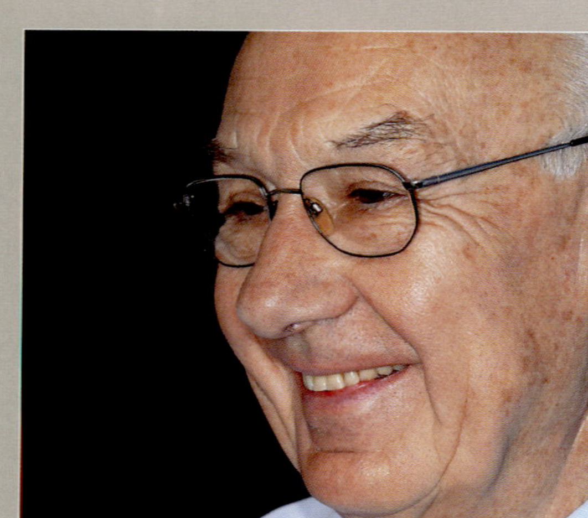

Oblique facial view of patient at 10-year recall.

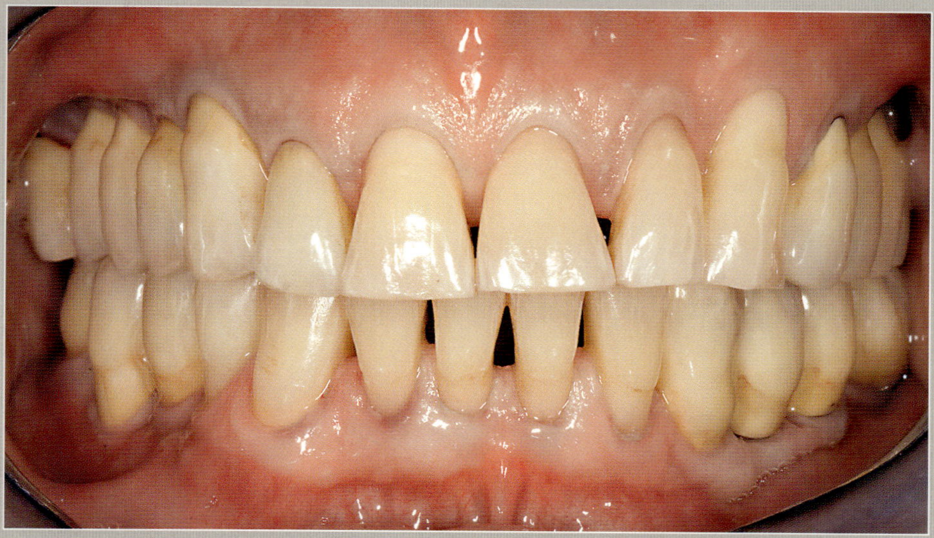

Frontal view of occlusion at 10-year recall.

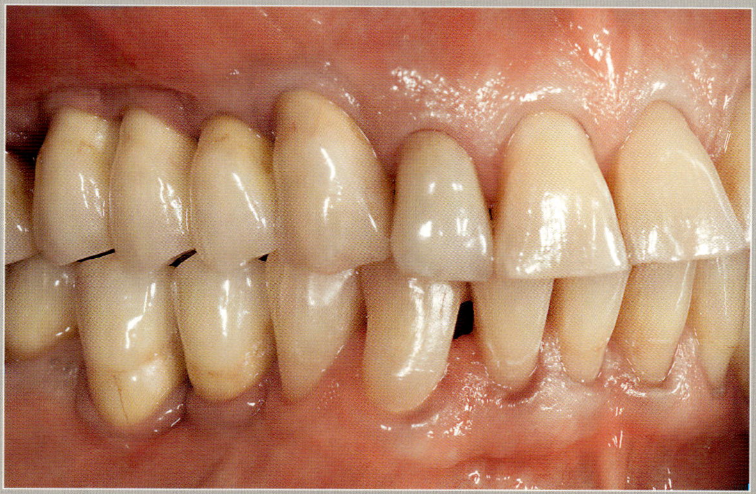

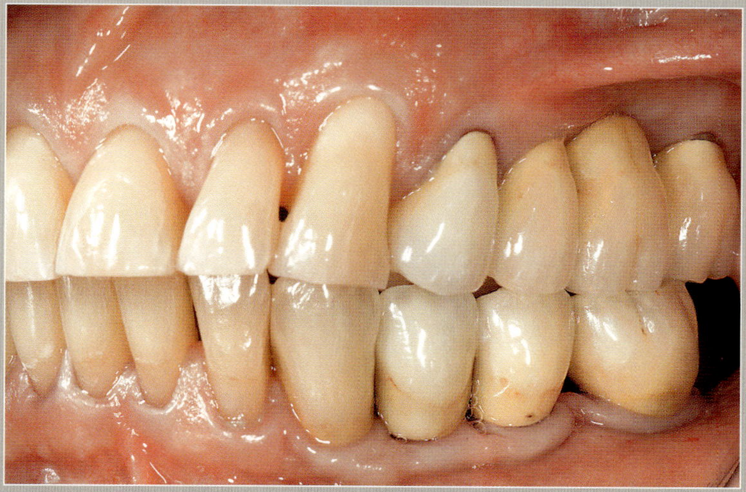

Lateral views of occlusion at 10-year recall.

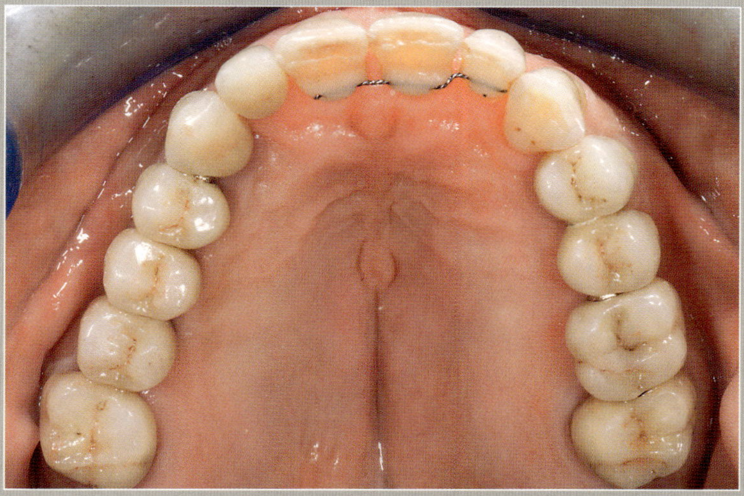

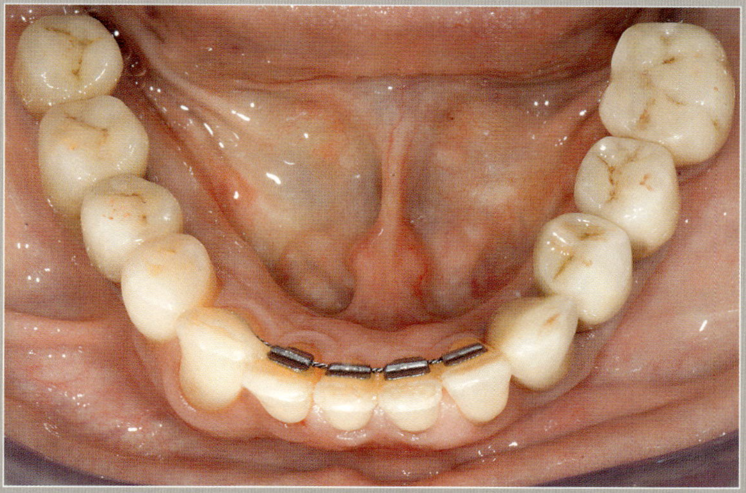

Occlusal views at 10-year recall.

You may now place the corresponding posttreatment overlay found in the separate folder over the pretreatment periodontal chart on page 7.

Commentary

Any time that a patient presents with a malocclusion, malpositioned teeth due to tooth migration resulting from missing teeth, and/or isolated bony defects, orthodontic therapy must be taken into consideration. Orthodontic therapy allows the restorative dentist to be more conservative and effective and, in many cases, leads to a higher-quality treatment outcome.

In speaking with many colleagues who perform restorative dentistry, I am surprised at the discovery of how seldom this approach is taken into consideration. The main argument voiced is that it is difficult to find an orthodontist who is knowledgeable on preprosthetic tooth movement in adult patients. Although this may be true, it should not be an excuse for avoiding what is undoubtedly the most prudent treatment approach in many clinical cases.

There is a need for orthodontists, periodontists, and restorative dentists to learn together and to communicate and collaborate on a regular basis because many of our adult patients present challenging situations that are of an interdisciplinary nature. The reality that most cases are restoratively driven naturally implies that either the restorative dentist or prosthodontist should take the lead in directing the interdisciplinary team during the course of treatment. This is the same individual who is usually responsible for keeping a watchful eye on the patient after the definitive restorations have been delivered and is likely to be the first to address a minor posttreatment problem before it becomes a major ordeal.

Aspects of this treatment that could be challenged

There are a number of questions related to this clinical case that may arise in the reader's mind. Some of these issues are addressed below.

- *Was orthodontic therapy necessary or could the same result have been achieved through restorative means only?* There is no doubt in my mind that we would not have been able to achieve the same treatment results without the inclusion of orthodontic therapy. The reasons were described above in Phase V of the Active Clinical Treatment section.

- *Is it safe to decrease VDO given the possible consequences at the joint level?* When the VDO is altered, whether it is increased or reduced, one can never assume that it will be well tolerated by the patient. Alteration of the patient's vertical dimension is a controversial approach that does not have strong scientific evidence to support its validity. However, there is also no scientific evidence that demonstrates that it cannot be done. Thus, it comes down to a decision determined by what is loosely defined as *prosthetic convenience:* If it is necessary or convenient to improve the maxillomandibular relationship while allowing or creating space for the restorative material without being excessively invasive, the operator can modify the maxillomandibular distance the minimum amount necessary using provisional restorations. It is essential to then observe the behavior of the patient over a reasonable period of time to assess whether he or she reacts favorably to this change. If the treating clinicians observe the onset of articular or muscular symptoms, phonetic impairment, or an increase in tooth mobility, after verifying the accuracy of the occlusal scheme developed, he or she has the ability to re-establish the original VDO.

- *Is the placement of an implant for each missing tooth justified?* No, the placement of an implant for each missing tooth is not necessarily justified, at least when the bone quality is satisfactory (type 1 to 3), the implant-crown ratio is favorable, and the occlusal scheme being developed has an efficient anterior guidance and properly sized posterior implant crowns in the correct occlusal relationship. In this specific case, in the mandible, my goal was to improve access for adequate oral hygiene, providing single units so that the patient could use regular floss. In the maxilla, however, splinted prosthetic units could not be avoided. Furthermore, because the anterior teeth were also splinted with extracoronal postorthodontic retainers, one could argue that it served no real purpose to have the mandibular posterior units separated and that it would only increase the cost of treatment. Had we planned for splinted units, we could have avoided placing one implant on each side.

- *Is it safe to leave neighboring implants as single units or is splinting necessary?* My current thinking is that it is safer to splint than to leave neighboring implants separated. However, research in this area is very controversial, and leaving the implants separated in this clinical situation has caused no harmful effects. There is an aspect that, in the past, may have influenced the decision whether to splint or not: the technical difficulty in achieving passive fit for a multi-unit implant prosthesis when fabricating it using traditional technologies (ie, casting and, eventually, soldering of multiple pieces). Modern manufacturing technologies (ie, computer-aided design/computer-assisted manufacturing [CAD/CAM], spark erosion, laser welding) have greatly reduced the complications, and a passive fit is more easily attainable even for complete-arch prostheses, provided that the proper impression technique is used. Whenever possible, it is recommended to use dental stone as an impression material for implants. In the case of a fully edentulous arch, it should be used as the only material. In the case of an arch with natural teeth and multiple adjacent implants, it can be used in combination with an elastomeric material by employing the modular custom impression tray technique.[18]

- *Can a group function occlusal scheme be achieved predictably without making a pantographic tracing and using a fully adjustable articulator?* Pantographic tracings and the use of fully adjustable articulators do not guarantee the uncomplicated and automatic development of an occlusal scheme that does not require any occlusal adjustments once the prostheses are tried in the mouth, even when canine guidance is the goal. As it was already pointed out in another publication,[1] many operator-related variables may adversely influence the possibility of obtaining in the laboratory an occlusal relationship between opposing arches that would be in harmony with the patient's oral system. If the cross-mounting procedure is employed (ie, mounting on the articulator the casts of the prepared abutments and the provisional restorations adjusted in the mouth, at the same vertical dimension and in the same spatial relationship), I feel that it is not necessary to record a pantographic tracing and use a fully adjustable articulator. Use of a semi-adjustable articulator set with values derived from the literature (see page 18) is adequate.

- *Can the use of ceramics be employed safely in a patient who has signs of severe tooth abrasion and a diagnosis of parafunction?* No, ceramics (regardless of whether they are supported by metal) cannot with any certainty be employed safely in a patient who has signs of severe tooth abrasion and a diagnosis of parafunction. However, if the patient's original wear is due to occlusal dysfunction, it is possible that with the rehabilitation of his or her mouth, occlusal hyperfunction will diminish or disappear, allowing occlusal surfaces to be developed in ceramic with a reasonably predictable long-term outlook. If, however, the diagnosis of parafunction is confirmed, then the only safe material from an occlusal standpoint, in my view, is metal (ie, gold alloy). This, however, has become unacceptable in most of our practices. We usually resort to informed consent in presenting the likely risks of ceramic chipping and fracture, possibly in short order. Regardless of the materials, precautions should always be taken to very carefully check the quality, number, and location of contacts in occlusion and during excursive movements at time of delivery and at regular intervals thereafter. The strategy of delivering a resin occlusal guard may be acceptable provided that the patient wears it regularly.

- *What could have been done differently?* In looking back at the treatment performed on this patient, there are four observations that can be made and that would possibly suggest a modification in the treatment plan and the treatment performed:

1. Tooth no. 12 could have been maintained intact if implants had been planned in the maxillary left quadrant (sites nos. 13 and 14) and a removable provisional appliance used once the existing partial denture was removed and tooth no. 14 extracted.
2. The removal of teeth nos. 30 and 31 could have been executed without performing the periodontal surgery in which they were hemisected. Once the mesial root of tooth no. 31 had been deemed unreliable and endodontic success on tooth no. 30 was not achievable, all the roots should have been removed and the three implants placed simultaneously. The patient was already wearing a removable provisional appliance to temporarily replace the teeth on the left side, and it would not have made any difference to him if a similar appliance had replaced the posterior teeth on the right side as well. This would have saved a few months of therapy.
3. Temporary anchorage devices (TADs) could have been employed to provide early anchorage for orthodontic movement of the anterior teeth to avoid having to wait for osseointegration of the implants that were used to support the provisional crowns. If successful, their use could have saved a few months of treatment time in both arches.
4. Immediate loading of implants in partially edentulous patients was not evidence-based practice at the time treatment was performed and remains controversial. However, in all three quadrants, implants were placed with an insertion torque of more than 40 Ncm. This degree of torque associated with the relatively high number of implants inserted (one per missing tooth) is thought to be a positive indicator for attempting immediate provisionalization.[19-22] If this had been implemented and no complications had occurred, the patient could have been spared the discomfort associated with the use of removable provisional appliances for several months and the 2-week period without them following implant surgery.

References

1. Gracis S. Clinical considerations and rationale for the use of simplified instrumentation in occlusal rehabilitation: Part I: Mounting of the models on the articulator. Int J Periodontics Restorative Dent 2003;23:57–67.
2. Roberts WE, Smith RK, Zilberman Y, Mozsary PG, Smith RS. Osseous adaptation to continuous loading of rigid endosseous implants. Am J Orthod 1984;86:95–111.
3. Roberts WE, Helm FR, Marshall KJ, Gongloff RK. Rigid endosseous implants for orthodontic and orthopedic anchorage. Angle Orthod 1989;59:247–256.
4. Turley PK, Kean C, Schur J, et al. Orthodontic force application to titanium endosseous implants. Angle Orthod 1988;58:151–162.
5. Linder-Aronson S, Nordenram A, Anneroth G. Titanium implant anchorage in orthodontic treatment. Eur J Orthod 1990;12:414–419.
6. Ödman J, Lekholm U, Jemt T, Thilander B. Osseointegrated implants as orthodontic anchorage in the treatment of partially edentulous adult patients. Eur J Orthod 1994;16:187–201.
7. Smalley WM. Implants for tooth movement. Determining implant location and orientation. J Esthet Dent 1995;7:26–36.
8. Smalley WM. Clinical and laboratory procedures for implant anchorage in partially edentulous dentitions. In: Higuchi K (ed). Orthodontic Applications for Osseointegrated Implants. Chicago: Quintessence, 2000:33–69.
9. Renouard F, Rangert B. Risk Factors in Implant Dentistry: Simplified Clinical Analysis for Predictable Treatment, ed 2. Paris: Quintessence, 2008.
10. Guichet N, Yoshinobu D, Caputo AA. Effect of splinting and interproximal contact tightness on load transfer by implant restorations. J Prosthet Dent 2002;87:528–535.
11. Huang HL, Huang JS, Ko CC, Hsu JT, Chang CH, Chen MY. Effects of splinted prosthesis supported a wide implant or two implants: A three-dimensional finite element analysis. Clin Oral Implants Res 2005;16:466–472.
12. Misch C. Consideration of biomechanical stress in treatment with dental implants. Dent Today 2006;25(5):80,82,84–85.
13. Bergkvist G, Simonsson K, Rydberg K, Johansson F, Dérand T. A finite element analysis of stress distribution in bone tissue surrounding uncoupled or splinted dental implants. Clin Implant Dent Relat Res 2008;10:40–46.
14. Naert I, Koutsikakis G, Quirynen M, Duyck J, van Steenberghe D, Jacobs R. Biologic outcome of implant-supported restorations in the treatment of partial edentulism. Part 2: A longitudinal radiographic study. Clin Oral Implants Res 2002;13:390–395.
15. Grossmann Y, Finger IM, Block MS. Indications for splinting implant restorations. J Oral Maxillofac Surg 2005;63:1642–1652.
16. Morneburg TR, Pröschel PA. In vivo forces on implants influenced by occlusal scheme and food consistency. Int J Prosthodont 2003;16:481–486.
17. Gracis S. Clinical considerations and rationale for the use of simplified instrumentation in occlusal rehabilitation. Part II: Setting of the articulator and occlusal optimization. Int J Periodontics Restorative Dent 2003;23:139–145.
18. Massironi D, Pascetta R, Romeo G. Precision in Dental Esthetics: Clinical and Laboratory Procedures. Chicago: Quintessence, 2007:300–306 .
19. Szmukler-Moncler S, Piattelli A, Favero GA, Dubruille JH. Considerations preliminary to the application of early and immediate loading protocols in dental implantology. Clin Oral Implants Res 2000;11:12–25.
20. Hui E, Chow J, Li D, Liu J, Wat P, Law H. Immediate provisional for single-tooth implant replacement with Brånemark system: Preliminary report. Clin Implant Dent Relat Res 2001;3:79–86.
21. Testori T, Galli F, Capelli M, Zuffetti F, Esposito M. Immediate nonocclusal versus early loading of dental implants in partially edentulous patients: 1-year results from a multicenter, randomized controlled clinical trial. Int J Oral Maxillofac Implants 2007;22:815–822.
22. Galli F, Capelli M, Zuffetti F, Testori T, Esposito M. Immediate non-occlusal vs. early loading of dental implants in partially edentulous patients: A multicentre randomized clinical trial. Peri-implant bone and soft-tissue levels. Clin Oral Implants Res 2008;19:546–552.

2

Functional Considerations in Treatment Planning the Biomechanically Compromised Dentition

Ariel J. Raigrodski, DMD, MS
Yen-Wei Chen, DDS, MSD

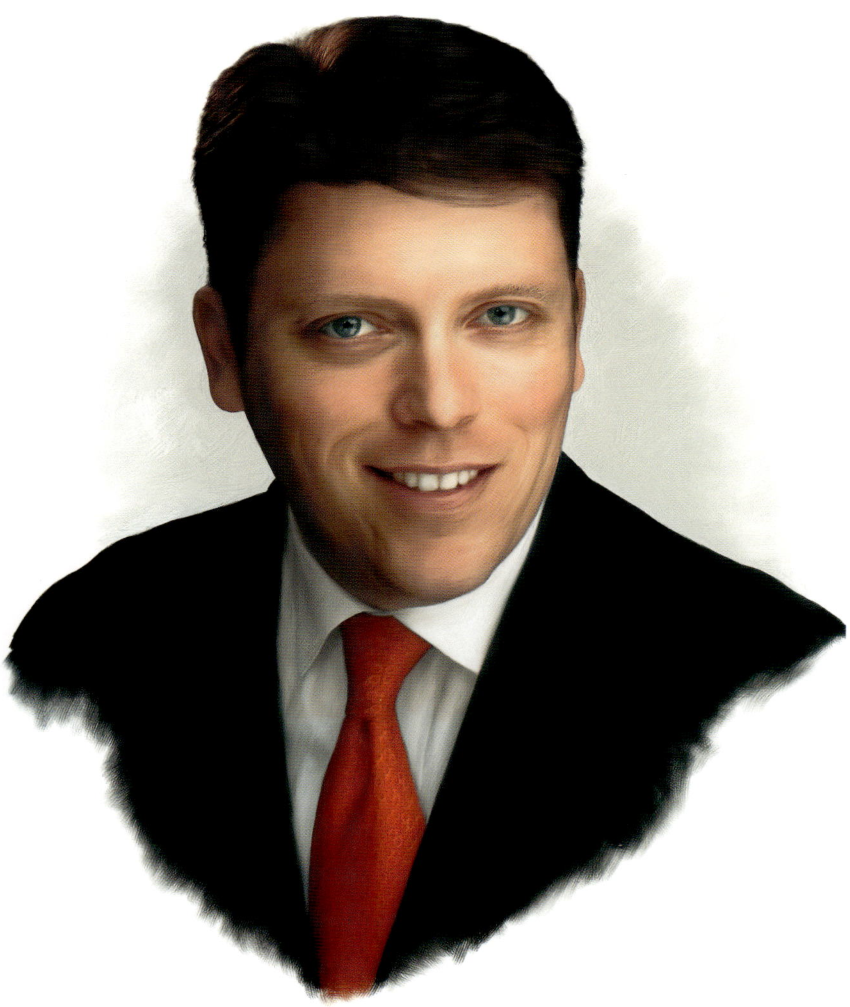

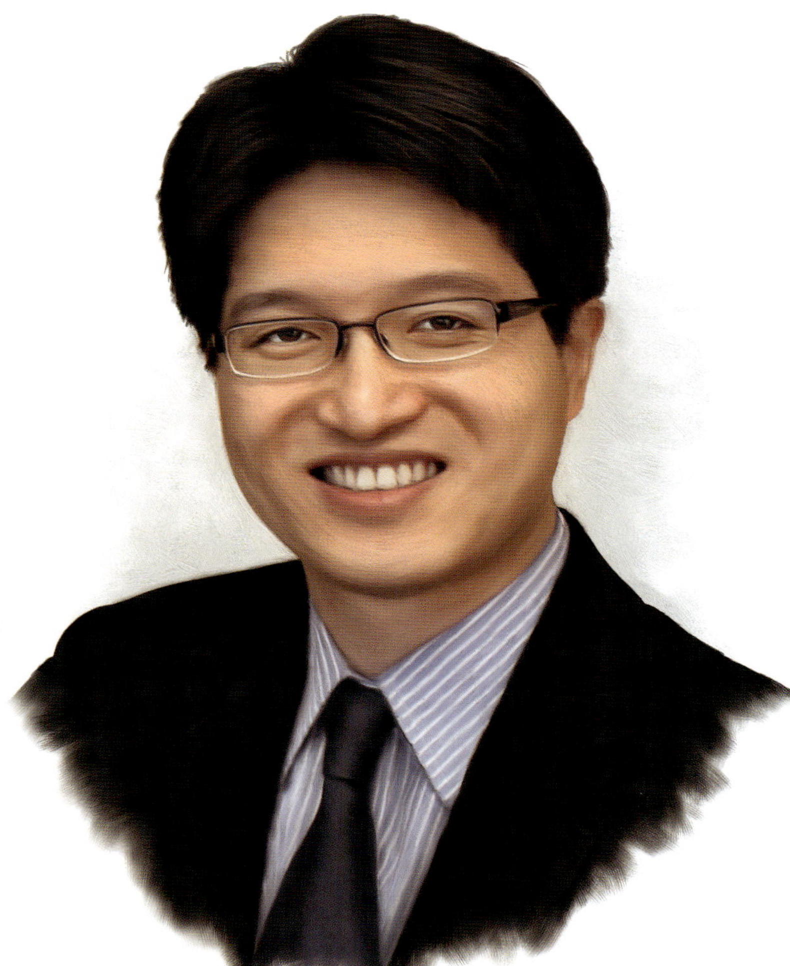

When planning treatment for patients with a biomechanically compromised dentition, the incorporation of functional considerations is critical in setting the stage for predictable long-term treatment success.

Philosophy and Background

Treating patients who have a severely biomechanically compromised dentition and are in need of complete-mouth fixed reconstruction is a significant challenge in our private practice and in the graduate prosthodontics program at the University of Washington. Such patients usually present with additional functional issues such as occlusal dysfunction and parafunction. A major dilemma in contemporary dental practice is whether such teeth should be restored at all cost or extracted to allow restoration with implant-supported prostheses.

Biomechanics is the study of the mechanical laws relating to the movement or structure of living organisms.[1] In dentistry, *biomechanics* is the relationship between the biologic behavior of oral structures and the physical influence of a dental restoration.[2] Biomechanical risk assessment is concerned with the degree to which the existing tooth structure is compromised.[3] Intact dentitions are considered most sound in terms of biomechanics and thus have the potential to best withstand functional as well as parafunctional forces. Loss of tooth structure may be related to normal physiologic processes that occur slowly and continuously throughout life. However, if the rate of tooth structure loss becomes accelerated and the degree of destruction becomes excessive, it may result in biomechanical, functional, and esthetic challenges.[4]

Numerous factors may increase the tooth's biomechanical risk. Such factors may be classified into five major groups:

1. Developmental disorders
2. Regressive alterations
3. Trauma
4. Dental caries
5. Pre-existing restorations

Developmental disorders such as amelogenesis and dentinogenesis imperfecta, enamel hypoplasia, and dentinal dysplasia may cause a reduction in the quality and quantity of tooth structure and may predispose the dentition to further mechanical and chemical breakdown.[5]

Regressive alterations in tooth structure are related mainly to tooth wear.[6–8] Excessive wear may be the result of:

- Mechanical causes (including attrition and abrasion, which may be the result of occlusal dysfunction or parafunctional habits)
- Chemical erosion (caused by consumption of acidic foods and beverages, gastroesophageal reflux disease, eating disorders, and chronic regurgitation such as that often seen with alcoholism)

Most often patients present with a combination of several such causes, which may have a synergistic effect and exacerbate tooth structure loss.

In the context of compromised tooth structure, trauma may cause not only coronal tooth structure loss or crown-root fracture but also incomplete root formation. This may result in either a short root with a poor crown-root ratio or a wide canal with thin dentinal walls, which may make the tooth more susceptible to root fracture.[9,10]

The inability to adequately manage and control dental caries may ultimately result in progressive tooth structure loss with or without pulpal disease. Additional loss of tooth structure occurs with caries removal and cavity preparation as well as endodontic therapy procedures when needed. The balance between demineralization and remineralization of tooth structure determines dental caries progression or reversal. Pathologic factors such as cariogenic bacteria, inadequate saliva quality and quantity, and exposure to fermentable carbohydrates resulting in low pH all contribute to caries progression. In contrast, adequate salivary flow and composition, topical fluoride application, use of xylitol, and extrinsic antibacterial agents are protective factors that contribute to caries reversal.[11] Caries management by risk assessment (CAMBRA) is an important instrument for potential reversal of early caries as well as disease prevention.[12,13] Such an assessment plays a major role in evaluating a patient for a comprehensive complete-mouth rehabilitation.[14]

Finally, restoration-related tooth structure loss and further weakening may be the result of one or more of the following causes:

- Fabrication of foundation restorations for crowns and fixed partial dentures (FPDs), such as dowels and cores and cores with or without pins
- Tooth preparation for direct, indirect intracoronal, and indirect extracoronal partial and complete coverage restorations
- Occlusal adjustment and reshaping

An extensive preparation design will result in increased tooth structure loss and increased biomechanical compromise.[15,16]

Although clinicians may lack an objective, quantifiable tool for making a definitive decision regarding the restorability of a tooth with a complete-coverage restoration and must mainly rely on their clinical experience, a major factor in such a decision is the residual tooth ferrule.[17,18] This ferrule (1.5 to 2 mm) can be detrimental to the longevity of a biomechanically compromised restored tooth. Orthodontic extrusion or surgical crown lengthening procedures may be used to improve the ferrule and facilitate the longevity of a definitive restoration. However, such decisions cannot be made independent of the following considerations, which will affect the definitive treatment plan:

- Tooth position relative to the patient's face, desired incisal edge position, and prospective occlusal plane
- Periodontal health as well as the prospective gingival levels, which may also be related to the gain of additional ferrule without severely compromising the crown-root ratio
- Susceptibility to dental caries and chemical erosion as related to the patient's medical and dental history and diet
- Esthetic requirements
- Patient acceptance of the cost of the treatment

In addition, functional considerations, which may include the presence or absence of muscle or joint disorders, occlusal dysfunction, and parafunctional habits, may profoundly affect the decision regarding whether the biomechanically compromised dentition may be restored with adequate prospects for longevity or whether an alternative mode of treatment should be considered.[19] The etiology of bruxism (which may occur while the patient is awake or asleep) is mainly related to stress and anxiety, central nervous system and sleep disorders, genetics, and occlusal disturbances.[20] This habit represents a significant liability after restorative therapy has been successfully completed and may result in future fracture and failure of both the restoration and the underlying dentition.

Thus, we as clinicians must ask ourselves the following questions: Is the tooth located in a favorable arch position? Is the tooth required to support a single crown? Is it planned to support a short- or long-span FPD or will it serve to bear a tooth-supported or a tissue-tooth–supported removable partial denture?

The case presentations that follow demonstrate the application of a principle we use in treating patients with severely biomechanically compromised dentitions: *Long-term treatment predictability in restoring the biomechanically compromised dentition is dependent on the presence of muscular, joint, or occlusal dysfunction, as well as parafunctional habits and the ability of the patient and the treating team to address and manage over time the etiology of tooth structure loss.* To apply this principle, clinicians must ask the following questions: Can we gain adequate ferrule for the prospective abutment teeth? Can the etiology of tooth structure loss be addressed and managed over time? Does the patient demonstrate signs or symptoms of occlusal dysfunction or parafunctional habits? If the etiology of tooth structure loss can be managed over time and the patient has no history of dysfunction or parafunctional habits, then the patient may be restored predictably, as presented in the first case. If the patient presents with functional concerns, the likelihood of restoration and tooth fracture may increase, and the course of treatment must be cautiously determined. Alternative treatment with an implant-supported prosthesis may be considered with the intention of having a contingency plan addressing a prospective need to manage prosthetic complications over time. This treatment initiative relates to the second case presented in this chapter.

Case Presentation 1

Treating clinicians
Prosthodontist: Yen-Wei Chen, DDS, MSD
Periodontist: Michelle Lee, DMD, MSD
Prosthodontist: Ariel J. Raigrodski, DMD, MS

Clinical Treatment Planning

Age at initial presentation: 59 years
Initial presentation: November 2005
Active treatment completed: June 2008

Introduction and background

A 59-year-old woman presented with the chief complaint of the "loosening" of her maxillary left central incisor. She was initially seen by her general dentist and referred to the University of Washington for extraction and replacement of the tooth with an implant-supported restoration. She recollected that "bumps had formed and disappeared at the gums around my upper teeth for about 3 years." The maxillary left central incisor had drifted coronally and labially over that period. The patient presented with an extensive restorative treatment history. She had neglected her dental care for years because of financial issues. With the understanding of her current dental condition and the improvement of her financial status, the patient was motivated to improve her oral health and dental esthetics and pursue comprehensive treatment.

Medical history

- Controlled hypertension for 10 years
- An aneurysm in the left cerebral hemisphere (1994) caused residual effects: slight paralysis/numbness in the right side and a problem with spelling
- Pacemaker placement in 2003
- History of chronic ear infections, causing 80% hearing loss in the right ear
- Glaucoma
- Current medications: hydrochlorothiazide 12 mg/day, atenolol 100 mg/day, latanoprost 2 drops (3.0 μg)/day, ranitidine 150 mg/day
- No known drug allergies

Diagnostic findings

Extraoral and facial findings

- Convex facial profile with ovoid facial form
- Commissural line slants downward to the right side with respect to the interpapillary line, which is parallel to the horizon
- Asymmetric lip mobility; the upper and lower lips on the left side elevate higher than on the right side
- Appproximately 90-degree nasolabial angle
- The upper lip is 2 mm posterior to the E-line and the lower lip touches the E-line slightly
- With the exception of the maxillary left central incisor, which is supraerupted, the incisal plane follows the curvature of the lower lip during smiling
- In lateral view, the maxillary incisors, except the left central incisor, remain inside the wet-dry line of the lower lip
- Facial midline does not coincide with the maxillary dental midline; the maxillary dental midline deviates 1 mm to the right side
- At rest, 80% of the maxillary incisors and 30% of the mandibular incisors are displayed
- During a complete smile, the maxillary incisors are completely displayed along with 3 to 4 mm of gingiva

TMJ and mandibular range of motion

- No pain or tenderness demonstrated in the muscles of mastication and facial expression
- Range of motion within normal limits

Pretreatment

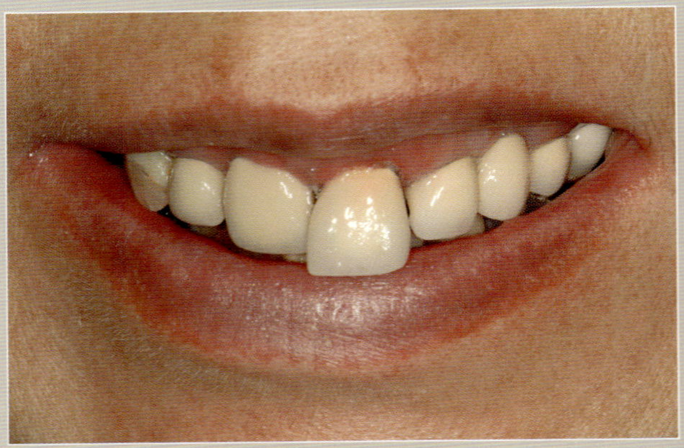

Close-up of the smile.

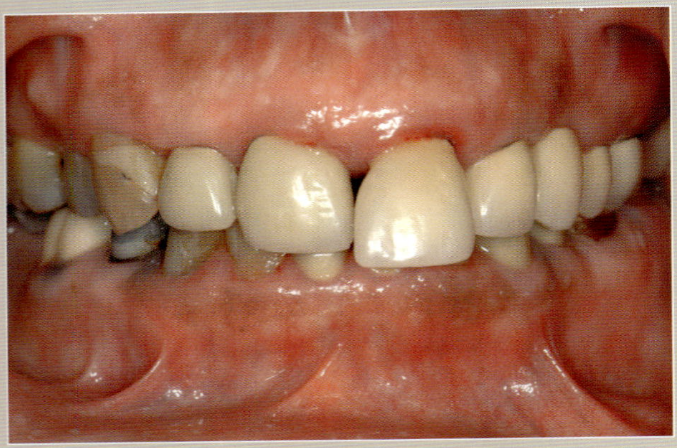

Frontal view in centric occlusion.

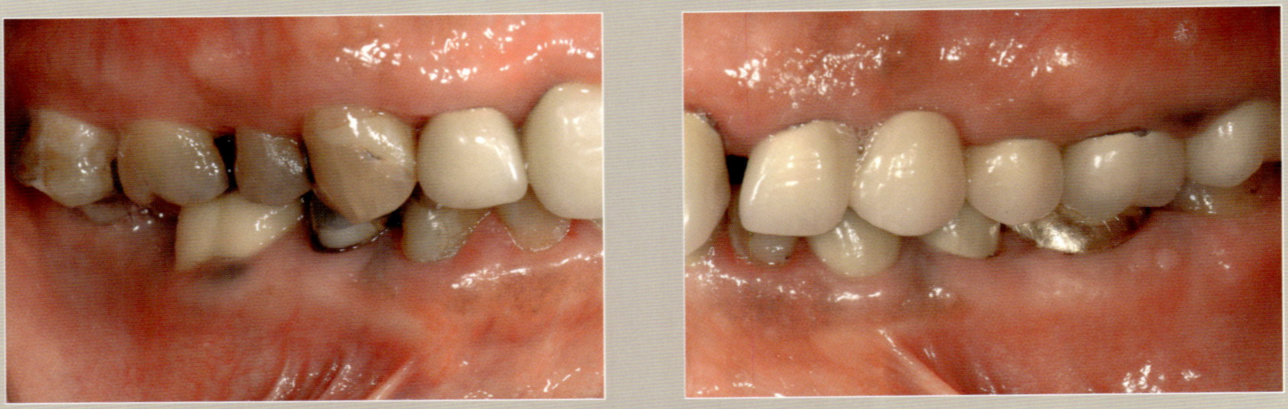

Right and left lateral views in centric occlusion.

Intraoral findings

Soft tissue and oral mucosa

- Soft tissue of the lips, cheeks, tongue, and oral mucosa and pharyngeal tissues were all within normal limits
- Saliva flow rate: resting, 0.3 mL/min; stimulated: 1.5 mL/min

Dental

- Dental arch forms: tapered, asymmetric maxilla; U-shaped, symmetric mandible
- Tooth form: square
- Generalized teeth discoloration
- Short clinical crowns
- Unfavorable width-to-length proportion of the maxillary incisors, which ranges from 91% to 107%
- Missing teeth nos. 1, 5, 11, 12, 16, 17, 21, 28, 31, and 32
- Defective composite resin restorations on teeth nos. 6, 23, 26, 27, and 29
- Defective amalgam restorations on teeth nos. 2, 3, 4, 6, 18, 27, and 29
- Overcontoured complete-cast metal and metal ceramic crowns on teeth nos. 7 to 9, 14, 15, 19, 20, 22, 24, 25, and 30
- An overcontoured metal ceramic FPD on teeth nos. 10 to 13
- Carious lesions on teeth nos. 6 to 10, 13 to 15, 18 to 20, 22 to 25, 27, 29, and 30
- Open margins and a severe carious lesion at the cervical aspect of the metal ceramic crown of tooth no. 9
- Generalized mild occlusal and palatal wear

Periodontal

- Fair oral hygiene with moderate plaque accumulation and minimal amounts of calculus
- Generally inflamed and edematous gingiva with bleeding upon probing
- Probing depths ranging from 2 to 4 mm with deeper measurements on teeth nos. 2, 3, 7, 9, 13 to 15, 18 to 20, 27, 29, and 30
- Disparate gingival levels
- Thick gingiva with moderate scallop
- Wide band of keratinized tissue
- Attached gingiva pigmented
- Amalgam tattoos present in the gingiva at the sites of teeth nos. 14, 15, 18 to 20, 22, 27, 29 to 31
- Gingival recession on tooth no. 30
- Chronic gingival inflammation around the maxillary central incisors
- Horizontal residual alveolar ridge resorption at the sites of teeth nos. 11 and 31
- Class III mobility of tooth no. 9

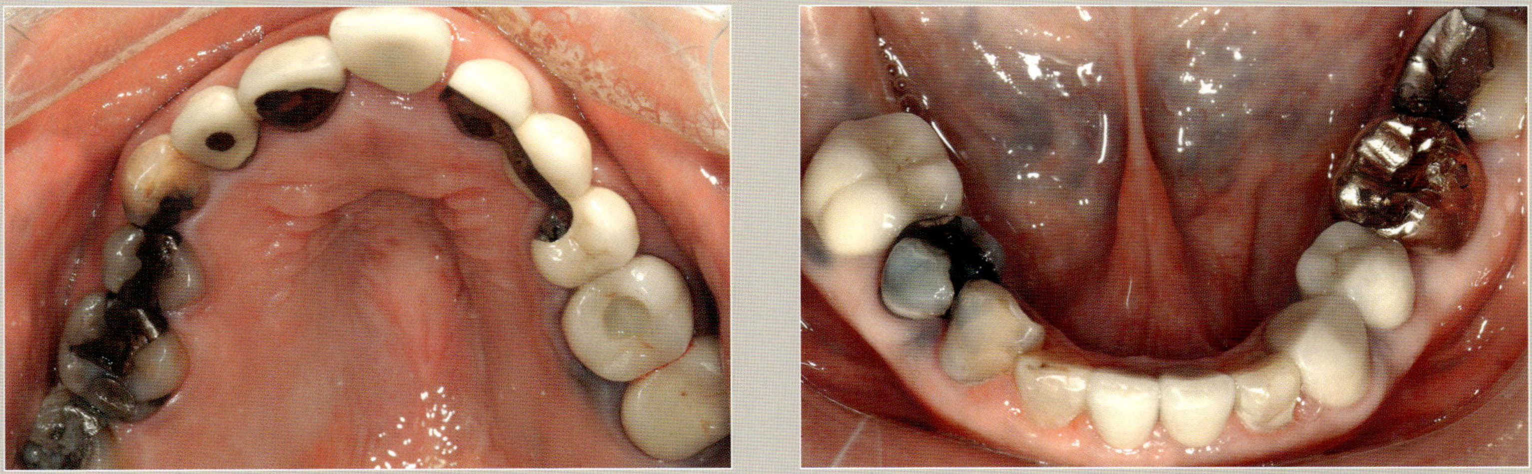

Intraoral occlusal views.

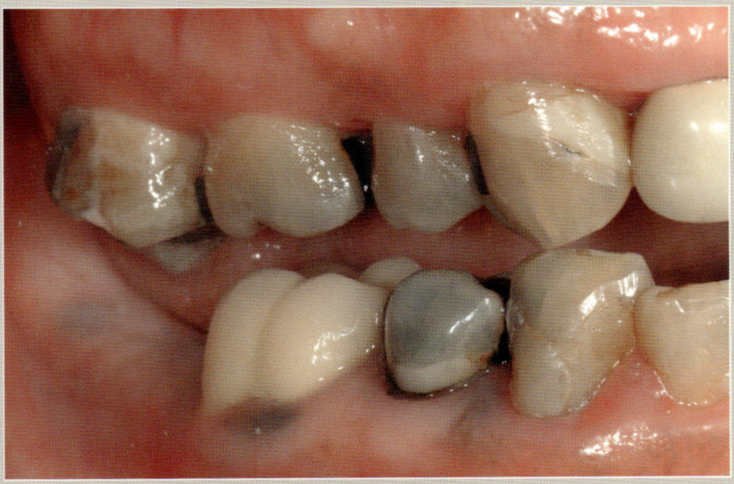

Canine guidance in right working movement.

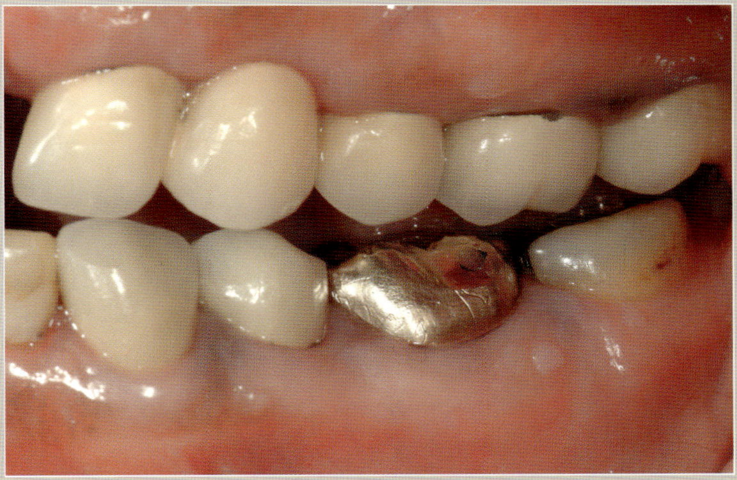

Canine and lateral guidance in left working movement.

Occlusal notes

- Centric occlusion coincided with MIP
- No history of parafunctional habits
- Vertical overlap: 4 mm (tooth no. 9 has a vertical overlap of 6 mm)
- Horizontal overlap: 4 mm (tooth no. 9 has a horizontal overlap of 7 mm)
- Bilateral Class I canine and molar relationships
- Right lateral excursive contacts: canine-protected articulation
- Left lateral excursive contacts: teeth nos. 10 and 22 and nos. 11 and 20
- Protrusive anterior group function excursive contacts: teeth nos. 7 and 27, 8 and 25/26, 9 and 23/24, and 10 and 22
- Uneven maxillary and mandibular incisal planes
- Uneven posterior occlusal planes
- Supraeruption of teeth nos. 2 and 9
- Fremitus on tooth no. 9

Radiographic findings

- Degenerative change of the left condyle (flat eminence and condyle)
- Cloudiness of the left maxillary sinus
- Generalized mild horizontal bone loss
- Localized severe horizontal and vertical bone loss on tooth no. 9
- General crown-root ratio of 1:2
- Periapical lesions on teeth nos. 9 and 14
- External root resorption on tooth no. 9
- Radiopacities in the mandible at sites nos. 31 and 32
- Radiopacities from the residual amalgams around the sites of teeth nos. 19, 20, and 29 to 31
- Incomplete/failing endodontic therapy with dowel and core placement on teeth nos. 7 to 9
- Overcontoured restorations on teeth nos. 8 to 10, 13 to 15, 19, 20, 24, 25, and 30

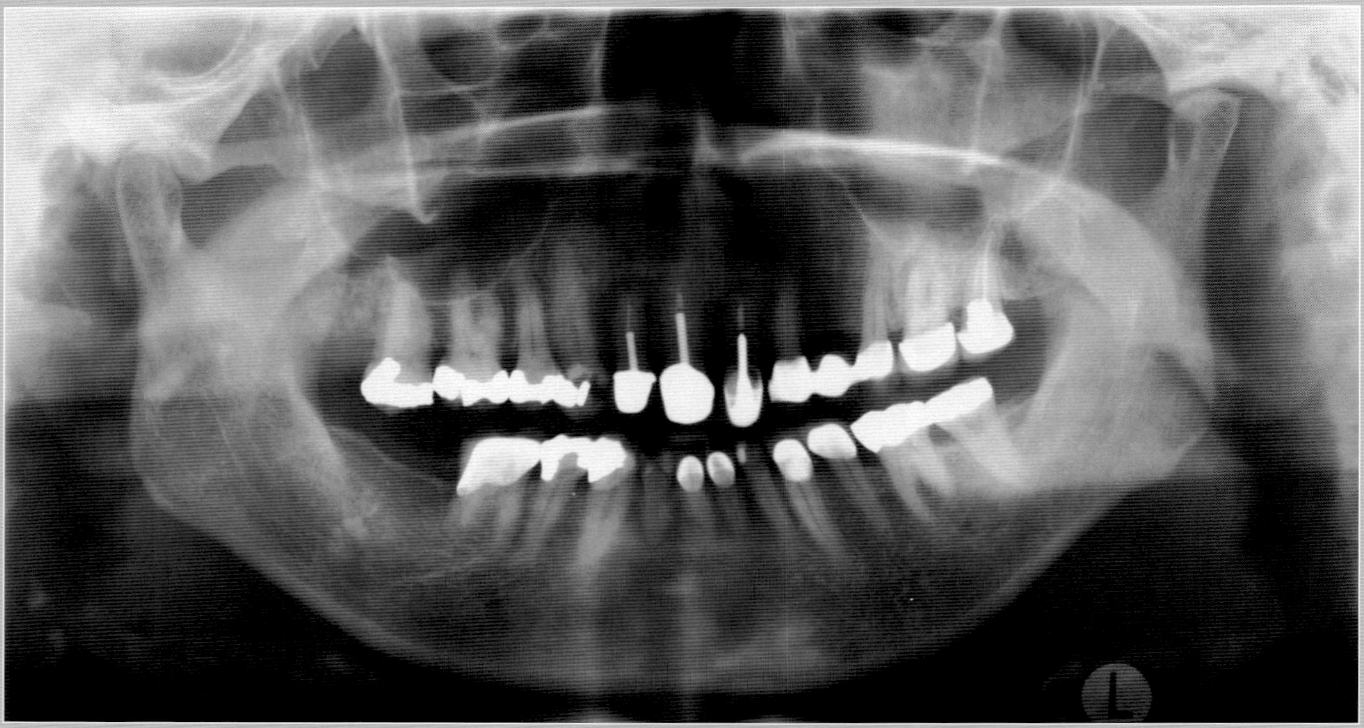

Panoramic radiograph.

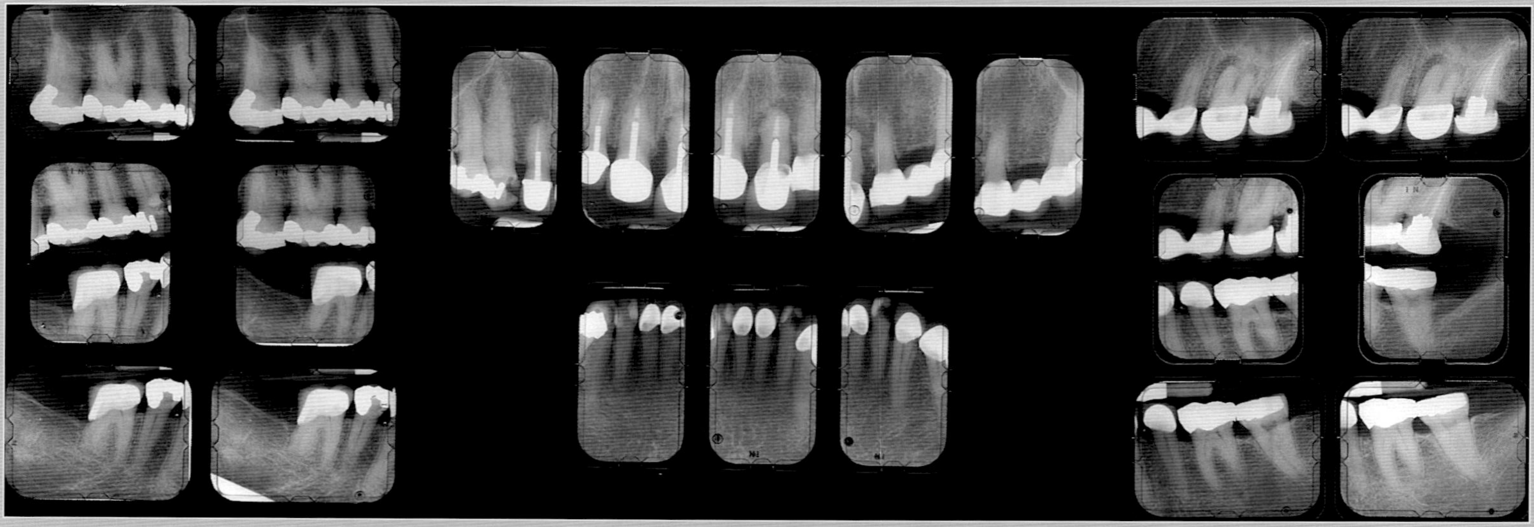

Complete-mouth radiographs.

Diagnosis

- Generalized mild with localized severe chronic periodontitis
- Dental caries
- Chronic periradicular periodontitis at teeth nos. 9 and 14
- Partial edentulism
- Defective restorations
- Class I malocclusion
- Siebert Class I ridge deficiencies
- Degenerative joint disease (asymptomatic)
- Poor esthetics

Prognosis

- Periodontal: good
- Biomechanical: guarded/poor
- Functional: good
- Esthetic: guarded

Summary of concerns

1. Would the amount and quality of residual tooth structure after removal of pre-existing restorations and caries be sufficient to allow good biomechanics?
2. Which teeth are restorable and which teeth need to be replaced?
3. Where should implants be placed to achieve functional and esthetic results?
4. How will we manage the incisal edge position of the maxillary anterior teeth and the occlusal plane?
5. Will resolving gingival level disparities increase the ferrule of compromised teeth?
6. How will we be able to provide the patient with functional and esthetic provisional restorations during transitional periods of the treatment?
7. Will we be able to satisfy the patient's esthetic concerns?
8. Will we be able to achieve a mutually protected articulation?
9. Can we achieve a long-lasting, restoratively successful outcome?

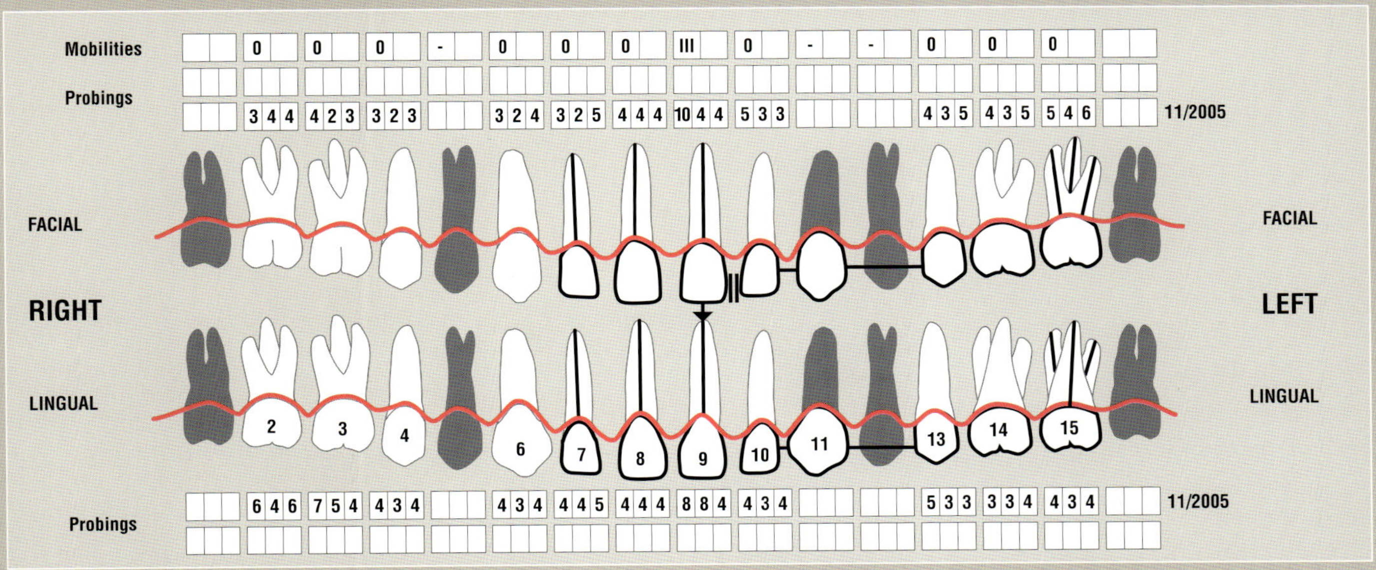

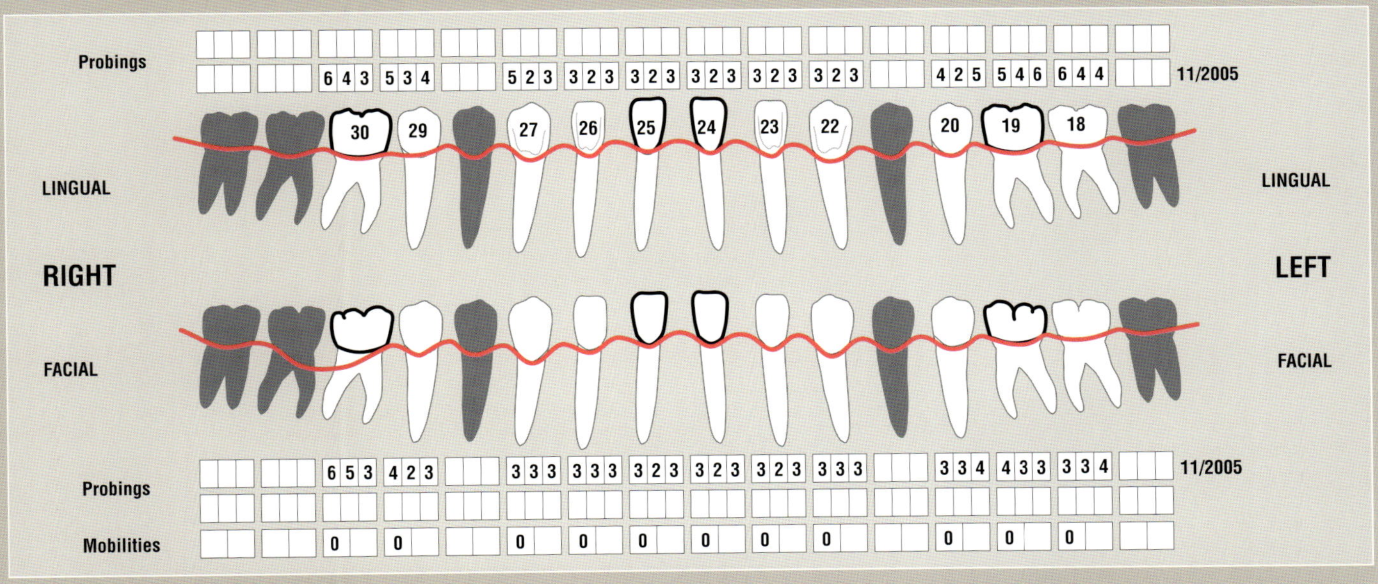

As a learning exercise, you may now outline goals/objectives of treatment and a treatment plan.

Proposed Treatment Plan

Goals/objectives of treatment

- Eliminate infection
- Improve oral hygiene
- Eliminate caries with long-term caries control
- Manage the structurally compromised teeth and ensure adequate residual tooth structure, ferrule, and foundation restorations for prospective complete coverage restorations where possible
- Replace nonrestorable and missing teeth with either an implant-supported prosthesis or an FPD
- Determine the ideal incisal edge position of the maxillary incisors and develop an ideal occlusal plane
- Establish a mutually protected articulation
- Provide a pleasing esthetic result
- Determine an effective maintenance protocol that is likely to improve longevity of the results

Phase I: Initial therapy

1. Medical and dental history review
2. Assessment of infected teeth nos. 9 and 14
3. Plaque control and initial periodontal therapy including scaling and root planing
4. Caries management by risk assessment, including oral hygiene and dietary instructions, chlorhexidine gluconate rinses, and fluoride and xylitol supplementation

Phase II: Diagnostics

5. Complete data collection, including diagnostic impressions, facebow transfer, centric relation record, mounted diagnostic casts, complete-mouth periapical and panoramic radiographs, and clinical photos
6. Caries risk assessment (bacterial, salivary, and dietary analyses)
7. Dentofacial/esthetic analysis
8. Endodontic consultation to assess teeth nos. 7, 8, 10, 14, and 15
9. Consultation with the periodontist to evaluate implant placement and crown lengthening procedures
10. Consultation with the specialist regarding the left TMJ
11. Fabrication of a diagnostic wax-up
12. Consultation with the patient to discuss tentative options for treatment
13. Fabrication of the radiographic and surgical guides for implant placement and crown lengthening procedures
14. Fabrication of preparation guides and shells for the second set of provisional restorations based on the diagnostic wax-up
15. Duplication of the existing dentition in the diagnostic casts for fabricating the first set of acrylic resin shell provisional restorations

Phase III: Caries control and first provisional restoration

16. Removal of pre-existing restorations, elimination of caries, evaluation of residual tooth structure, determination of the restorability of the teeth based on the prospective gingival levels (obtained from the diagnostic wax-up), and placement of new foundation restorations as needed
17. Reline and delivery of the first set of provisional restorations with the same pre-existing occlusal scheme and with improved cervical contours
18. Consultation with the patient to confirm the definitive treatment plan

Phase IV: First surgical treatment

19. Extraction of tooth no. 9, ridge preservation, and provisionalization with an ovate pontic to maintain soft tissue contours
20. Surgical crown lengthening procedures in the maxillary posterior segments and pocket reduction procedures where indicated
21. Implant placement at site no. 9 and additional sites as deemed necessary
22. Fabrication and placement of custom provisional abutments on the implants to create the desired gingival contours

Phase V: Second surgical treatment

23. Surgical crown lengthening procedures in the mandible
24. Implant placement as needed in the mandible
25. Surgical crown lengthening procedures in the maxillary anterior segment to create harmonious gingival levels

Phase VI: Second provisional restoration

26. Preparation of the maxillary and mandibular tooth abutments for complete coverage restorations
27. Reline and delivery of the prefabricated shells of the complete-arch provisional restorations with the new vertical dimension of occlusion and mutually protected articulation based on the diagnostic wax-up

Phase VII: Definitive restoration

28. Fabrication and delivery of definitive complete-coverage metal ceramic and all-ceramic restorations as needed with mutually protected articulation

Phase VIII: Maintenance

29. Fabrication and delivery of a heat-processed, clear acrylic resin maxillary occlusal appliance providing mutually protected articulation
30. Establishment of a maintenance regimen of 3-month recall intervals with in-office and home fluoride supplementation

Active Clinical Treatment

Review of the goals/objectives of treatment

The patient's chief complaint was the loose maxillary tooth with surrounding inflamed gingiva. She presented with numerous compromised restorations and active dental caries. There was no recorded history of parafunctional habits and also a lack of evidence of any significant tooth wear for the patient's age. She was motivated to pursue comprehensive treatment to improve her oral health and prevent further breakdown of her compromised dentition. The following treatment goals were determined:

- Eliminate infection and improve oral hygiene
- Manage the structurally compromised teeth and the dental caries
- Restore the dentition with fixed restorations to provide adequate esthetics and achieve a mutually protected articulation
- Establish a maintenance protocol to facilitate longevity of the restorations

Phase I: Initial therapy

The initial phase of the treatment started with infection control. A series of caries management procedures were performed, including dietary consultation, chlorhexidine gluconate rinses, and fluoride supplementation. Initial periodontal therapy was performed, including root planing, scaling, and oral hygiene instructions. A complete evaluation of the infected teeth nos. 9 and 14 was performed. The prognosis for tooth no. 9 was determined to be hopeless because of the crown-root fracture with associated severe bone loss. It was decided to extract the tooth and then perform a thorough socket curettage and ridge preservation procedure. The endodontic therapy for tooth no. 14, which was diagnosed with periradicular chronic periodontitis, was performed after the tooth had been deemed restorable.

Phase II: Diagnostics

The diagnostic work-up began with a comprehensive clinical examination and data collection.

Periodontally, the patient presented with generalized gingival inflammation with moderate plaque accumulation. There was mild bone loss except for teeth nos. 9 and 30, which presented with severe and moderate bone loss, respectively. The patient presented with a thick gingival consistency and a wide band of keratinized tissue. Extensive restorative work in both arches suggested that the patient was historically susceptible to dental caries. A systemic caries risk assessment, including a dietary analysis, cariogenic bacterial assessment, and an evaluation of salivary flow and buffering capacity, was carried out. It was confirmed that the patient was at high caries risk. Accordingly, the first step in caries control included oral hygiene instruction and reinforcement, cariogenic bacteria management, and dietary instructions.

The patient presented with generalized short clinical crown length, which compromised not only the esthetic appearance of the prospective restorations but also their biomechanical foundation. The average crown lengths of the posterior teeth were 4.5 mm. In general, 1.5 to 2 mm of occlusal clearance is recommended for complete-coverage metal ceramic and all-ceramic restorations. To gain the adequate retention and resistance form, 4-mm and 3-mm minimum preparation heights for the posterior and anterior tooth abutments, respectively, were suggested. To lessen the amount of the occlusal reduction, the decision was made to increase the interarch distance 1 mm at the second molars.

The patient was subsequently referred to the endodontist to assess the previous endodontic therapy at teeth nos. 7, 8, and 10 and to evaluate tooth no. 14. The remaining tasks were to determine which teeth were restorable and to provide the patient with a definitive treatment plan.

Functionally, according to the clinical findings and the patient report, there was no evidence or history of parafunctional habits. The mild attrition of the dentition was regarded as physiologic tooth wear, considering the years the teeth had been in function, possibly in combination with prior occlusal adjustments via occlusal reshaping. The flat left condyle, shown on the panoramic radiograph, was diagnosed by a specialist as degenerative joint disorder with no contraindications for proceeding with the process of complete-mouth reconstruction.

Dentofacial and esthetic analyses determined that the patient displayed 8 mm of her maxillary right central incisor with the lips at rest, which is considered more than the average amount for her age and sex. The patient presented with a high smile line, displaying the maxillary anterior teeth and 4 mm of gingival tissues. In addition, the patient presented with uneven gingival levels. The maxillary anterior teeth presented with a short and wide appearance, with the width-length proportion ranging from 91% to 107%. These clinical findings contributed to the challenge of restoring the anterior dentition with an acceptable esthetic result.

A diagnostic wax-up was fabricated according to the dentofacial analysis with the aim of providing the patient with a

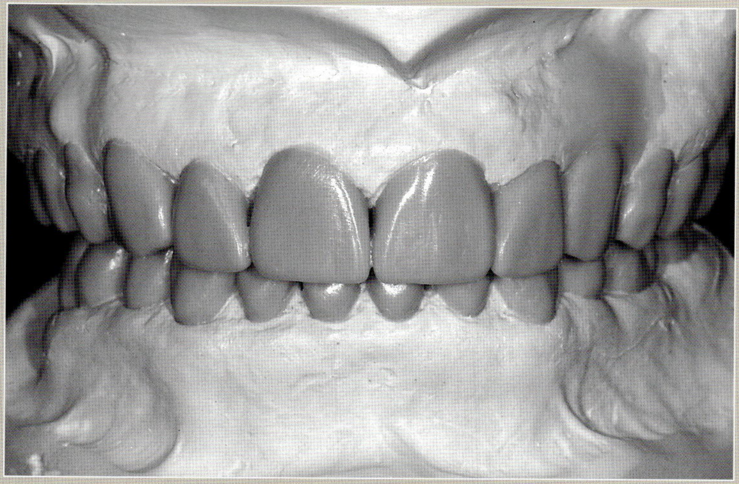

Frontal view of the diagnostic wax-up.

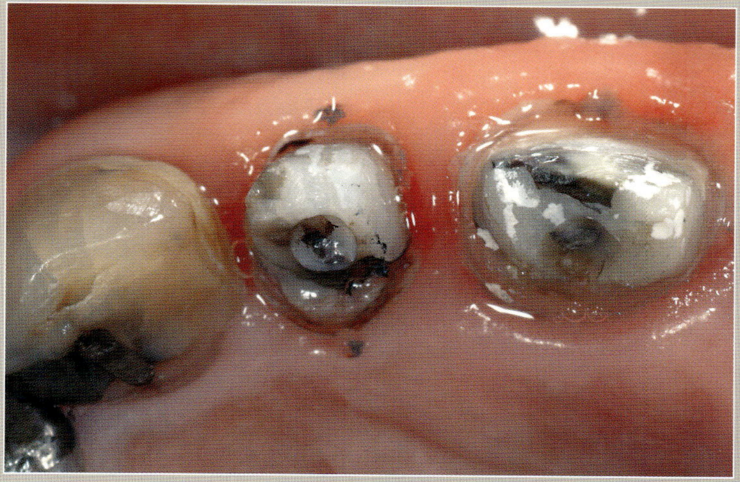

Occlusal view of the maxillary right anterior segment after the removal of crowns.

mutually protected articulation. The first step of the wax-up was to gain adequate width-length proportions for the maxillary anterior teeth. Given the restriction of the dental arch, lengthening the tooth was the only way to improve the width-length tooth proportion. It was decided that, for esthetic purposes, the maxillary incisors should be lengthened 2 mm to enhance the width-length proportions. The amount of the incisor display within the lip frame dictates whether the teeth should be lengthened coronally or cervically. Lengthening the teeth coronally would increase the amount of incisal display with the lips at rest. Because the patient's incisal display had been beyond the average measurements, it was decided to surgically elongate the maxillary anterior teeth cervically by 2 mm.

Radiographic guides for the computed tomographic scan were fabricated based on the diagnostic wax-up to assess the proposed implant sites. The patient was referred to the periodontist for evaluation prior to implant placement and surgical crown lengthening procedures.

Phase III: Caries control and first provisional restoration

Because the patient presented with an extensively restored dentition, it was challenging to determine the definitive treatment plan without exploring the integrity of the tooth structure under the pre-existing restorations. The caries under the pre-existing defective restorations needed to be completely explored, not only to prevent the compromised tooth structure from continuing to breakdown but also to determine which teeth were restorable and to finalize a treatment plan.

Subsequent to the caries control at the initial therapy, the second step of caries control was to eliminate the existing carious lesions and to provide new foundation restorations over the compromised tooth structure. It was decided to provide the patient with two sets of provisional restorations during the transitional periods of treatment.

The first set of provisional restorations was delivered after removal of the pre-existing complete-coverage restorations. The shells of the first provisional restorations were made of autopolymerizing acrylic resin using duplicated diagnostic casts of the pre-existing dentition with improved cervical contours and adequate incisal edge position for tooth no. 9.

The pre-existing complete-coverage restorations on teeth nos. 7, 8, 10 to 12, 14, 15, 19, 20, 22, 24, 25, and 30 were removed. The defective pre-existing restorations with suspected secondary caries on teeth nos. 18, 23, and 26 to 28 were removed as well. Caries was subsequently removed and completely eliminated with the aid of caries detection agents. Each tooth was re-evaluated, and the tentative treatment plan was modified accordingly. Composite resin foundation restorations were built up, and initial preparations were made. The previously fabricated shells were relined over the preparations with autopolymerizing acrylic resin to immediately restore the patient with the pre-existing occlusal scheme.

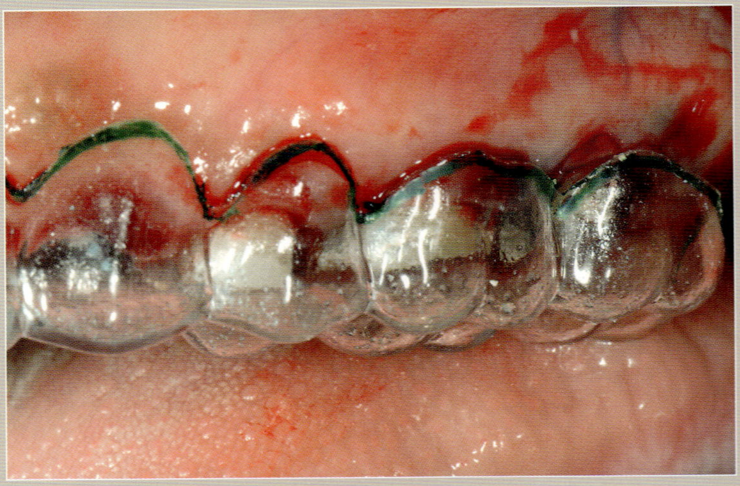

Surgical guide in place for crown lengthening procedures.

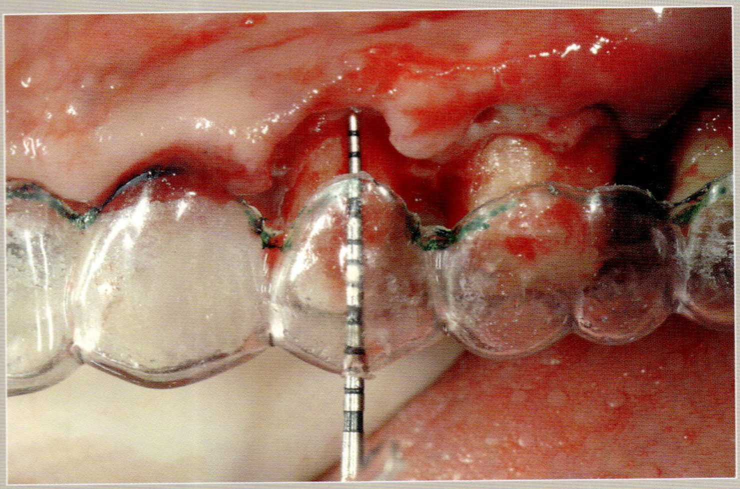

After flap reflection.

Phase IV: First surgical treatment

The decision was made to extract tooth no. 9 because of the extent of caries and infection, the severe bone loss, a poor crown-root ratio, and the suspected resorption and fracture. After extraction and a thorough socket debridement, a ridge preservation procedure was performed. The prospective implant site no. 9 was then gradually developed with an ovate pontic made with the first provisional restoration. Acrylic resin was added at the pontic site of tooth no. 9 to create an ideal ovate pontic shape based on the diagnostic wax-up. The ovate pontic extended 2.5 mm into the socket with facial undercontour to provide adequate support for the facial free gingival margin and the interproximal papillae.

After removal of the pre-existing direct and indirect restorations, the remaining clinical crowns were revealed to have an average length of 2 mm, which was not sufficient to ensure adequate tooth preparation height and ferrule for prospective complete-coverage restorations with adequate retention and resistance form. In addition, recurrent caries and defective foundation restorations were noted adjacent to the free gingival margins, which prevented finish line placement on sound tooth structure without biologic width violation. Thus, a decision was made to perform complete-mouth surgical crown lengthening procedures based on both esthetic and biomechanical concerns. Consequently, crown lengthening also reduced periodontal pocketing that remained following initial therapy.

A surgical guide was fabricated through duplication of the diagnostic wax-up. The template was tried in intraorally to ensure stability. Sounding of the alveolar crest was accomplished under local anesthesia to determine the height of the supracrestal gingival tissue, which averaged 3 mm facially and 4.5 mm interproximally. An internal beveled, scalloped surgical incision was outlined following the surgical guide from teeth nos. 2 to 4 and 12 to 15. Full-thickness buccal and palatal flaps were reflected. Ostectomy and osteoplasty were performed to expose the required tooth structure and to create a positive osseous architecture. The surgical guide was reseated after ostectomy to re-evaluate the results. After the planned dimensions were achieved, the flap was sutured with 4-0 silk vertical mattress interrupted sutures.

Three months after the atraumatic extraction and subsequent ridge preservation procedure at site no. 9, a decision was made to place implants on the edentulous ridge at the sites of teeth nos. 9 and 11. Due to the nonrestorability of tooth no. 7, the plan included the extraction of this tooth and immediate placement of a dental implant. The splinted provisional restorations from teeth nos. 6 to 12 were removed. The residual root of tooth no. 7 was atraumatically removed to preserve both the osseous and soft tissue architecture. A narrow-platform straight implant (NobelReplace 3.5 × 11.5 mm) was immediately placed at the site of tooth no. 7. Primary implant stability was achieved by engaging the palatal wall and bone approximately 4 to 5 mm beyond the apex of the extraction site. Two regular-platform straight implants (NobelReplace 4.3 × 11.5 mm) were subsequently placed using a single-stage surgical protocol at sites nos. 9 and 11. The implants were placed without flap reflection to minimize the risk of inducing significant tissue architecture changes. The implant placements were performed with a surgical guide made from the diagnostic wax-up. The depth of the implant platform was 3 mm apical to the prospective free gingival margin, as dictated by the surgical guide.

Because the preservation of the pre-existing tissue topography may be less of a challenge than its re-creation, custom provisional abutments were fabricated and placed immediately after implant placement to prosthetically guide optimal healing and adaptation of the soft tissues. Prefabricated provisional abutments were first placed onto the implants to assess the need for alteration. The abutments were removed, and laboratory-processed composite resin (Sinfony, 3M ESPE) was added to the subgingival area to capture the cervical gingival emergence at sites nos. 7 and 9 to initiate formation of the subgingival contour at site no. 11. The provisional abutments were subsequently tried in again to assess the tissue support and subgingival emergence contour of the added material. The abutments were then removed and shaped to provide ideal tissue support and subgingival contour. Once the proper tissue contour was established, the provisional abutments were seated, marking the outline of the gingival margin. The abutments were removed and prepared extraorally according to the fundamentals of traditional prosthetic crown preparation. The abutments were then connected to the implants and torqued to 15 Ncm. The pre-existing provisional restorations from teeth nos. 6 to 12 were then relined and provisionally cemented. The provisional restoration was adjusted to eliminate contacts in MIP and during eccentric movements.

Phase V: Second surgical treatment

Given the biomechanically compromised nature of the mandibular teeth after caries removal, surgical crown lengthening procedures were performed on all the mandibular teeth to expose additional sound tooth structure. It also was decided to remove tooth no. 30 because of extensive subgingival caries on the distal root. Four months after extraction, following bone graft maturation at site no. 30, a wide-diameter straight implant (NobelReplace 5.0 x 10 mm) was placed following a single-stage surgical protocol.

Tooth no. 2 was extracted because of supraeruption and lack of opposing tooth support after the placement of the second provisional restoration. In addition, it was decided to extract tooth no. 10 because of the unfavorable crown-root ratio and lack of adequate ferrule. Tooth no. 10 had served as a provisional abutment during the integration period of the implants at sites nos. 7, 9, and 11. It was used to share the load of the occlusal force and to minimize the potential flattening of the papillae architecture. After a 6-month integration period, the soft tissue around the implants exhibited a more favorable gingival architecture. The newly developed gingival levels became a reference for the crown lengthening procedure on teeth nos. 6 and 8 to facilitate harmonious gingival levels. Tooth no. 10 was extracted, and a ridge preservation procedure was performed. The pre-existing provisional restorations were modified at the site to create an ovate pontic to prosthetically support the anatomical gingival profile.

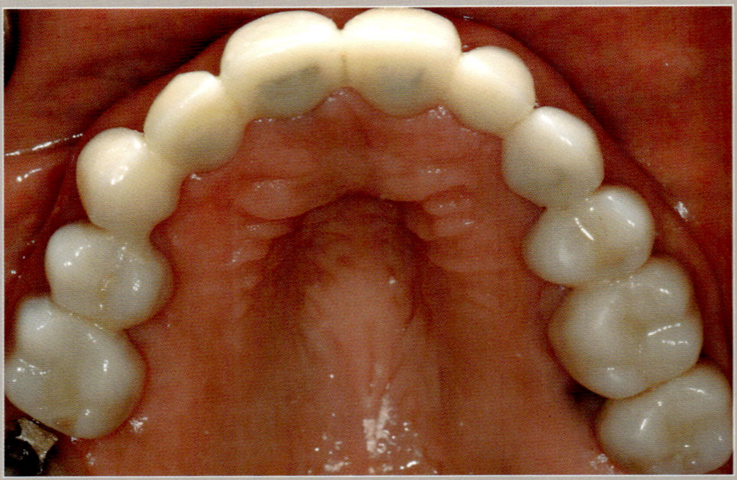

Maxillary occlusal view of the second set of provisional restorations.

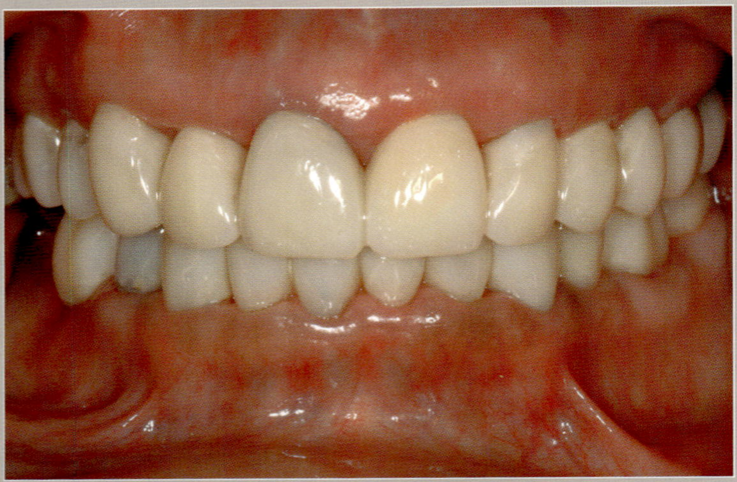

Frontal view of the second provisional restorations in centric occlusion.

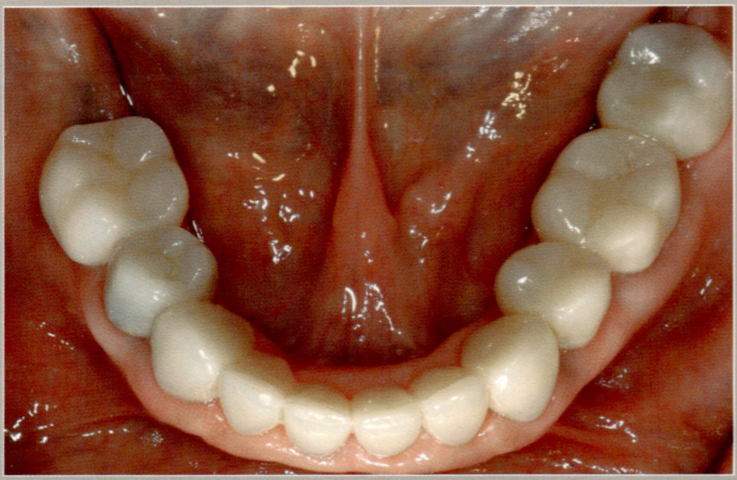

Mandibular occlusal view of the second set of provisional restorations.

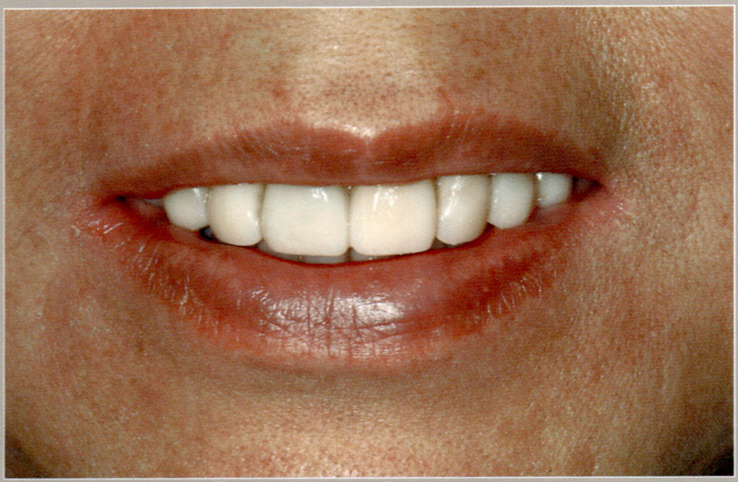

Close-up of the patient's smile with the second set of provisional restorations.

Phase VI: Second provisional restoration

The pre-existing amalgam restorations on teeth nos. 2, 3, and 4 were removed. The cavities were cleaned and prepared for the new composite resin foundation restorations. The first set of provisional restorations on teeth nos. 6 to 15 and in the mandibular arch were retrieved. Tooth preparations on the maxillary and mandibular dentition were refined according to the diagnostic wax-up with the assistance of vacuum-formed clear preparation guides. The second set of provisional shells for the maxilla, made from a duplicate of the diagnostic wax-up, was fabricated with bisphenol glycidyl methacrylate (bis-GMA) composite resin (Protemp, 3M ESPE). It was tried in the patient's mouth to verify correct placement at the proposed incisal edge position and occlusal plane. It was then airborne-particle abraded to roughen the intaglio surface and relined with polymethyl methacrylate (PMMA) acrylic resin. The excessive resin beyond the provisional restoration margins was trimmed to gain ideal marginal integrity. The provisional shell of the mandibular arch was subsequently relined in a similar manner to articulate with the maxillary provisional in centric occlusion at the predetermined vertical dimension of occlusion. The esthetics and phonetics of the incisal edge position and lingual contours of the maxillary anterior teeth were validated. All biologic, functional, and esthetic objectives were achieved with the secondary provisional restorations.

Phase VII: Definitive restoration

The prospective prosthetic recipient sites were well developed following the sculpting of the subgingival emergence contour around the implants with the custom provisional restorations. Ideally, the definitive restorations follow the soft tissue

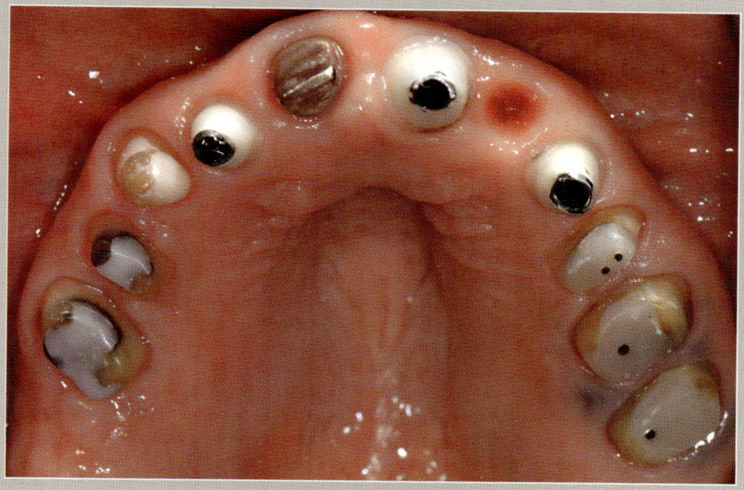

Occlusal view of the maxilla prior to making the master impression with custom provisional abutments in place.

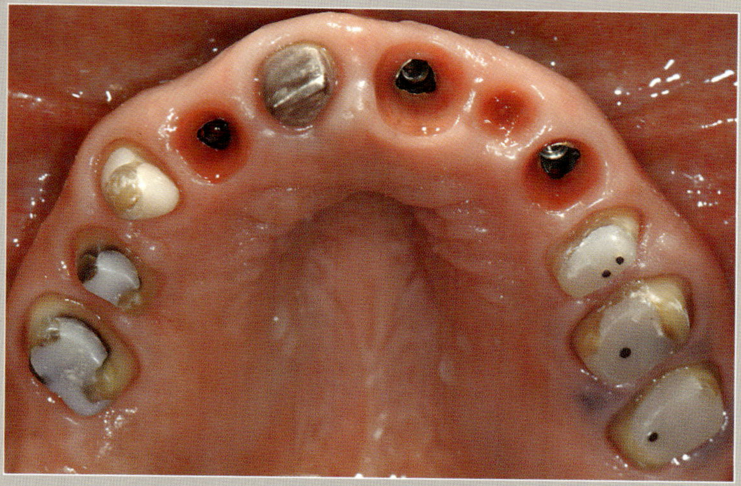

Occlusal view of the maxilla after removal of the provisional abutments.

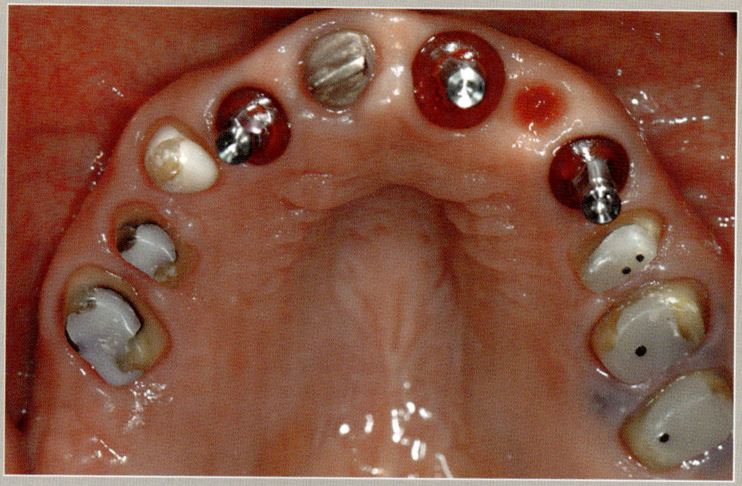

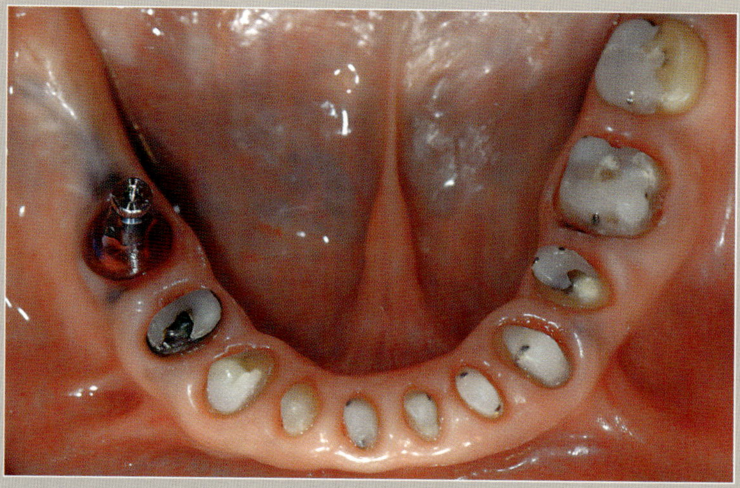

Occlusal views with custom impression copings in place.

modifications established intraorally with the custom provisional restorations. These soft tissue contours include those of the peri-implant soft tissue and the soft tissue under the ovate pontic sites, which should be transferred to the definitive cast via the master impression.

Implant laboratory analogs were first fixed with fast-set plaster in a small plastic cup. The custom provisional abutments at the sites of teeth nos. 7, 9, 11, and 30 were retrieved. Vinyl polysiloxane occlusal registration material was immediately placed on the peri-implant soft tissue to prevent its collapse. The custom provisional abutments were connected with the corresponding implant laboratory analogs. Vinyl polysiloxane impression material was injected around the custom provisional abutments to capture the contour of the emergence profile. After the impression material set, the provisional abutments were retrieved and repositioned on the implants intraorally. Impression copings were then attached to the implant analogs. A mixture of PMMA acrylic resin (Pattern Resin, GC) was placed into the vinyl polysiloxane mold to duplicate the cervical contours of the customized provisional abutments. The excessive resin was trimmed after setting, and the custom impression copings were formed.

The provisional restorations on the maxillary and mandibular arches were retrieved. After refining the preparations, the retraction cords were placed using the double-cord technique (Ultrapak #000 and #0, Ultradent). The custom provisional abutments on teeth nos. 7, 9, 11, and 30 were removed, and the custom impression copings were placed on the corresponding implants. Vinyl polysiloxane master impressions of the maxillary and mandibular arches were made with the double-mix one-step impression technique (Imprint III, 3M ESPE). A facebow transfer and centric relation records were made with the maxillary provisional restoration. Impressions of the maxillary and mandibular provisional restorations were also made for cross mounting with the definitive casts. Mounting of the cast of the maxillary provisional restoration against the cast of the mandibular provisional restoration,

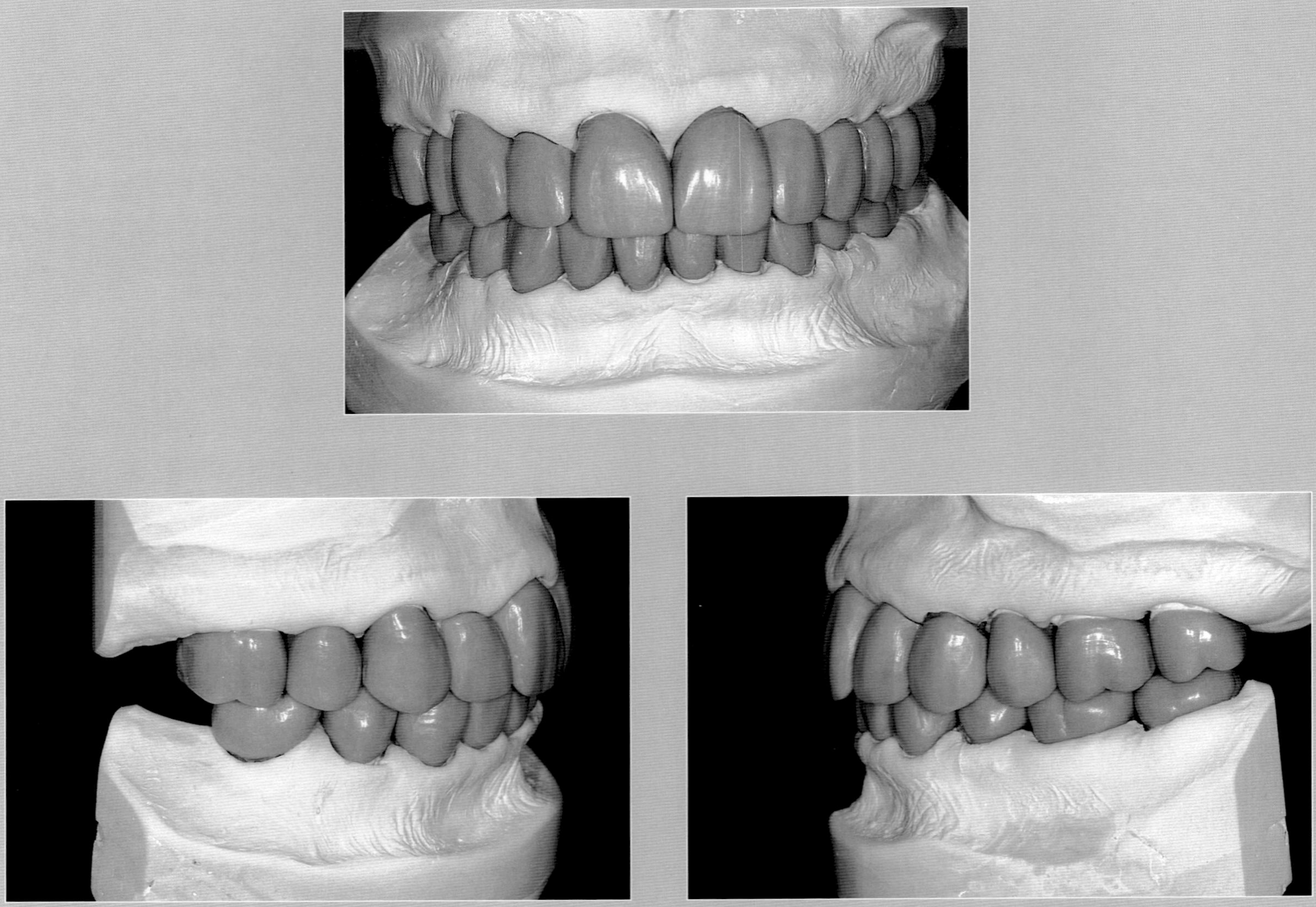

Full-contour wax-up on the solid casts.

the cast of the maxillary provisional restoration against the cast of the mandibular definitive restoration, and the cast of the mandibular definitive restoration against the cast of the maxillary definitive restoration provided crucial information for all subsequent working steps during the definitive prosthetic phase.

A full-contour wax-up was made on the definitive casts based on the provisional restorations. This was a critical step for adequately designing the definitive restorations in terms of the proposed occlusal scheme and the required three-dimensional space for the restorative materials. Subsequently, a silicone matrix was made to serve as a guide for fabricating the definitive abutments and frameworks. The wax patterns of the custom abutments for the sites nos. 7, 9, 11, and 30 were fabricated following the established subgingival emergence contours around the implants. They were then scanned using a Procera Forte scanner (Nobel Biocare) to generate custom zirconia abutments for sites nos. 7, 9, and 11 and a custom titanium abutment for site no. 30.

The definitive casts were then scanned with an optical scanner (Lava, 3M ESPE), and crown copings and an FPD framework were virtually designed for the zirconia-based restorations on teeth nos. 4, 6 to 10, 13, 20, 22 to 27, and 29. Cast metal copings were fabricated for metal ceramic crowns on teeth nos. 3, 14, 15, 18, 19, and 30. At the try-in appointment for the copings and FPD frameworks, a soft tissue pickup impression of the no. 9 pontic site was made with the zirconia framework. The emergence profile developed with the ovate pontic provisional restoration was captured and transferred to the definitive cast. The maxillary and mandibular definitive restorations were subsequently completed by the dental ceramist. The definitive restorations were tried in to verify fit, occlusion, and esthetics. Implant abutments were torqued to 35 Ncm, and all the restorations were cemented with dual-cured composite resin cement with a translucent shade (RelyX Unicem, 3M ESPE).

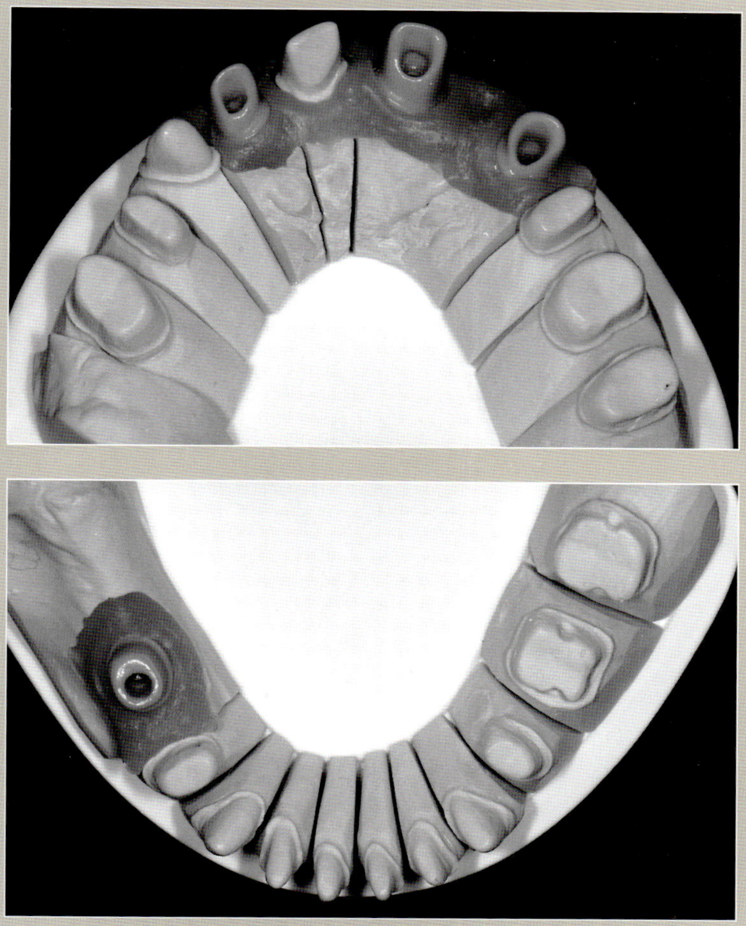

Occlusal views of the definitive casts.

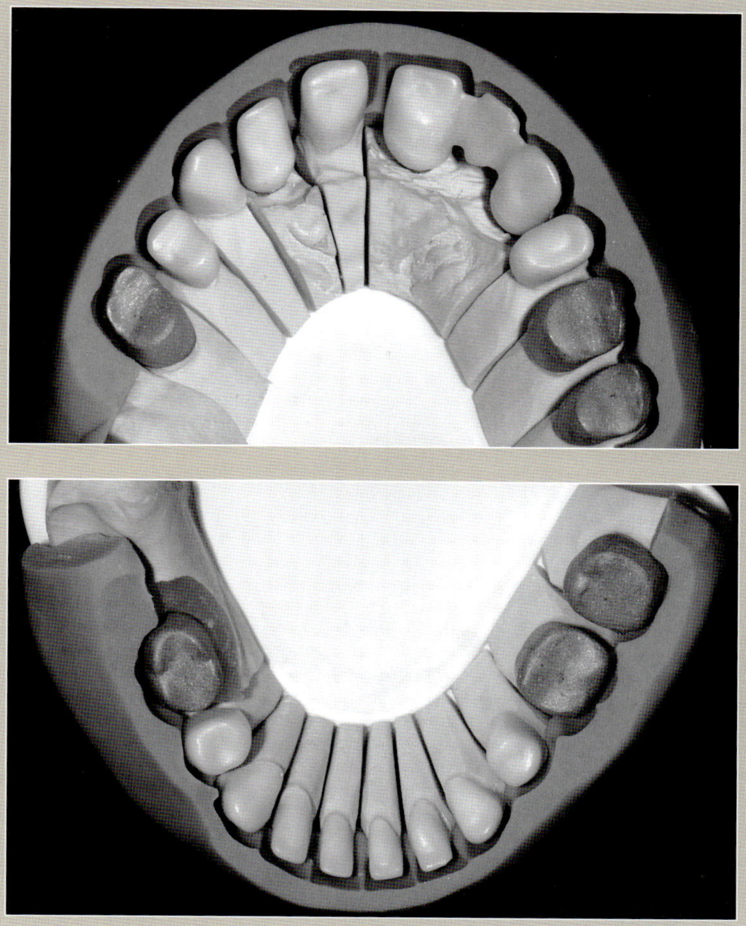

Occlusal views of the definitive casts with the zirconia and high-noble alloy infrastructures.

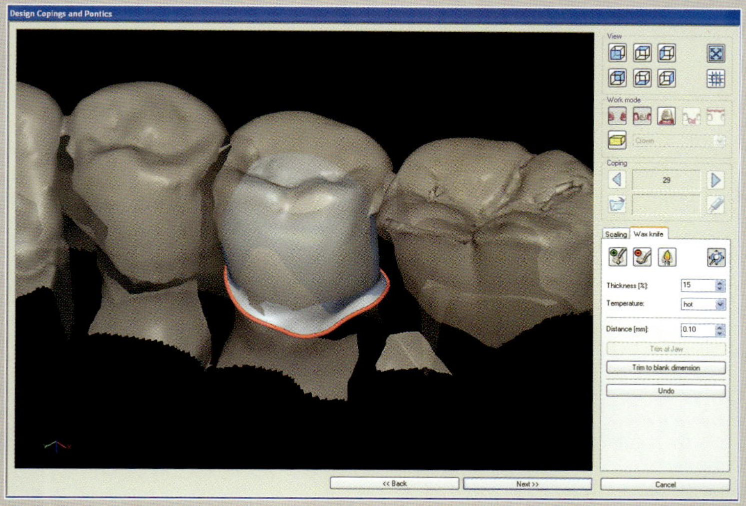

CAD design of a zirconia coping with the superimposed wax-up.

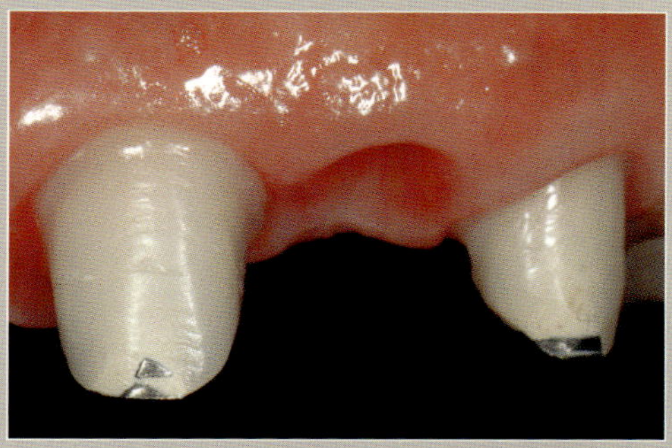

Custom provisional abutments for the maxillary anterior FPD.

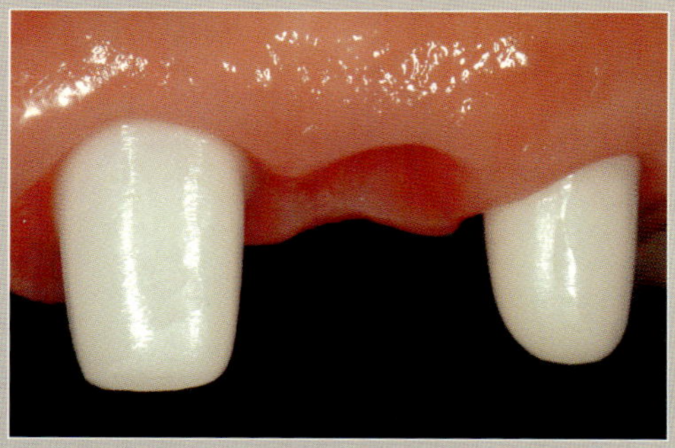

Definitive zirconia abutments for the maxillary anterior FPD.

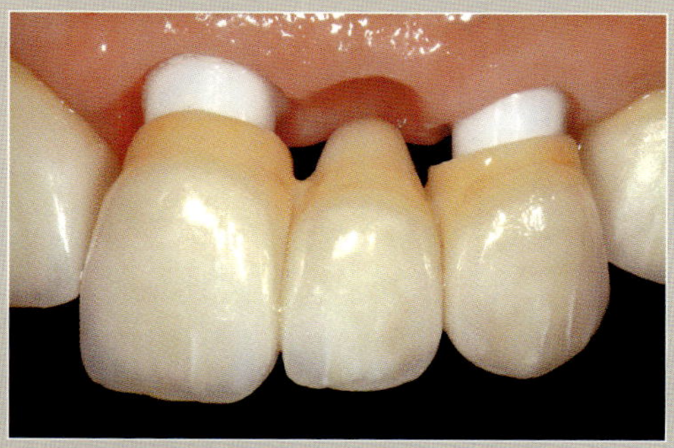

Try-in of the anterior maxillary FPD.

Posttreatment

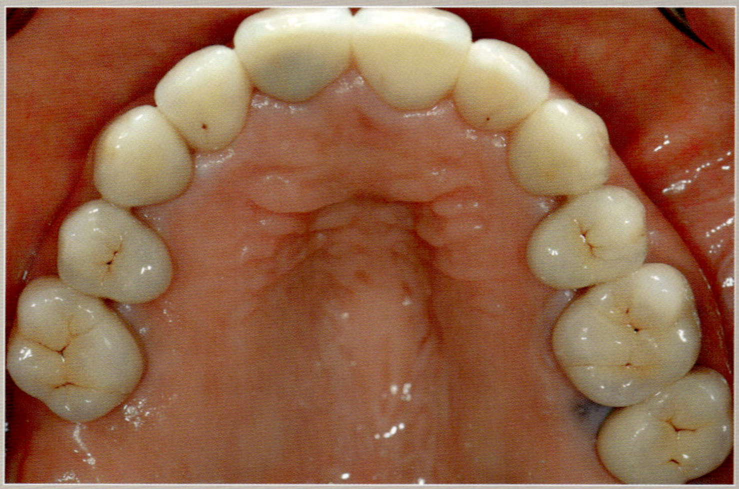

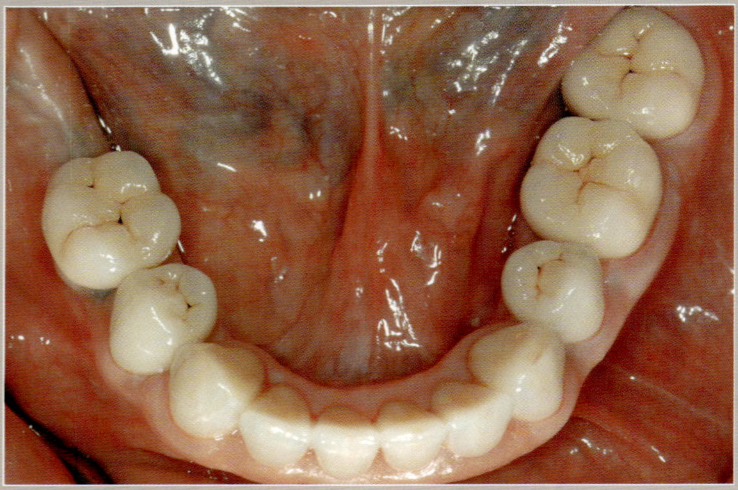

Occlusal views of the definitive restorations.

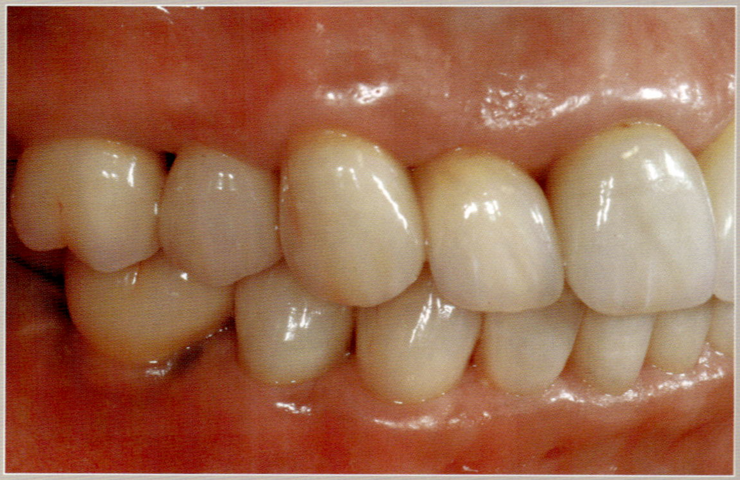

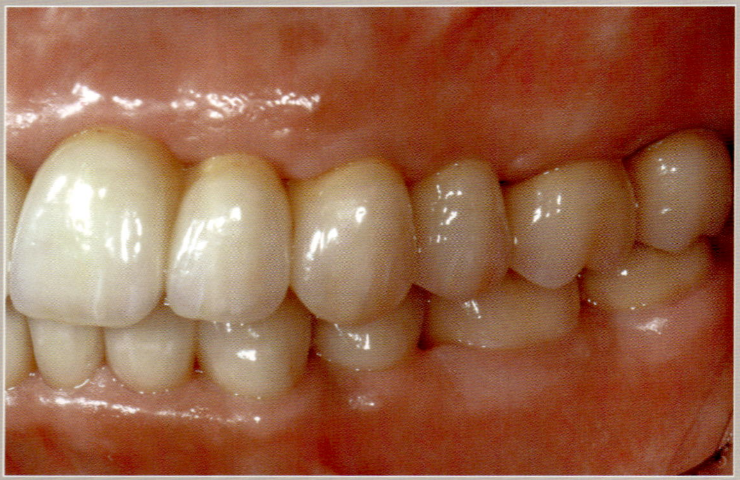

Lateral views of the definitive restorations in centric occlusion.

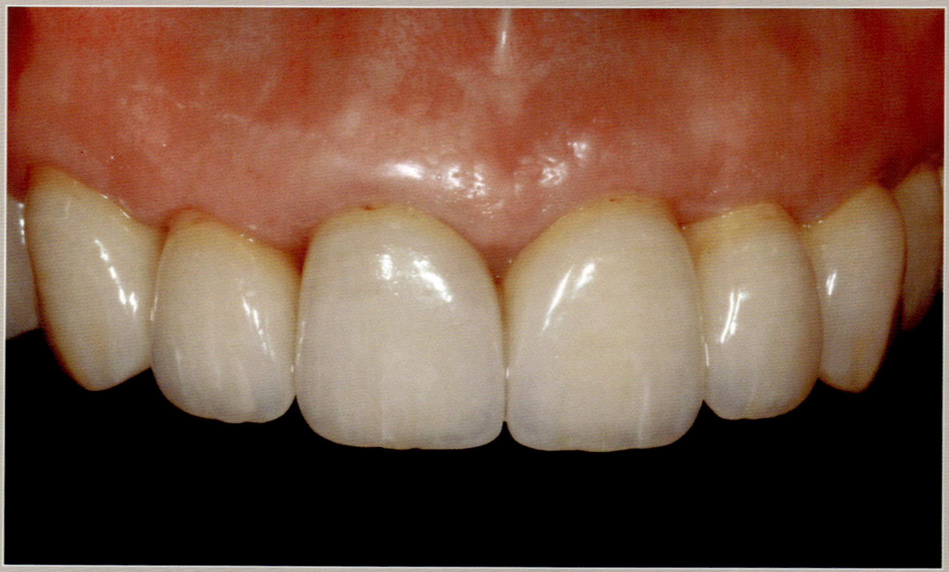

Frontal view of the maxillary anterior definitive restorations.

Phase VIII: Maintenance

The importance of maintaining a high standard of oral hygiene was stressed to the patient, and oral hygiene instructions were reinforced. A heat-processed clear acrylic resin maxillary occlusal device providing a mutually protected articulation was fabricated and delivered. The patient was placed on a maintenance regimen at 3-month recall intervals with in-office and home fluoride supplementation.

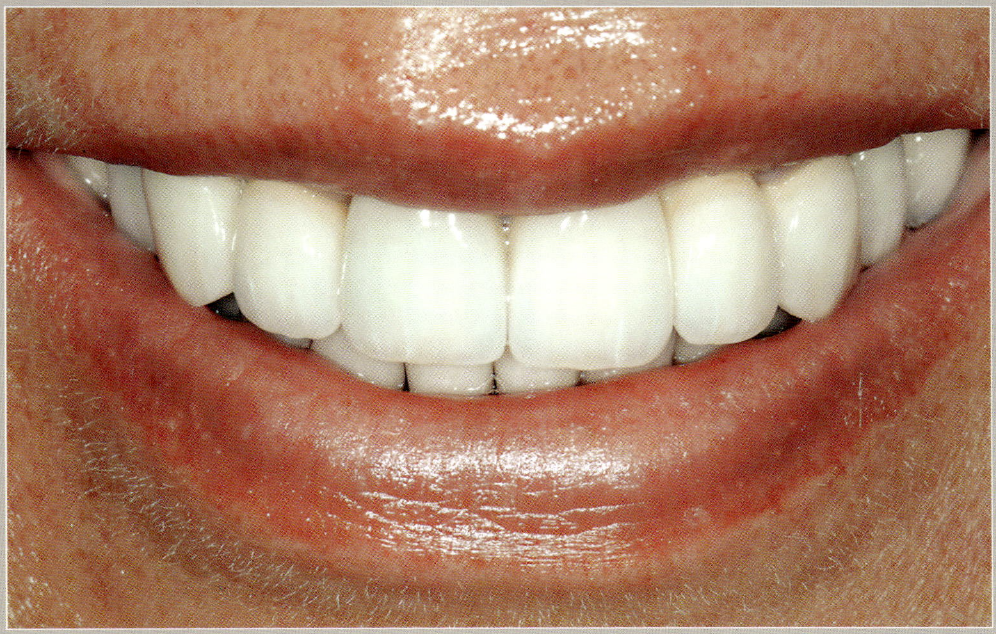

Facial view of the smile.

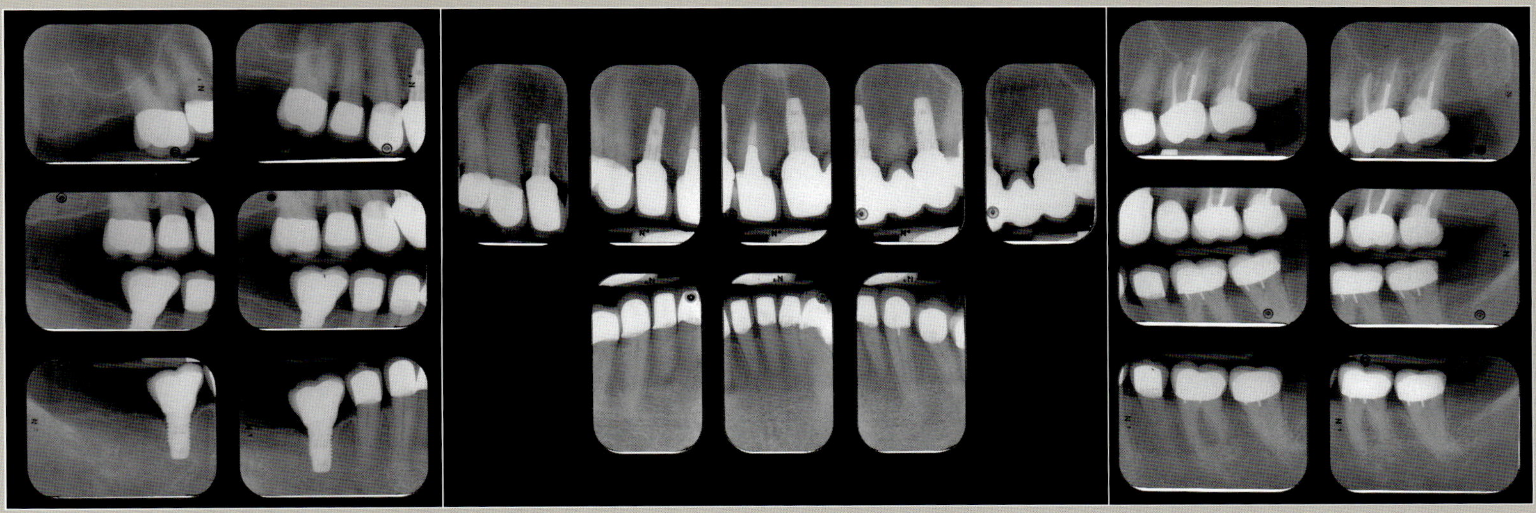

Complete-mouth radiographs.

You may now place the corresponding posttreatment overlay found in the separate folder over the pretreatment periodontal chart on page 35.

Case Presentation 2

Treating clinicians
Prosthodontist: Ariel J. Raigrodski, DMD, MS
Periodontist: Michael Cohen, DDS, MSD

Clinical Treatment Planning

Age at initial presentation: 65 years
Initial presentation: March 2007
Active treatment completed: August 2009

Introduction and background

The patient's chief complaint was: "I have sensitivity to cold and hot as well as pain when I chew on the lower right back tooth. I also have sensitivity when I bite on my front teeth. I had a lower removable partial denture made, which functioned well for several years and then broke about 10 years ago. It has not been replaced ever since. I would like to be able to chew better, and I would also like to improve my smile. I am embarrassed with how my teeth look, especially when I spend time with my grandchildren."

The patient was concerned about his level of discomfort on the mandibular right side and the prospect of restoring his dentition after many years of neglect and avoidance of comprehensive treatment. He was also concerned about the possibility of improving his smile, which he felt had been severely compromised for many years. The patient had noticed continuous wear of his dentition for quite some time. He reported daytime and sleep bruxing and clenching habits. In addition, he stated that he frequently consumed citrus fruits and soda pop. The patient had a history of smoking one pack of cigarettes a day for 40 years but had ceased smoking in 1999. His most recent annual dental checkup and cleaning occurred 6 years prior to the initial examination. He felt that time and financial constraints, as well as procrastination, prevented him from seeking treatment in the past. He was searching for treatment options that would provide affordable fixed restorations. He was now willing to invest the time and a "reasonable" amount of money toward this objective.

Medical history

- Mild ulcerative colitis
- Benign prostate hypertrophy
- No known drug allergies
- Medications and supplements: balsalazide disodium 750 mg/day, tamsulosin hydrochloride 0.4 mg/day, aspirin 81 mg/day, fish oil, calcium, and daily multivitamins
- Dietary considerations: Daily consumption of citrus fruit and soda pop

Diagnostic findings

Extraoral and facial findings

- No palpable lymph nodes
- No facial asymmetries
- Facial midline coincident with the maxillary dental midline
- Lip mobility and thickness were within normal limits
- Maxillary tooth display was 0 mm with lips at rest and 2 to 3 mm during smile
- Mandibular tooth display was 0 mm with lips at rest and during smile

TMJ and mandibular range of motion

- Muscles of mastication, muscles of facial expression, and TMJs were asymptomatic
- Mandibular range of motion was within normal limits, with maximum opening of 45 mm

PRETREATMENT

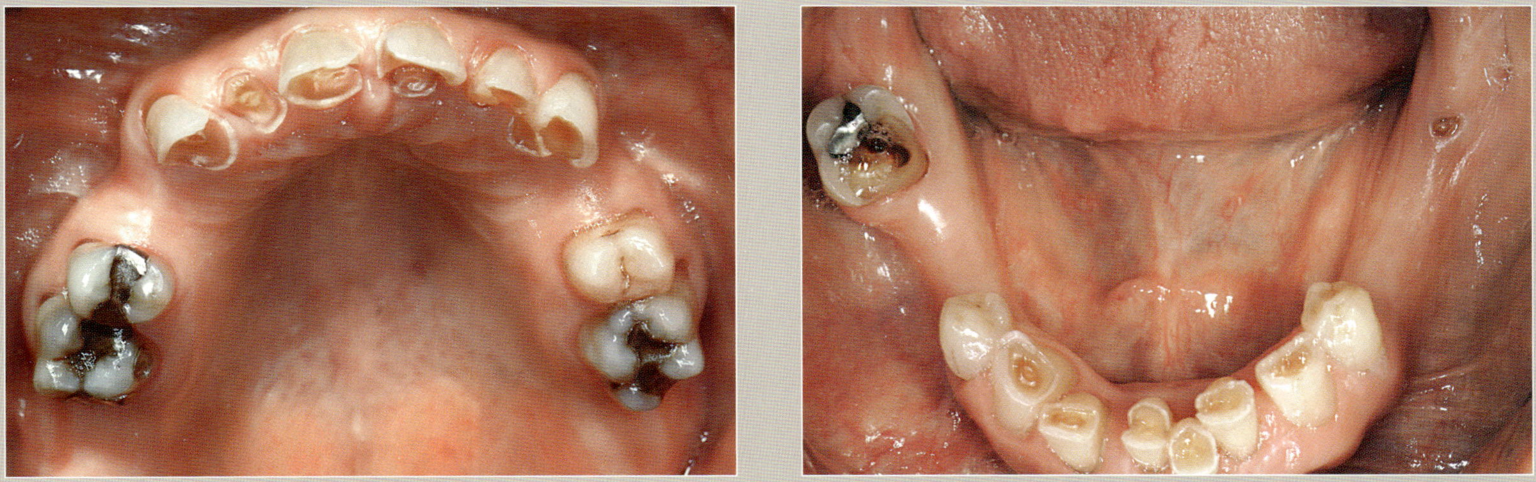

Occlusal views.

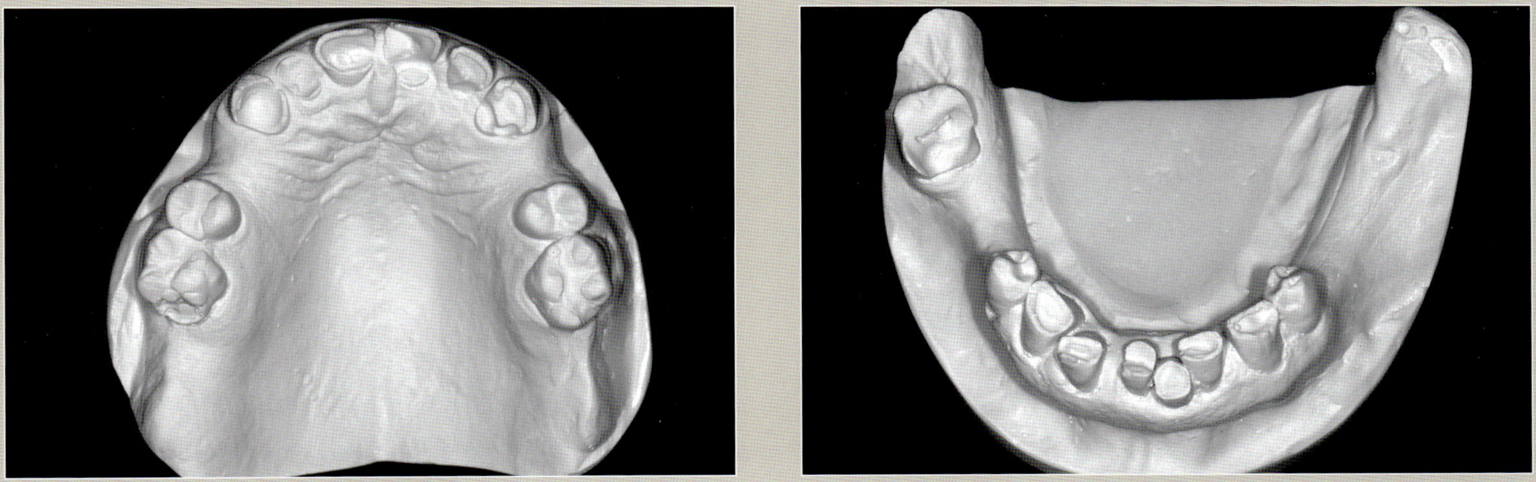

Occlusal views of diagnostic casts.

Intraoral findings

Soft tissue and oral mucosa

- Soft tissue of the lips, buccal mucosa, vestibule, frena, soft palate, hard palate, oropharynx, tongue, and floor of mouth were all within normal limits
- Salivary glands were not enlarged; saliva was thick and copious and flowed freely

Dental

- U-shaped arches
- Mandibular dental midline deviated 1 mm to the right side
- Severe wear on both maxillary and mandibular anterior segments with exposure of the pulp chambers
- A carious lesion and fractured amalgam restoration as well as fractured cusps on tooth no. 31
- Failing restorations on teeth nos. 3 and 14
- Cervical carious lesions on teeth nos. 3, 4, 6, 14, and 28
- Occlusal and palatal carious lesions on teeth nos. 6, 7, 8, 9, 11, 22, 26, and 27
- Tooth no. 7 worn and fractured to the level of the free gingival margin
- Intact amalgam restoration on tooth no. 4
- Open interproximal contacts between all maxillary anterior teeth
- Open interproximal contacts between teeth nos. 22 and 23 and nos. 25 and 26
- Mandibular anterior crowding
- Missing teeth nos. 1, 2, 5, 12, 15, 16, 17 to 20, 29, 30, and 32

- Horizontal residual alveolar ridge deficiencies in the maxillary arch
- Horizontal and vertical residual alveolar ridge deficiencies in the mandibular arch
- Residual root tip from tooth no. 18

Periodontal

- Level of oral hygiene: fair
- Gingiva generally pink with a thick consistency and scalloped form
- Generally a wide band of keratinized tissue
- Disparate gingival levels
- Generalized bleeding upon probing
- Periodontal probing depths ranging between 2 and 9 mm
- Multiple areas of gingival recession and evidence of attachment loss (teeth nos. 3, 4, 6, 14, 28, and 31)
- Class II furcation on tooth no. 31
- Class II tooth mobility for teeth nos. 24 to 26

Occlusal notes

- Centric occlusion did not coincide with maximal intercuspal position (MIP), with less than 1 mm horizontal and vertical discrepancies
- Right and left working group function articulation in lateral excursions, with a posterior nonworking interference on the right side (teeth nos. 3 and 31)
- Protrusive contacts on teeth nos. 9 and 23 and nos. 10 and 22
- Horizontal overlap: 1 mm
- Vertical overlap: 7 mm
- No fremitus noted
- Matching wear facets on both the anterior and posterior segments
- Canine Class II malocclusion on right and left sides
- Extensive supraeruptions in both the anterior and posterior segments

Radiographic findings

- Condyles appear normal
- Clear and pneumatized maxillary sinuses
- Generalized moderate to moderately advanced horizontal and vertical bone loss with localized areas displaying more advanced periodontal breakdown
- Residual fractured root tip from tooth no. 18
- Localized severe bone loss around tooth no. 31
- Root proximity between teeth nos. 6 and 7, 10 and 11, 22 and 23, 23 and 24, and 27 and 28
- All crown-root ratios at least 1:1
- Carious lesions on teeth nos. 3, 9, 11, 14, 22, and 31

Diagnosis

- Generalized moderate periodontitis with localized severe periodontitis
- Dental caries
- Partial edentulism
- Bruxism and clenching
- Erosion
- Malocclusion
- Siebert Class I ridge deficiencies in the maxilla
- Siebert Class III ridge deficiencies in the mandible
- Poor esthetics

Prognosis

- Periodontal: fair
- Biomechanical: poor
- Functional: guarded/poor
- Esthetic: good

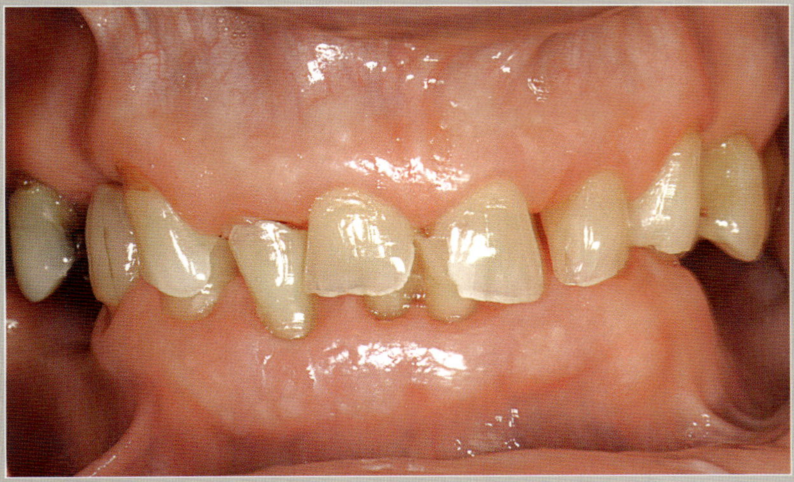

Frontal view in MIP.

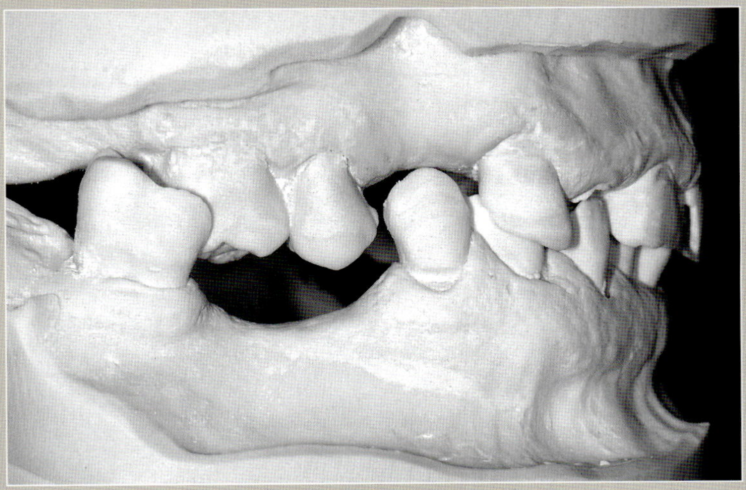

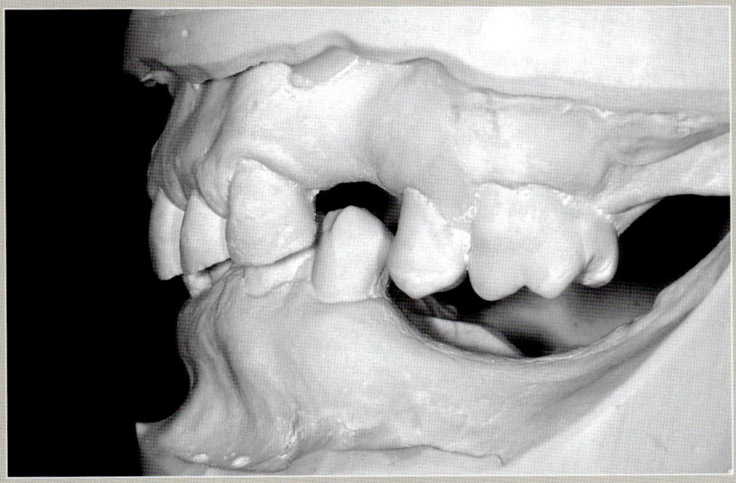

Lateral views of mounted diagnostic casts in centric occlusion.

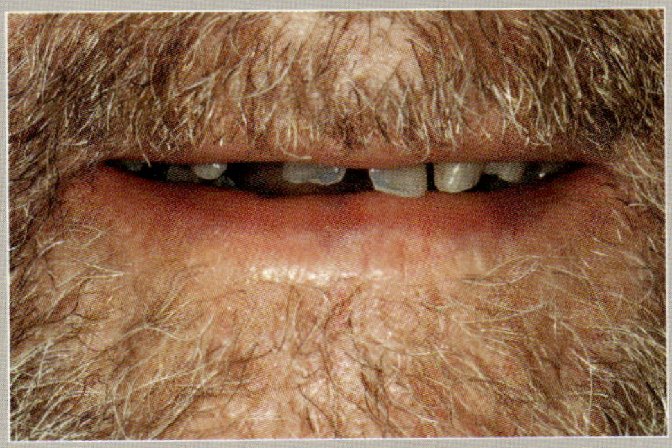

Frontal view of smile.

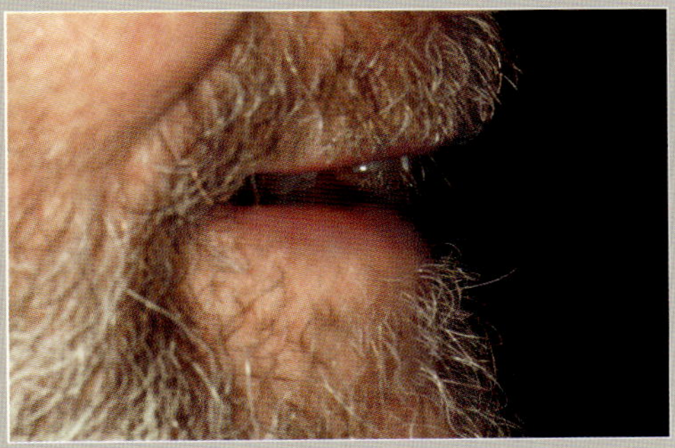

Lateral view of smile.

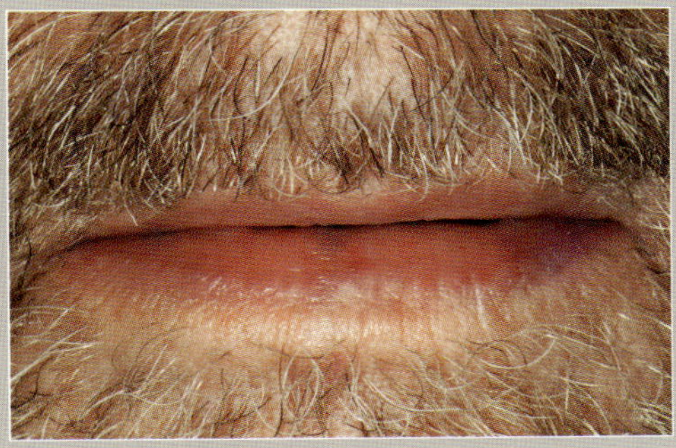

Frontal view at rest.

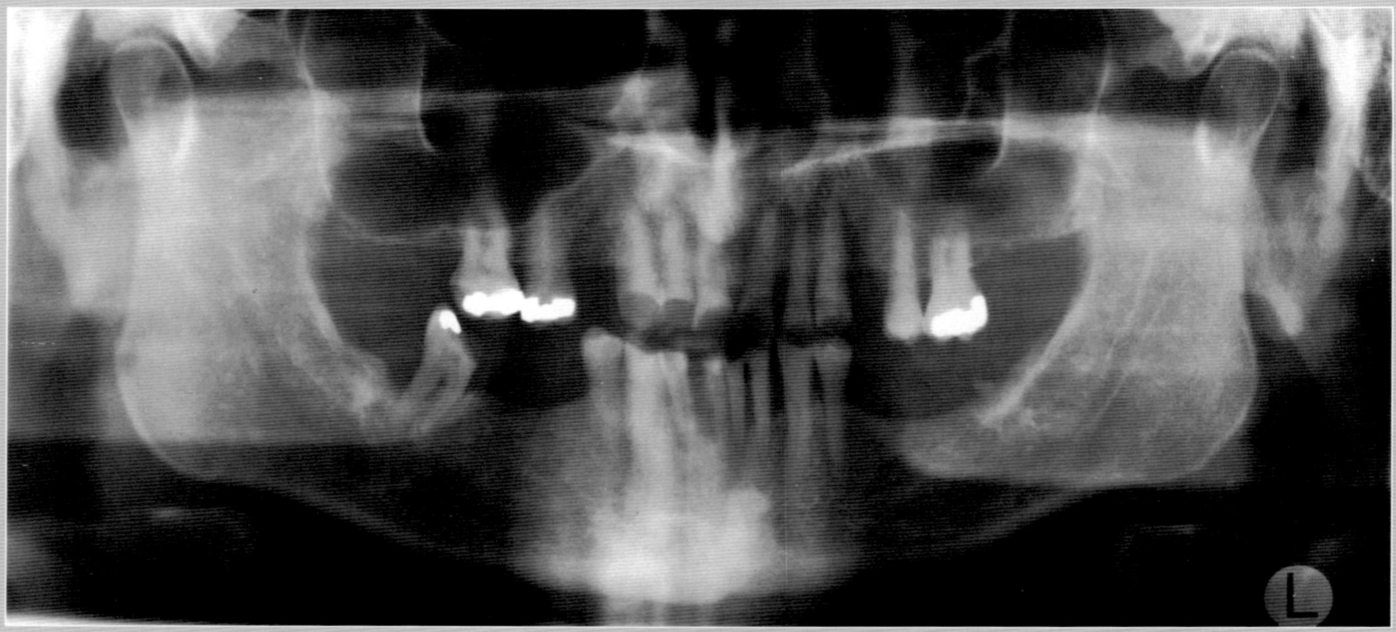

Panoramic radiograph.

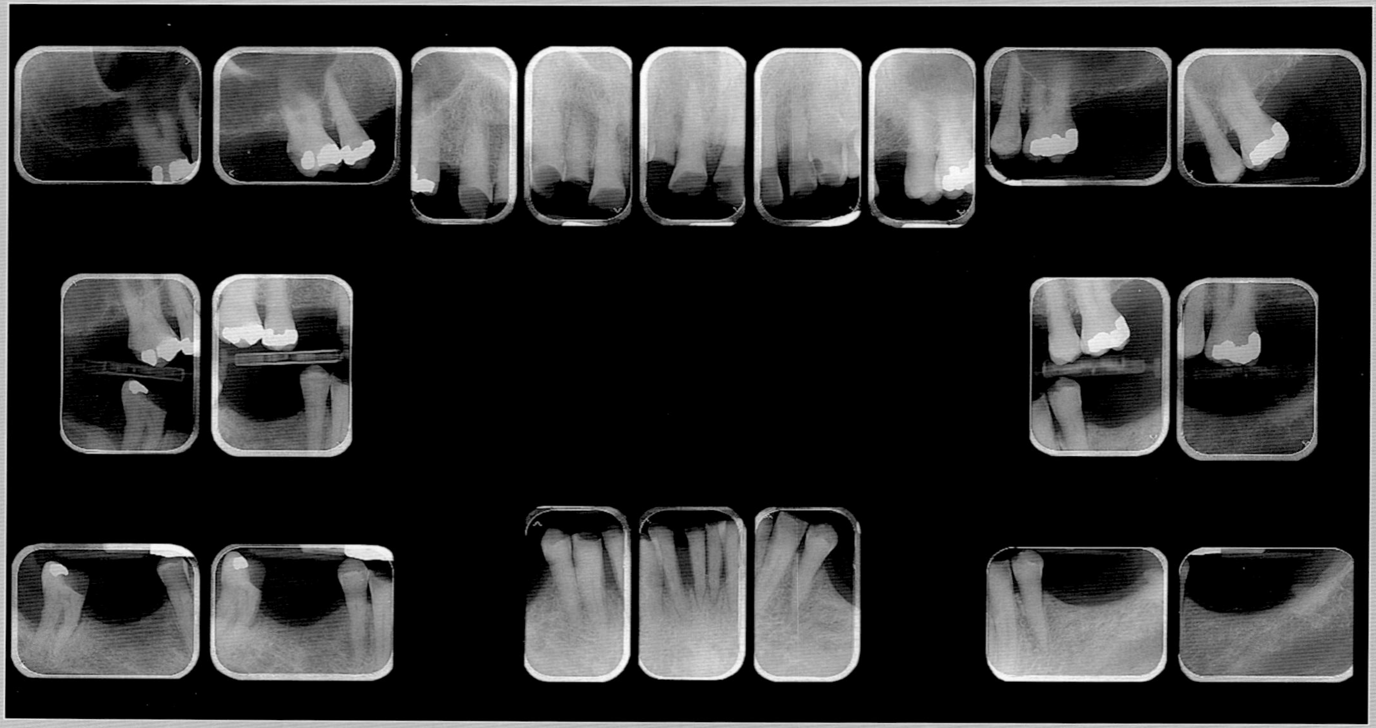

Complete-mouth radiographs.

Summary of concerns

1. What cautions in treatment planning and treatment should be taken for this patient, who presents with a biomechanically compromised dentition?
2. Considering the patient's somewhat limited resources and history of parafunction and severe wear, how can we provide a long-term solution that will provide both retrievability and flexibility should there be future breakage?
3. Considering the patient's diet, which consists of acidic components (eg, soda pop) that are known to cause chemical erosion, and his history of caries (in particular cervical caries), can we achieve longevity for his dentition?
4. How do we manage the extensive supraeruptions and malocclusion and achieve a stable occlusal scheme?
5. How can we provide the patient with a relatively low-cost fixed restoration while meeting his expectations for a highly esthetic result?
6. Ultimately, can this patient be successfully restored with long-term predictability?

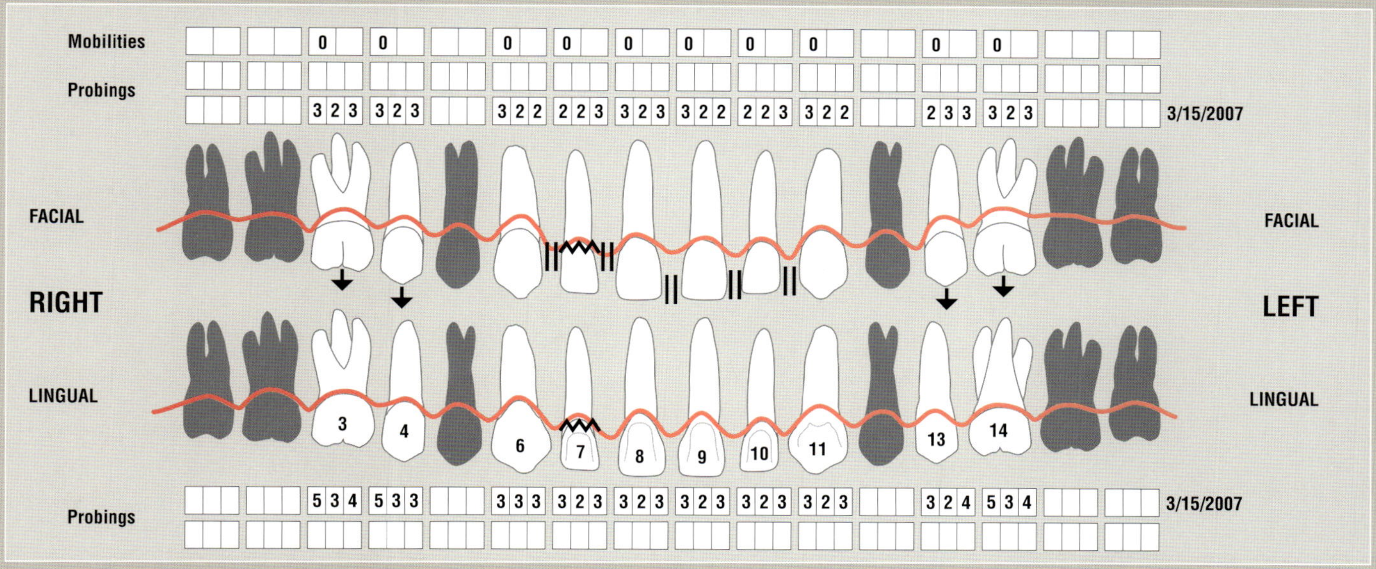

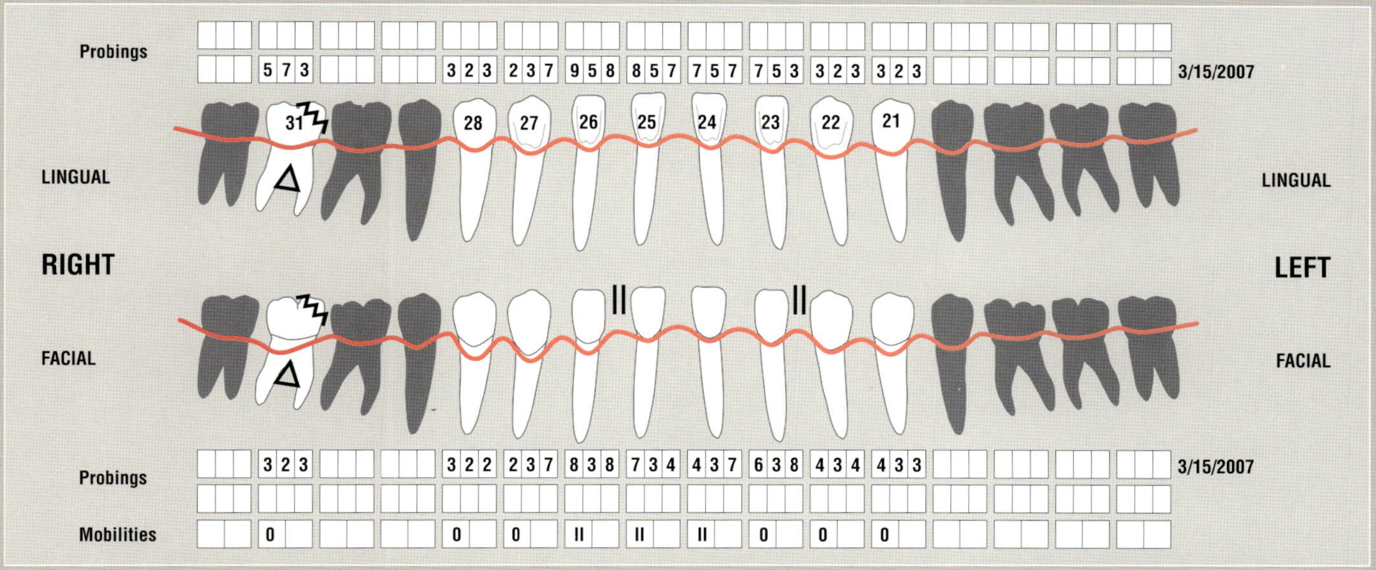

As a learning exercise, you may now outline goals/objectives of treatment and a treatment plan.

Proposed Treatment Plan

Goals/objectives of treatment

- Improve oral hygiene
- Eliminate infection
- Determine ideal incisal edge position and ideal occlusal plane as related to the patient's face and lips
- Manage a bruxer with a severely biomechanically compromised dentition with fixed restorations
- Determine maintenance protocol to facilitate the longevity of the restorations
- Achieve an esthetically pleasing result with fixed restorations while considering somewhat limited finances

Phase I: Initial therapy

1. Oral hygiene instruction and initial periodontal therapy.

Phase II: Diagnostics

2. Clinical and radiographic data collection, including clinical photographs. Make diagnostic impressions, a facebow transfer, and a centric relation record, and then perform a dentofacial and esthetic analysis.
3. Fabrication of an esthetic diagnostic mock-up for determining the maxillary incisal edge position and the anterior occlusal plane and evaluating lip support.
4. Evaluation of the prospective vertical dimension of occlusion.
5. Consultation with the periodontist to determine the sequence for maxillary and mandibular extractions in conjunction with insertion of immediate dentures. Evaluate the prospective dental implant positions for a mandibular fixed-detachable prosthesis and a maxillary implant-supported overdenture without palatal coverage. Also discuss and plan the surgical steps, including extractions, alveoloplasty, ridge augmentation, and maxillary sinus elevation.
6. Fabrication of complete maxillary and mandibular trial setups that will be used to make immediate dentures and surgical guides for implant placement.

Phase III: First surgical treatment

7. Extraction of all the maxillary and mandibular teeth with minor alveoloplasty in the mandibular anterior segment to allow for adequate vertical space for all restorative components and materials.
8. Delivery of maxillary and mandibular immediate complete dentures.
9. Postoperative functional and esthetic evaluation with minor chairside reline as needed 24 hours after surgery.
10. Continued observation with minor adjustments to the dentures as necessary.

Phase IV: Re-evaluation

11. Evaluation of the newly established vertical dimension of occlusion as well as the occlusal scheme, esthetics, and phonetics.
12. Observation of the healing of the residual alveolar ridges.

Phase V: Second surgical treatment

13. Two months after extraction of the mandibular teeth, placement of four dental implants between the mental foramina using a one-stage surgical protocol.
14. Relief and chairside reline of the mandibular immediate denture, engaging the mandibular healing abutments, 1 week after surgery.
15. Six months after extraction of the maxillary teeth (anterior to the maxillary sinuses), placement of six dental implants using a two-stage surgical protocol.
16. Relief and chairside reline of the maxillary immediate denture as needed.
17. Four to five months after placement of the maxillary implants, a second-stage surgery and placement of healing abutments.
18. Relief and chairside reline of the mandibular immediate denture, engaging the maxillary healing abutments, 1 week after surgery.

Phase VI: Definitive restorations

19. Fabrication and delivery of a mandibular fixed-detachable prosthesis with a titanium computer-aided design/computer-assisted manufacture (CAD/CAM) framework.
20. Fabrication and delivery of a maxillary implant-supported overdenture with a titanium CAD/CAM milled infrastructure bar, a titanium CAD/CAM superstructure, and a metal denture base.
21. Fabrication and delivery of a second maxillary implant-supported overdenture with a titanium CAD/CAM superstructure without a metal base to serve as a provisional restoration while the definitive maxillary prosthesis is maintained (such as replacement of worn acrylic resin teeth).
22. Fabrication and delivery of a soft mandibular occlusal guard to protect the mandibular teeth and the maxillary infrastructure bar at night while the implant-supported prosthesis is kept out of the patient's mouth.

Phase VII: Maintenance

23. Recall every 3 months for prophylaxis and implant/prosthodontic evaluation for the first year and subsequently on a 6-month basis.
24. Replacement of worn denture teeth as needed.

Active Clinical Treatment

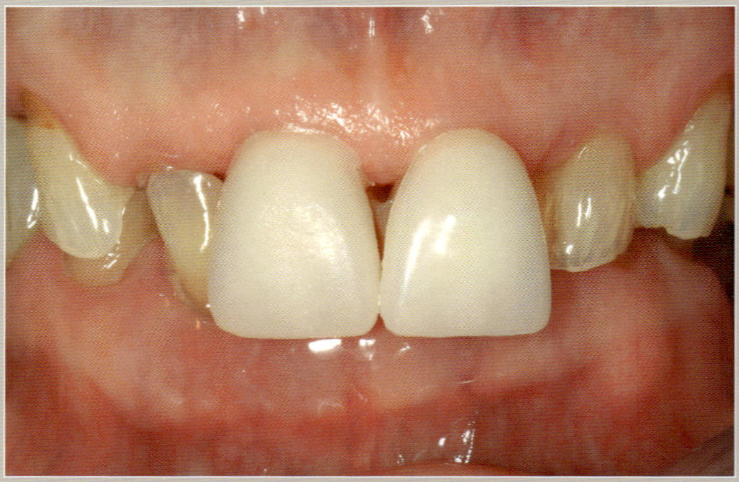

Diagnostic mock-up tried in the patient's mouth.

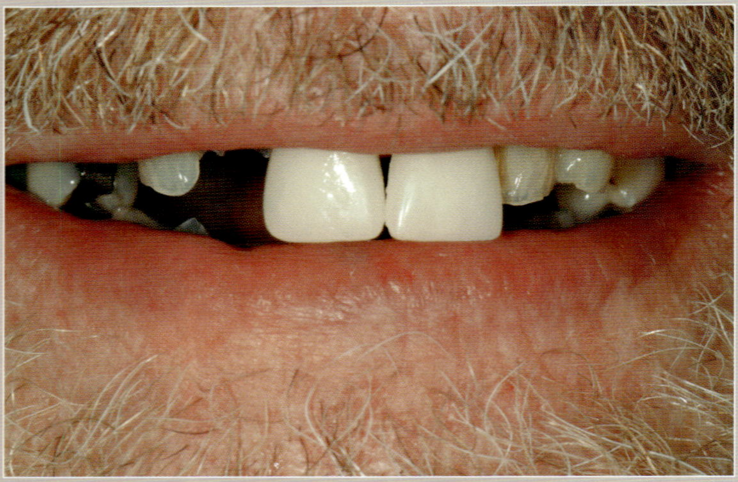

Frontal view of smile with diagnostic mock-up.

Review of the goals/objectives of treatment

The patient had major concerns about the appearance of his teeth and expressed a desire to improve his smile. He reported clenching his teeth and displayed evidence of bruxism, exhibiting generalized severe occlusal and incisal wear. Untreated dental caries and chemical erosion had also resulted in significant loss of tooth structure. The patient wanted a fixed restoration but did not wish to deplete all of his savings to accomplish this. The following were the treatment goals established for this patient:

- Improve oral hygiene and eliminate infection
- Provide an ideal anterior and posterior occlusal plane as related to the patient's face and lips
- Restore the patient's function and esthetics with fixed restorations that may be maintained in a relatively simple manner considering his severe parafunctional habits
- Provide the patient with a relatively low-cost fixed restoration
- Determine an effective maintenance protocol to facilitate the longevity of the restorations

Phase I: Initial therapy

Oral hygiene instruction and initial root planing and scaling procedures were performed to improve periodontal health. At the onset of therapy, numerous treatment alternatives were presented, some of which included saving teeth. Until the treatment plan was finalized, the patient was treated to maintain teeth and minimize periodontal problems.

Phase II: Diagnostics

Clinical and radiographic data were collected. Diagnostic impressions were made, and diagnostic casts were mounted on a semi-adjustable articulator with the aid of a facebow transfer and a centric relation record.

Using a duplicate of the maxillary diagnostic cast, an esthetic diagnostic mock-up simulating the ideal dimensions of the maxillary central incisors, as well as the ideal labiopalatal and apicocoronal position, was fabricated. It was tried in to determine the maxillary incisal edge position and anterior occlusal plane, to facilitate the development of the posterior occlusal plane, and to assess upper lip support. Clinical frontal and profile photographs at rest and with full smile were taken, and an additional diagnostic impression was made with the composite resin mock-up in the patient's mouth. It was cross-mounted with the diagnostic mandibular cast on the semi-adjustable articulator.

The vertical dimension of occlusion was evaluated, and it was determined that because of the severe wear, supraeruption of the teeth, and the uneven occlusal plane, the vertical dimension of occlusion could be increased by 3 mm in the incisor area. In addition, surgical crown lengthening was considered to allow for ideal vertical tooth position, resistance, and retention form. However, because of the extensive loss of tooth structure resulting from the severe wear, tooth fractures, and caries, this approach would have also resulted in less-than-adequate crown-root ratios for the remaining dentition. There possibly would be a need for endodontic therapy on multiple teeth, which may require dowels for the retention of foundation restorations with further biomechanical compromise.

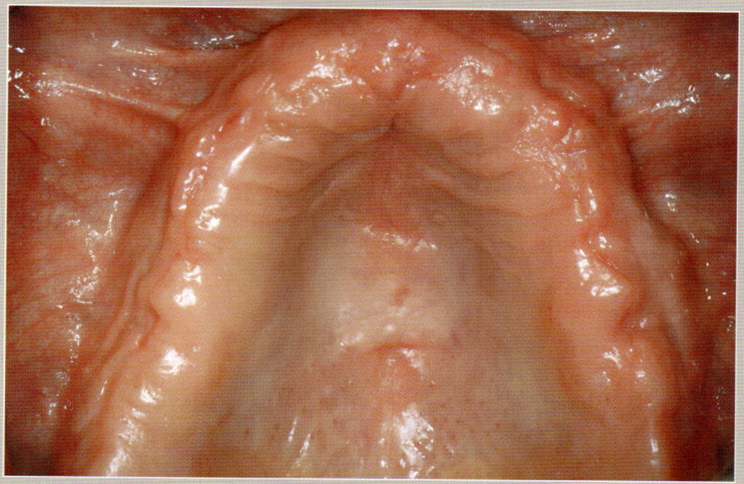 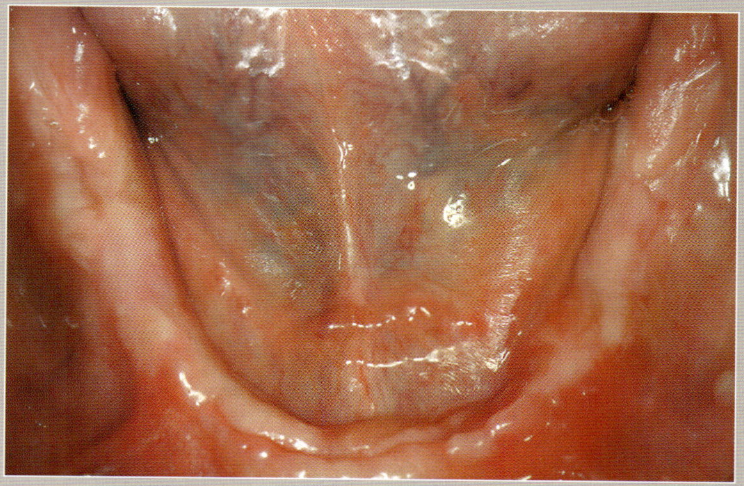

Occlusal views 3 months after extractions.

In addition, the patient was not in favor of pursuing orthodontic treatment. With a biomechanically compromised dentition in a patient with severe parafunction, it was concluded that this approach would likely result in a significantly shortened lifespan for the remaining dentition.

After multiple consultations with the patient and great deliberation, the decision was made by the treatment team and patient to extract the remaining teeth followed by delivery of immediate dentures. Subsequently, the patient would receive implant-supported fixed-removable prostheses.

A consultation with the periodontist determined the prospects for and position of dental implants for a mandibular fixed-detachable prosthesis and a maxillary implant-supported overdenture without palatal coverage. This maxillary prosthesis would provide the patient with a fixed sensation while providing him with adequate lip support and phonetics. These restorations would lend themselves well to a simplified oral hygiene maintenance program. To avoid a sinus elevation procedure, the implants were placed anterior to the maxillary sinus.

Subsequently, based on all collected data as well as the dentofacial and esthetic analyses, complete maxillary and mandibular trial teeth setups were fabricated and used for both the fabrication of the immediate dentures and for the fabrication of surgical guides for alveoloplasty and dental implant placement.

Phase III: First surgical treatment

All maxillary teeth were extracted, and minor alveoloplasty was performed to allow for adequate vertical space for all restorative materials. Because of the location of the roots of tooth no. 14 and an open communication to the maxillary sinus postsurgically, a flap was designed to gain primary closure in the area.

The maxillary denture was delivered, and an occlusal adjustment via selective grinding was performed. Tooth no. 30, which had severe decay, was extracted as well. The following day postoperative functional and esthetic evaluation was performed, including a minor chairside soft reline.

After 2 months, all mandibular teeth were extracted, and minor alveoloplasty was performed to allow for adequate vertical space in the anterior mandible for the dental implants and for restoration. The mandibular denture was delivered, creating with the opposing maxillary denture a new vertical dimension of occlusion and a lingualized occlusion for stability. The following day, a postoperative occlusal functional and esthetic evaluation was performed, along with a minor chairside soft reline.

Phase IV: Re-evaluation

The newly established vertical dimension of occlusion and the new occlusal scheme of the dentures were evaluated and adjusted as needed. The healing of the residual alveolar ridges was evaluated, and soft relines were made as needed. The patient expressed his satisfaction with his new esthetic appearance and his excitement about the functional improvement he was expecting following dental implant placement.

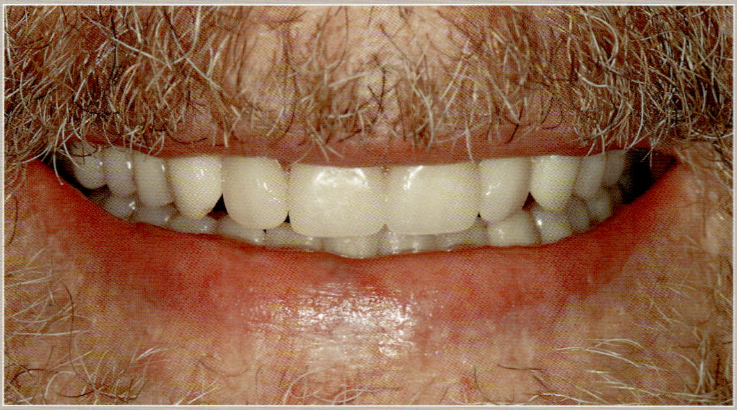

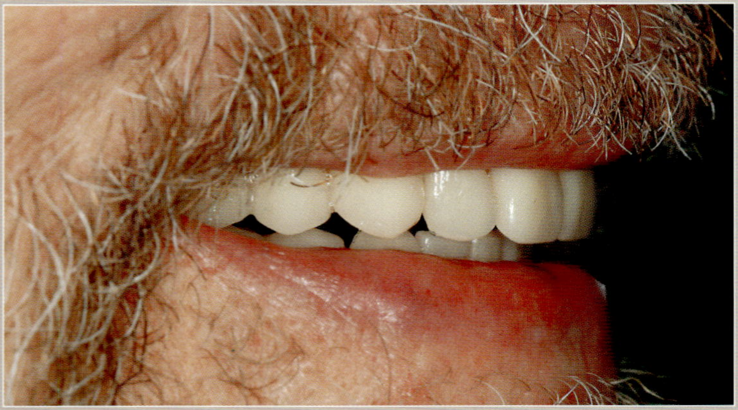

Frontal view of smile with dentures.

Lateral view of smile with dentures.

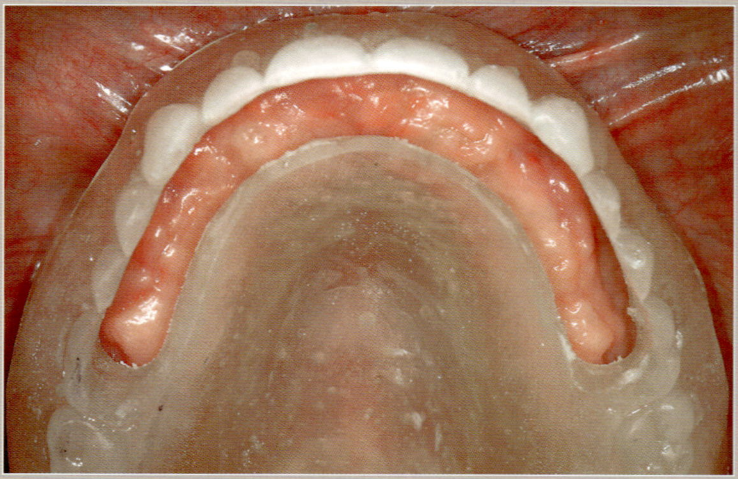

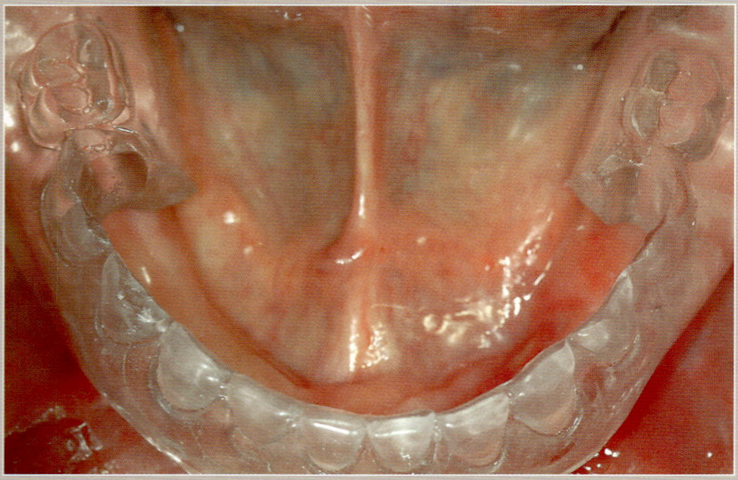

Occlusal views of surgical guides for implant placement.

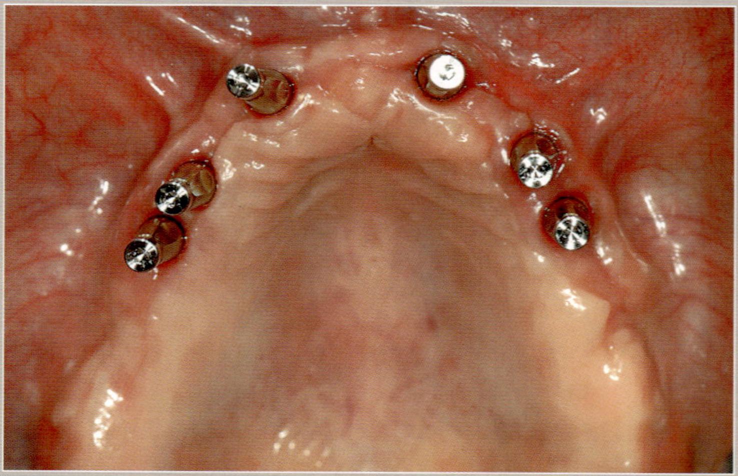

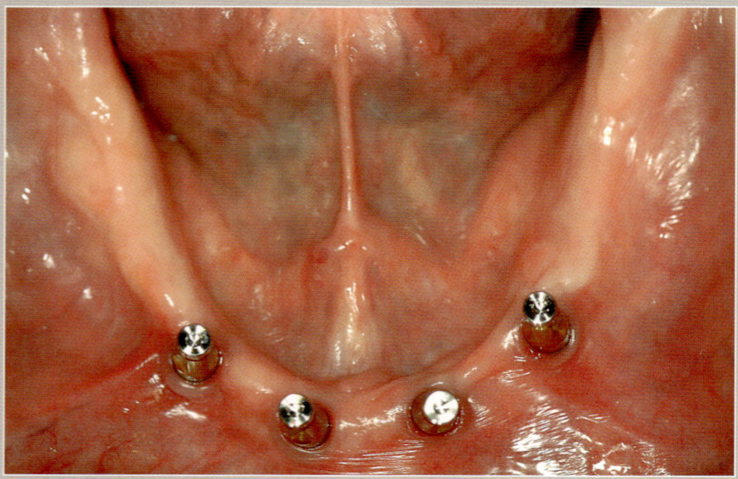

Occlusal views of closed-tray transfer copings.

Phase V: Second surgical treatment

Six months after the extractions in the mandible, four dental implants (NobelReplace RP, Nobel Biocare) were placed between the mental foramina using a one-stage surgical protocol. One week after surgery, the mandibular denture was redelivered, and a chairside soft reline was performed to engage the mandibular healing abutments, enhancing the stability of the denture. Subsequently, six dental implants (NobelReplace RP) were placed in the maxilla using a two-stage surgical

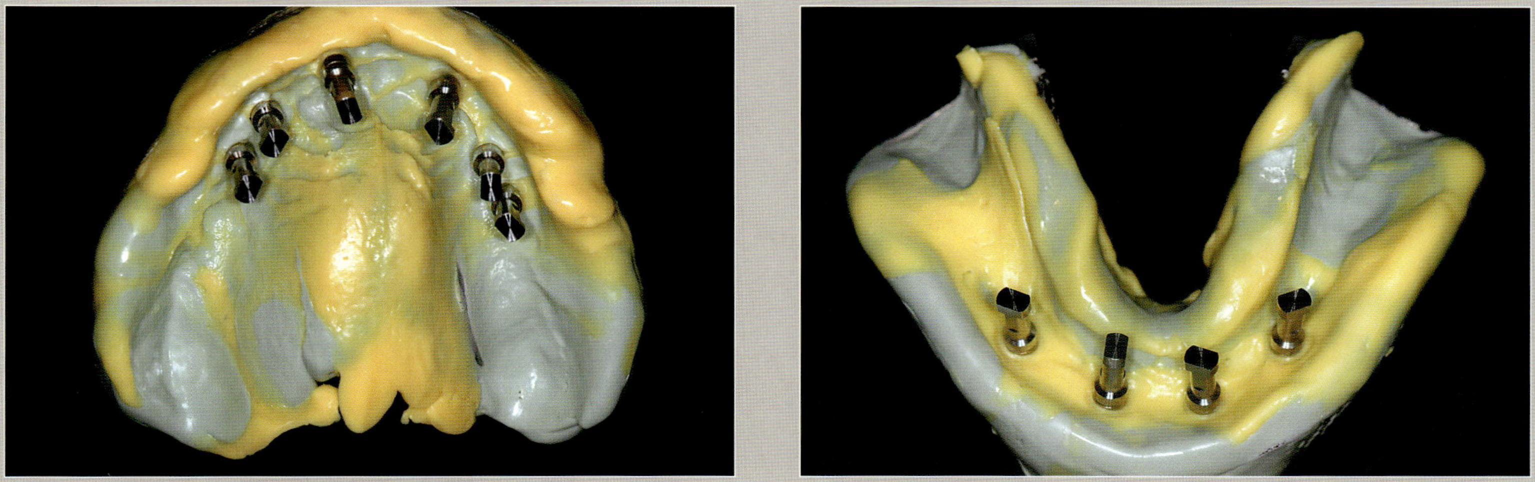

Occlusal views of the closed-tray preliminary impressions.

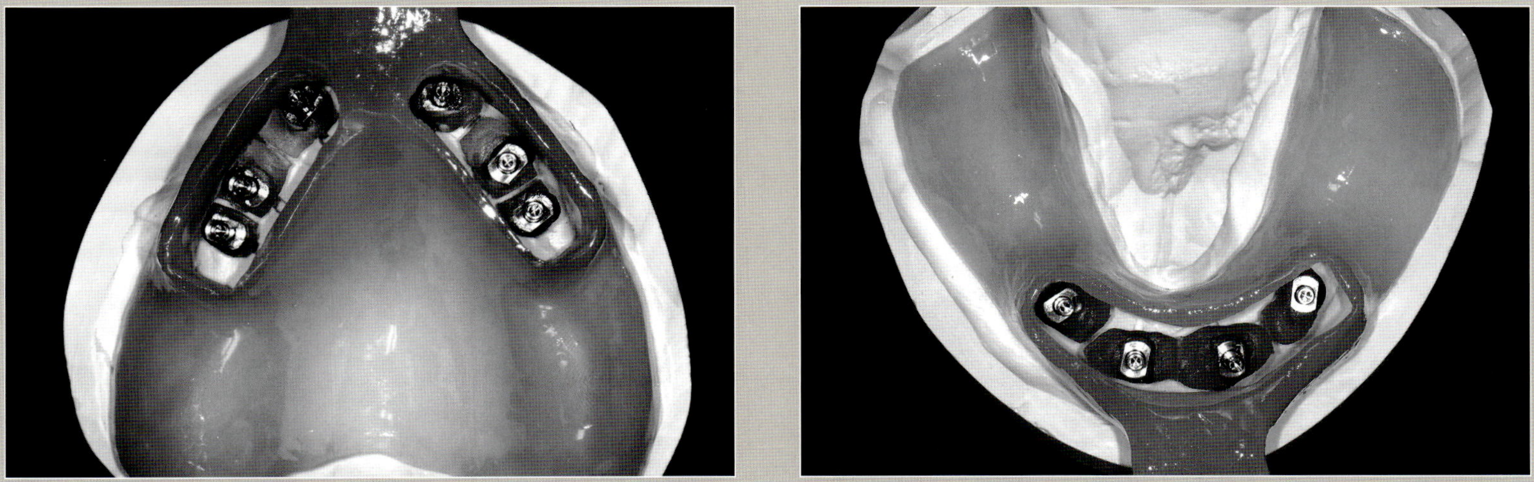

Occlusal views of the preliminary casts with custom open trays and open-tray pickup copings built up with self-curing acrylic resin.

protocol. A week after maxillary implant placement, the maxillary denture was redelivered and relined chairside.

Five months after maxillary implant placement, a second-stage surgery was performed, and healing abutments were placed. The maxillary denture was relieved and relined chairside to engage the healing abutments for improved stability.

Phase VI: Definitive restorations

Once the soft tissue healed, the patient presented for master impressions. Because it was decided to use titanium CAD/CAM frameworks for both the maxillary and mandibular prostheses, the importance of accurate master impressions and accurate definitive casts could not be overemphasized. Thus, a two-stage approach was used, commencing with a closed-tray transfer impression with vinyl polysiloxane followed by an open-tray vinyl polysiloxane impression using the splinted open-tray pickup impression technique.

Closed-tray transfer impression copings were secured to the implants in the patient's mouth, and preliminary vinyl polysiloxane transfer impressions were made with a closed stock tray for both the maxillary and mandibular arches. The impressions were poured in dental stone with the transfer impression copings and analogs in place.

Open-tray pickup impression copings were secured to the implant analogs on the casts and then splinted together with autopolymerizing acrylic resin (Pattern Resin, GC). The acrylic resin was sectioned with a 1-mm thin diamond disk, and the pickup impression copings were numbered. Custom open trays were fabricated to allow for master pickup impressions.

The healing abutments were removed, and the pickup impression copings were placed in the patient's mouth at

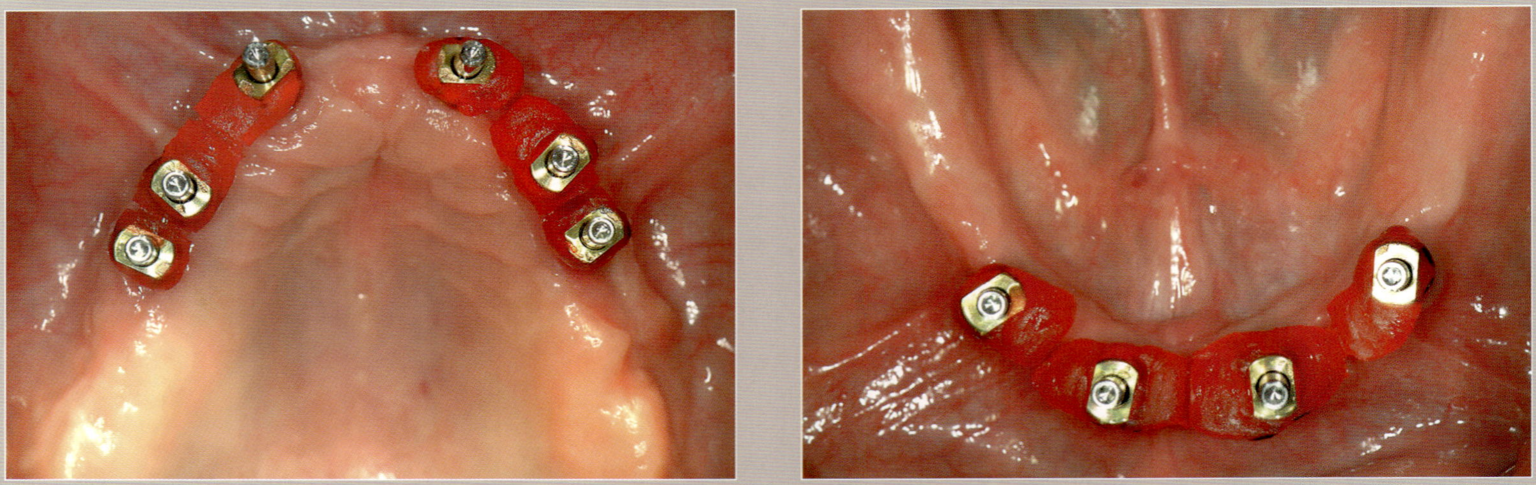

Intraoral occlusal views of the splinted open-tray pickup copings.

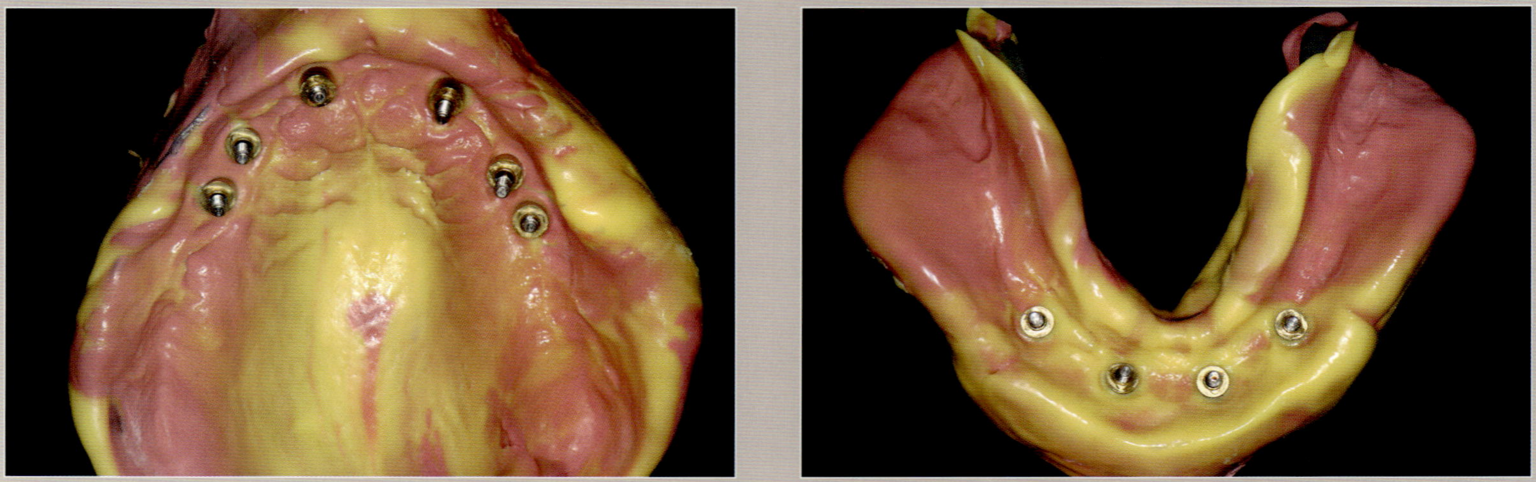

Occlusal views of the master open-tray impressions.

the positions corresponding to their numbers, one arch at a time. Autopolymerized acrylic resin was used to reconnect the impression copings prior to impression making. Once polymerized, master impressions were made first for the maxillary and then for the mandibular arch.

The definitive casts were poured with soft tissue simulation. Maxillary and mandibular verification jigs were made using temporary abutments and autopolymerized acrylic resin. These were tried in the patient's mouth, and fit was verified clinically using the one-screw test.

Subsequently, record bases and occlusion rims were fabricated while the patient's healing abutments were placed on the definitive casts. Once resecured in the mouth, the healing abutments facilitated the stability of the record bases and occlusion rims while the maxillomandibular relationship was evaluated. A facebow transfer was made to mount the maxillary definitive cast, the vertical dimension of occlusion and the occlusal plane were assessed, and a centric relation record was made.

The shade and mold of teeth were selected according to the patient's preferences. A trial denture setup was made and tried in the patient's mouth to evaluate the esthetics and phonetics and to reassess the prospective occlusal scheme, centric relation, and the vertical dimension of occlusion. Once verified, maxillary and mandibular matrices were made to re-evaluate the space available for the restorative components and materials and to mark tooth positions for the definitive setup.

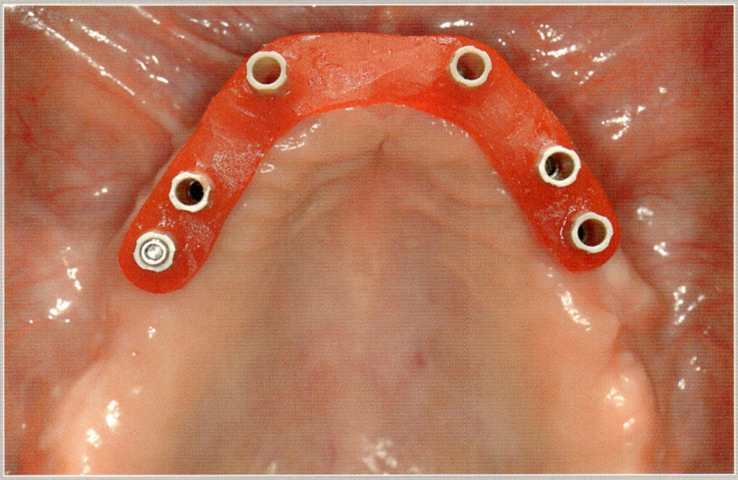
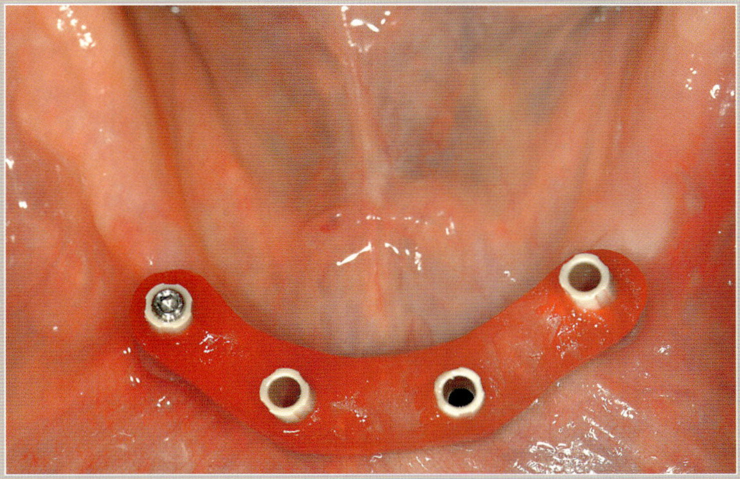

Intraoral occlusal views of verification jigs.

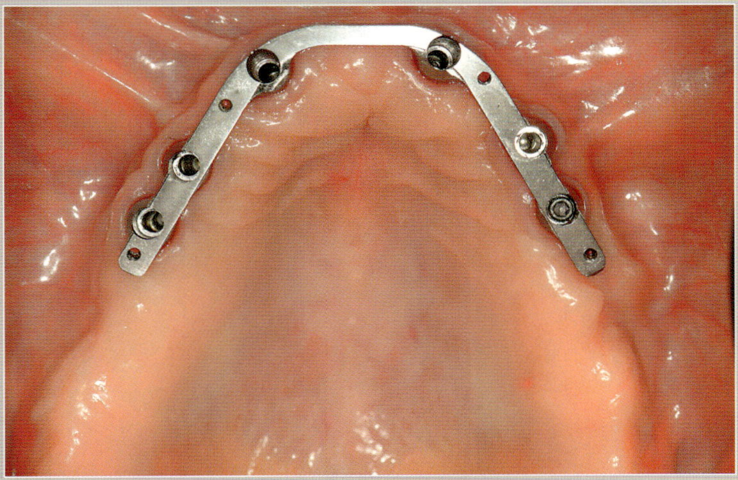
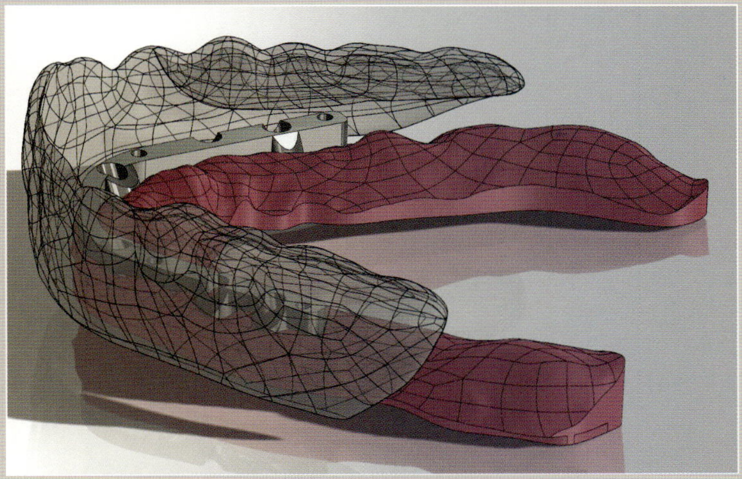

Occlusal view and CAD design of the primary bar of the maxillary infrastructure.

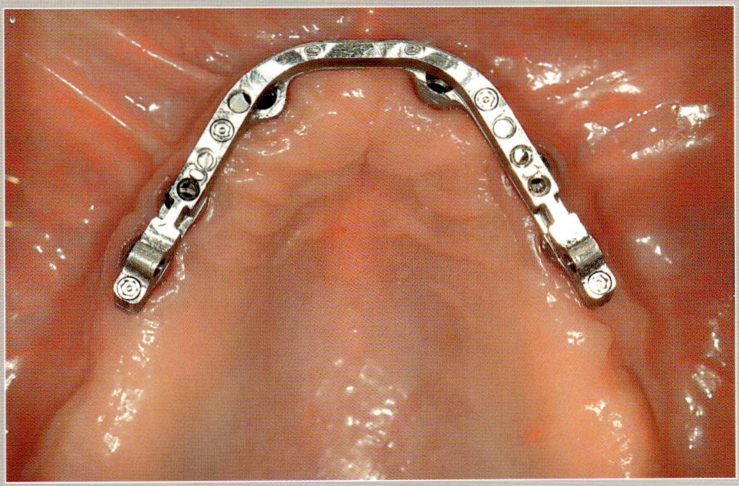
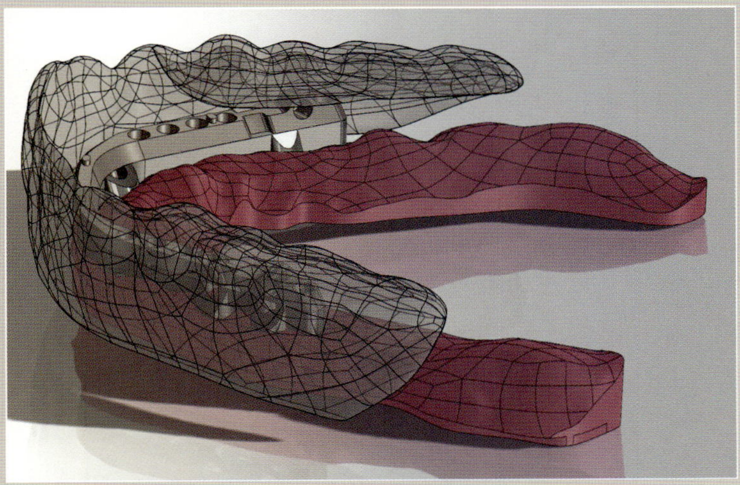

Occlusal view and CAD design of the secondary bar of the maxillary infrastructure.

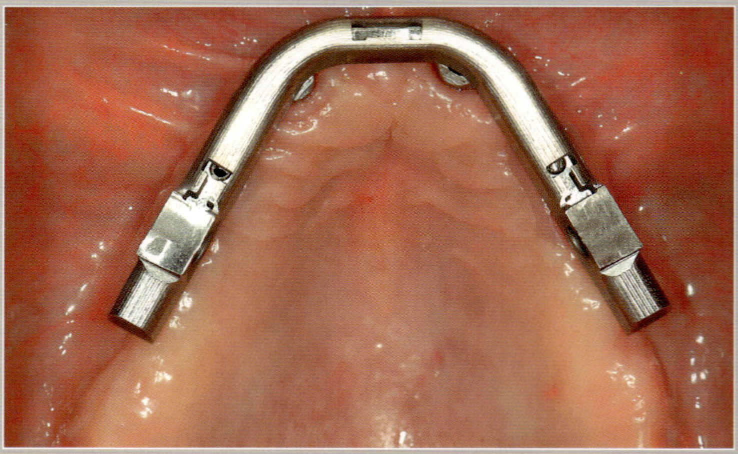

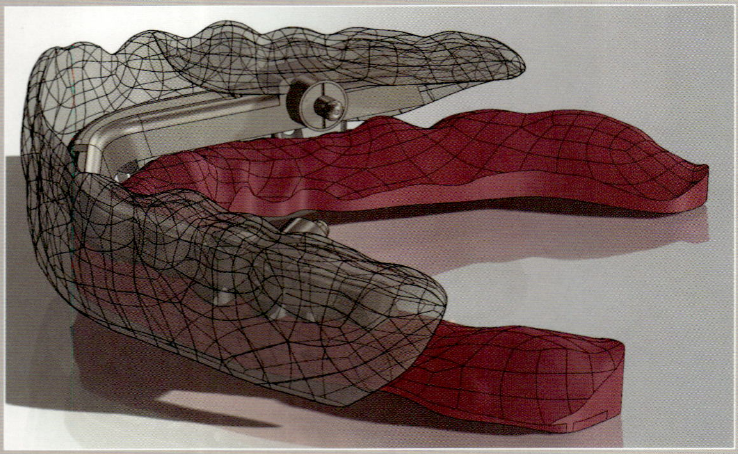

Occlusal view and CAD design of the maxillary superstructure to be embedded in the overdenture.

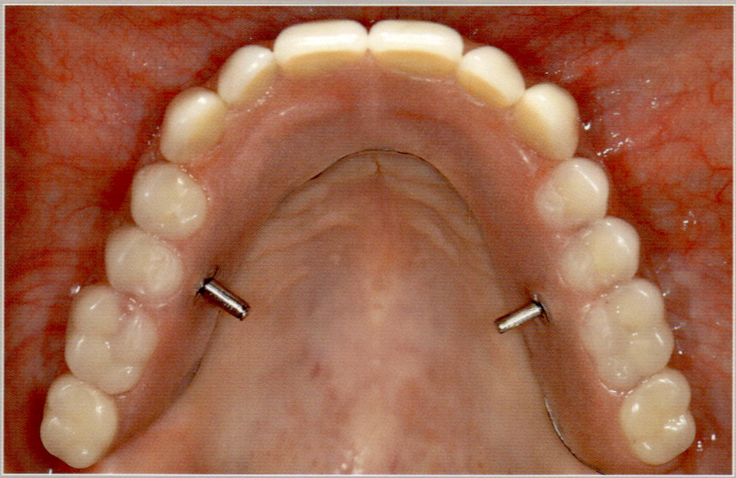

Occlusal view of the maxillary complete prosthesis with the attachments set for overdenture removal.

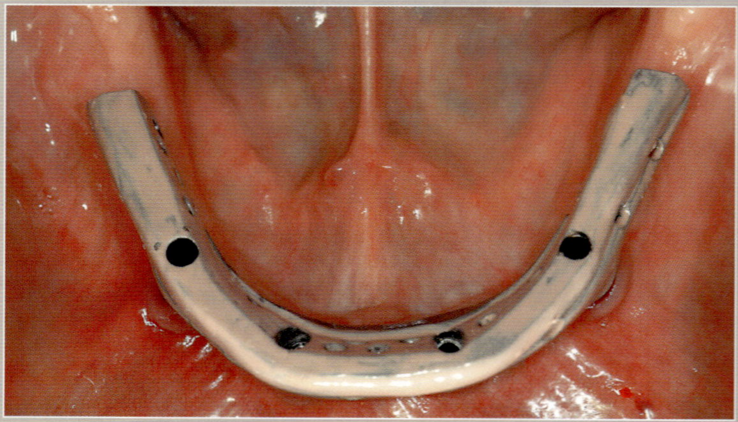

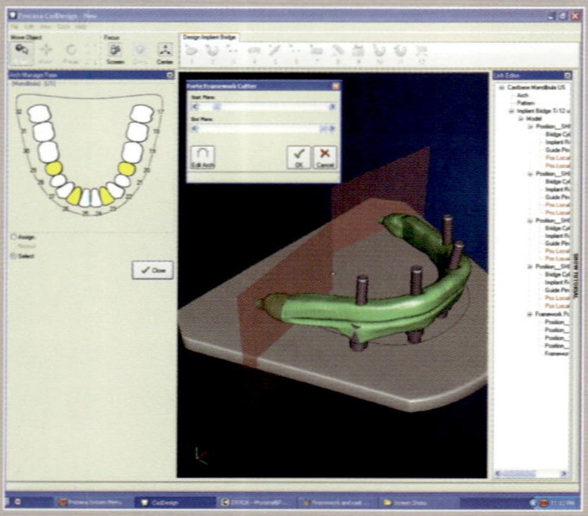

Occlusal view and CAD design of the titanium framework for the mandibular fixed-detachable prosthesis after initial opaque application.

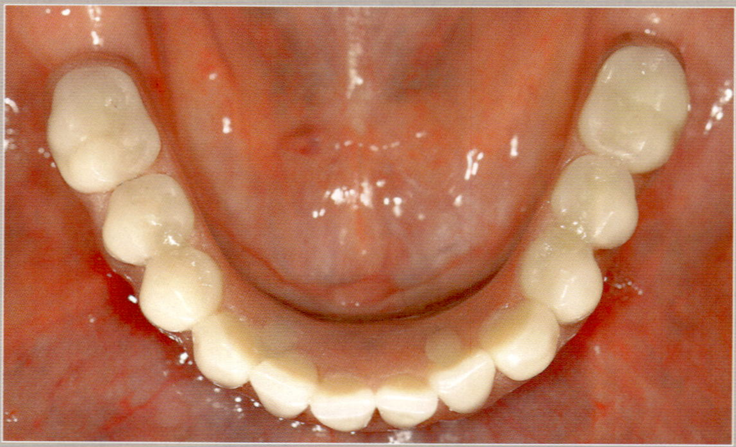

Occlusal view of the mandibular fixed-detachable prosthesis.

Posttreatment

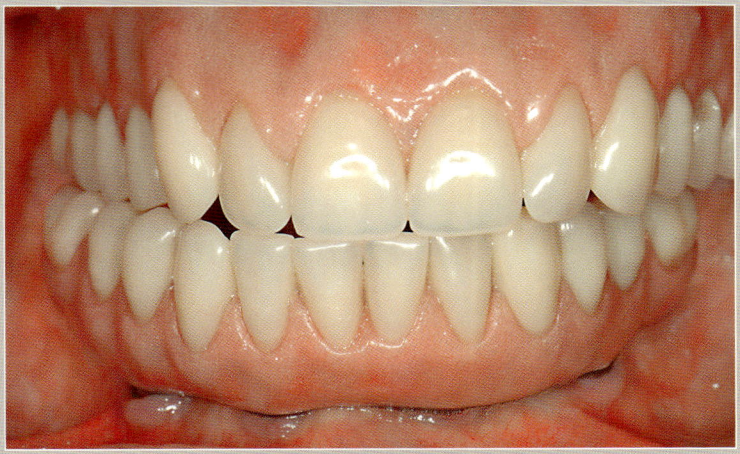
Prostheses in right lateral excursion.

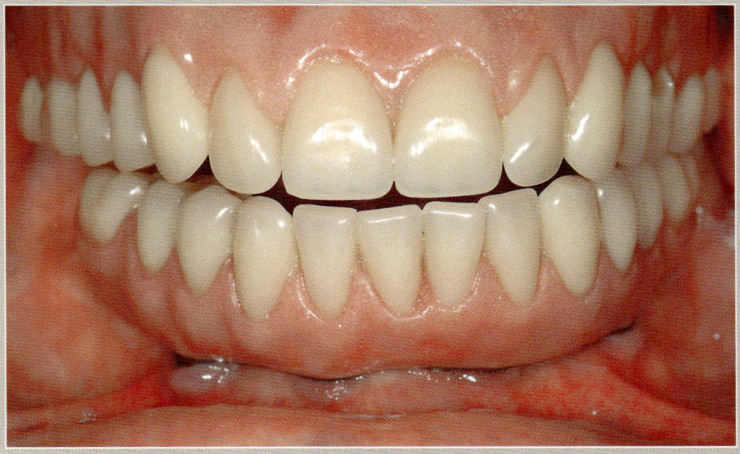
Prostheses in left lateral excursion.

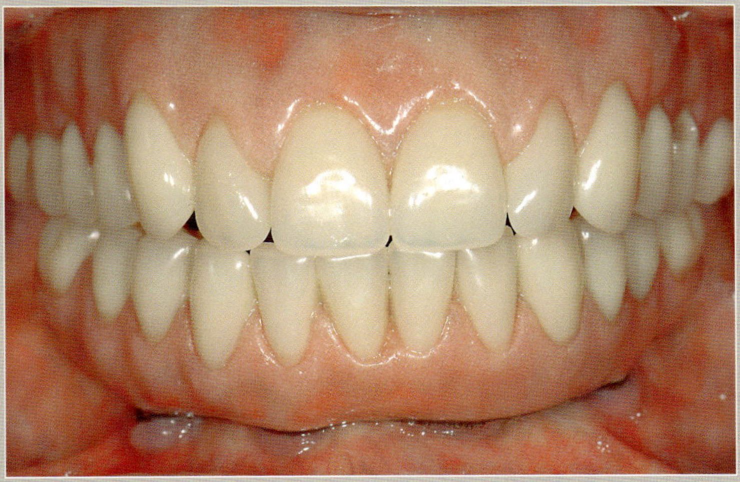
Prostheses in centric occlusion.

For the mandibular fixed-detachable framework, an autopolymerizing acrylic resin pattern was fabricated and scanned with the Procera system (Nobel Biocare) for the fabrication of a CAD/CAM titanium framework. For the maxillary implant-supported overdenture, a CAD/CAM titanium infrastructure comprising two bars and a titanium superstructure were made (ie, the Marius bridge system). Both mandibular and maxillary titanium frameworks were evaluated in the patient's mouth using the one-screw test, and passivity of fit was verified. The maxillary titanium superstructure was fabricated to fit the maxillary infrastructure and was embedded with modified MK 1 plunger attachments (Attachments International) in the metal-based maxillary overdenture.

A wax try-in was made to re-evaluate esthetics, phonetics, and occlusion, and the prostheses were processed and completed. The maxillary infrastructure and the mandibular fixed-detachable prosthesis were secured to the implants and torqued to 35 Ncm according to the manufacturer's instructions. Subsequently, the maxillary overdenture was delivered, and a minor occlusal adjustment was performed.

An impression of the mandibular fixed-detachable prosthesis was made, and a soft occlusal guard was fabricated. This occlusal guard was designed to be worn at night after removal of the maxillary overdenture to protect the maxillary titanium infrastructure from parafunctional habits. The patient was given oral hygiene instructions and scheduled for a 1-week re-evaluation.

Phase VII: Maintenance

The importance of maintaining a high level of oral hygiene was stressed to the patient. Instruction was given on the use of floss and a floss threader to maintain both the mandibular fixed-detachable prosthesis and the area under the maxillary infrastructure. The patient returned at 1 and 4 weeks for an occlusal analysis and for soft tissue evaluation and was placed on a 6-month recall schedule.

The patient reported absolute satisfaction with the esthetics, function, and comfort of the prosthesis and was very content with his new smile.

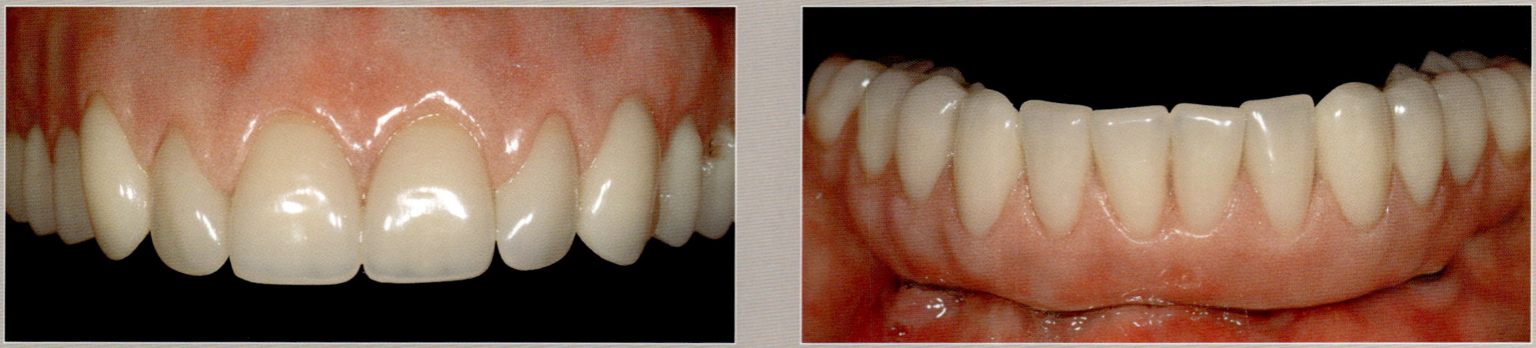

Frontal views of the complete prostheses.

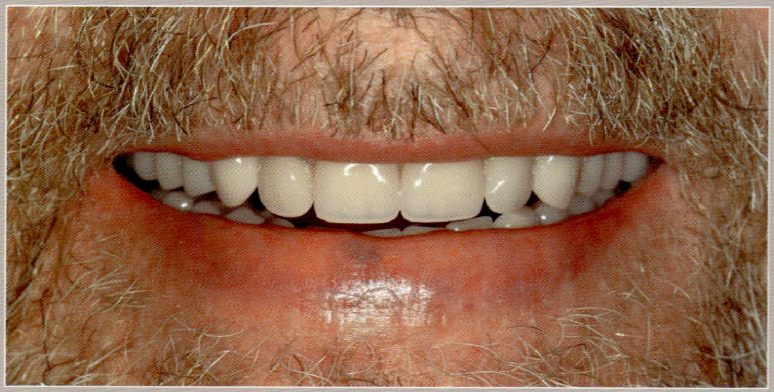

Frontal view of smile.

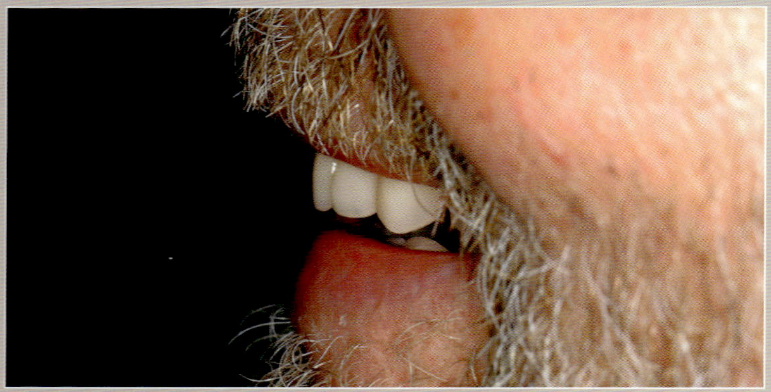

Lateral view of smile.

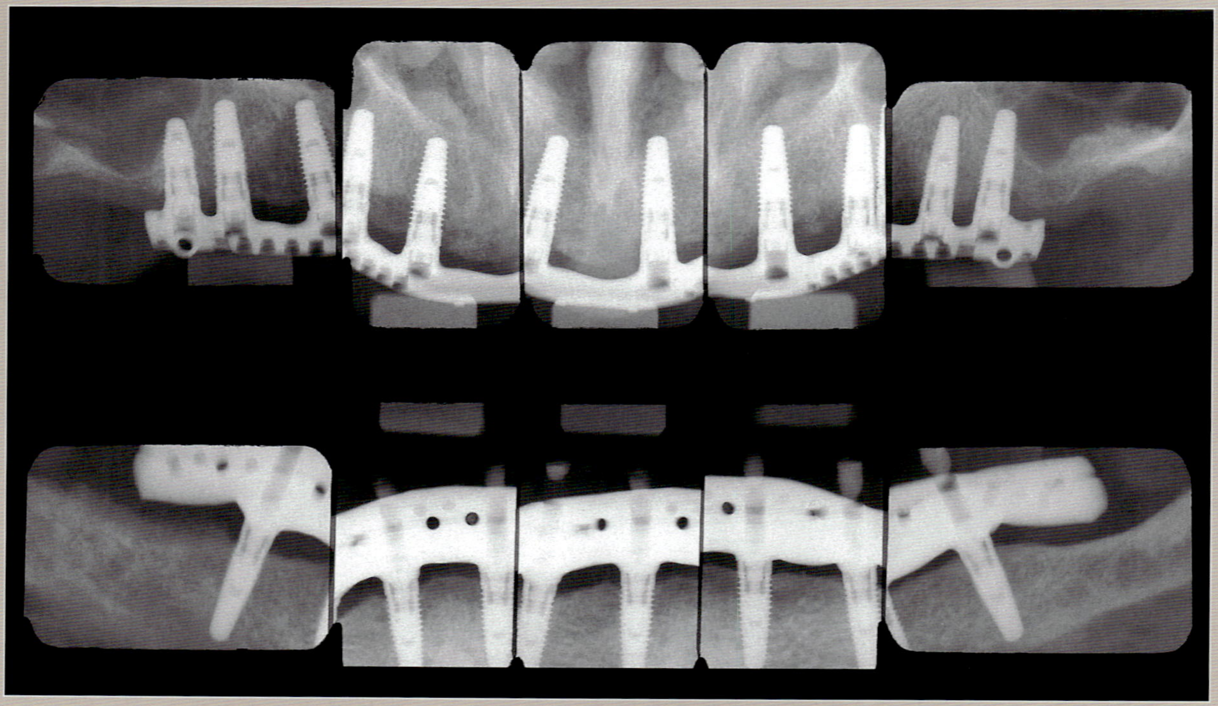

Complete-mouth radiographs.

You may now place the corresponding posttreatment overlay found in the separate folder over the pretreatment periodontal chart on page 53.

Commentary

In this chapter, we emphasized the interaction between biomechanical and functional considerations with the goal of treatment planning patients for fixed restorations while enhancing function, esthetics, and longevity. Both patients described presented with many treatment dilemmas. Although they both presented with biomechanically compromised dentitions, they differed in terms of their functional risk. Consequently, their treatment planning and execution proceeded in opposite directions in terms of preservation of their dentition and the types of restorations and restorative materials used.

The first patient was determined to have fundamental biomechanical risks. However, the patient presented with no history of parafunction or excessive tooth wear for her age. Therefore, a relatively low functional risk led the treating clinicians to retain many of the compromised teeth and use fixed metal ceramic and all-ceramic restorations. A comprehensive treatment plan was provided to manage biomechanical risk, determine the restorability of the teeth, and prevent further breakdown of compromised but still adequate tooth structure.

With the extensive amount of restorative dentistry performed in the past, it was inadvisable to determine a definitive treatment plan without first exploring the integrity of the dentition. Therefore, it was decided to provide two provisional restorations during the transitional phases of the process. The first provisional restorations were delivered after the removal of the pre-existing restorations and caries and assessment of residual tooth structures (ferrule, resistance and retention form). These restorations were used to give the uncovered teeth mechanical protection and to provide reasonable esthetics and function based on the pre-existing occlusion during the transitional stage with better cervical contours. In this patient, the diagnostic wax-up was made with altered cervical gingival levels, and during the first provisional phase, it helped to determine if the teeth were restorable based on the residual tooth structure in relation to the prospective gingival levels.

After complete removal of the carious lesions, compromised tooth structure was evident in both the anterior and posterior teeth. Two major aspects, the biomechanical and the esthetic, were taken into consideration in determining if the teeth should be retained or replaced. In the posterior segments, surgical crown lengthening procedures were performed to provide adequate ferrule and retention and resistance form to address the biomechanical concerns.[21,22] For the teeth in the esthetic zone, the esthetic perspective was equally crucial in the decision-making process.[23–25]

Because the patient initially presented with a high caries risk, management of the cariogenic bacteria and alteration of her diet, as well as fluoride and xylitol supplementation, were important factors in facilitating long-term success. The patient's commitment to cooperate fully and to follow instructions, as well as to maintain a strict oral hygiene regimen, are all key elements for a predictable long-term prognosis.

The major concern with treatment of the second patient was achieving longevity in terms of biomechanics and function while providing the patient with fixed restorations at a reasonable cost. The dentition was severely compromised from a biomechanical standpoint because of excessive mechanical and chemical wear, caries, and dental neglect. In addition, this patient presented with high functional risk due to severe parafunctional habits. The synergistic effect of both high biomechanical and functional risk greatly influenced the decision not to restore the existing dentition but rather to proceed with complete-mouth extractions, followed by the fabrication of implant-supported prostheses. Although one may argue that some of the teeth (eg, maxillary anterior) could have been restored, this would have required orthodontic extrusion or surgical crown lengthening followed by endodontic therapy, dowel and core buildups, and complete-coverage restorations. All of this would have been accomplished with little assurance that the restorations would last over the long term.

Because severe bruxism is very difficult to manage and because of the lack of proprioception present with implant-supported restorations, it was decided to use acrylic resin rather than ceramics as the restorative material. It was explained to the patient that replacement of the acrylic resin teeth would be a relatively low-cost treatment. A contingency plan was incorporated into the treatment by designing a weak link within the restoration that can be managed in a relatively simple and cost-effective manner when a complication occurs.

In summary, when planning treatment for patients with a biomechanically compromised dentition, the incorporation of functional considerations is critical in setting the stage for predictable long-term treatment success. If, as in the first case, the etiology of tooth structure loss is addressed and managed over time and the patient demonstrates no signs or symptoms of dysfunction or parafunctional habits, then clinicians may be able to successfully restore the biomechanically compromised dentition. However, if, as in the second case, in addition to the high biomechanical risk the patient presents with functional concerns, then the likelihood of restoration and tooth fracture may be increased and alternative treatment solutions should be considered. A variety of implant-supported restorations may be considered, which may be managed in a relatively simple and cost-effective manner when complications occur.

Acknowledgments

The authors would like to express their sincere appreciation to Harald Heindl, MDT, Aesthetic Dental Creations, Mill Creek, Washington, for fabricating the restorations presented in the first case in this chapter. In addition, the authors would like to thank Bob Williams, CDT, Techsource, Plano, Texas, for the fabrication of the zirconia copings and framework.

The authors also would like to express their sincere appreciation to Ruth Bourke, CDT, RE Bourke Prosthodontic Art & Technology, Redmond, Washington, for fabricating the restorations presented in the second case in this chapter. In addition, the authors would like to thank Dr Yves Fortin for the fabrication of the Marius bridge infra- and superstructure.

References

1. "Biomechanics." Oxford English Dictionary, ed 11. Oxford: Oxford University Press, 2004:135.
2. "Biomechanics." The Glossary of Prosthodontics Terms, ed 8. J Prosthet Dent 2005;84:18.
3. Bakeman EM, Kois JC. Maximizing esthetics/minimizing risk: The line of predictable success. Inside Dent 2005;1:16–24.
4. Litonjua LA, Andreana S, Bush PJ, Cohen RE. Tooth wear: Attrition, erosion, and abrasion. Quintessence Int 2003;34:435–446.
5. Shafer WG, Hine MK, Levy BM. Developmental disturbances in tooth structure. In: Textbook of Oral Pathology, ed 4. Philadelphia: Saunders, 1983:51–64.
6. Shafer WG, Hine MK, Levy BM. Regressive alterations of the teeth. In: Textbook of Oral Pathology, ed 4. Philadelphia: Saunders, 1983:318–323.
7. Bardsley PF. The evolution of tooth wear indices. Clin Oral Investig 2008;12(suppl 1):S15–S19.
8. Verrett RG. Analyzing the etiology of an extremely worn dentition. J Prosthodont 2001;10:224–233.
9. Tsukiboshi M. Crown fracture. In: Treatment Planning for Traumatized Teeth. Chicago: Quintessence, 2000:21–34.
10. Tsukiboshi M. Crown-root fracture. In: Treatment Planning for Traumatized Teeth. Chicago: Quintessence, 2000:35–45.
11. Featherstone JD. The science and practice of caries prevention. J Am Dent Assoc 2000;131:887–899.
12. Steinberg S. Adding caries diagnosis to caries risk assessment: The next step in caries management by risk assessment (CAMBRA). Compend Contin Educ Dent 2009;30:522–528.
13. Featherstone JD, Domejean-Orliaguet S, Jenson L, Wolff M, Young DA. Caries risk assessment in practice for age 6 through adult. J Calif Dent Assoc 2007;35:703–707,710–713.
14. Featherstone JD, Singh S, Curtis DA. Caries risk assessment and management for the prosthodontic patient. J Prosthodont 2011;20:2–9.
15. Edelhoff D, Sorensen JA. Tooth structure removal associated with various preparation designs for posterior teeth. Int J Periodontics Restorative Dent 2002;22:241–249.
16. Edelhoff D, Sorensen JA. Tooth structure removal associated with various preparation designs for anterior teeth. J Prosthet Dent 2002;87:503–509.
17. Libman WJ, Nicholls JI. Load fatigue of teeth restored with cast posts and cores and complete crowns. Int J Prosthodont 1995;8:155–161.
18. Pereira JR, de Ornelas F, Conti PC, do Valle AL. Effect of a crown ferrule on the fracture resistance of endodontically treated teeth restored with prefabricated posts. J Prosthet Dent 2006;95:50–54.
19. Dawson PE. Functional Occlusion: From TMJ to Smile Design. St Louis: Mosby, 2007:259–264.

20. Lavigne GJ, Khoury S, Abe S, Yamaguchi T, Raphael K. Bruxism physiology and pathology: An overview for clinicians. J Oral Rehabil 2008;35:476–494.
21. Goodacre CJ, Campagni WV, Aquilino SA. Tooth preparations for complete crowns: An art form based on scientific principles. J Prosthet Dent 2001;85:363–376.
22. Smukler H, Chaibi M. Periodontal and dental considerations in clinical crown extension: A rational basis for treatment. Int J Periodontics Restorative Dent 1997;17:464–477.
23. Vig RG, Brundo GC. The kinetics of anterior tooth display. J Prosthet Dent 1978;39:502–504.
24. Simon JF. Retain or extract: The decision process. Quintessence Int 1999;30:851–854.
25. Belser UC, Schmid B, Higginbottom F, Buser D. Outcome analysis of implant restorations located in the anterior maxilla: A review of the recent literature. Int J Oral Maxillofac Implants 2004;19(suppl):30–42.

3

Managing Treatment for the Restorative Patient with Significant Maxillary Anterior Bone Loss

Vincent G. Kokich, DDS, MSD
Vincent O. Kokich, DMD, MSD

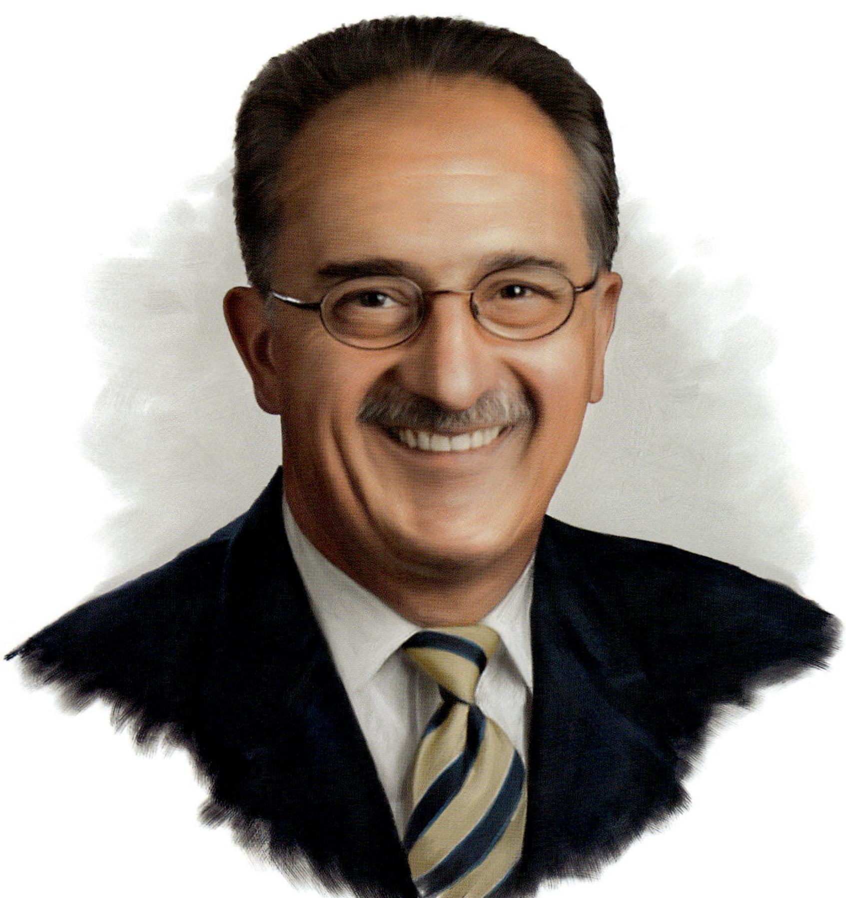

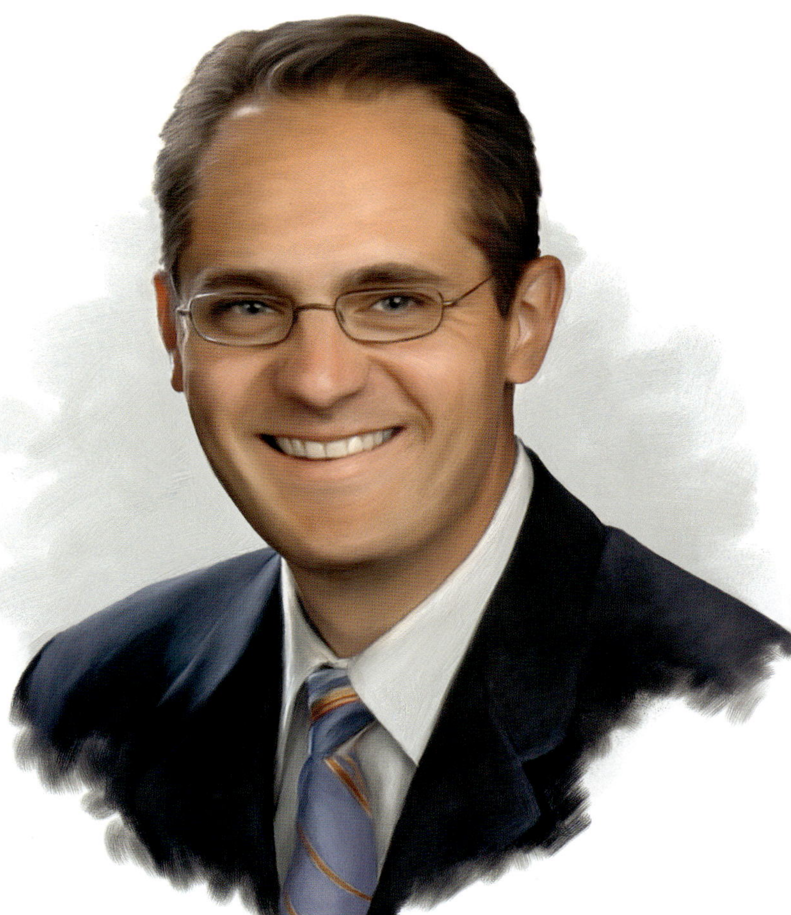

In some cases, the beneficial opportunities of interdisciplinary collaborative tooth movement are critical and yet subtle.

Philosophy and Background

As orthodontists, we believe that orthodontics should be an integral part of any periodontal-restorative treatment plan in which tooth malposition and occlusal discrepancies are fundamental obstacles to providing optimal treatment. In most interdisciplinary cases, the need for orthodontics is readily apparent. However, in other cases, the beneficial opportunities for collaborative tooth movement are subtle. The patient presented in this case report would fall into the latter category.

The patient's chief complaint was the unesthetic appearance of her smile. However, as the diagnostic findings show, she has significant periodontal bone loss around the maxillary incisors. When the restorative dentist dismantles the previous restorations, how will the team avoid creating an esthetic nightmare? The second subtle problem that exists is that her maxillary midline is deviated significantly because of a missing maxillary lateral incisor. How should the interdisciplinary team deal with the midline discrepancy? Should space be opened for a maxillary lateral incisor implant? How will the bone loss affect implant esthetics? Finally, she has an asymmetric posterior malocclusion with bilateral Angle Class II molar and canine relationships that are worse on one side than the other. How should the team solve this occlusal discrepancy? Should posterior arch symmetry be created?

While working through the diagnosis, identifying the problem list, establishing treatment objectives, and thoroughly weighing all treatment options, remember one important concept: evidence-based dentistry. Is there clinical research published in peer-reviewed journals that would substantiate all the decisions made to correct her problems? If not, how can the treatment plan be justified? The treatment of this patient could be extremely complicated and involve several different disciplines, including orthognathic surgery, or it could be very straightforward. The key to discovering the appropriate treatment plan for this patient is to correct only those problems that could adversely affect the long-term outcome of treatment. Good luck, and enjoy this intellectual challenge in interdisciplinary treatment planning.

Case Presentation

Treating clinicians
Orthodontists: Vincent G. Kokich, DDS, MSD and Vincent O. Kokich, DMD, MSD
Periodontist: David P. Mathews, DDS
Prosthodontist: Rodger A. Lawton, DDS

Clinical Treatment Planning

Age at initial presentation: 41 years
Initial presentation: August 2001
Active treatment completed: June 2005

Introduction and background

This 41-year-old woman was primarily concerned about the appearance of her maxillary anterior teeth. She had porcelain crowns on many of her teeth, most of which had been in place for over a decade. She had seen a periodontist 3 years prior, who had recommended a comprehensive approach to solving her problems. However, she had been postponing her treatment for financial reasons. Her financial situation improved, and at the time of initial presentation she had sufficient funds to pursue a comprehensive treatment plan. She had been a smoker in the past but had not smoked for 10 years.

Medical history

- Noncontributory

Diagnostic findings

Extraoral and facial findings

- Reasonable facial profile
- Maxillary midline deviated to the left
- Canting of the maxillary incisal plane
- 3-mm gingival display on smiling

TMJ and mandibular range of motion

- No joint sounds
- No history of locking or limited range of motion
- No history of muscle pain

Dental cast analysis

- Angle Class II molar and canine relationships
- Maxillary midline deviated 3 mm to the left

Intraoral findings

- Missing teeth nos. 3, 10, 19, and 30; spaces have closed
- Previous extensive restoration of most teeth
- Patient unhappy with the esthetics of the existing anterior crowns
- Gingival inflammation in many areas

Radiographic findings

- Moderate periodontal bone loss around maxillary anterior teeth
- Short maxillary incisor roots
- Acceptable bone support in the maxillary and mandibular posterior areas
- Extensive restoration of most teeth
- Endodontic therapy previously performed on nine teeth, with large endodontic posts in both maxillary central incisor root canals
- Periapical lesions around root apices of teeth nos. 7 and 25

Cephalometric analysis

- Class I skeletal pattern
- Slightly convex facial profile
- Normal facial proportions
- Maxillary incisal edges positioned 2 mm below upper lip

Summary of concerns

1. When the restorative dentist removes the crowns from the maxillary anterior teeth, will there be any tooth structure left to restore?
2. With the previous root canal therapy and short roots of the maxillary incisors, will these teeth provide good support for new porcelain crowns?
3. If implants are chosen to replace the maxillary incisors, how should the bone level be enhanced to support implants and facilitate excellent esthetics?
4. Should the maxillary midline deviation be corrected, and if so, how?
5. Should space be opened for an implant at site no. 10?
6. Should orthognathic surgery be employed in the maxilla to eliminate the "gummy smile" and correct the canted incisal plane?
7. Will the patient require orthognathic surgery or tooth extraction to correct the Angle Class II molar and canine relationships?
8. Can tooth no. 25 be salvaged with further endodontic therapy, or would it be better to extract this tooth (and if so, when)?

PRETREATMENT

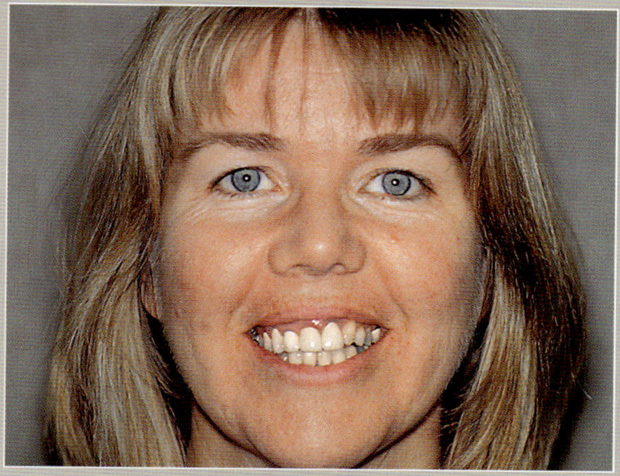
Facial view of smile.

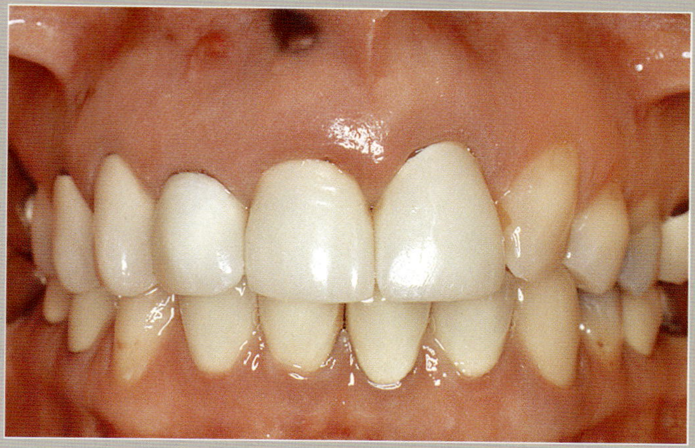
Intraoral frontal view.

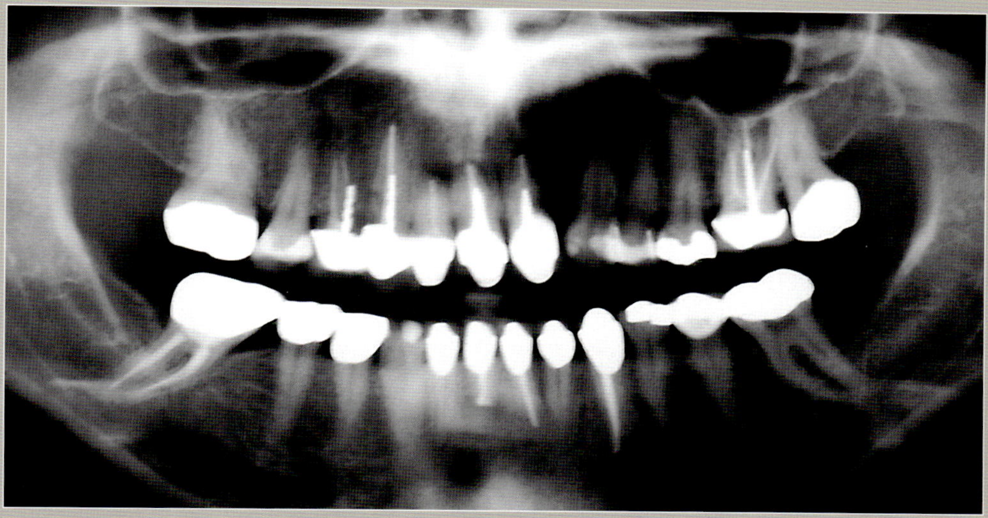
Pretreatment panoramic radiograph, August 2001.

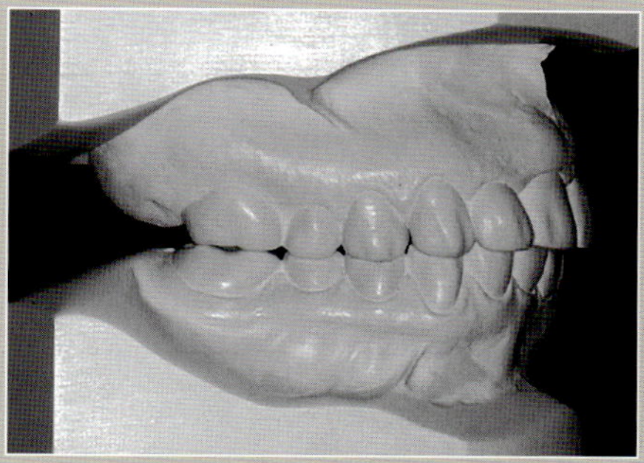
Right lateral occlusion.

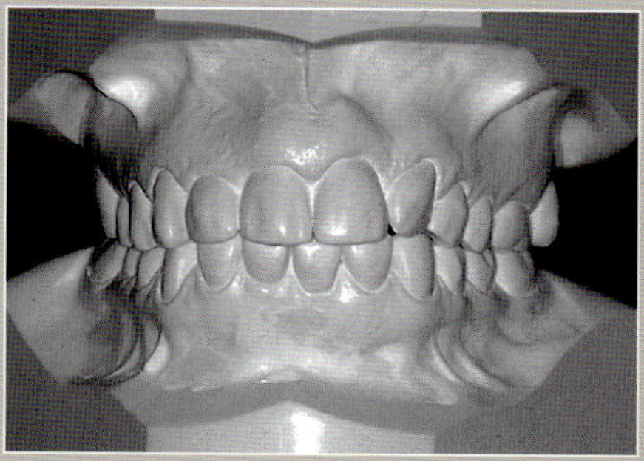
Frontal occlusion.

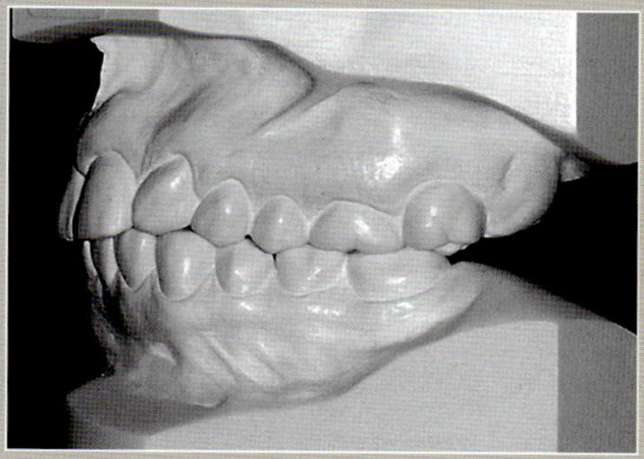
Left lateral occlusion.

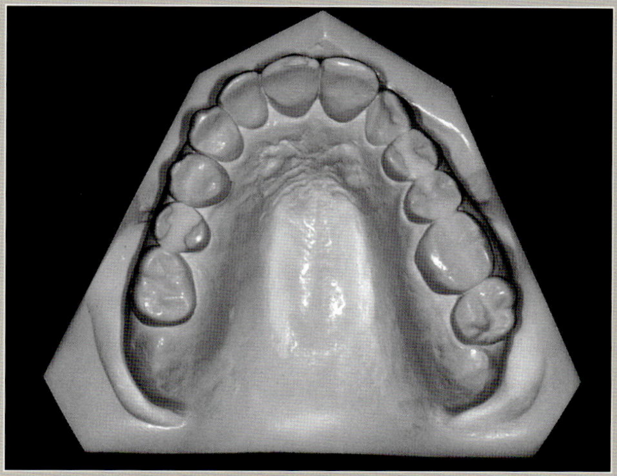
Maxillary occlusal view.

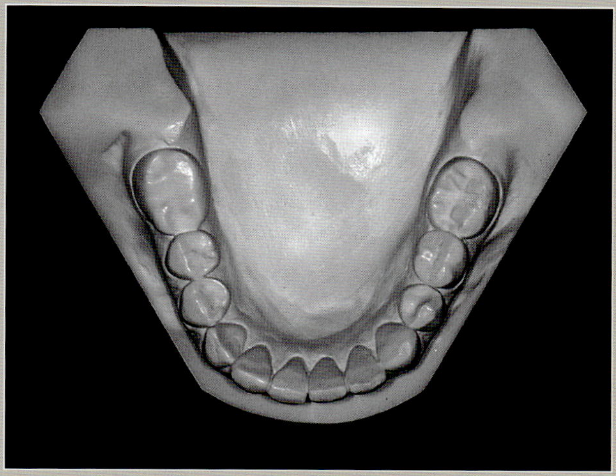
Mandibular occlusal view.

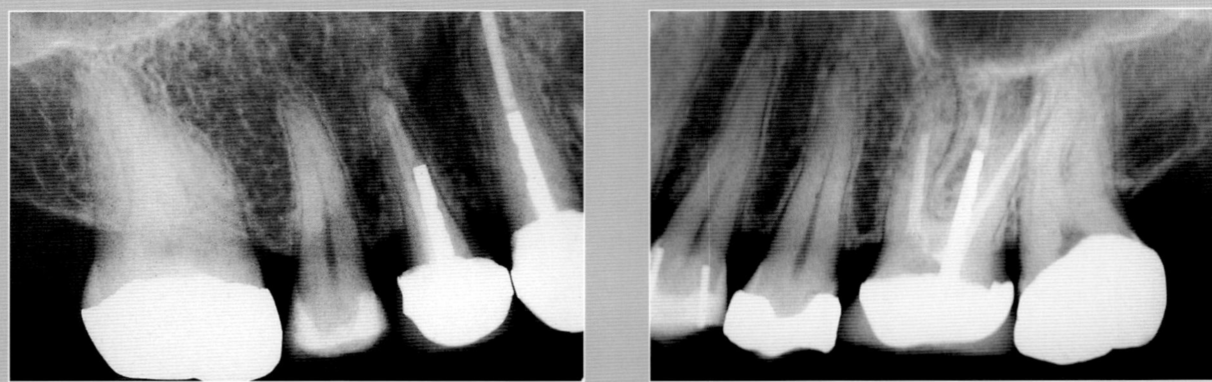

Radiographs of the maxillary posterior regions.

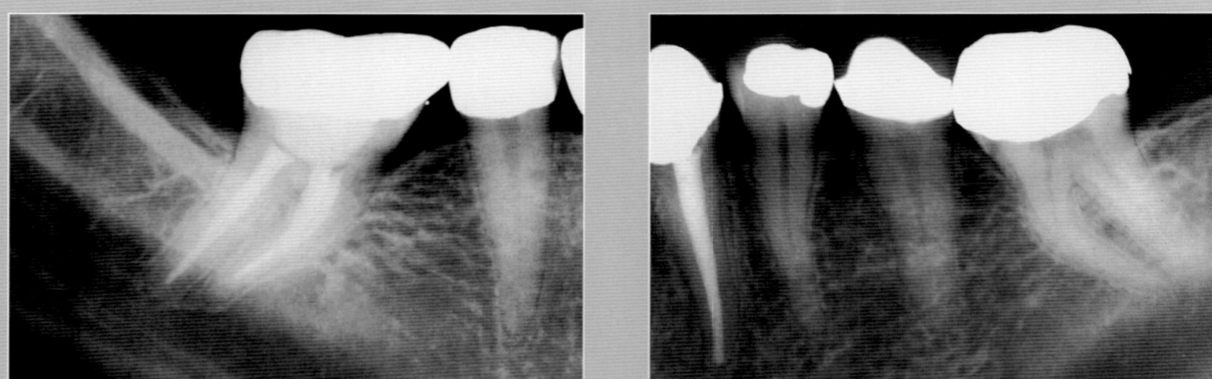

Radiographs of the mandibular posterior regions.

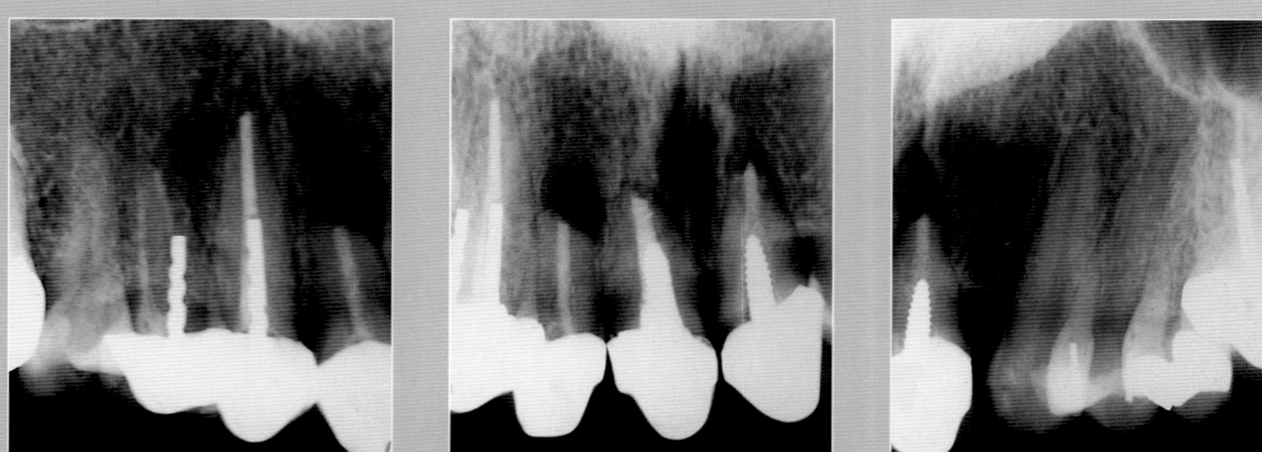

Radiographs of the maxillary anterior region.

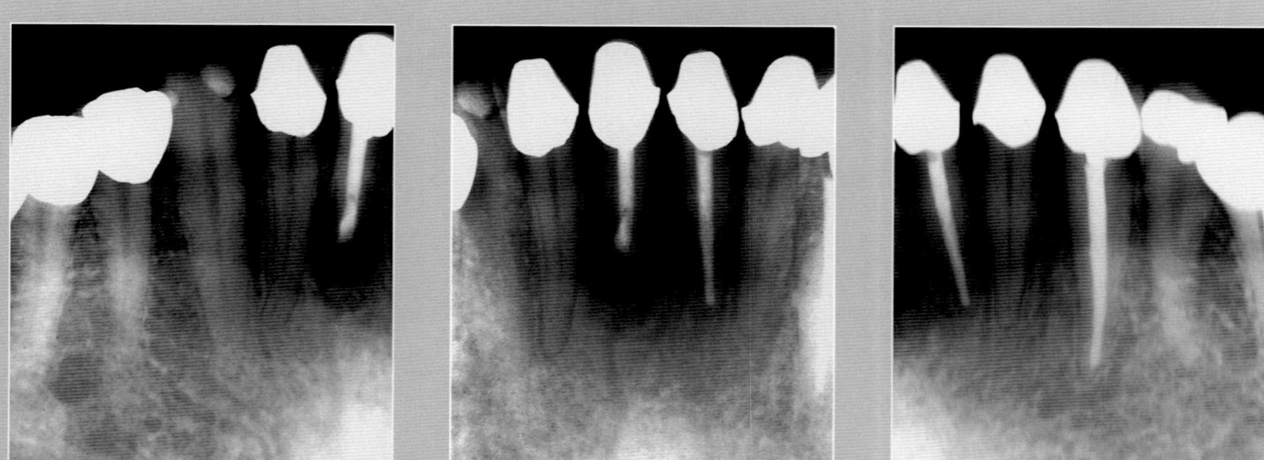

Radiographs of the mandibular anterior region.

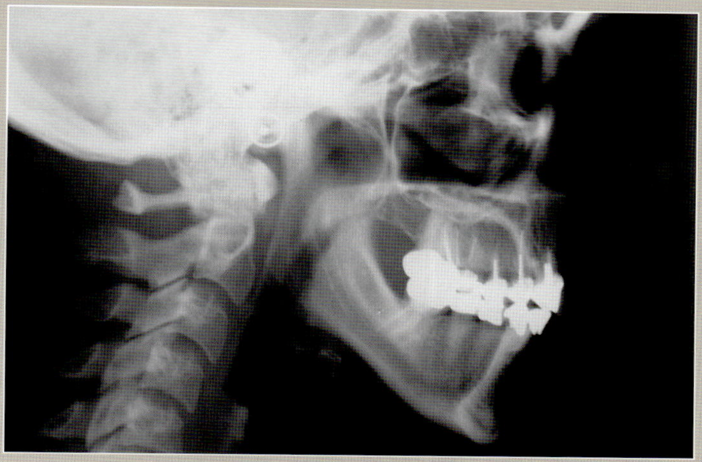

Lateral cephalometric radiograph.

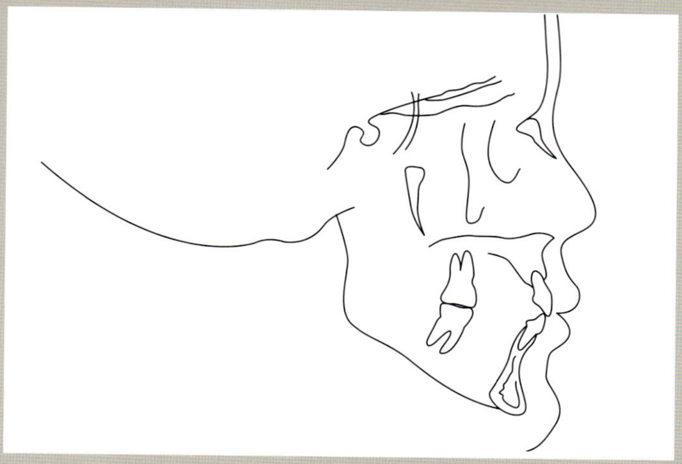

Lateral cephalometric tracing.

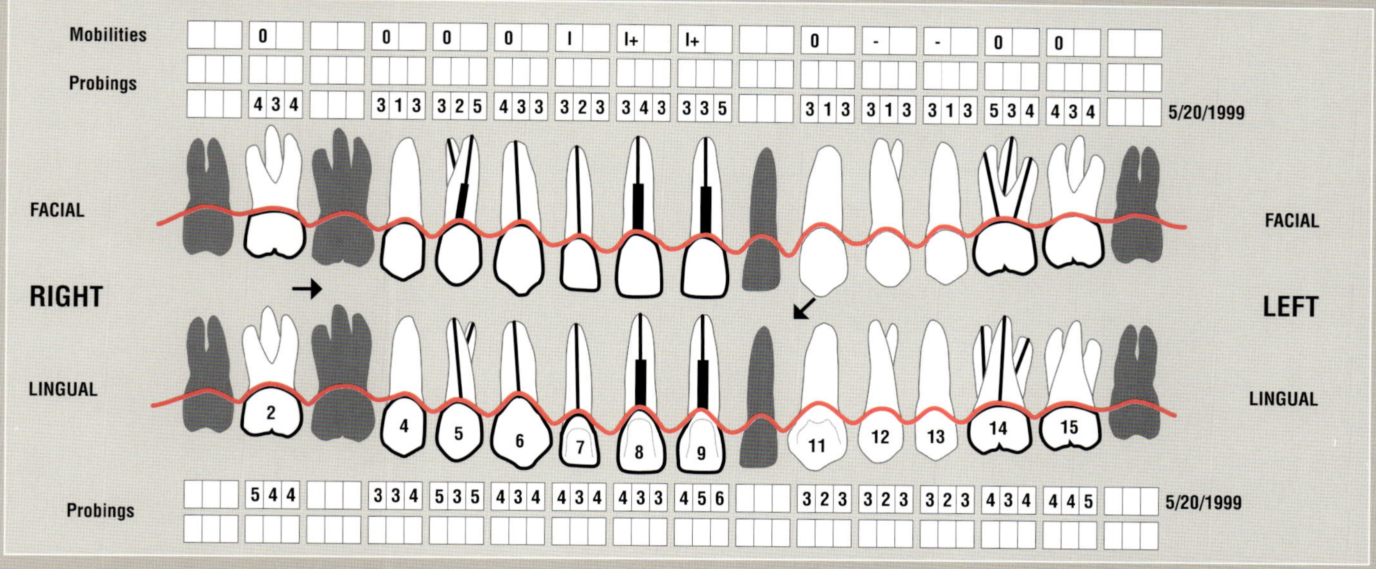

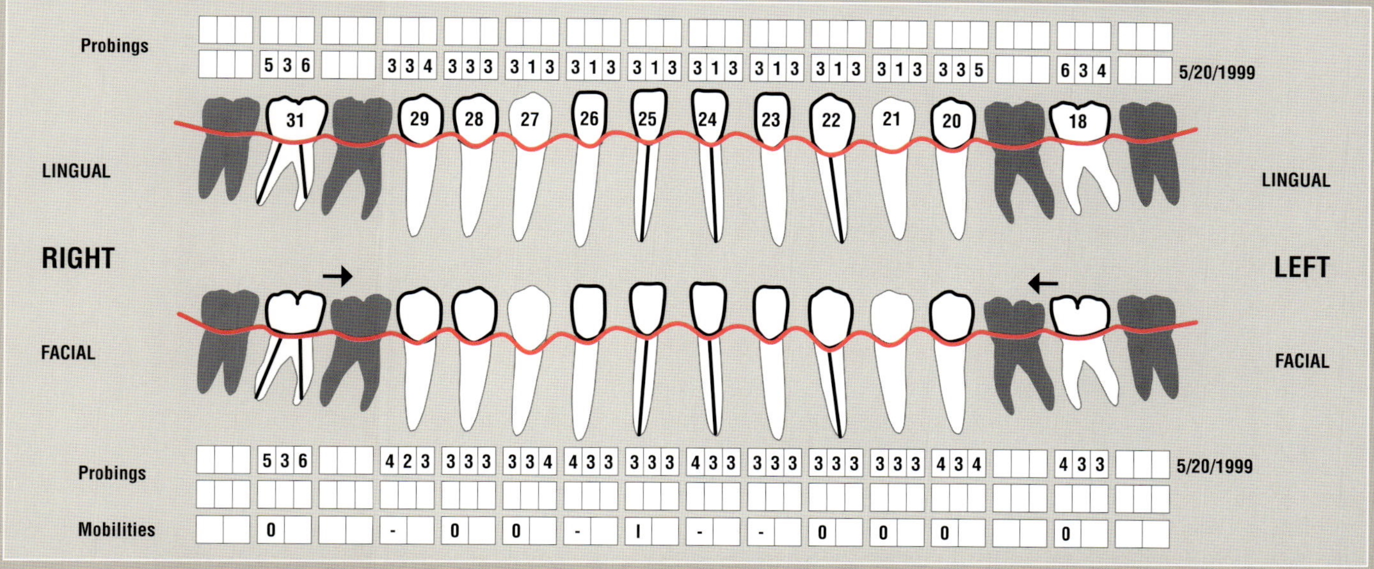

As a learning exercise, you may now outline goals/objectives of treatment and a treatment plan.

Proposed Treatment Plan

Goals/objectives of treatment

The key to achieving this patient's goals is to establish realistic treatment objectives. Once realistic objectives have been established, the alternatives for treatment can be explored.

- How should the midline deviation be addressed? Is there evidence in the literature that a 3-mm midline deviation would be regarded as unattractive by the lay public? Previous studies have shown that the midline deviation would not be an esthetic compromise, so we chose not to correct that problem.
- Should a space be opened for a maxillary lateral incisor implant? Because the midline would not be corrected, and because orthodontics could level the gingival margins, it was decided to leave the canine in the lateral incisor position and restore it as a lateral incisor.
- Does the patient need orthognathic surgery to correct her gummy smile? Orthognathic surgery is contraindicated because the patient shows 2 mm of her incisal edges at rest, which is normal for her age. Maxillary impaction surgery would overly intrude her incisors and eliminate any incisal display at rest.
- Does the posterior occlusion need to be corrected to an Angle Class I relationship? She has no TMJ problems, she is not a bruxer, and she has little evidence of tooth wear. There is nothing in the literature to suggest that altering her posterior occlusion will be of any significance to the outcome of her treatment.

Based on an assessment of the evidence, our team engaged in realistic treatment planning that addressed only those problems that required correction to achieve the patient's goals. Therefore, the objectives were to:

- Level the gingival margins with orthodontics
- Level the maxillary incisal plane with restorations
- Improve the maxillary anterior bone levels for implants with controlled orthodontic extrusion/extraction of the incisors
- Place maxillary implants to restore anterior esthetics
- Replace all existing restorations to harmonize the esthetic result

Phase I: Initial therapy

1. Interdisciplinary team meeting between the orthodontists, periodontist, endodontist, and restorative dentist
2. Construction of diagnostic wax-up to create the vision of the result
3. Patient consultations with all four practitioners
4. Root planing and scaling prior to orthodontics
5. Replacement of maxillary incisor crowns with acrylic provisional restorations
6. Evaluation of existing endodontically treated teeth

Phase II: Orthodontic therapy

7. Bracket placement on maxillary and mandibular teeth
8. Extrusion of maxillary incisors 5 mm to develop more ideal bone heights and sites for dental implant placement

Phase III: Incisor extraction and implant placement

9. Extraction of teeth nos. 7 to 9
10. Immediate placement of implants in sites nos. 8 and 9
11. Placement of three acrylic teeth on maxillary archwire

Phase IV: Completion of orthodontics

12. Orthodontic detailing as implants integrate
13. After bracket removal, placement of provisional restorations
14. Decision regarding whether to maintain or replace tooth no. 25

Phase V: Definitive restorations

15. One year after orthodontic treatment, porcelain crown placement on all teeth
16. Placement of heat-processed nightguard on maxillary teeth
17. Routine periodontal maintenance every 3 to 6 months

Active Clinical Treatment

Review of the goals/objectives of treatment

- Level the gingival margins with orthodontics
- Even out the maxillary incisal plane with restorations
- Alter the maxillary anterior bone levels for the placement of implants with controlled orthodontic extrusion/extraction of the incisors
- Use maxillary implants to replace missing teeth and restore anterior esthetics
- Replace all existing restorations to enhance and harmonize the final esthetic result

Phase I: Initial therapy

Initially, the team (prosthodontist, periodontist, endodontist, and orthodontists) met to identify the problems and determine realistic objectives for treatment. We collectively decided to leave the midline deviation and not to correct the Class II posterior occlusion because neither was causing any problems, nor would either interfere with the successful esthetic reconstruction of this case. Our primary objectives centered on the controlled orthodontic extrusion and extraction of the remaining maxillary incisors to help develop more ideal vertical bone levels in the maxillary incisor region for implant placement. The plan also included extruding tooth no. 11 to help level the gingival margin of that tooth, which would eventually be restored as a lateral incisor.

Phase II: Orthodontic therapy

A round archwire was used to extrude teeth nos. 7 to 9. During the extrusion process, the incisal edges of the provisional crowns were reduced in proportion to the amount of extrusion that was being accomplished. The endodontist confirmed the adequacy of all previous root canal therapy except for that performed at tooth no. 25. It was decided to extract this tooth after orthodontics and replace it with a pontic as part of a three-unit fixed partial denture.

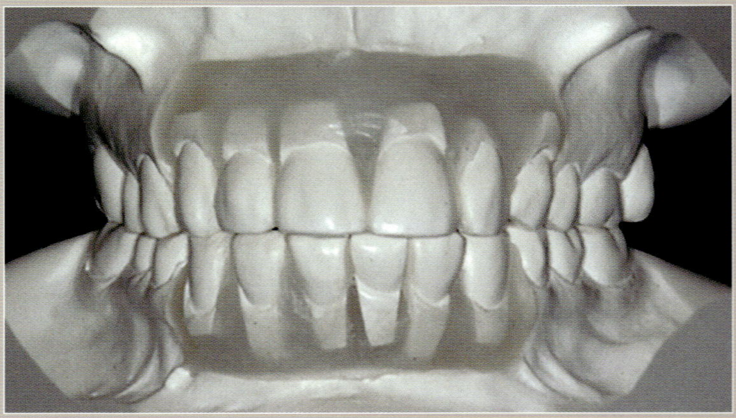

Frontal view of diagnostic wax-up.

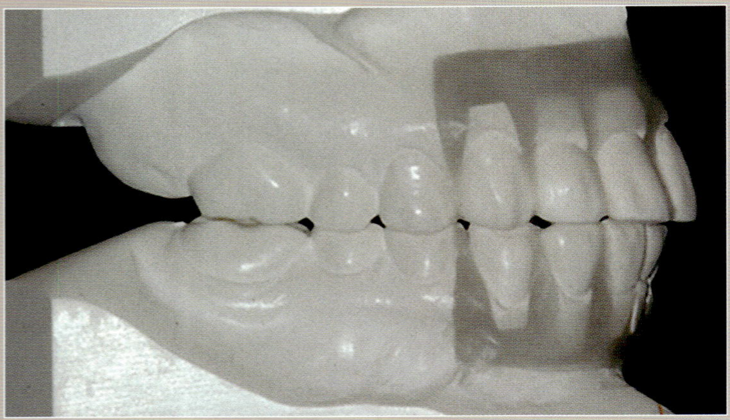

Right lateral view of diagnostic wax-up.

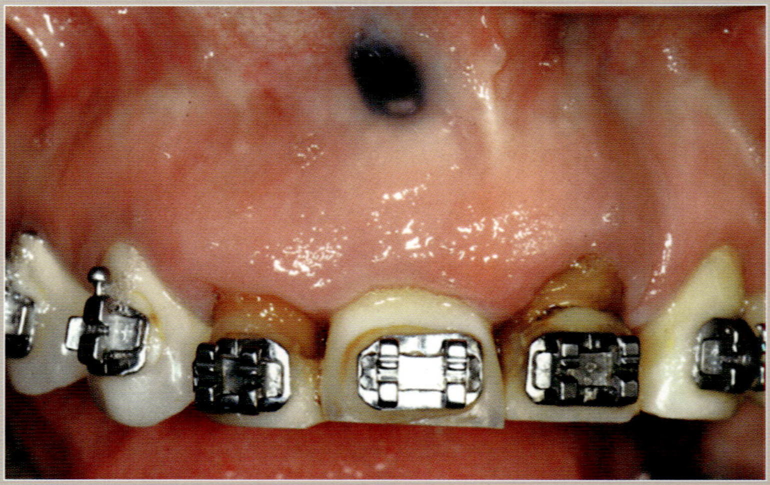

Orthodontic extrusion of maxillary incisors.

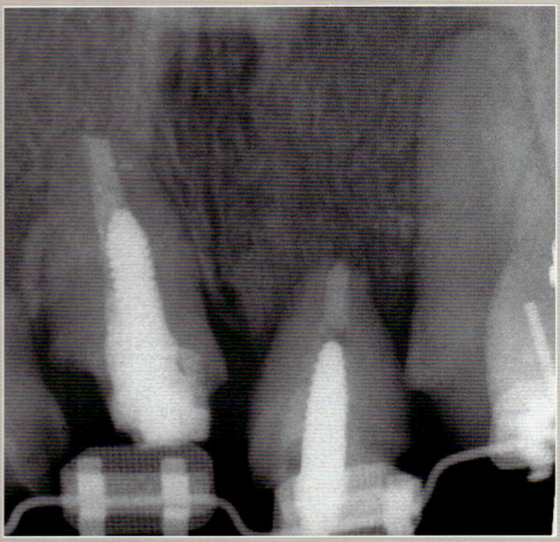

Radiographic view of orthodontically extruded maxillary incisors.

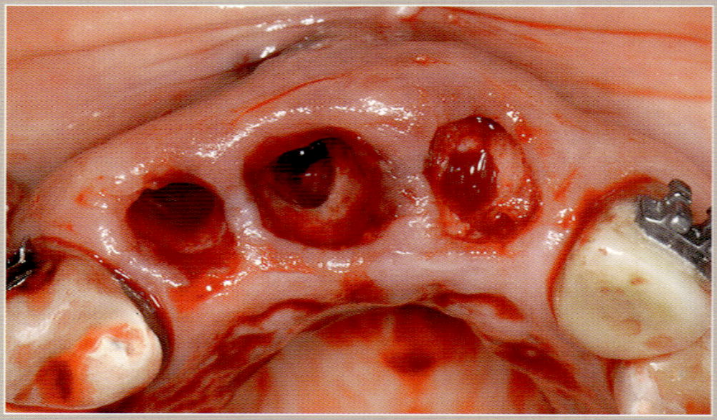

Occlusal view following extraction of teeth nos. 7 to 9.

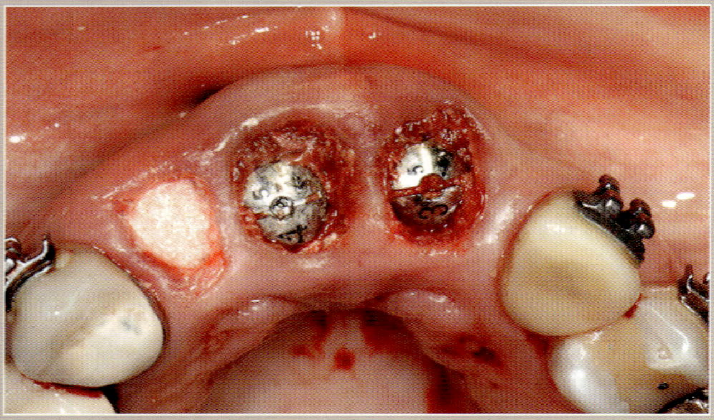

Occlusal view following immediate implant placement in sites nos. 8 and 9 and placement of freeze-dried cadaver bone in site no. 7.

Phase III: Incisor extraction and implant placement

When teeth nos. 7 through 9 had been extruded 5 mm, periapical radiographs were taken to determine the bony response. The periodontist decided that this was the right time to extract these teeth. An impression was made of the maxillary arch prior to extraction so that the laboratory could construct an acrylic segment of three teeth that could be placed on the archwire after extraction to replace the missing teeth.

Following extraction of the incisors, two implants were immediately placed in the sockets of teeth nos. 8 and 9, and the socket of tooth no. 7 was filled with freeze-dried cadaver bone to preserve the height of bone for a future pontic site. The archwire was replaced, and the segment of teeth helped to maintain the space while the implants were integrating.

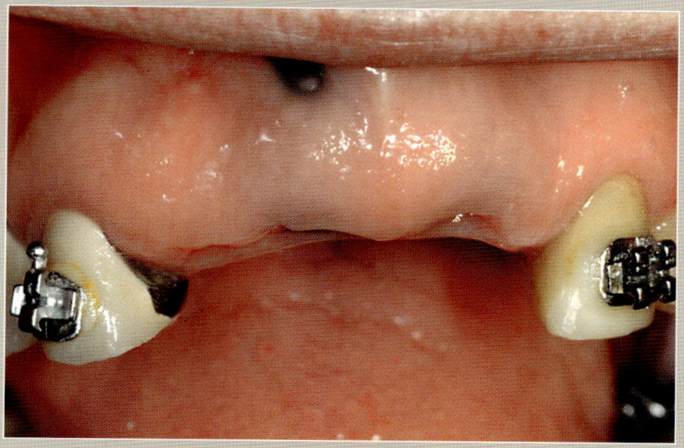

Frontal view following extraction and implant placement.

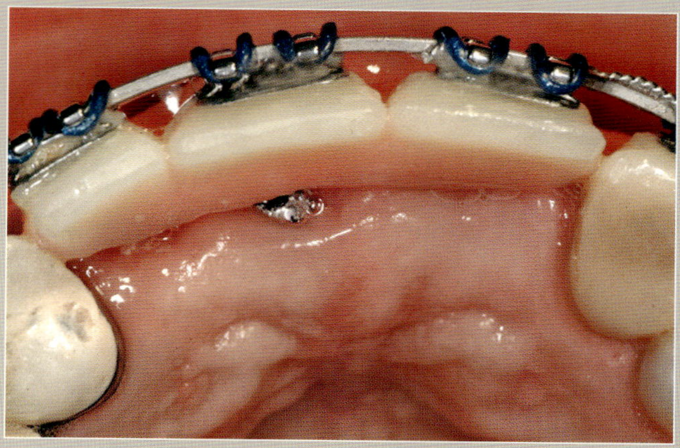

Occlusal view of artificial teeth on archwire.

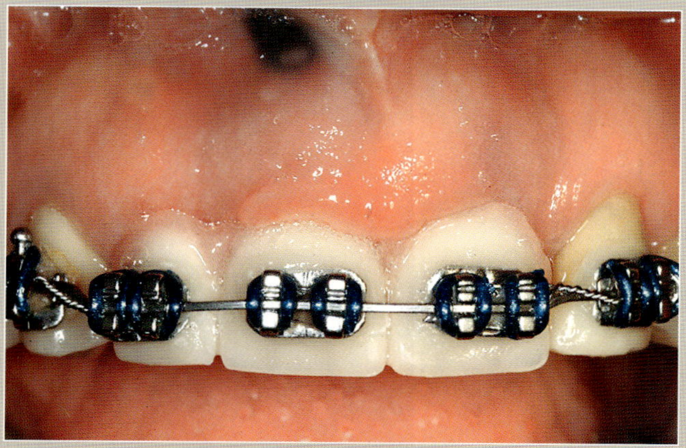

Frontal view of artificial teeth on archwire.

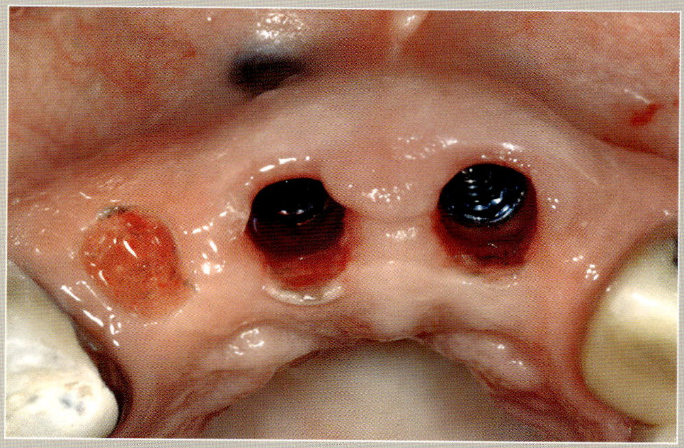

Occlusal view at completion of orthodontics and implant integration.

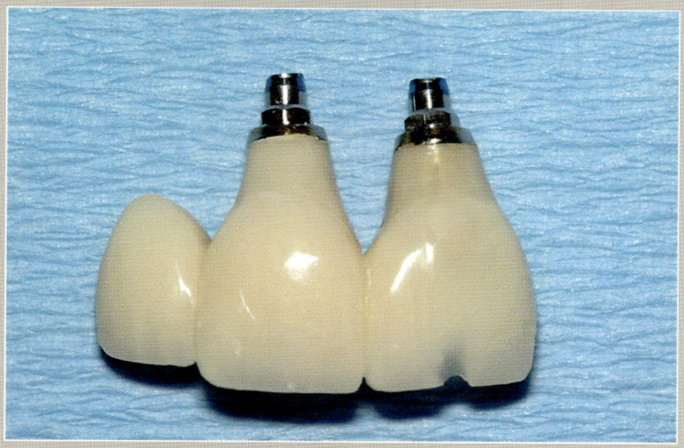

Provisional restorations.

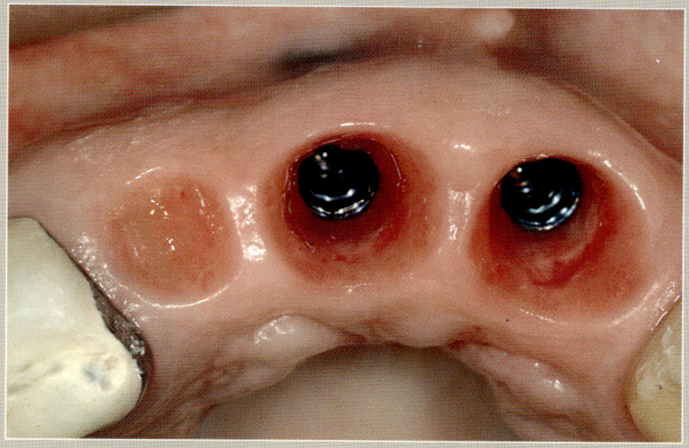

Occlusal view following tissue conditioning.

Phase IV: Completion of orthodontics

Four months after implant placement, the orthodontic appliances were removed, and the prosthodontist and periodontist began developing the tissue form around the central incisor implants using provisional restorations.

Posttreatment

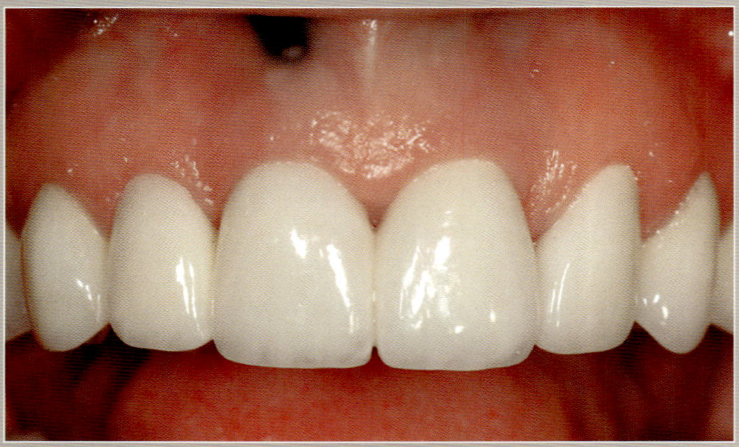

Frontal view of definitive restorations.

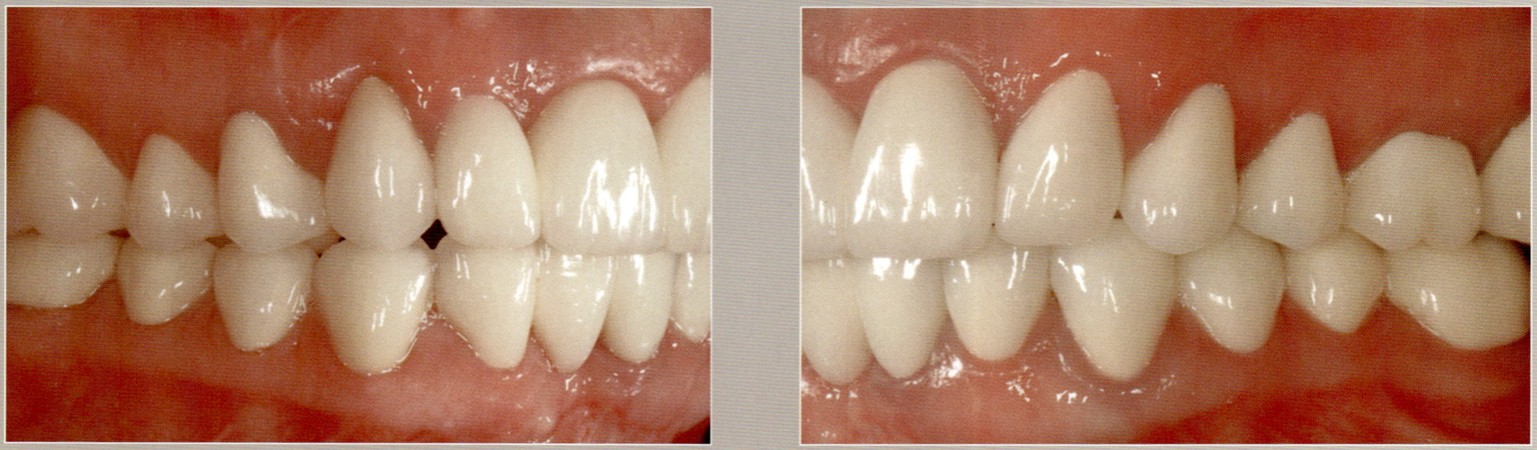

Lateral views of definitive restorations.

Phase V: Definitive restorations

Definitive restorations were placed on all teeth. The implant crowns at sites nos. 8 and 9 were splinted with a cantilevered pontic at site no. 7. Tooth no. 11 was restored as a lateral incisor. All existing crowns were replaced, and tooth no. 25 was extracted and replaced with a pontic on a three-unit fixed partial denture (teeth nos. 24 to 26).

Phase VI: Follow-up

The radiographs and intraoral photographs taken 3 years after restoration show that the tissue and bone levels achieved with controlled orthodontic extrusion have been maintained without resorption or apical migration of the gingival margins. The periodontist performed crown lengthening on tooth no. 12 to make it look more like a canine. The patient was pleased with the esthetic result, and her periodontal health has improved significantly.

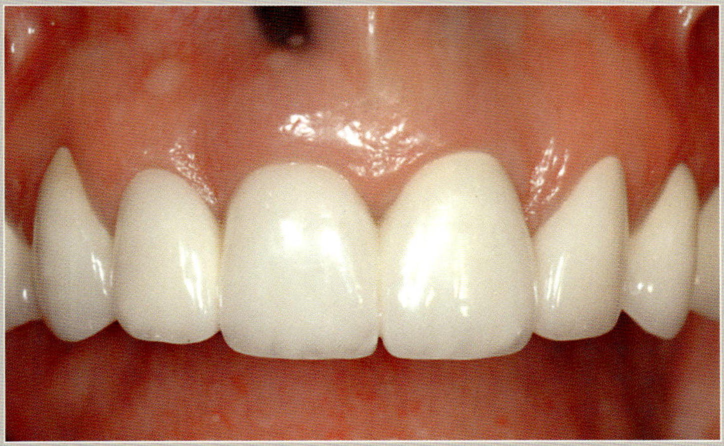

Frontal view 3 years after restoration.

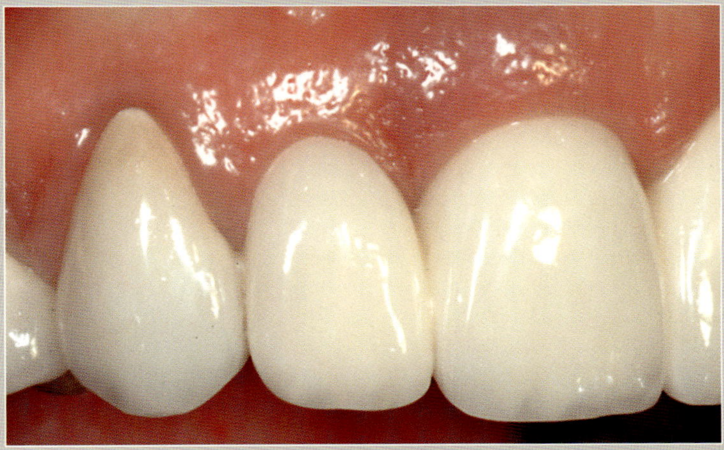

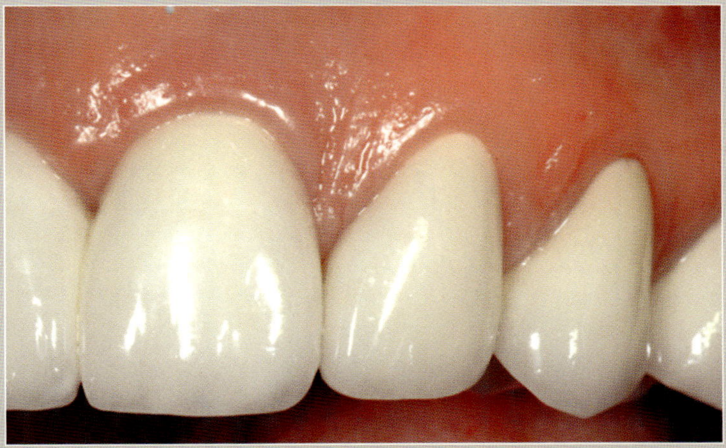

Lateral anterior views 3 years after restoration.

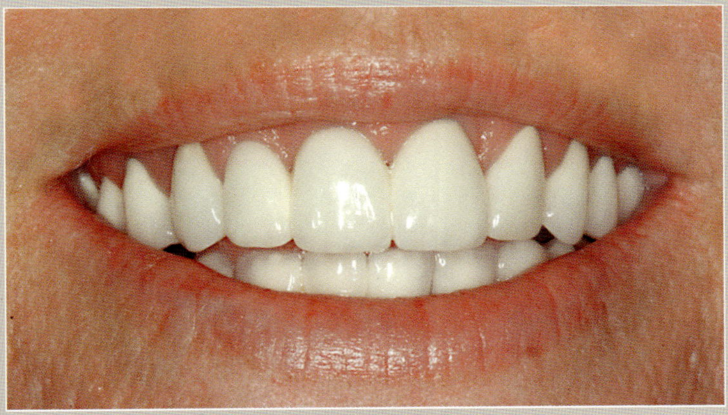

Smile 3 years after restoration.

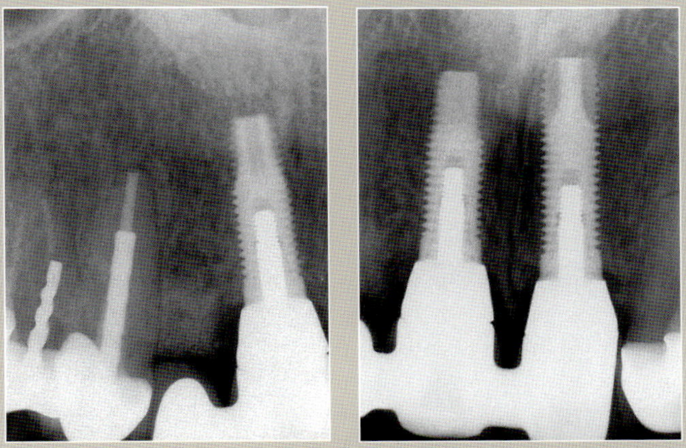

Radiographs of the anterior maxillary region 3 years after restoration.

You may now place the corresponding posttreatment overlay found in the separate folder over the pretreatment periodontal chart on page 75.

Commentary

This section further elucidates the thought processes and steps that combined to make this treatment plan successful.

Problems left untreated

There were three major pretreatment problems that we chose not to address: the midline deviation, the gummy smile, and the posterior Class II malocclusion.

Midline deviation

Several studies have surveyed dentists and laypersons to ascertain whether a midline deviation is perceived as unattractive.[1-3] The results of these studies show that a 3-mm midline discrepancy is not regarded as unattractive by either dentists or laypersons. The most important factor is not the midline deviation but the orientation of the interproximal contact between the central incisors relative to the occlusal plane and to the long axis of the patient's face. When the interproximal contact is oriented perpendicular to the occlusal plane and parallel to a patient's facial long axis, then the midline deviation is not apparent to lay observers. However, when the orientation of the contact is deviated to the right or left relative to the occlusal plane and facial long axis, it is readily perceived as unattractive. Therefore, it was important for the prosthodontist to make certain that the interproximal contact between the two central incisor implants was oriented perpendicular to the occlusal plane and parallel to the long axis of the patient's face, but the midline deviation did not need to be corrected.

Gummy smile

We chose not to correct the patient's gummy smile by either intruding the maxillary teeth orthodontically or performing orthognathic surgery to impact the maxilla because it was not caused by maxillary alveolar vertical excess. The key diagnostic feature that verifies this conclusion is the distance from the patient's incisal edge to her lip at rest prior to treatment. That distance was 2 mm. This was ideal for her age. Therefore, her gummy smile was due to a hyperfunctional or hypermobile lip. A solution for this problem would be to inject the elevator muscles of the upper lip with botulinum toxin type A (Botox, Allergan) to prevent the lip from moving excessively. Recent clinical studies[4,5] in the surgical and orthodontic literature have shown successful, albeit temporary, amelioration of gummy smiles using this technique.

Posterior Class II malocclusion

The third pretreatment problem that we did not correct was the Angle Class II malocclusion. Typically, orthodontists would attempt to fix this problem in an adult either through tooth extraction or orthognathic surgery. However, this patient had no TMJ symptoms, nor did she have a bruxing habit. In other words, this patient had lived with her existing malocclusion for more than 25 years without any detrimental effects on her TMJ health. Therefore, there was no reason to change her posterior occlusion. There is extensive evidence in the literature that shows that a posterior Class II malocclusion has no correlation with temporomandibular disorders.[6,7]

Controlled orthodontic extrusion

Probably the most remarkable accomplishment in this case was the creation of 5 mm of vertical bone and tissue height through orthodontic extrusion of the maxillary incisors. Controlled orthodontic extrusion is a useful tool in implant site development, but it is not always indicated or successful. There are four criteria that we evaluate to determine whether the patient would be a good candidate for controlled extrusion. The first is the need to move the gingival margins of the maxillary anterior teeth coronally. In this patient, the gingival margins of the maxillary left central incisor and left canine definitely needed to be moved coronally in order to make them appear harmonious with the contralateral teeth. The second criterion is the necessity of moving the crestal bone level coronally, which also applied to this patient.

The third criterion, which is often overlooked but is perhaps the most important for predictable success, is the vertical orientation of the teeth to be extruded. When the central incisors are perpendicular to the maxillary occlusal plane, the extrusive movement of the teeth will be oriented vertically, and the expansion of the alveolar crestal bone will follow the teeth. This was true for our patient, and that is why the bony response to extrusion was so successful. However, if her crowns were proclined labially, the teeth would have been extruded labially and away from the alveolus. In this situation, the alveolar bone labial to the root tends to dehisce and not follow the teeth.

The fourth and final criterion to evaluate when contemplating controlled extrusion for implant site development is good periapical health of the teeth. Radiographs should be taken to check for periapical radiolucencies indicating active infection in the area. When an inflammatory process is occurring, the bone will not follow the teeth as they are extruding because the intervening inflammatory process prevents the periodontal ligament from stretching and stimulating bone formation. In our patient, the maxillary right lateral incisor had a periapical inflammatory lesion. Therefore, we did not expect a favorable bony response in this area. In fact, that is why we decided to place the implants in the central incisor sites with a cantilevered right lateral incisor pontic rather than place the implants in the right lateral and left central incisor sites with the pontic at the right central incisor site.

Another key to successful implant site development when extruding hopeless teeth is the speed of extrusion. We prefer slow to fast extrusion because when teeth are extruded rapidly, a red margin appears around the extruded tooth, signaling the eversion of the nonkeratinized sulcular epithelium. The problem with this is not the lack of keratinization; it is the loss of the sulcus. When the sulcus is eliminated, the stretching of the periodontal ligament at the alveolar crest proceeds at such a rapid pace that the deposition of crestal bone becomes jeopardized. As a result, the labial plate of bone, which is critical in an anterior implant case, is difficult to maintain. This will result in a less-than-ideal esthetic gingival margin position in the definitive restoration. We prefer to extrude the teeth slowly, approximately 0.5 mm per month. In this case, it took 10 months to extrude the incisors 5 mm. This rate of extrusion gave the alveolar crestal bone an opportunity to keep up with the extruding teeth. In order to determine whether the tooth is being extruded too rapidly, the orthodontist should probe the sulcus at every appointment. As long as a probeable sulcus is maintained, then the tooth is most likely being extruded at an appropriate rate.

Canine substitution for lateral incisor

For this patient, we chose to leave the maxillary left canine in the lateral incisor position. Some clinicians would criticize this decision for several reasons. First, the canine does not look like a lateral incisor because of its length and shape. Although this is true, in this case the left canine was extruded and equilibrated in order to relocate the gingival margin coronally and create a shorter tooth that could be crowned and closely simulate a lateral incisor. Another reason canines are not substituted for lateral incisors is that it leaves the patient without a canine-protected occlusion on the affected side. Although this objection seems reasonable, there are several studies that have shown that there are no untoward occlusal or temporomandibular consequences of leaving a canine in the lateral incisor position.[8–10]

Summary

This patient presented with a challenging set of pretreatment problems. The key to successful management of this case was being able to focus on realistic treatment objectives that corrected the most important problems while not addressing the problems that, according to evidence-based analysis, did not affect the comprehensive management of this patient.

References

1. Kokich VO, Kiyak HA, Shapiro PA. Comparing the perception of dentists and lay people to altered dental esthetics. J Esthet Dent 1999;11:311–324.
2. Kokich VO, Kokich VG, Kiyak HA. Perceptions of dental professionals and laypersons to altered dental esthetics: Asymmetric and symmetric situations. Am J Orthod Dentofacial Orthop 2006;13:141–151.
3. Ker AJ, Chan R, Fields HW, Beck M, Rosenstiel S. Esthetics and smile characteristics from the layperson's perspective: A computer-based survey study. J Am Dent Assoc 2008;139:1318–1327.
4. Polo M. Botulinum toxin type A in the treatment of excessive gingival display. Am J Orthod Dentofacial Orthop 2005;127:214–218.
5. Polo M. Botulinum toxin type A (Botox) for the neuromuscular correction of excessive gingival display on smiling (gummy smile). Am J Orthod Dentofacial Orthop 2008;133:195–203.
6. Gesch D, Bernhardt O, Kocher T, John U, Hensel E, Alte D. Association of malocclusion and functional occlusion with signs of temporomandibular disorders in adults. Angle Orthod 2004;74:512–520.
7. Gesch D, Bernhardt O, Mack F, John U, Kocher T, Alte D. Association of malocclusion and functional occlusion with subjective symptoms of TMD in adults. Angle Orthod 2005;75:183–190.
8. Nordquist GG, McNeill RW. Orthodontic versus restorative treatment of the congenitally absent lateral incisor—Long-term periodontal and occlusal evaluation. J Periodontol 1975;46:139–143.
9. Zachrisson BU. Improving the esthetic outcome of canine substitution for missing maxillary lateral incisors. World J Orthod 2007;8:72–79.
10. Rosa M, Zachrisson BU. Integrating space closure and esthetic dentistry in patients with missing maxillary lateral incisors. J Clin Orthod 2007;41:563–573.

4

The Papilla Between Adjacent Implants: Treatment Planning to Optimize Esthetic Outcomes

Sonia S. Leziy, DDS
Brahm A. Miller, DDS

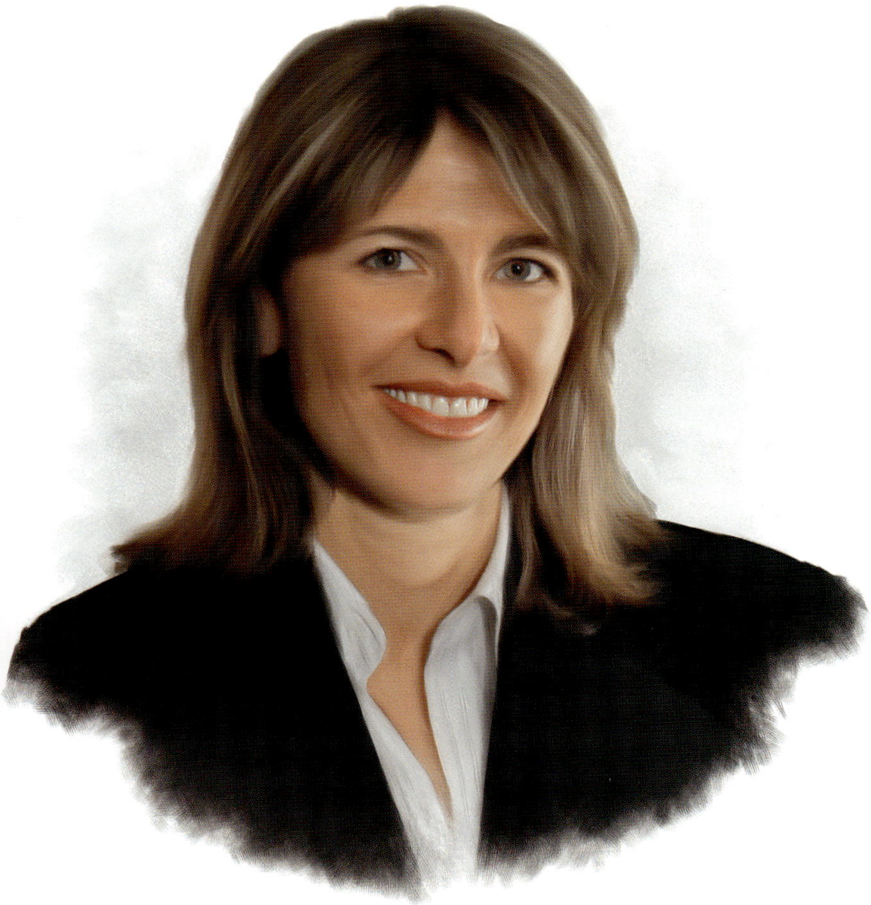

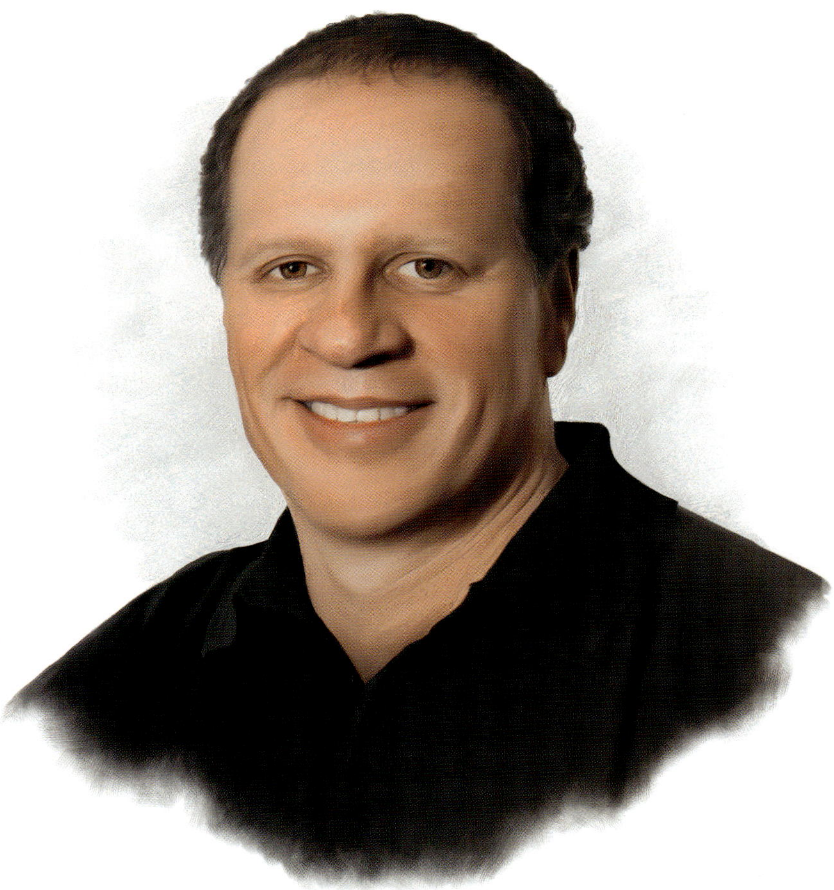

What initially may seem to be an "easy" or straightforward case is rarely so when it comes to the esthetic zone.

Philosophy and Background

We are excited to have the opportunity to participate in this second venture into interdisciplinary treatment planning. In the chapter we contributed to the first volume of *Interdisciplinary Treatment Planning,*[1] we presented an overview ("blueprint") of our treatment-planning process and considerations related to implant treatment in the esthetic zone. We concluded with a case presentation that explored the challenges of adjacent implants and the treatment plan that we ultimately pursued. In the interim, we have continued to seek better solutions to this common esthetic challenge through our ongoing education, reading, and daily clinical practices, culminating in the development of a format for categorizing and treating patients requiring adjacent implants, particularly in the maxillary anterior region. This has been our quest: to help our patients achieve the most natural, esthetic appearance possible at the end of treatment.

What initially may seem to be an "easy" or straightforward case is rarely so when it comes to the esthetic zone. With this in mind, we have selected an esthetically challenging case that will explore and illustrate our treatment-planning process and protocol for managing the challenges of adjacent tooth replacement with implants. Diverging slightly from the format of most of the other chapters in this book, we compare the outcome of our principle case to three similar cases treated in our clinic by different approaches in order to highlight our views on the difficulty of controlling tissue around teeth and implants and especially between implants. This is particularly enlightening because it demonstrates that although individual cases present with their own unique set of circumstances, it is possible to classify adjacent implant cases and effectively treat our patients by following one of these four treatment approaches.

Implant treatment in the esthetic region presents unusual challenges that often do not have to be considered as acutely in the treatment of posterior teeth simply because patients can see everything in the front of their mouths and less in the back. Osseointegration itself is no longer the primary focus of treatment given the high implant and prosthesis survival and success rates clearly documented in the literature; however, with long-term follow-up, the high incidence of biologic and technical complications has become apparent.[2,3] Instead, the esthetic outcome of treatment in the anterior dentition has become an issue of intense interest, and controlling soft tissue levels around and between adjacent implants in a highly visible area has become the subject of many clinical reports and trials.[4–11] It is widely accepted that labial gingival tissues over implants are at risk for recession of up to 1 mm following restoration and that papillae between implants are often difficult to maintain or to develop compared with those adjacent to single-implant restorations or natural teeth.[12–18] This issue becomes even more critical and potentially more complex to manage when procedures such as tooth extraction, implant placement, and restoration are performed simultaneously.

Compromised tissue anatomy around adjacent implant restorations is common, and the etiology, which is often multifactorial, may include any one or a combination of the following causes:

- *Anatomical or ridge deficiencies that exist before tooth removal or that occur as a result of tooth extraction.* The loss of multiple and adjacent teeth will typically result in reduced ridge height and ridge width with a corresponding loss of the physiologic soft tissue form that is far more significant than that seen with single-tooth extraction cases.[19–21]
- *Potential space restrictions along with flawed treatment planning, which can result in implant placement with inadequate tooth-implant and interimplant spacing and negatively affect papilla architecture.* Problems or errors in three-dimensional implant positioning generally result in some degree of bone remodeling that impacts the soft tissue outcome.[8,22–25]

- *Crestal bone remodeling around implants (ie, bone saucerization), which typically occurs around conventional two-piece implant and abutment designs.* The relatively constant relationship between bone anatomy and soft tissue form must be considered when adjacent implants are being planned. Increasingly, there is support for the positive impact of platform-switched or -shifted implant designs on crestal bone stability and hence their potential to improve soft tissue outcomes[26-28] and to reduce the number of disruptions at the implant-abutment junction associated with implant restoration.[29,30]
- *The association between thin tissue and compromised implant esthetics and gingival health.* Although such an association is weakly documented at this time, some literature suggests that thin peri-implant tissues are more prone to gingival recession and poor transmucosal tissue color following restoration, affecting soft tissue esthetics.[31-33]

To begin, we explore a typical clinical situation that involves rehabilitation of a failed maxillary anterior partial denture (maxillary right central incisor to canine) that involves the loss of one of the abutments (maxillary right central incisor). The scenario of missing adjacent central and lateral incisors represents one of the most significant esthetic challenges that we face and has its own unique problems, including space concerns, asymmetry resulting in easily discernable esthetic differences from one side of the maxillary anterior area to the other, and the lack of an incisive papilla, which can sometimes give the illusion of a papilla form as seen between the central incisors or restorations spanning this area. Achieving ideal soft tissue outcomes is rarely achievable unless unique preoperative clinical parameters support effective outcomes, as illustrated in a previously published case report in which we used a scalloped implant design coupled with specific surgical and restorative protocols.[34] In this chapter, our selected approach and treatment outcome is contrasted with three other anterior cases requiring different treatment plans. The rationale for considering various approaches is reviewed, and the esthetic outcomes in terms of soft tissue esthetics are critiqued.

In the Commentary section at the end of the Active Clinical Treatment, we present our views on the merits and limitations of each approach. Our principle case exemplifies the challenges of implant placement in a site that requires management of an anatomically deficient ridge for esthetic reasons. The rationale for the selected surgical and restorative protocol is discussed. The results of this case are predictable and exemplify the persistent challenge of regenerating bone in moderate to advanced defects and the considerable impact this has on the esthetic outcome. The subsequent three cases, as noted earlier, emphasize the impact of differing implant placement procedures and the potential effect on bone and soft tissue outcomes. Our goal is to sensitize the reader to the implant placement protocols that can be considered depending on the preoperative clinical findings. Most cases fit into one or more of the four treatment approaches presented; hence, these cases provide guidelines for implant placement strategies and restoration protocols. The first of the cases used for comparison illustrates a less complex scenario in which the preoperative ridge anatomy is initially more favorable. This case was selected to emphasize that the complexity of the treatment is reduced with appropriate implant timing or early intervention relative to extraction, thereby allowing the use of more conservative techniques that may enhance hard and soft tissue stability. The next case illustrates management of two periodontally compromised central incisors with advanced probing depths, treated with extraction and a brief period of healing to alter the local bacterial flora and to improve soft tissue volume, followed by early implant placement. The final case illustrates a less commonly used treatment approach in which staged adjacent implant placement is used in the replacement of adjacent failing teeth. The rationale for sequencing implant placement centers on stabilizing interproximal tissues through progressive treatment. This case is similar to the one presented in our chapter in the first volume of *Interdisciplinary Treatment Planning.*[1]

Case Presentation

Treating clinicians
Periodontist/implant surgeon: Sonia S. Leziy, DDS
Prosthodontist: Brahm A. Miller, DDS

Clinical Treatment Planning

Age at initial presentation: 48 years
Initial presentation: November 2007
Active treatment completed: June 2009

Introduction and background

Our patient's primary concern related to her failing maxillary anterior partial denture (teeth nos. 6 to 8). Her dentist had remade this partial denture approximately 4 years previously. One of the abutment teeth had recently become sore, and her gingiva had become increasingly red and swollen. She was informed that one of the supporting teeth had developed a root fracture.

Based on our discussions with the patient, her treatment expectations were assessed to be reasonable, and she was presented with treatment options to replace this partial denture, bearing in mind the short- and long-term functional and esthetic challenges associated with each solution.

She also commented that she might consider implants in the future to replace her mandibular left missing teeth. Failing implants in the sites nos. 19 and 20 were removed 5 years previously in our clinic because of peri-implantitis. They had been in function for approximately 13 years prior to their removal. Re-treatment was delayed for financial reasons and because of the patient's misgivings related to the success of implant treatment.

The patient was compliant with dental treatment and adhered to a routine recall program and supportive periodontal therapy with her general dentist.

Medical history

- Medication: levothyroxine (Synthroid, Abbott)
- No significant issues limiting potential dental or surgical procedures

Diagnostic findings

Extraoral and facial findings

- No significant extraoral findings

Intraoral findings

Calcitek (Zimmer) endosseous implants were placed in sites nos. 19 and 20 in 1992. The patient was seen for supportive periodontal therapy aimed at controlling the peri-implantitis condition in sites nos. 19 and 20 between 2002 and 2004. The implants ultimately failed and were removed (site no. 20 in 2004 and no. 19 in 2006) using limited surgical access and trephines. The sites healed uneventfully, but the remaining residual ridge anatomy was considered unfavorable for implant replacement without ridge augmentation procedures.

Other findings included:

- High lip line and dynamics
- Failing partial denture spanning teeth nos. 6 to 8, with advanced bone loss at tooth no. 8 associated with a vertical root fracture

Pretreatment

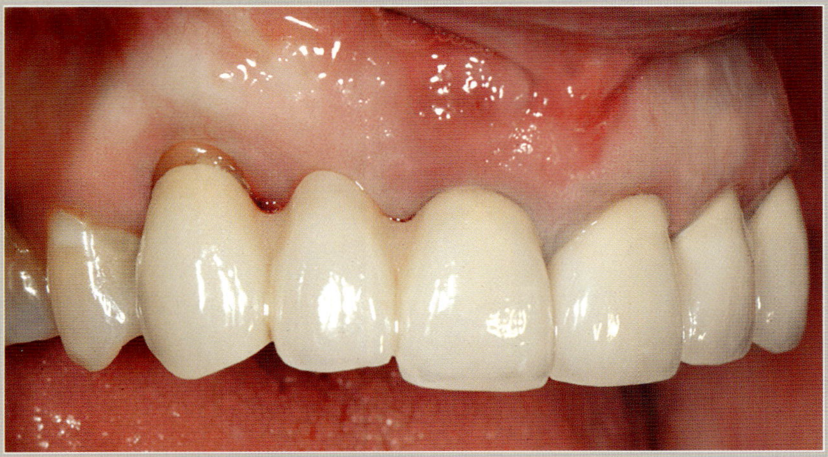

Intraoral right oblique view.

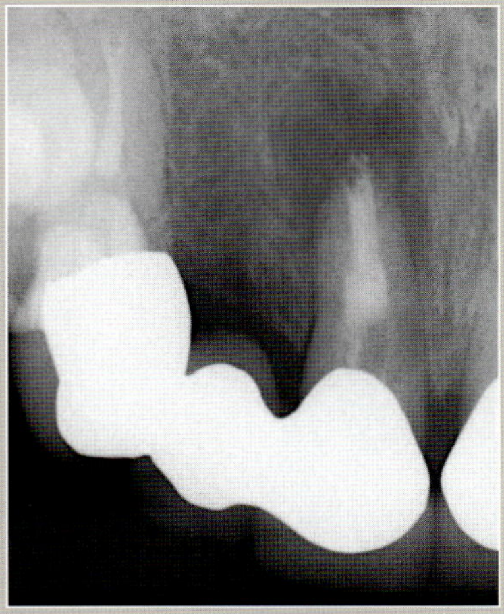

Periapical radiograph of teeth nos. 6 to 8 provided at the time of consultation.

- Missing teeth: nos. 1, 3, 7, 16, 18 to 20, 29, and 32
- Mesially tipped molars: teeth nos. 2, 17, 30, and 31
- Deficient restorations: teeth nos. 6, 9, 10, 11 (poor esthetics, biologic width violation), and 12 (recession and margin exposure)
- Fixed partial dentures: teeth nos. 6 to 8 and 28 to 30
- Crowns: teeth nos. 9, 10, 11, and 12
- Restorations: teeth nos. 2, 4, 5, 13, and 14
- Unrestored edentulous spaces: sites nos. 2 and 18 to 20
- Favorable gingival phenotype
- Moderate gingival scallop
- Oral hygiene: good; less than 10% of tooth surfaces with plaque using a plaque disclosing agent

Occlusal notes

- Class I malocclusion
- Overbite: 60%
- Overjet: 3 mm
- Posterior simultaneous contacts and canine guidance with posterior disocclusion
- No temporomandibular joint problems or muscle pain
- No obvious wear faceting as a result of parafunctional activity

Radiographic findings

- Missing teeth as noted clinically
- Mesially tipped molars: teeth nos. 2, 17, 30, and 31
- Advanced bone loss around tooth no. 8

Diagnosis

- Severe ridge resorption at sites nos. 19 and 20
- Vertical root fracture of tooth no. 8 and associated bone loss negatively impacting the gingival architecture
- Molar tipping due to prior tooth loss
- Otherwise good periodontal health
- Numerous failing and/or deficient crown restoration margins
- Evidence of clinical adjustment of the maxillary anterior crowns from teeth nos. 6 to 11

Prognosis

- Periodontal: hopeless for tooth no. 8, but otherwise good
- Restorative: challenging due to a high lip line along with significant bone loss associated with the maxillary right central and lateral positions

Summary of concerns

1. The high esthetic risk of treatment was primarily related to severe bone loss and active infection in site no. 8 and the anticipated negative bone level changes following the extraction of this tooth, particularly because tooth no. 7 was previously extracted. Contributing factors included:
   - The significant tissue display during smiling, speaking, and natural facial expressions.
   - The level of postextraction vertical bone loss in the anterior edentulous area. Although horizontal ridge augmentation is highly predictable, vertical ridge augmentation presents challenges that have not been overcome with current surgical treatment protocols.[35] In this case, vertical and horizontal bone and soft tissue regeneration was considered essential to achieve an acceptable treatment outcome.
2. The tissue phenotype and moderate scallop were deemed favorable for long-term tissue stability following restoration. The tissue was determined to have a thick phenotype (> 1 mm) as assessed by the absence of tissue color change when a metal periodontal probe was placed in the gingival sulci of adjacent teeth.[15,36] Based on this assessment, altering or enhancing the gingival phenotype was not required.
3. Restorative options to manage the edentulous area included a new, larger-span fixed partial denture, a single implant in either site no. 7 or 8 with a corresponding cantilevered pontic, or adjacent implants in sites nos. 8 and 9. The deep overbite and the patient-perceived ease of maintenance led to the decision to consider adjacent implant placement. This option increased the esthetic challenge for the following reasons:
   - Acceptable but limited space for two implants was available, demanding high precision in terms of three-dimensional placement, specifically in terms of interimplant spacing. Correct three-dimensional implant placement is essential to support and stabilize soft tissue levels.
   - Optimal gingival scalloping was assessed as impossible to re-create because of the preoperative soft tissue architecture. Placing adjacent implants could further compromise papilla form should additional bone remodeling occur between the implants.
4. Prior restoration failures and tooth loss were related primarily to endodontic treatment failures and tooth preparation with inadequate ferrule. Restoratively, this patient was deemed to be at fairly low risk for material failure even with an all-ceramic solution based on the restorative success of prior treatment and absence of parafunctional habits.
5. Prior late implant failures in the left mandibular quadrant were presumed to be the result of problematic surface technology of the implants and not caused by patient risk factors

Treatment-planning considerations

- Soft tissue display when smiling and talking
- Anticipated significant vertical bone loss after extraction
- Limited space for adjacent implants, requiring precise placement
- Poor initial soft tissue architecture in the area to be treated

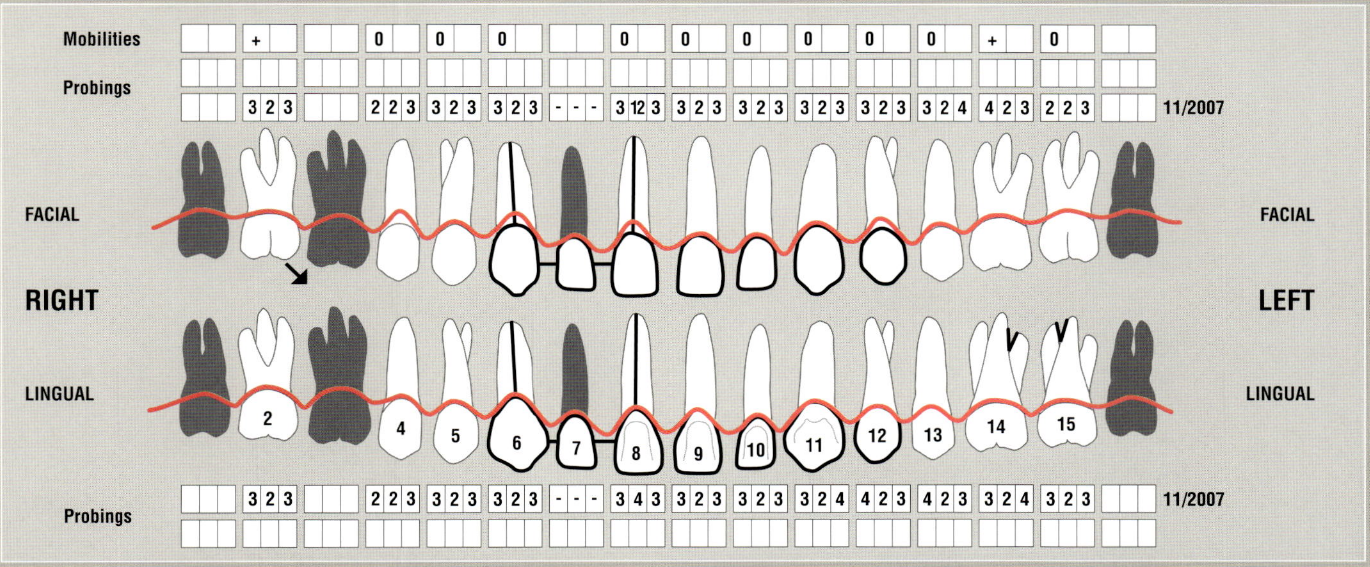

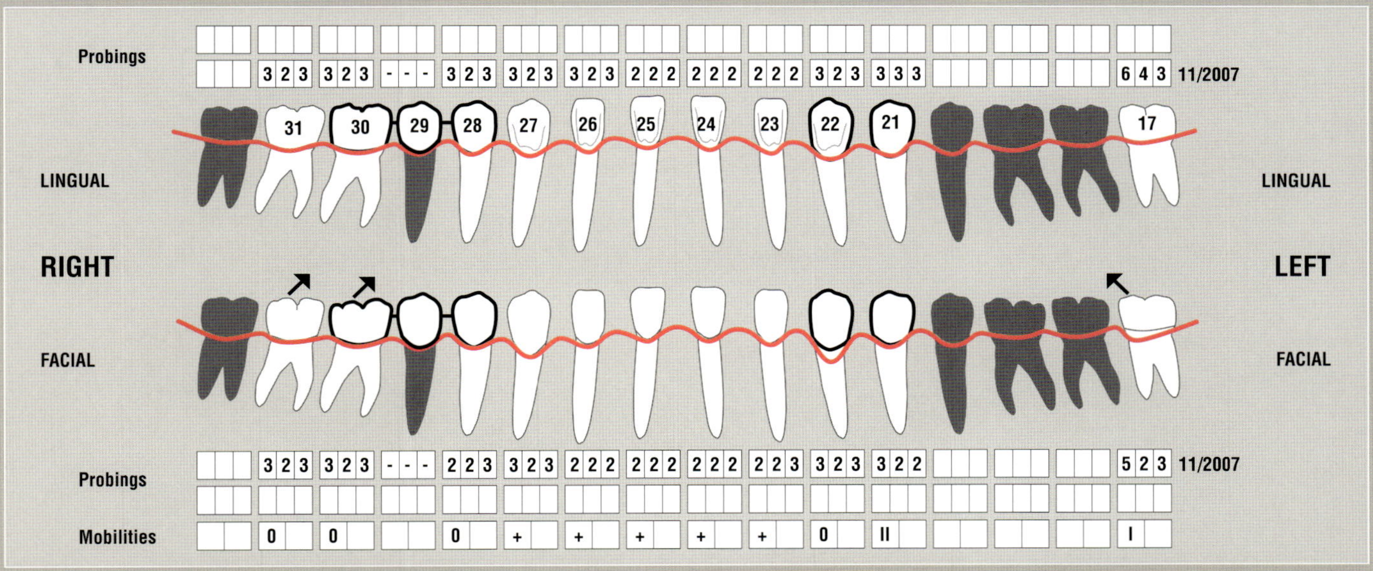

As a learning exercise, you may now outline goals/objectives of treatment and a treatment plan.

Proposed Treatment Plan

The patient indicated that she was receptive to treatment of the maxillary arch and would consider restoring the mandibular arch at a later date.

Goals/objectives of treatment

The objective of treatment focused on the replacement of the missing maxillary right central and lateral incisors with a fixed restoration and esthetic improvement of the adjacent restorative treatment. The goal was to offer the patient an esthetic treatment outcome centered on efforts to re-create a framework of natural-looking soft tissues.

Phase I: Restoration of the maxillary arch

1. The initial clinical and radiographic evaluations identified severe bone loss associated with a failed endodontic treatment and vertical root fracture in tooth no. 8. The acute infection was treated with a broad-spectrum antibiotic. Extraction of tooth no. 8 was planned, along with a ridge preservation procedure to minimize postextraction resorption. The area would be restored transitionally with an Essix splint until the treatment-planning phase was completed with the dentist and prosthodontist.
2. Diagnostic records: prosthodontic referral, periodontal charting, study casts, diagnostic wax-up, and a cone beam computed tomography (CBCT) scan to evaluate the ridge anatomy and plan for additional bone grafting and implant surgery (including implant position and size).
3. Block bone graft procedure to improve the ridge height and width in the region of teeth nos. 7 and 8. Bone grafting prior to implant placement was proposed because simultaneous vertical ridge augmentation and implant success is unpredictable.
4. Review of transitional restoration options: Essix splint, removable partial denture, or lab-processed provisional partial denture spanning teeth nos. 6 to 9.
5. Consideration of options for definitively replacing teeth nos. 7 and 8, including:
   —Fixed partial denture spanning teeth nos. 6 to 9 (and possibly tooth no. 10)
   —Two implants (nos. 7 and 8) to support individual restorations (risk: potential interimplant space limitation and difficulty in creating ideal papilla anatomy)
   —One implant (no. 8) to support a cantilevered pontic into site no. 7 (risk: existing deep overbite increases the risk for restoration complications or implant overload)
6. Restoration of teeth nos. 6, 9, 10, and 11.

Phase II: Restoration of the mandibular arch

7. Restoration of the mandibular left edentulous span, involving ridge augmentation and delayed implant placement; the crown-implant ratio was deemed unfavorable for the use of short implants
8. Replacement of the mandibular right posterior fixed partial denture
9. Supportive periodontal therapy to continue at 6-month intervals with the referring dentist
10. Restorative recall at 6- to-12 month intervals

ACTIVE CLINICAL TREATMENT

Review of the goals/objectives of treatment

The objective of treatment focused on the replacement of the missing maxillary right central and lateral incisors with a fixed restoration and esthetic improvement of the adjacent restorative treatment. The goal was to offer the patient an esthetic treatment outcome centered on efforts to re-create a framework of natural-looking soft tissues.

Treatment progress

The patient was given a prescription for amoxicillin 500 mg three times a day for 7 days and instructed to perform warm salt water rinses to control the active infection associated with tooth no. 8.

A decision was made to section the partial denture and extract tooth no. 8 as soon as possible. This was completed under local anesthesia within 2 weeks of the initial consultation. After site debridement, the extraction socket was grafted with a particulate allograft (Puros, Zimmer) and a Bio-Gide membrane (Geistlich) in an effort to minimize the postextraction ridge resorption. The facial flap was mobilized, and the flap was closed with 5-0 coated Vicryl Plus antibacterial sutures (Ethicon). The partial denture was transitionally replaced with an Essix splint to minimize pressure on the surgical site.

The patient was examined by the treating prosthodontist, and record collection was completed. Postextraction healing was uneventful, but negative vertical hard and soft tissue changes were evident in the ensuing 3 months of observation. The horizontal ridge volume appeared acceptable from the clinical assessment. In order to address the ridge height deficiency in view of the high lip line, further ridge augmentation was recommended using a block graft of autogenous origin (chin or ramus) or a block allograft (Puros). A decision was made with the patient to consider the allograft material. The potential advantage of using an allograft was the elimination of graft donor site morbidity. Preliminary evidence from recent case reports and clinical investigations on the use of allograft blocks as an alternative to autogenous grafts provides encouraging evidence for this alterative treatment protocol.[37–39]

Bone grafting with block and particulate allograft in the proximal voids was completed under local anesthesia. The block was rehydrated in saline and modified extraorally with a round carbide bur with a clean technique. The recipient site was prepared to receive the block with numerous perforations to create a regional acceleratory phenomenon and minor buccal plasty to mortise the block. The block was adapted and stabilized with two fixation screws (Bone Block Fixation, Straumann). Mineralized cortical allograft particles were used to fill voids between the block and receptor site. A resorbable Bio-Gide membrane was used to contain the particulate graft, to delay soft tissue ingress, and to reduce block resorption.[40,41]

Minor surgical crown lengthening of teeth nos. 9 to 12 was completed at the time of bone grafting to visually harmonize the anterior gingival display, to address the inflammation resulting from biologic width violation in sites nos. 9, 10, and 11, and to apically reposition the gingiva. A 1.0- to 1.5-mm ostectomy was completed using specific carbide burs (Crown Lengthening Kit, Brasseler).

A vestibular release was prepared to mobilize the facial tissues in order to achieve passive closure over the block graft. Nonresorbable Cytoplast polytetrafluoroethylene (PTFE) sutures (Osteogenics Biomedical) were used in a combination of interrupted and horizontal mattress suturing tech-

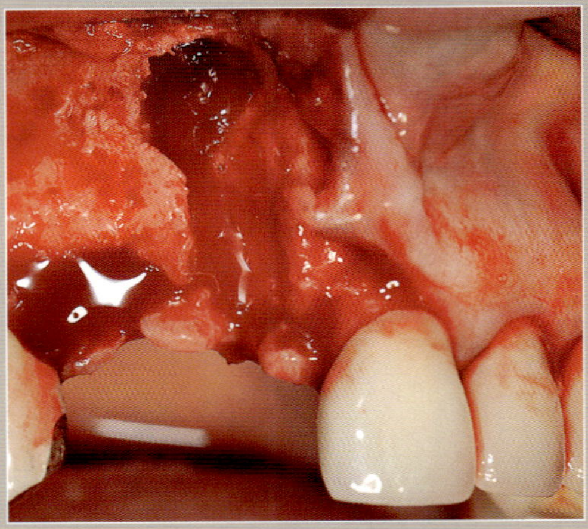

After sectioning of the fixed partial denture and extraction of tooth no. 8.

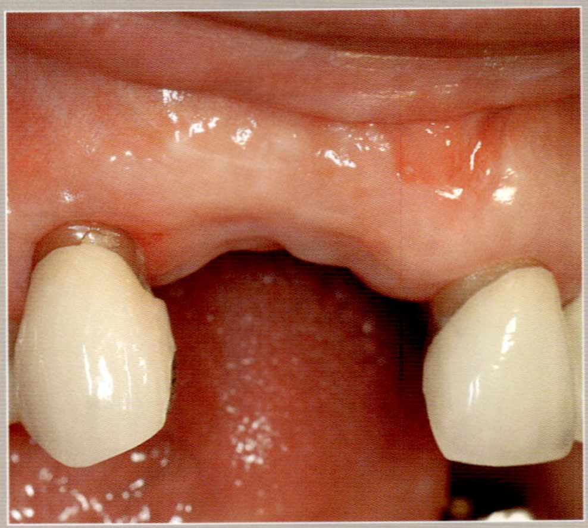

Condition of the ridge 3 months after extraction.

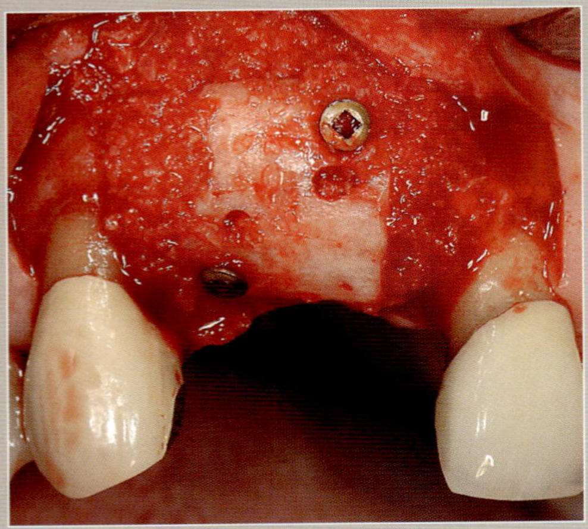

Stabilized block allograft and surrounding particulate material.

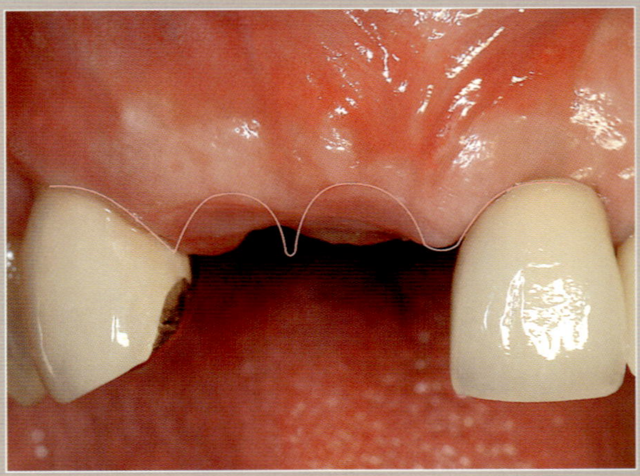

Healed ridge 4 months after augmentation. Note the missing soft tissue architecture in the area between where the implants are anticipated to be placed.

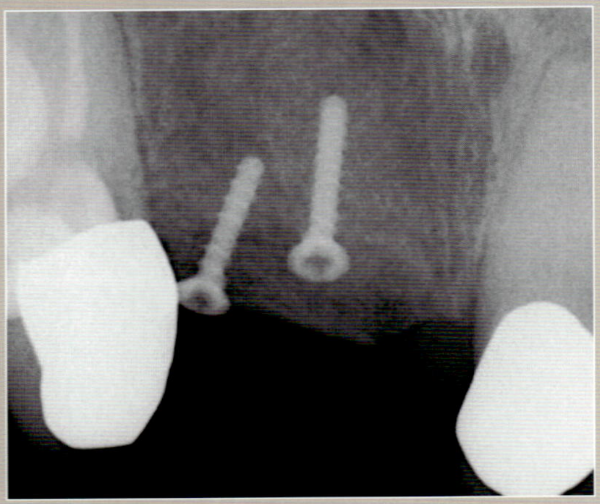

Periapical radiograph 4 months after augmentation.

niques. The area was allowed to heal for 4 months. The ridge height was significantly enhanced relative to the postextraction tissue level, but an outline of the desired gingival tissue architecture revealed a deficiency in the future papilla area of sites nos. 7 and 8. Radiographic assessment at 4 months of healing included a periapical radiograph indicating uneventful healing of the bone allograft, and a CBCT confirmed favorable three-dimensional ridge anatomy.

The patient elected to proceed with placement of two implants in sites nos. 7 and 8. This could easily be criticized because the literature on implant soft tissue esthetics points to better papillary architecture development between an implant and a tooth or pontic than between two implants.[42] With this in mind, implants with a platform-shifted design (NobelActive, Nobel Biocare) were selected based on the potential for enhanced crestal bone stability

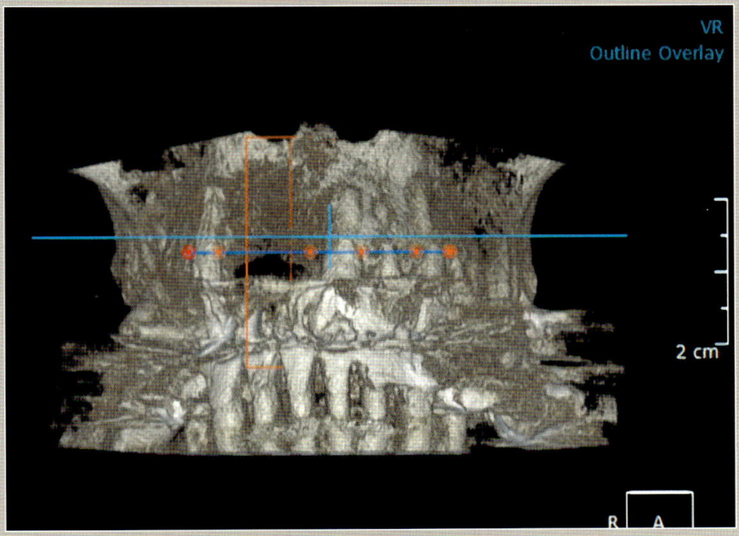

CBCT 4 months after augmentation.

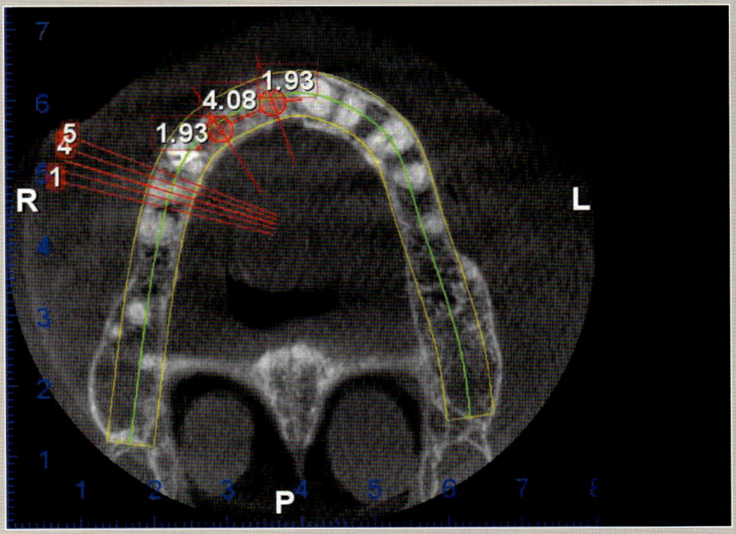

CBCT axial scout view prior to implant placement.

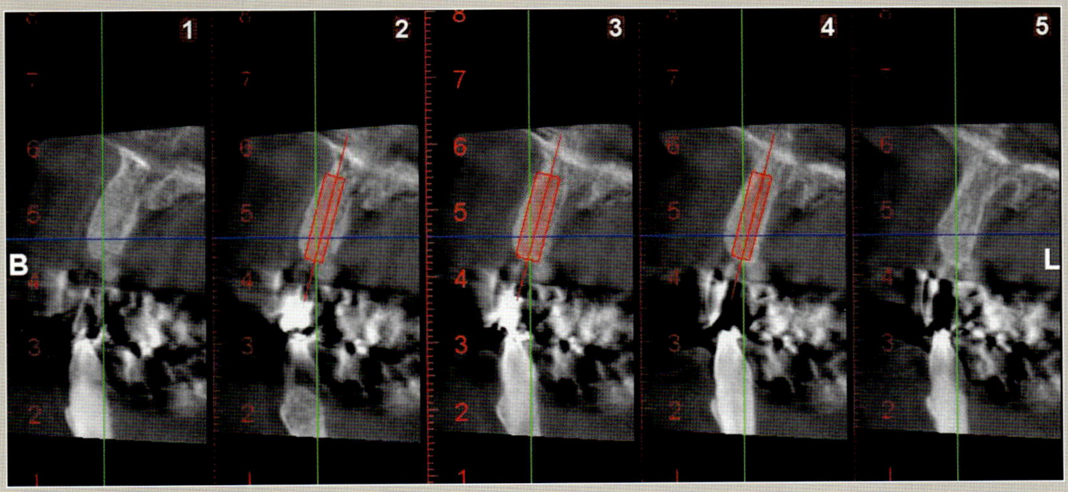

CBCT cross-sectional views with proposed implant positions.

due to reduced bone remodeling around the implants. The subject of marginal bone level changes and the impact of platform-switched implants compared with conventional matched abutments and implants was recently reviewed by Atieh et al.[43] The unique benefits of this implant design also include exceptional primary stability due to a unique body and thread design; its back-tapered collar that potentially enhances crestal bone volume, which would improve the soft tissue stability and volume; and a bone density–based drilling protocol that reduces the amount of bone removal during the preparation of the implant osteotomy. Regardless of the potential positive impact of implant design on bone stability, a key point to note in this case and our subsequent comparative cases is that three-dimensional spacing, both

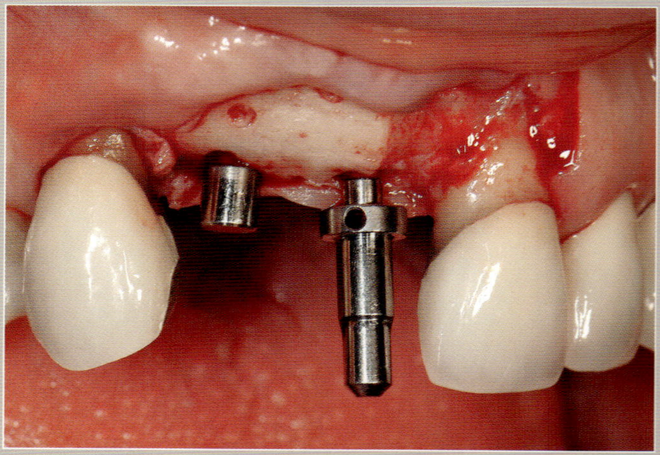

Implant site preparation with direction indicators in place.

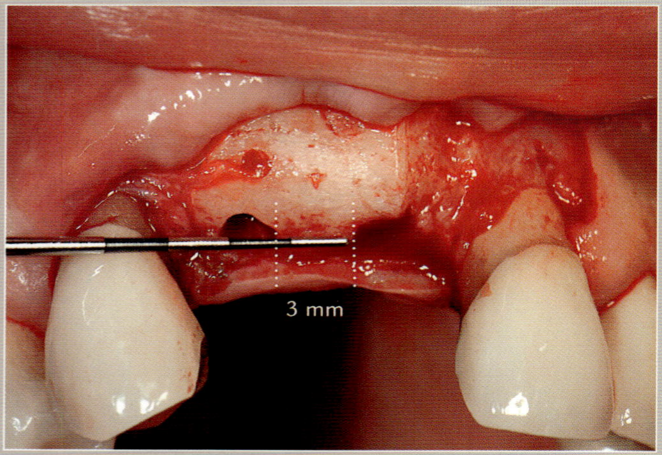

Measurement of spacing between implants on completion of the osteotomies.

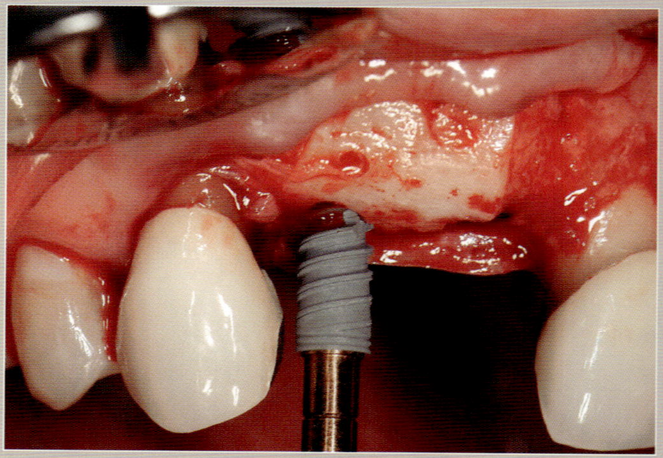

Implant placement at site no. 7.

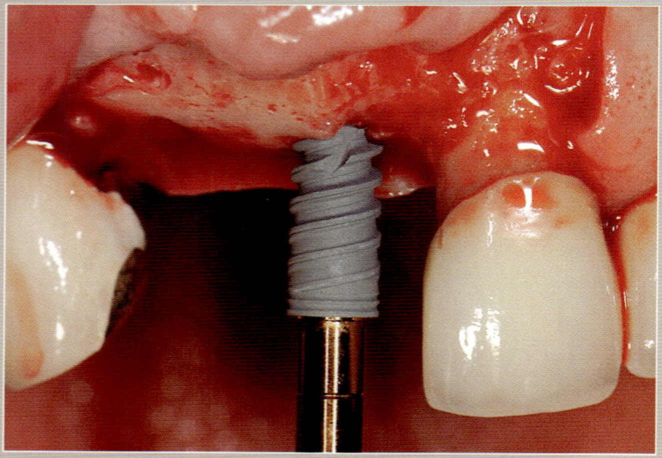

Implant placement at site no. 8.

between an implant and an adjacent tooth as well as in the interimplant area, significantly contributes to crestal bone stability. An implant-tooth distance of close to 1.5 mm and an interimplant distance of 3 to 4 mm should be allowed. Some of the literature suggests that implants of a platform-switched design can be placed closer together without negative impact on crestal remodeling.[26,27] Our views on this issue are discussed in our concluding remarks.

Under local anesthesia, the ridge was visualized and accessed with minimal palatal exposure and adequate labial exposure to access and remove the two block fixation screws. Osteotomies were prepared using the recommended protocol for bone of medium density, and three-dimensional positioning was initially confirmed at the precision drill step in site no. 7 and at the 2-mm pilot drill step in site no. 8. Two 3.5 × 13-mm implants were placed with insertion torques of 70 Ncm. Intra- and postoperative radiographs were taken to confirm mesiodistal positioning. An implant-level impression was taken at the time of implant placement for the fabrication of provisional restorations that would be delivered after a 10- to 12-week integration period. The tissues were closed with coated Vicryl FS-2 undyed, braided 5-0 interrupted sutures. The tissues were contoured using 3-mm biopsy punches around narrow, 3-mm-high healing abutments. The patient was given complete hygiene instructions and asked to dab around the implant sites with 0.12% chlorhexidine rinse twice daily. The area was monitored at 10 days (suture removal), 21 days, and 3 months.

Although implants with favorable primary stability theoretically can be provisionalized at the time of placement, this step was delayed for 10 weeks because the implants were placed in a large volume of grafted bone, and the deep over-

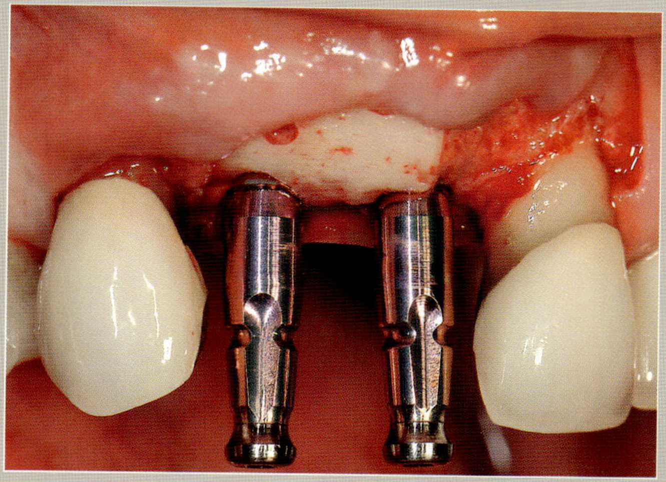

Impression copings in place for implant-level impression.

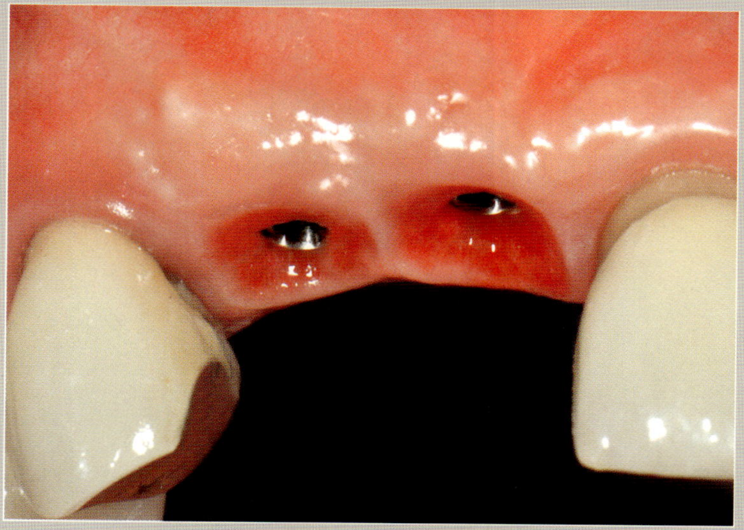

Gingival architecture 3 months after provisionalization.

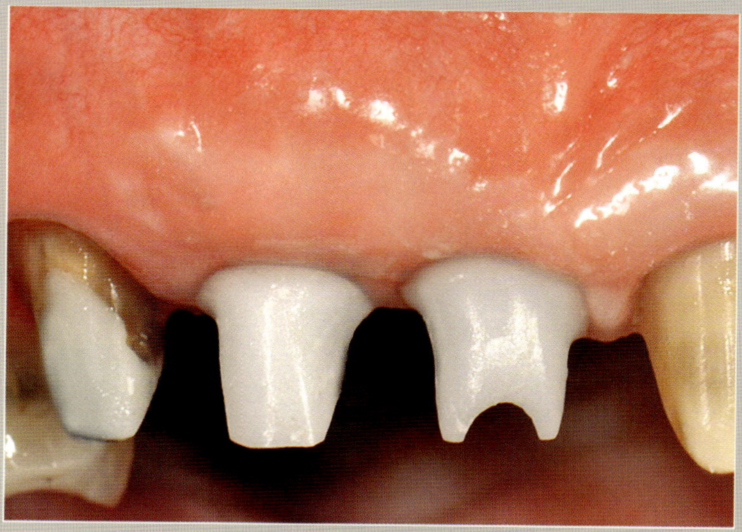

Custom zirconia abutments.

bite could potentially compromise integration as a result of occlusal overload. A fixed provisional restoration was judged to be the ideal transitional restoration because the adjacent teeth required restoration replacement; however, the patient chose to continue to use the Essix splint fabricated for the emergency extraction procedure. Based on subsequent cases treated with similar materials and approaches, provisionalization of the implants at the time of surgery could have been considered.

The implants were restored 3 months after the implant surgery with screw-retained implant head–level provisional restorations to develop the peri-implant tissue emergence profile prior to definitive restoration. At 6 weeks after delivery of the provisional restorations, the gingival profile showed minimal scalloping, in particular in the interimplant area. Final impressions were completed after a 4-month period.

All-ceramic restorations were selected for the implants and adjacent teeth. Customized zirconia abutments (NobelProcera, Nobel Biocare) were placed on the implants at sites nos. 7 and 8, and core buildup was performed on tooth no. 6. Ceramic crowns (e.max, Ivoclar Vivadent) were placed on the implants and adjacent natural dentition and cemented with RelyX Luting Plus Cement (3M ESPE).

The clinical appearance of the definitive all-ceramic restorations shows that despite successful horizontal and vertical ridge augmentation, the papilla form is blunted in the interimplant area between nos. 7 and 8. However, the relatively draping lip line diminishes the impact of the gingival asymmetry. Favorable bone levels were found around the implants at the radiographic follow-up 14 months after definitive restoration.

Posttreatment

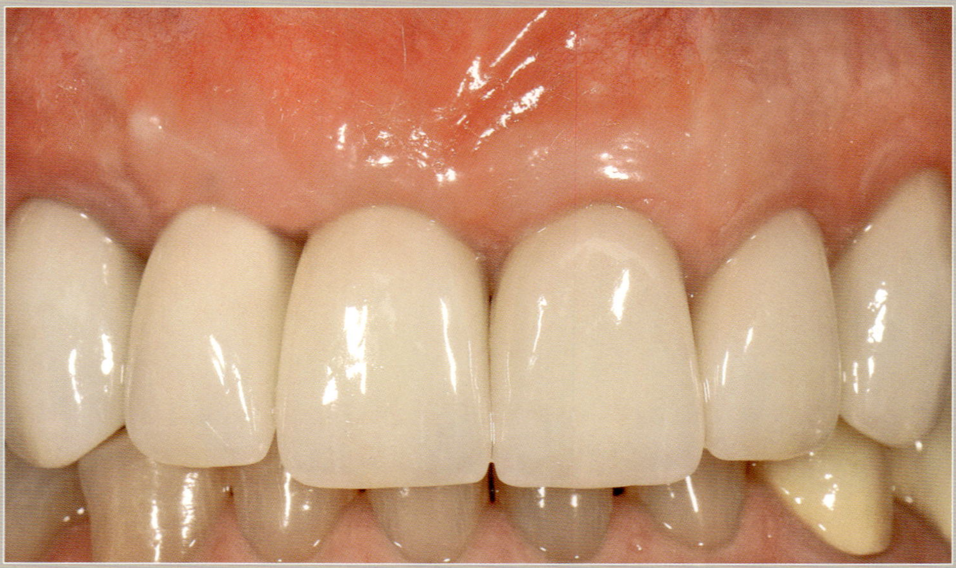

Definitive all-ceramic restorations. Note the lack of an interimplant papilla between nos. 8 and 9.

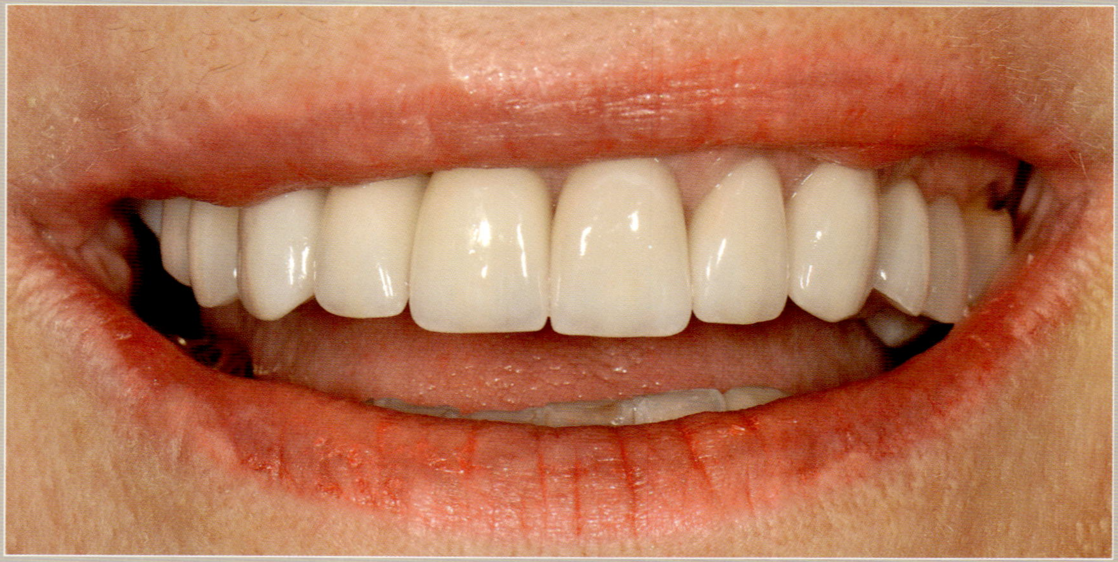

A forgiving smile reveals the soft tissue on the other side of the mouth.

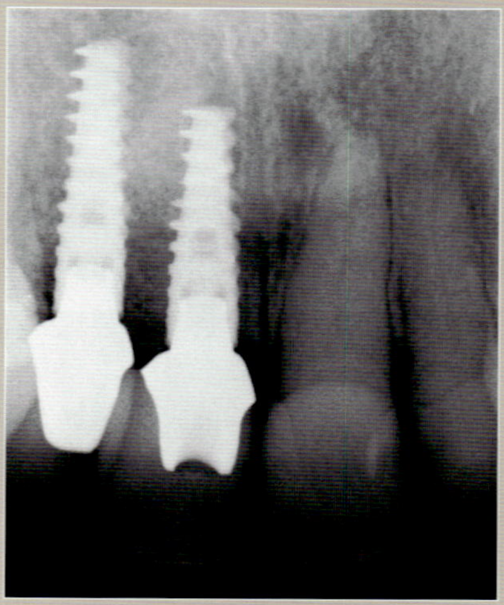

Radiograph 10 months after delivery of the definitive restorations.

You may now place the corresponding posttreatment overlay found in the separate folder over the pretreatment periodontal chart on page 91.

Case Comparisons

Following are three case presentations that demonstrate the impact of different implant placement and restoration protocols on the esthetic outcomes of treatment.

Comparative case 1. Immediate implant restoration: Defining tissue architecture through the engineering of hard and soft tissues

This 35-year-old healthy man presented for consultation approximately 4 months following the extraction of fractured teeth nos. 8 and 9 and ridge preservation procedures; an acrylic partial denture had been fabricated by the patient's general dentist to transitionally replace these teeth. The patient had been functioning acceptably with this prosthesis but wanted information about a fixed treatment alternative. He had no other treatment requirements.

Diagnostic findings included:

- No significant intraoral or dental findings
- High smile line: displays the peaks of papillae and the facial gingival margins during natural smile and speech
- Occlusion: Class I malocclusion, 20% overbite, 1-mm overjet
- Mild vertical ridge resorption (< 3 mm) with associated loss of papillae height in the edentulous area and at the proximal tooth surfaces
- Favorable (thick) gingival tissue phenotype; moderately high gingival scallop
- Fair oral hygiene: 18% of surfaces with plaque coverage at the preliminary assessment

After several discussions, the patient's esthetic expectations were assessed as reasonable, with a clear understanding of the limitations of fully redeveloping interimplant and implant-tooth papillae heights.

Based on the clinical examination, the ridge width was determined to be favorable at the start of treatment, with almost no resorption of the buccal plate, which was confirmed with the tomographic assessment. This case was suitable for a minimally invasive implant placement protocol with limited flap reflection. NobelGuide (Nobel Biocare) was used to perform virtual implant placement, including planning of the interimplant and implant-tooth distances based on the selected implant sizes.

Vertical hard and soft tissue loss was evident, with blunting of the papilla in the region from the mesial aspect of tooth no. 7 to the mesial aspect of tooth no. 9. Bone loss at the proximal surfaces of teeth nos. 7 and 9 and loss of bone scallop were noted radiographically. Vertical ridge augmentation through bone grafting was not possible because bone regeneration at the proximal root surfaces cannot be achieved. As a result, a decision was made to accept the existing ridge level and optimize the tissue anatomy through correct three-dimensional implant positioning and soft tissue architecture enhancement during provisionalization. The tissue phenotype was thick; therefore, a soft tissue graft was not required. Definitive restoration with custom zirconia abutments and all-ceramic restorations after a 4-month hard and soft tissue integration period was planned.

Record collection included periodontal charting, restorative needs assessment, study casts, a diagnostic wax-up, and a CBCT to assess the edentulous ridge architecture. With the information provided, the patient chose an implant-based method of restoration.

Adjacent implant placement was proposed for the replacement of teeth nos. 8 and 9. Implants with a platform-switched design (NobelActive) were selected based on the potential for enhanced crestal bone stability as previously discussed.

Under local anesthesia, the ridge crest was accessed using minor flap reflection. Surgical access was limited to a midcrestal incision and the use of 4-mm biopsy punches to discard crestal tissue plugs. Using a surgical guide, two 4.3 × 13-mm implants were placed with insertion torques of 70 Ncm. The implant collars were positioned approximately 1.5 mm subcrestally in order to develop space for the desired restoration contours. Interestingly, it has been suggested that subcrestal implant placement may positively impact crestal bone stability.[44] A comparison of equicrestal and subcrestal implant placement showed better maintenance of bone levels between implants that were submerged.

Provisionalization after implant surgery is still often accomplished with removable appliances, but immediate restoration has long been recognized as an appropriate treatment option in certain clinical scenarios and may be advantageous in terms

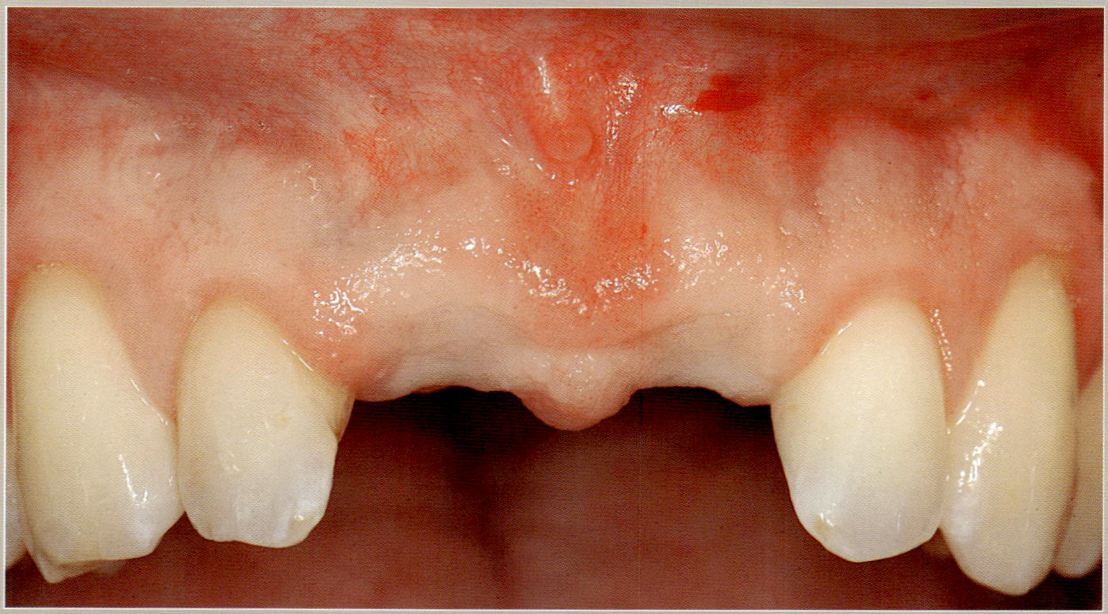

Initial presentation: Intraoral facial view.

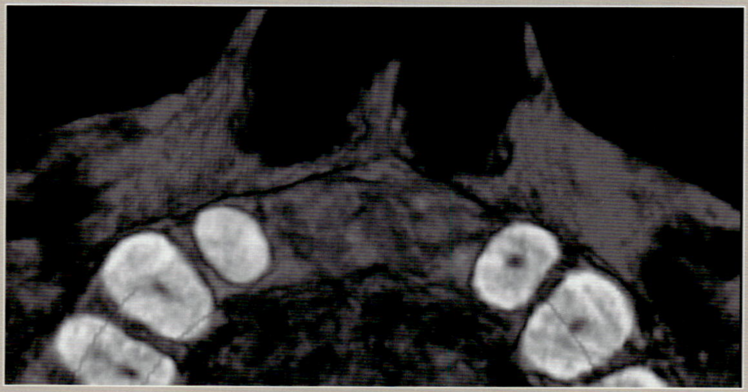

CBCT arch reconstruction.

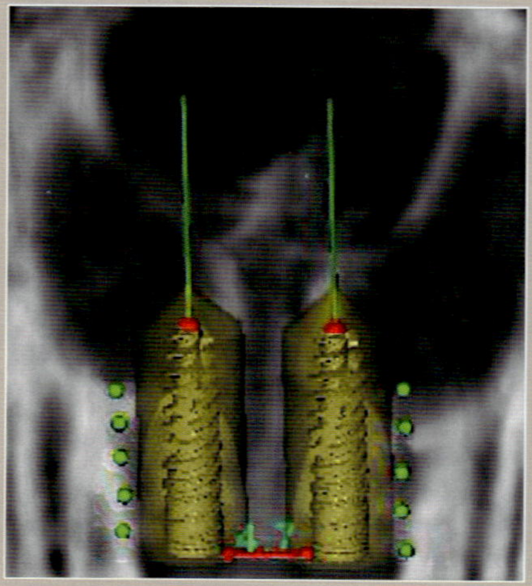

Virtual implant placement planning.

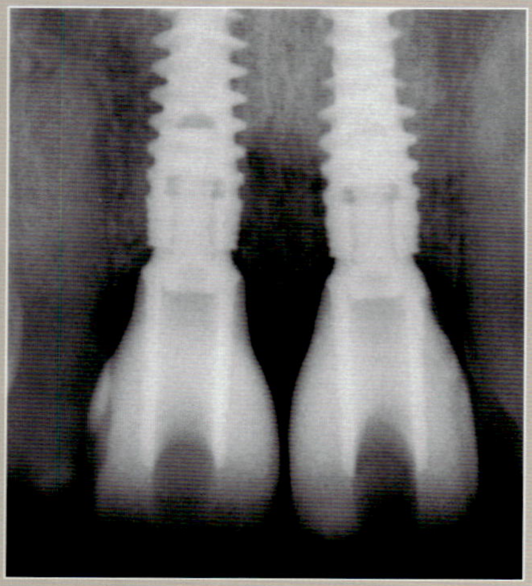

Radiograph showing subcrestal implant placement.

of developing both facial and proximal tissue levels and form. In a prospective study by Block et al,[45] support of the gingival margin with a provisional restoration resulted in 1-mm superior facial gingival margin position compared with the delayed restoration group. De Rouck et al[46] also found that, in the case of single implants, delayed restoration resulted in initial papilla loss requiring up to 1 year to achieve comparable height as immediately restored implants, while midfacial recession was 0.75 mm greater when restoration was delayed compared to the immediately restored implant at 1-year post-restoration. In a study by Kourkouta et al,[17] it was found that interproximal tissue dimensions between adjacent implants were 1 mm superior when fixed restorations were used compared to removable prostheses.

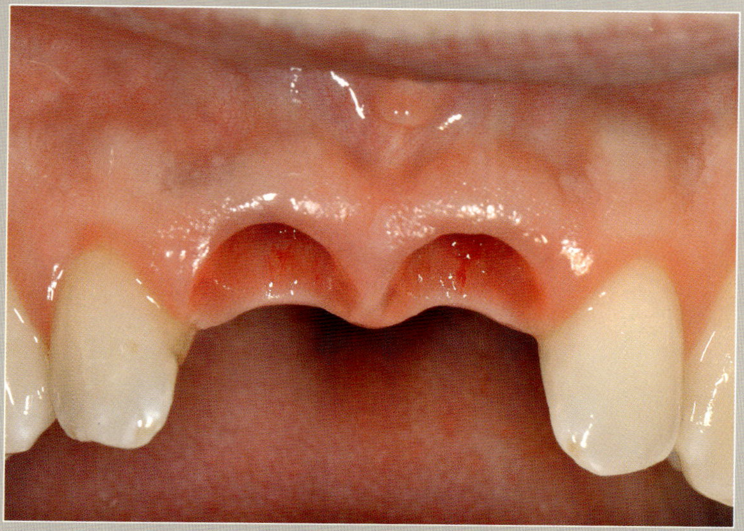

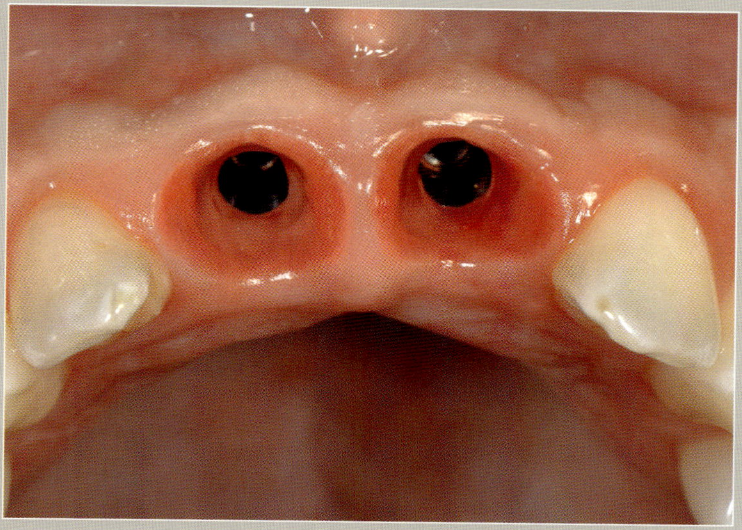

Subgingival anatomy and marginal gingival form following removal of the provisional restorations.

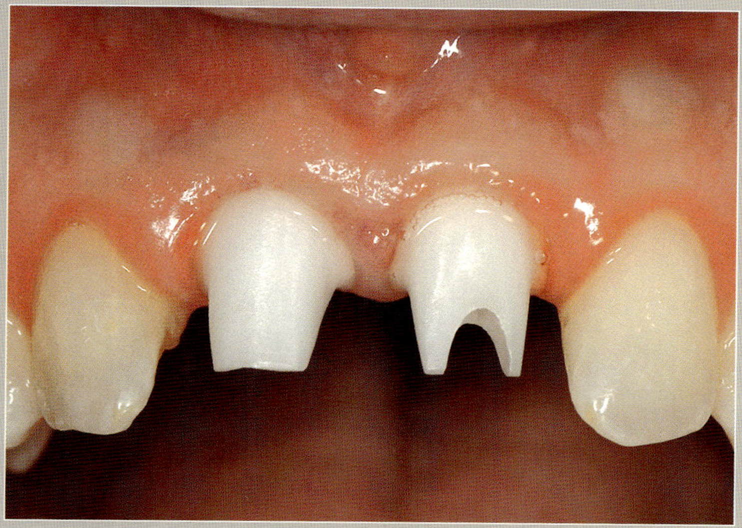

Intraoral frontal view following placement of custom zirconia abutments.

In this case, immediate implant restoration was considered appropriate because of the high primary stability of the implants and favorable overbite-overjet relationship. Two individual screw-retained provisional restorations were fabricated chairside; lab-processed shells were indexed intraorally and adapted to provisional titanium abutments with acrylic. The subgingival provisional restoration contours were developed and finished extraorally. The patient understood that restricted function on the implants was necessary in the first 6 weeks after surgery. The restorations were inserted and torqued to 35 Ncm. Palatal access cavities were sealed with cotton pellets and Fermit (Ivoclar Vivadent).

After 4 months of healing, an impression was taken using stock impression copings. Radiographs were completed to verify full seating of the impression copings. A vinyl polysiloxane material was used (Imprint 3, 3M ESPE) to register the implant positions along with the developed peri-implant tissue contours.

Zirconia abutments (NobelProcera) were designed to specifically position the cement lines approximately 0.5 to 1.0 mm subgingivally circumferentially. The abutments were torqued to 35 Ncm. To help deflect cement from the gingival sulcus, Ultrapak #000 cord (Ultradent) was gently placed apical to the cement lines. Two all-ceramic zirconia restora-

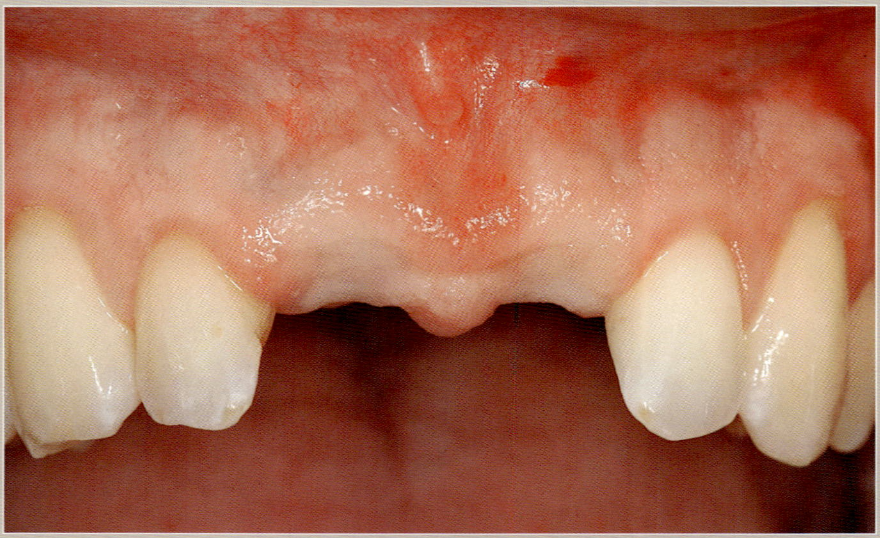

Pretreatment intraoral facial view.

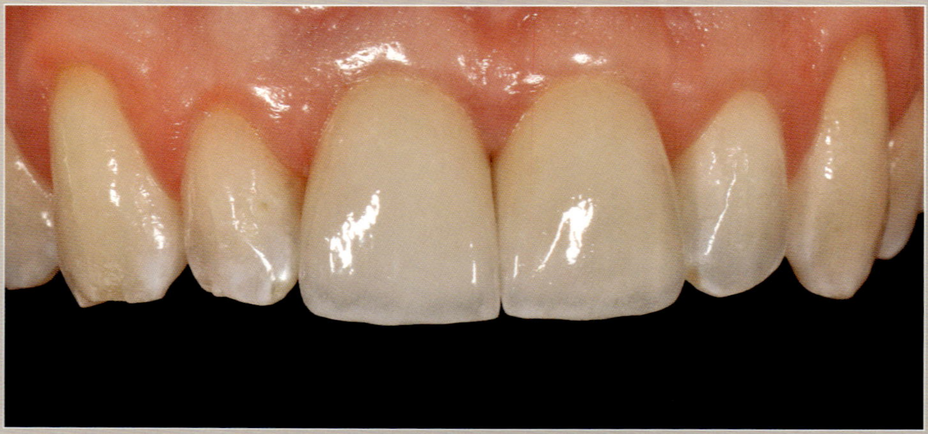

Intraoral facial view of the definitive restorations.

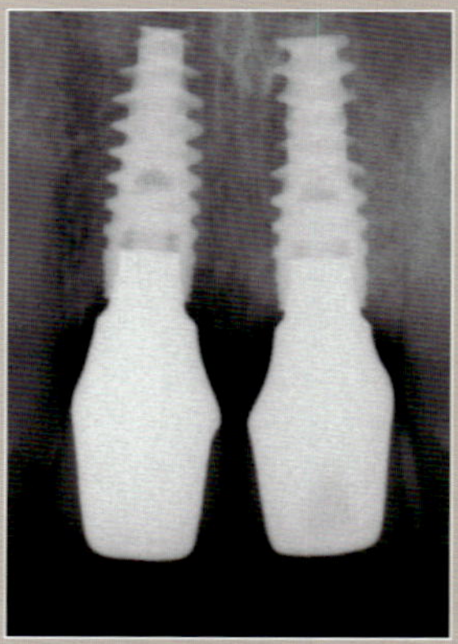

Radiograph taken at
25-month follow-up.

tions (NobelProcera) veneered with Noritake were cemented with a 10-methacryloyloxydecyl dihydrogen phosphate (MDP)–type dual-cure cement (Clearfil Esthetic Cement and DC Bond, Kuraray). Excess cement was removed, and complete cement removal was confirmed through clinical and radiographic inspection.

This case has been followed for 26 months since the delivery of the definitive restorations. Clinical and radiographic follow-ups have been uneventful.

This is a clinical situation we see routinely; the patient presents with missing adjacent teeth due to a variety of reasons, including trauma or prior disease. The decision regarding how to treat this case was primarily based on the remaining bone and soft tissue volume and quality.

First, if the roots remain (which is a rare advantage), then atraumatic extraction followed by either immediate implant placement or ridge preservation is recommended. If the roots have been removed prior to the patient presentation, then

Things to Keep in Mind

Papilla height

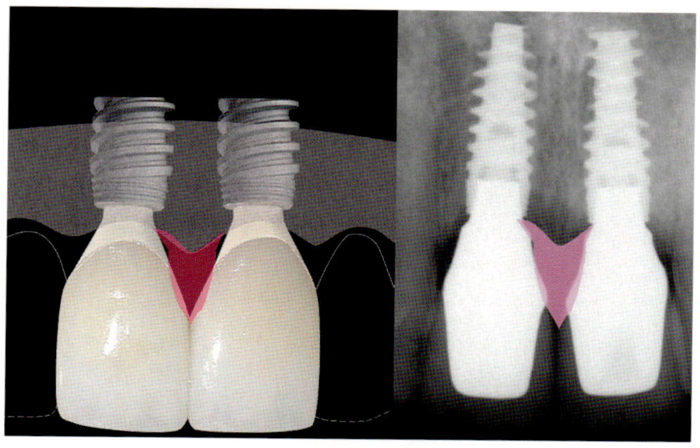

The papilla height between implants averages 3.4 mm; this is shorter than the papilla height between natural teeth.

Contact point

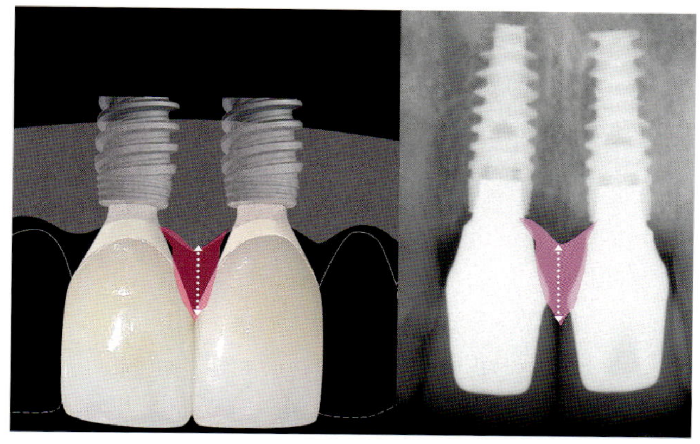

The contact area between the crowns ideally should be 3 to 4 mm from the bone crest. This crest should be "sounded" or, if possible, measured radiographically and the information relayed to the technician.

Spacing between implants

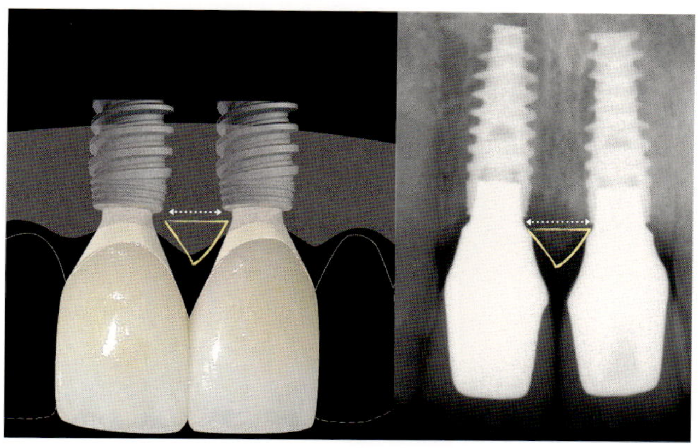

Spacing between implants should be a minimum of 3 to 4 mm. Perhaps in the future, with the use of platform-switched implant and abutment designs or implant surface configurations such as LaserLok, we may have more consistent reporting of stable bone levels right to the top of the implant, in which case implants could be placed closer together more confidently and even closer to natural teeth where space is limited.

Depth of implant placement

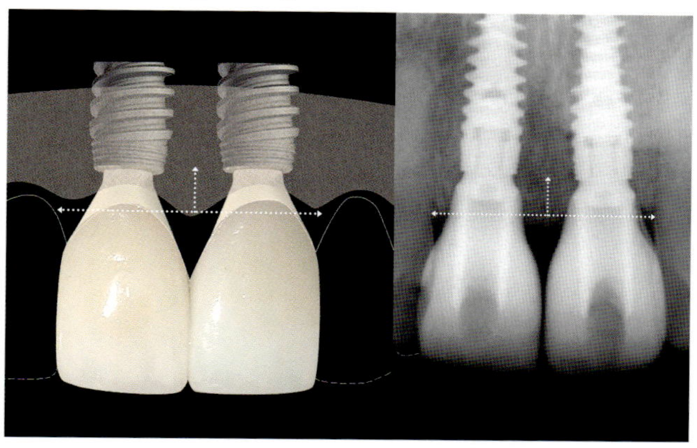

Our results have suggested that placing platform-shifted implants slightly more subcrestal has resulted in less crestal bone resorption.

ideally bone grafting materials are placed in the sockets. When teeth are extracted, ridge preservation procedures will reduce the degree of post-extraction ridge resorption. Generally, when this is not done, three-dimensional bone loss and a flattened ridge are expected, necessitating some form of bone and/or soft tissue augmentation procedure. In this case, the sockets had been grafted and the ridge anatomy was favorable.

Second, we need to determine if the soft tissue levels are favorable. If the patient has a removable partial denture, was it made with ovate pontics? Where are the gingival levels with respect to the remaining teeth? In this case, we had a decent starting position and some soft tissue definition maintained by a properly shaped partial denture.

In comparison with the main case presentation, there is more room available for adjacent implant placement because the missing teeth are both central incisors rather than a central and lateral incisor. Therefore, this is a comparatively straightforward situation, unlike the main case, which had ongoing disease associated with significant bone destruction.

Comparative case 2. Early implant placement (8 weeks postextraction): Altering the bacterial flora and enhancing soft tissue volume

When this 37-year-old woman presented for treatment, she was taking thyroxine but was otherwise healthy. At the preliminary consultation, she reported an achy feeling in the area of the maxillary central incisors. Both teeth were fractured when she was 8 years old and were restored with composite restorations; crowns were placed on the teeth when she was 21 years old. A sinus tract developed on two occasions on the maxillary left central incisor in the year prior to her referral and each time had been managed with a course of antibiotic therapy. At the preliminary consultation, both central incisors showed advanced bone loss with probing depths ranging up to 9 mm with radiographic evidence of complex and advanced bone loss patterns, bleeding, and suppuration upon probing. There were root proximity problems between the central and lateral incisors that were considered a risk factor for tissue change with any intervention. Her dental health status was otherwise stable and noncontributory.

Diagnostic findings included:

- High lip line and lip dynamics
- Occlusion: Class I, 20% overbite, 1- to 2-mm overjet
- High gingival scallop and moderately thick or fibrous phenotype as assessed visually and through probing
- Good oral hygiene

The patient's treatment expectations were high. She was advised that the risk for negative gingival tissue architecture changes was significant, with a high probability of blunt papillae with a conventional partial denture approach or with implant-based treatment. Based on the information presented and the understanding of the potential flattening of the ridge after healing, the patient nevertheless decided that she would prefer implants to a fixed partial denture.

Active periodontal disease affecting teeth that must undergo extraction presents a considerable risk and potentially affects subsequent implant success. Numerous studies have suggested that implants can be successfully used in the rehabilitation of a periodontally compromised patient but that bone levels may be prone to greater change over time.[47–50] In this case, the added risk of adverse soft tissue changes associated with adjacent immediate implant placement had to be considered in view of the high lip line and pronounced lip dynamics. The report of Hürzeler et al[51] illustrated the increased esthetic complications that may occur with multiple adjacent extractions and immediate implant placement. One can speculate that this type of tissue change may be more significant in the periodontally affected patient.

A comprehensive periodontal examination to evaluate the periodontal status of the remaining dentition was scheduled, along with a restorative assessment of the remaining teeth, study casts, and a diagnostic wax-up. Impressions were taken to fabricate an immediate acrylic partial prosthesis to replace the central incisors.

Unlike Comparative case 1, this patient presented with compromised teeth that required extraction with delayed adjacent implant placement. Hard and soft tissue augmentation would be required as part of the implant procedure. Because of the degree of bone destruction and active periodontal disease, ridge preservation was not planned, with a preference for allowing the ridge to heal briefly (6 to 8 weeks) to change the local flora and grafting the remaining bone defects in conjunction with implant placement. Although the phenotype was moderately fibrous, a decision to use a connective tissue graft on the labial aspect was considered in order to further enhance the stability of the facial tissue and the papilla.

The central incisors were extracted under local anesthesia, and the sockets were debrided. Bone graft products were not placed in the sockets. A transitional partial denture was modified to support the soft tissues and delivered at the extraction appointment.

Eight weeks later, the implants were placed using punch access, and granulation tissue was removed, followed by a standard drilling protocol. NobelPerfect implants (Nobel Biocare) were inserted with favorable primary stability. Healing abutments were placed, Bio-Oss (Geistlich) was added into the residual horizontal defect on the labial aspect of the implants, and a buccal split-thickness flap preparation was made for simultaneous connective tissue graft adaptation. A partial denture was used for the 10- to 12-week integration period following surgery.

Preliminary impressions of the implants were taken, and 2 weeks later implant head–level, screw-retained provisional restorations were delivered. They remained in place for an additional 16 weeks to develop and stabilize the gingival tissue architecture. At this point a final impression was taken.

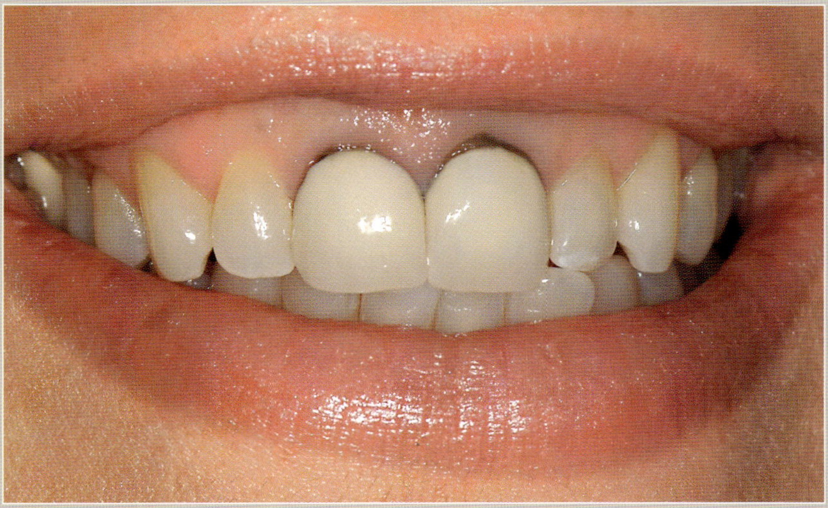

Initial presentation: Frontal view of the smile.

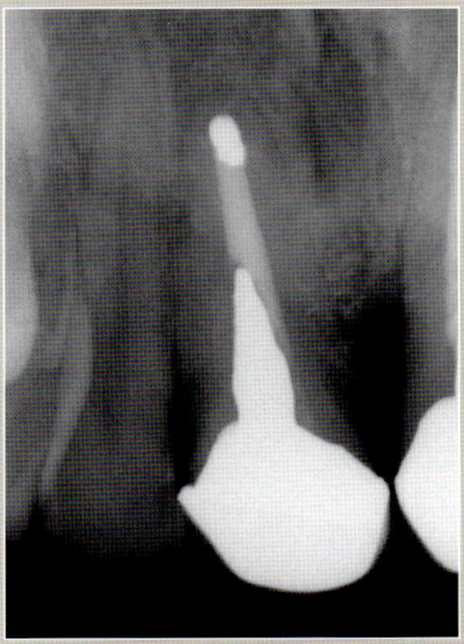

Radiograph of tooth no. 8.

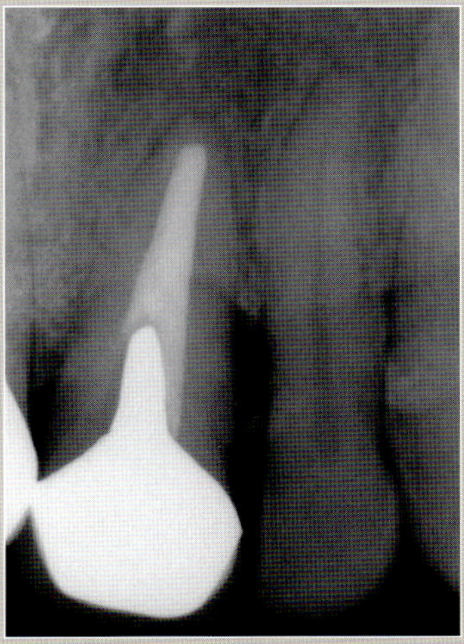

Radiograph of tooth no. 9.

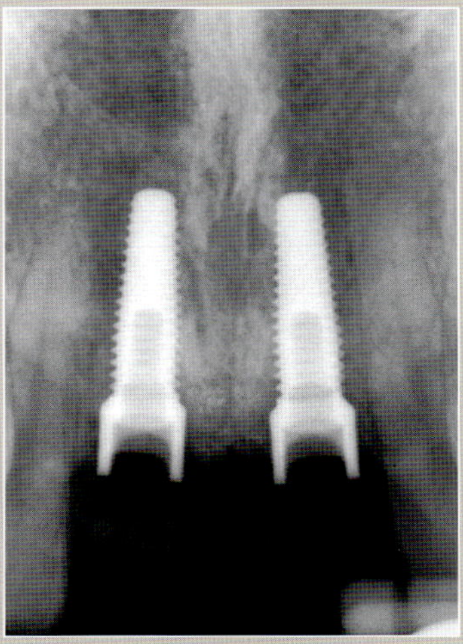

Radiographic view after implant placement.

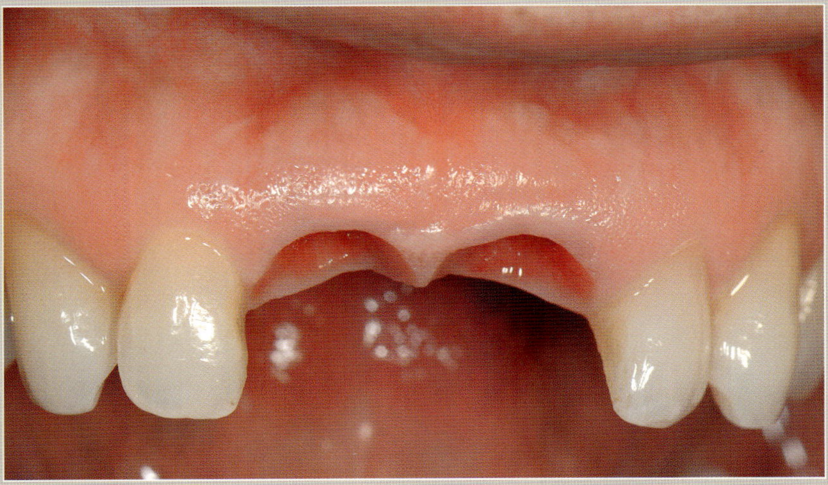

Gingival tissue form 4 months after placement of provisional restorations.

The impression procedures were fundamentally the same as previously described except that the implants used in this case had a scalloped design. Definitive restorations were cemented with a resin-modified glass ionomer (RelyX Unicem, 3M ESPE).

With the scalloped implant design, the abutment sits internally in the implant, and a crown is cemented both to the abutment and the head of the implant. The downside of this is a deep cement line that increases the risk for cement trapping and creates a risk of damaging the implant surface during the removal of the cement. To overcome this, definitive abutments were designed using CAD/CAM zirconia copings cemented extraorally over provisional titanium cylinders in order to achieve a better seal to the implant head and to move the definitive abutment margin coronally. The customized coping and abutment complex were inserted and torqued to 35 Ncm. When this approach is used, a deflective cord could be placed at the time of cementation to avoid subgingival cement retention.

This case has been followed for 5 years with annual recalls, including periapical radiographs and photographs. To date there have been no clinical and minimal radiographic changes. A robust interimplant bone crest can be attributed to the interimplant spacing of 4 mm and possibly to the scalloped implant design that has repositioned the implant-abutment microgap away from the ridge crest. The interimplant papilla has been fairly well maintained, although it is nominally deficient relative to the preoperative level.

Unlike Comparative case 1, this case involves missing central incisors associated with active disease and bone loss, which led to the decision to use an early placement protocol. The level of bone loss was such that augmentation could be accomplished at the time of implant placement. Provisional restorations could have been placed at the time of surgery. This decision is often made during the surgical procedure because the pattern of bone loss and number of exposed threads, amount of grafting required, and primary stability of the implants must all be considered. The volume of bone grafting required was deemed to be more significant than in Comparative case 1, supporting the decision to delay implant restoration.

It is interesting to note that although the scalloped implant design used in this case was anticipated to maintain crestal bone levels, some degree of bone remodeling toward the first major thread has been noted in this case. Despite this, the gingival tissue levels have been effectively maintained, emphasizing the effectiveness of this implant design for soft tissue support. This may be the result of its minimal submergence, which creates a physical scaffold for the gingival architecture.

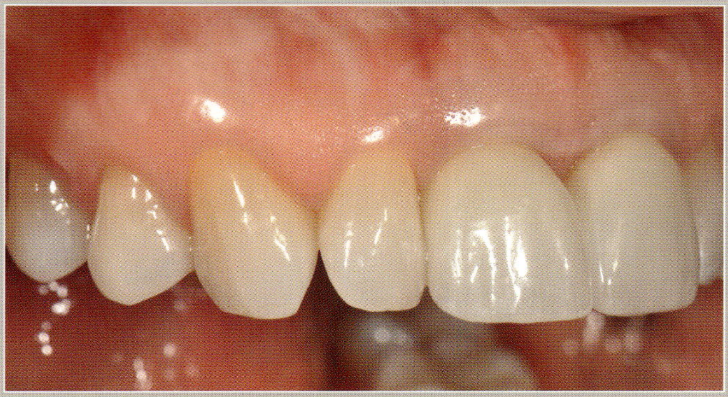

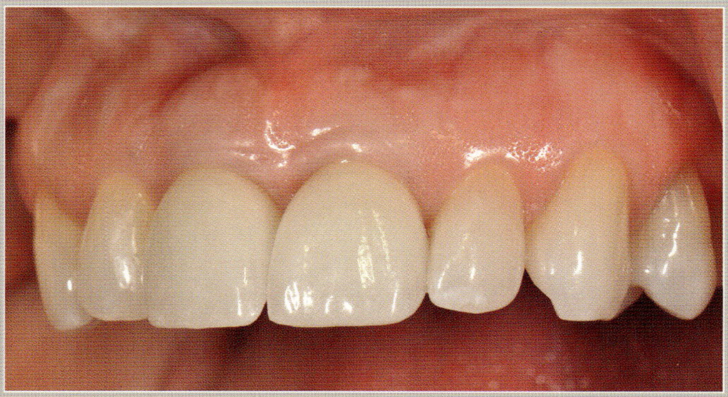

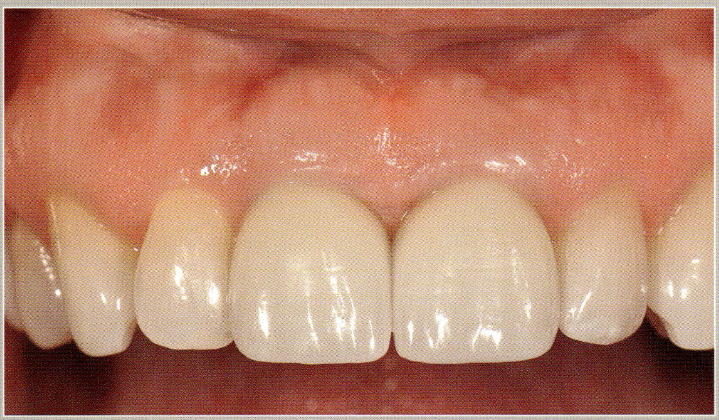

Clinical appearance 6 weeks after delivery of the definitive restorations.

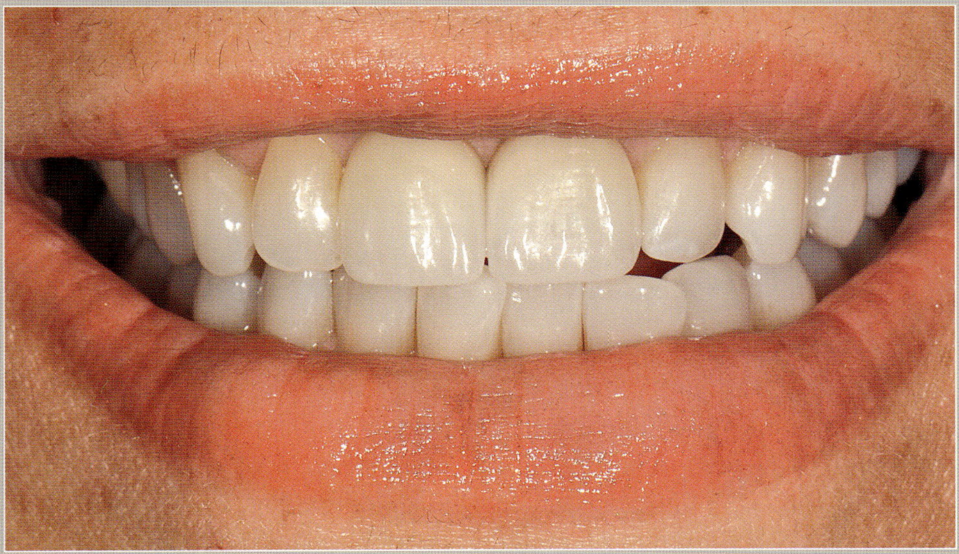

Smile after 5 years in function. Note improvement in the papilla architecture.

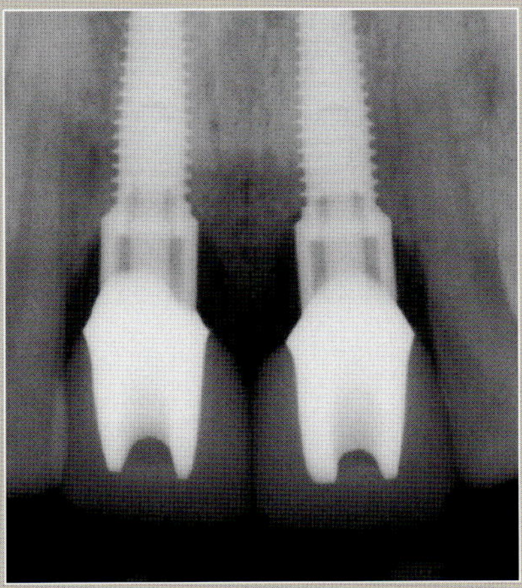

Radiographic view after 5 years in function.

Comparative case 3. Staged or sequenced implant placement: A strategy to improve interimplant bone and gingival form

This 38-year-old healthy man presented for treatment with a primary concern related to his failing maxillary central incisors—tooth no. 8 due to ankylosis and tooth no. 9 due to a deep palatal fracture. He was extremely unhappy with the poor esthetics of the teeth and the disparate gingival levels. He was frustrated by unsuccessful and prolonged ongoing efforts by his dentist to restore these teeth, both of which had been traumatized by a blow to the mouth many years before his consultation. The patient's dentist had attempted to extrude teeth nos. 8 and 9 in order to expose more tooth structure for restoration. Tooth no. 9 had been extruded to some degree, but the palatal fracture was still located 7 mm below the free gingival margin. Tooth no. 8 was ankylosed and could not be extruded. Other dental requirements included replacement of the missing tooth no. 19.

Diagnostic findings included:

- No significant intraoral findings
- High smile line that displays the papillae and free gingival margins
- Occlusion: Class I malocclusion; no overbite or overjet
- Moderate gingival scallop and favorable (thick) tissue phenotype
- Good oral hygiene

The patient's treatment expectations were high. He had consulted with several dentists and specialists prior to accepting treatment in our clinic. The case presented a high esthetic risk because of the high lip line and patient expectations as well as high risk for negative hard and soft tissue changes because of adjacent tooth extraction, with added risk due to the anticipated difficult extraction of tooth no. 8 as a result of ankylosis.

Record collection included periodontal charting, restorative needs assessment, study casts, a diagnostic wax-up, and a preoperative CBCT scan to evaluate the positions of the roots of teeth nos. 8 and 9 and the existing ridge architecture.

Both central incisors were deemed to be unrestorable, tooth no. 8 due to ankylosis and early signs of resorption and tooth no. 9 due to the depth of the palatal fracture. With the information provided, the patient agreed to the extraction of teeth nos. 8 and 9 and their replacement with implants. He was not prepared to consider the preparation of his adjacent teeth nos. 7 and 10 for a fixed partial denture.

Kan and Rungcharassaeng[52] suggested that sequenced implant placement and provisionalization (ie, placement of one implant at a time, with allowance for an osseointegration healing period for the first implant prior to placement of the second) could stabilize the future interimplant papilla when adjacent implant placement is necessary. Their report of six cases suggested promising results with high papilla indices according to Jemt's classification.[53]

We explored this concept in the previous volume of *Interdisciplinary Treatment Planning,*[1] reviewing a case that involved the replacement of adjacent failing central incisors due to horizontal root fractures and associated bone loss. The esthetic results were encouraging, with good tissue form around the implant restorations, including the interimplant papilla. However, this approach has the disadvantage of prolonged treatment time and costs, and, based on this comparative review of four treatment approaches, the results of staged extractions and implant placement are not superior to those of other methods.

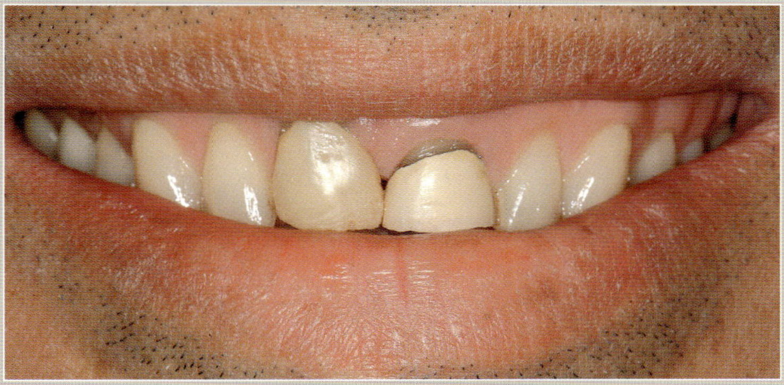

Preoperative view at initial presentation.

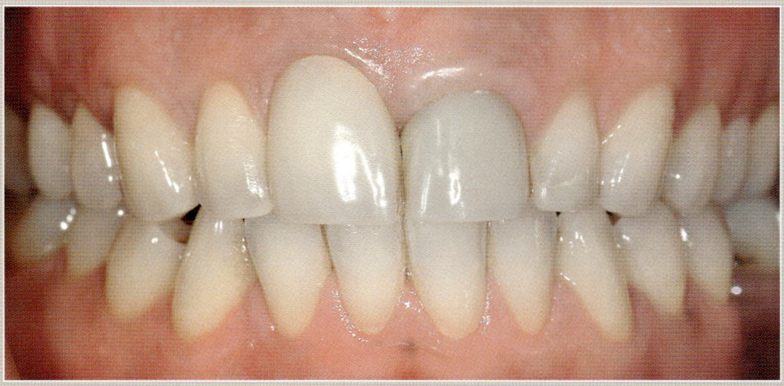

Intraoral view after initial provisionalization.

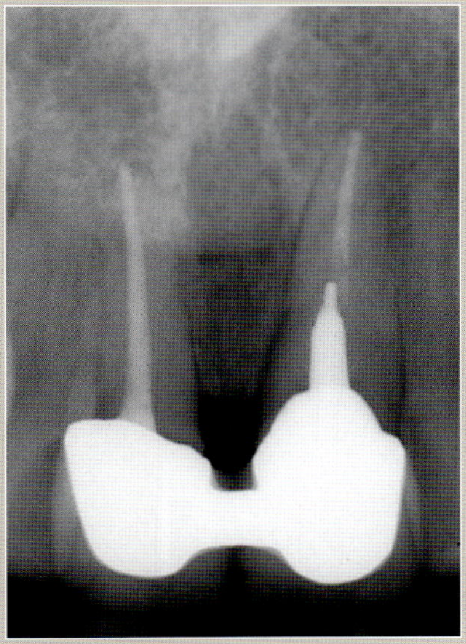

Radiograph taken prior to orthodontic extrusion.

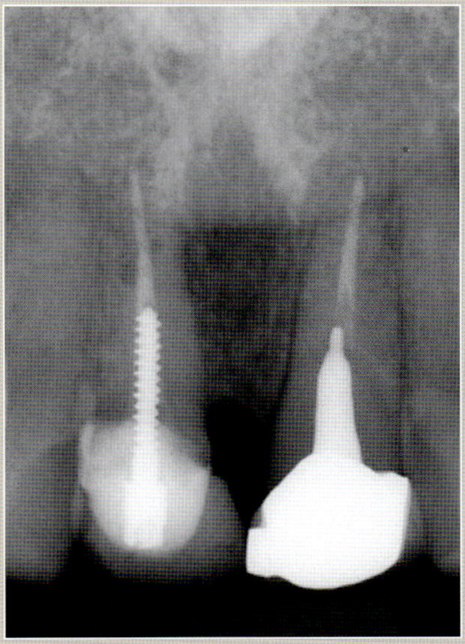

Radiograph taken after orthodontic extrusion but prior to referral.

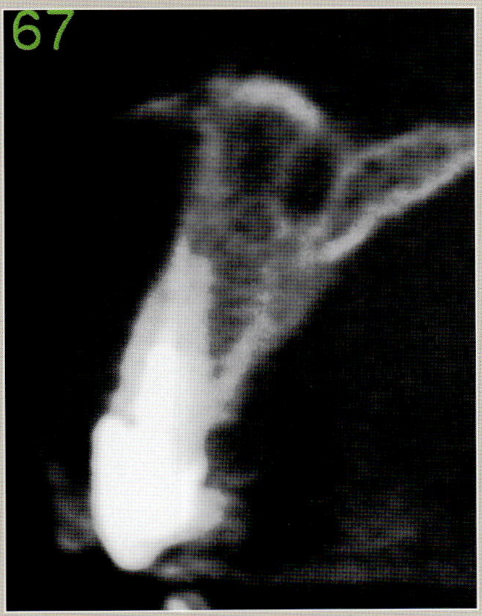

Cross-sectional CBCT image of tooth no. 8.

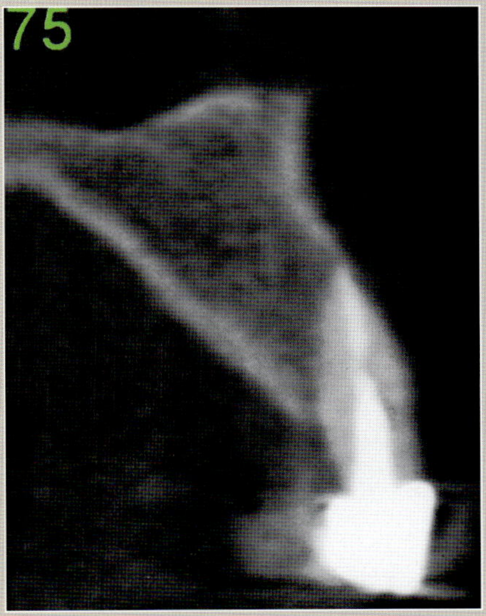

Cross-sectional CBCT image of tooth no. 9.

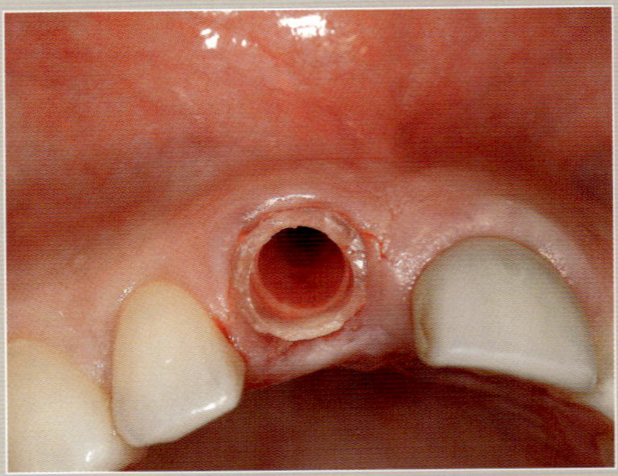

Hollowing of the root of tooth no. 8.

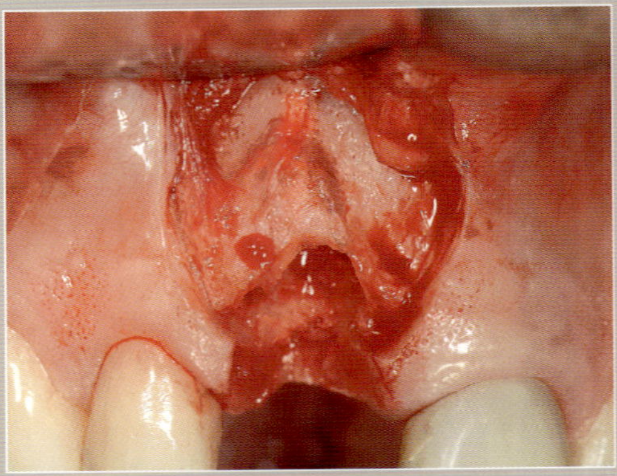

Flap elevation to expose labial aspect of root.

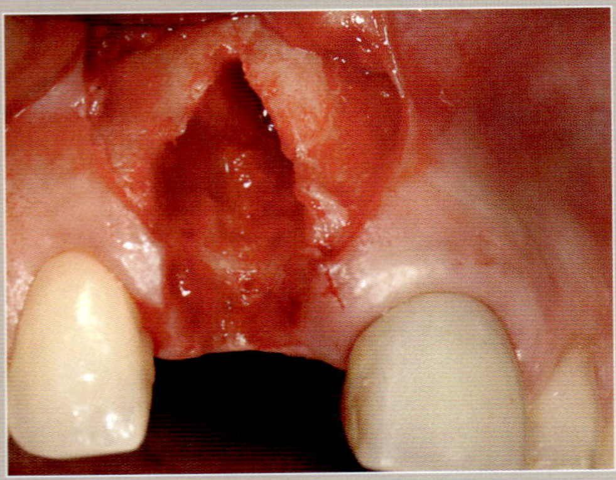

Labial dehiscence resulting from extraction.

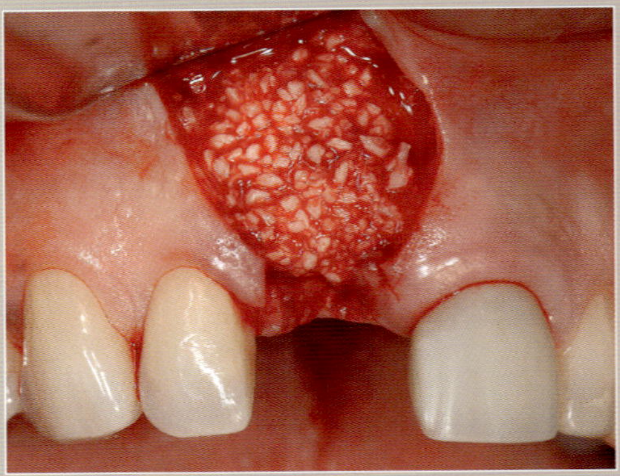

Ridge preservation using a mineralized particulate bone allograft.

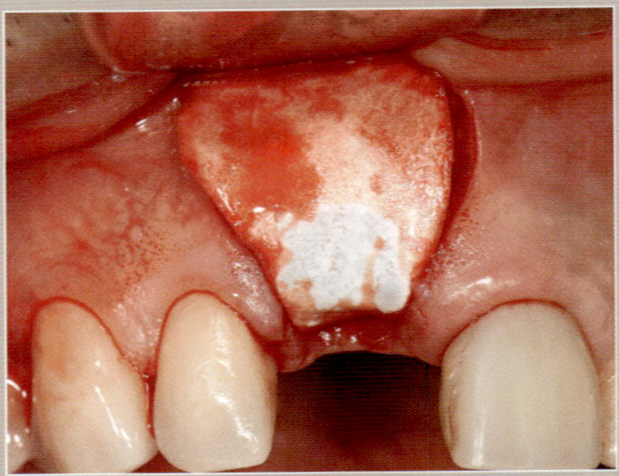

Placement of a resorbable membrane.

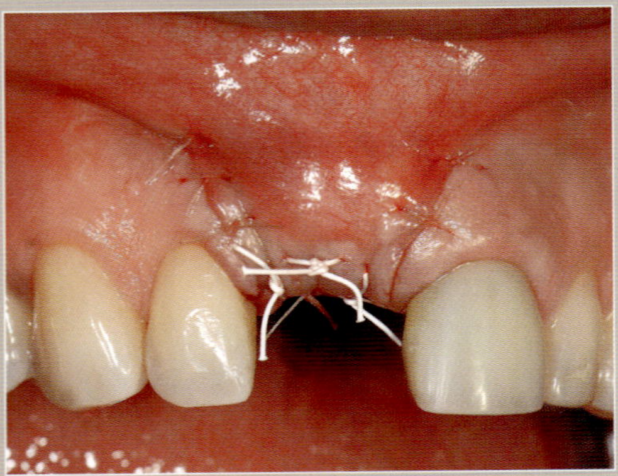

Connective tissue graft adaptation and passive closure of the flap.

Tooth no. 8 was extracted first. The rationale for this was the anticipated difficulty of extraction and risk for adverse bone level changes that could occur with extraction of the ankylosed tooth. The extraction was initiated by hollowing the root using tapered implant drills. When the root structure was sufficiently reduced, the residual walls were infractured using root tip elevators, and all segments were removed. Ultimately, elevation of a flap was necessary because the labial aspect of the root could not effectively be distinguished from bone. A labial dehiscence resulted from the removal process. A ridge preservation procedure was performed to minimize bone changes using a procedure similar to that described by Wang and Tsao.[54] A connective tissue graft was used to seal the socket and to further enhance the phenotype. The crown of tooth no. 8 was modified and splinted as a transitional restoration. The site healed uneventfully during the subsequent 4 months.

Using a conventional preparation protocol, a drilling approach based on medium bone quality, and a conservative flap procedure, a 4.3-mm-wide NobelActive implant was placed. Because the primary implant stability was favorable (70-Ncm insertion torque), a screw-retained restoration was fabricated chairside and torqued to 35 Ncm at the time of surgery. The access hole was sealed with a cotton pellet and flowable composite (Filtek Supreme, 3M ESPE).

After a 3-month integration period for stabilization of the bone and gingival tissues, the adjacent tooth no. 9 was extracted, a 4.3-mm-wide NobelActive implant was placed immediately, and the residual horizontal defect was grafted with Bio-Oss. A screw-retained provisional restoration was placed on the implant. Healing in this site was also uneventful over the next 3 months. At removal of the screw-retained provisional crowns, the development of the gingival architecture could be observed.

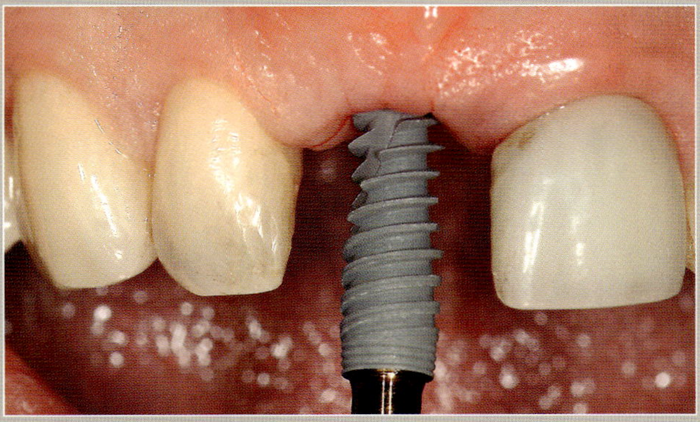

Implant placement in site no. 8.

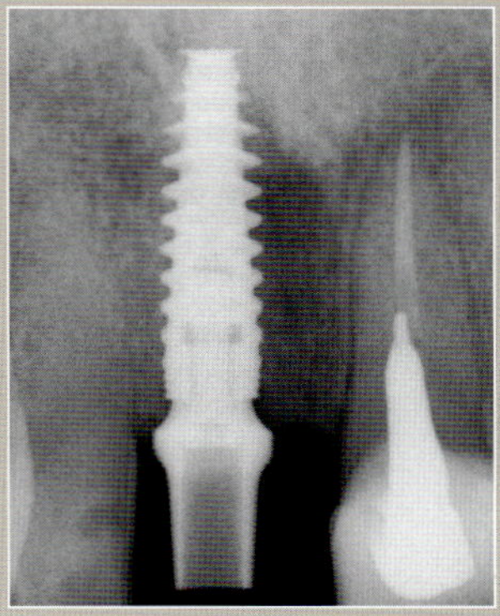

Radiograph following implant placement in site no. 8.

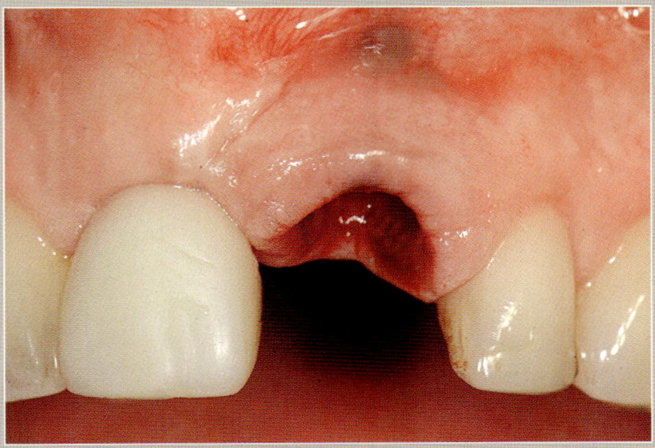

Implant placement in site no. 9.

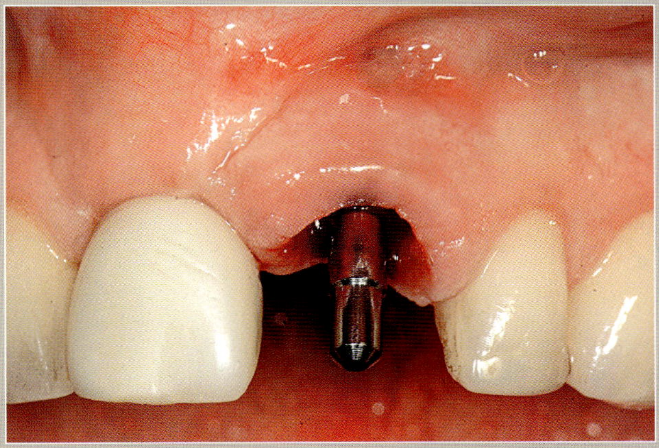

Direction indicator to verify site preparation and projected position of implant.

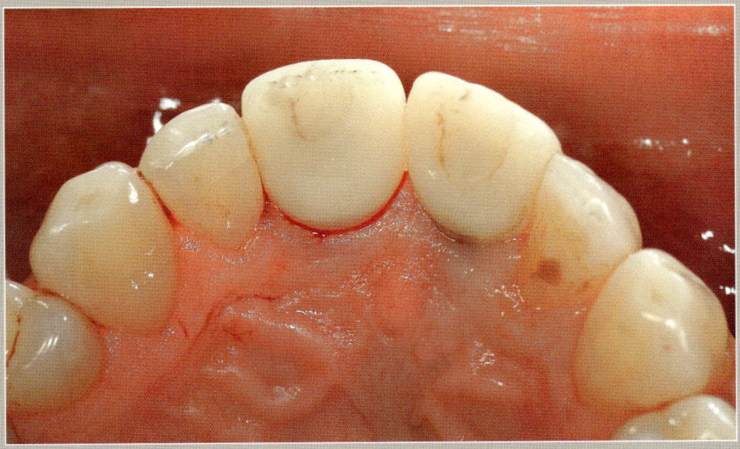

Palatal view immediately after placement of provisional restoration in site no. 9.

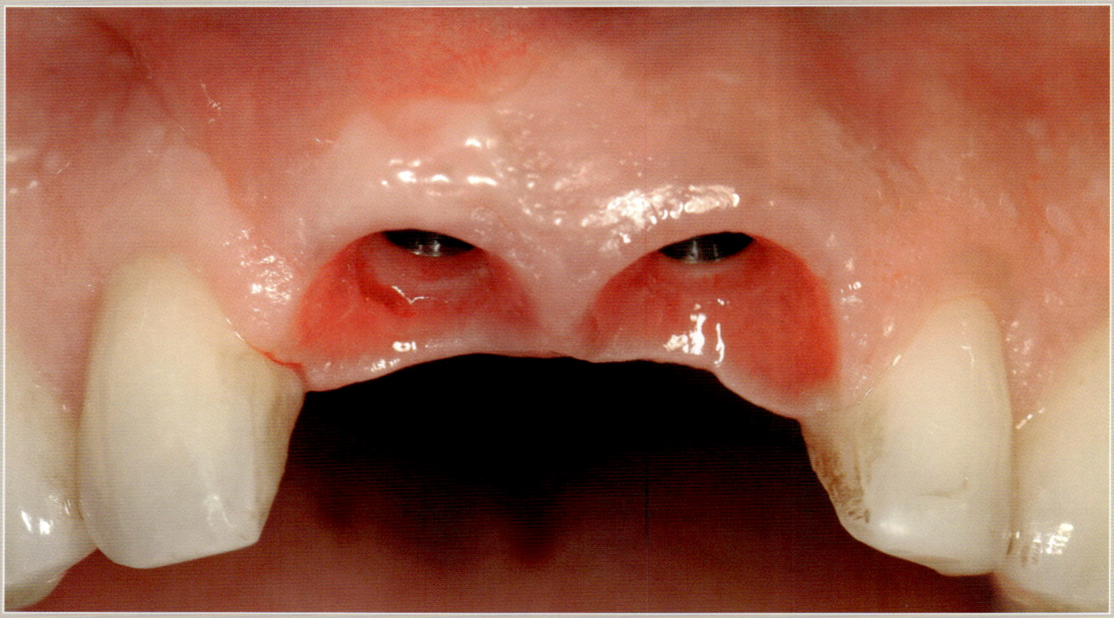

Developed tissue architecture at 12 weeks after placement of second implant.

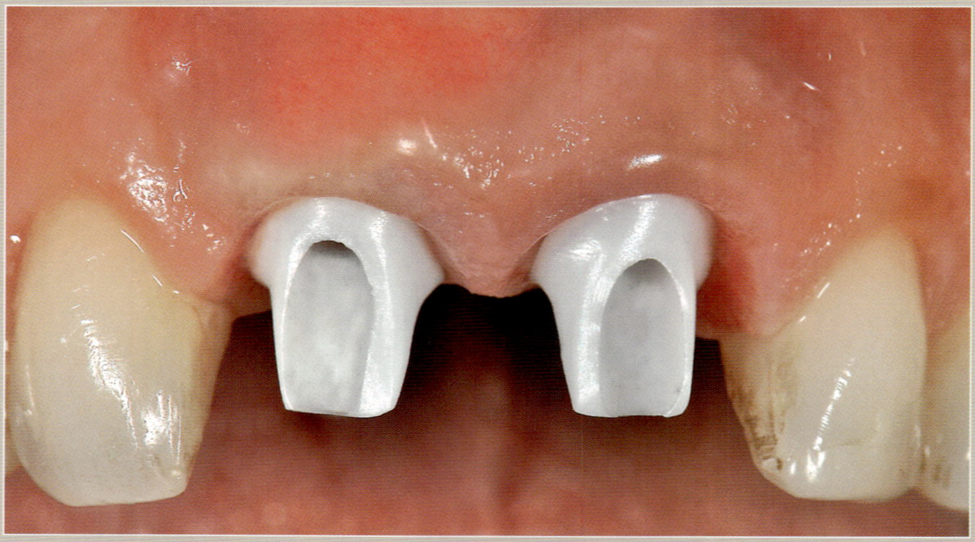

Custom zirconia abutments in position.

Customized impression copings were made for impression of the implants and the developed transmucosal gingival architecture following the integration of the second implant. Custom zirconia abutments and NobelProcera zirconia crowns were made and inserted 4 weeks later. Both were cemented with GC FujiCEM cement (GC) using the cord-deflection technique previously described.

These implants have been monitored uneventfully for more than 3 years. The missing tooth no. 19 has also since been replaced with an implant. It has been monitored for 18 months, again without significant findings. An esthetically acceptable outcome was achieved.

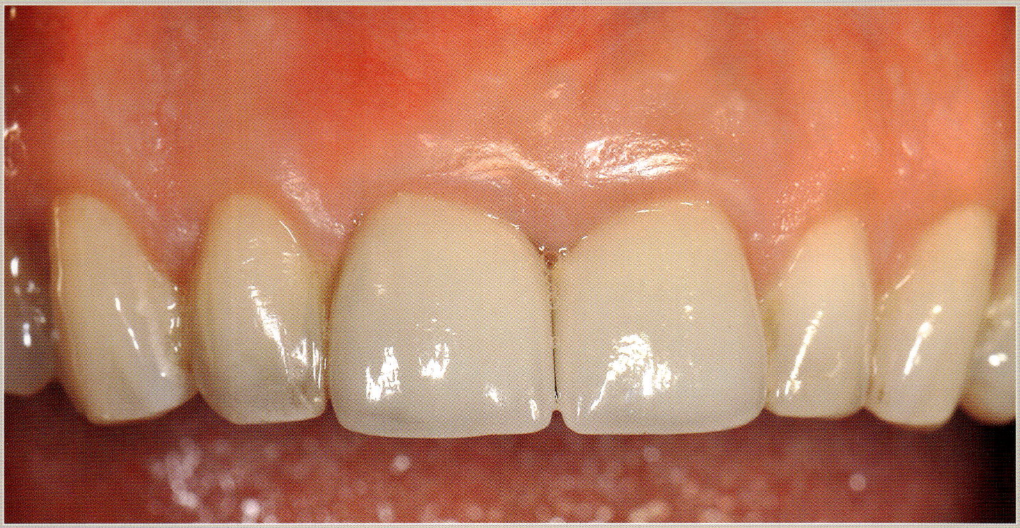

Intraoral view of definitive restorations at the 12-month follow-up.

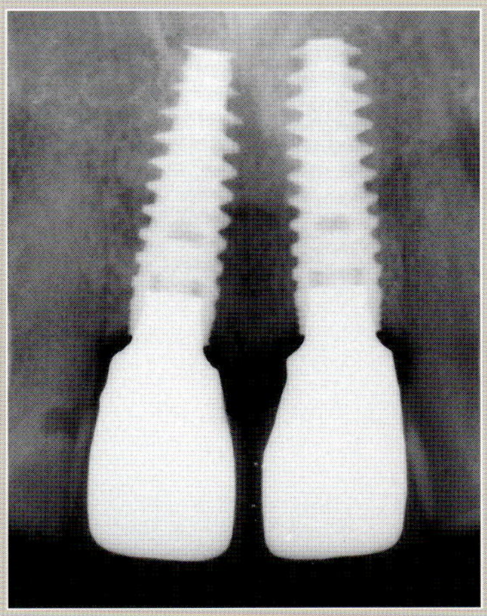

Radiographic view of definitive restorations at the 18-month follow-up.

Unlike Comparative cases 1 and 2, decisions on implant timing were made primarily based on the anticipated difficulty of the extraction of tooth no. 8 and a desire to determine whether a staged approach would preserve the interimplant bone tissue more effectively than extracting both central incisors at the same time. The concept is based on the fact that only one ligamentous area would be disrupted at a time; the bone would be allowed to stabilize around the first implant before the second tooth was removed. What is important to remember is that when extracted teeth are relatively healthy, every effort should be made to preserve the tissue anatomy, regardless of implant placement strategy. This also emphasizes the important role of provisionalization in supporting the gingival tissue framework.

Commentary

Below we summarize our knowledge and understanding of five factors that have a critical impact on the outcome of treatment to replace adjacent teeth with implants in the esthetic zone.

1. Healing of extraction sites

Several studies have shown that extraction site healing includes both resorption of the labial wall of the socket and bone fill within the socket. In a clinical report by Schropp et al,[19] it was reported that the ridge underwent 50% reduction buccolingually and a vertical reduction of up to 2 to 4.5 mm with adjacent tooth extraction. The majority of these changes occurred in the first 4 months postextraction at the buccal aspect of the extraction site. The actual amount of vertical and horizontal ridge resorption is generally greater in multiple adjacent extraction situations compared with the loss of a single tooth.

It becomes clear through the review of these four implant placement and restoration treatment approaches that we have intentionally avoided simultaneous extraction and implant placement in adjacent sites in order to minimize the esthetic complications associated with the increased probability of hard and soft tissue remodeling. Although immediate implant placement and immediate restoration protocols have been shown to be highly successful from an esthetic perspective in single-tooth sites, this approach is less predictable in multiple extraction cases where dimensional changes of greater magnitude are anticipated because an adjacent attachment apparatus is not present. In the case of adjacent implant placement into fresh extraction sockets, there is a lack of predictability in papilla preservation because what happens between the implants is not controlled by the attachment level on adjacent teeth.

2. Delayed, early, immediate, and sequenced implant placement protocols

In the cases presented, we made significant efforts to minimize postextraction ridge changes. In our main case and Comparative case 3, ridge preservation was incorporated into the treatment plans because delayed implant placement protocols were deemed appropriate. In Comparative case 2, early implant placement was carried out 8 weeks postextraction, potentially minimizing the bone remodeling associated with longer healing periods of 4 to 6 months and potentially benefiting from the osteogenic activity of the early healing period. In Comparative case 1, in which immediate implant placement was incorporated in the protocol, an anorganic bone graft was placed in the residual horizontal defect with the goal of reducing the resorption of the labial bone following extraction.

There are advantages and disadvantages for each of the treatment protocols assessed. Each patient must be assessed independently, and risk assessment should be based in part on the projected esthetic outcome.

3. Phenotype and its impact on implant esthetics and tissue stability

Kan and Rungcharassaeng[52] reported more tissue recession following implant restoration in patients with highly scalloped and thin tissues. A retrospective study by Zigdon and Machtei[36] reported on tissue stability following restoration as well as degrees of inflammation and probing depths around implants in tissues of different phenotypes. Their results showed twice as much recession, lower inflammatory mediator levels, and shallower probing depths in cases with thin phenotypes. In contrast, Chen et al[55] found little association between phenotype and labial tissue recession.

In all four treatment plans presented, the phenotype was a factor that was considered, and where it was characterized as thin to moderately thick, connective tissue grafts were incorporated in the surgical protocol with the view that this could improve gingival tissue volume and stability. We worked under the premise that this is even more important when adjacent extractions are necessary and underlying bony volumetric changes are more substantial.

4. Interimplant spacing and implant designs for tissue stability

Gastaldo et al[23] retrospectively assessed the impact of spacing of adjacent implants on the presence of papilla (part or complete fill) versus absence of papilla. They found that spacing of 3 mm, 3.5 mm, and 4 mm between implants resulted in papilla fill, but when the distance was 2 mm or 2.5 mm, the papilla was absent 100% of the time. Other articles suggest that less interimplant spacing may support stable bone levels as evaluated through radiographic follow-up but do not address the impact on papilla architecture postrestoration.[27]

Grunder et al[25] stressed that adequate spacing is a key issue to maintaining an interimplant bone peak to support the papilla but suggest that this can be compensated for, to some degree, by thickening the facial bone to a minimum of 2 mm but optimally up to 4 mm, compensating for the normal crestal saucerization around conventional implants. They also comment that innovative implant designs that incorporate the concept of platform switching are promising for enhancing crestal bone stability. If this promising concept is supported with clinical findings and corroborating research, the issue of adequate interimplant spacing and volume of facial bone will need to be reviewed and modified.

In all four clinical scenarios presented, implants with features that may contribute to enhanced marginal bone stability were used, with greater emphasis on the use of platform-switched implants. In one case, a scalloped implant design was used. Although we have had success with this implant design overall, we discontinued using this implant several years ago because its design resulted in challenging cement removal, and in approximately 25% of our cases, it failed to produce bone levels that were superior to conventional implant designs. In the cases using platform-switched implants, crestal bone stability and elimination of saucerization to the first major implant thread was more consistently noted, with a small number of cases still illustrating crestal bone remodeling. In all cases, interimplant spacing of a minimum of 3 mm was maintained because we felt that the scientific evidence supporting reduced spacing is inadequate at this time.

5. Immediate versus delayed restoration protocols

The nonsubmerged implant placement protocol involves either exposure of a healing abutment to the oral cavity or the placement of an immediate provisional restoration. As discussed earlier, several articles point to the positive role of fixed provisional restorations in the degree of soft tissue development and stability after restoration in comparison with removable appliances, especially when they are delivered at the time of implant placement.

Single-tooth replacement with immediate or delayed implant placement and immediate provisionalization has several requisites that should be considered, including surgical experience and skill, primary stability in a healthy site, and a favorable occlusion to allow for minimal stresses during healing. Thus far, the literature seems to support nonfunctional immediate restoration of single or small edentulous sites, although very few long-term studies are available.[46,56]

Implant placement (delayed or immediate) coupled with immediate restoration was shown in two of our cases to effectively guide soft tissues, resulting in pleasing esthetic results. Patients prefer immediate restoration of implants because this obviates the need for transitional removable appliances; in addition, we find that the high functional and esthetic predictability and progressively shortened healing period are benefits of immediate surgical and restorative treatment protocols in implant therapy.

Conclusion

The selected cases represent commonly used implant placement and restoration protocols in our clinical practice. Bone and soft tissue grafting procedures are routinely incorporated into the surgical phase of treatment because it has been rare to find situations in which bone and gingival quality and quantity are optimal at the start of treatment as a result of damage caused by disease, trauma, or previous treatment. Our conclusion is that there is not one superior treatment methodology over another. Patient health, the clinical and radiographic presentation, and patient expectations must be assessed, weighing the risks for treatment in each of these areas: the perceived risk for ridge resorption as it relates to extraction, the effect on implant stability, and the requirements for adjunctive regenerative procedures on implant placement timing, as well as the impact of occlusion, parafunction, and patient cooperation on the selection of a restoration protocol.

What we have come to appreciate is that most anterior adjacent implant cases will fit into at least one of these four protocols or permutations of them, provided that a careful initial diagnosis is made. Several years ago, the replacement of a single missing anterior tooth was a demanding treatment. Today, when the clinician has an intimate understanding of the literature, single implant placement in the maxillary esthetic zone where adjacent teeth have healthy periodontium represents far less of a challenge, given adherence to several key steps. However, adjacent implants still represent the most difficult clinical scenario in terms of normalizing the interimplant papilla form with current surgical and restorative concepts, implant designs, and treatment plan options. Recognizing the indications and limitations of each treatment approach discussed in this chapter will help guide the clinician in the decision-making and treatment processes. This is precisely how we treatment plan each case.

ACKNOWLEDGMENTS

Our most sincere thanks for the tireless efforts of our incredibly talented technicians Hans Forssander, David Choo, Steve Mori, and Aki Miyazaki. We also want to thank our remarkable primary assistants Christine Thirlwell and Stacey Esau, who work closely with us every day.

REFERENCES

1. Leziy S, Miller B. Esthetics in implant therapy: A blueprint for success. In: Cohen M (ed). Interdisciplinary Treatment Planning: Principles, Design, Implementation. Chicago: Quintessence, 2008:81–122.
2. Simonis P, Dufour T, Tenenbaum H. Long-term implant survival and success: A 10–16-year follow-up of non-submerged dental implants. Clin Oral Implants Res 2010;21:772–777.
3. Jung RE, Pjetursson BE, Glauser R, Zembic A, Zwahlen M, Lang NP. A systematic review of the 5-year survival and complication rates of implant-supported single crowns. Clin Oral Implants Res 2008;19:119–130.
4. Belser UC, Buser D, Hess D, Schmid B, Bernard JP, Lang NP. Aesthetic implant restorations in partially edentulous patients—A critical appraisal. Periodontol 2000 1998;17:132–150.
5. Kois JC. Predictable single tooth peri-implant esthetics: Five diagnostic keys. Compend Contin Educ Dent 2001;22:199–206.
6. Kan JY, Rungcharassaeng K, Umezu K, Kois JC. Dimensions of peri-implant mucosa: An evaluation of maxillary anterior single implants in humans. J Periodontol 2003;74:557–562.
7. Belser UC, Schmid B, Higginbottom F, Buser D. Outcome analysis of implant restorations located in the anterior maxilla: A review of the recent literature. Int J Oral Maxillofac Implants 2004;19(suppl):30–42.
8. Buser D, Martin W, Belser UC. Optimizing esthetics for implant restorations in the anterior maxilla: Anatomic and surgical considerations. Int J Oral Maxillofac Implants 2004;19(suppl):43–61.
9. Evans CD, Chen ST. Esthetic outcomes of immediate implant placements. Clin Oral Implants Res 2008;10:73–80.
10. Meijer HJA, Stellingsma K, Meijndert L, Raghoebar GM. A new index for rating aesthetics of implant-supported single crowns and adjacent soft tissues—The Implant Crown Aesthetic Index. Clin Oral Implants Res 2005;16:645–649.
11. Fürhauser R, Florescu D, Benesch T, Haas R, Mailath G, Watzek G. Evaluation of soft tissue around single-tooth implant crowns: The pink esthetic score. Clin Oral Implants Res 2005;16:639–644.
12. Choquet V, Hermans M, Adriaenssens P, Daelemans P, Tarnow DP, Malevez C. Clinical and radiographic evaluation of the papilla level adjacent to single-tooth dental implants. A retrospective study in the maxillary anterior region. J Periodontol 2001;72:1364–1371.
13. Oates TW, West J, Jones J, Kaiser D, Cochran DL. Long-term changes in soft tissue height on the facial surface of dental implants. Implant Dent 2002;11:272–279.
14. Tarnow D, Elian N, Fletcher P, et al. Vertical distance from the crest of bone to the height of the interproximal papilla between adjacent implants. J Periodontol 2003;74:1785–1788.
15. Lee DW, Park KH, Moon IS. Dimension of keratinized mucosa and the interproximal papilla between adjacent implants. J Periodontol 2005;76:1856–1860.

16. Cardaropoli G, Lekholm U, Wennström JL. Tissue alterations at implant-supported single-tooth replacements: A 1-year prospective clinical study. Clin Oral Implants Res 2006;17:165–171.
17. Kourkouta S, Dedi KD, Paquette DW, Mol A. Interproximal tissue dimensions in relation to adjacent implants in the anterior maxilla: Clinical observations and patient aesthetic evaluation. Clin Oral Implants Res 2009;20:1375–1385.
18. Chow YC, Wang HL. Factors and techniques influencing peri-implant papillae. Implant Dent 2010;19:208–219.
19. Schropp L, Wenzel A, Kostopoulos L, Karring T. Bone healing and soft tissue contour changes following single tooth extraction: A clinical and radiographic 12-month prospective study. Int J Periodontics Restorative Dent 2003;23:313–323.
20. Araújo MG, Lindhe J. Dimensional ridge alterations following tooth extraction. An experimental study in the dog. J Clin Periodontol 2005;32:212–218.
21. Nevins M, Camelo M, De Paoli S, et al. A study of the fate of the buccal wall of extraction sockets of teeth with prominent roots. Int J Periodontics Restorative Dent 2006;26:19–29.
22. Tarnow DP, Cho SC, Wallace SS. The effect of inter-implant distance on the height of inter-implant bone crest. J Periodontol 2000;71:546–549.
23. Gastaldo JF, Cury PR, Sendyk WR. Effect of the vertical and horizontal distances between adjacent implants and between a tooth and an implant on the incidence of interproximal papilla. J Periodontol 2004;75:1242–1246.
24. Spray RJ, Black CG, Morris HR, Ochi S. The influence of bone thickness on facial marginal bone response: Stage 1 placement through stage 2 uncovering. Ann Periodontol 2000;5:119–128.
25. Grunder U, Gracis S, Capelli M. Influence of the 3-D bone-to-implant relationship on esthetics. Int J Periodontics Restorative Dent 2005;25:113–119.
26. Becker J, Ferrari D, Herten M, Kirsch A, Schaer A, Schwarz F. Influence of platform switching on crestal bone changes at non-submerged titanium implants: A histomorphometrical study in dogs. J Clin Periodontol 2007;34:1089–1096.
27. Rodriguez-Ciurana X, Vela-Nebot X, Segala-Torres M, et al. The effect of interimplant distance on the height of the interimplant bone crest when using platform-switched implants. Int J Periodontics Restorative Dent 2009;29:141–151.
28. Kielbassa AM, Martinez-de Fuentes R, Goldstein M, et al. Randomized controlled trial comparing a variable-thread novel tapered and a standard tapered implant: Interim one-year results. J Prosthet Dent 2009;101:293–305.
29. Abrahamsson I, Berglundh T, Lindhe J. The mucosal barrier following abutment dis/reconnection. An experimental study in dogs. J Clin Periodontol 1997;24:568–572.
30. Leziy SS, Miller BA. Prefabricated zirconia abutments: Surgical advantages, indications and handling considerations. Quintessence Dent Technol 2008;31:95–104.
31. Jung RE, Sailer I, Hämmerle CH, Attin T, Schmidlin P. In vitro color changes of soft tissues caused by restorative materials. Int J Periodontics Restorative Dent 2007;27:251–257.
32. Watkin A, Kerstein RB. Improving darkened anterior peri-implant tissue color with zirconia custom implant abutments. Compend Contin Educ Dent 2008;29:238–240.
33. Koutayas SO, Vagkopoulou T, Pelekanos S, Koidis P, Strub JR. Zirconia in dentistry: Part 2. Evidence-based clinical breakthrough. Eur J Esthet Dent 2009;4:348–380.
34. Leziy S, Miller B. Replacement of adjacent missing anterior teeth with scalloped implants: A case report. Pract Proced Aesthet Dent 2005;17:331–338.
35. Esposito M, Grusovin MG, Felice P, Karatzopoulos G, Worthington HV, Coulthard P. The efficacy of horizontal and vertical bone augmentation procedures for dental implants—A Cochrane systematic review. Eur J Oral Implantol 2009;2:167–184.
36. Zigdon H, Machtei EE. The dimensions of keratinized mucosa around implants affect clinical and immunological parameters. Clin Oral Implants Res 2008;19:387–392.
37. Wallace S, Gellin R. Clinical evaluation of a cancellous block allograft for ridge augmentation and implant placement: A case report. Implant Dent 2008;12:151–158.
38. Nissan J, Mardinger O, Calderon S, Romanos GE, Chaushu G. Cancelllous bone block allografts for augmentation of the anterior atrophic maxilla. Clin Implant Dent Relat Res 2011;13:104–111.
39. Wassdorp J, Reynolds MA. Allogenic bone onlay grafts for alveolar ridge augmentation: A systematic review. Int J Oral Maxillofac Implants 2010;25:525–531.

40. Simion M, Masitano U, Salvato A. Treatment of dehiscences and fenestration around dental implants using resorbable and non-resorbable membranes associated with bone autografts: A comparative clinical study. Int J Oral Maxillofac Implants 1997;12:159–167.
41. Beitlitum I, Artzi Z, Nemcovsky CE. Clinical evaluation of particulate allogeneic with and without autogenous bone grafts and resorbable collagen membranes for bone augmentation of atrophic alveolar ridges. Clin Oral Implants Res 2010;21:1242–1250.
42. Salama MA, Ishikawa T, Salama H, Funato A, Garber D. The advantages of root submergence technique for pontic site development in esthetic implant therapy. Int J Periodontics Restorative Dent 2007;27:521–527.
43. Atieh MA, Ibrahim HM, Atieh AH. Platform switching for marginal bone preservation around dental implants: A systematic review and meta-analysis. J Periodontol 2010;81:1350–1366.
44. Novaes AB Jr, Barros RR, Muglia VA, Borges GJ. Influence of interimplant distances and placement depth on papilla formation and crestal resorption: A clinical and radiographic study in dogs. J Oral Implantol 2009;35:18–27.
45. Block MS, Mercante DE, Lirette D, Mohamed W, Ryser M, Castellon P. Prospective evaluation of immediate and delayed provisional single tooth restorations. J Oral Maxillofac Surg 2009;67(11 suppl):89–107.
46. De Rouck T, Collys K, Wyn I, Cosyn J. Instant provisionalization of immediate single-tooth implants is essential to optimize esthetic treatment outcome. Clin Oral Implants Res 2009;20:566–570.
47. Wennström JL, Ekestubbe A, Gröndahl K, Karlsson S, Lindhe J. Oral rehabilitation with implant-supported fixed partial dentures in periodontitis-susceptible subjects. A 5-year prospective study. J Clin Periodontol 2004;31:713–724.
48. Karoussis IK, Salvi GE, Heitz-Mayfield LJ, Brägger U, Hämmerle CH, Lang NP. Long-term implant prognosis in patients with and without a history of chronic periodontitis: A 10-year prospective cohort study of the ITI Dental Implant System. Clin Oral Implants Res 2003;14:329–339.
49. Mengel R, Flores-de-Jacoby L. Implants in regenerated bone in patients treated for generalized aggressive periodontitis: A prospective longitudinal study. Int J Periodontics Restorative Dent 2005;25:331–341.
50. Alves CC, Correia AR, Neves M. Immediate implants and immediate loading in periodontally compromised patients—A 3-year prospective clinical study. Int J Periodontics Restorative Dent 2010;30:447–455.
51. Hürzeler MB, Fickl S, Zuhr O, Wachtel H. Clinical failures and shortfalls of immediate implant procedures. Eur J Esthet Dent 2006;1:128–140.
52. Kan JY, Rungcharassaeng K. Interimplant papilla preservation in the esthetic zone: A report of six consecutive cases. Int J Periodontics Restorative Dent 2003;23:249–259.
53. Jemt T. Regeneration of gingival papillae after single-implant treatment. Int J Periodontics Restorative Dent 1997;17:326–333.
54. Wang HL, Tsao YP. Histologic evaluation of socket augmentation with mineralized human allograft. Int J Periodontics Restorative Dent 2008;28:231–237.
55. Chen ST, Darby IB, Reynolds EC. A prospective clinical study of non-submerged immediate implants: Clinical outcomes and esthetic results. Clin Oral Implants Res 2007;18:552–562.
56. Esposito M, Grusovin MG, Polyzois IP, Felice P, Worthington HV. Interventions for replacing missing teeth: Dental implants in fresh extraction sockets (immediate, immediate-delayed and delayed implants). Cochrane Database Syst Rev 2010;8(9):CD005968.

5

Smile Design: From Digital Treatment Planning to Clinical Reality

Christian Coachman, DDS, CDT
Eric Van Dooren, DDS
Galip Gürel, MSc
Cobi J. Landsberg, DMD
Marcelo A. Calamita, DDS, MSD, PhD
Nitzan Bichacho, DMD

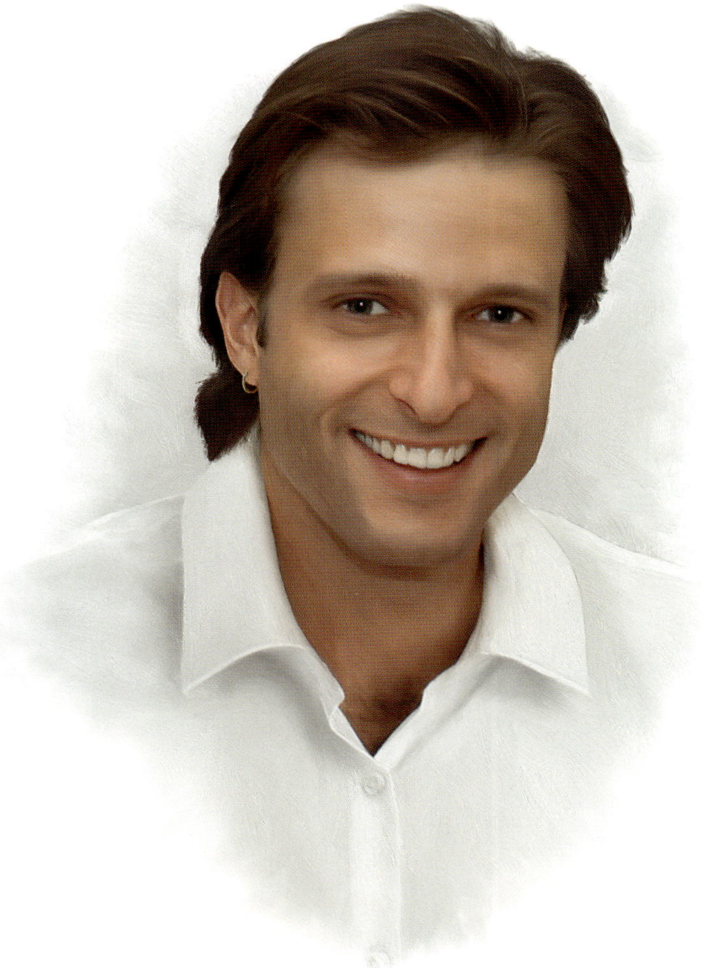

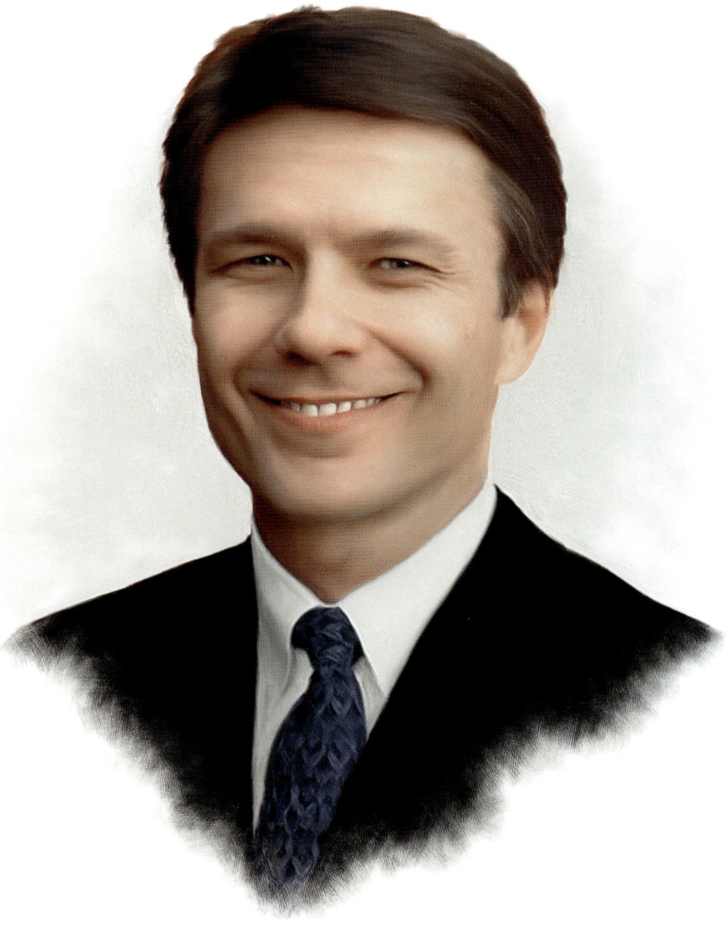

Editor's Introduction

One of dentistry's most challenging dilemmas relates to whether or not we can actually meet or exceed patients' expectations for treatment in the esthetic zone. The world's most prominent clinician-lecturers would have you believe so. Dental publications, advertisements, and media saturation also dramatically increase patient expectations. The reality is that this may not be the case.

Professional audiences are dazzled by bone and soft tissue augmentation procedures that result in exquisite dental outcomes and engaging smiles. But are these results reproducible chairside each and every day? Are there limits to what is actually achievable? What can we promise our patients, if anything?

This chapter addresses severe deformities and failure in the esthetic zone. There are no "magic bullets" here. Compromise is an integral part of the treatment landscape, and part of this process is setting realistic expectations with the patient before any treatment is instituted. And yet, with new diagnostic methodologies, the introduction of digital treatment planning, and masterful laboratory procedures, even compromise can result in stunning results and delighted patients.

The suite of cases presented in this chapter by three master clinicians and a dedicated team of master laboratory technicians all have been designed with compromise in mind, readily accepting that the "ideal" is not readily achievable or even possible. Practicality prevails, and with some ingenuity (use of the concept of "smile design"), effective communication in a collaborative team setting, and an understanding patient, treatment results can be quite gratifying.

Drs Christian Coachman and Marcelo Calamita first introduce the reader to the concept of smile design. Drs Bichacho, Landsberg, Gürel, and Van Dooren then offer cases for the reader to treatment plan, incorporating the concept of smile design into their presentations. Finally, Drs Coachman and Calamita describe in the Commentary section the practical aspects and workflow of digital smile design (DSD). Dr Coachman provided the laboratory support for all of the treatment-planning cases. He has been the conceiver and link to the treatment modality employed by each clinician in achieving these remarkable outcomes.

Authors' Introduction

With the increasing demand for highly customized treatment in contemporary esthetic dentistry, it is paramount to incorporate tools that can strengthen our diagnostic vision, improve the communication between the team members, and create predictable systems throughout the smile design process and treatment.

In order to obtain consistent outcomes, the design of the restorations should be defined as soon as all diagnostic data is gathered, guiding the subsequent phases of the rehabilitation.[1] Every work of art requires an initial visualization: In architecture, painting, or sculpture, it is necessary to make use of plans, drafts, or prototypes. They are two-dimensional (2D) or three-dimensional (3D) representations of the final outcome, and once developed, they will guide the processes of drawing, modeling, and building. Similarly, in dentistry, all of the patient's needs and desires and functional and biologic issues must be scientifically incorporated into the esthetic treatment design and serve as a frame of reference for all of the treatment that will be performed.[2,3]

The aim of this chapter is to present a unique concept of 2D DSD, which will provide important parameters to guide an effective 3D diagnostic wax-up. The DSD is based on the use of high-quality digital images—static and dynamic—that are essential for analysis, documentation, and communication in contemporary esthetic dentistry[4] and can also be used as a basis to perform a series of diagnostic procedures, adding critical data to the process of treatment planning.

Prior to treatment planning the cases in this chapter, the reader should understand the concept and diagnostic rationale of DSD. DSD allows a gradual discovery of many critical factors involved in simple or complex restorative cases that might have been overlooked during the clinical, photographic, or study cast evaluation. The drawing of reference lines and shapes over high-quality images on a computer screen following a predetermined sequence widens the diagnostic vision and helps the team measure limitations and risk factors such as asymmetries, disharmonies, and violations of esthetic principles. Choosing the appropriate technique is easier once the problem has been identified and the solution clearly visualized.

The DSD protocol is characterized by effective communication between the interdisciplinary team members, including the dental technician. It is also an amazing tool for communication with patients, enabling them to better visualize the issues and possible solution, balancing their expectations, and increasing their commitment to and trust in the team. By increasing understanding of the issues involved, the clinician can better explain the treatment plan, transforming future retrospective excuses into prospective explanations. Team members can identify and highlight discrepancies in soft or hard tissue morphology, discussing—with the aid of digitally magnified and measured images on the monitor—the best possible solutions for the case. Every team member can add information directly on the slides, in writing or using voiceover, simplifying the process even more. All team members can access this information whenever necessary, changing or adding new elements during the diagnostic and treatment phases. The use of the DSD can make the diagnosis more effective and the treatment planning more complete, and the effort required to implement it is rewarded as the treatment sequence becomes more logical and straightforward, time and materials are saved, and the costs of treatment are reduced.

The following cases have been chosen for treatment planning in this chapter because they present significant challenges in achieving optimal esthetic outcomes. Compromise was accepted in all of these cases, and yet with meticulous and careful analysis of the diagnostic information and some extremely well-organized and creative planning, exceptional outcomes were achieved. Compromise is not necessarily akin to defeat. It should be considered an opportunity to achieve gratifying treatment results using alternative methods. Each case has its own unique lessons to be shared with the reader.

The first case presentation focuses on the advantages of performing a precise esthetic analysis through digital photography and digital design. The lines and drawings clearly illustrate the challenges and provide very important insights into potential solutions. The patient's focus was short treatment duration because her wedding was scheduled in 3 months.

The second case presentation shows the advantages of performing a white and pink mock-up to communicate to the patient the esthetic issues to be faced in treatment. This case also addresses the importance of understanding both tooth morphology for proper shaping of the teeth as well as gingival design. The patient's main objective was to achieve the best possible esthetic outcome despite past negative dental experiences.

The third and final case presentation shows the importance of the diagnostic wax-up in guiding treatment planning and in visualizing the defect and the challenges that the clinician is going to face. The wax-up also guides the fabrication of acceptable provisional restorations and surgical stents. The patient's focus was minimally invasive treatment because of previous traumatic dental experiences.

Prosthetic Challenges Associated with the Implant-Supported Restoration in a Deficient Ridge

Nitzan Bichacho, DMD
Cobi J. Landsberg, DMD

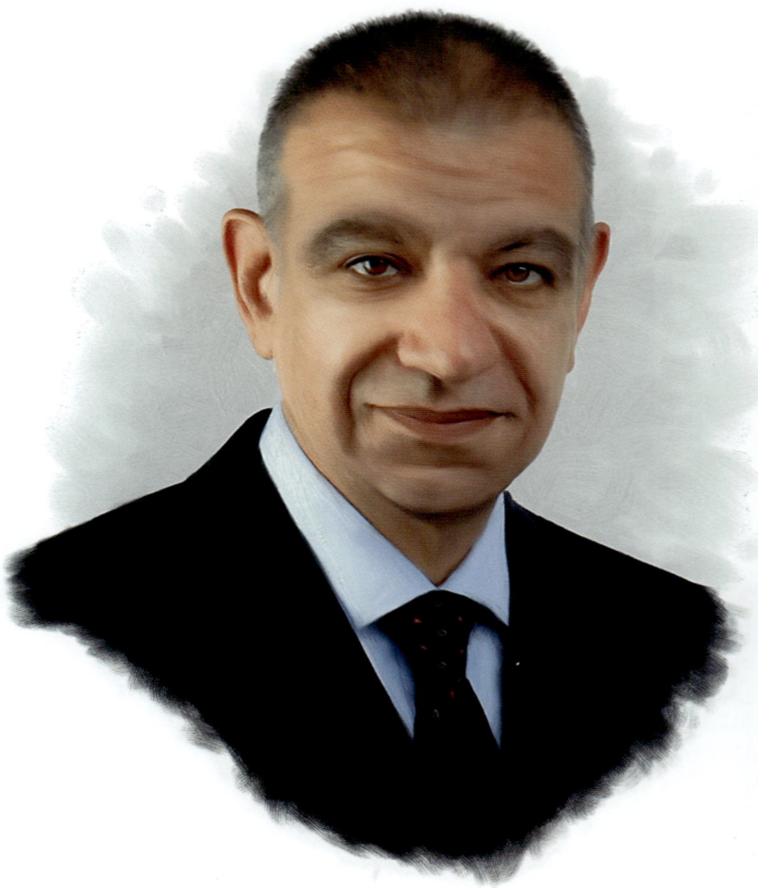

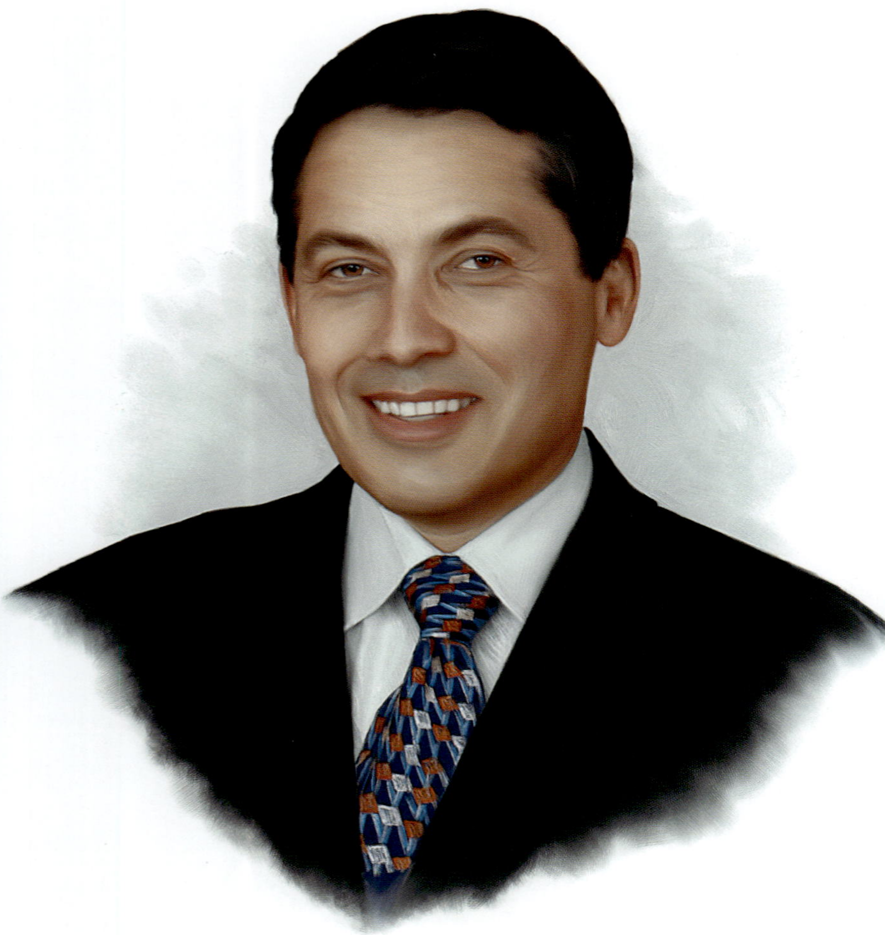

Treating missing teeth in the esthetic zone is always a challenge when improved function and a natural appearance are the primary goals. When the supporting tissue foundation is impaired, the risks associated with the treatment become much higher and the outcomes considerably more speculative.

We chose this case because it exemplifies realistic clinical quandaries that we confront in practice every day. It also represents what is possible when obstacles are formidable and options few.

This case presentation combines some initial treatment that was performed in the late 1990s with more recent dental implant therapy and underscores the attendant challenges with ridge deficiencies in the esthetic zone. The treatment of three missing maxillary incisors with implant-supported restorations is described and analyzed. The surgical and prosthetic phases of the treatment resulted in a compromised outcome, and 10 years later the treatment site was prosthetically re-treated.

Case Presentation 1

Treating clinicians
Prosthodontist: Nitzan Bichacho, DMD
Periodontist and implant surgeon: Cobi J. Landsberg, DMD
Dental laboratory and smile designer: Christian Coachman, DDS, CDT

Clinical Treatment Planning

Age at initial presentation: 17 years
Initial presentation: November 1998
Active treatment completed: August 2010

Introduction and background

A 17-year-old girl presented to the clinic unhappy with her appearance after prolonged orthodontic treatment. She was in a car accident a year earlier that resulted in a fracture of the right condyle, loss of tooth no. 8, and intrusive luxation and mesial displacement of tooth no. 9. This tooth had not lost its vitality. After a year of intensive dental care she was quite discouraged by the orthodontic result, making her reluctant to smile.

Medical history

- Noncontributory

Diagnostic findings

Extraoral and facial findings

- High lip line
- Maxillary midline shifted to the right
- Noticeable anterior ridge deficiency where tooth no. 8 had been lost

Intraoral findings

Dental

- Tooth no. 9 apically displaced
- Open occlusal relationship in the central incisor area
- Disproportionate sizes of the one remaining maxillary central incisor and the pontic that had replaced missing tooth no. 8 and was attached to the archwire
- Missing tooth no. 8 and significantly reduced tissue volume
- Apically displaced tooth no. 9 shifted and tilted to the right, with a disproportionately large tooth crown compared with the other natural teeth

Periodontal

- Generally healthy periodontium
- Significant ridge resorption in tooth no. 9 area

Occlusal notes

- Not able to accurately assess centric relation (CR) and centric occlusion (CO) due to previous orthodontic therapy
- Tongue thrust evident upon swallowing
- Moderate vertical and horizontal overlap evident with exception of apically displaced tooth no. 9

Radiographic findings

- Apically positioned tooth no. 9 exhibited a short root with presentation of a minimal periodontal ligament space and appeared ankylosed
- Tooth no. 7 showed a short root with internal and external cervical resorption
- Tooth no. 8 missing

Pretreatment

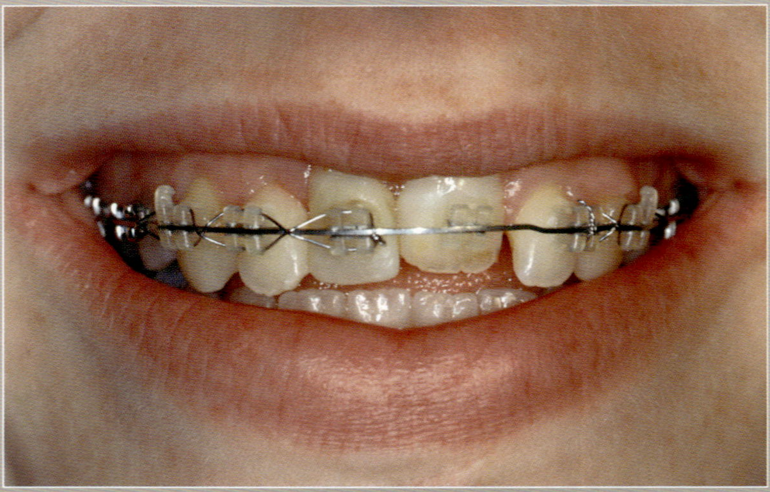

Smile view.

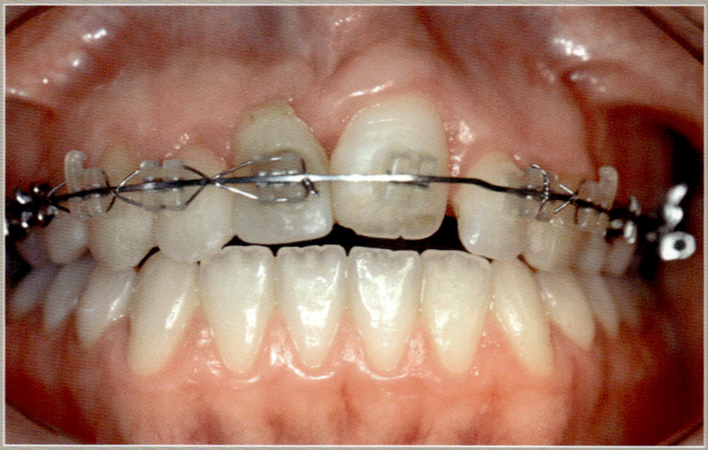

Intraoral frontal view.

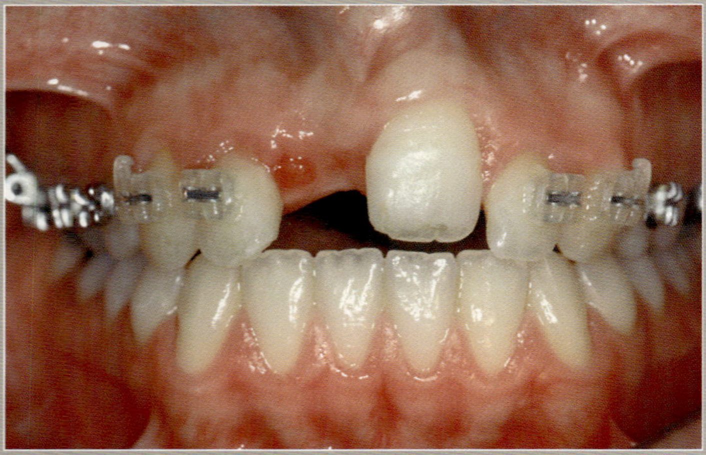

Removal of the archwire and pontic.

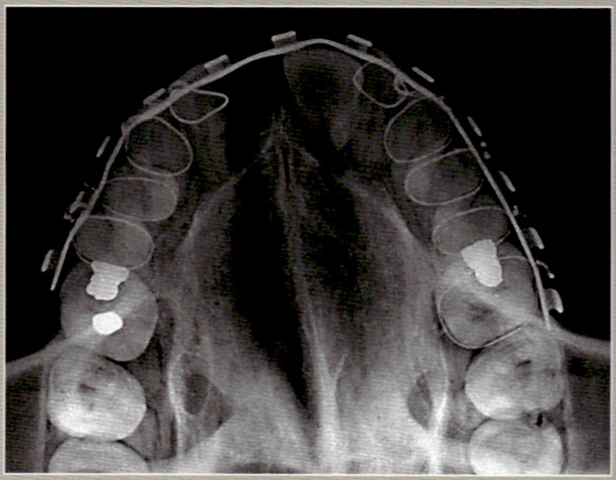

Occlusal radiograph of the maxilla.

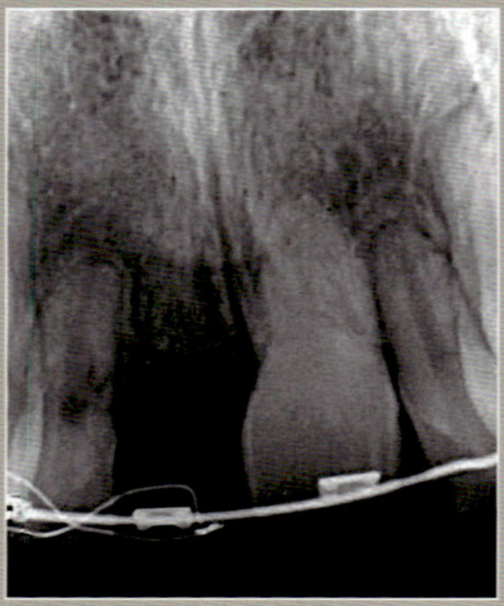

Periapical radiograph of maxillary anterior teeth.

Diagnosis and prognosis

- AAP Type II
- Tooth no. 7: hopeless because of a short root and cervical root resorption
- Tooth no. 8: missing with residual ridge defect
- Tooth no. 9: hopeless from a restorative perspective because it is ankylosed and malpositioned
- Tongue thrust

Summary of concerns

1. With the anterior ridge deficiency in the area of tooth no. 9 and the prospect of possible esthetic compromise, would the treating clinicians be able to meet or exceed the patient's treatment expectations?
2. How much could realistically be gained from vertical ridge augmentation and would it be possible to reconstruct the edentulous ridge to reestablish all that had been lost from the traumatic injury?

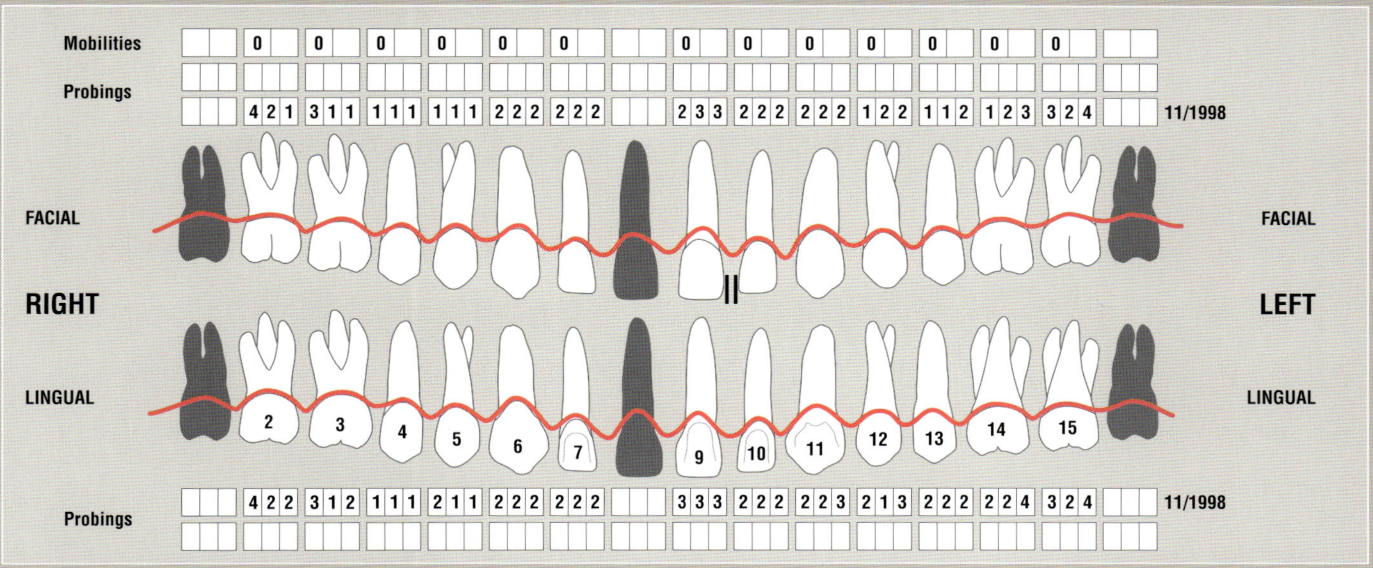

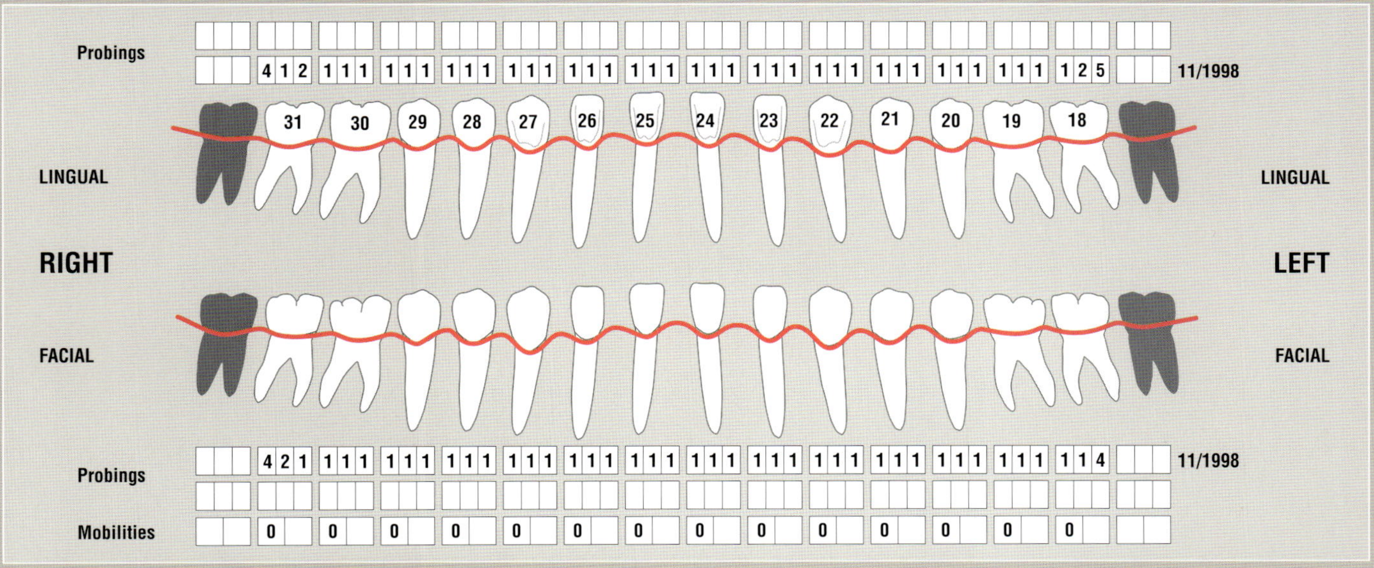

As a learning exercise, you may now outline goals/objectives of treatment and a treatment plan.

Proposed Treatment Plan

Goals/objectives of treatment

The clinicians opted to treat the affected site without involving the adjacent teeth. The patient declined any plan that would include a removable appliance. This applied to any provisional restorations as well. An implant-supported restoration would be designed; however, a number of treatment choices could still be considered:

1. Three implants to replace missing tooth no. 8 and the two adjacent teeth, which would be extracted
2. An anterior implant-supported fixed partial denture on teeth nos. 7 to 9 with a pontic in the no. 8 site
3. Two implants to replace missing tooth no. 8 and soon-to-be-extracted tooth no. 9, with the no. 7 position treated as a cantilevered pontic extending from the implant in site no. 8

Before establishing which treatment option to use, it was important to lay out the esthetic goals and objectives because this could help to determine which choice would most likely meet everyone's expectations. The three esthetic goals were to:

1. Rebuild the deficient horizontal volume
2. Create a harmonious gingival line with the adjacent natural dentition
3. Create scalloping of the gingival line confluent with the interproximal papillae

The treatment team evaluated the three options in terms of achieving the above goals and did not find any of the choices to be significantly superior to any of the others. Ultimately, it was decided that three implant placements would result in blunted or shortened papillae and probably the most compromised esthetic outcome. With two implant placements, the best choice seemed to be using sites nos. 8 and 9. The pontic area of site no. 7 would be the smallest and most likely subject to the least amount of vascular compromise following soft tissue augmentation. There would also be a positive influence on tissue height from the mesial of natural tooth no. 6. Therefore, the plan was to place implants in the nos. 8 and 9 areas and fabricate a cantilevered pontic in the no. 7 location.

Phase I: Provisional endodontic treatment of tooth no. 7

This would involve pulp extirpation and filling with calcium hydroxide. Although it is somewhat unusual to perform root canal therapy on a tooth planned for extraction, this was considered necessary because of the length of time required for this tooth to act as an abutment in a provisional adhesive fixed partial denture while the central incisor sites were being developed and osseointegration was taking place.

Phase II: Extraction of tooth no. 9 with socket preservation

Phase III: Implant placement with guided bone regeneration

After waiting 6 months, two implants would be placed in the nos. 8 and 9 locations.

Phase IV: Implant exposure following osseointegration

After waiting 6 months for osseointegration, the implants would be exposed.

Phase V: Extraction of tooth no. 7 with socket preservation and ridge augmentation

After waiting approximately 8 weeks, tooth no. 7 would be extracted with simultaneous socket preservation and ridge augmentation.

Phase VI: Fabrication and seating of a provisional screw-retained acrylic fixed partial denture

Phase VII: Definitive restoration

Prosthetic rehabilitation with a screw-retained, implant-supported cantilevered fixed partial denture.

Active Clinical Treatment

Review of the goals/objectives of treatment

This patient was discouraged by the proposed solutions and treatment immediately following her traumatic injury. She was emphatic about not wanting a removable appliance but was open to any treatment plan that would restore her smile and self-esteem.

Due to the unsightly anterior ridge defect that was caused by the traumatic injury, there were some very specific goals and objectives set in addition to restoring the patient's overall morale. They included:

- Rebuilding the maxillary ridge to restore 3D hard and soft tissue volume
- Re-creating a normal scalloped gingival appearance in harmony with the adjacent natural teeth
- Achieving overall esthetic enhancement

Phase I: Provisional endodontic treatment of tooth no. 7

Because this tooth was to be removed at a later stage in treatment, the pulp was extirpated and calcium hydroxide placed. Glass ionomer was introduced and forced through the canal in an attempt to block the resorption defect.

Phase II: Extraction of tooth no. 9 with socket preservation

Tooth no. 9, which was partially ankylosed, was carefully removed by hollowing out the internal aspect of the tooth until a thin shell remained. This shell was then infractured and remaining pieces of the tooth removed. A thin plate of buccal bone remained. After an analysis of the anatomy of the area, a decision was made to augment the ridge in two steps. Initially an attempt to preserve the socket dimensions was made using an expanded polytetrafluoroethylene (e-PTFE) membrane only. During a 4-month healing period, a six-unit adhesive partial denture was fabricated for the patient. At this time, the edentulous ridge, as anticipated, had not gained the adequate buccolingual dimensions for implant placement; however, the soft tissue covering the ridge was more than adequate to set the stage for a guided bone regeneration (GBR) procedure with simultaneous implant placement.

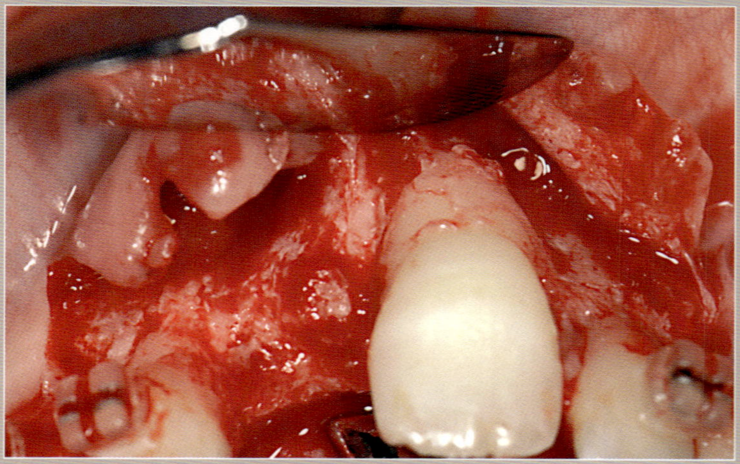

Tooth no. 9 just prior to extraction.

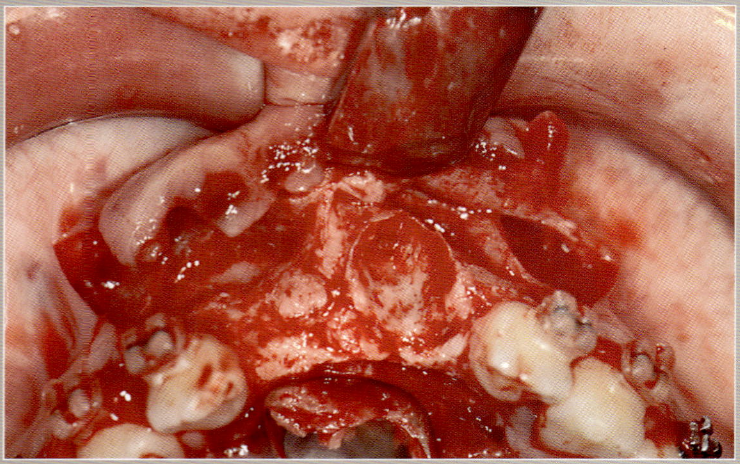

Immediately following extraction of tooth no. 9.

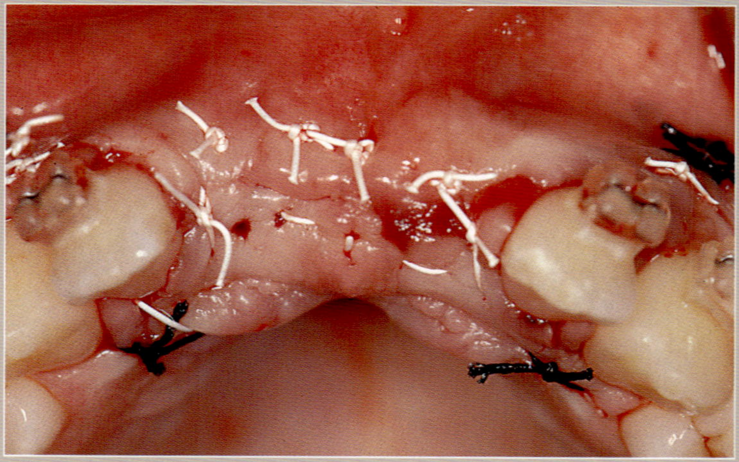

Suturing following placement of e-PTFE membrane for socket preservation.

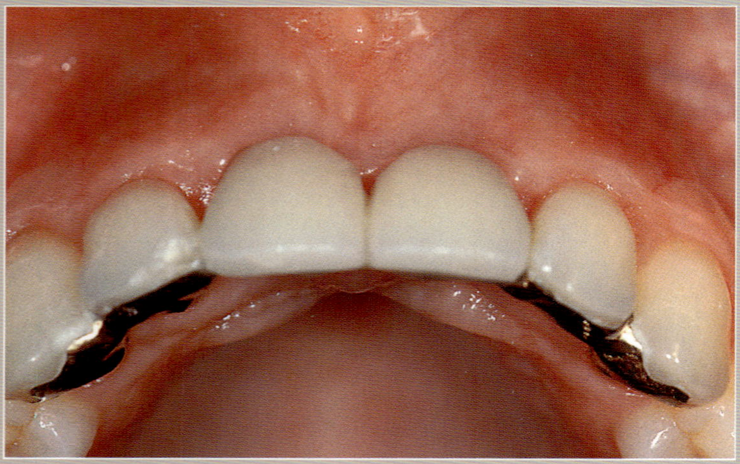

Occlusal view of six-unit adhesive provisional partial denture.

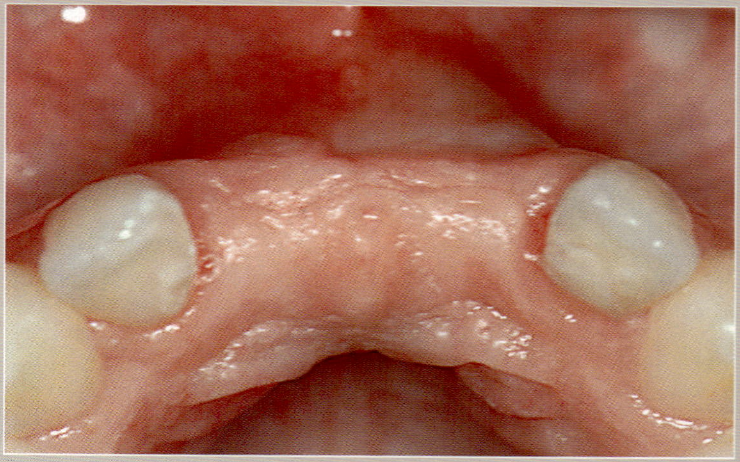

Occlusal view of sites nos. 8 and 9 after 4 months of healing.

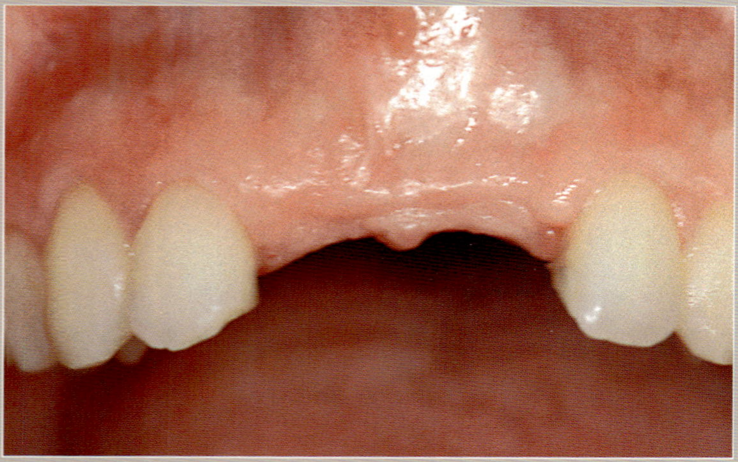

Frontal view of sites nos. 8 and 9 after 4 months of healing.

Phase III: Implant placement with guided bone regeneration

Four months following socket preservation, the e-PTFE membrane (W. L. Gore) was uncovered and found intact with a typical sheath of connective tissue underneath. The ridge was fully exposed, and two implants (Steri-Oss external hex, 3.4-mm diameter; Nobel Biocare) were placed in sites nos. 8 and 9. The ridge was simultaneously augmented with autogenous bone chips harvested from the chin as a first graft layer and deproteinized bovine (Bio-Oss, Geistlich) as a second layer. An e-PTFE membrane was fixed and adapted to cover the augmented ridge. The membrane was fully concealed by primary closure of the flaps with a combination of simple and mattress sutures.

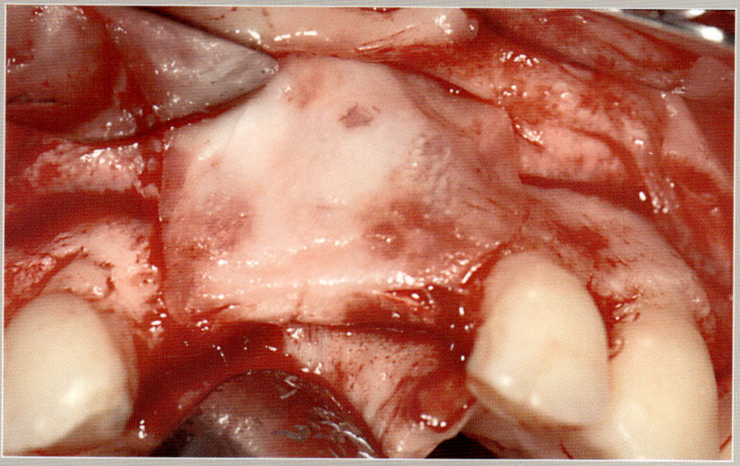

Uncovering of e-PTFE membrane.

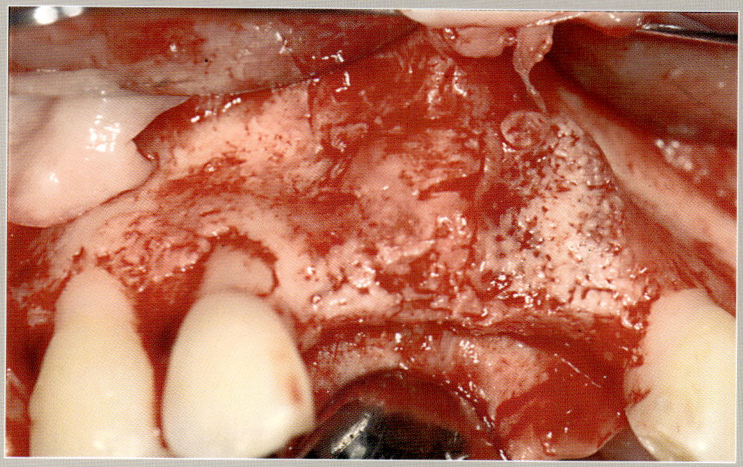

Full exposure of ridge immediately prior to implant placement.

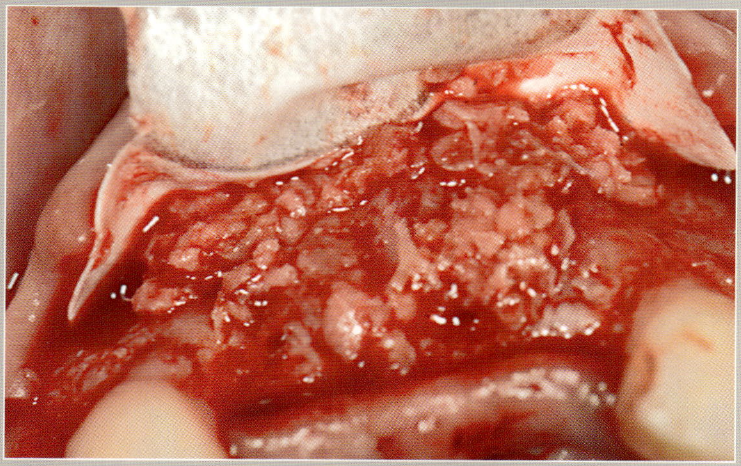

Placement of autogenous bone chips after implant placement.

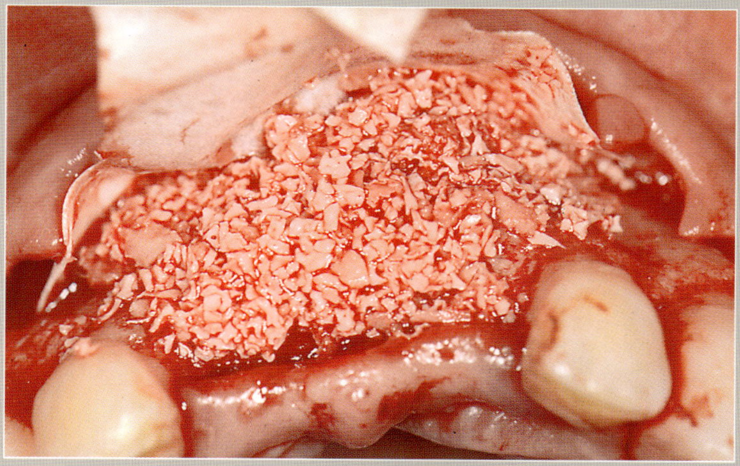

Placement of Bio-Oss as second graft layer.

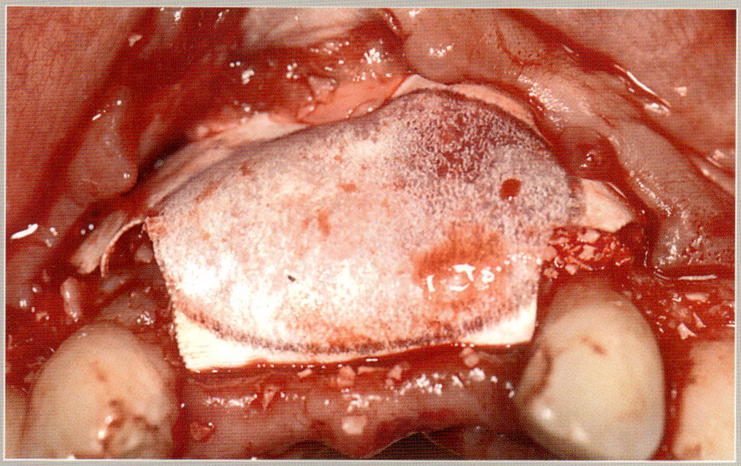

Adaptation of e-PTFE membrane.

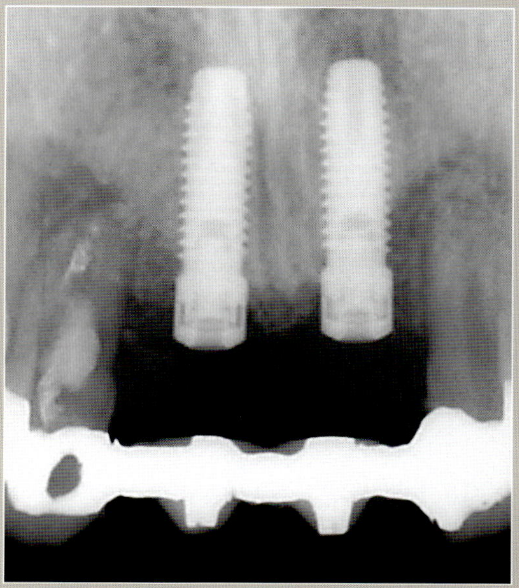

Radiograph following implant placement.

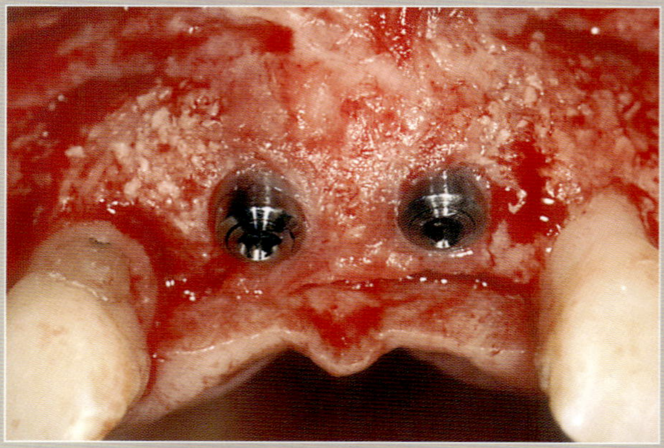

Exposure of implants 6 months after placement.

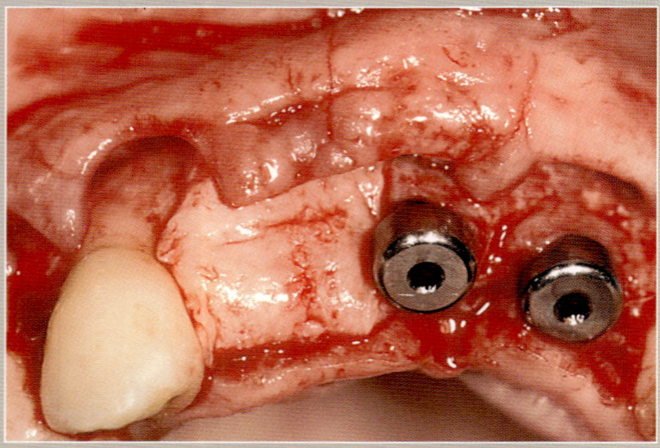

Placement of connective tissue graft following extraction of tooth no. 7.

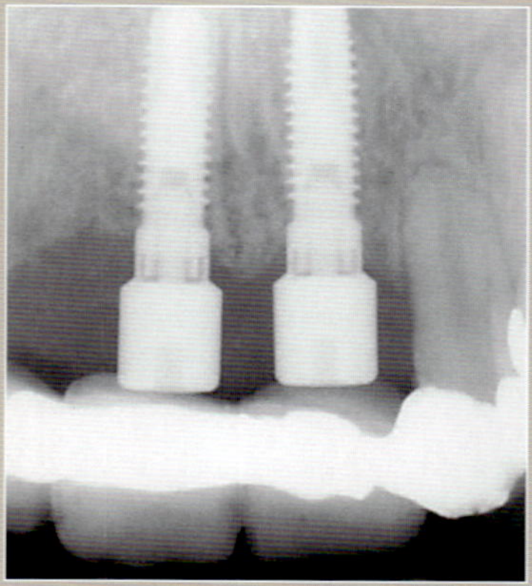

Radiograph of healing abutments and new adhesive fixed partial denture.

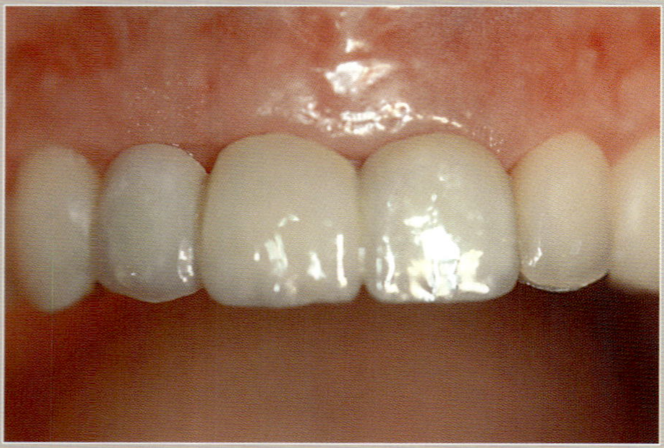

Intraoral frontal view of adhesive provisional partial denture with three pontics.

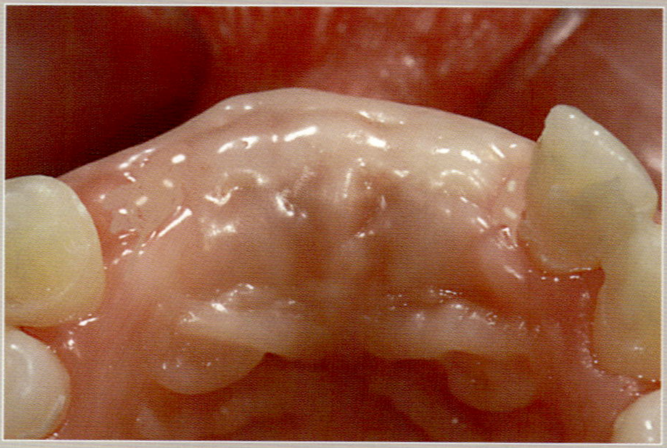

Occlusal view of edentulous ridge after 3 months of healing.

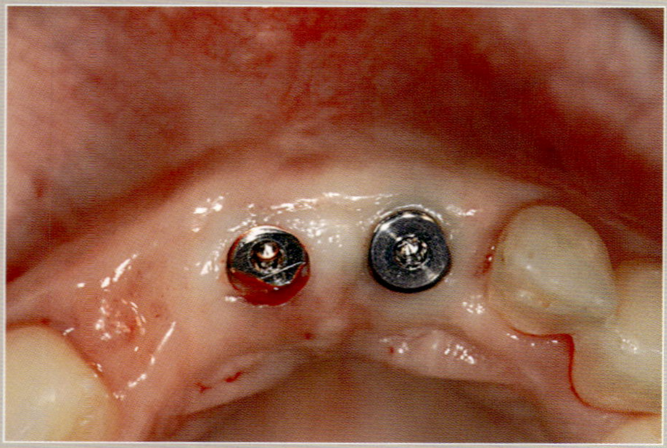

Following tissue punch exposure of implants.

Phase IV: Extraction of tooth no. 7 and socket preservation and ridge augmentation

Six months later, the membrane was removed, and the implants in sites nos. 8 and 9 were exposed. Two healing abutments (4 mm in height) were connected, and the buccal flap was advanced to fully cover them. Tooth no. 7 was extracted at the same time, and the extraction site was filled with bovine bone to help preserve as much of the ridge as possible. A connective tissue graft was placed as an onlay over the grafted bone. The buccal flap, which covered the abutments, was also advanced to cover the extraction site. During a healing period of 3 months, a new adhesive partial denture with three pontics was bonded to the adjacent teeth.

Phase V: Implant exposure at site no. 7

At 3 months, because the edentulous ridge (no. 7 site) had gained sufficient volume, it was found suitable to expose the implants using a biopsy punch without the need for flap elevation.

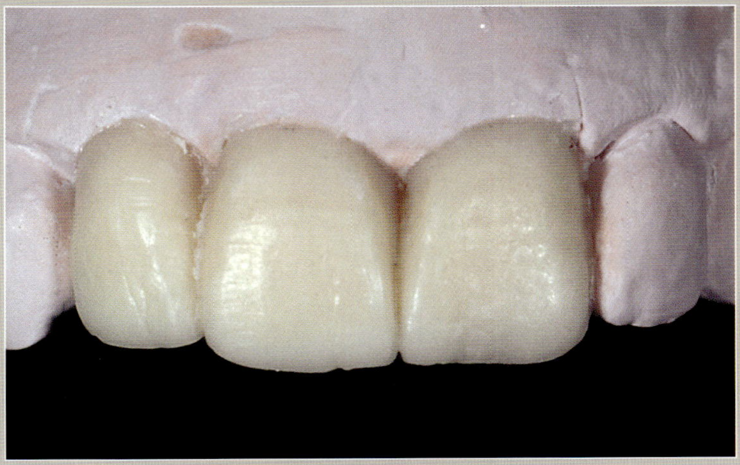

Diagnostic wax-up.

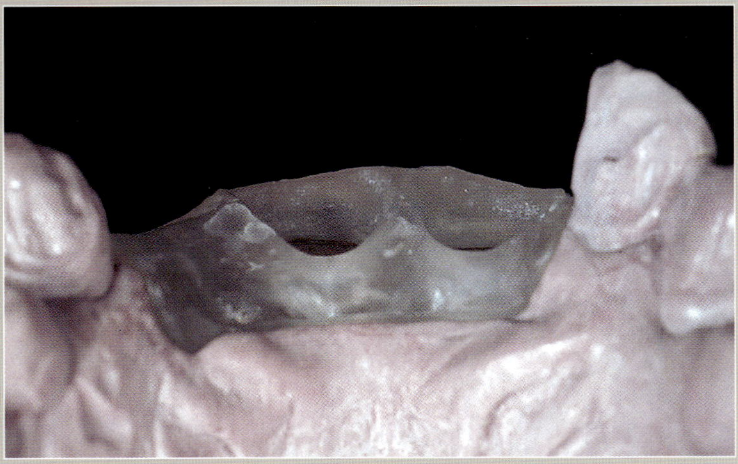

Redesign of the peri-implant mucosa on the working cast.

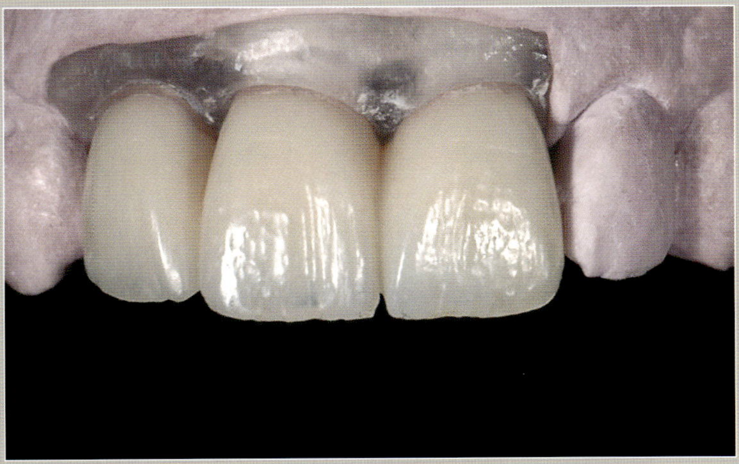

Provisional acrylic restoration connected to implant replicas.

Phase VI: Fabrication and seating of a provisional screw-retained acrylic fixed partial denture

It was decided to restore the missing teeth with a three-unit, screw-retained (UCLA-type) fixed partial denture to avoid the negative consequences of excess cement entrapment apical to the crown-abutment margins that might occur with a cement-retained fixed partial denture over screw-retained abutments.

A conventional method for taking impressions was used for the implants and adjacent tissues. Narrow impression transfers were used with an open-tray method, and a stone master cast was poured. A diagnostic wax-up was used to assess the optimal tooth dimensions and the curvature of the gingival line of the teeth to be restored.

The authors' experience has shown that the most predictable and efficient way to achieve optimal esthetic integration of the implants with the soft tissues (in cases of delayed placement and restoration) is by implementing a cervical contouring concept. A prerequisite for this technique is having excess soft tissue that can be prosthetically manipulated surrounding the head of the implant. The replica of the peri-implant mucosal envelope is redesigned to its desired 3D configuration on the laboratory master cast. Then the transmucosal prosthetic component is designed to match and support the desired new "mucosal" configuration. Subsequent intraoral connection of the prosthetic component will force the surrounding mucosa into its predesigned optimal configuration.

Redesign of the peri-implant mucosa was created on the working cast in a removable clear acrylic resin in the desired shape to match the diagnostic wax-up. A three-unit provisional fixed partial denture (metal-reinforced acrylic resin) was created to match the tooth form of the diagnostic wax-up and the newly scalloped mucosa replica. The submergence profiles of the implant provisional crowns were designed with convex proximal contours to support the papillae, whereas the buccal submucosal aspect was made relatively flat in order to avoid excessive pressure on the labial mucosa. The provisional fixed partial denture blended naturally with the adjacent teeth and the surrounding mucosa.

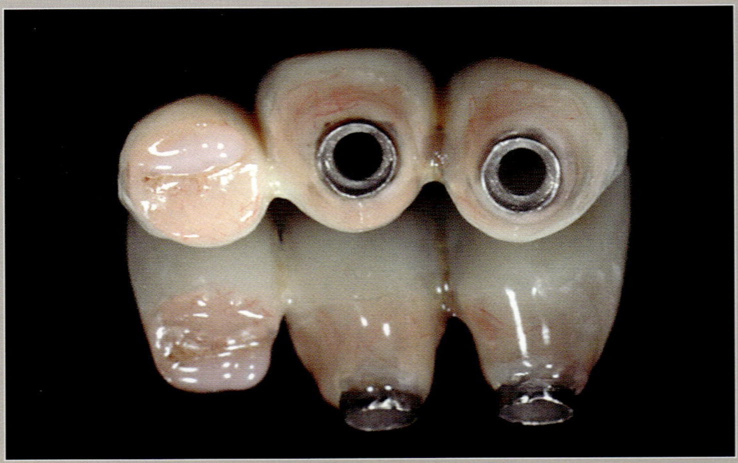

Implant provisional crowns with convex proximal contours and flat buccal submucosal aspects.

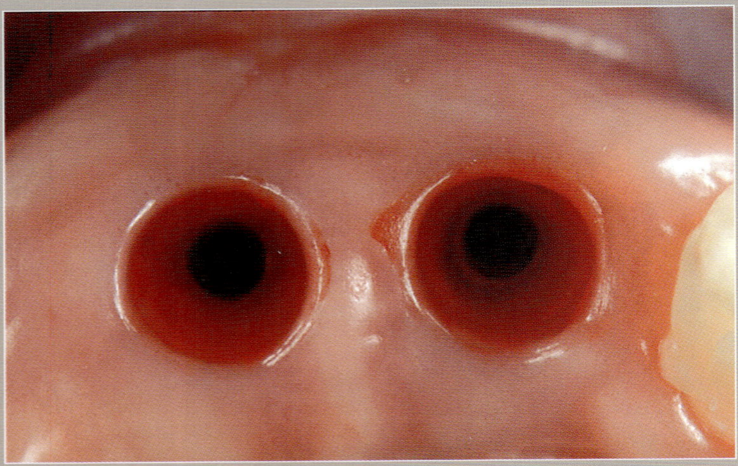

Occlusal view of implant heads and peri-implant mucosa following removal of healing abutments.

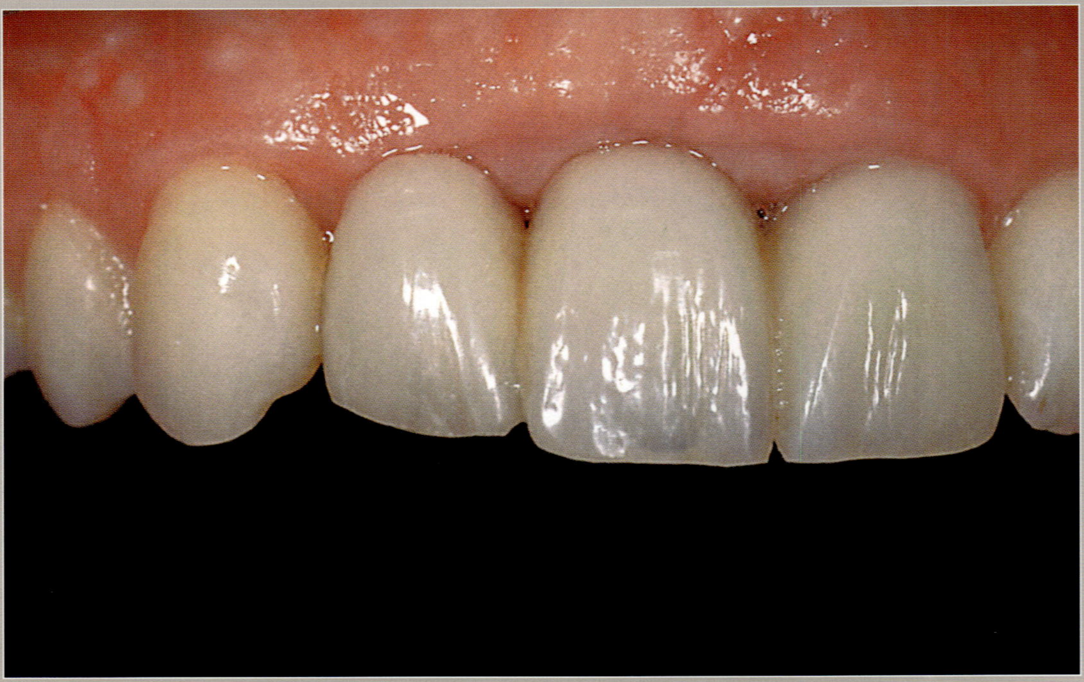

Provisional fixed partial denture in place.

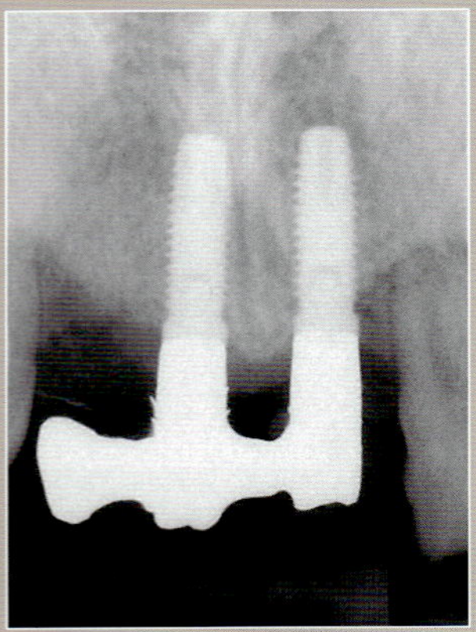

Radiograph with provisional fixed partial denture in place.

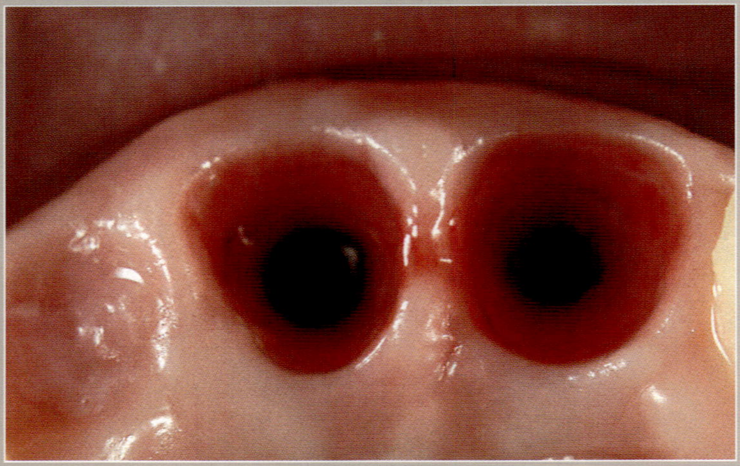

Occlusal view of peri-implant mucosa and pontic sites following removal of provisional restoration.

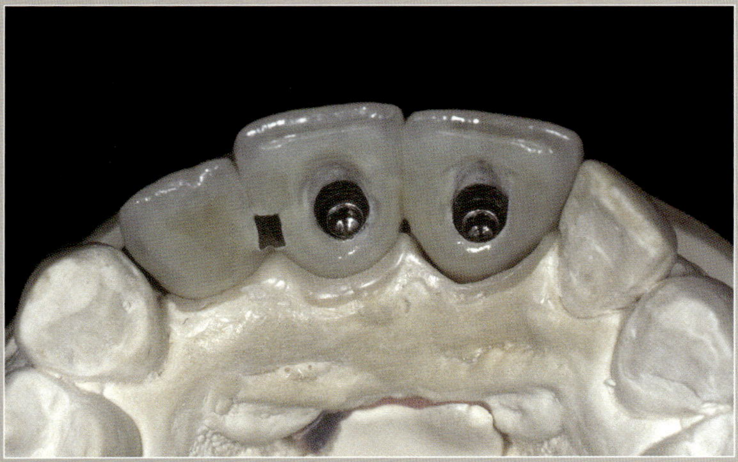

Occlusal view of definitive restoration on the cast.

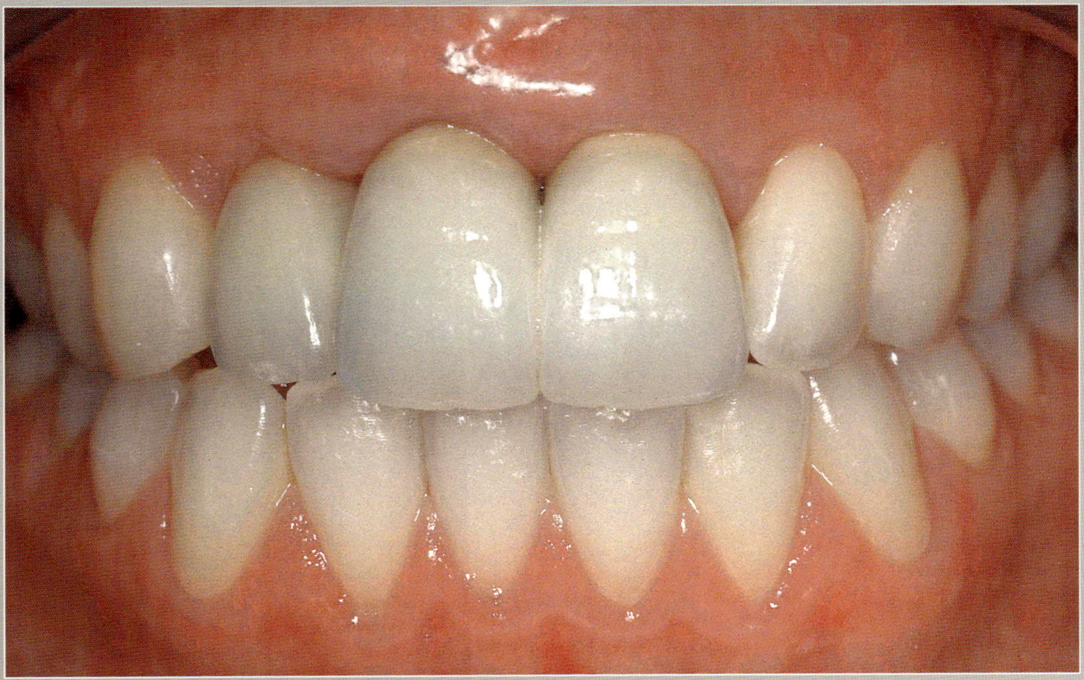

Intraoral frontal view of the definitive restoration.

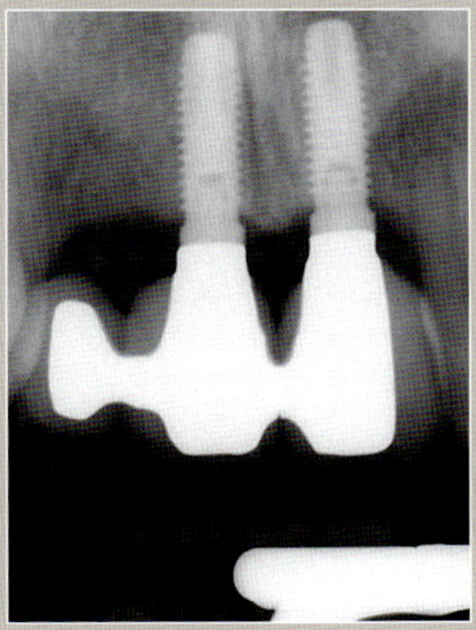

Radiograph with the definitive restoration in place.

Phase VII: Definitive restoration

Three months after the provisional restoration was fabricated, the treating clinicians verified that both esthetics and function were acceptable and initiated the steps toward definitive restoration. Following removal of the provisional restoration, it was determined that the peri-implant mucosa and the pontic site configuration matched the design that had been made on the master cast. Therefore, the same design was used for fabrication of the definitive restoration. For porcelain buildup, a plaster cast was used.

Because the soft tissue adaptation to the submucosal prosthetic configuration of the provisional restoration was acceptable, even though it did not duplicate the master cast design exactly, the same design could be used for fabrication of the definitive restoration. This would ensure identical shape, contour, and appearance of the provisional and definitive restorations. In cases where the provisional restoration has been modified intraorally and is no longer a blueprint of the mucosal design of the cast, an additional impression of the modified intraoral mucosa must be taken to serve as the template for the definitive restoration design.

A three-unit, screw-retained porcelain-fused-to-gold restoration was fabricated. The patient was 19 years old at the time treatment was completed.

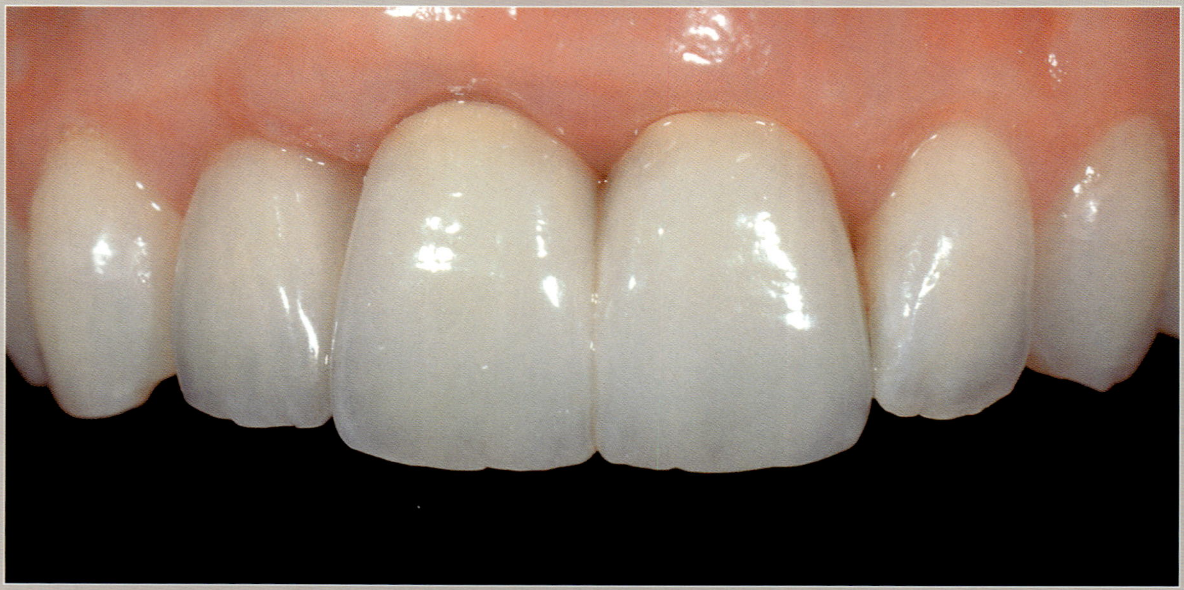

Intraoral frontal view of maxilla at 2-year posttreatment re-evaluation.

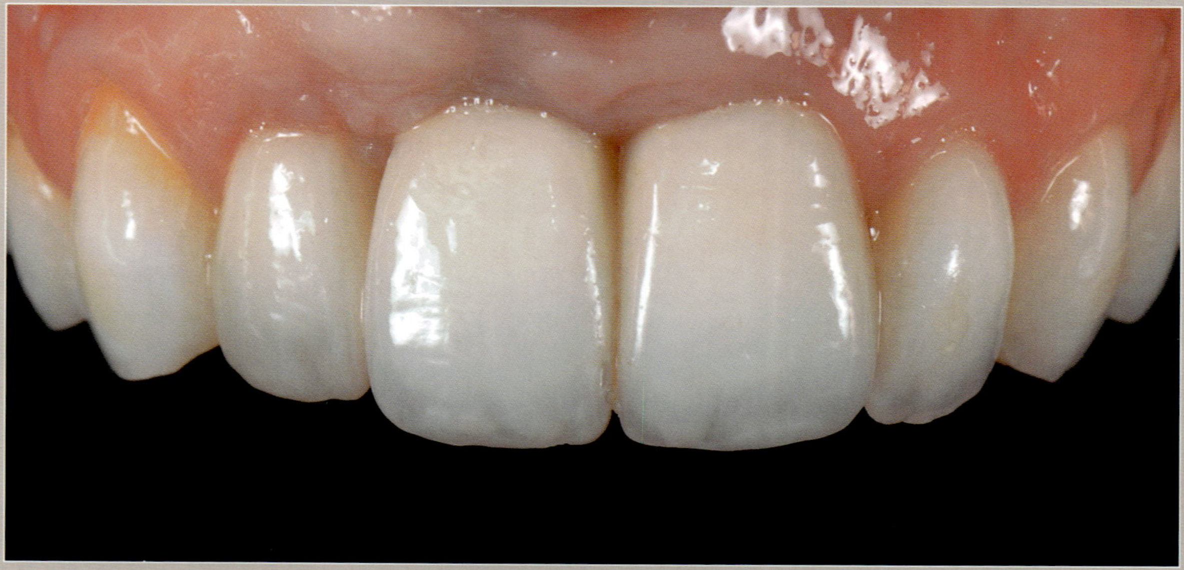

One year after modification of crowns to close gaps.

Phase VIII: Two-year posttreatment re-evaluation

The patient returned for examination and complained of saliva and air bubbles readily passing through the gingival embrasures between her crowns. She requested that the gaps be closed because this had become quite bothersome. Changing the crown contours to close the spaces might make the patient more comfortable but also would result in the oval shape of her crowns becoming more square in form and the scalloping of the gingival line becoming flatter, altering her appearance. However, the patient insisted on making these alterations.

One-year follow-up of the modified crowns revealed a flat and more apical gingival line, and the patient was still complaining of bubbles in the gaps between the crowns. At this stage, the patient relocated without additional treatment.

Phase IX: Seven-year posttreatment re-evaluation

The patient returned for examination and consultation 4 years later at the age of 26. During this time, some changes had occurred:

- Tooth no. 6 had moved buccally.
- The mandibular anterior teeth had also moved buccally and had become crowded.
- Gingival recession was noted on the facial aspects of some anterior teeth.

The patient accepted a recommendation for orthodontic treatment to reposition and realign the mandibular anterior teeth and tooth no. 6. The Invisalign system (Align Technology) was used.

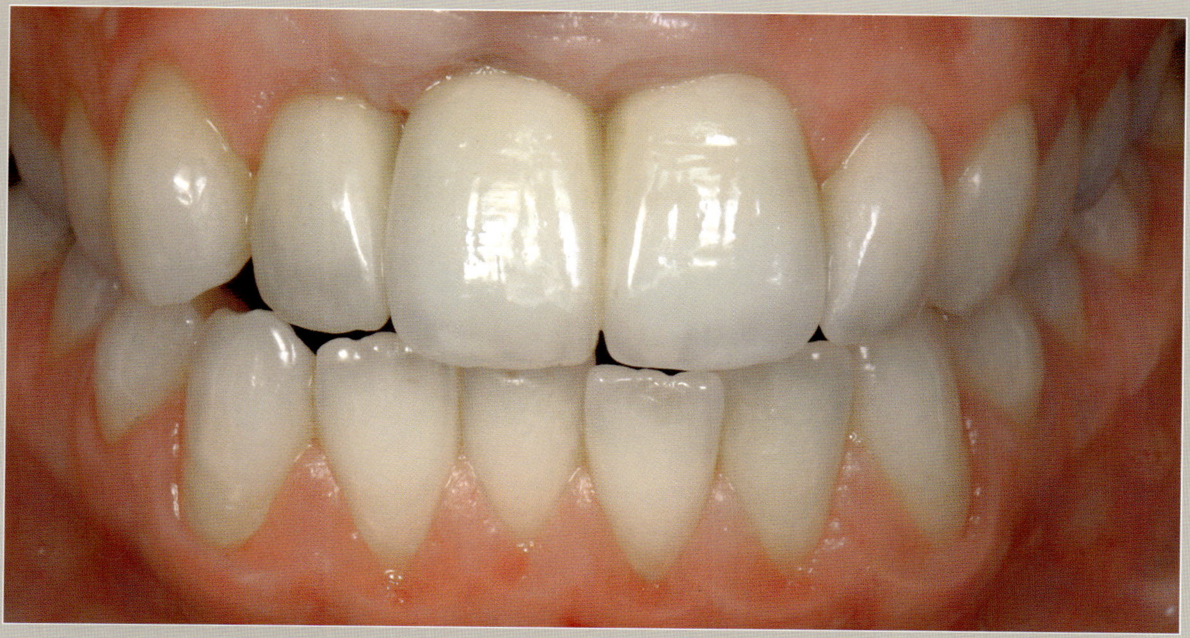

Intraoral frontal view at 7-year posttreatment re-evaluation.

After orthodontic treatment, the patient returned with some esthetic concerns. She was unhappy with the tooth form and her appearance when smiling. She wanted to know if there was anything else we could do to improve her smile.

The key objective at this point was to determine the exact cause of her unattractive appearance. Envisioning the ideal form and three-dimensional position of the teeth aided in distinguishing between this and any other deviation such as soft tissue discrepancies.

Ridge augmentation procedures are designed to re-establish lost hard and soft tissue volume. Unfortunately, many of these procedures fall short of the restorative dentist's clinical expectations. Lack of papilla volume is a common postoperative deficiency. Even when ridge grafting fills most of the defect (eg, 90%), the problem is that usually the most critical portion of the void still remains. The final missing 10% is exactly what would be required to allow for fabrication of natural-looking crowns. This 10% usually includes the papillae and gingival margins—the framework for the future restoration.

This is exactly what had happened with our patient. There was a soft tissue discrepancy that was affecting the shape and position of the crowns, and this was responsible for the unattractive appearance of her smile.

Morphologic and esthetic problems when restoring a deficient ridge

Maxillary anterior tooth loss generates a bone resorption process in the direction and inclination of the roots, shortening the height of the ridge and the perimeter of the arch form. In order to reconstruct this vertical loss of the ridge and gingiva, the surgeon will typically first execute grafts to gain the essential height, hopeful that this will re-create satisfactory papilla form for the restorative phase. What we have seen most often is a horizontally shortened arch with vertically re-established height but with unsatisfactory papilla and gingival esthetics. This is the worst-case scenario for the ceramist. Usually in these situations, if the restorative dentist and ceramist opt for a conventional partial denture, ie, without prosthetic gingiva, we can expect the problems below:

- Narrower teeth due to less mesiodistal circumference and arch space.
- Longer teeth toward the apical aspect due to the ridge height that remains inadequate, even following surgical augmentation.
- Inverted smile line: Because the crown is longer apically, the technician typically must compensate by shortening the incisal edges of the anterior teeth, trying to keep reasonable

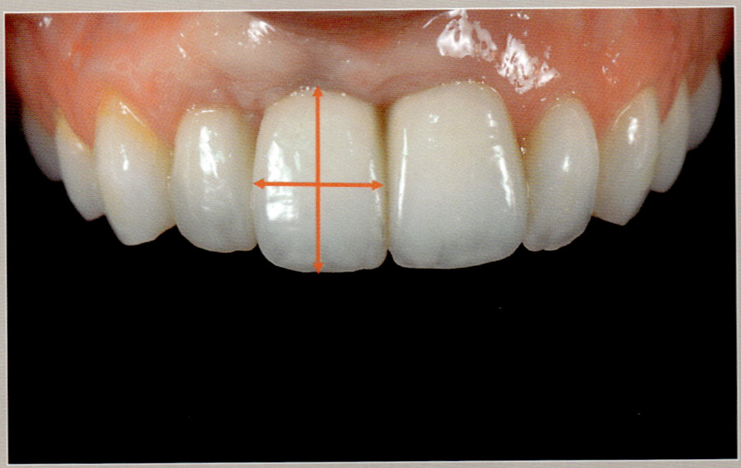

Incorrect dental proportion (long and narrow teeth).

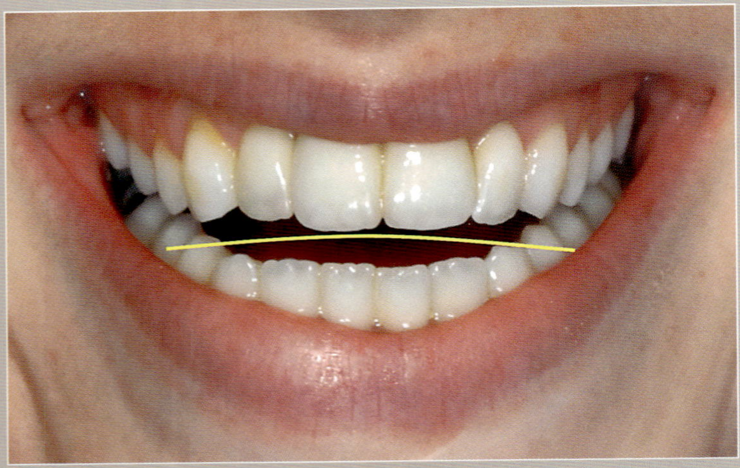

Short incisal edge of the crowns and inverted smile line.

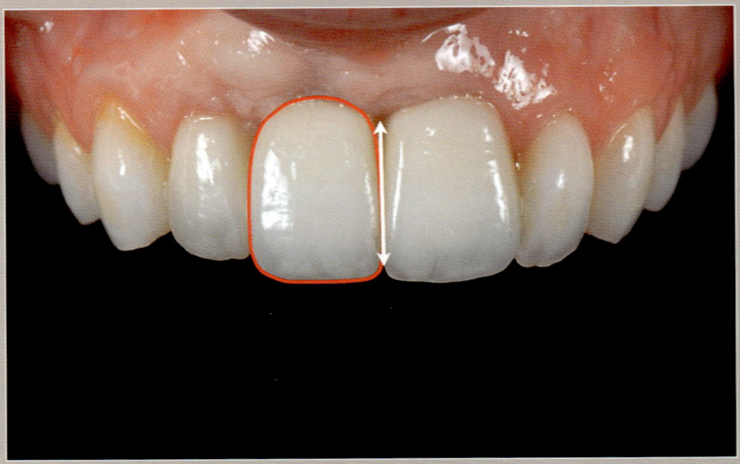

Rectangular teeth and long contacts.

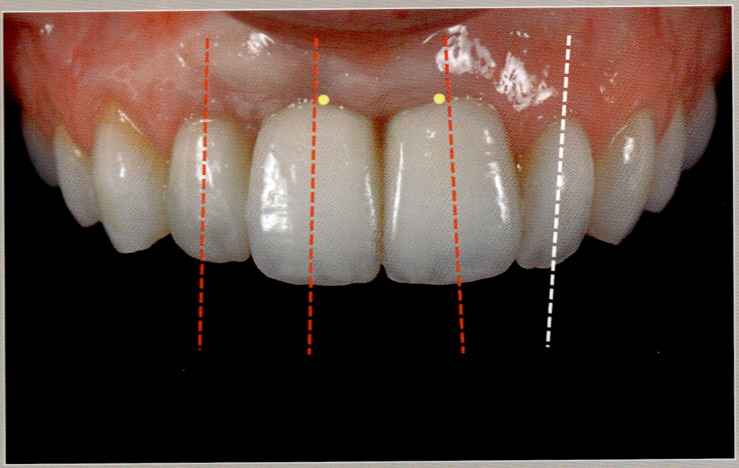

Incorrect tooth axis and zenith position.

tooth proportions. That will make the anterior teeth shorter than ideal and lead to poor lip-tooth esthetic form.

- Rectangular teeth without natural tooth anatomy due to extended contact points in the interproximal area: Lack of papilla volume often requires the ceramist to create these longer contact areas in an effort to avoid the black holes interproximally.
- Inversion of the tooth axes: Instead of converging toward the incisal half of the tooth, the tooth axes will diverge. This is typically observed when conventional partial dentures are fabricated over resorbed ridges. This occurs when the ceramist tries to keep the incisal third on the occlusal plane, guided by the mandibular teeth, and at the same time tries to take the cervical third of the tooth form toward the reduced ridge, modifying the natural tooth axis. It is interesting to note that when the correct modifications are made on the crowns to give them the proper axis, spaces for the artificial papillae are naturally opened. The correct positioning of the crowns in the arch will therefore lead to the need for prosthetic gingiva.
- Unsupported upper lip: When fabricating a partial denture with lack of adequate arch perimeter, we lose appropriate support, and the upper lip will tend to move down and backwards. Consequently, the patient shows less of the maxillary teeth, which creates an aged appearance.

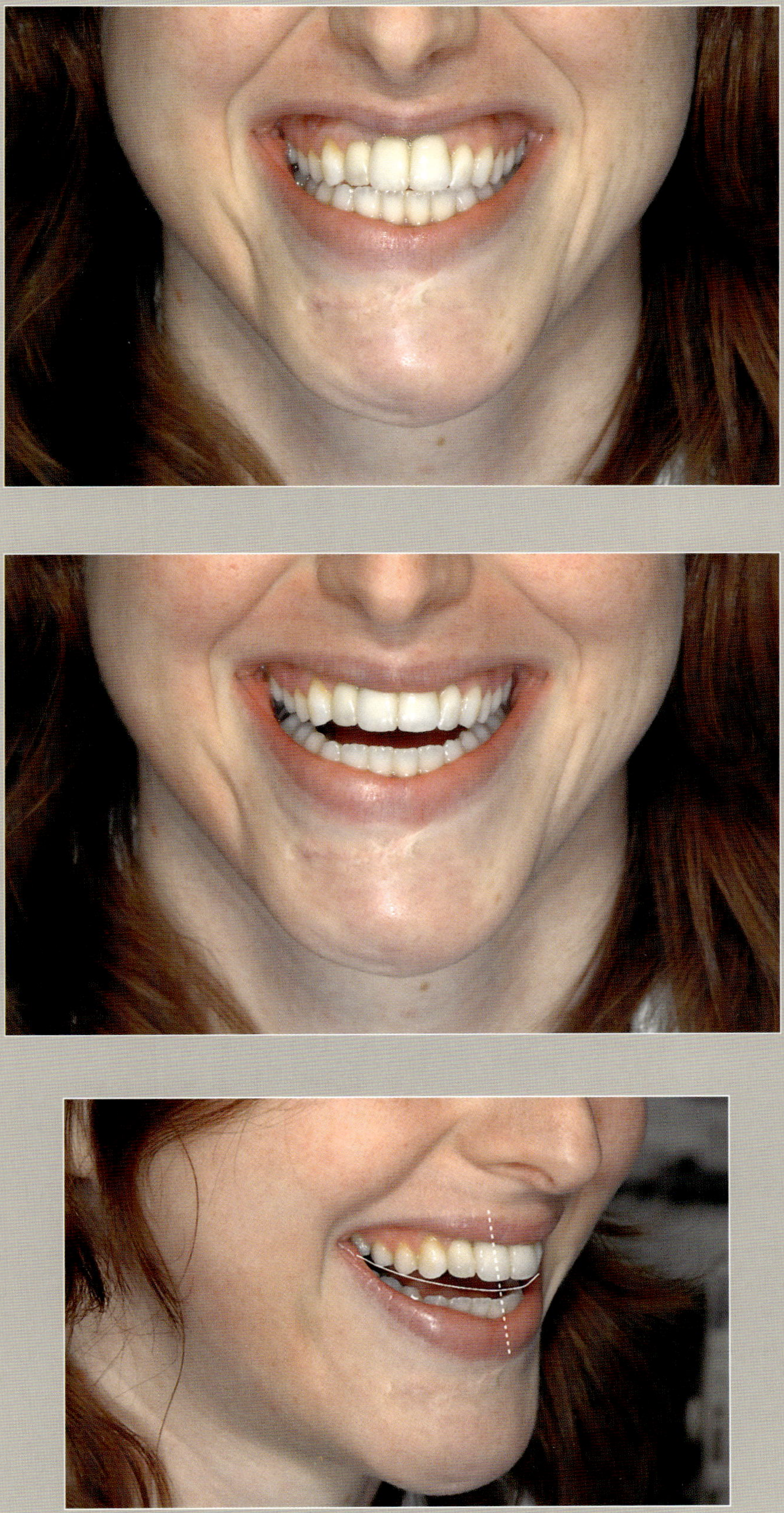

Facial views of the patient's smile for the DSD.

Phase X: Digital smile design

Initially, a full digital photographic series was taken. A Keynote presentation (Apple) was created with the photos, and the facial analyses were completed. The facial midline and horizontal plane were determined. The two main guidelines (vertical midline and horizontal line) were transferred to the smile photo, and the ideal incisal edge position was designed. The lines then were transferred to the intraoral photo, allowing us to better visualize the proposed treatment outcome in relation to the face. After creating the intraoral photo with the two main guidelines and incisal edge position, we could then develop the dentogingival design.

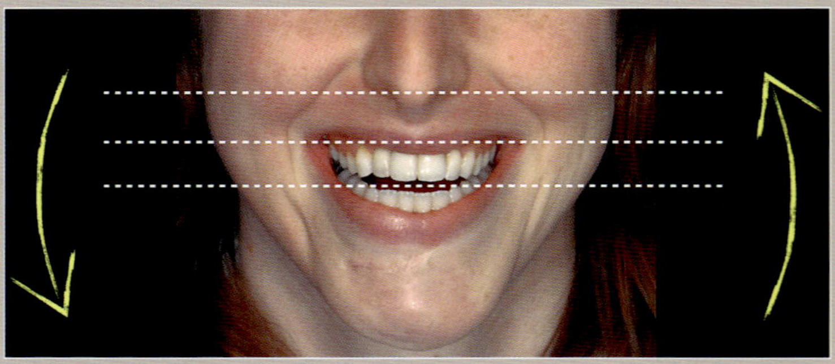

Determining the ideal facial position according to the horizontal plane of reference.

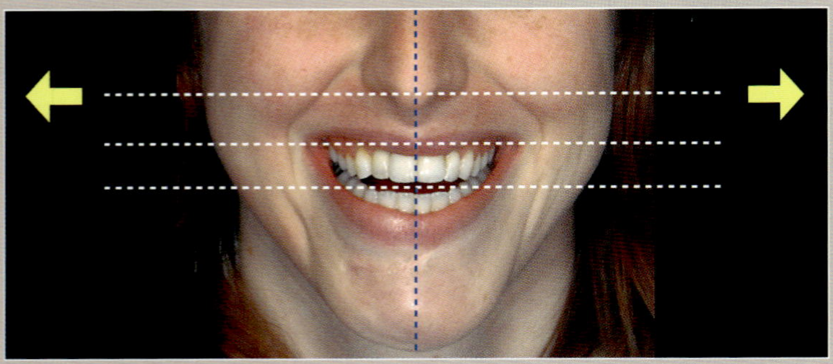

Determining a harmonious midline position.

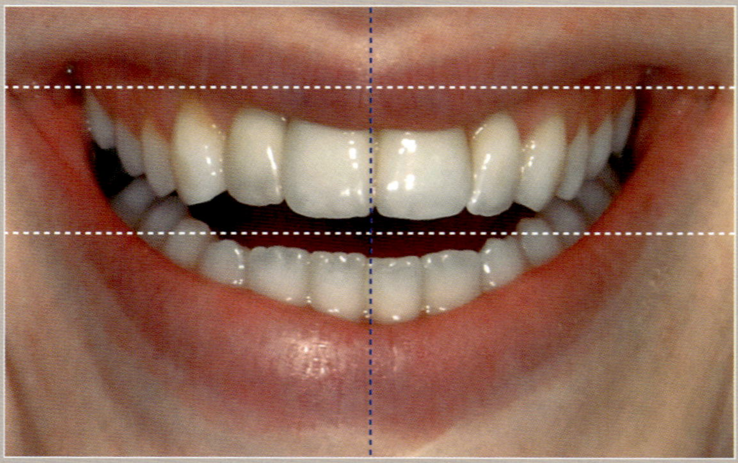

Close-up of the smile with midline and horizontal lines marked.

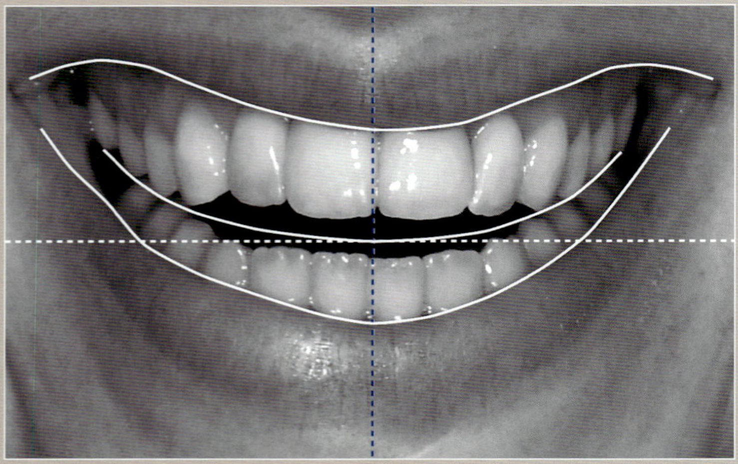

Black and white version of photograph with lip lines for determination of ideal incisal edge position.

Phase XI: White and pink mock-up

The decision was made to prepare a white and pink mock-up to evaluate the problem. The mock-up design was guided by the DSD. The mock-up was fabricated with the white and pink composite directly added to the existing implant partial denture. The white composite was added first to alter the position of the teeth, and then the pink was added, filling in the interproximal spaces to re-create the ideal gingival esthetics.

The following steps were taken to complete the mock-up:

1. Lengthening incisally to fix the inverted smile line
2. Adding cervical volume to both central incisors to position the teeth perpendicular to the occlusal plane and eliminate the flared out appearance
3. Adding distobuccal volume on the lateral incisor to correct the tooth axis, mimicking the contralateral tooth that converges (instead of diverging) towards the incisal
4. Reshaping the interproximal spaces to create good tooth form and appropriate interproximal contact appearance and opening ideal space for natural-looking papillae
5. Adding pink composite and repositioning the papillae ideally to match the remaining natural papillae
6. Recreating ideal zenith position and gingival margin design

After the mock-up was finished, photos were taken (face, smile, and intraoral) to best communicate the new design to the patient. The patient approved the design and had great confidence that this approach would solve her problem.

Prior to initiating treatment, the team had to answer some very important questions:

- Many treatment paths existed. Which would provide the most predictable, esthetically pleasing outcome?
- Would additional surgery to augment the ridge enhance the final esthetic outcome or would this add an additional element of risk? For instance, was there a risk of additional recession?
- In lieu of a surgical reconstruction, would it be more prudent to consider reconstructing the defect prosthetically?
- What would be the drawbacks of a nonsurgical prosthetic reconstruction?

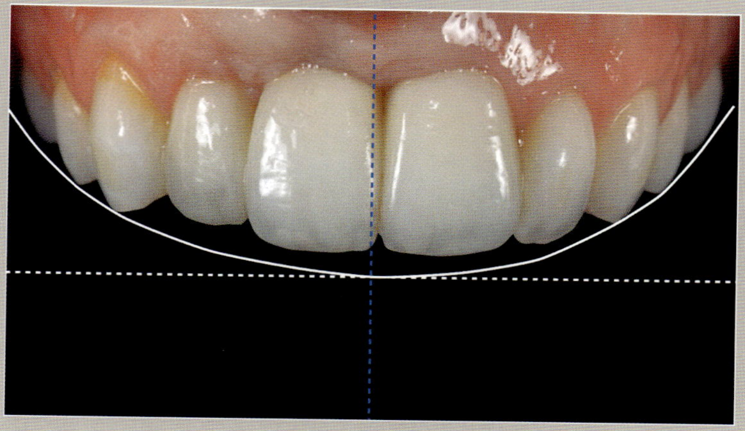

Intraoral photo with facial lines transferred.

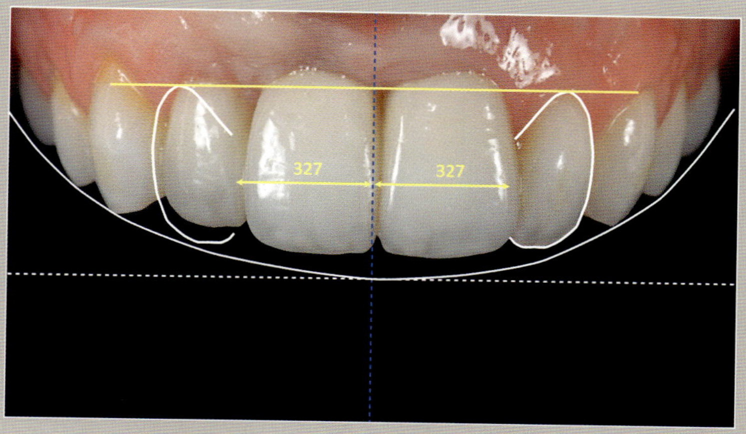

Outline of tooth no. 10 duplicated, flipped, and repositioned equidistant to the midline during the dentogingival design process.

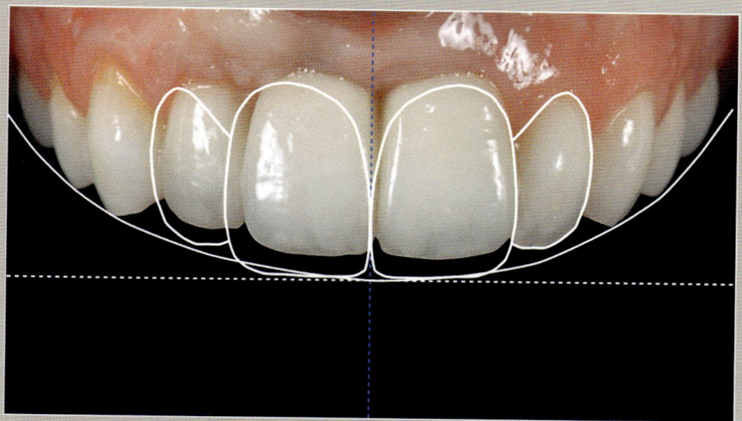

Design and position of the central incisors according to the reference lines.

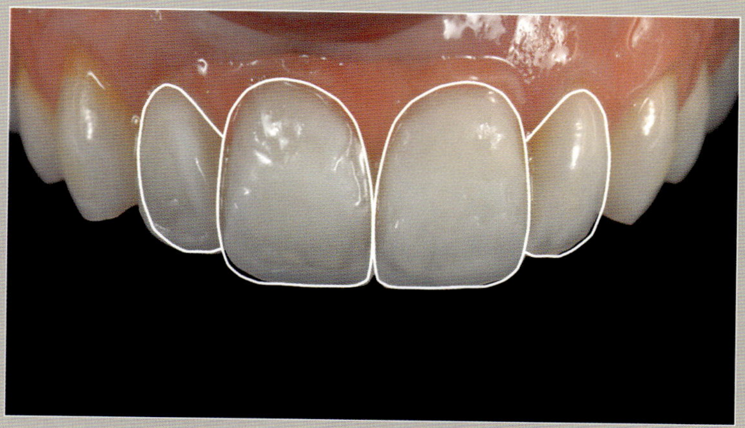

Photograph of mock-up overlapping the intraoral DSD photograph.

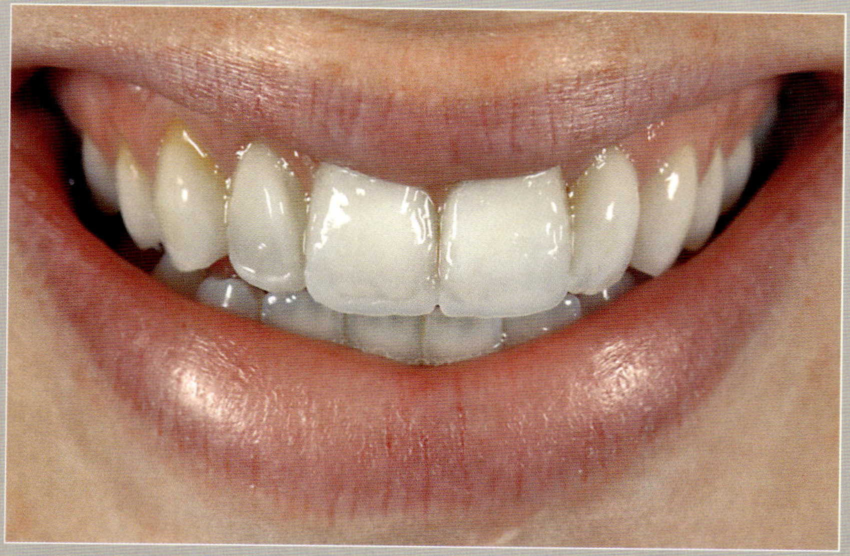

Photograph of smile with mock-up in place.

The treatment team, in accordance with the patient's wishes, decided to institute a nonsurgical, prosthetically driven treatment plan.

The rationale for this decision was as follows:

- Additional surgery to reconstruct the ridge area could still fall short of what would be necessary to ensure an esthetically pleasing result. Although a purely prosthetic approach might also fall short of patient expectations, it would be far less invasive, thus giving the patient one less reason to be unhappy.
- This patient had a very negative and stressful dental history and we wanted to minimize the risk of this continuing.
- This patient was very difficult and demanding, and we wanted to minimize the number of visits necessary to complete treatment.
- The patient was getting married in a few months, which presented time constraints.

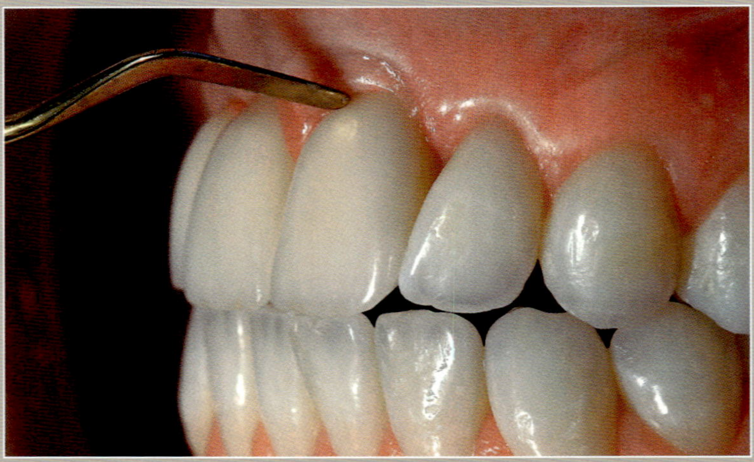

Direct addition of pink composite resin over the pink ceramics of the definitive three-unit implant partial denture.

The decision was made to create a new implant fixed partial denture with artificial gingiva. The technique of choice was the so-called pink hybrid restoration. The main advantage of this approach is that we could re-create pink and white esthetics predictably without extra surgery. The main disadvantage would be the need for constant care and maintenance.

Phase XII: Fabrication and placement of the pink hybrid restoration

Using the mock-up as a guide, a zirconium frame was fabricated, and a ceramic buildup was performed. The crowns were ideally located to receive the artificial gingiva.

The pink hybrid restoration consists of an implant partial denture with ceramics providing the white esthetics (teeth) and the pink esthetics (the base). After the ceramic part of the restoration was completed, the pink base was treated so that pink composite material could be bonded intraorally.

The seating process was achieved in two different appointments. The first appointment focused on the white esthetics and soft tissue conditioning. The partial denture was tried in prior to application of the pink composite. After all of the esthetic parameters involved were checked and all of the necessary adjustments were made, the partial denture was glazed and screwed back in. The condition of the soft tissues was not ideal at this time because of compression, bleeding, and blanching. This necessitated application of the pink composite at a separate appointment.

A few days later, after adequate healing of the soft tissue, the shape and color of the soft tissues was again stable, and we were able to add the pink composite material to the pink base. The implant partial denture was removed from the mouth. The gingival area was treated for bonding in the following sequence:

1. Creation of mechanical retention with a small, round diamond bur in multiple locations
2. Hydrofluoric acid etching
3. Application of a silane coupling agent
4. Application of a bonding agent
5. Application of the first layer of pink composite extraorally to guarantee good bonding (without the interference of saliva)
6. Reattachment of the implant partial denture and addition of the remainder of the pink composite, matching shape, color, and texture to the natural soft tissue of the patient

The key was to blend in the interface between the artificial and natural soft tissue, which is facilitated by the pink composite.

After the restoration was completed, the focus switched to oral hygiene maintenance. Very specific hygiene instruction was given in order to adequately maintain this unique type of restoration. This is essential for long-term success.

The most important aspect of this restoration is that it has to be retrievable. The pink hybrid restoration is designed to be screw retained for maintenance purposes. The patient was scheduled for a checkup 3 months after seating to confirm that hygiene was being performed correctly. After this, at every 6-month hygiene appointment, the partial denture will be removed to check the peri-implant and periodontal status and to examine the adjacent teeth to confirm that the artificial pink extensions are not causing any harm to the soft tissues. The screws will require replacement every year (after two rounds of insertion and removal).

Posttreatment

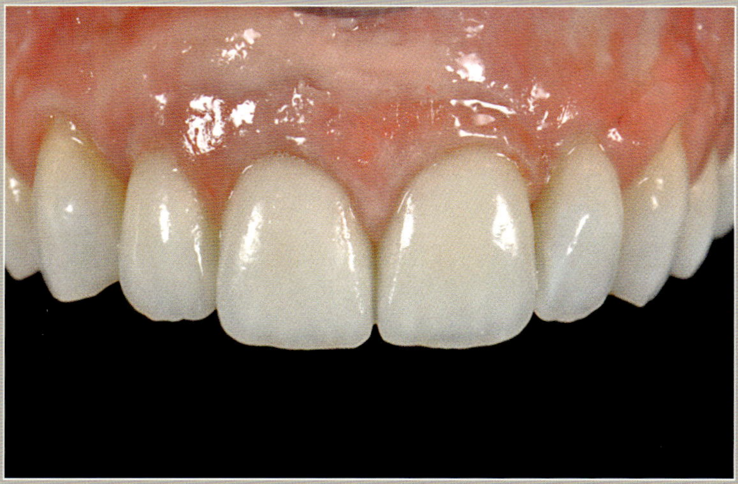

Intraoral frontal view of the anterior maxilla.

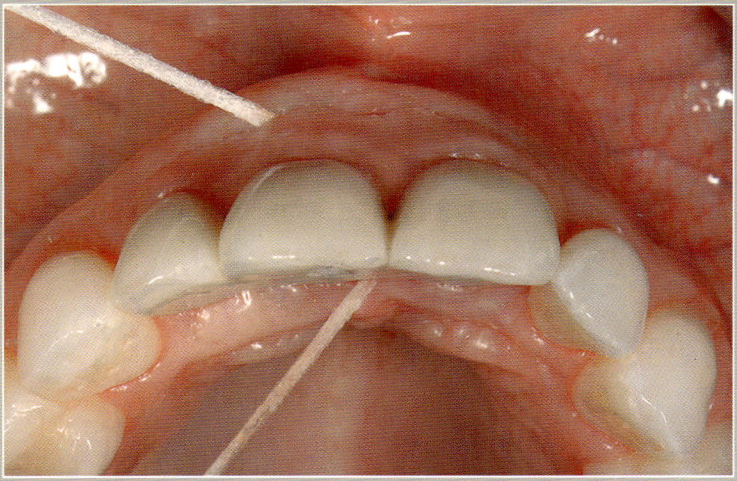

Occlusal view of essential hygiene procedures.

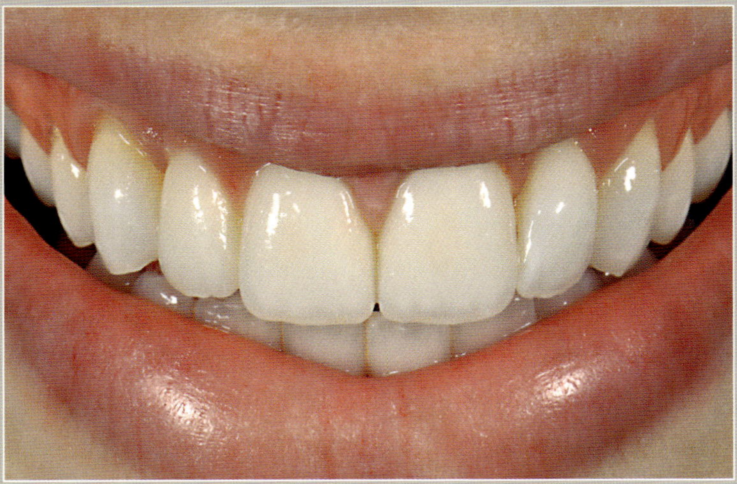

Smile view.

You may now place the corresponding posttreatment overlay found in the separate folder over the pretreatment periodontal chart on page 125.

Overcoming Incorrect Implant Inclinations

Galip Gürel, MSc

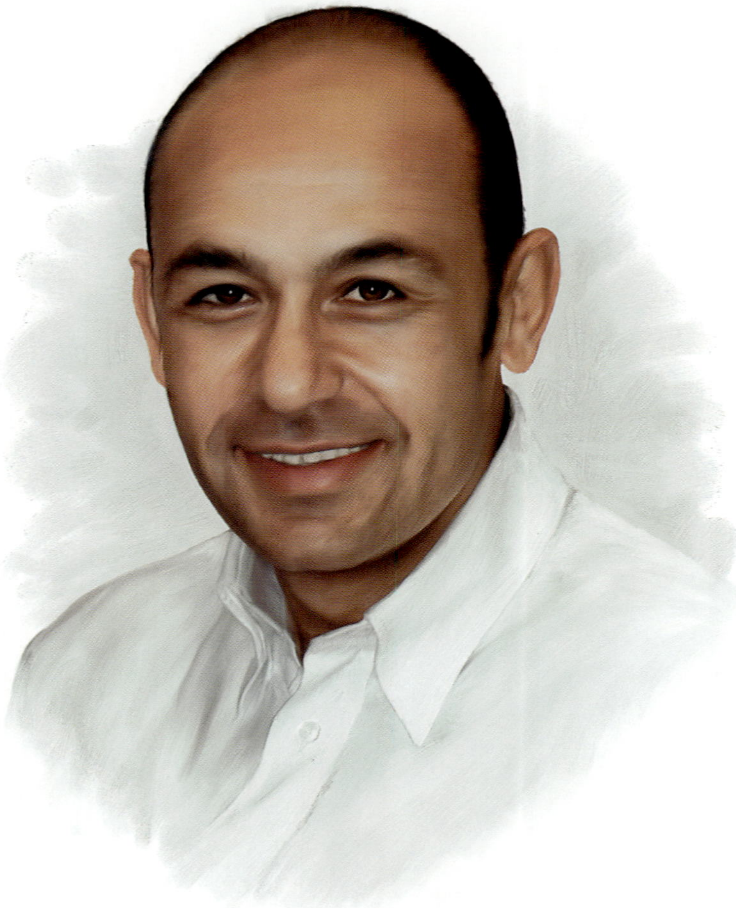

Despite recent advances in periodontal and peri-implant surgical regenerative procedures, predictably re-establishing hard and soft tissue contours remains a formidable challenge in cases with 3D ridge deficiencies.

This case was chosen because it presents a reliable and consistently predictable alternative in prosthetically compromised cases in which patients are unwilling to undergo regenerative surgical procedures. As already shown, the pink hybrid restoration[5-8] represents a remarkable innovation because it ensures an extremely close match between the prosthetic and natural gingiva with simplicity and dependability while still providing easy maintenance.

The main issue in this case was to overcome the implant angulations, which were inappropriate for a pink restoration. The implants, already placed, had a buccal inclination not allowing for a one-piece, screw-retained framework, which is ideal for the pink hybrid restoration.

Case Presentation 2

Treating clinicians
Prosthodontist: Galip Gürel, MSc
Dental laboratory and smile designer: Christian Coachman, DDS, CDT

Clinical Treatment Planning

Age at initial presentation: 30 years
Initial presentation: December 2007
Active treatment completed: June 2008

Introduction and background

This patient had been in an automobile accident approximately 3 years before her presentation for examination in our office. She had lost five anterior teeth (nos. 7 to 11) and had undergone numerous surgical procedures to correct the facial and intraoral defects that resulted from the traumatic injury. She presented with facial asymmetry and a large depression on the left side of her upper lip. Previous treatment was directed toward correcting these deficiencies by augmenting the intraoral defect with hard and soft tissue grafts and placing three implants. The augmentation procedures did not provide enough new bone volume to fill the defect completely and compromised the definitive restorative outcome. Although there was some esthetic improvement extraorally, the patient was very disappointed with the shape and proportions of her new teeth as well as their relation to her gingival tissues. The traumatic injury, multiple surgeries, hundreds of hours in the dental chair with lost work time, and an enormous financial investment had resulted in depression and complete loss of self-esteem. She had given up hope and had severed her relationship with the previous dental surgeon.

At initial presentation, the patient complained about the appearance of her teeth and the minor facial asymmetry that still existed due to the lack of bone support for her upper lip. She was tired of treatment and was adamant about not proceeding with any additional surgical procedures. The only option remaining to improve esthetics and to help this patient feel better about herself was to use a minimally invasive prosthetic approach.

Medical history

- Noncontributory

Diagnostic findings

Extraoral and facial findings

- Normal profile with visible depression on the upper lip
- Asymmetric facial appearance due to the loss of lip support, mainly on the left side
- Flared incisal edges of the anterior teeth
- Lack of papillary display when smiling, resulting in longer-looking teeth

TMJ and mandibular range of motion

- Normal range of motion
- No joint sounds with external palpation
- No muscle tenderness
- No pain on opening or with lateral movement
- Very easy manipulation
- No signs or symptoms of temporomandibular disorders

Intraoral findings

- Porcelain-fused-to-metal (PFM) partial denture extending from teeth nos. 5 to 13
- Long proximal contact areas on the anterior teeth
- Incisal edges flared out
- Asymmetric gingival levels
- Lack of interproximal papillae in the maxillary left anterior segment

Pretreatment

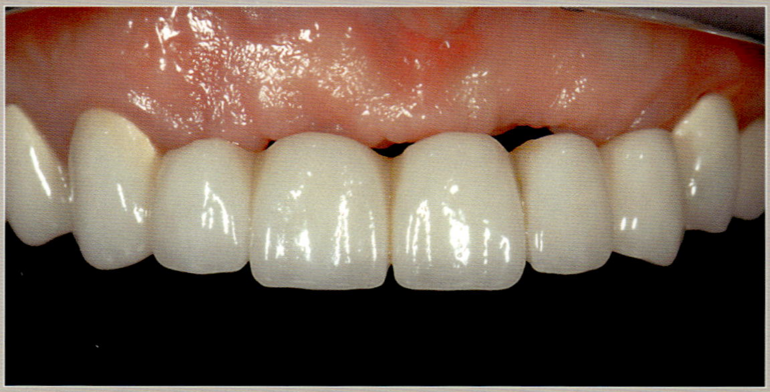

Intraoral frontal view of maxilla with existing fixed partial denture, which was trimmed at the cervical aspect and used as a provisional.

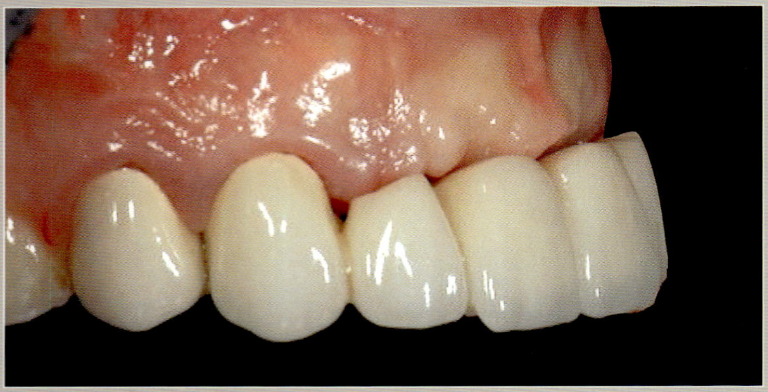

Intraoral lateral view of maxilla with existing fixed partial denture.

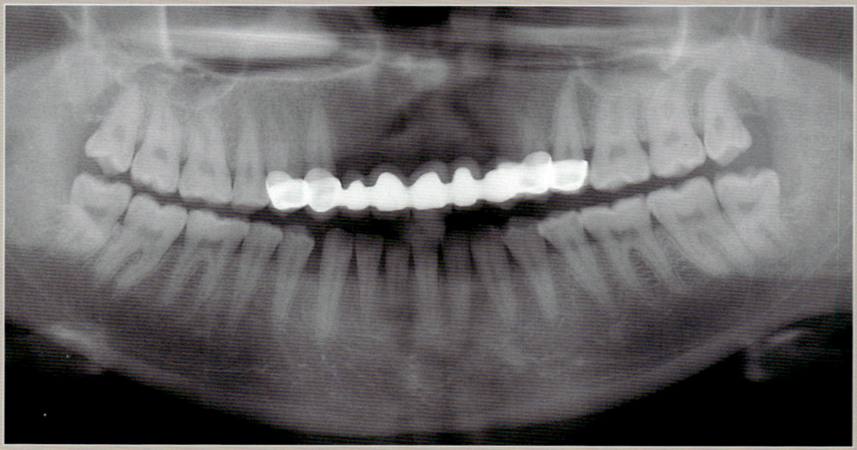

Panoramic radiograph taken before implant placement.

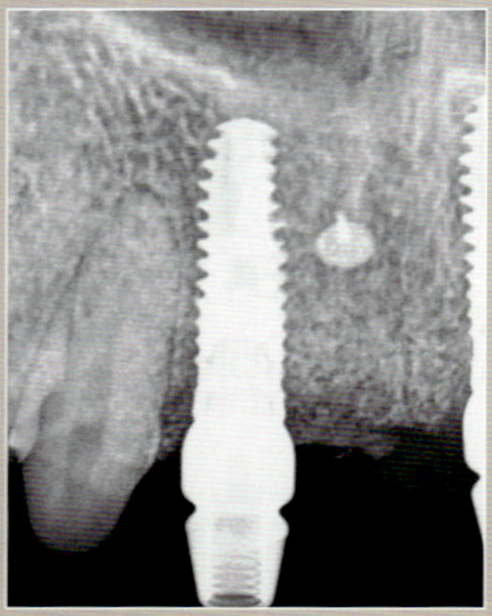

Radiograph of implant at site no. 7.

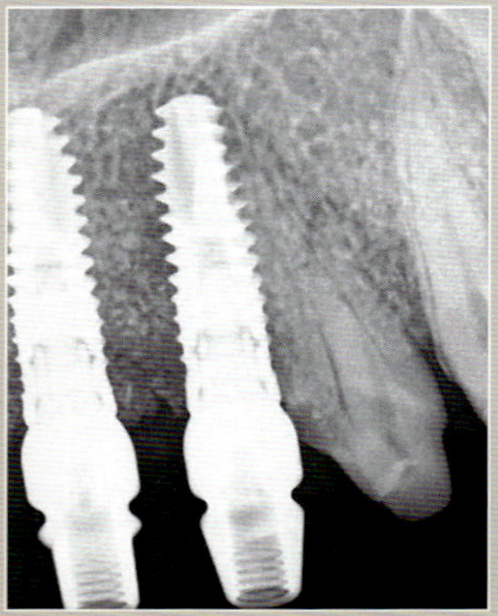

Radiograph of implants at sites nos. 9 and 11.

Dental

- Missing teeth nos. 7 to 11
- No active caries on the remaining teeth
- Diastema between teeth nos. 27 and 28
- No significant wear or attrition

Periodontal

- Acceptable plaque control and oral hygiene
- Isolated areas with slight gingival inflammation
- Healthy and stable periodontium with minimal periodontal pocketing
- Little or no tooth mobility
- Furcation areas intact

Occlusal notes

- Class I canine and molar relationships
- Slight CR-CO shift on closing
- 1-mm horizontal and 1-mm vertical overlap

Radiographic findings

- Good bone levels with exception of anterior bony defect
- Implants replacing missing teeth nos. 7, 9, and 11
- No sign of caries

Diagnosis and prognosis

- AAP Type I
- Healthy periodontium
- Excellent prognosis for all teeth

Summary of concerns

1. How would we address all of the following issues: facial asymmetry; asymmetry of gingival levels; loss of the papillae; long, unsightly interproximal contact areas; flared-out incisal edges; and inverted smile line?
2. How could we achieve a pleasing result that would meet or exceed the patient's expectations?
3. Could we re-create the missing papillae and ridge volume with additional surgical procedures?
4. Could we comply with the patient's wishes and achieve this result without performing any surgery?

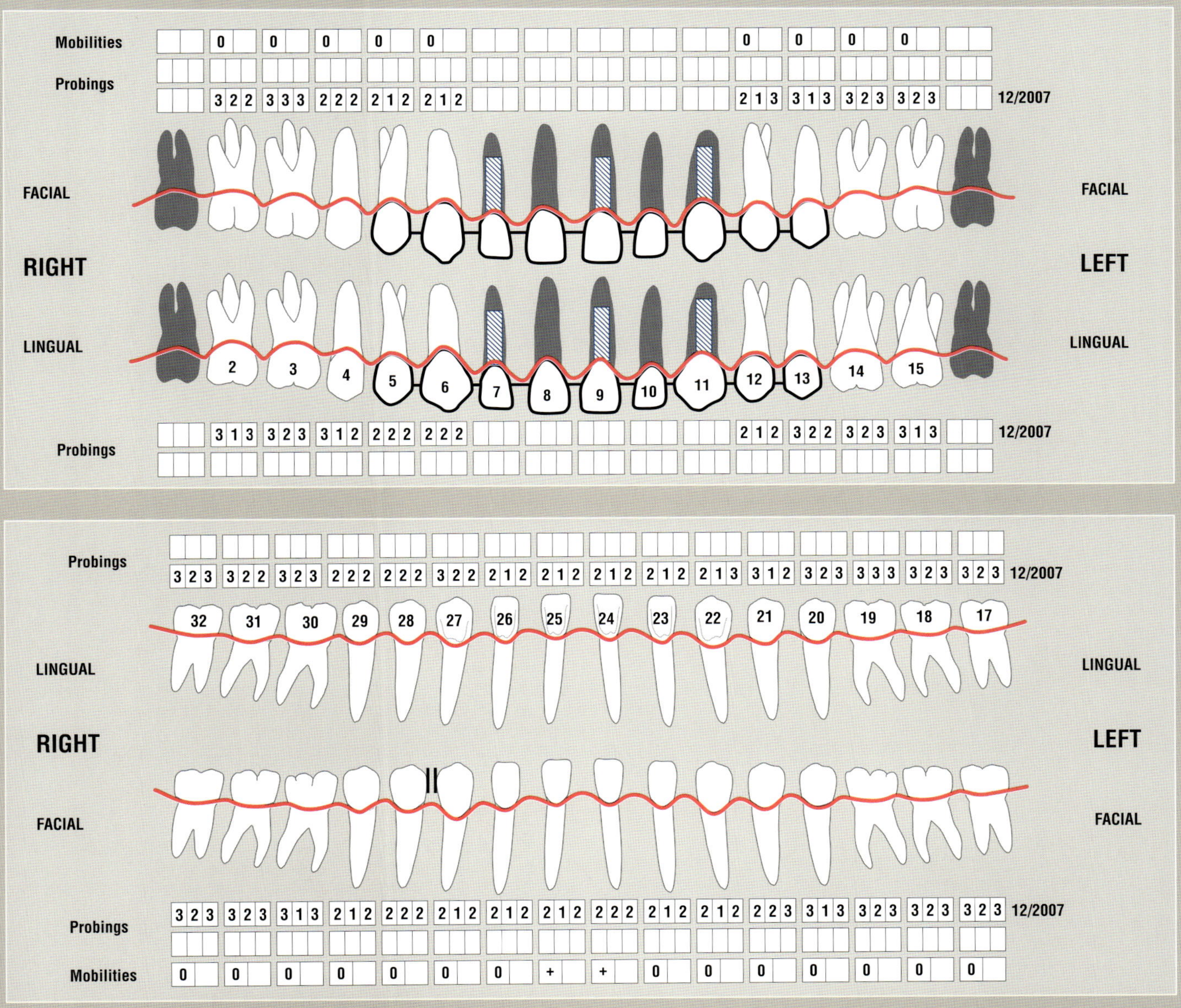

As a learning exercise, you may now outline goals/objectives of treatment and a treatment plan.

Proposed Treatment Plan

Goals/objectives of treatment

Our plan was to accomplish the following:

- Gain white and pink esthetic harmony with a smile design that complements the patient's facial features
- Restore the teeth and implants that had already been placed
- Restore the lost horizontal volume
- Gain lip support and correct the facial asymmetry
- Correct the papillary and gingival levels
- Correct the buccolingual axis of the anterior teeth
- Correct the inverted smile line

Phase I: Initial therapy

1. Comprehensive examination and consultation
2. Pretreatment photographic series
3. Prophylaxis, root planing and scaling, oral hygiene instruction

Phase II: Smile design test drive

4. Clinical and photographic analysis
5. White and pink mock-up to re-create an attractive smile design, support the upper lip, and level the papillae
6. Records taken
7. Finalization of treatment plan and presentation to the patient

Phase III: Definitive restoration

8. Final precision implant impression
9. Fabrication of master casts
10. Maxillomandibular relationship record
11. Framework design
12. Definitive design and implementation of white esthetics
13. Try-in
14. Definitive design and implementation of pink esthetics
15. Finishing
16. Hygiene test
17. Seating of definitive restoration

Phase IV: Follow-up/recall

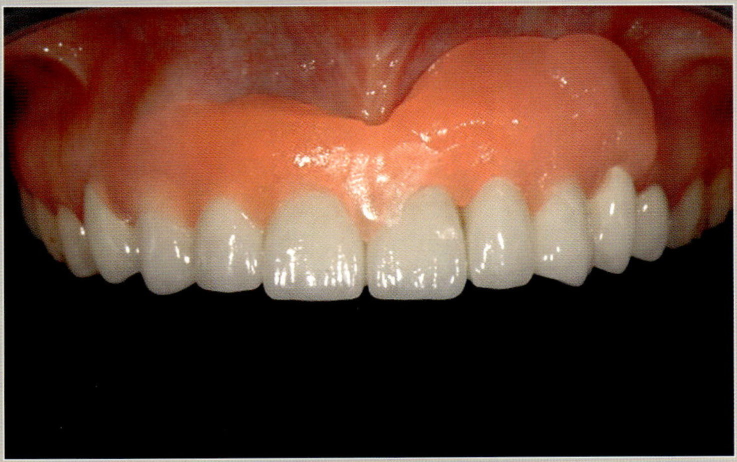

Pink wax placed over the ridge defect to check for interference with upper lip support.

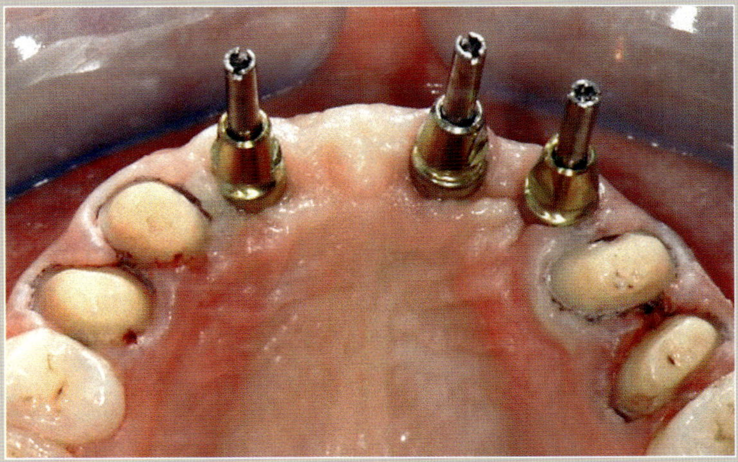

Occlusal view of the maxilla prior to taking open-tray impressions of the teeth and implants.

Review of the goals/objectives of treatment

- Gain white and pink esthetic harmony with a smile design that complements the patient's facial features
- Restore the teeth and implants that had already been placed
- Restore the lost horizontal volume
- Gain lip support and correct the facial asymmetry
- Correct the papillary and gingival levels
- Correct the buccolingual axis of the anterior teeth
- Correct the inverted smile line

Phase I: Initial therapy

At the initial examination, it became quite clear that we would have to address this patient's discontent with her past dental experiences and her appearance before we could consider moving forward with any treatment. Although an examination was scheduled for the first appointment, this was not initiated. Instead, a great deal of time was spent simply listening, acknowledging that her concerns were valid, and expressing a commitment to helping this patient improve her appearance and ultimately her self-esteem. No promises were made other than to explore all treatment possibilities and to decide together what would be the most reasonable approach.

The patient was willing to go through more surgeries if that was the only way to improve her appearance, even though she was very traumatized by previous treatment. Her only hesitation was related to the uncertainty of the treatment outcome even with surgical intervention.

Possible limitations were discussed and realistic expectations set. This appointment cleared the way for developing a good relationship with this patient and gaining an ally in moving forward with treatment.

At the following appointment, a comprehensive examination was performed and a photographic series taken. The patient was then appointed for initial root planing and scaling procedures and oral hygiene instruction.

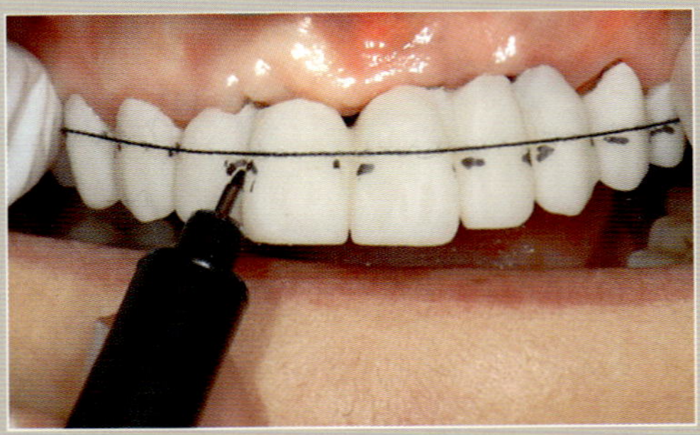

Marking the ideal position of the papillae on a new acrylic provisional restoration.

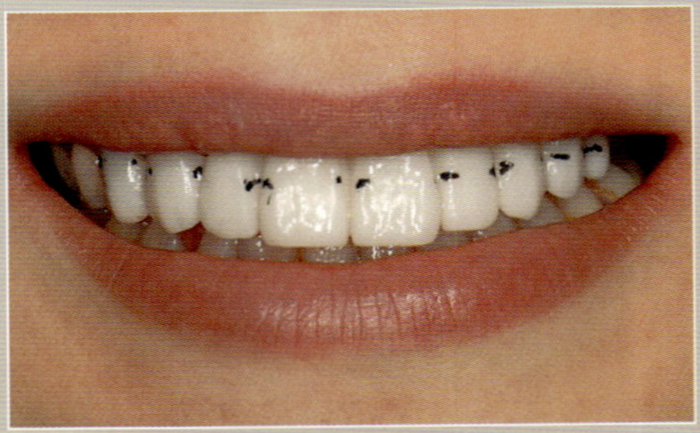

Analyzing and comparing the position of the papillae with the lips.

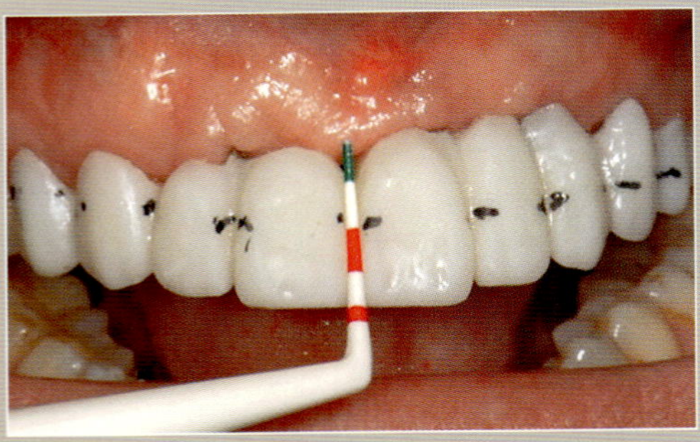

Checking the size of the vertical component of the defect with a probe. Note 5-mm vertical soft tissue deficiency.

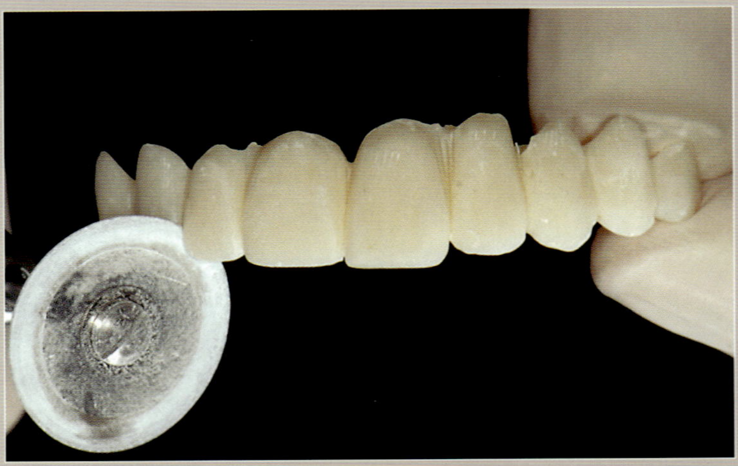

Shaping the partial denture.

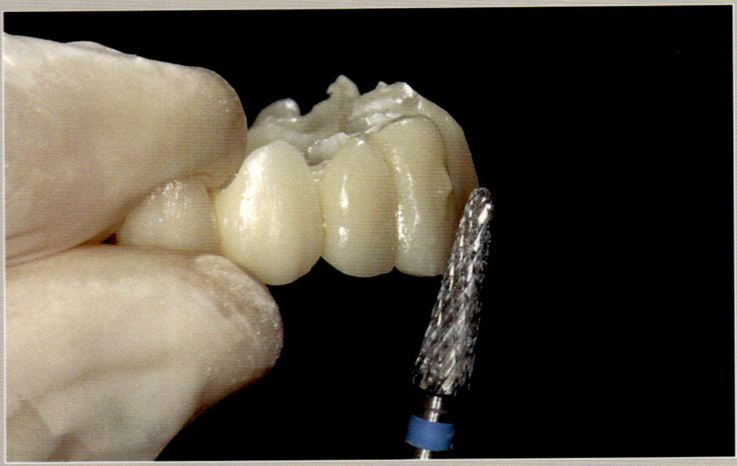

Reducing the incisal third to decrease flaring.

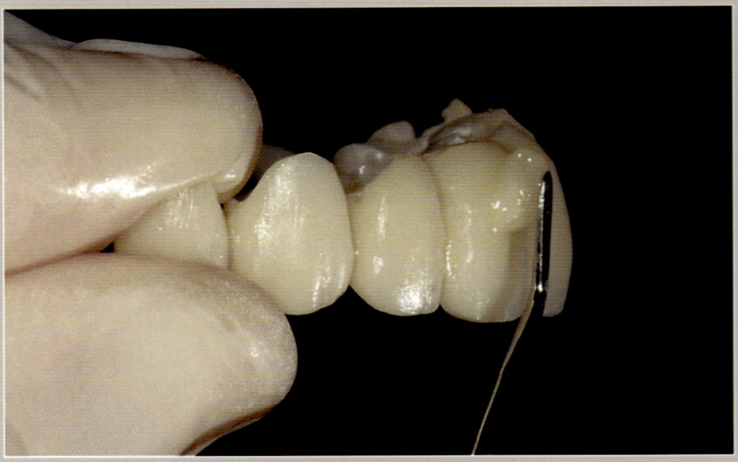

Increasing the cervical volume.

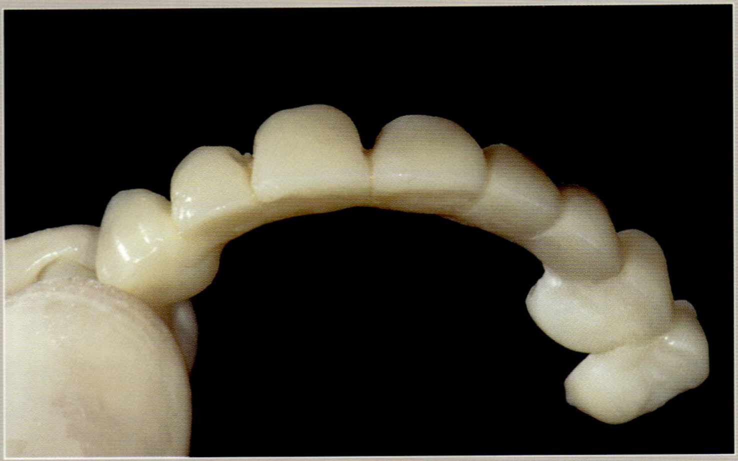

Occlusal view of restoration showing the difference between the side with increased cervical volume and the side that was not modified.

Phase II: Smile design test drive

The main goal of the test drive phase was to more clearly assess the actual dimension of the defect and then be able to determine the most optimal solution, whether it be surgically or prosthetically driven. During this phase of treatment, the first step was to remove the old fixed partial denture and replace it with a new acrylic provisional restoration. This partial denture was seated, and an initial esthetic evaluation was made. The objective was to reposition the anterior teeth into an ideal 3D position, which would complement the face and lips, ignoring the existing ridge defect and its distance from the

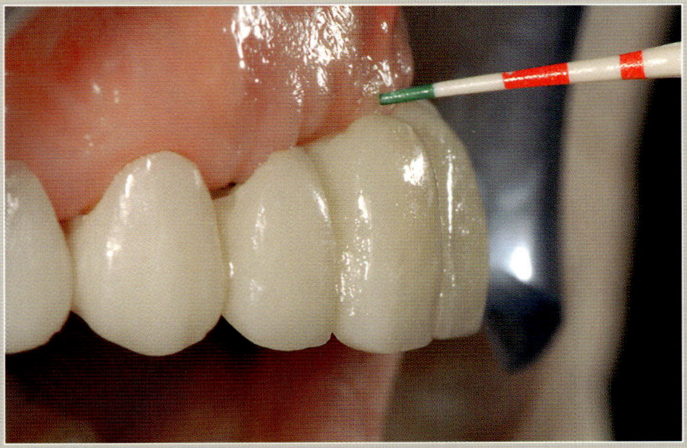

Intraoral lateral view of acrylic provisional restoration showing the horizontal component of the ridge defect (minimum 3 mm).

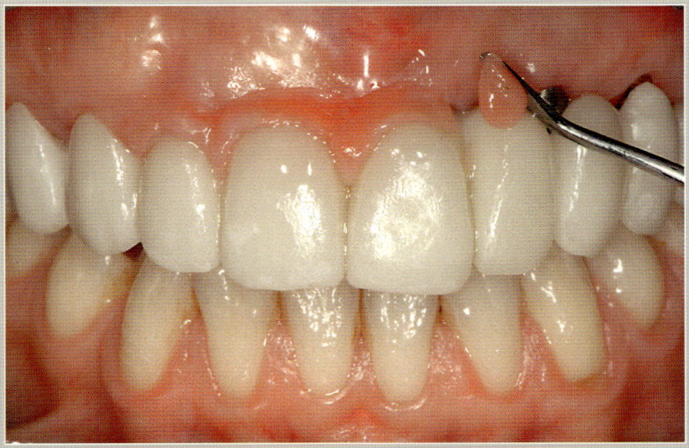

Intraoral addition of pink composite to replace the missing soft tissues.

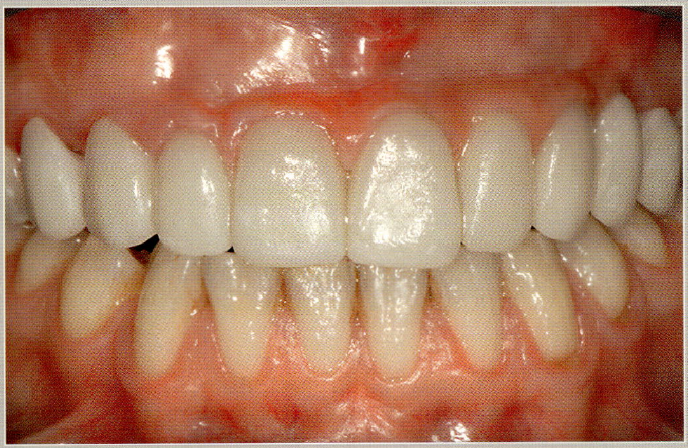

Intraoral frontal view of provisional restoration after placement of the pink composite. Note the correct proportions of the teeth as defined by the new papillae shapes and horizontal pink composite addition.

new location of the teeth. To create the most ideal position, composite material was added on the buccal of the acrylic partial denture to position the teeth anteriorly and incisally, improving the overall esthetic display, reversing the inverted smile line, and correcting the flaring of the anterior teeth. An emphasis was also placed on properly shaping the interproximal areas to create natural tooth morphology and opening space for the future addition of artificial pink material. The shape of the interproximal area is the most critical and challenging part of designing an anterior partial denture. Ideal management of this area allows for the individualization of each crown, creating the illusion of separation among splinted crowns. The interproximal area will also determine the tooth silhouette, which is so important in creating the illusion of tooth shape and proportion. Understanding how to shape this area is a key factor in being able to create natural-looking artificial papillae.

After this first step was completed, the partial denture was seated in the mouth, and the deficient soft tissue space was filled in with pink composite material, re-creating ideal gingival design. The objective was to use the unaffected adjacent gingiva as a guide in shaping the pink composite so that it would blend well with the existing soft tissues. This was most important in the area of the distal papilla of the maxillary right canine and in harmonizing the artificial gingiva with the upper lip.

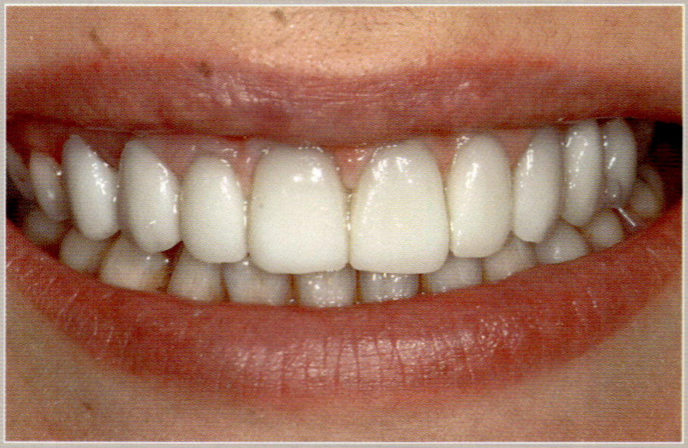

Frontal view of smile with the provisional restoration.

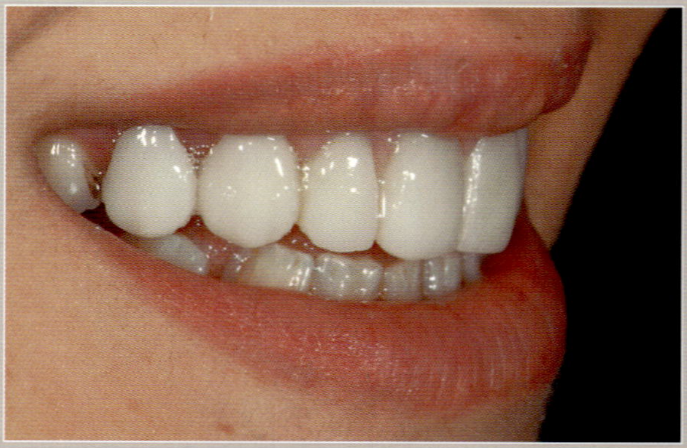

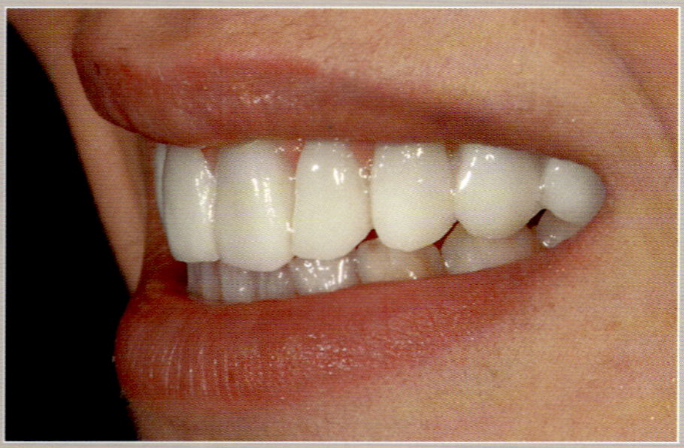

Lateral views of the smile with the provisional restoration.

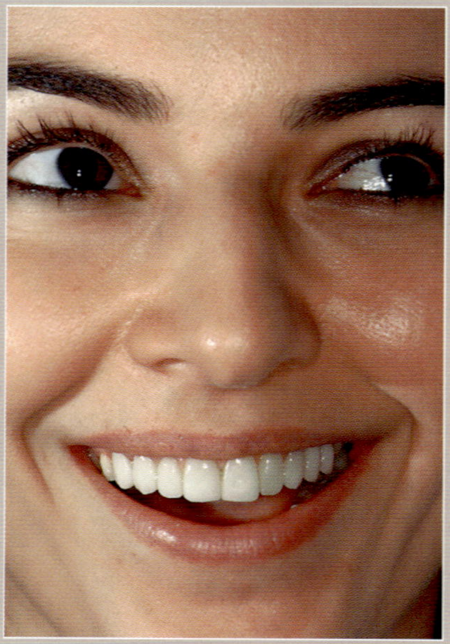

Facial view of smile with the provisional restoration.

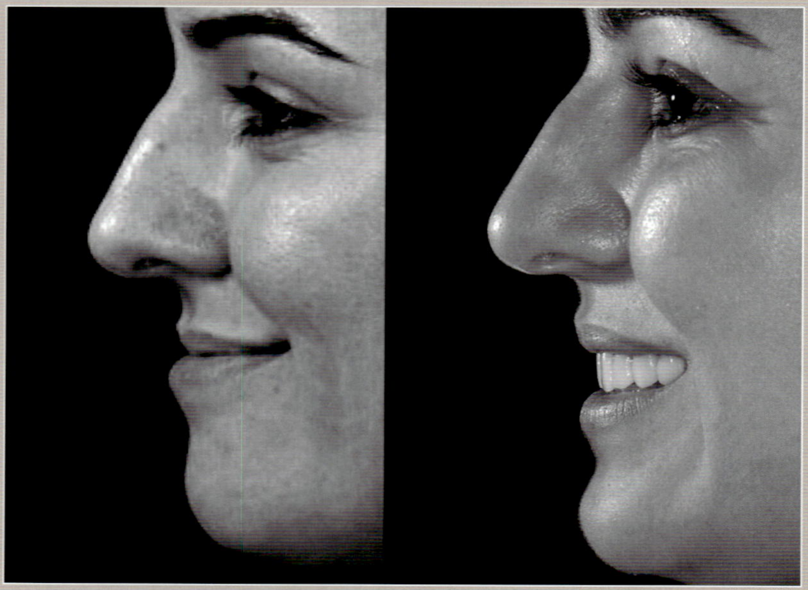

Comparison of facial profiles with the old fixed partial denture *(left)* and the new provisional partial denture *(right)*.

Communicating the proposed definitive esthetic outcome of the smile design test drive with the patient was essential. Photos were taken with the mock-up in the mouth, and final adjustments were made to achieve the best esthetic design for the patient. After this was achieved, an alginate impression was made, and photos were taken to serve as a guide for the definitive restoration.

When comparing the photos of the face with the old fixed partial denture to the new mock-up, the patient was very excited about gaining additional lip support and, most importantly, improving her entire dental and facial appearance.

After analyzing the mock-up clinically and reviewing the photos, it was apparent that a surgical approach would not result in achieving our goals. The patient was informed of this, and an alternative plan was considered. We decided to use the implants placed and fabricate a pink hybrid partial denture. The plan was to design a framework that would allow a retrievable restoration.

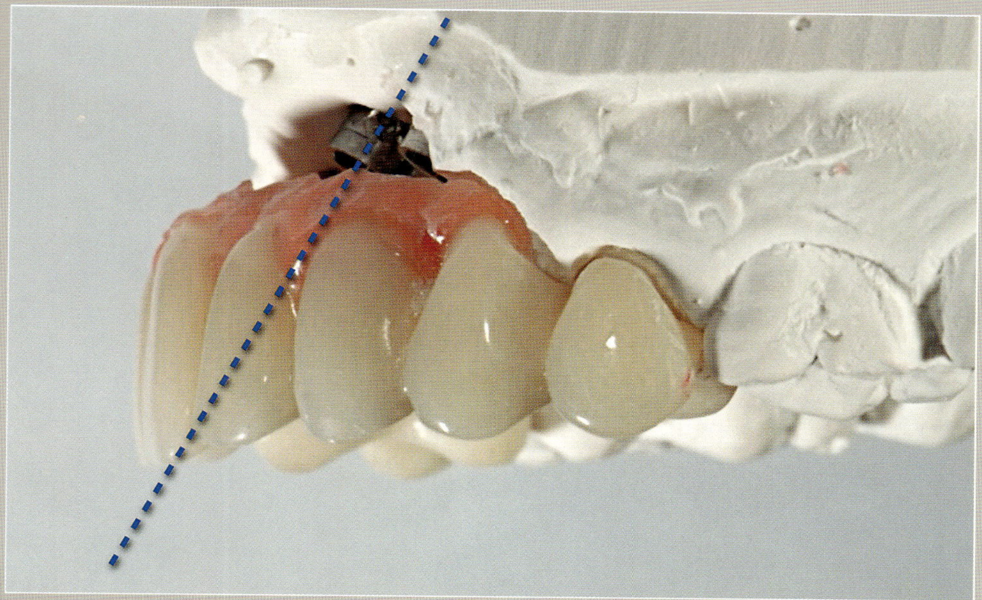

Provisional restoration placed on the cast, showing the implant axis *(dashed line)*, which does not allow lingual screw access.

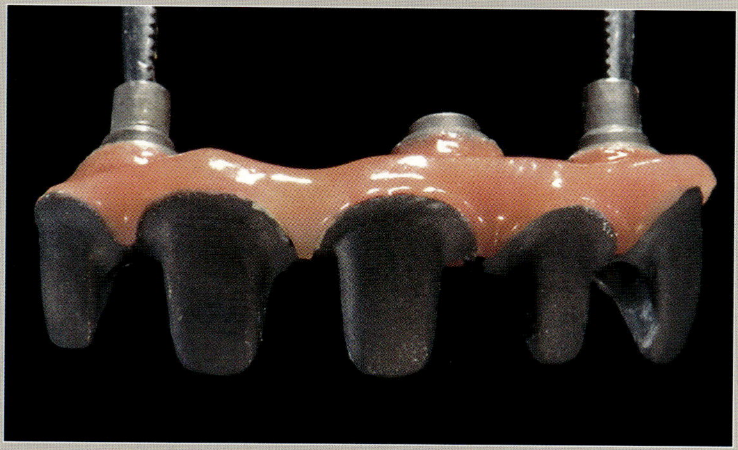

Infrastructure with pink ceramics.

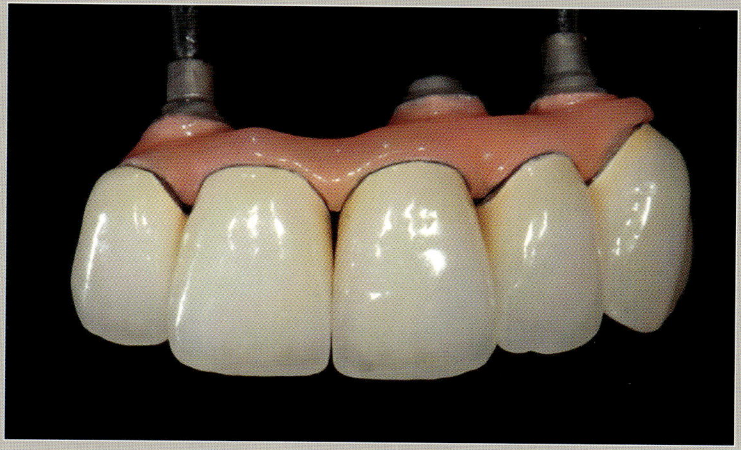

Single crowns on the infrastructure.

Phase III: Definitive restoration

Framework design

There are many advantages to a pink hybrid restoration. These include remarkable esthetic outcomes considering the extent of the hard and soft tissue defects present and retrievability should anything fail in the future. However, there are drawbacks as well. These are related to the design of the restoration, which makes it difficult to perform adequate home care and provide adequate soft tissue conditioning. The solution, interestingly enough, is also found in the design of the restoration, in that it is removable by the dentist to allow for any necessary adjustments, hygiene maintenance, and the addition of restorative material in the future to maintain intimate contact with the soft tissues as recession occurs.

When implant placements are anticipated, we always plan for lingual screw access so that a one-piece, implant-level partial denture can be fabricated. If implants already exist, their locations and/or angulations may not allow for this, and we may have to create alternative solutions, with retrievability still in mind.

In this case, the three implants were emerging from the facial aspect of the future restorations. This would not allow for lingual screw access and presented a formidable challenge. Ultimately, a solution was found. The plan was to develop an infrastructure that would receive the pink material and be screwed over the implants. This infrastructure was made out of dental alloy. The framework would also have the shape of preparations toward the level of the crowns. Then single crowns could be cemented on top of this with provisional cement, allowing us to access the screws when necessary.

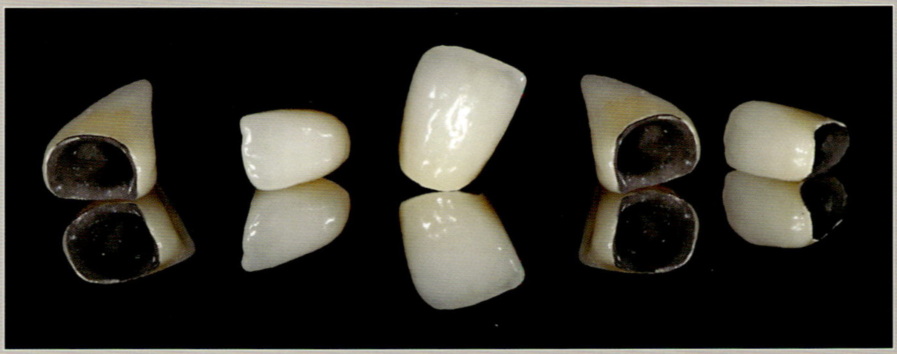

Single PFM restorations.

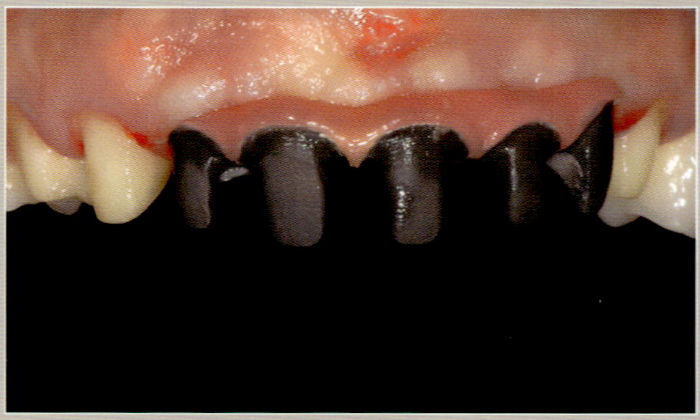

Infrastructure screwed in intraorally.

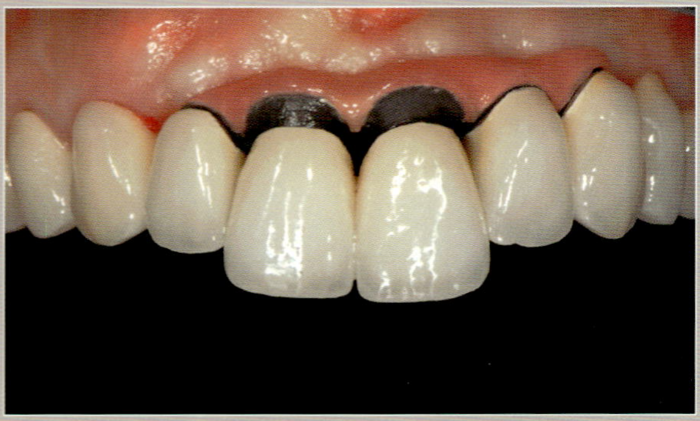

Try-in of the crowns.

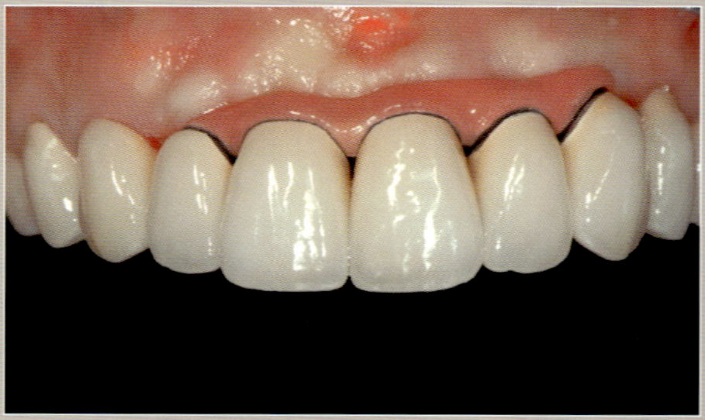

Intraoral frontal view of the crowns in position.

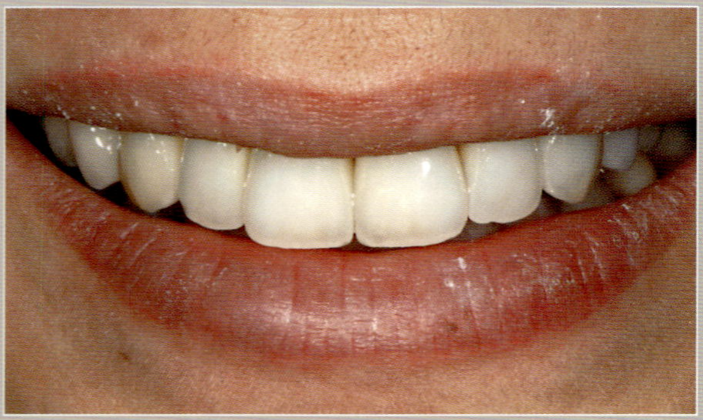

Smile view of the crowns.

White esthetics

Single dental alloy–ceramic restorations were fabricated on top of the infrastructure, following the white esthetic principles developed on the mock-up.

Try-in

The infrastructure was screwed in the mouth. The crowns were seated in position, and the white esthetic evaluation was made. After the necessary final adjustments, the crowns were glazed.

Pink esthetics

The infrastructure was then removed and the pink ceramics treated to be able to receive the pink composite when reseated intraorally. The frame was then reseated, crowns were cemented provisionally on top of it, and the pink composite was added, following the pink esthetic principles developed on the mock-up.

Finishing

The partial denture was unscrewed following removal of the crowns. The pink composite was refined at the laboratory bench, with the undercuts and thin edges removed, followed by a final light curing cycle and polishing of the restoration.

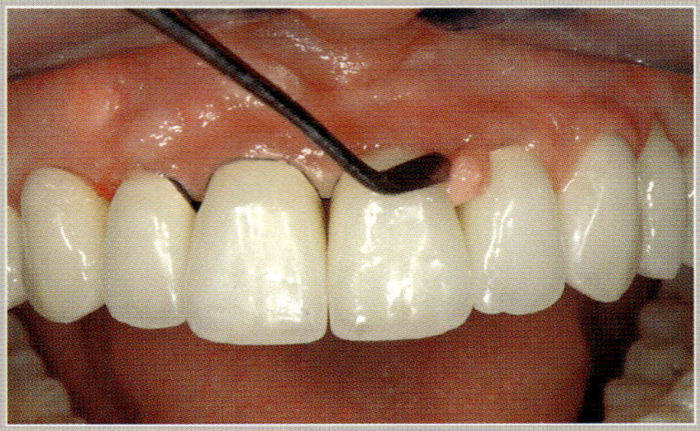

Incremental addition and light curing of the pink composite intraorally.

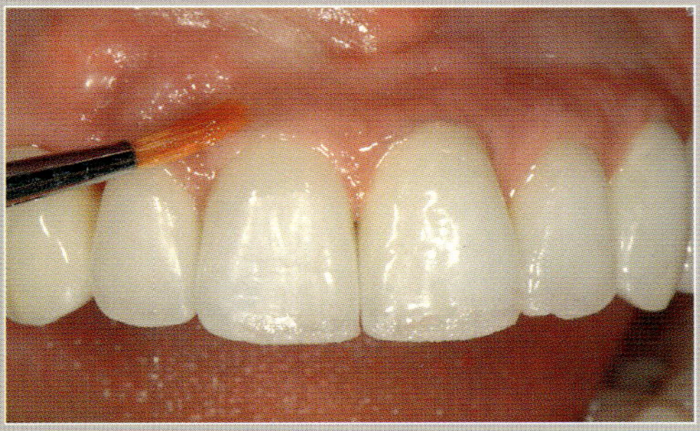

A brush is used to apply stains, the edges are blended, and texture is created.

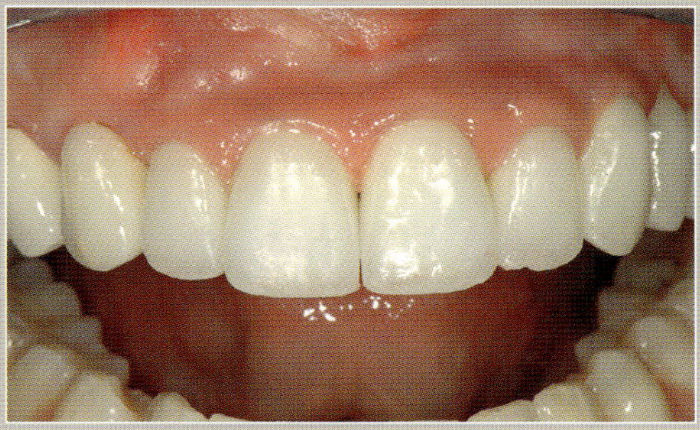

Intraoral frontal view after completion of direct pink composite.

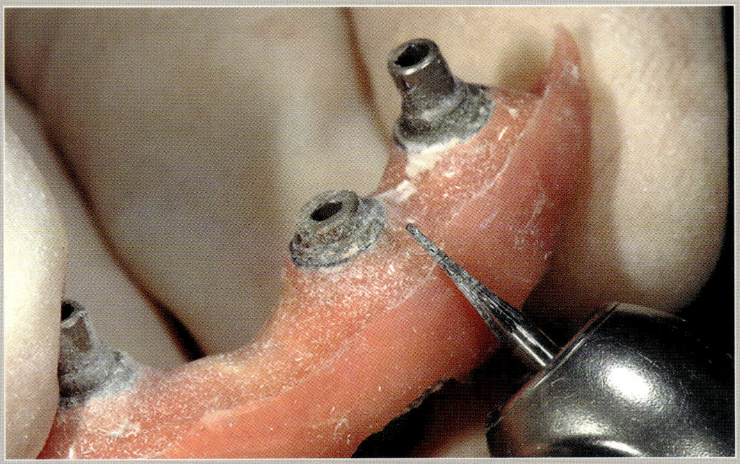

After removal of the crowns and infrastructure from the mouth, the edges of the pink composite are smoothed with a carbide bur.

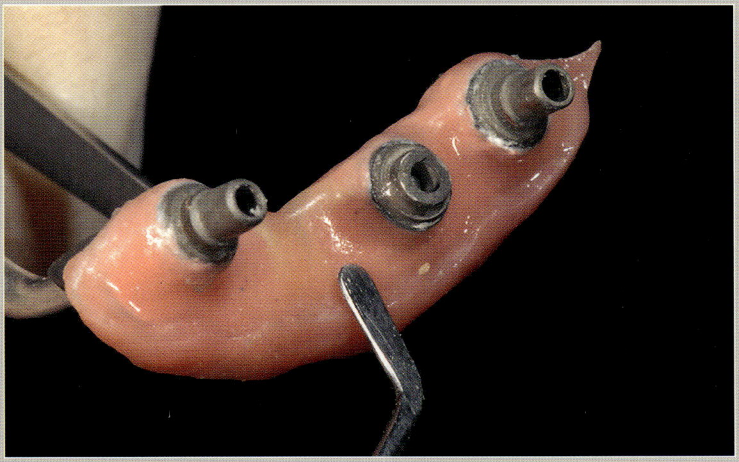

Addition of pink composite to improve the emergence profile and fill in undercuts.

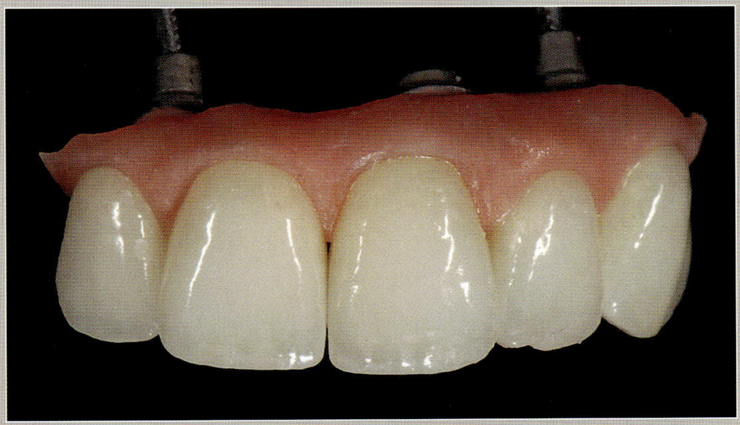

Definitive partial denture ready for the last try-in.

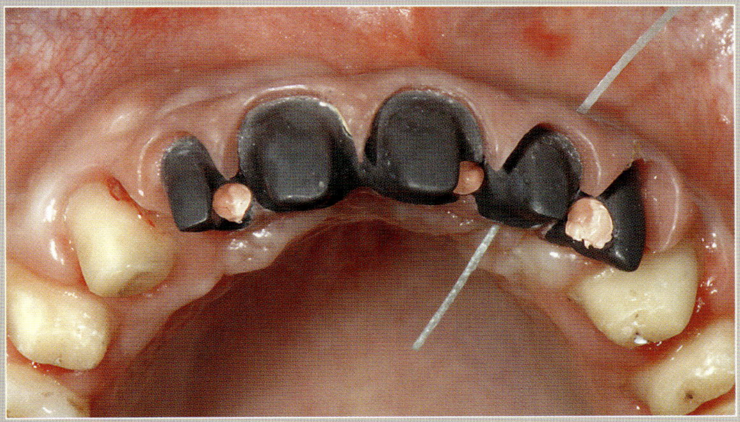

Occlusal view of flossing procedures around the infrastructure.

Hygiene test

The infrastructure was placed back in the mouth, and the flossing procedure was tested. The entire interface between artificial and natural gingiva should be cleansable. If some spots are difficult to reach, adjustments can be made on the restoration to improve access for ideal home care. The process should be tested by the clinician and then explained and demonstrated very carefully to the patient.

Final seating

After final evaluation of access for adequate oral hygiene and the condition of the soft tissue, the infrastructure was screwed down definitively, and the single crowns were seated with cement.

Follow-up

The patient was scheduled for a 3-month postoperative reevaluation, at which we planned to evaluate the soft tissue condition and the patient's level of oral hygiene. Oral hygiene reinforcement and instruction would be implemented if necessary.

Posttreatment

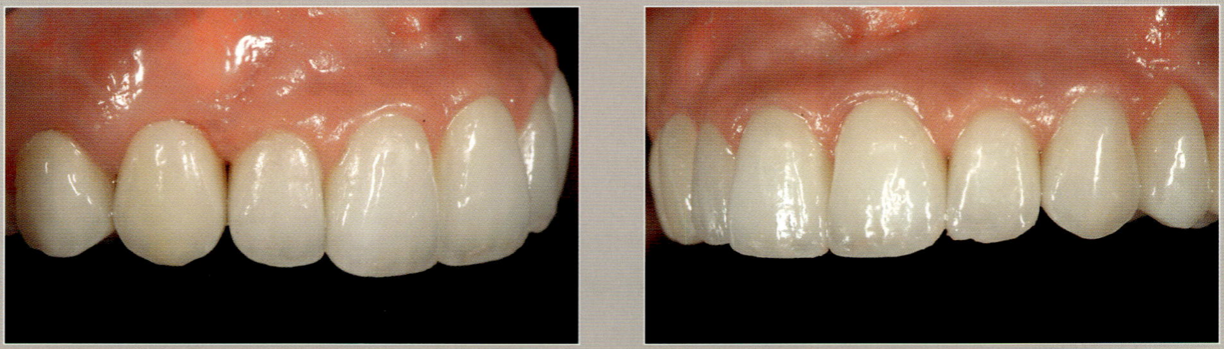

Intraoral lateral views of definitive restoration.

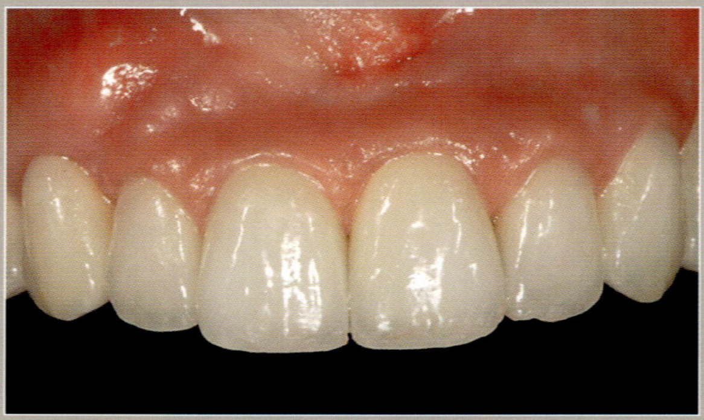

Intraoral frontal view.

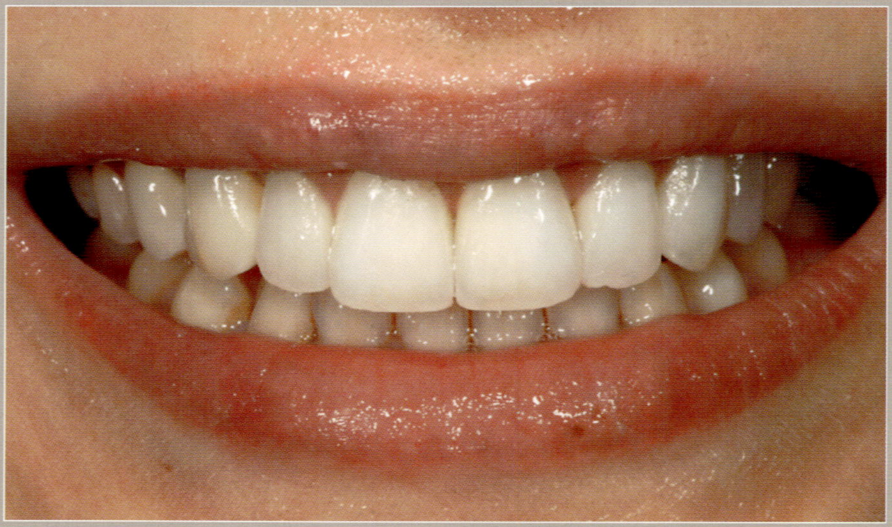

Frontal smile view.

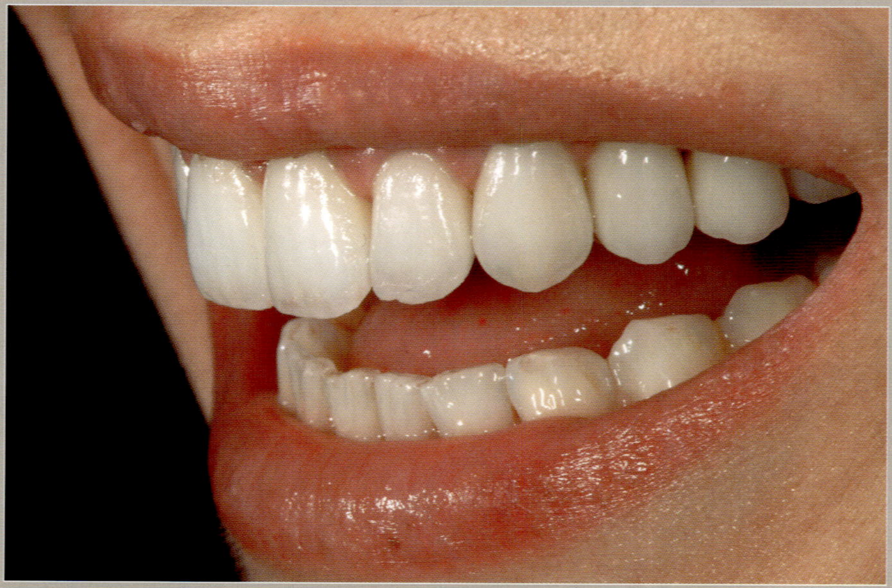

Oblique left lateral smile view.

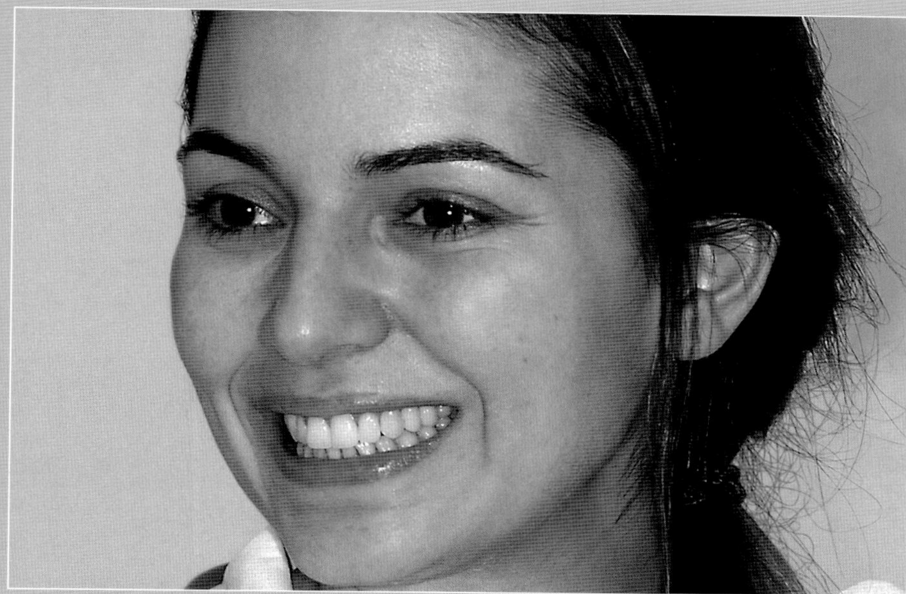

Facial view of smile.

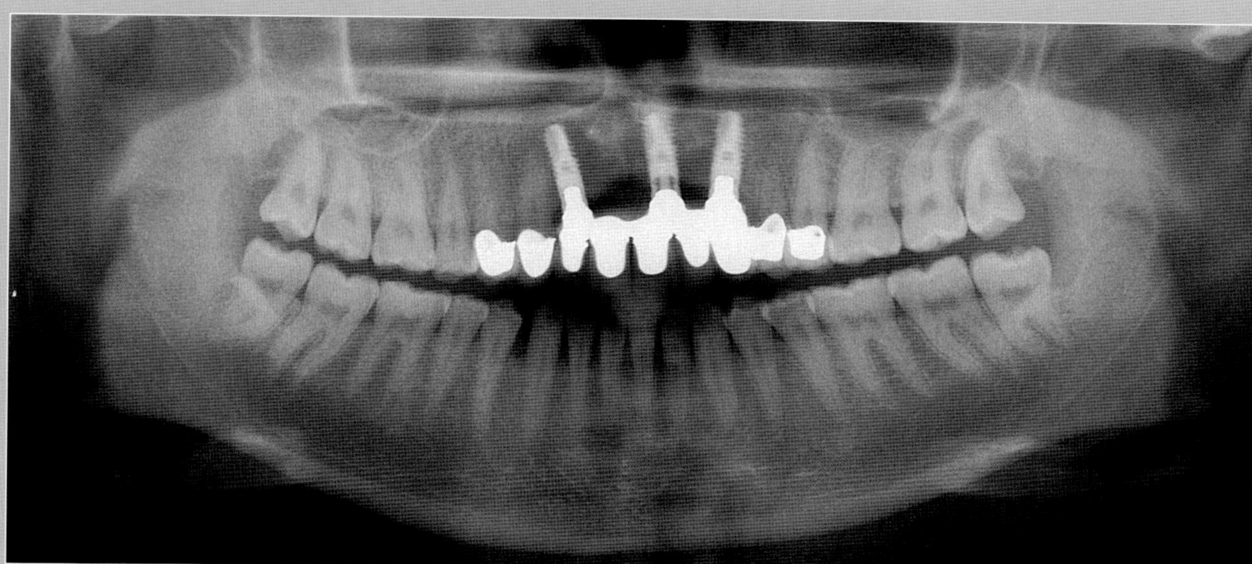

Panoramic radiograph.

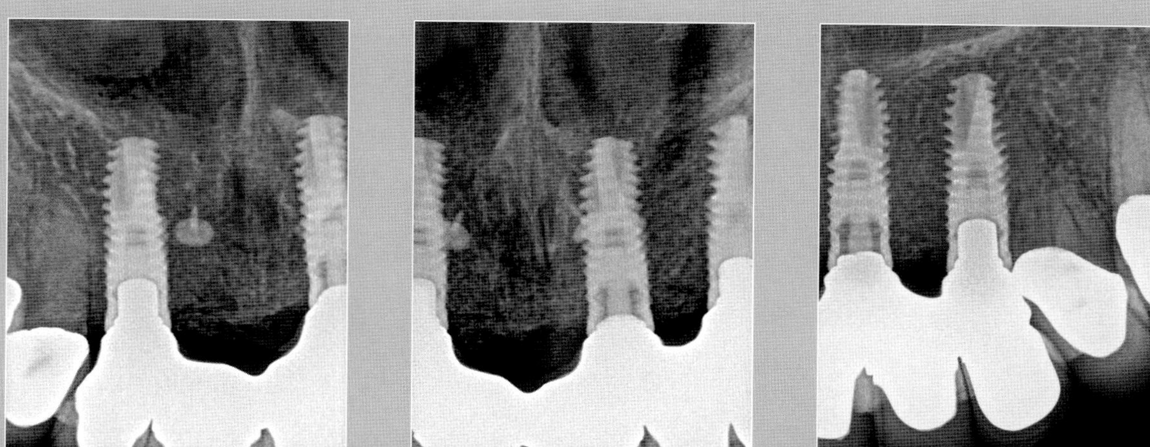

Radiographs of implants at sites nos. 7, 9, and 11.

You may now place the corresponding posttreatment overlay found in the separate folder over the pretreatment periodontal chart on page 145.

A Novel Design for Overcoming Bone Loss

Eric Van Dooren, DDS

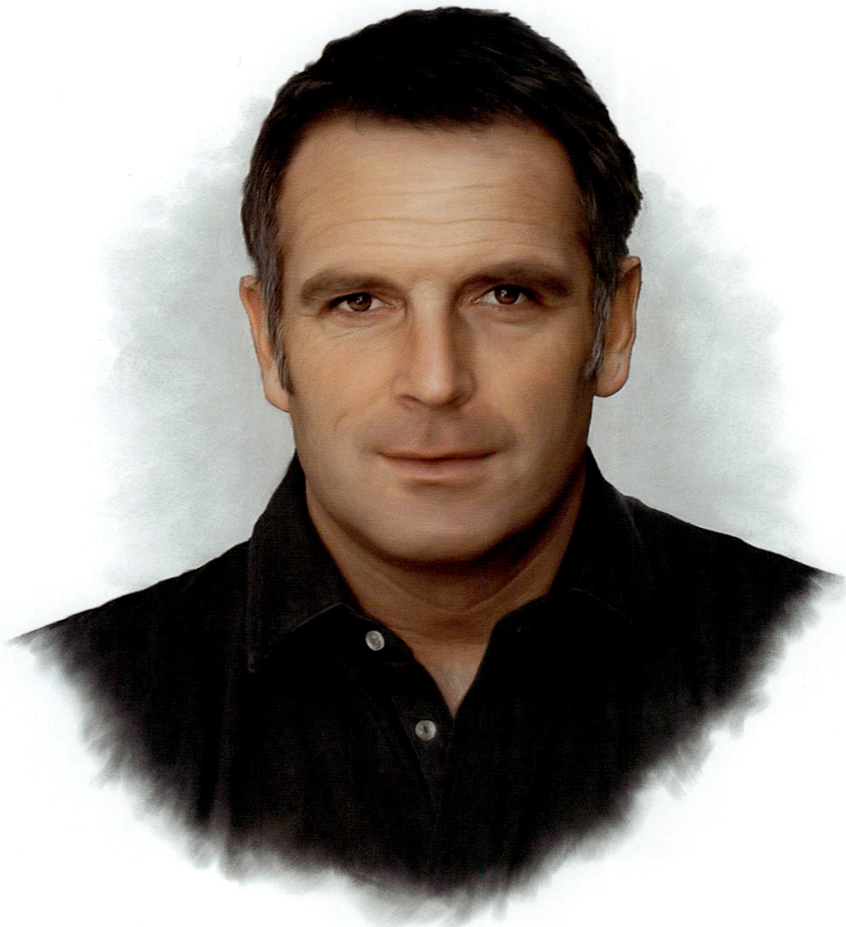

The "new world" of esthetic dentistry has created a great burden for the practicing clinician. Media-centered advertising would have one believe that anyone and everyone can buy the "perfect" smile. Although most of us recognize that this is not the case, this global hype has created a number of negative consequences:

- Patients present for treatment with unrealistic expectations.
- Many dentists are misguided into thinking that they should be able to meet or exceed patient esthetic expectations in all cases. Many of these clinicians feel inadequate if they cannot achieve the results that they see in monthly dental journals and magazines and online resources.
- Some cosmetic dentists are focusing more on patient "wants" than on patient "needs" and are not availing themselves of a comprehensive approach to treatment.

This case was chosen because it is does not exemplify ideal treatment. It is not a treatment plan that the present-day cosmetic dentist would necessarily want to implement. And it is not a plan that the treating clinicians would consider as a first or even second choice of therapy. However, it is a very realistic and practical plan, considering the amount of bone loss present in the esthetic zone. It is novel in its design and relatively straightforward in implementation. This plan was minimally invasive and simple in concept, and the treatment outcome was esthetically pleasing.

Case Presentation 3

Treating clinicians
Prosthodontist, periodontist, and implant surgeon: Eric Van Dooren, DDS
Orthodontist: Ralph Lemmens, DDS
Dental laboratory and smile designer: Christian Coachman, DDS, CDT

Clinical Treatment Planning

Age at initial presentation: 42 years
Initial presentation: August 2007
Active treatment completed: February 2009

Introduction and background

A 42-year-old woman presented with an esthetic problem associated with a failing implant restoration. The previous treatment, which was necessitated by trauma resulting from a car accident, was performed 7 years prior to the initial examination. Extensive bone grafting was performed at that time in order to restore the anterior ridge defect. Two implants had been placed in the areas of the missing teeth nos. 9 and 10. This patient's main complaint was an unpleasing smile. She was not in favor of re-treating the area surgically but stated that she might consider this option if it was minimally invasive. She also insisted that any solution be relatively simple and limited to as few procedures as possible.

Medical history

- No notable findings
- Smokes 10 cigarettes/day

Diagnostic findings

Extraoral and facial findings

- Patient attempts to conceal teeth when smiling but displays teeth with full smile.

Intraoral findings

Dental

- Crowding of the mandibular anterior teeth
- Supraeruption of teeth nos. 23 to 26
- Porcelain cracked and failing on teeth nos. 6 and 11
- Caries on tooth no. 8

Periodontal

- Thin gingival phenotype
- Generalized slight gingival inflammation
- Generalized periodontal probing depths of 2 to 3 mm
- Generalized moderate scalloping of gingival margins
- Generalized slight gingival recession
- Slight localized gingival recession on facial of previously restored teeth, especially tooth no. 6
- Extensive ridge deficiency in the area of teeth nos. 9 and 10
- Slight facial gingival excess on teeth nos. 2, 3, 7, 12, and 13
- Fair to good home care with minimal to moderate amounts of plaque present

Occlusal notes

- Angle Class II occlusion
- Horizontal overlap: 2.0 mm
- Vertical overlap: 2.5 mm
- Mandibular range of motion within normal limits

Radiographic findings

- Advanced bone loss between implants at sites nos. 9 and 10
- Subgingival cement trapped between implants at sites nos. 9 and 10
- Open margins and imprecise fit of full crown on implant at site no. 9

Pretreatment

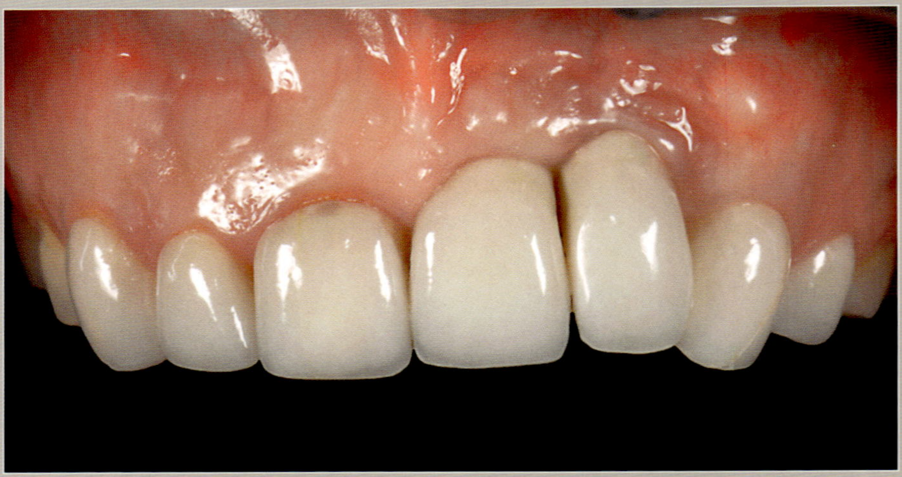

Intraoral frontal view of maxilla.

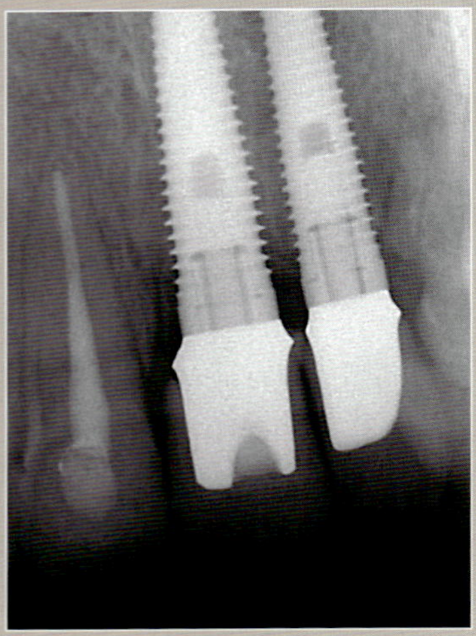

Radiograph of implants.

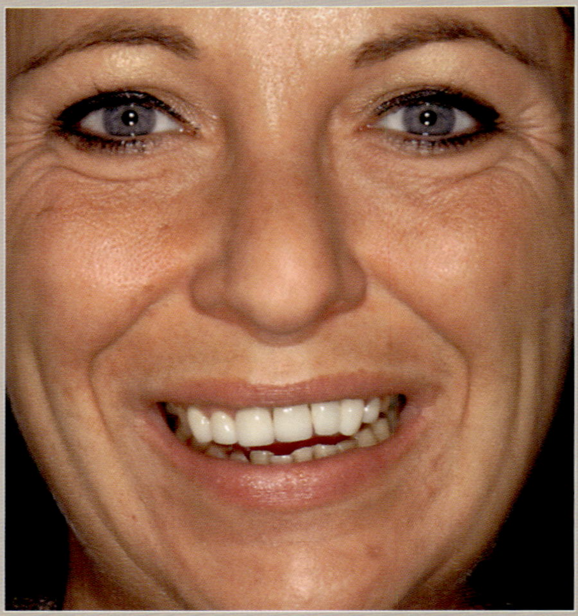

Facial view of smile.

Diagnosis

- Generalized slight marginal gingivitis
- Advanced bone loss around implants at sites nos. 9 and 10
- Severe soft tissue deformity in area of implants at sites nos. 9 and 10

Prognosis

- General: excellent
- Implants at sites nos. 9 and 10: poor

Treatment-planning considerations

- This patient was very apprehensive about treatment because of negative past dental experiences and expressed interest in a noninvasive, nonsurgical approach to treatment. She qualified her wishes by stating that if surgery was absolutely unavoidable to achieve a successful esthetic result, it should be minimal and limited to a single surgical procedure.
- The patient expressed some concerns about her smile, especially regarding the midline, inclination of the incisal plane, and lack of symmetry in the length and form of her anterior teeth.
- This patient wanted to focus on the failing implants and did not want any of her other teeth to be treated. On the other hand, she understood that in order to improve tooth proportions and to create more esthetic harmony and balance, additional teeth may require treatment.

Summary of concerns

1. Even if the patient consents to surgical soft and hard tissue augmentation, are there any surgical techniques that would predictably and fully restore the anterior ridge to its original state? Is it advisable to propose surgery, even with qualifications, and possibly create unrealistic expectations?
2. Considering that this patient is hesitant to proceed with any surgical treatment, if a decision is made to replace the existing crowns and to try to restore harmony and balance to the face and smile, how can this be accomplished with minimally invasive procedures?
3. Recognizing that we may be limited in the amount of vertical ridge augmentation that can be achieved, how will we be able to compensate for this restoratively to meet or exceed the patient's treatment expectations?

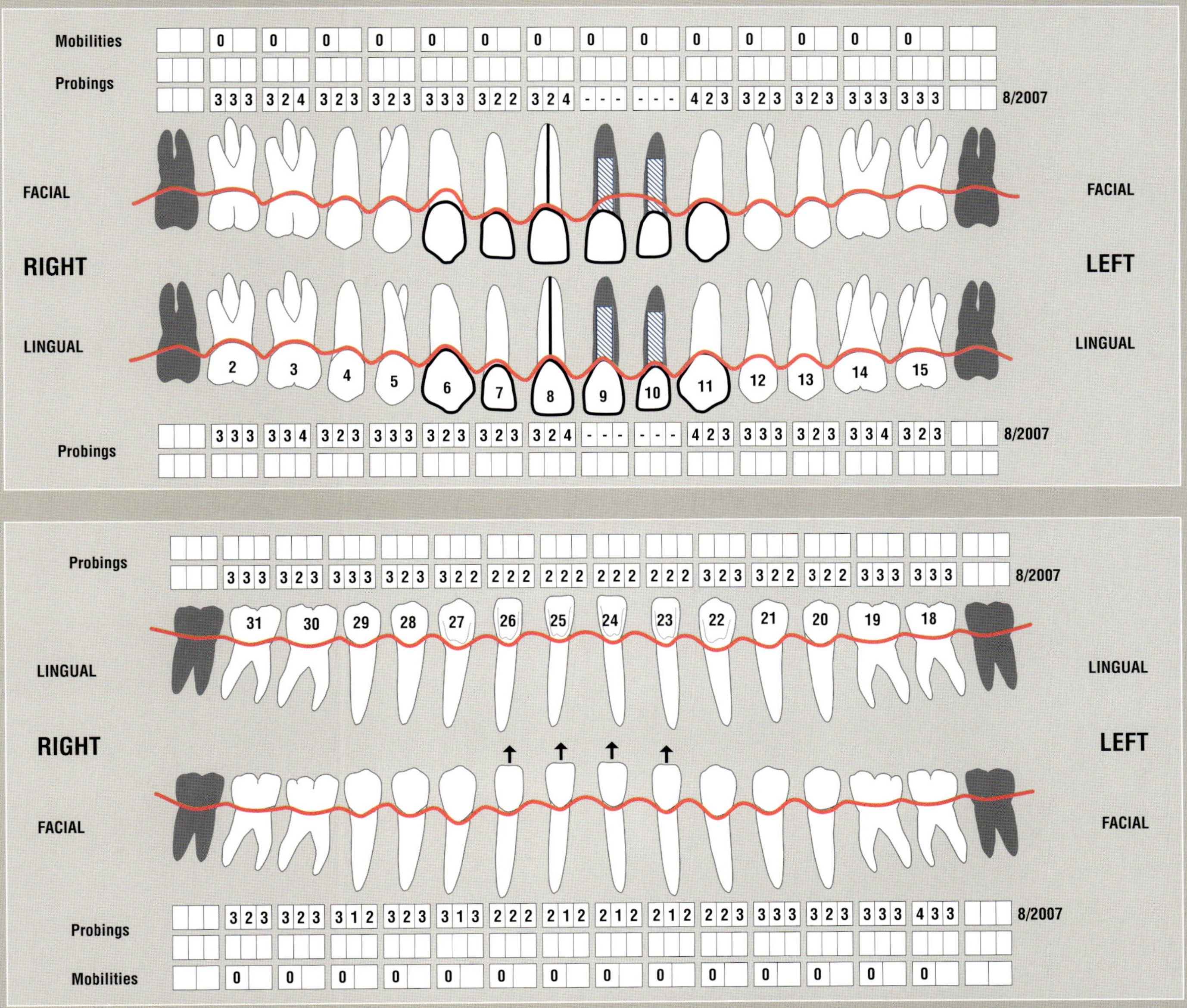

As a learning exercise, you may now outline goals/objectives of treatment and a treatment plan.

Proposed Treatment Plan

Goals/objectives of treatment

- Accomplish a fixed method of rehabilitation without involving nonrestored teeth
- Achieve optimal esthetics

Phase I: Data gathering and digital planning

1. Intraoral and full-face digital photos are captured in order to establish:

    - Proper incisal edge position
    - Appropriate midline position and angulation
    - Ideal tooth proportions and gingival contours

Photographic documentation is transferred to the computer for digital planning. The first step would be to relate the full-face smile photo to the horizontal reference line. The most common reference line used is the interpupillary line; however, the nasal or commissural lines can also be used. The midline is then projected onto the horizontal line, and digital planning is initiated. The treatment plan is evaluated, modified, and related to the DSD.

Phase II: Transfer of digital wax-up to the master cast

2. The digital plan is transferred to the master cast.
3. Tooth form is copied from the digital forms.
4. White esthetics are optimized.
5. Pink esthetics are optimized.
6. The 3D defect around the implants is filled with pink wax, which allows us to evaluate the vertical and horizontal components of the ridge deficiency.

Phase III: Fabrication of intraoral mock-up and provisional partial denture

7. The digital project or intraoral smile design is evaluated.
8. Old restorations are removed, and tooth locations and form are evaluated. Anterior provisional partial denture is fabricated.
9. DSD is evaluated and minor changes in form are made, if necessary, by applying flowable composite. The size of the anterior ridge defect is visualized by both the patient and the dentist.
10. Decisions are made as to whether and to what extent the anterior defect can be managed and how this will affect the definitive restoration. Much of the decision making occurs based on careful 3D evaluation of the soft tissue contours, with special focus on the papilla heights and volume.
11. Esthetic and functional evaluation is performed to establish incisal edge position, soft tissue contours, altered midline inclination, lip support, and tooth form, which should provide overall facial balance and harmony.
12. Patient approval is obtained.
13. The treatment plan is finalized.

Phase IV: Establishing the definitive treatment plan

14. Any final changes to the treatment plan are made, taking into consideration patient preferences. Final adjustments are also made to maximize soft tissue harmony, gain optimal soft tissue contours (compensating for the ridge deficiency), and optimize selection of prosthetic materials.
15. The definitive digital and intraoral concept is translated into the definitive treatment plan.

Phase V: Orthodontic therapy

16. Orthodontic treatment is initiated in the mandibular arch to realign the mandibular anterior teeth and to intrude the incisors to aid in reducing the existing vertical overlap.

Phase VI: Surgical treatment

17. Surgical therapy is performed, including possible clinical crown lengthening to attain adequate biologic width in the maxillary anterior segment.
18. Connective tissue grafting is performed where indicated to augment the anterior ridge.
19. Postoperative care is provided, and healing is allowed to occur.

Phase VII: Definitive restorations

20. Minimally invasive definitive tooth preparation is performed.
21. Final impressions are taken, and the master cast is fabricated.
22. Definitive restorations are fabricated.
23. All restorations are tried in.
24. The definitive restoration is cemented.

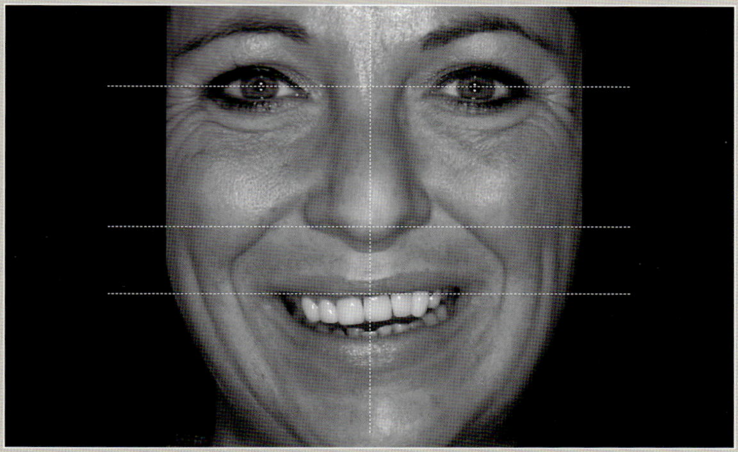

Digital determination of the facial midline and horizontal reference plane on the facial photograph.

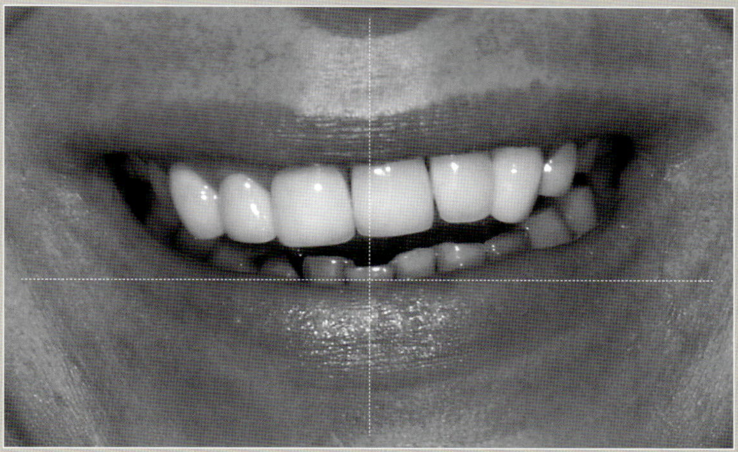

Close-up of smile from facial photograph with facial reference lines.

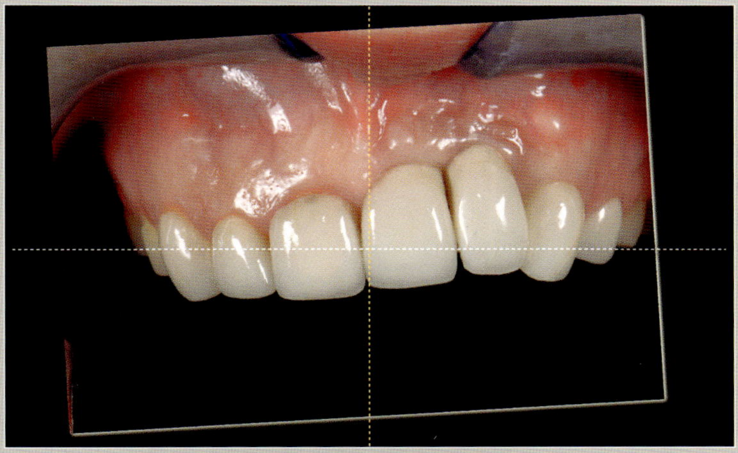

Transfer of the reference lines to the intraoral situation.

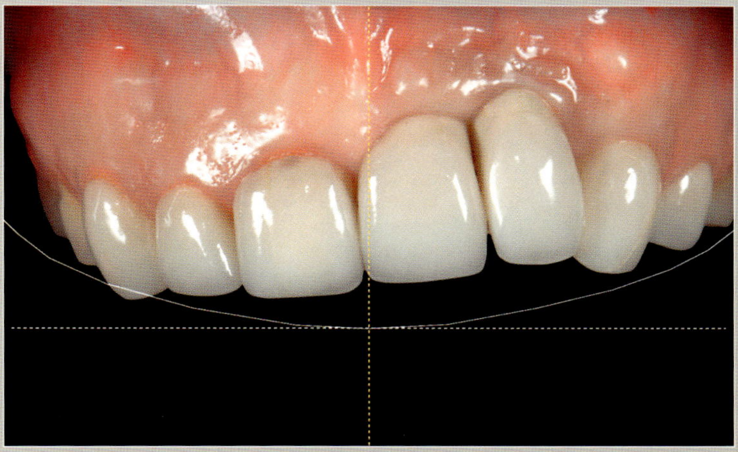

Incisal edge guideline.

Review of the goals/objectives of treatment

- The goals and objectives of treatment for this patient were to accomplish a fixed method of rehabilitation without involving nonrestored teeth and to achieve optimal esthetics. The patient limited possible therapeutic options by insisting that treatment be performed with the fewest number of minimally invasive procedures.
- Digital treatment planning would be used in designing the most practical approach to achieving esthetic success considering the extent of the anterior alveolar ridge deficiency present.

Phase I: Data gathering and digital planning

A protocol was established to be able to transfer the clinical and digital findings into a digital treatment plan. Photographic and dynamic video data were gathered on the patient. Intraoral and full-face smile images were taken. This data would be important for establishing proper incisal edge position, midline position and angulation, tooth preparation, and gingival contours.

The photographic information was transferred to a computer so that digital planning could be initiated by relating the full-face smile image to the horizontal reference line. It was evident that digital planning with only an intraoral photo would make it extremely difficult to correctly analyze these parameters because of the lack of any facial horizontal reference.

The interpupillary line should be the first reference used to establish the horizontal plane, but it should not be the only one. We have to analyze the face as a whole and then determine the best horizontal reference that will result in the most harmonious facial outcome. Other facial lines, such as the nasal line, commissure line, and mandibular angle, should be analyzed. Determining the horizontal plane of reference is a much more subjective and artistic decision than an objective exercise. We have found that it is easier to determine this esthetic reference digitally rather than relying on a facebow or any other device. The static image of the patient on the computer screen and the addition of the lines is the most

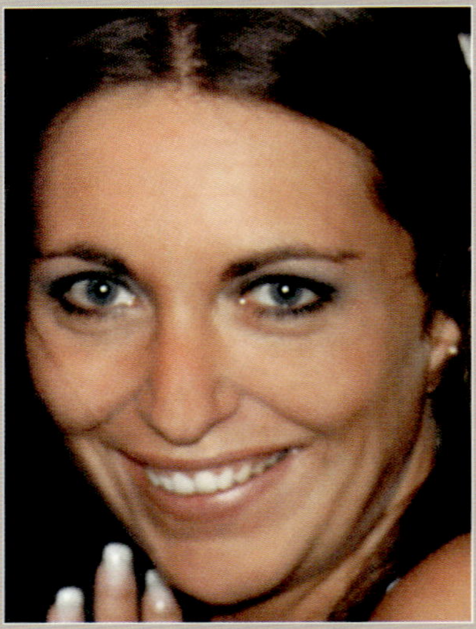

Photograph of the patient taken before the accident with the natural dentition intact.

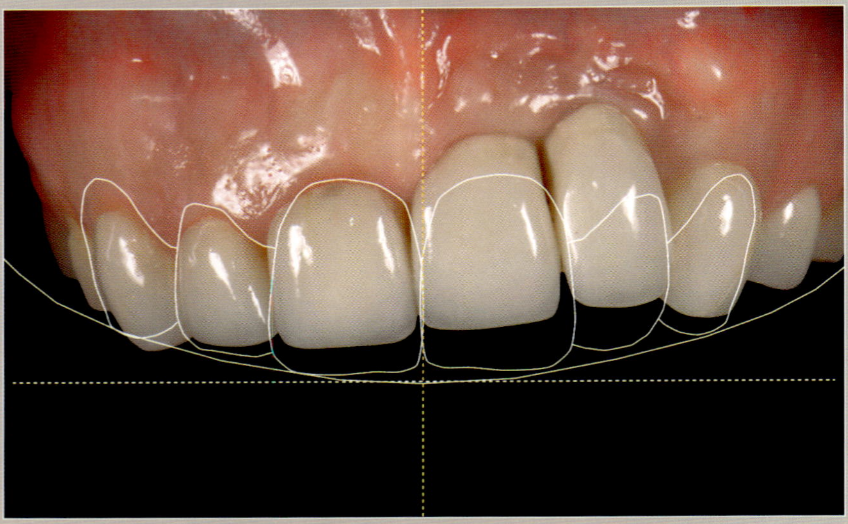

Outlines of the teeth accomplished using Keynote software.

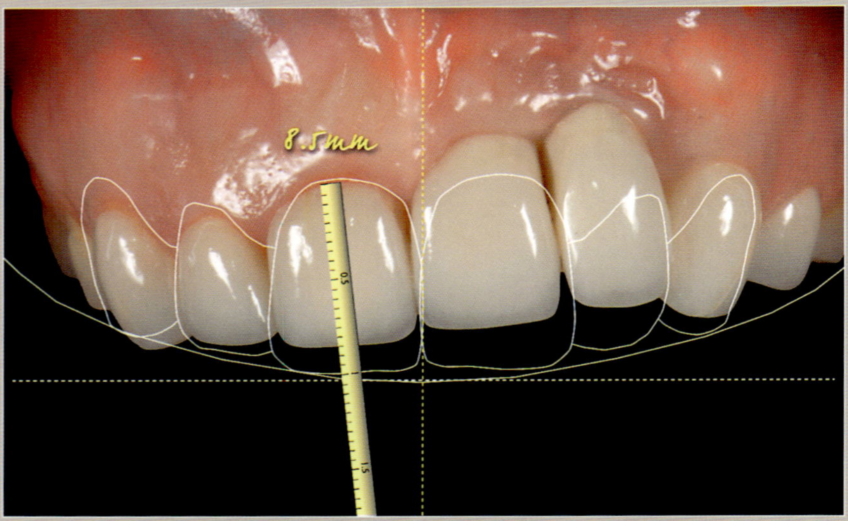

Digital ruler used to make initial measurements.

precise way to determine this horizontal plane. Then this digital information must be transferred to the master cast, which is accomplished using the digital ruler and a real caliper. Once the horizontal reference has been established, the midline can then be projected onto the horizontal line.

It became quite evident that in this particular case the midline was significantly canted and the incisal edge position and length were incorrect. Tooth no. 6 appeared disproportionately long, and excessive gingival display was present around teeth nos. 4 to 7, 12, and 13.

After relating the intraoral to the full-face photograph, keeping the same angulation, we initiated digital planning. First the incisal length of one of the central incisors was determined digitally by outlining the correct tooth proportions and ideal form. This image was then mirrored, and from this point a digital setup could be completed. A facial photo that was taken before the accident was very helpful at this stage. We considered this a virtual mock-up, allowing us to relate the digitally created forms to the existing clinical situation and the face. At this point, the clinical treatment plan for the patient needed to be adjusted and related to the DSD.

By evaluating the distance from the digitally determined ideal incisal edge position of tooth nos. 9 and 10 to the existing marginal soft tissue level, it was apparent that surgical ridge augmentation would not accomplish what was necessary to significantly improve the esthetic outcome. After evaluating the buccal soft tissue level of tooth no. 10 as it related to the buccal placement of the implant (followed by apical soft tissue shifting) and the papilla height defect between teeth nos. 9 and 10, it became clear that this area was not surgically restorable. Limitations of vertical augmentation procedures, especially for papilla augmentation, should be recognized early and then assessed to determine the most prudent treatment approach if compromise is going to be accepted.

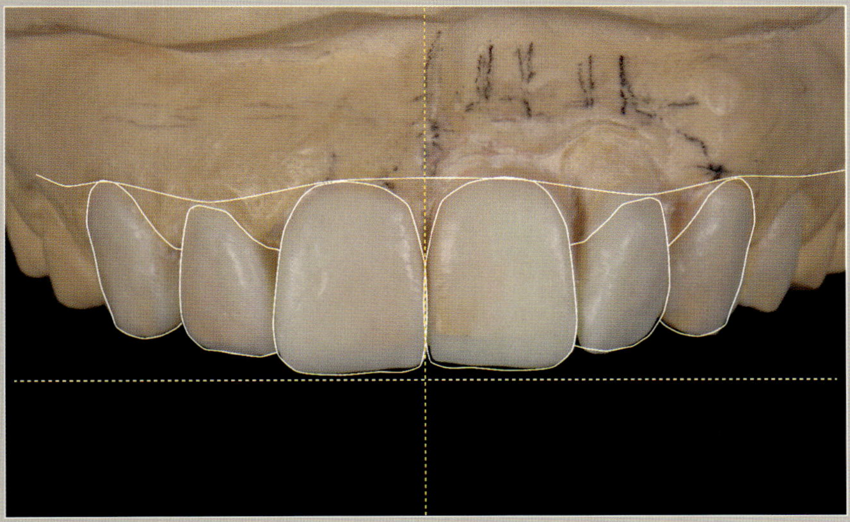

Information and measurements transferred to the study cast.

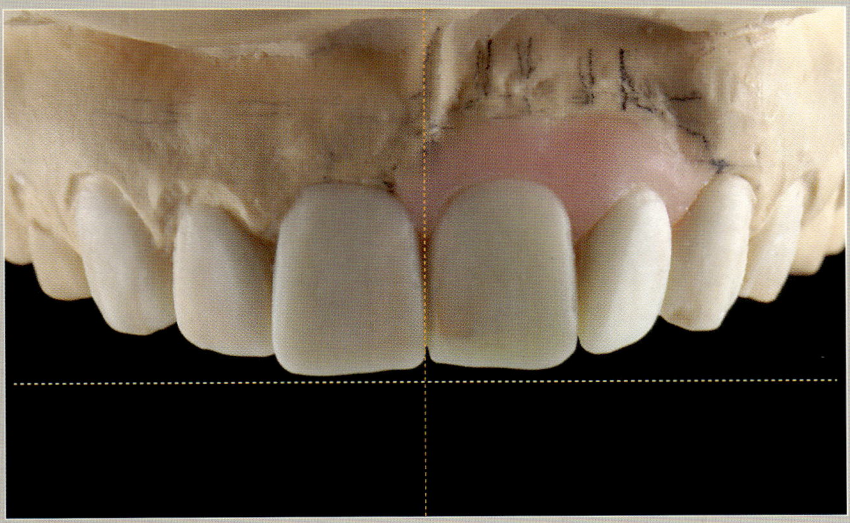

Addition of pink wax to create the ideal gingival outline.

By designing the incisal contours, relating them to the horizontal line, and correcting the interincisal line, it became evident that the patient would benefit from plastic periodontal surgery and surgical crown lengthening.

Phase II: Transfer of digital wax-up to the master cast

At this point, we needed to transfer the digital plan to the master cast. It was important to position the cast in the articulator with the same inclination as was established in the digital planning. Digital measurements are made on the computer and then transferred to the cast with a caliper. First the horizontal plane and then all other measurable information are transferred from digital form to the cast with a pencil. The information transferred to the cast will act as a guide in the wax-up procedure. Drawing a horizontal line, keeping the cast in hand, and comparing it visually with the digital inclination aided in accomplishing this. Tooth form was copied from the digital forms. At this point, the dental technician focused on ideal tooth form.

After white esthetics were optimized, ideal pink esthetics were established by filling the 3D defect around the implants with pink wax. This would again allow us to evaluate the vertical and horizontal component of the ridge deficiency. With careful pre-evaluation of an ideal white and pink wax-up by the surgical team, there would be a better understanding of the 3D topography of the ridge defect and its effect on smile design. From this wax-up, we could produce a silicone index that would enable us to intraorally fabricate an exact copy of the wax-up.

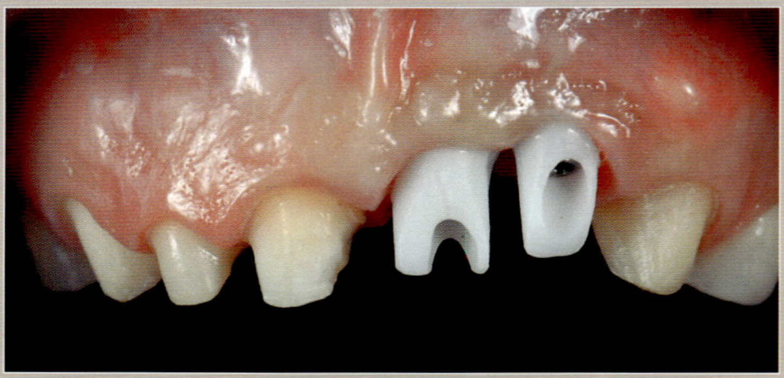

Intraoral view after removal of the old crowns.

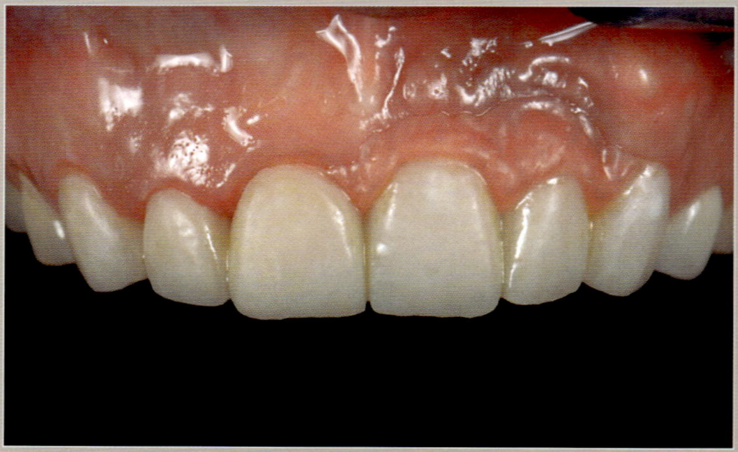

Intraoral view of provisional partial denture with pink composite.

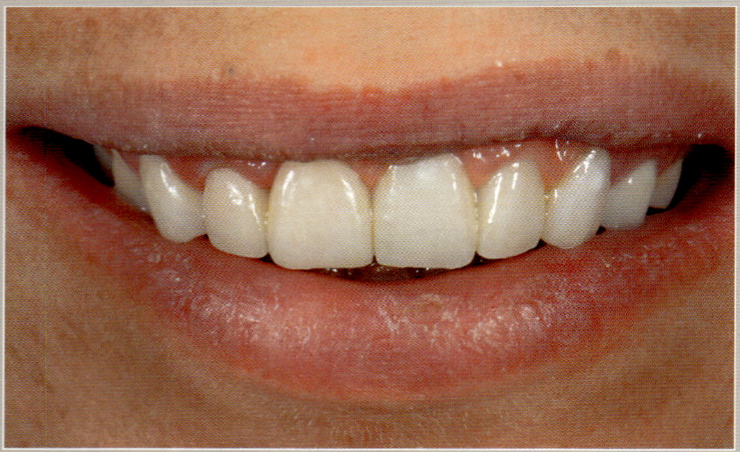

Smile view of provisional partial denture.

Phase III: Fabrication of intraoral mock-up and provisional partial denture

In the next phase, we evaluated the DSD intraorally. The old restorations were removed. It became evident that the implant in tooth position no. 10 was in significant labioversion. A silicone index (related to the final tooth forms on the wax-up) guided the preparation of the provisional restorations. At this point, an acrylic material (Outline, Anaxdent) was injected in the silicone index and applied intraorally. The provisional partial denture was seated and adjusted.

At this stage, the digital plan was evaluated, and a flowable composite was used to visualize the size and extent of the soft tissue and bony defects. As previously anticipated, the defect was going to be unmanageable surgically, and we would not be able to restore the ridge to its original dimensions.

To better conceptualize the size of the defect, a pink composite provisional material was applied to the provisional partial denture. While the optimal tooth form was the guide for this provisional pink application, care was taken to establish the ideal 3D soft tissue contours, focusing on the papilla heights and volume. This step led to the conclusion that the defect was affecting not only the vertical and horizontal components of the ridge but also the papilla height and volume on the mesial aspect of tooth no. 8 and distal aspect of tooth no. 11. At this time, it was apparent that the most optimal esthetic and functional restoration would be an artificial prosthetic gingival restoration.

The papilla height of the natural teeth on the contralateral side was used as a reference in order to establish proper gingival contours in the area of the defect. Many times it is easier to establish the papilla design digitally first by taking a photograph of the provisional partial denture and designing the soft tissue contours on the computer screen in an Apple Keynote presentation. This makes it easier to transfer the DSD concept to the oral environment.

At this time, we performed an esthetic and functional evaluation. The objective was for the incisal edge position, soft tissue contours, altered midline inclination, lip support, and tooth form to create an overall balance and facial harmony. Once the projected esthetic outcome was approved by the patient, the final treatment plan was established.

Hygiene instruction was provided because it is crucial for all artificial prosthetic gingival restorations, including the provisional restorations.

Phase IV: Establishing the definitive treatment plan

When it was time to translate the digital intraoral concept into a final treatment plan, we contemplated what we could do to maximally enhance the definitive esthetic and functional outcomes, considering that the patient wanted little or no surgery and that the existing ridge deficiency could not be restored surgically if we wanted any symmetry in soft tissue levels and papilla heights.

The following ideas were considered:

- We would improve soft tissue harmony and achieve a better balance in soft tissue levels by performing surgical clinical crown lengthening on teeth nos. 4 to 8, 12, and 13. The patient was reluctant but willing to undergo this procedure.
- We would fabricate a pink hybrid restoration to compensate for the extremely compromised ridge. There were two options considered to achieve this:

1. Use the two natural teeth (nos. 8 and 11) as abutments for a four-unit fixed partial denture. With this approach, the implants would be submerged or eventually removed.
2. One or both implants would be incorporated into the hybrid restoration.

Using the natural teeth as abutments for a fixed partial denture would not be ideal because the pink interface between natural and artificial gingiva would not be esthetically pleasing. Moreover, there would be limited retrievability should the restorative material need to be replaced in the future. Therefore, the hybrid concept was chosen.

The decision was also made to incorporate only one implant as an abutment in supporting the hybrid restoration because it would provide easier access for hygiene maintenance. Also, with a cantilever it would be easier to achieve optimal esthetics with the artificial gingiva. We decided to use the implant in the no. 9 position and to submerge the implant in the location of tooth no. 10. A connective tissue graft procedure was performed to augment the buccal aspect of the ridge defect at the time that the implant was submerged. This resulted in easier and better adaptation of the artificial gingiva material.

- We would endeavor to optimize the prosthetic materials. All-ceramic single crowns (e.max Press, Ivoclar Vivadent) were to be fabricated on teeth nos. 6 to 8, 11, and 12. A PFM, two-unit, palatally screw-retained, cantilevered partial denture would be fabricated on the implant at site no. 9. The challenge for the technician would be to match the two-unit, PFM partial denture to the all-ceramic, single-tooth restorations.

Phase V: Orthodontic therapy

Once the treatment plan had been finalized, orthodontic therapy was initiated to intrude and align the mandibular anterior teeth. This took approximately 6 months to complete, was uneventful, and did not interfere with any treatment being performed simultaneously in the maxillary arch.

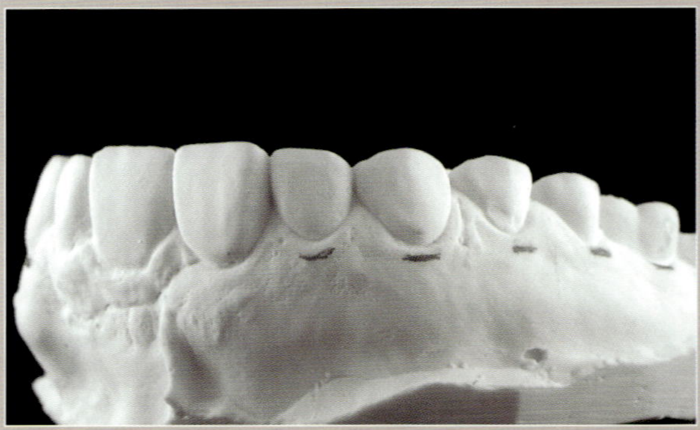

Crown lengthening suggested on the digital design transferred to the cast for fabrication of surgical stent.

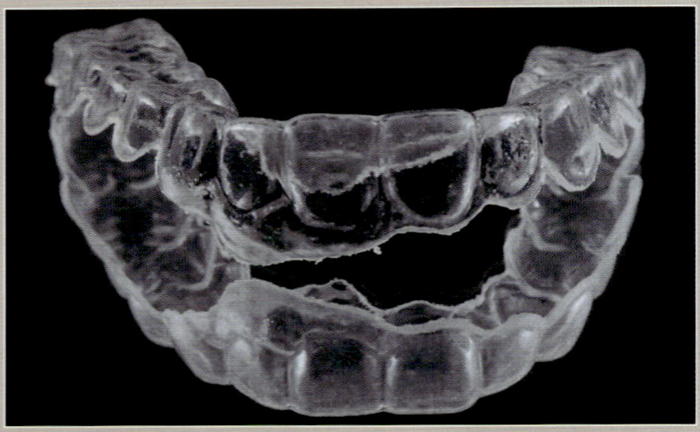

Crown lengthening surgical stent.

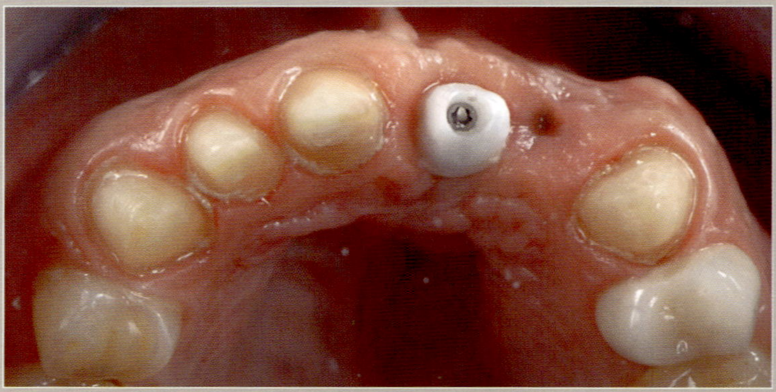

Occlusal view of anterior maxilla before surgery.

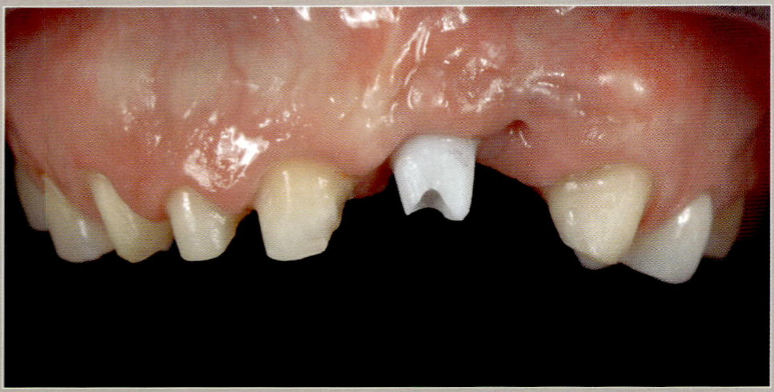

Intraoral frontal view of maxilla before surgery and after removal of the zirconia abutment of tooth no. 10.

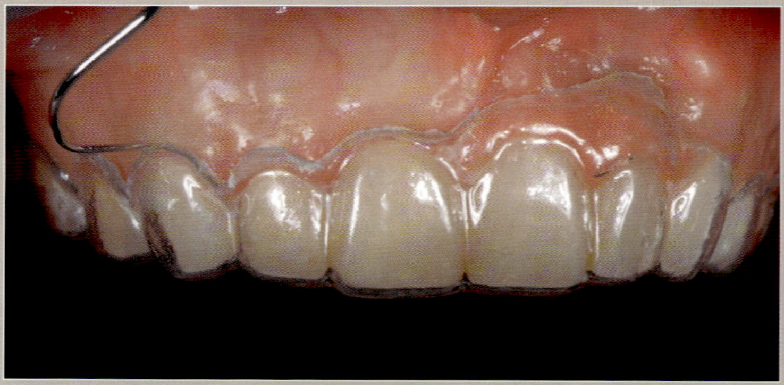

Marking the soft tissue with the explorer with the crown lengthening surgical stent in place.

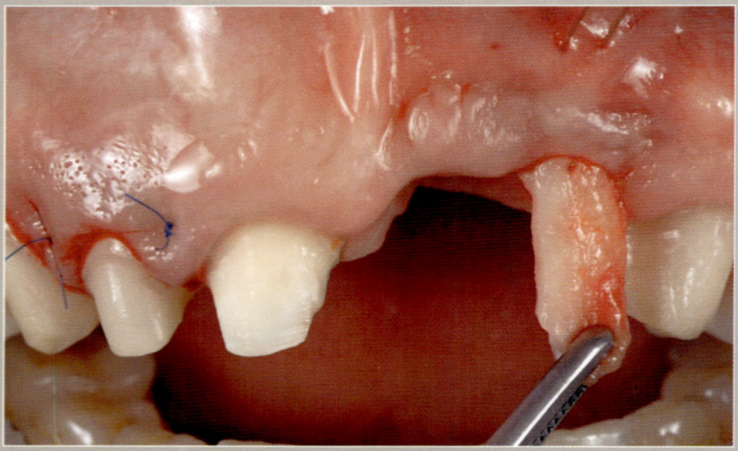

Connective tissue graft for submergence of the implant at site no. 10 and to improve the horizontal aspect of the defect.

Phase VI: Surgical treatment

Surgical treatment was guided by a surgical stent designed and fabricated from the cast made with the approved provisional fixed partial denture.

Clinical crown lengthening via osseous resection was performed on teeth nos. 4 to 7 and 11 to 13, making sure that at least 3 mm of functional, attached gingiva was maintained. Adequate biologic width was also created. A connective tissue graft was placed as an onlay to the ridge (covering the implant) and in a buccal pouch at site no. 10. Healing was uneventful, and sutures were removed after 1 week.

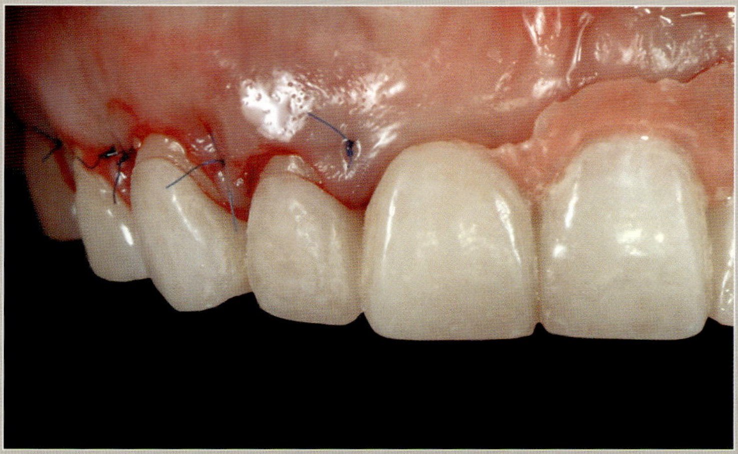

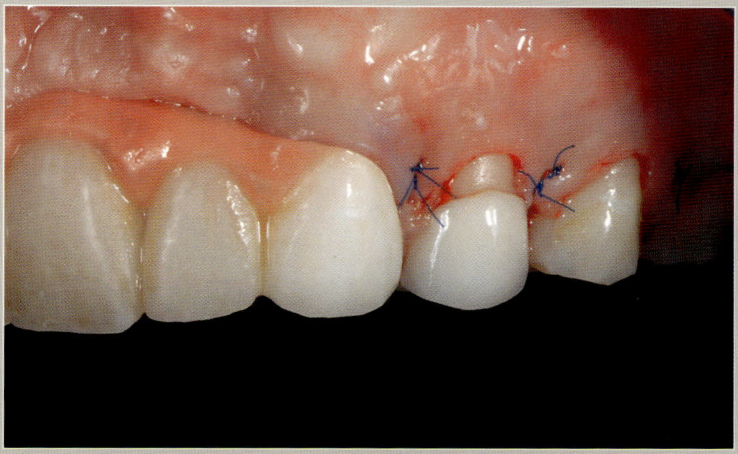

Intraoral lateral views of the maxilla after crown lengthening.

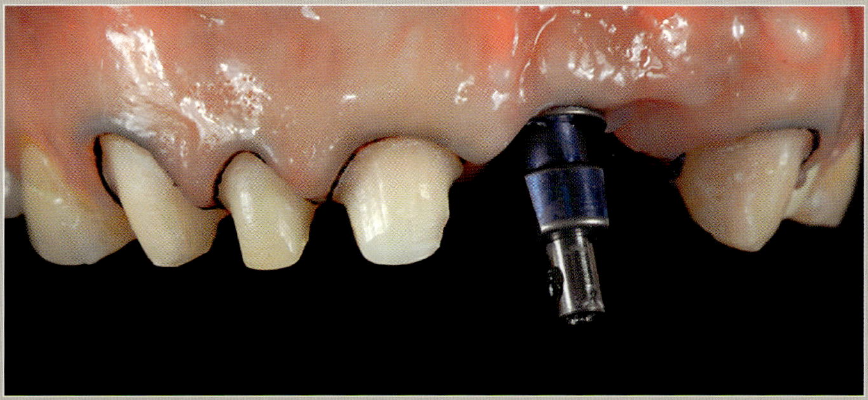

Intraoral frontal view of maxilla prior to final impression taking.

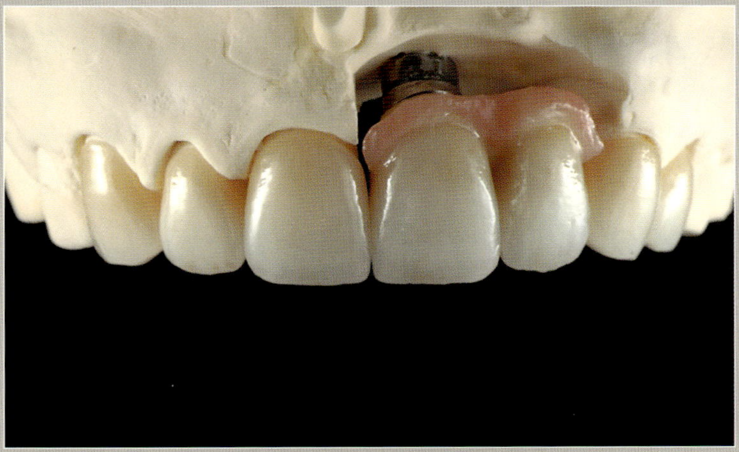

Definitive restorations on the cast.

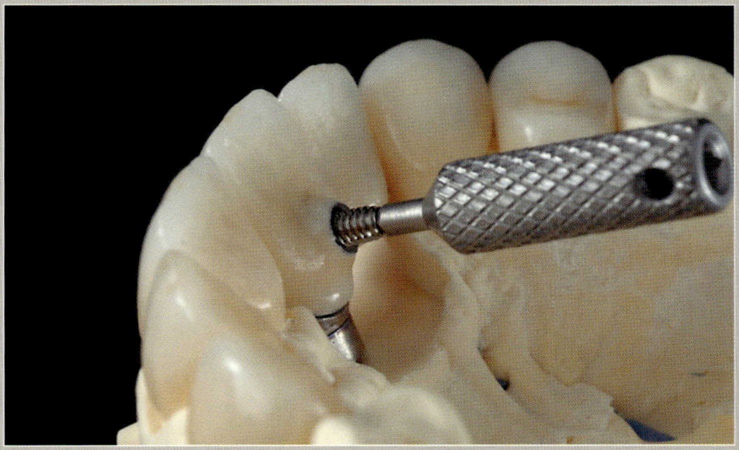

Placement of palatal screw.

Phase VII: Definitive restorations

At 4 months postoperative, final tooth preparation was initiated. Care was taken to maintain a minimally invasive approach and to achieve biologically compatible preparations and impressions. A silicone index (related to the tooth forms of the provisional design) was used to guide our final preparations. Impressions were taken, and the master cast was fabricated.

Ideally, for the pink hybrid restoration,[5-8] an implant-supported restoration should be retrievable. Because the implant in site no. 9 was placed buccally, a custom abutment was required to allow for adequate retention of the palatal screw. All-ceramic single crowns and a two-unit PFM partial denture (IPS d.Sign, Ivoclar Vivadent) were fabricated. The two-unit partial denture was already provided with a palatal layer of pink porcelain, which allowed for intraoral application and finishing with pink composite material (Anaxgum, Anaxdent).

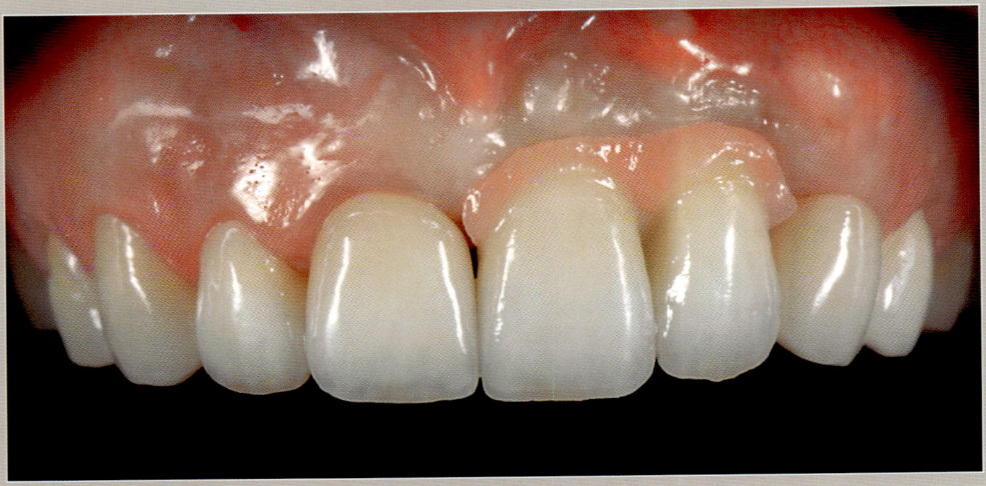

Intraoral frontal view of maxilla at try-in.

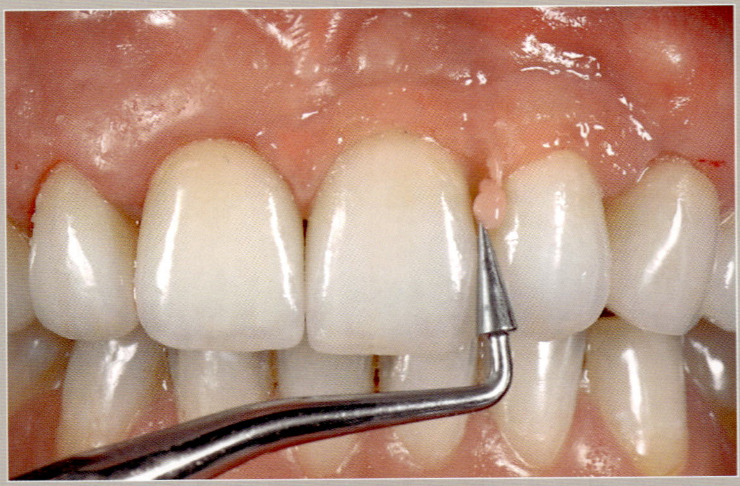

Intraoral application of the pink composite layer.

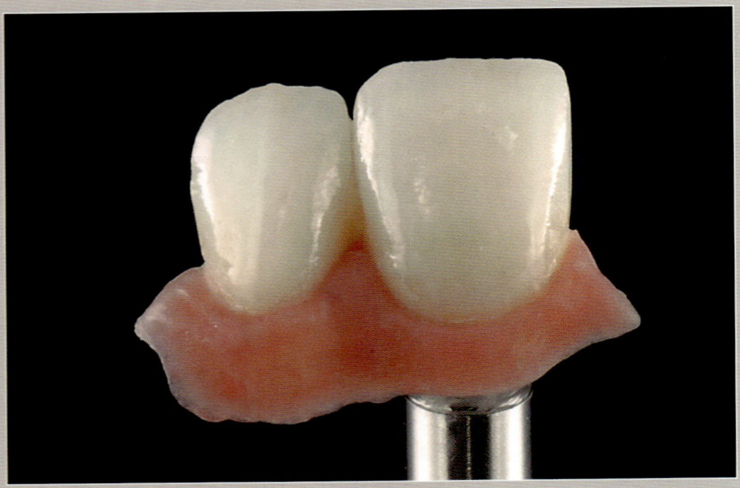

Partial denture with finished pink composite removed for final shaping, polishing, and glazing.

At this stage, all prosthetic components and crowns were tried in, and minor modifications were made. Tight adaptation with some light ischemia was visible around the pink porcelain at the try-in.

All single e.max crowns were adhesively cemented, which was followed by intraoral application of the pink composite layer. Prior to this, in the lab, the usual protocol of steaming, sandblasting, etching, silanization, bonding, and application of the first layer of flowable pink composite was used to ensure effective and strong bonding between the pink porcelain and the first layer of pink composite.

The color of the gingiva on the right side was used to select the most ideal color of pink composite. Different shades and tints were used to enhance the esthetic outcome. Surface texture and polish of the pink composite were optimized, and after final polymerization and polishing in the lab, the two-unit partial denture was cemented. Occlusion and hygiene were checked. The patient was seen on a 6-month maintenance program.

The 18-month postoperative pictures demonstrate a very acceptable and pleasing esthetic and functional result. When comparing the before and after pictures, a dramatic change could be observed. It is clear that diagnosis and treatment planning, using digital technology, can assist in evaluating ridge deficiencies, visualizing potential treatment solutions, and achieving predictable esthetic and functional outcomes.

Posttreatment

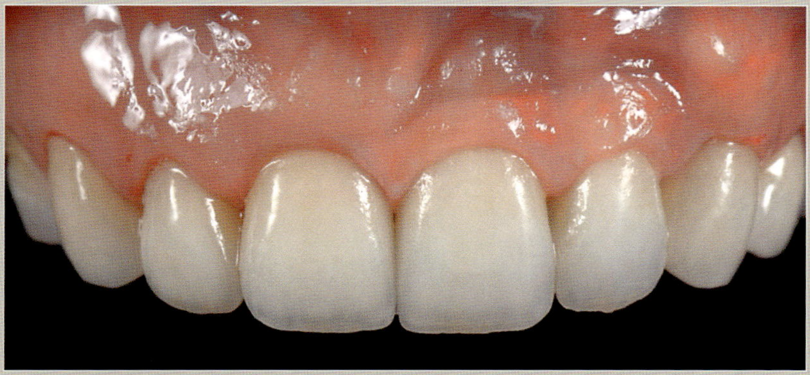

Intraoral frontal view of maxilla at the end of treatment.

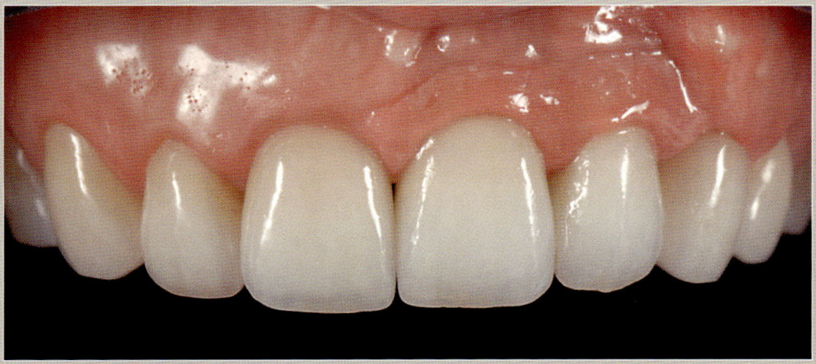

Intraoral frontal view of maxilla 18 months after treatment.

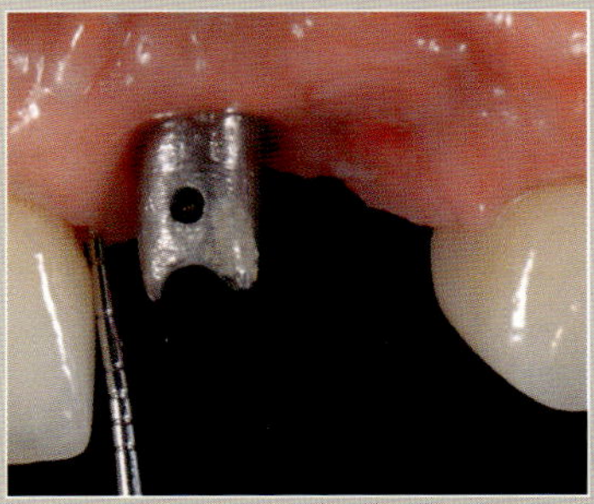

Removal of partial denture to check the soft tissue condition at 18-month checkup.

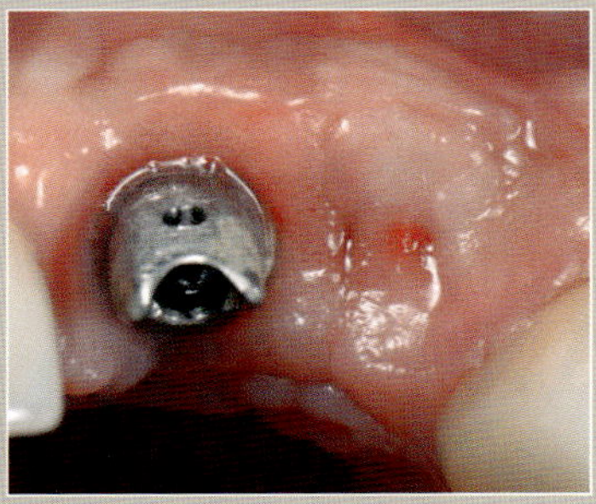

Occlusal view of healthy soft tissues at 18-month recall.

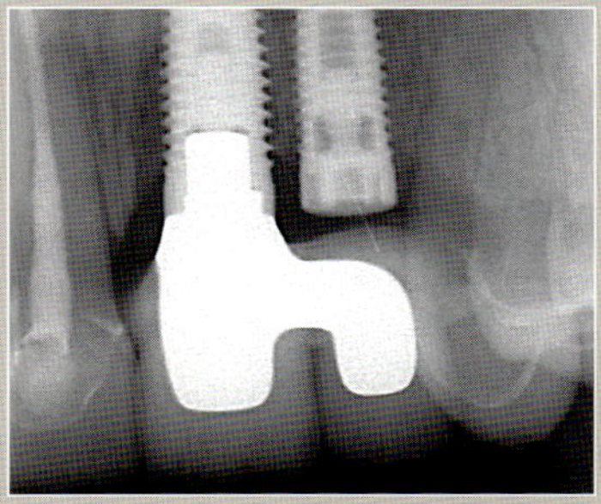

Radiograph at 18-month recall.

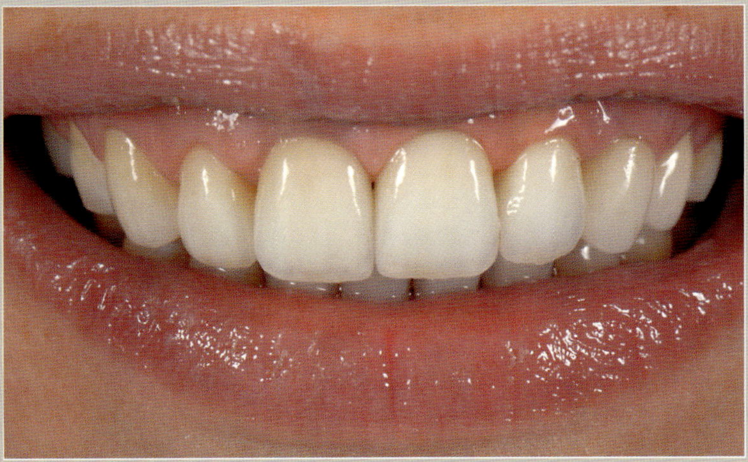

Smile view at 18 months posttreatment.

You may now place the corresponding posttreatment overlay found in the separate folder over the pretreatment periodontal chart on page 159.

Commentary

Communication

The dental literature has highlighted the importance of the smile design, although it has been vague regarding how the information ideally should be gathered and implemented. The importance of gathering the diagnostic data through forms and checklists[9–14] is emphasized. However, many of these pieces of information may be lost if their real meaning is not transferred in an adequate way to the design of the rehabilitation.

Traditionally, the smile design has been instituted by the dental technician, who performs the restorative wax-up, creates shapes and arrangements in accordance with limited information, and follows instructions and guidelines provided by the clinician in writing or by phone. In many cases, the technician is not given enough information to use his or her skills to their maximum potential, and the opportunity to produce a restoration that will truly satisfy the patient is missed.

When the treatment coordinator or another member of the restorative team who has developed a strong personal relationship with the patient takes the responsibility for the smile design, the results are likely to be far superior. This individual has the ability to communicate the patient's personal preferences and/or morphopsychologic features to the laboratory technician, providing information that can elevate the quality of the restoration from one that is adequate to one that is viewed by the patient as exceptional.[14,15]

With this valuable information and that from the 2D DSD in hand, the dental technician will be able to develop a 3D wax-up more efficiently, focusing on developing anatomical features within the parameters provided, such as planes of reference, facial and dental midlines, recommended incisal edge position, lip dynamics, basic tooth arrangement, and the incisal plane.

Transferring this information from the wax-up to the test-drive phase is achieved through a mock-up or a provisional restoration.[11,13,16] The design of the definitive esthetic restorations should be developed and tested as soon as possible, guiding the treatment sequence to a predetermined esthetic result. Efficient treatment planning results in the entire treatment team being able to better identify the challenges they will face and helps expedite the initiation and completion of treatment.[1]

Assessment, feedback, and learning

The DSD allows a precise re-evaluation of the results obtained in every phase of treatment. With the drawings and reference lines created, it is possible to perform simple comparisons between the before and after pictures, determining if they are in accordance with the original planning or if any other adjunctive procedures are necessary to improve the outcome. The dental technician also gains feedback related to tooth shape, arrangement, and color so that definitive refinements can be made. This constant double-checking of information ensures that a higher-quality product will be delivered from the laboratory and also provides a great learning tool for the entire interdisciplinary team.

Education

In many cases, patients are not satisfied with their appearance but really do not understand which contributing factors are responsible. When the clinician is able to clearly illustrate the elements present that deviate from ideal esthetic principles, the patient is more likely to appreciate the treatment challenges ahead and the potential compromises that may ensue. In an educational presentation, the clinician can explain the severity of the case, introduce strategies for treatment, discuss the prognosis, and make case management recommendations.

Case Presentation

The DSD makes the treatment-planning presentation much more effective and clear because it allows patients to see and better understand the combined multiple factors that are responsible for their orofacial issues. The case presentation is effective and dynamic because the problem list is superimposed over the patient's own photographs, increasing the credibility, trust, and acceptance of the proposed plan.

Digital smile design workflow

The proposed DSD technique is performed by the authors using Apple Keynote; however, other similar software, such as Microsoft PowerPoint, can also be used with minor adjustments in the technique. Keynote allows simple manipulation of the digital images and the addition of drawings, lines, shapes, and measurements over the clinical and laboratory images. The main steps of the DSD are described and illustrated below.

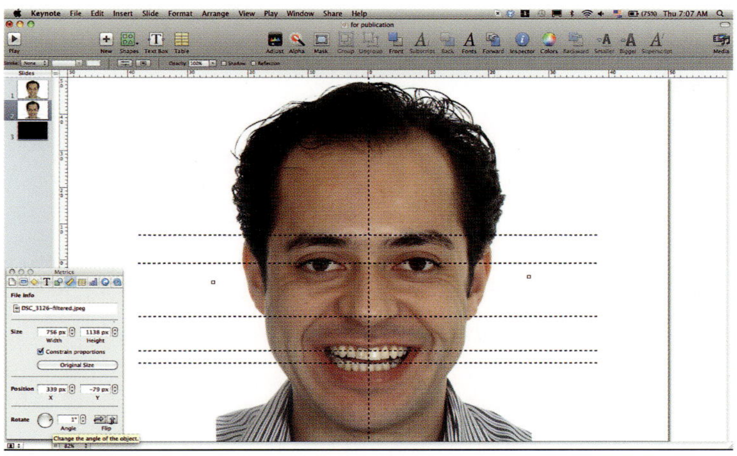

1. Digital facebow: Determining adequate horizontal plane of reference and facial midline by moving and turning the photo behind the lines.

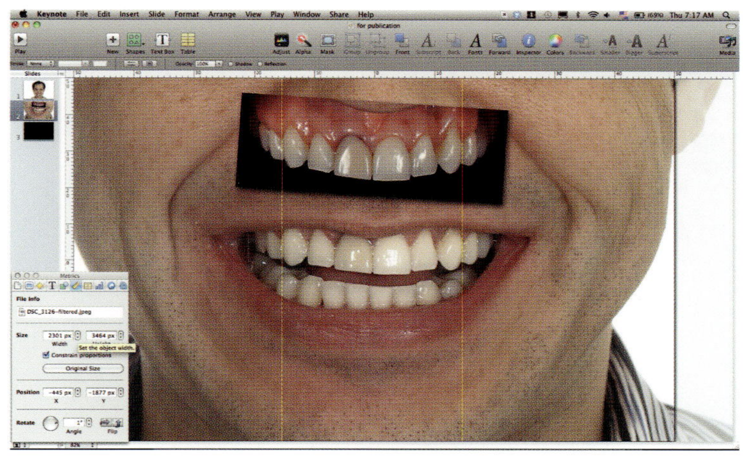

2. Transferring the facial lines to the intraoral situation by grouping the lines and overlapping the photos. Matching the dimensions of the photos by using the two vertical lines on the distal of the canines as a reference.

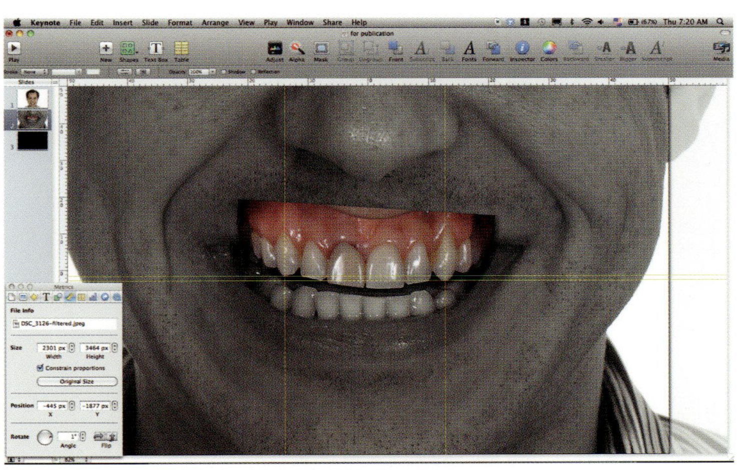

3. Leveling the canting of the incisal edges by taking as a reference the tips of the canines. The black background of the intraoral photo is removed to facilitate the process.

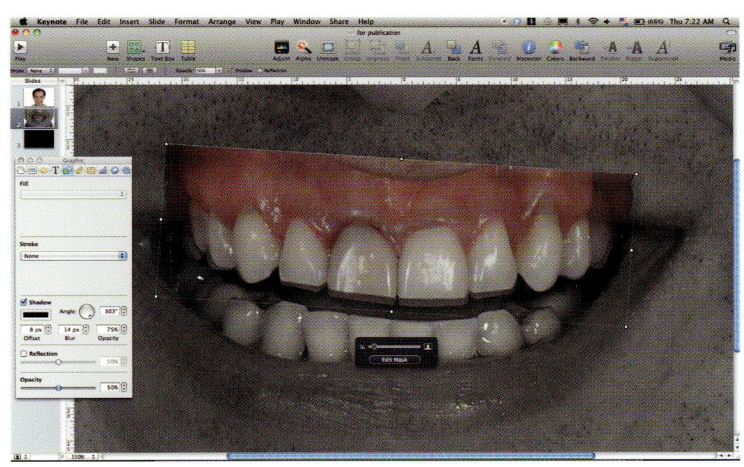

4. Matching the dental midlines by moving the photo left and/or right. The opacity of the intraoral photo is decreased (50%) to facilitate the process.

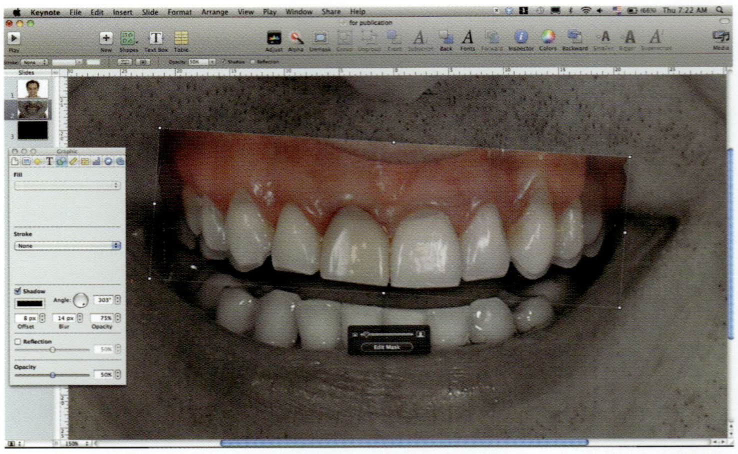

5. Matching the incisal edge of the central incisors by moving the intraoral photo up and/or down.

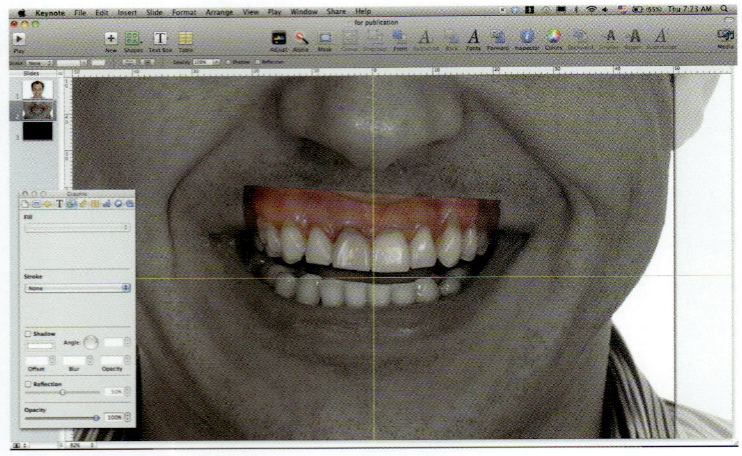

6. The intraoral photo is then completely adjusted to the facial reality.

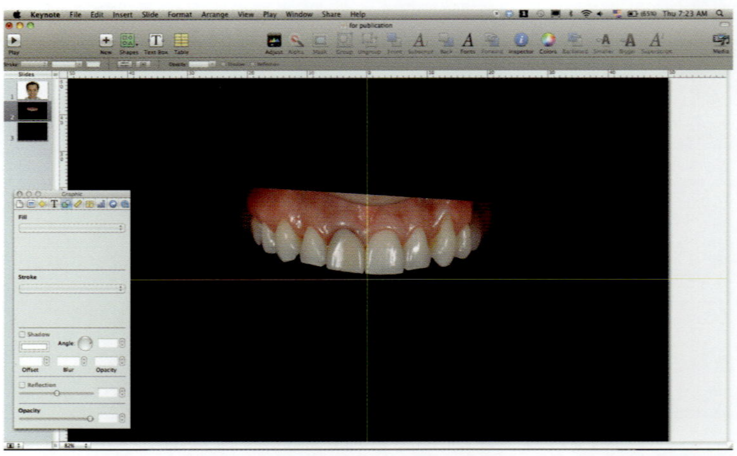

7. Deleting the facial photo and analyzing the intraoral photo according to the two main facial guidelines.

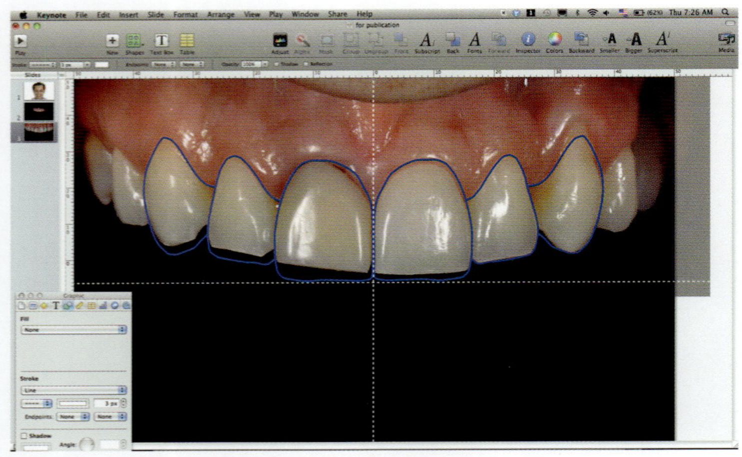

8. Digital mock-up: Designing the teeth on the screen following the guidelines. Analyzing the discrepancies and possible solutions.

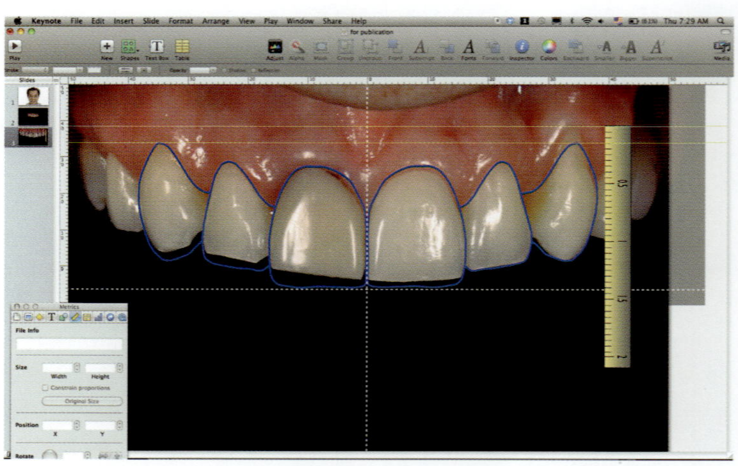

9. Digital ruler: Making all the digital measurements necessary to transfer the guidelines to the working cast. Before measurement, the ruler needs to be calibrated by measuring the real size of the central incisor on the stone cast.

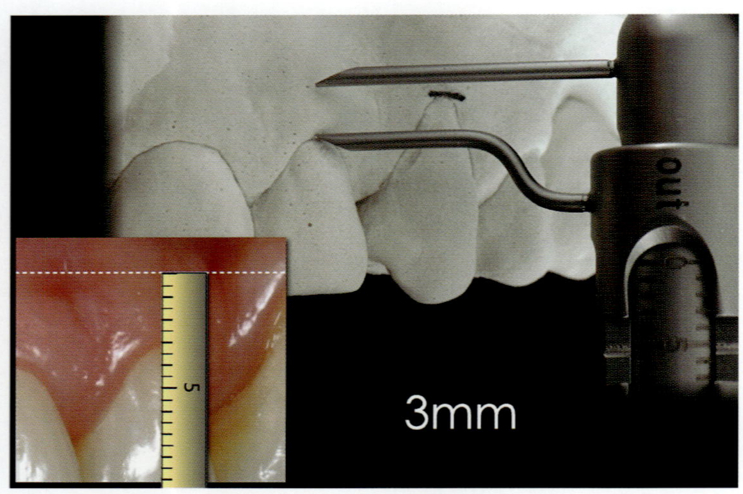

10. Transferring the measurements to the working cast using a caliper.

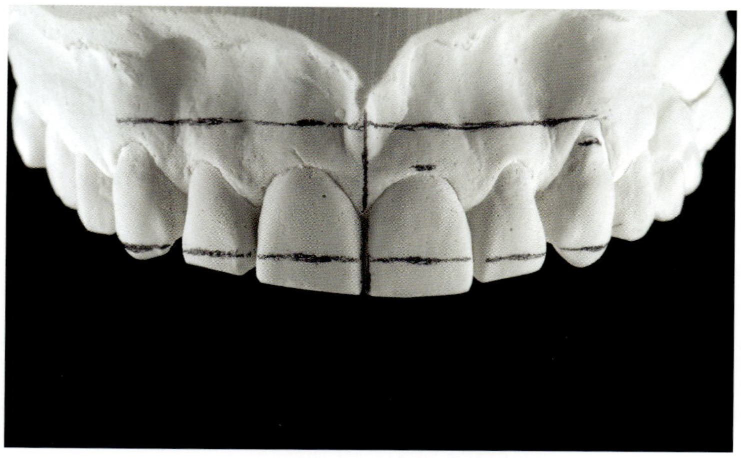

The cast is ready for a guided, precise, and predictable wax-up that will be in harmony with the patient's face and smile.

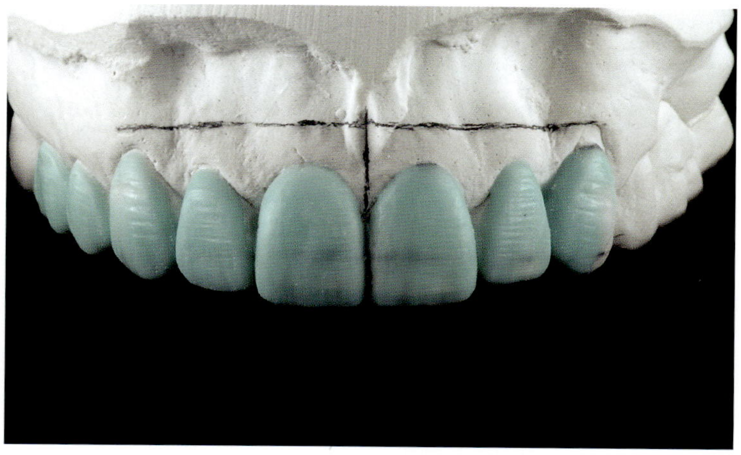

11. Performing a guided wax-up.

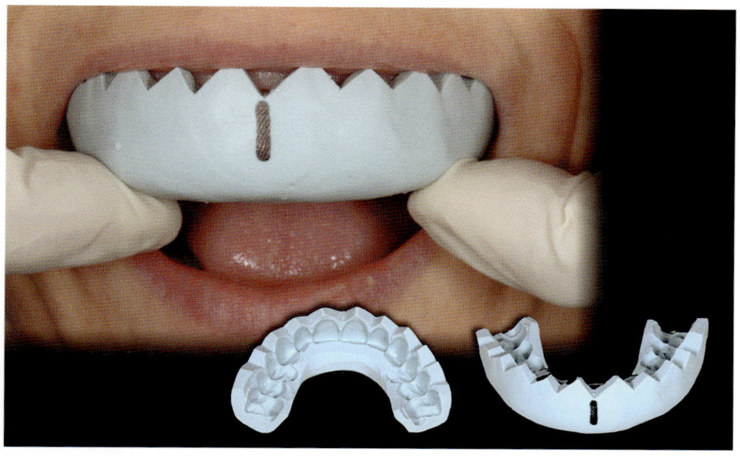

12. Testing the whole project by transforming the wax-up into a mock-up using silicone indices and resin.

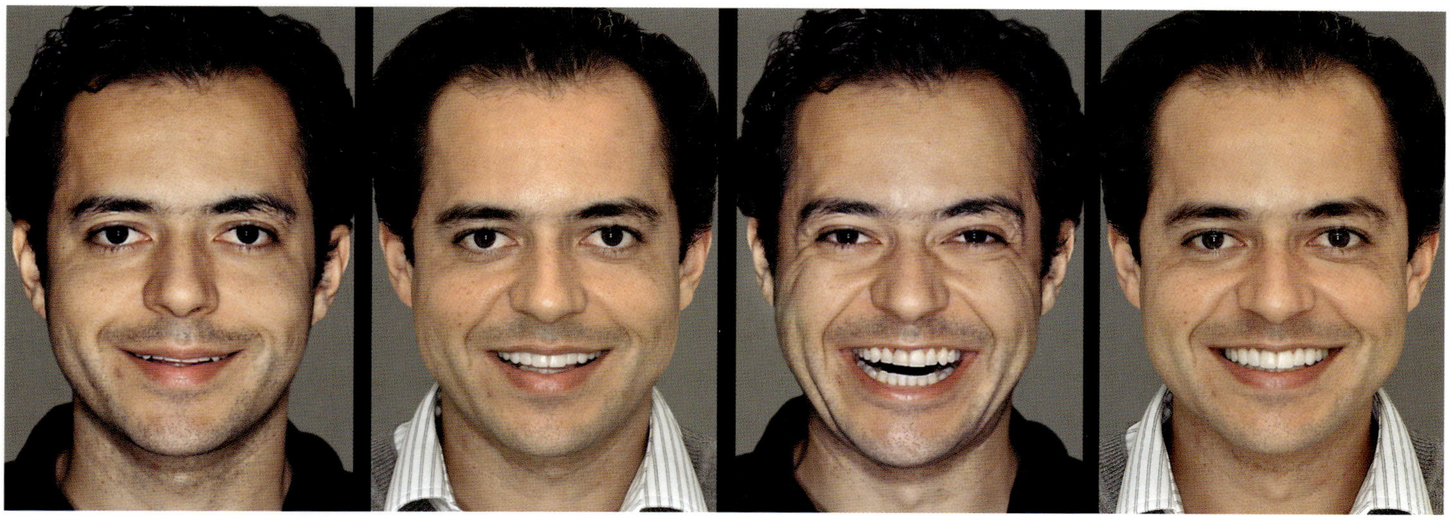

13. Using photographs and videos to analyze the mock-up and communicate with the patient to determine the final project for the new smile design.

Living with Compromise

The cases presented for treatment planning in this chapter all challenge our willingness to accept compromise. The concept of compromise sometimes can be hard to swallow, and yet the treatment outcomes in all three cases suggest that falling short of the ideal should not necessarily be taken as defeat. Treatment success is most important and is subject to the interpretation of the patient. Patient satisfaction trumps the clinician's view of the ideal outcome every time that the two are not the same. As previously proposed in the Editor's Introduction to this suite of cases, compromise should be considered an opportunity to achieve exceptional treatment results using alternative treatment modalities. The treating clinicians and laboratory technicians in all three cases are well versed in ideal dentistry and yet feel that the outcomes in situations like these are the most fulfilling and rewarding. All three patients expressed their gratitude and appreciation for treatment that far exceeded their expectations. They were thrilled with the results, and is this not the reason that we engage in our profession each day?

References

1. Dawson PE. Functional Occlusion: From TMJ to Smile Design. St Louis: Mosby, 2007.
2. Spear FM. The maxillary central incisor edge: A key to esthetic and functional treatment planning. Compend Contin Educ Dent 1999;20:512–516.
3. Kois JC. Diagnostically driven interdisciplinary treatment planning. Seattle Study Club J 2002;6(4):28–34.
4. Terry DA, Snow SR, McLaren EA. Contemporary dental photography: Selection and application. Compend Contin Educ Dent 2008;29:432–440.
5. Coachman C, Van Dooren E, Gürel G, Calamita MA, Calgaro M, Souza Neto J. Minimally invasive reconstruction in implant therapy: The prosthetic restoration. Quintessence Dent Technol 2010;33:61–75.
6. Coachman C, Salama M, Garber D, Calamita M, Salama H, Cabral G. Prosthetic gingival reconstruction in a fixed partial restoration. Part 1: Introduction to artificial gingiva as an alternative therapy. Int J Periodontics Restorative Dent 2009;29:471–477.
7. Coachman C, Salama M, Garber D, Calamita M, Salama H, Cabral G. Prosthetic gingival reconstruction in the fixed partial restoration. Part 2: Diagnosis and treatment planning. Int J Periodontics Restorative Dent 2009;29:573–581.
8. Coachman C, Salama M, Garber D, Calamita M, Salama H, Cabral G. Prosthetic gingival reconstruction in the fixed partial restoration. Part 3. Int J Periodontics Restorative Dent 2010;30:18–29.
9. Goldstein RE. Esthetics in Dentistry: Principles, Communication, Treatment Methods. Ontario: Decker, 1998.
10. Chiche GJ, Pinault A. Esthetics of Anterior Fixed Prosthodontics. Chicago: Quintessence, 1996.
11. Magne P, Belser U. Bonded Porcelain Restorations in the Anterior Dentition: A Biomimetic Approach. Chicago: Quintessence, 2002.
12. Fradeani M. Esthetic Rehabilitation in Fixed Prosthodontics, Vol 1. Esthetic Analysis: A Systematic Approach to Prosthetic Treatment. Chicago: Quintessence, 2004.
13. Gürel G. The Science and Art of Porcelain Laminate Veneers. Berlin: Quintessence, 2003.
14. Rufenacht CR. Fundamentals of Esthetics. Chicago: Quintessence, 1990.
15. Paolucci B. Visagismo e odontologia. In: Hallawell P. Visagismo integrado: Identidade, estilo e beleza. São Paulo: Senac, 2009:243–250.
16. Gürel G, Bichacho N. Permanent diagnostic provisional restorations for predictable results when redesigning smiles. Pract Proced Aesthet Dent 2006;18:281–286.

6

Autotransplantation to Replace an Ankylosed Maxillary Anterior Tooth in a Young Patient

Greggory A. Kinzer, DDS, MSD
Jim Janakievski, DDS, MSD

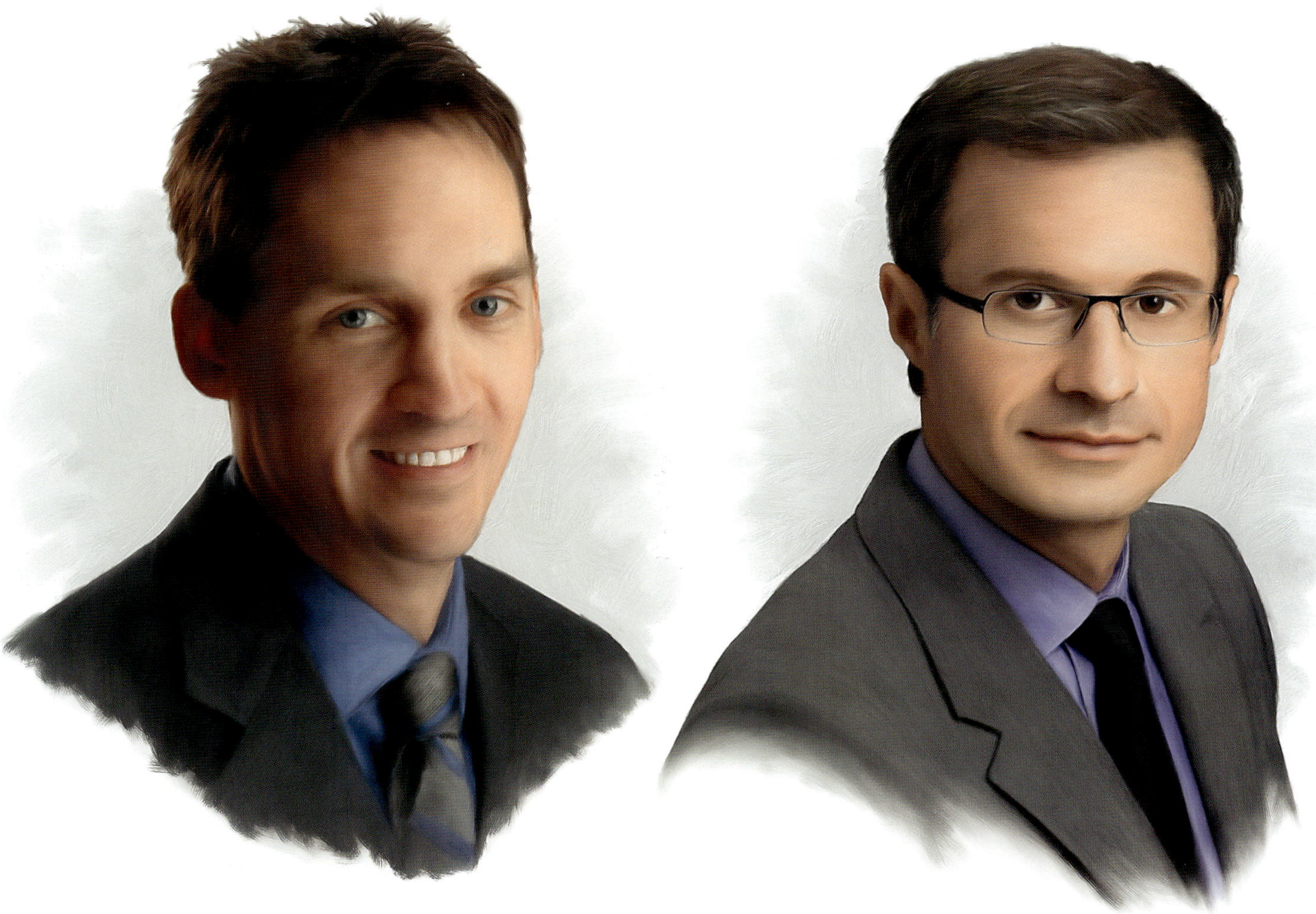

The transplanted tooth allows for the continued development of the alveolar ridge during growth and development while providing a natural tooth replacement in the esthetic zone.

Philosophy and Background

Managing young patients that have experienced an injury to the maxillary anterior dentition can be a challenge. Trauma to these teeth can result in avulsion, subsequent ankylosis, and the inability to restore the tooth. If a tooth is avulsed and replanted, it can often become ankylosed. Ankylosis of the traumatized tooth interferes with normal growth and development of the alveolar ridge; therefore, the most judicious treatment option is usually extraction. If the root shows significant evidence of replacement resorption, another option is decoronation. If an avulsed tooth is not replanted, treatment should be directed at developing the alveolar ridge through orthodontically guided tooth eruption of the adjacent teeth into the edentulous site. Regardless of the treatment option chosen, the primary goal is to manage the alveolar ridge to minimize the anticipated deficiency in bone volume.

Given that most traumatic injuries to anterior teeth occur between the ages of 9 and 12 years, what treatment options are available to restore these patients? The primary treatment plan is to restore the edentulous site with a single-tooth implant, thereby conserving the adjacent teeth. However, in young patients, this often means waiting several years for growth to be completed prior to implant placement. If the patient is male, the waiting period may be greater than 10 years. During this growth period:

- How is the edentulous space held?
- How should the interim tooth replacement be managed?
- How does the bone in the edentulous space change during this time period?

The answers to these questions can significantly influence the treatment required once growth is completed.

Looking back at the many treatment challenges we have faced when managing patients who had lost a central incisor at a young age, we began searching for new treatment options. Was there an option that we could offer these patients that would provide an immediate functional and natural tooth replacement so they wouldn't have to wait until they were 20 years old to have an implant placed? One often-overlooked treatment option that we discovered was tooth autotransplantation. This involves transplanting a developing premolar to a maxillary incisor position and then restoring it to change the tooth morphology. The use of autotransplantation has been studied most extensively in Scandinavia.[1–5] The results of a recently published long-term review (follow-up range of 17 to 41 years) of patients treated with autotransplantation[6] showed a success rate similar to that of an implant-supported restoration. By transplanting a tooth to the edentulous site, no future implant treatment will be required. In addition, the transplanted tooth allows for the continued development of the alveolar ridge during growth and development while providing a natural tooth replacement in the esthetic zone.

Following is a challenging and yet fairly predictable case to treatment plan. Although autotransplantation is clearly the treatment we chose, there were several factors that had to be taken into consideration when planning this approach.

- Selection of the tooth: Which tooth is best suited for transplantation to a central incisor position?
- Stage of root development: Can the premolar be harvested at any stage of root development? Will the root continue to develop? Will the pulp survive?
- Recipient site: How is this site prepared? How is the transplanted tooth stabilized?

Studies have been performed to evaluate all of these factors, and the results will be summarized in the case presentation.

Case Presentation

Treating clinicians
Prosthodontist: Greggory A. Kinzer, DDS, MSD
Periodontist: Jim Janakievski, DDS, MSD
Orthodontist: Rafael Hernandez, DDS

Clinical Treatment Planning

Age at initial presentation: 10 years
Initial presentation: January 2005
Active treatment completed: June 2006

Introduction and background

Six months prior to presentation, the patient was playing in the family pool when he suffered a traumatic injury to the maxillary incisors that resulted in avulsion of the maxillary left central incisor. The tooth was found at the bottom of the pool 1 hour later and was reimplanted 2 hours after the injury at the office of his general dentist. It was noted by the general dentist that at approximately 6 months after reimplantation, the maxillary left central incisor became ankylosed and was in infraocclusion. The parents of this patient were eager for the clinicians involved to "address the ankylosed tooth with the most appropriate treatment to restore both function and esthetics."

Medical history

- Noncontributory; good overall health
- No current medications
- No known drug allergies

Diagnostic findings

Extraoral and facial findings

- Brachycephalic facial form
- Good facial symmetry
- Average lip mobility with a low to average smile line

TMJ and mandibular range of motion

- No joint sounds with external palpation
- No joint pain with palpation, upon loading, or with movement
- Range of motion within normal limits
- Easy manipulation

Intraoral findings

General
- Intraoral soft tissues within normal limits
- Negative cancer screen

Dental
- All teeth present at different stages of eruption
- Retained primary tooth K (tooth no. 20 not yet erupted)
- Teeth nos. 1, 2, 15, 16, 17, 18, 20, 29, 31, and 32 are unerupted
- Ankylosed tooth no. 9 is in infraocclusion

Periodontal
- Generalized slight gingival inflammation
- Plaque index approximately 50% with home care fair at best
- Probing depths generally $\leq$ 3 mm
- Tooth mobility within normal limits with exception of ankylosed tooth no. 9

Occlusal notes

- Angle Class I molar relationship
- Overbite: 0%
- Overjet: 1 mm

PRETREATMENT

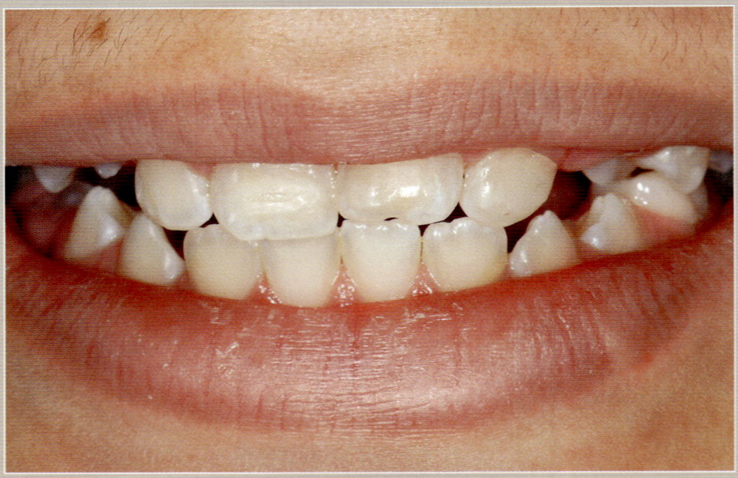

Smile.

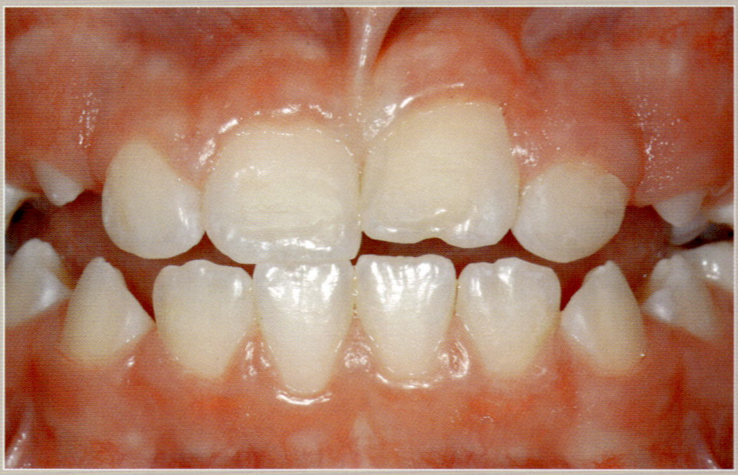

Frontal view of occlusion.

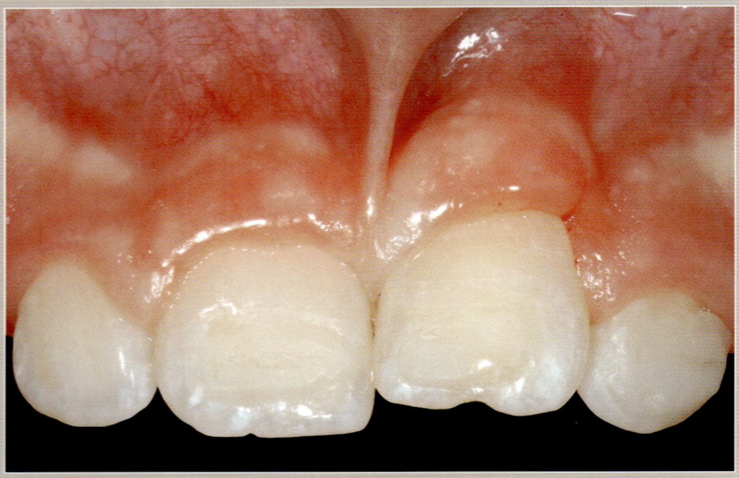

Anterior maxilla.

Radiographic findings

- Nonexistent to minimal alveolar bone loss
- Tooth no. 9 lacks a periodontal ligament with evidence of early replacement resorption

Diagnosis and prognosis

- Ankylosed tooth no. 9
- Prognosis for tooth no. 9: poor
- General esthetic, functional, biomechanical, and periodontal prognosis: good

Summary of concerns

1. When should the ankylosed tooth be extracted?
2. After the ankylosed tooth is extracted, how should we replace the missing tooth?
3. What will happen to the bone in the edentulous site if the tooth is extracted and the space is left edentulous until the patient completes growth and an implant can be placed?
4. How will the appropriate mesiodistal spacing be maintained in the edentulous site if the tooth is extracted?
5. How do we manage tooth replacement until a permanent solution can be implemented?

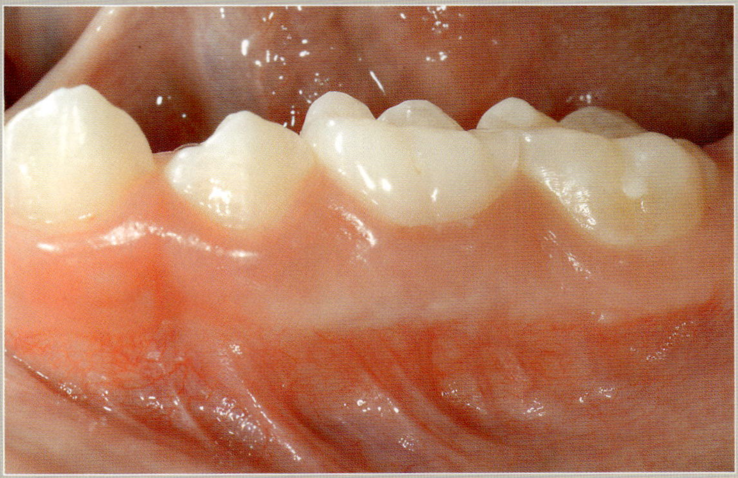

Buccal view of mandibular left posterior area.

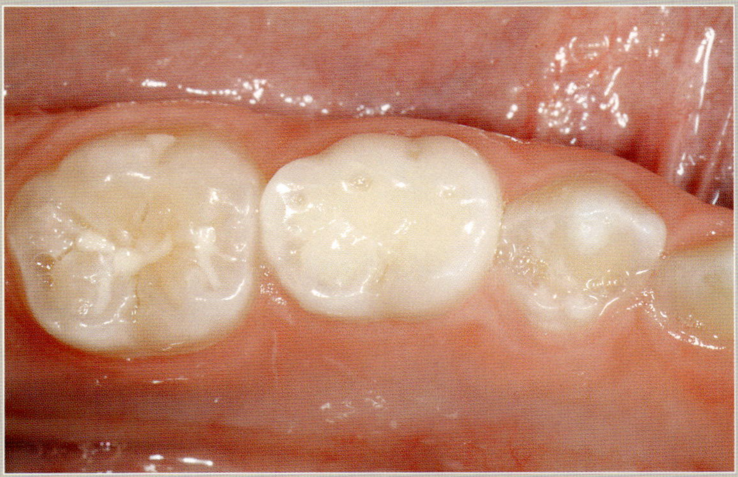

Occlusal view of mandibular left posterior area.

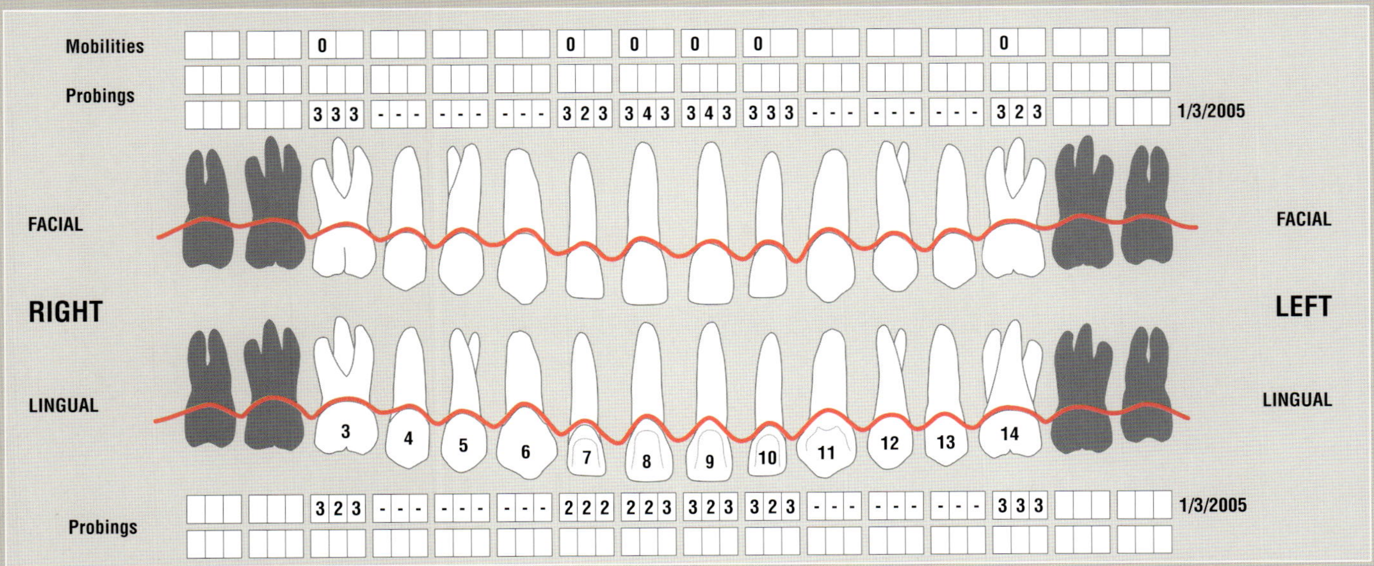

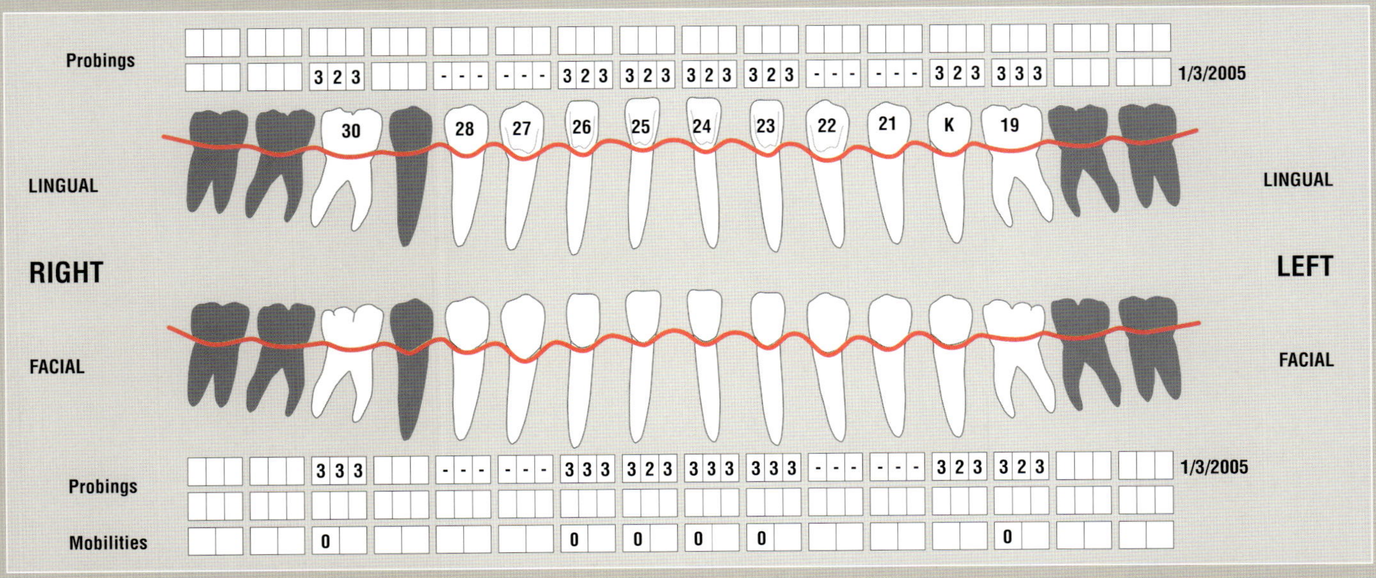

As a learning exercise, you may now outline goals/objectives of treatment and a treatment plan.

Proposed Treatment Plan

Goals/objectives of treatment

The goal of treatment is to extract the ankylosed tooth no. 9 and provide immediate replacement using autotransplantation of developing tooth no. 20. The treatment will allow for continued alveolar ridge development as well as restoration of natural esthetics and function.

Phase I: Data gathering

1. Comprehensive oral evaluation
2. Pretreatment photographic series
3. Referral to the periodontist for autotransplantation evaluation
4. Referral to the orthodontist for orthodontic evaluation

Phase II: Surgical treatment and postoperative follow-up

5. Extraction of tooth no. 9
6. Extraction of primary tooth K
7. Harvesting of tooth no. 20
8. Immediate transplantation of tooth no. 20 into the no. 9 site

Phase III: Orthodontic treatment

9. Three to four months after autotransplantation surgery, initiation of orthodontic treatment to align the transplanted premolar and facilitate veneer placement

Phase IV: Restorative treatment

10. Preparation and impression of transplanted premolar for a composite laminate veneer
11. Indirect fabrication of composite laminate veneer
12. Seating of composite laminate veneer

Phase V: Completion of orthodontic treatment

Active Clinical Treatment

Review of the goals/objectives of treatment

The main treatment goal expressed by the patient's parents at the beginning of treatment was to address the ankylosed tooth with the most appropriate treatment to restore proper function and esthetics. The treatment objectives for this patient were established as follows:

- To extract the ankylosed central incisor
- To provide immediate replacement of the extracted maxillary central incisor with the autotransplantation of the developing mandibular left second premolar
- To allow for continued alveolar ridge development in the central incisor site and restore natural esthetics and function

Phase I: Data gathering

In order to gather the appropriate data for the treatment of tooth no. 9, the patient was referred for orthodontic (Dr Rafael Hernandez) and surgical (Dr Jim Janakievski) evaluation. Given the age of the patient, as well as the stage of root development for tooth no. 20, the treatment plan for the patient was to extract the ankylosed tooth no. 9, extract the primary tooth K, and harvest the developing tooth no. 20 for immediate transplantation into the no. 9 site. This treatment will allow for continued alveolar ridge development and the restoration of natural esthetics and function.

Phase II: Surgical treatment and postoperative follow-up

To prepare the recipient site, the ankylosed central incisor was extracted carefully, preserving the surrounding socket wall. Any residual ankylosed root remnants were removed during the osteotomy process. The recipient site was prepared with rotary instruments and sized to the root dimension of the premolar planned for transplantation.

To harvest the developing tooth no. 20, tooth K was extracted and a mucoperiosteal flap was raised to gain access to the buccal bone. Ostectomy of the alveolar bone followed to expose the follicle surrounding the crown of the premolar. The transplant tooth was carefully harvested, with care taken to avoid contact with the periodontal ligament, and transferred to the anterior maxilla. The transplanted tooth was positioned passively at a level similar to its harvest position. The tooth was stabilized for several weeks with mattress sutures (a wire splint also could have been used).

The flap at the donor site was repositioned and sutured. Over the next 3 months, healing was monitored both clinically and radiographically. The premolar began to erupt through the follicle in the area of the central incisor, and there was radiographic evidence of continued root formation.

Phase III: Orthodontic treatment

Development of a periodontal ligament was confirmed before orthodontic tooth movement was initiated, which occurred 4 months after the transplantation procedure. In order to facilitate the subsequent placement of a composite laminate veneer on the transplanted premolar, specific instructions were given for positioning the transplanted tooth within the no. 9 space:

- *Apicocoronally:* The transplant tooth was positioned to align its cementoenamel junction (CEJ) with the CEJ of the adjacent central incisor.
- *Mesiodistally:* The transplant tooth was positioned mesial of center, leaving one-third of the remaining space on the mesial and two-thirds of the remaining space on the distal.
- *Labiopalatally:* The transplant tooth was positioned slightly palatally on the ridge to allow the restorative treatment to be performed additively with minimal removal of tooth structure.

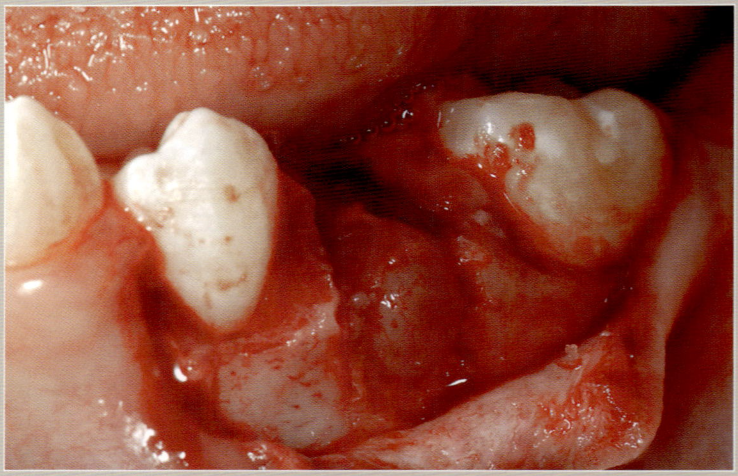

Buccal bone removed to gain access to the developing premolar.

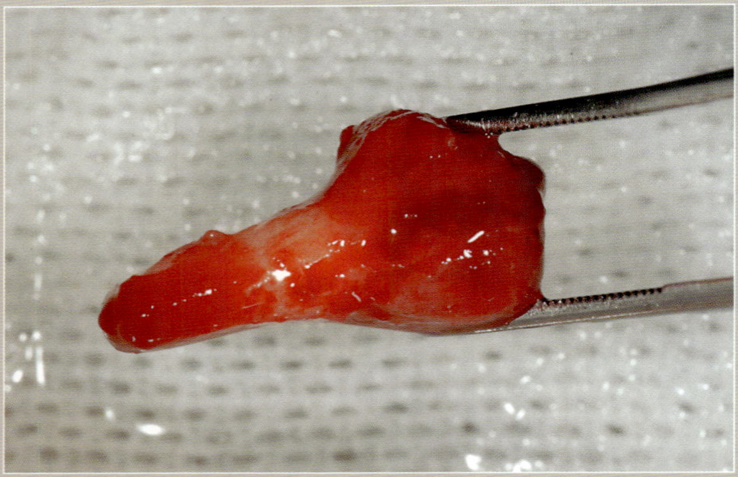

Extracted tooth no. 20 ready for transplantation.

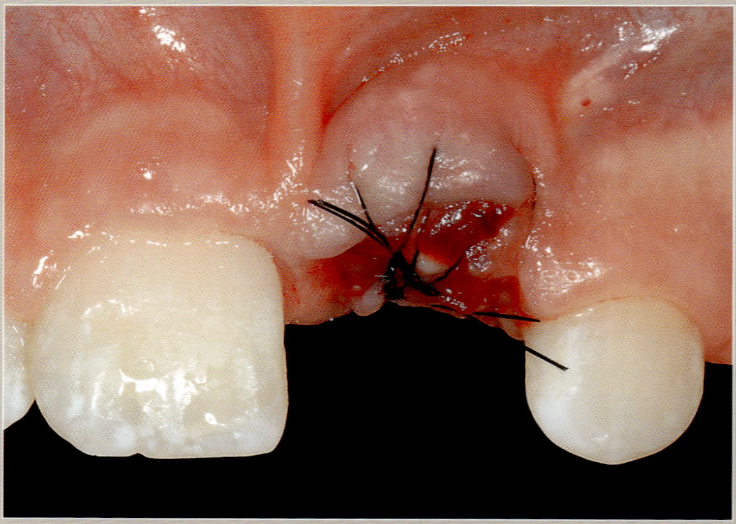

Transplanted tooth placed in the central incisor socket.

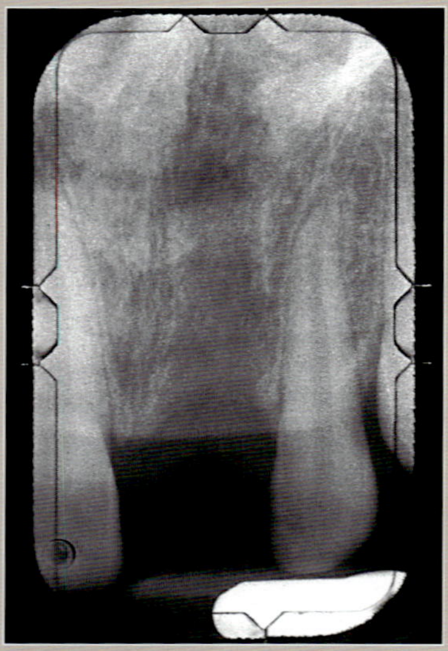

Radiograph following extraction of tooth no. 9.

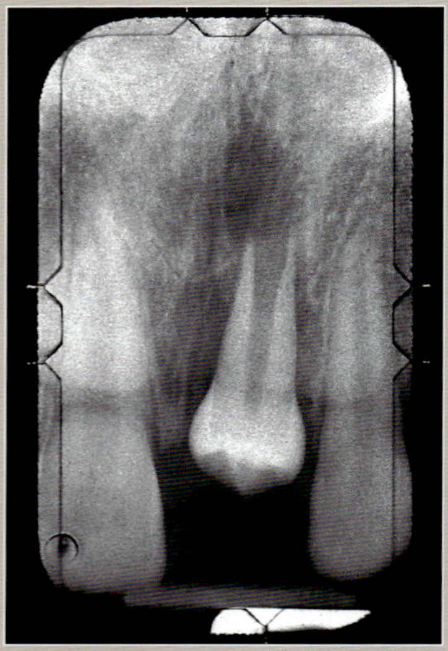

Radiograph immediately following transplantation.

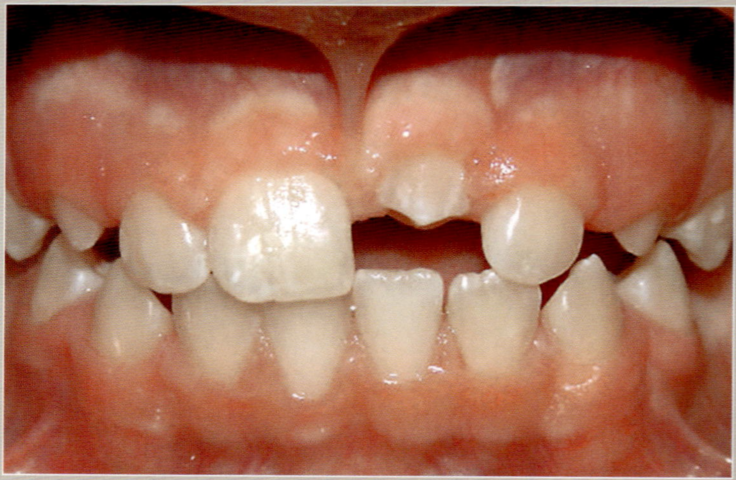

Frontal view 3 months after transplant, prior to orthodontic treatment.

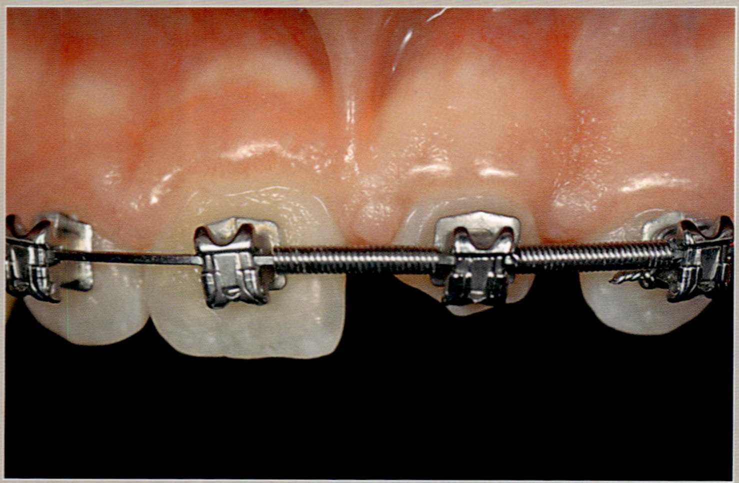

Orthodontic progress 12 months after transplant.

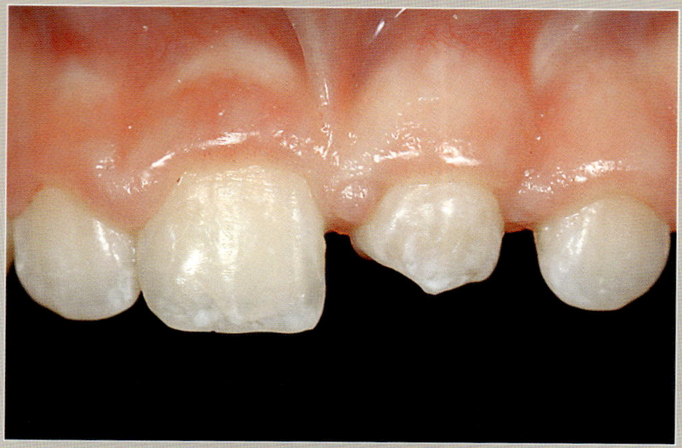

Transplanted tooth before preparation.

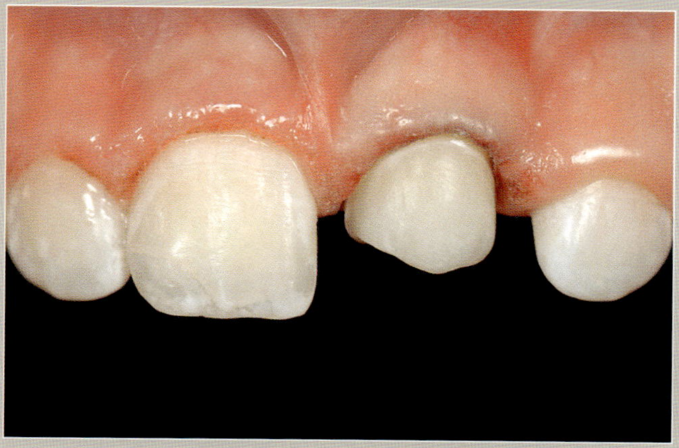

Frontal view of prepared transplanted tooth.

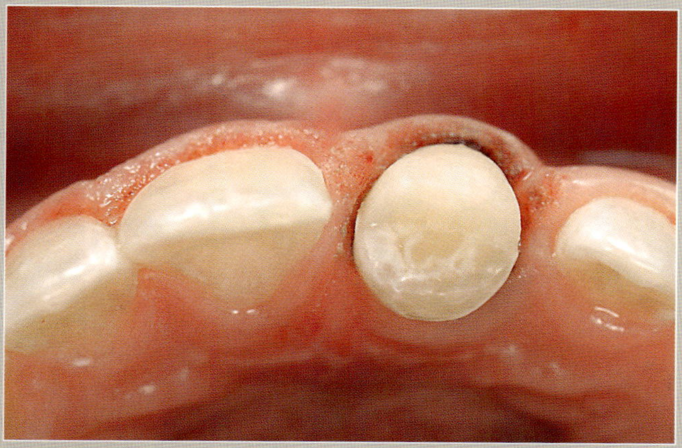

Occlusal view of prepared transplanted tooth.

Phase IV: Restorative treatment

Once the above positioning criteria were met, restorative treatment was initiated. Gingivectomies were performed on the transplanted tooth and the adjacent central incisor with a laser (Waterlase MD, Biolase) to improve the tissue symmetry prior to preparation. The transplanted tooth was minimally prepared to decrease the thickness at the cervical height of contour and create a slight finish line. A silicone impression was taken, and the cast was poured in type IV dental stone. The composite veneer (Miris 2, Colténe Whaledent) was fabricated directly on the cast. The restoration was tried in to verify fit, occlusion, and esthetics and adjusted as needed. Prior to cementation, the preparation was microabraded, etched with phosphoric acid, and treated with a dentin adhesive (Single Bond, 3M ESPE). The restoration was bonded with a resin cement (RelyX Veneer Cement, 3M ESPE). After light curing, the excess cement was removed, and the restorative margins were finished. A post-cementation radiograph was taken to verify complete cement removal.

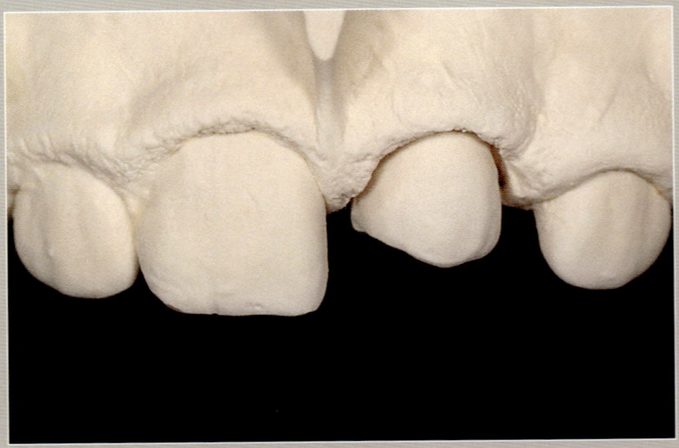

Cast of tooth preparation.

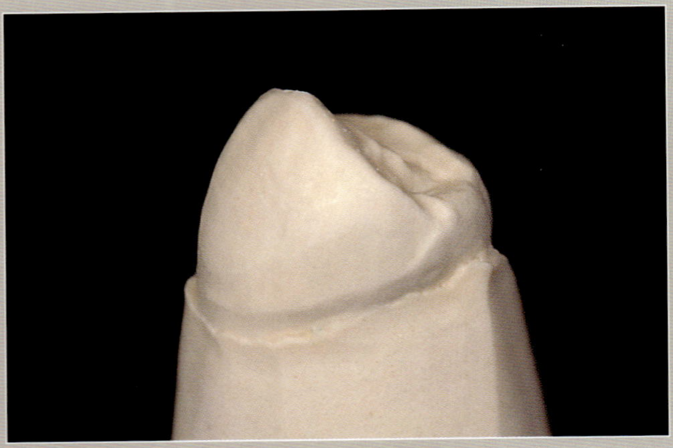

Close-up of stone die cast of tooth preparation.

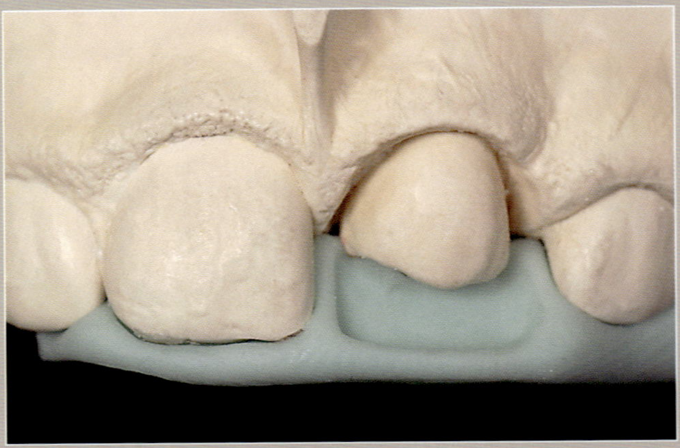

Cast of tooth preparation with palatal index.

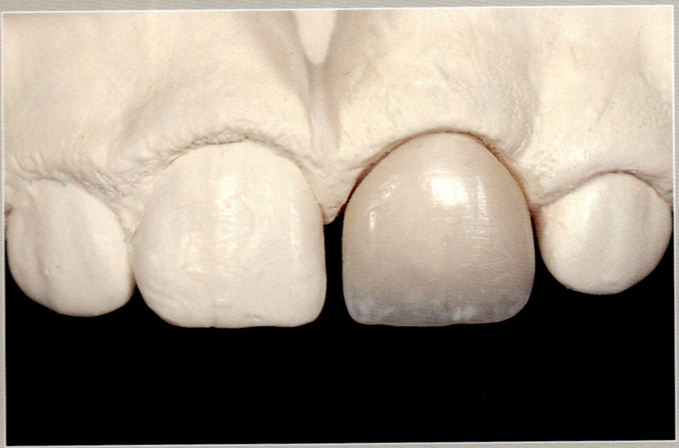

Composite veneer on cast.

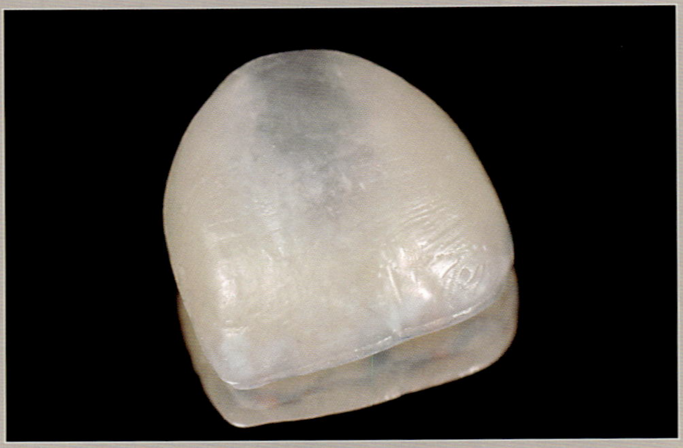

Composite veneer.

Phase V: Completion of orthodontic treatment

The transplanted tooth was initially placed slightly too labially on the ridge, and this necessitated a change in the restorative plan. Veneer preparation should be minimally invasive, and this would not have been possible if the objective was to gain ideal alignment between the two central incisors. Instead, minimal tooth structure was removed from the facial surface in preparation for the veneer, resulting in the transplanted tooth being positioned facial to the adjacent central incisor. This would ultimately be corrected with some additional orthodontic treatment to reposition the transplant tooth palatally. The patient was referred to the orthodontist for the completion of orthodontic treatment.

Posttreatment

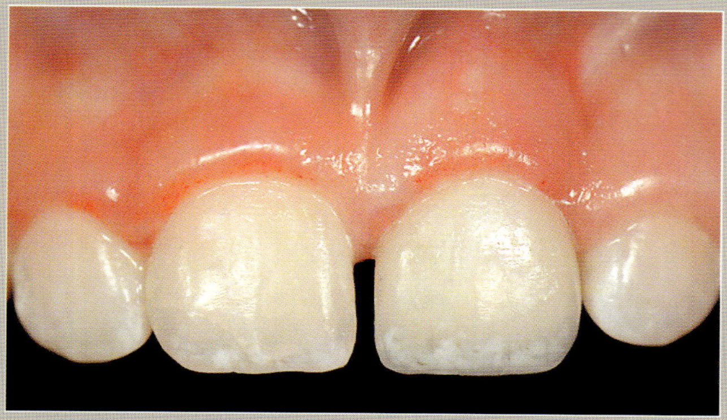

Composite veneer after placement.

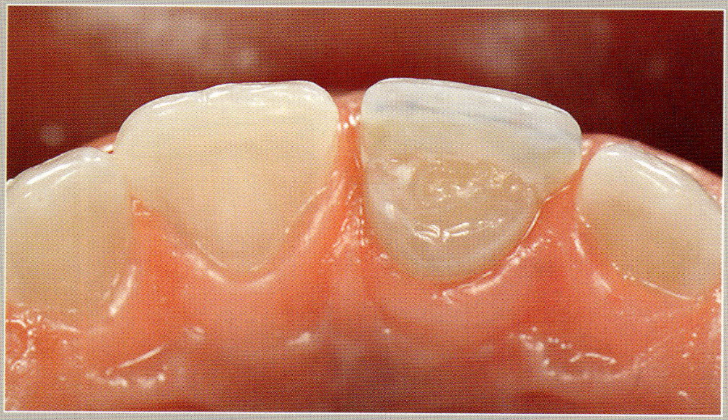

Occlusal view of composite veneer.

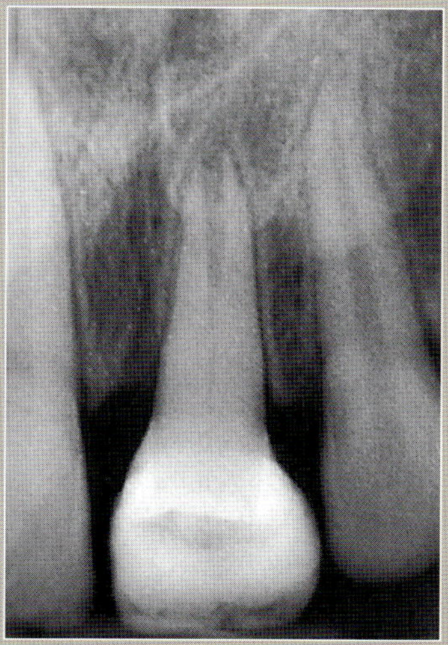

Radiograph of cemented composite veneer.

You may now place the corresponding posttreatment overlay found in the separate folder over the pretreatment periodontal chart on page 179.

Commentary

Surgical considerations

There are several surgical considerations when planning for the autotransplantation of teeth. The first consideration is the choice of tooth. The mandibular first and second premolars as well as the maxillary second premolar can be considered for autotransplantation. The maxillary first premolar is not preferred because the buccal root would be too prominent in the anterior maxilla. Because the mandibular second premolar has the greatest mesiodistal width, it is often the most appropriate choice to replace a central incisor.

The second consideration when planning for autotransplantation is the stage of root development. Studies that have evaluated autotransplantation of teeth with regard to root growth and pulpal healing recommend harvesting the transplant tooth when the root is between two-thirds to fully developed and has an open apex. It has been shown that 21% of the transplanted teeth will continue to grow to normal root length, 65% will partially arrest, and 14% will fully arrest.[7] This arrested root development is attributed to trauma to the root sheath, which can occur during the transplantation process. This reinforces the importance of meticulous surgical treatment.

Space closure at the harvest site

The remaining edentulous space at the harvest site is typically closed by unilateral protraction of the posterior teeth using either traditional or mini-implant anchorage mechanics. This eliminates the need for future tooth replacement in this space. In other situations, it may be beneficial to maintain the edentulous site and restore it with a single-tooth implant at the completion of growth.

Clinical and radiographic evaluation of the transplanted tooth determines the success of the procedure and gives guidance to the orthodontist. Healing of a transplanted tooth differs from that of a replanted tooth. An avulsed and replanted tooth typically has an intimate fit within its original socket, which is lined with a periodontal ligament. A transplanted tooth is placed within a surgically created socket and requires more time for granulation tissue formation and development of a periodontal ligament. It typically takes 3 to 4 months for autotransplanted teeth to develop periodontal ligament attachment to the new socket. After that time, the orthodontist can be instructed to proceed with tooth movement.

Orthodontic positioning

Historically, in order to have the transplanted mandibular second premolar more closely match the mesiodistal dimensions of the central incisor, transplanted teeth were turned 90 degrees. Although the mesiodistal width of the premolar when rotated is closer to the width of the central incisor, the interproximal scallop of the CEJ on the rotated premolar is located on the facial surface and scallops in the reverse direction compared with the facial gingival margin. Therefore, the facial margin of the veneer restoration must be placed on the root surface rather than remain on enamel. Given this situation, the transplanted tooth should not be rotated 90 degrees; restorative treatment can compensate for any difference in the mesiodistal dimension.

Timing of restorative treatment

In the process of deciding when the transplanted tooth should be restored, two options exist:

1. The tooth can be restored early in the orthodontic phase of treatment, ie, prior to definitive positioning.
2. The tooth can be restored later in the orthodontic treatment, ie, after the tooth is positioned more ideally with respect to the apicocoronal, mesiodistal, and buccolingual positioning criteria.

Given that the goal of the restorative treatment is to create a restoration that mirrors the adjacent central incisor, positioning the tooth more ideally prior to beginning the restorative process can significantly ease the visualization and creation of the restoration.

In this case, the transplanted tooth was positioned too far labially; therefore, the plan had to be modified at the time of restorative treatment. Given that the restorative goal is one of minimal tooth preparation that should never involve the exposure of dentin, the restoration was fabricated into a more facial position relative to the adjacent central incisor. The tooth could then be moved palatally with additional orthodontic therapy into a more ideal position.

Restorative contouring of the transplanted tooth

In this case, excess space was created mesially and distally around the transplanted tooth to facilitate the fabrication, seating, and finishing of the restoration. The restoration was fabricated to match the mesiodistal dimensions of the adjacent central incisor, adding one-third of the additional contour to the mesial and two-thirds of the additional contour to the distal. The rationale for this distribution of the additional contour is to enable the restoration to more closely resemble a natural central incisor, which has a relatively straight mesial contour and a more convex distal contour. If too much space were to be left on the mesial, the restoration would have to be designed with more convexity on the mesial aspect to allow for space closure, avoiding the creation of a black space. Although this can be done, it negatively influences the shape of the papilla, thereby detracting from the symmetry of the soft tissue.

Type of restorative material

The restoration can be fabricated using either ceramic or composite material. The benefits of ceramic are esthetics and material strength. However, ceramic is usually associated with a higher cost and is more difficult to repair if it fractures. Composite on the other hand can also be highly esthetic, is associated with a lower treatment cost, and although the strength is less than ceramic, it is easy to repair if it fractures. For young patients, given their activities and the likelihood of additional trauma to their dentition, composite is our restorative material of choice. An additional benefit of composite is that with continued active and passive eruption of the teeth, any future staining of the facial restorative margin can be easily remedied.

Fabrication of a composite veneer

While the fabrication of the composite veneer requires a degree of clinical artistry on the part of the clinician, the real challenge arises when trying to create the proper proximal contours. Given the mesiodistal size differential between the transplanted tooth and the natural central incisor (typically about 2 mm), build up of the restoration must begin subgingivally. This enables the creation of contours that resemble the natural central incisor and can be easily cleaned. Working with composite material subgingivally in the mouth can be extremely difficult. To enable more control of the subgingival contours, an impression was taken with Aquasil Ultra (Dentsply Caulk), and the composite restoration was fabricated on the cast.

We are often asked what should be done with the lingual cusps of the transplanted tooth, and our answer is to leave them the way they are. Given the apicocoronal size differential between the transplanted tooth and the central incisor and the fact that the orthodontist has control over the amount of overbite that is created, the lingual cusps are not a concern from an occlusal standpoint. In addition, young patients are most often unaware that the additional lingual contour is atypical, and they rarely report a problem. However, consideration should be given to sealing the occlusal grooves.

Long-term treatment

The composite veneer restoration can be considered definitive treatment for the transplanted tooth. Once the patient has completed growth and the gingival tissue position is stable, the restoration can be re-evaluated. If the patient desires a change in the esthetics, the composite restoration can be removed and replaced with a porcelain veneer.

If the transplanted tooth itself were to fail in the future, then it will still have served its purpose of influencing the development of the ridge and maintaining the bone in the area to allow single-tooth implant placement when growth is completed.

REFERENCES

1. Andreasen JO, Paulsen HU, Yu Z, Bayer T, Schwartz O. A long-term study of 370 autotransplanted premolars. Part II. Tooth survival and pulp healing subsequent to transplantation. Eur J Orthod 1990;12:14–24.
2. Andreasen JO, Paulsen HU, Yu Z, Schwartz O. A long-term study of 370 autotransplanted premolars. Part III. Periodontal healing subsequent to transplantation. Eur J Orthod 1990;12:25–37.
3. Kristerson L, Lagerström L. Autotransplantation of teeth in cases with agenesis or traumatic loss of maxillary incisors. Eur J Orthod 1991;13:486–492.
4. Kugelberg R, Tegsjö U, Malmgren O. Autotransplantation of 45 teeth to the upper incisor region in adolescents. Swed Dent J 1994;18:165–172.
5. Czochrowska EM, Stenvik A, Zachrisson BU. The esthetic outcome of autotransplanted premolars replacing maxillary incisors. Dent Traumatol 2002;18:237–245.
6. Czochrowska EM, Stenvik A, Bjercke B, Zachrisson BU. Outcome of tooth transplantation: Survival and success rates 17–41 years posttreatment. Am J Orthod Dentofacial Orthop 2002;121:110–119.
7. Paulsen HU, Andreasen JO, Schwartz O. Pulp and periodontal healing, root development and root resorption subsequent to transplantation and orthodontic rotation: A long-term study of autotransplanted premolars. Am J Orthod Dentofacial Orthop 1995;108:630–640.

7

Anterior Wear: Orthodontic and Restorative Management

John C. Kois, DMD, MSD

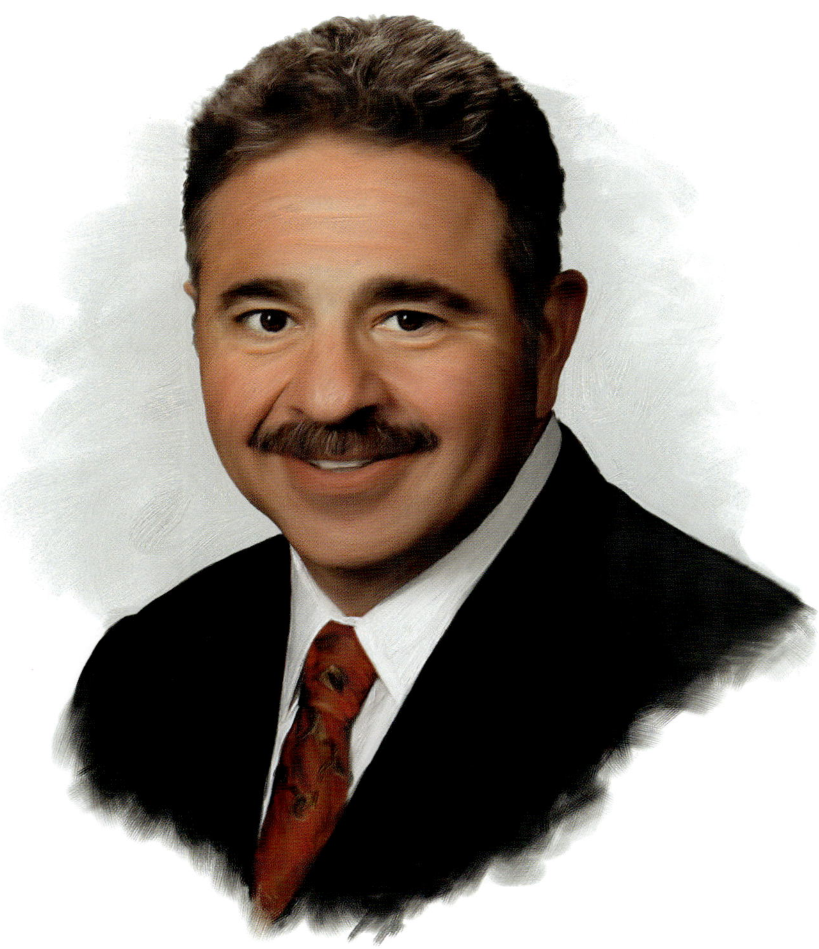

Ultimately, what becomes most critical is how we measure the outcome of treatment.

PHILOSOPHY AND BACKGROUND

Treatment-planning decisions require an evaluation of the patient's health status, extent of existing disease, and risk of impending disease. Most clinicians tend to focus on the first two issues only. However, managing a patient's dental health concerns always involves asking three very important questions:

1. *What?*
   - What are the facts?
   - What happened?
   - What is the problem? (diagnosis)
2. *So what?*
   - What does this mean?
   - What do I expect? (risk assessment)
3. *Now what?*
   - What care do I provide?
   - What will I continue to provide? (treatment)

The case presentation in this chapter addresses concerns commonly seen in any dental practice. This patient is resistant to periodontal disease and caries but continues to manifest occlusal problems and esthetic challenges in spite of previous treatment *(What?)*.

The patient is at risk of ongoing physical disability from the occlusion and psychologic disability mediated through the perceived stigma of a compromised smile *(So what?)* if treatment is not provided.

The required treatment *(Now what?)* created some interesting challenges in terms of managing a new orthopedic position of the jaw, creating a new tooth position that could account for the replacement of lost tooth structure, and developing normal tooth proportions. In addition, it was critical to provide a minimally invasive protocol that allowed the laboratory technician to create natural-looking teeth.

Ultimately, what becomes most critical is how we measure the outcome of treatment. There is a difference between a surrogate outcome, such as a laboratory or physical clinical measurement, and a true outcome, which is a clinically meaningful endpoint that measures directly how a patient feels, functions, or survives and reflects unequivocal evidence of tangible patient benefit. True endpoints include quality-of-life measures and should continue to be the ultimate goal in our treatment planning.

Case Presentation

Treating clinicians
Prosthodontist: John C. Kois, DMD, MSD
Orthodontist: Brett C. Fidler, DDS, MSD
Laboratory technician: Leon Hermanides, NHD, CDT

Clinical Treatment Planning

Age at initial presentation: 34 years
Initial presentation: March 2003
Active treatment completed: June 2006

Medical history

The patient presented with an unremarkable history, except for exercise-induced asthma. He was a healthy man taking no medications and therefore had no medical contraindications for dental treatment.

Dental history

The patient presented with several concerns about his dental health. Most significantly, he felt embarrassed to smile and was concerned that his maxillary anterior teeth were "thinning" and chipping on the edges. This had continued to occur even though he had worn a nightguard for years. He had experienced jaw problems for the last 10 years, including difficulty in opening wide. The patient had also suffered from tension headaches 1 week per month for 2 to 3 consecutive days at a time. He had often awakened with an "awareness" of his teeth, with some of them feeling sore. In addition, he voiced frustration with his previous dental care because attempts to equilibrate his teeth only made his situation worse. He expressed that, when he removed his nightguard in the morning, "my posterior teeth do not touch unless I squeeze them together to make them fit, because my front teeth are in the way."

Diagnostic findings

Extraoral and facial findings

- Cancer screen: negative
- Generally within normal limits

TMJ and mandibular range of motion

- Maximum opening of 44 mm with normal range of movement and no deviation upon opening
- Bilateral joint sounds: grade 1
- Load test: negative
- Immobilization test: negative

Intraoral findings

- Bilateral mandibular lingual tori approximately 10 mm × 5 mm
- Missing teeth nos. 1, 16, 17, and 32

Periodontal

- Mild chronic periodontitis; AAP II
- Probing depths within normal limits without bleeding on probing
- Radiographically, bone support within 2 mm of the cementoenamel junction (CEJ) without any infrabony defects
- Gingival architecture symmetric with the exception of tooth no. 9, which had 2 mm apical recession on the facial

Pretreatment

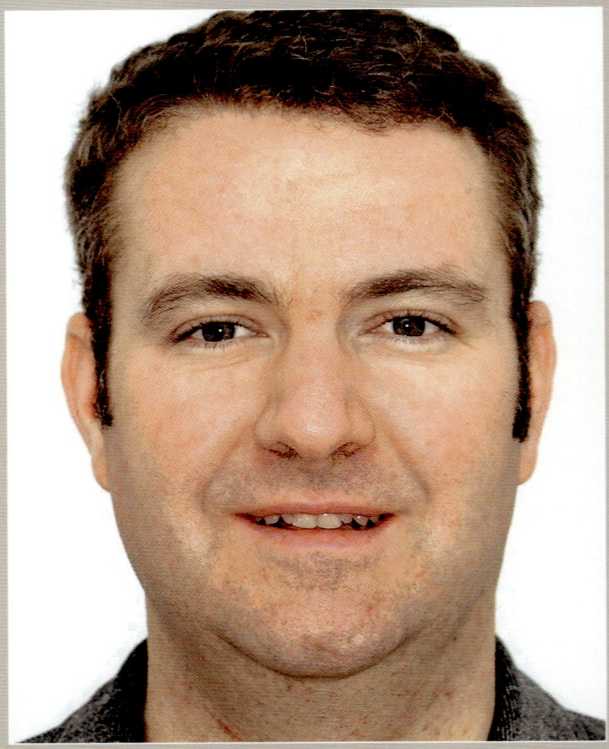

Facial view.

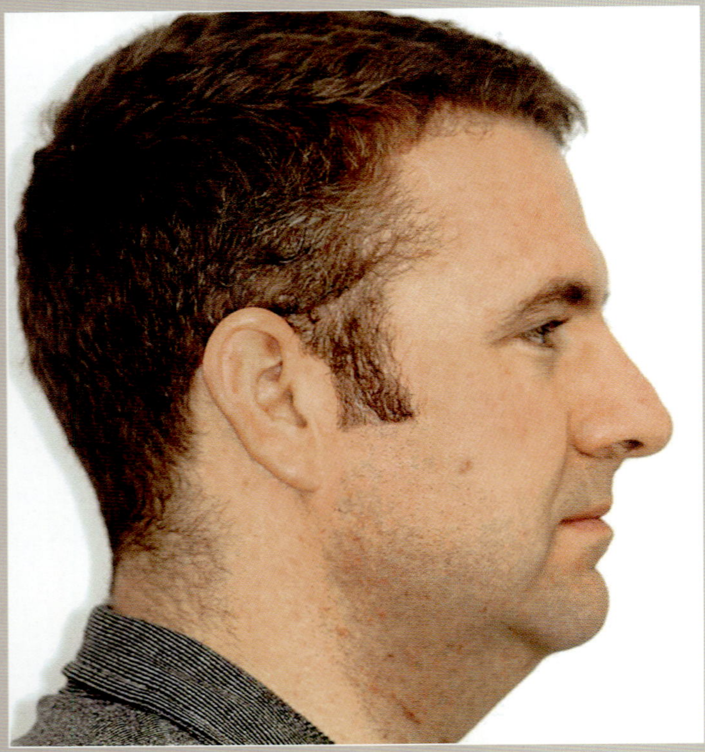

Profile view.

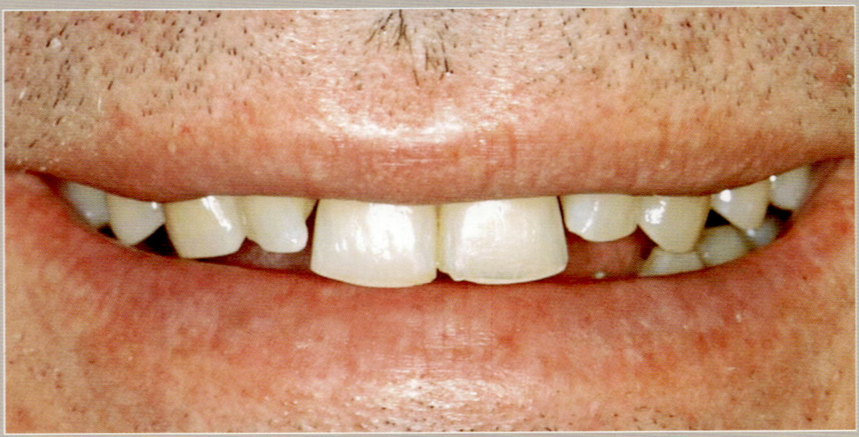

Close-up of full smile.

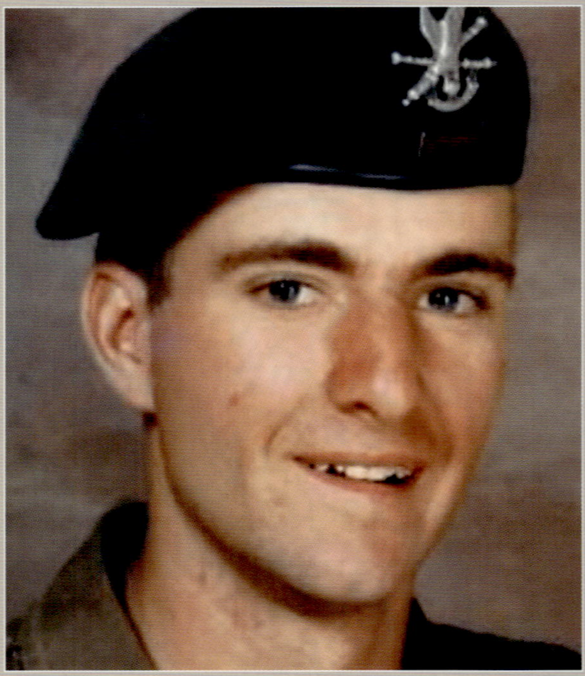

Historical photo used for comparative analysis.

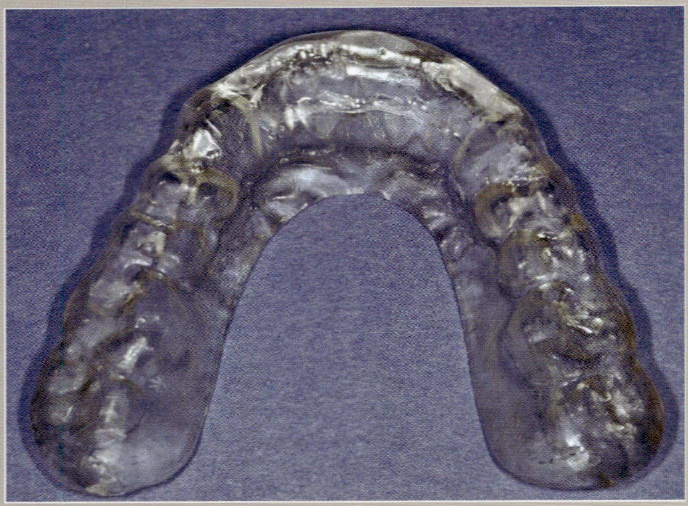

Evidence of wear on the maxillary occlusal nightguard confirms nighttime parafunctional activity.

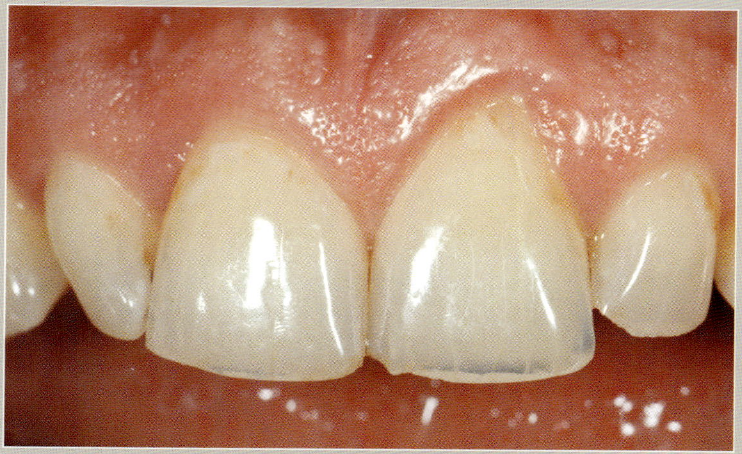

Frontal view of maxillary anterior teeth.

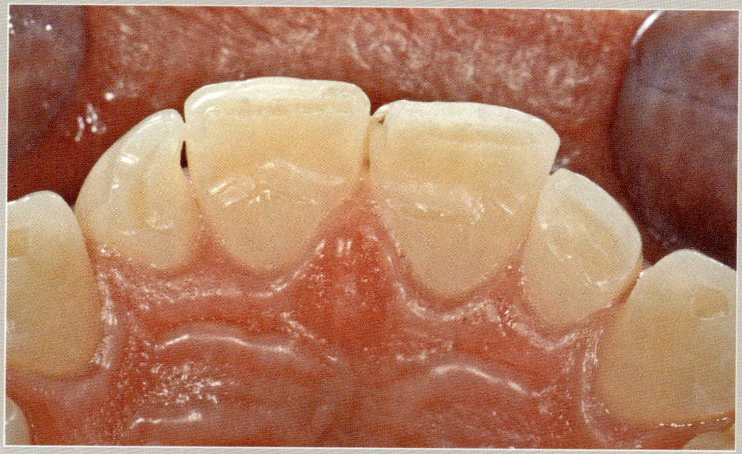

Lingual view of maxillary anterior teeth.

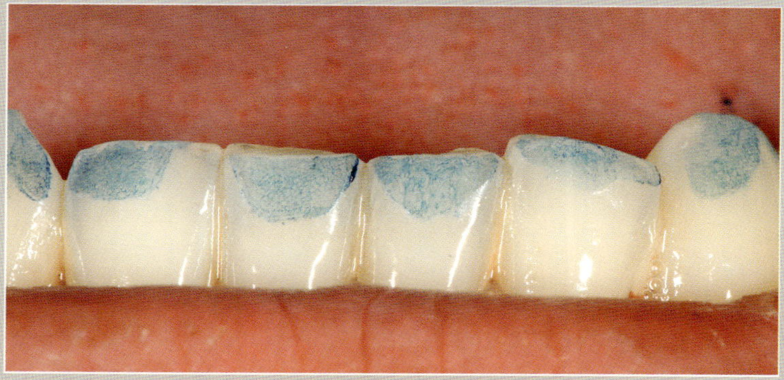

Frontal view of worn mandibular anterior teeth.

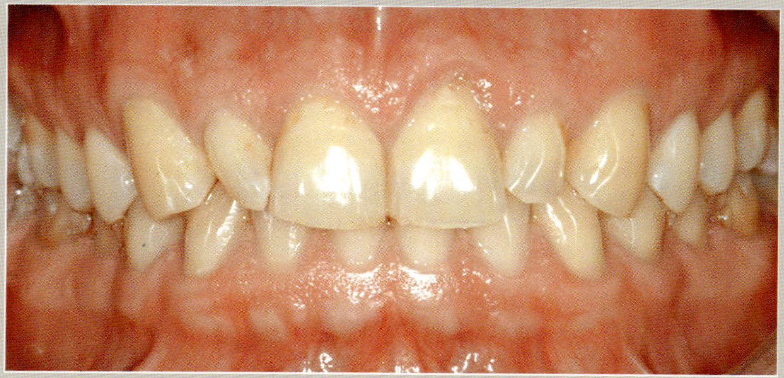

Frontal view in maximal intercuspal position.

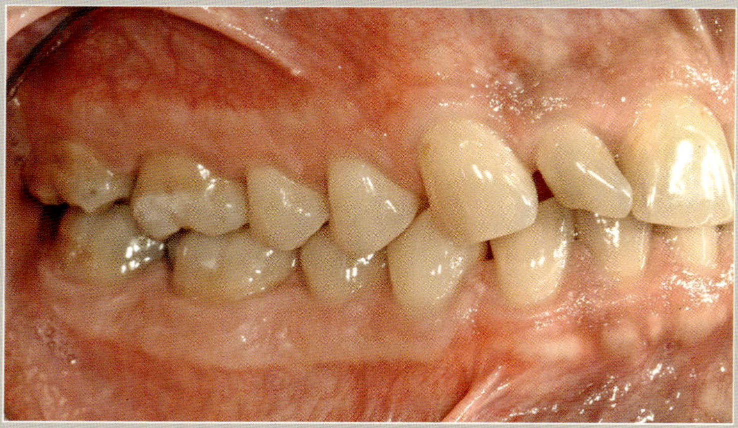

Right lateral view.

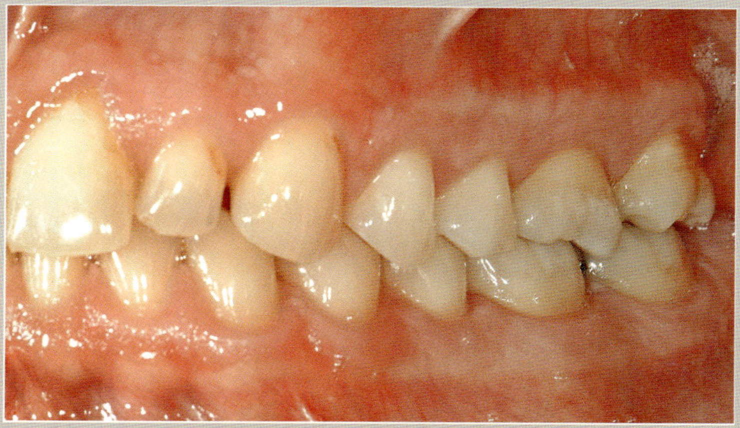

Left lateral view.

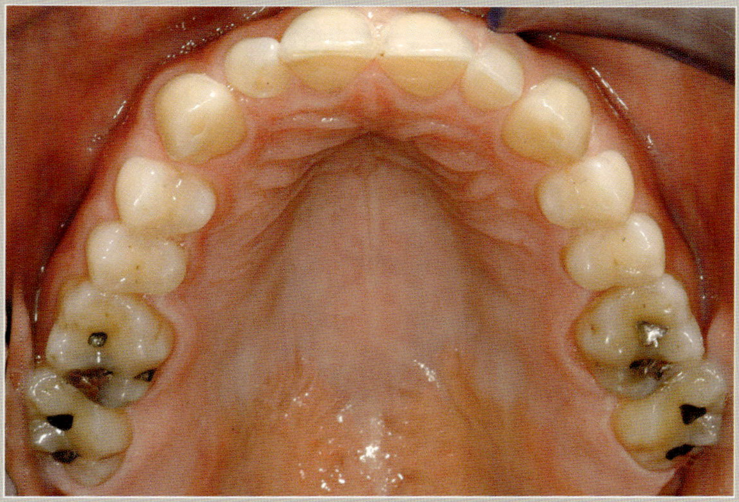

Maxillary occlusal view.

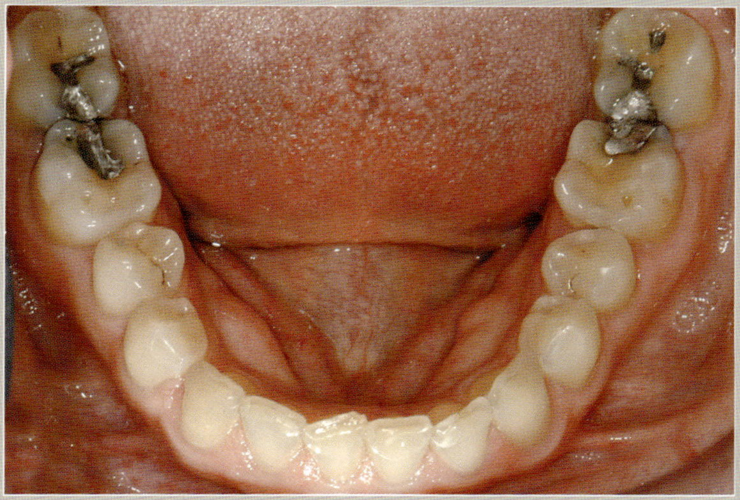

Mandibular occlusal view.

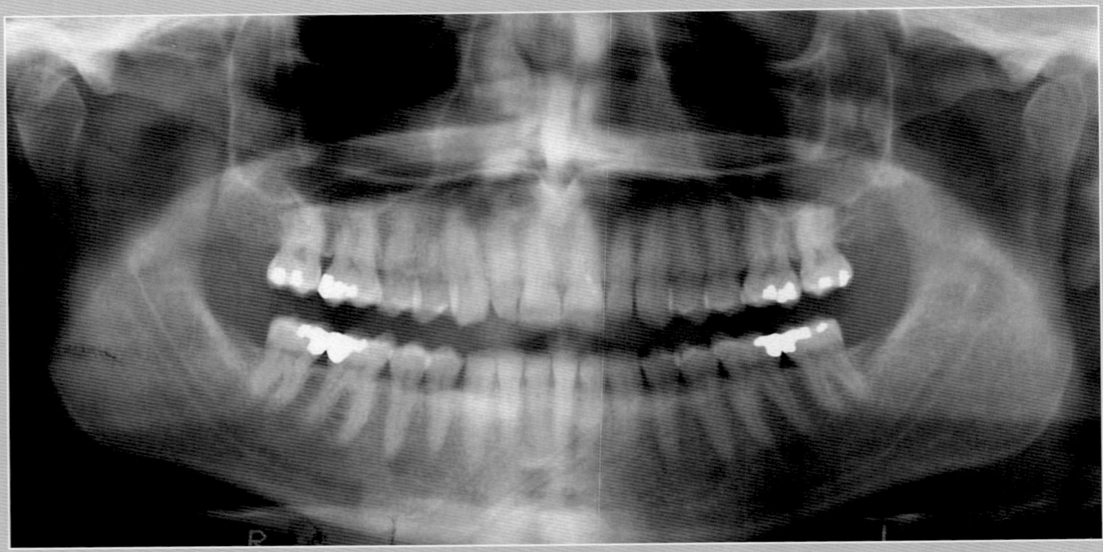

Panoramic radiograph.

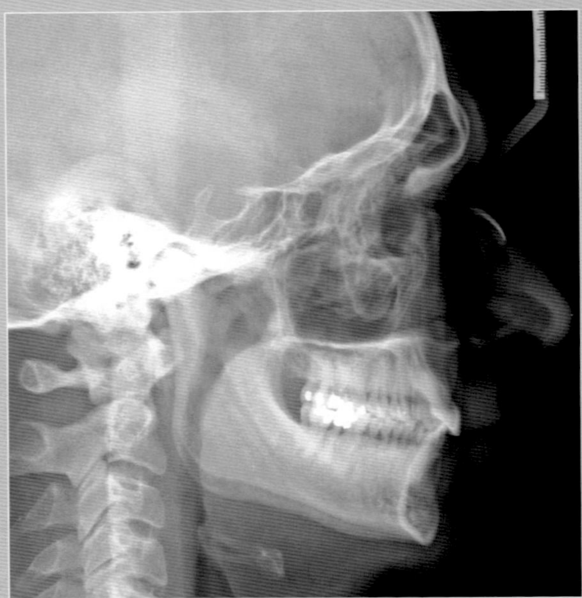

Cephalometric radiograph.

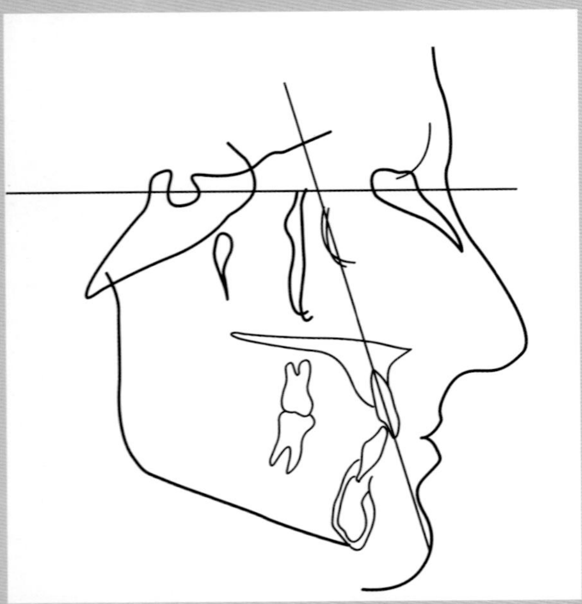

Cephalometric tracing.

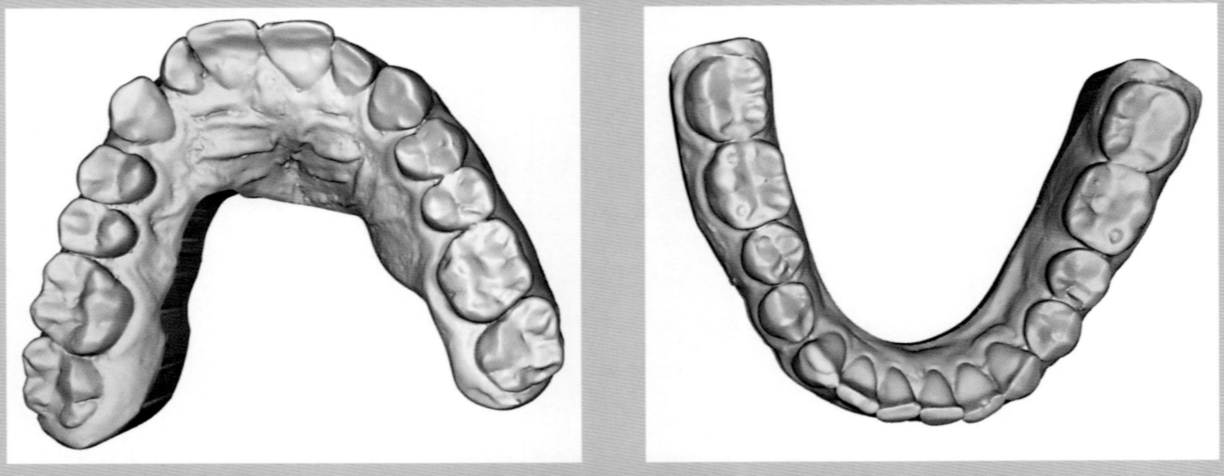

Maxillary and mandibular digital scans (Cadent, iTero).

Biomechanical

- No dental caries noted
- Minimal erosion on the occlusal surface of teeth nos. 19 and 30
- Multiple questionable alloy restorations

Functional

- Moderate lingual attrition on teeth nos. 6 to 11
- Moderate incisal/facial attrition on teeth nos. 22 to 27
- Evidence of constricted chewing pattern and nocturnal bruxism

Dentofacial

- Medium lip dynamics
- Unacceptable rotation of teeth
- Maxillary tooth size discrepancies
- Acceptable tooth color

Cephalometric findings

- SNA: 77 degrees (norm: 82 ± 3 degrees)
- SNB: 76.5 degrees (norm: 79 ± 3 degrees)
- ANB: 0.5 degrees (norm: 3 ± 2 degrees)
- SN–MP: 32 degrees (norm: 32 ± 5 degrees)
- UAFH/LAFH (N–ANS/ANS-Me): 0.8 (norm: 0.8)
- Maxillary incisor to SN: 100 degrees (norm: 103 ± 6 degrees)
- Mandibular incisor to MP: 92 degrees (norm: 90 ± 5 degrees)
- Interincisal angle: 142 degrees (norm: 135 ± 11 degrees)

Risk Assessment

An individual risk assessment is critical to determine the most appropriate treatment plan. Traditionally, we have collected data that assess the current state of disease (a reparative model); however, risk assessment expands our ability to determine the possibility of disease before it is actually expressed (a wellness model). In other words, risk assessment develops prognostic capability. Only when the composite of the diagnostic categories are considered simultaneously and risk is reduced or prognosis is improved can interdisciplinary treatment be rendered successfully with the most promising outcomes.

Dentofacial

There is moderate risk due to the medium lip dynamics, incomplete tooth display, and inability to display the gingival architecture. However, exceeding the patient's expectations is more likely than falling short of them, which makes treatment less difficult.

Functional

There is moderate to high risk due to the combination of constricted chewing patterns and nocturnal bruxism. This will require management of the occlusion to minimize ongoing friction and nighttime protection with appliance therapy for life.

Biomechanical

There is low risk due to previous minimal caries expression, minimally restored teeth with minimal structural compromises, and no other shared risk factors. However, if more tooth structure is reduced to allow space for restorative materials, this will result in removing more tooth structure than the patient may lose in his lifetime, even without treatment. Therefore, using an additive strategy rather than a subtractive one to achieve functional and esthetic goals is preferrable.

Periodontal

There is low risk due to minimal bone loss, no family history, and no other shared risk factors for periodontal disease.

Summary of concerns

1. How can the anterior teeth be managed to reduce the functional risk?
2. How can his esthetic concerns be addressed and resolved without increasing the biomechanical risk?

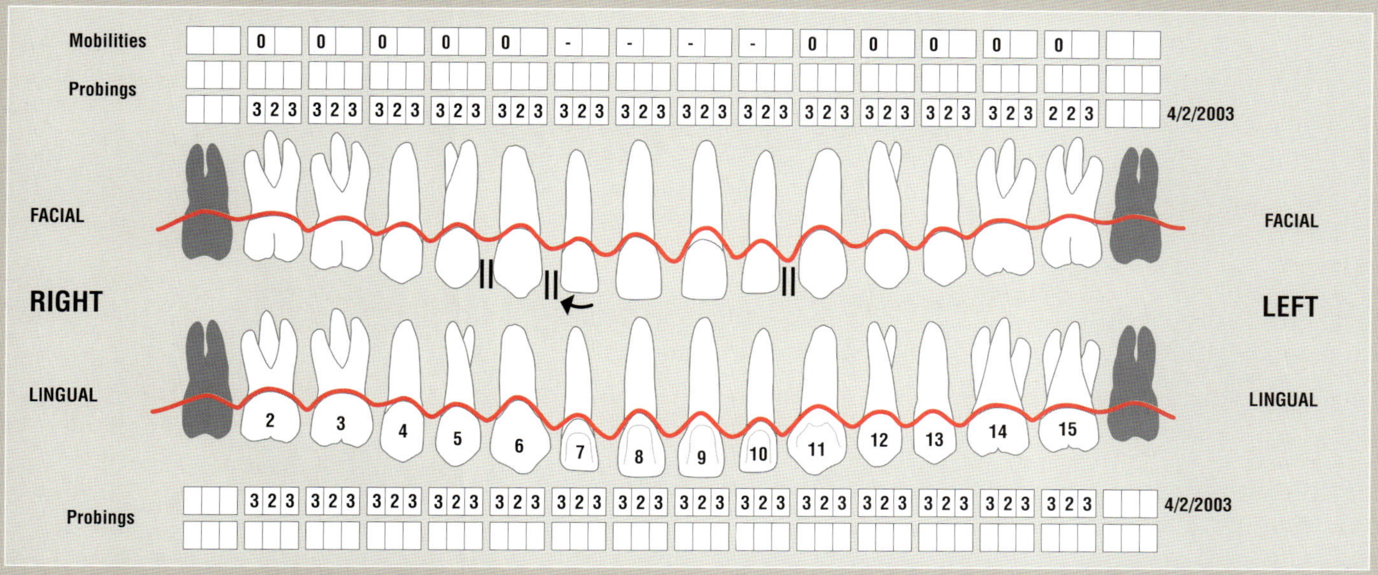

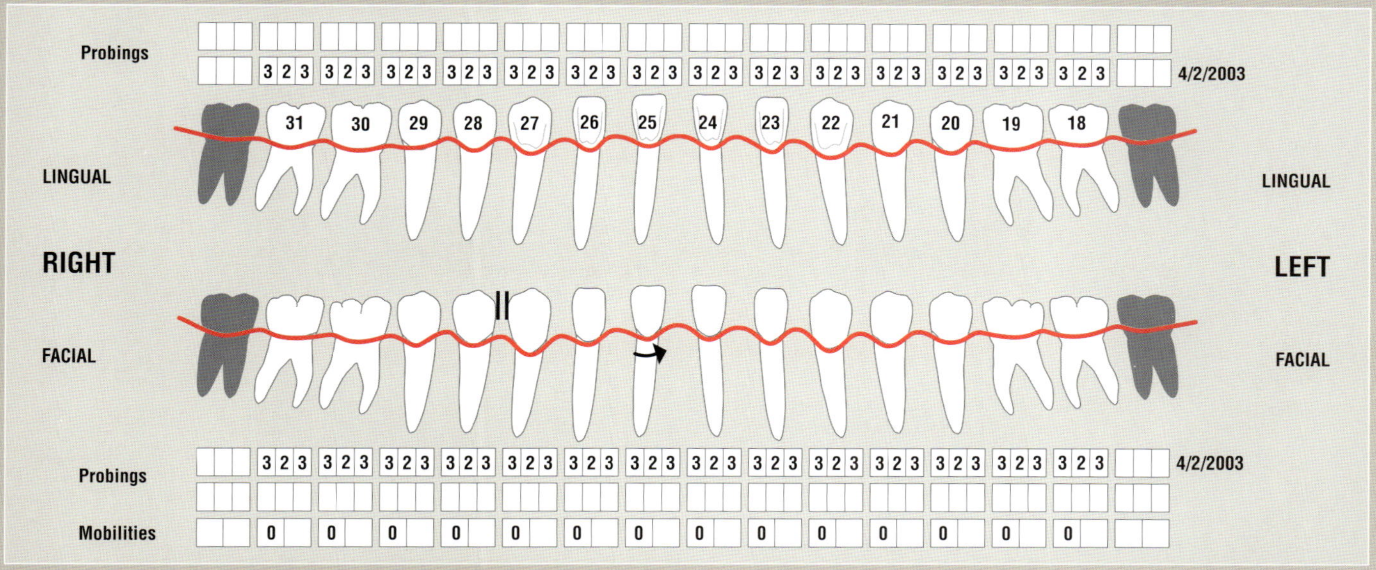

As a learning exercise, you may now outline goals/objectives of treatment and a treatment plan.

Proposed Treatment Plan

Goals/objectives of treatment

Managing the continued loss of anterior tooth structure, improving esthetics, and eliminating the existing symptoms were the patient's primary objectives. In order to minimize the compromises to the health of the teeth that did not require restorative dentistry and limit the restorative treatment to the anterior teeth only, orthodontics would be essential. Then occlusal management commensurate with veneers on teeth nos. 6 to 11 and 22 to 27 could be accomplished.

Phase I: Initial periodontal therapy

1. Scaling and root planing as appropriate
2. Home care review

Phase II: Orthodontic treatment

3. To minimize compromise to teeth that did not require restorative treatment and to limit the extent of treatment to the anterior teeth, orthodontic treatment would be necessary to create proper space appropriation and more favorable root inclinations to reduce the existing interincisal angle.
4. Specific orthodontic objectives were to provide 3 mm of labial crown torque to the maxillary incisors, level the deep curve of Spee, and intrude the worn mandibular anterior teeth to level the CEJs. This would create the necessary room for anterior restoration.

Phase III: Restorative treatment

5. Six-month stabilization period following the completion of orthodontic therapy to allow for reduction of orthodontically induced tooth mobilities
6. Anterior open bite maintained during this period of time with retainers
7. Occlusal equilibration in adapted centric posture position, retaining the anterior open bite
8. Provisional restorations fabricated and placed on teeth nos. 6 to 11 and 22 to 27
9. Definitive restorations, including veneers for teeth nos. 6 to 11 and 22 to 27
10. Minor occlusal adjustment
11. Insertion of maxillary occlusal nightguard

Active Clinical Treatment

Review of the goals/objectives of treatment

Managing the continued loss of anterior tooth structure, improving esthetics, and eliminating the existing symptoms were the patient's primary objectives. In order to minimize the compromises to the health of the teeth that did not require restorative dentistry and limit the restorative treatment to the anterior teeth only, orthodontics would be essential. Then occlusal management commensurate with veneers on teeth nos. 6 to 11 and 22 to 27 could be accomplished.

- Managing the continued loss of anterior tooth structure
- Improving esthetics
- Eliminating existing symptoms

Treatment options and goals were discussed with the patient.

Phase I: Initial periodontal therapy

Scaling and root planing procedures were performed as appropriate, along with a home care review.

Phase II: Orthodontics

The patient presented with a Class I malocclusion characterized by dental alignment irregularity, mild mandibular dental crowding, deep incisor overbite, moderate incisal attrition, low mandibular plane angle consistent with a brachycephalic facial type, strong perioral musculature, and a history of sleep bruxism.

Complete facial evaluation and cephalometric analysis were performed to determine the proper space appropriation for normal tooth proportions and more favorable root inclination to reduce the interincisal angle. This was necessary to allow the mandibular anterior teeth to move behind the maxillary anterior teeth without friction and improve the esthetic outcome. In order to determine the magnitude of the movement necessary, the mandibular orthopedic reference position needed to be established. Following the use of the Kois deprogrammer and the deprogramming protocol, it was determined that centric relation was actually anterior to the initial maximal intercuspal position (MIP). Once a stable centric relation was confirmed, the incisal edge of the maxillary anterior teeth would need to be positioned 3 mm facially. In addition, the tooth position had to satisfy the functional concerns for anterior guidance by allowing space for the restorative material with minimal to no further tooth preparation. Therefore, the mandibular anterior teeth also needed to be aligned and intruded.

Specific orthodontic treatment objectives were to provide 3 mm of labial crown torque to the maxillary incisors, level the deep curve of Spee, and intrude the worn mandibular anterior teeth to level the CEJs. This would create the necessary space for the anterior veneers.

Deprogramming hyperactive musculature and freeing the patient from a constricted chewing pattern allowed the condyles to assume a more balanced position in the glenoid fossa. The patient reported significant relaxation in the muscles of mastication and perioral musculature following the deprogramming phase. This alteration in muscle function is crucial as orthodontic treatment is initiated to significantly change occlusal relationships and establish a new MIP that is harmonious with the new centric relation.

Brackets were initially placed on the maxillary teeth, and the patient continued using the Kois deprogrammer while sleeping. After approximately 3 months, braces were added to the mandibular teeth, and the deprogrammer was placed with a palatal coverage anterior occlusion rim. The patient was initially instructed to wear the occlusion rim full-time. This opening of the occlusal vertical dimension provided the freedom to establish a new posterior occlusion. Following the leveling of the mandibular arch, the occlusion rim was only needed at night. A comparison of the pretreatment and postorthodontic/prerestorative cephalometric head films revealed more than 3 mm of maxillary labial crown torque, which created a decrease in the interincisal angle (from 142 to 130 degrees); 4 mm of overeruption of the mandibular premolars, which resulted in a leveling of the occlusal plane; and the creation of an anterior open occlusal relationship in preparation for minimally invasive restorations.

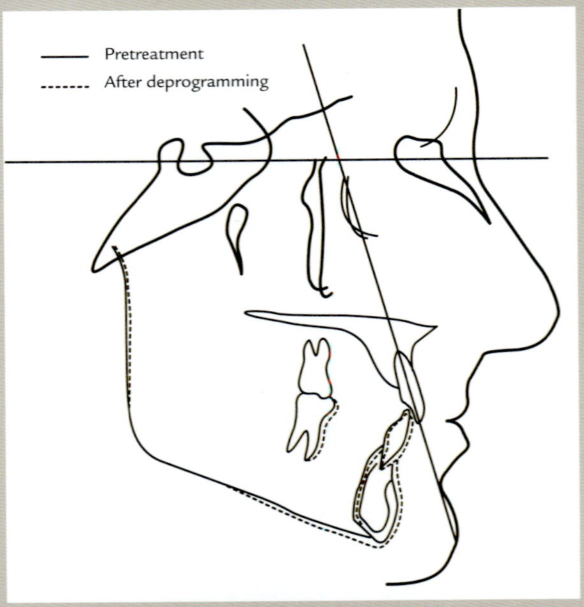

Cephalometric tracing following deprogramming, indicating a mandibular position anterior to MIP.

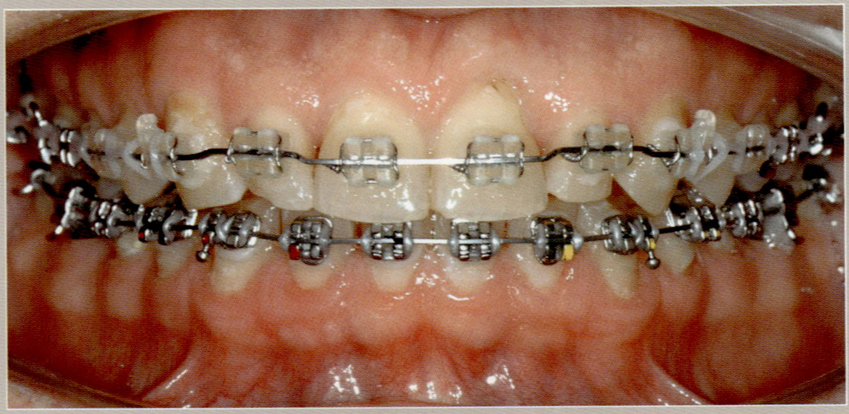

Frontal view at the beginning of orthodontic treatment.

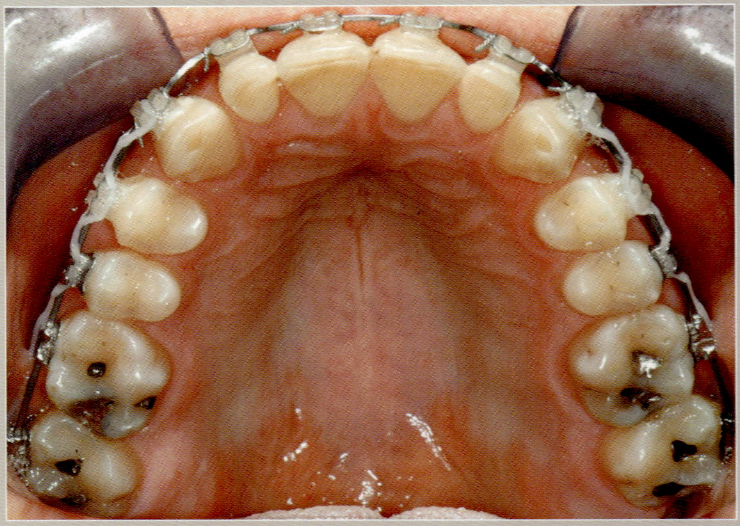

Maxillary occlusal view at the beginning of orthodontic treatment.

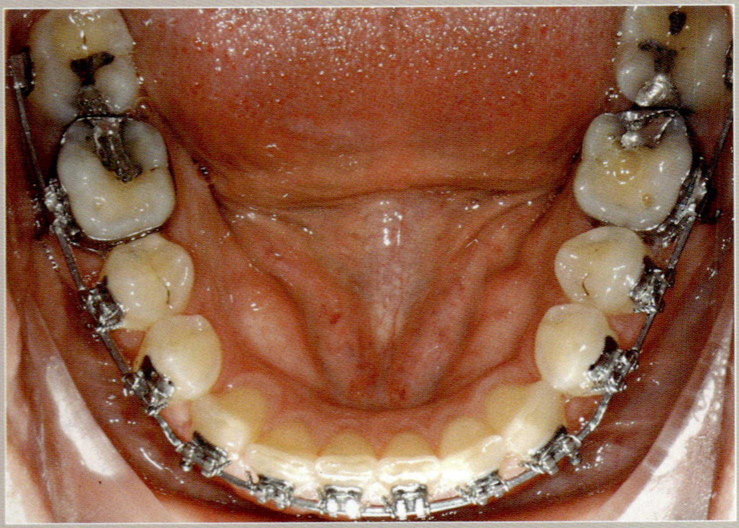

Mandibular occlusal view at the beginning of orthodontic treatment.

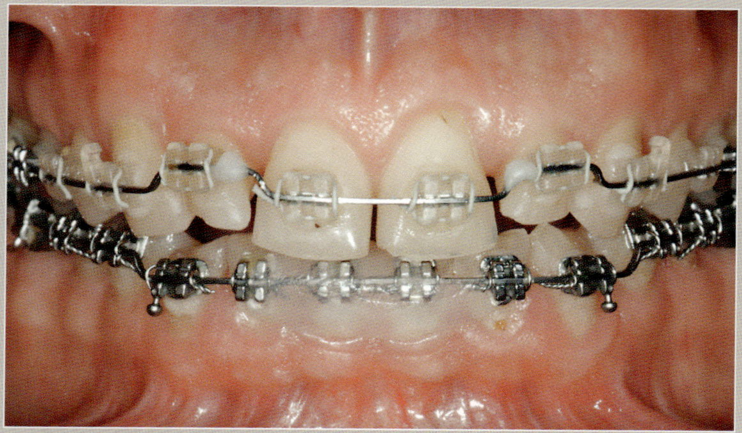

Frontal view after orthodontic treatment.

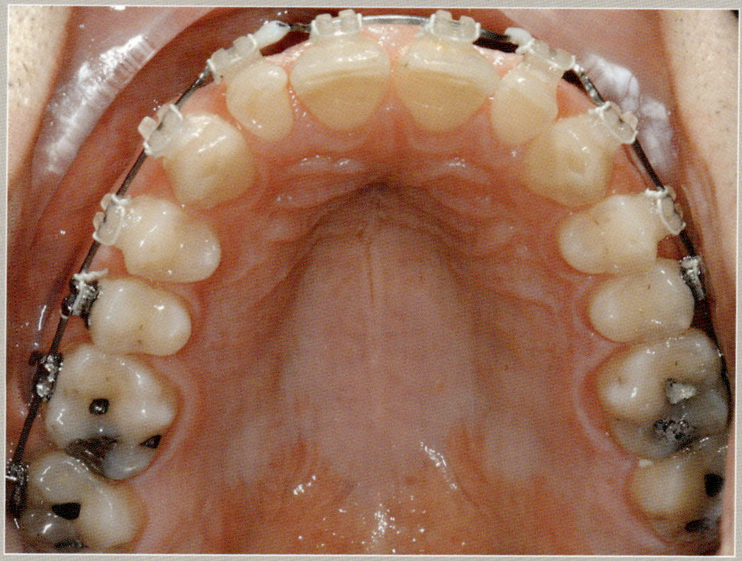

Maxillary occlusal view after orthodontic treatment.

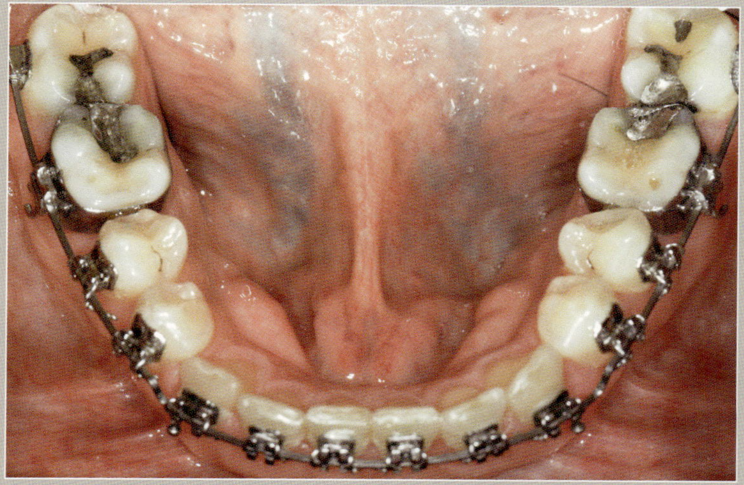

Mandibular occlusal view after orthodontic treatment.

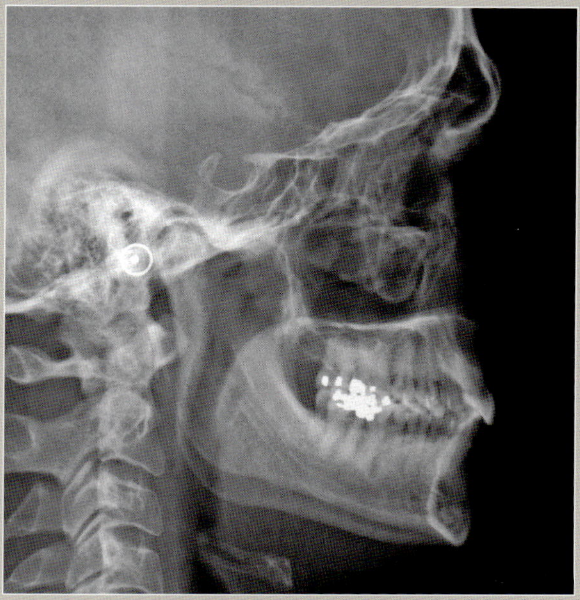

Postorthodontic cephalometric radiograph.

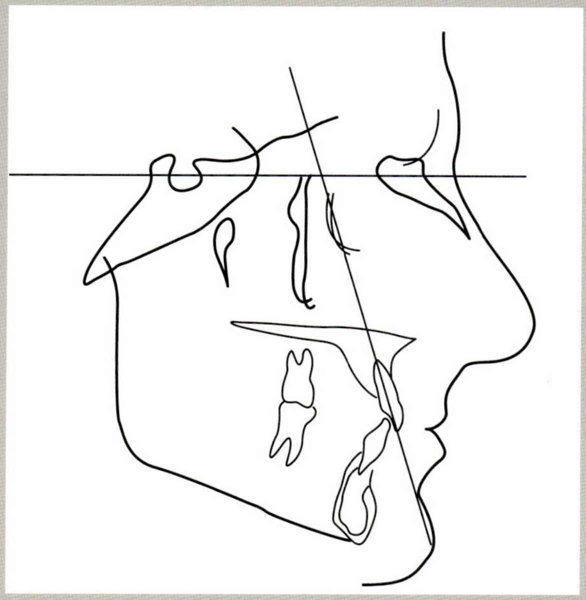

Postorthodontic cephalometric tracing.

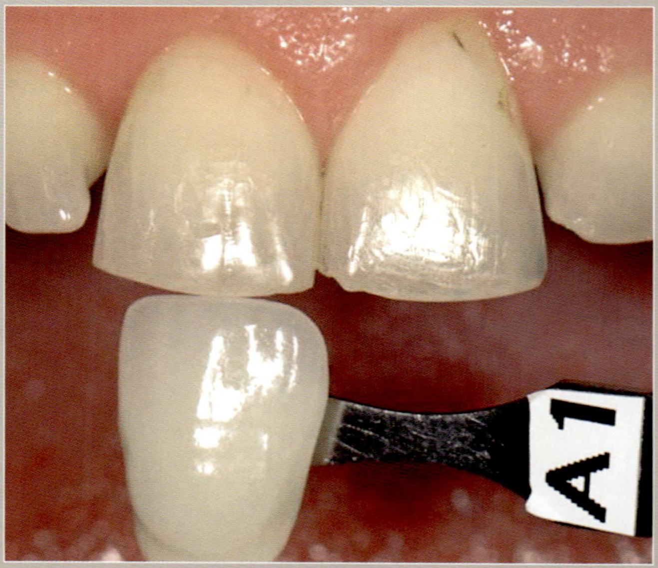

Shade communication with VITA shade tab A1 (Vita Zahnfabrik).

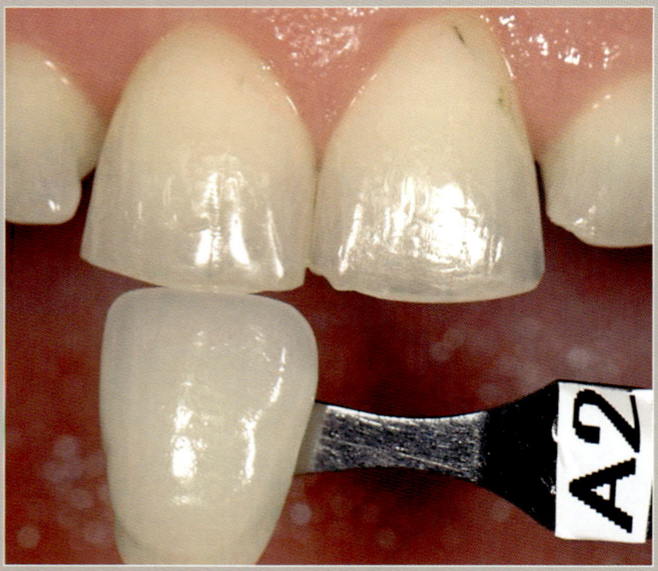

Shade communication with VITA shade tab A2.

Phase III: Restorative treatment

Following orthodontic therapy, a 6-month stabilization period was necessary to allow for the tooth mobility to resolve. It was necessary to maintain the anterior open occlusal relationship during this time with retainers. The patient was then equilibrated in the adapted centric posture position, Dawson Type II, retaining the anterior open occlusal relationship. The lingual of the maxillary anterior teeth would be managed with veneers on teeth nos. 6 to 11 and the incisal edges of the mandibular incisors with veneers on teeth nos. 22 to 27. The remaining tooth preparation was designed to meet the needs of the tooth, ie, replacing the missing tooth structure for esthetics, not the requirements of the restorative material. Otherwise, this would have unnecessarily increased the amount of tooth reduction and the biomechanical risk.

When the prepared tooth is not substantially discolored, a translucent all-ceramic restoration can be used with a good outcome. However, it is vital that the color of the prepared teeth be communicated to the ceramist, who will need to develop a ceramic layering strategy. The ceramist will be able to mask any underlying discoloration or use translucent materials to blend margins prepared supragingivally as appropriate. This communication is easily managed by taking a digital photograph of the prepared teeth with a matching shade tab.

Final impressions were made using a dual-phase, single-stage technique with light- and heavy-viscosity polyvinyl siloxane (Impressiv, Cosmedent) according to the manufacturer's instructions, and a stone cast was poured. Provisional restorations for teeth nos. 6 to 11 were made chairside with a methyl methacrylate (Temporary Crown and Bridge Resin, Dentsply Caulk) using an eggshell technique and subsequent direct reline. The direct provisional restorations for teeth nos. 22 to 27 were made chairside using a bisphenol glycidyl methacrylate (bis-GMA; Integrity, Dentsply Caulk). The Kois Dento-Facial Analyzer System (Panadent) was used to communicate essential functional and esthetic parameters for the mounting of the maxillary provisional cast. Jaw relation records were made in MIP, which had become coincident with the mandible in adapted centric posture, using Jet Bite (Colténe Whaledent). Records, casts, final impressions, and digital photographs were transferred to the laboratory technician for the fabrication of the maxillary and mandibular anterior veneers.

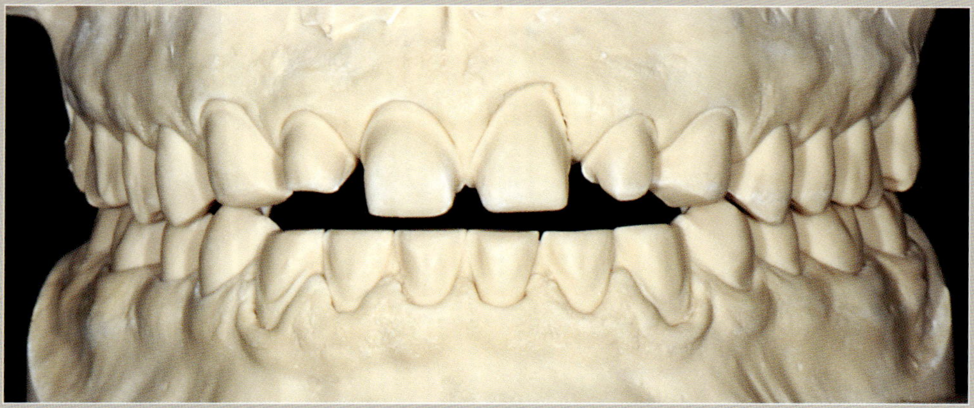

Maxillary and mandibular stone casts.

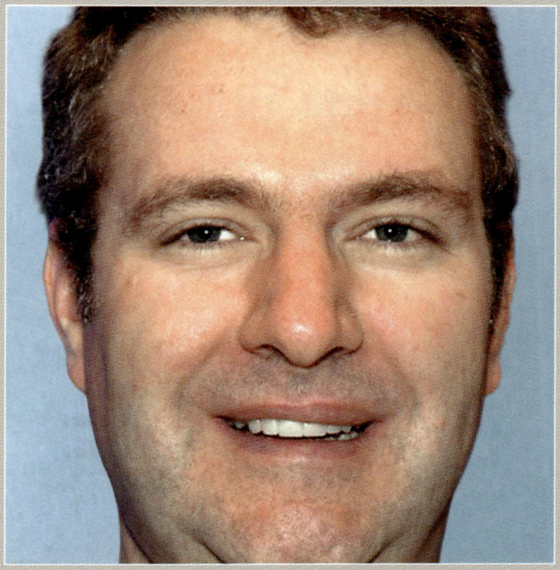

Facial view of smile with maxillary anterior provisional restorations.

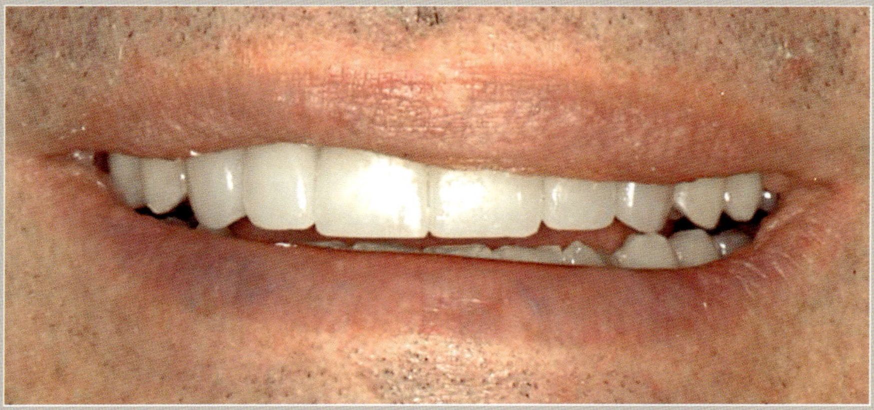

Close-up of smile with maxillary anterior provisional restorations.

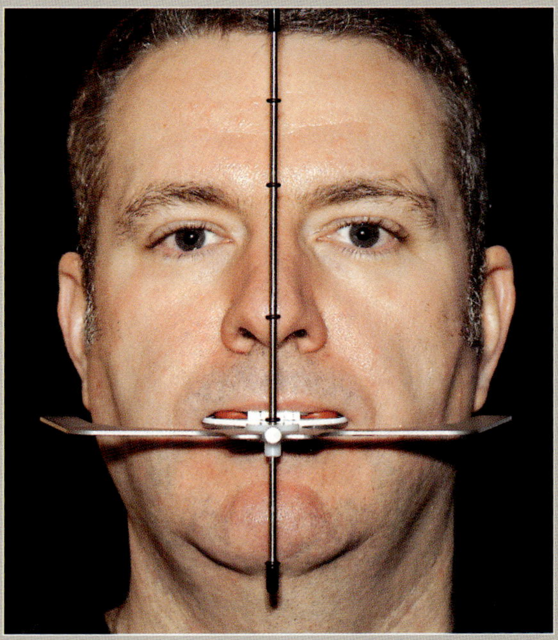

Frontal view of Kois Dento-Facial Analyzer System.

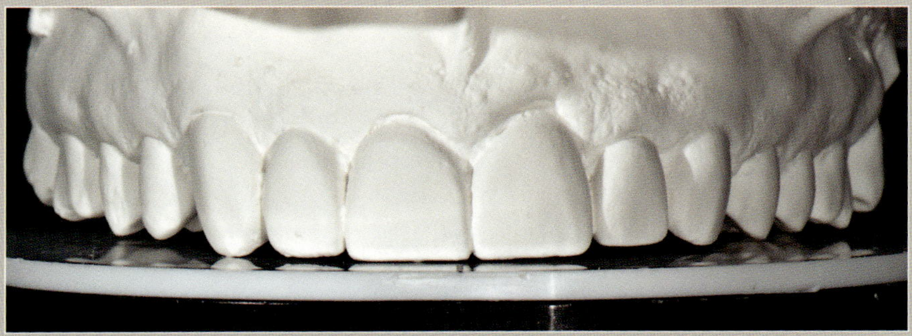

Maxillary cast with provisional restorations transfer on the Kois Dento-Facial Analyzer.

Laboratory communication and procedures

When a case is prepared for definitive restorations, a system is required to predictably communicate to the dental laboratory the esthetic expectations of the restorative dentist and patient. This communication includes two parts: the desired color of the restorations and the basic tooth shape and position. The most important esthetic and functional tooth position references are the vertical and horizontal position of the maxillary central incisors, the maxillary occlusal plane, and the facial midline. Traditionally, the provisional restorations have been used in conjunction with silicone matrices to communicate the tooth position and basic contours of the definitive restorations. This requires a fairly high degree of accuracy in the contours of the provisional restorations to ensure the references were accurately duplicated in the definitive restorations.

As this case demonstrates, with the use of the Kois Dento-Facial Analyzer System and a study cast of the provisional restorations, it is possible to communicate the most important tooth position references to the laboratory technician simply and predictably. As the esthetic information was transferred from the patient to the articulator, the platform on the articulator served as the natural head posture reference to ensure the symmetry of the incisal edge plane and horizontal and vertical tooth position. This system allows a technician to see the vertical and horizontal references on the articulator as they appear in the patient's face. When combined with digital photographs and the patient's esthetic concerns, the technician has all the esthetic information required to provide a symmetric smile. With this system, precise contouring of the provisional restoration becomes less critical because the ceramist can use the articulator and reference platform to make the definitive restorations closer to an ideal result while also incorporating artistic nuances and specific patient preferences.

Once the working casts and dies have been produced in the laboratory, the casts are articulated. The sequence of articulation and occlusal registration accuracy is critical; the study cast of the provisional restorations and the maxillary working cast need to be mounted on the articulator so they can be cross-mounted. This is vital for duplicating tooth position references in the definitive restorations. The sequence always begins with articulating the study cast of the provisional restorations; in this case, using the record made with the Dento-Facial Analyzer and the mounting/reference platform. Once the study cast is articulated, the mandibular opposing cast (or mandibular provisional cast) is mounted, and then the working cast of the prepared teeth is mounted. If this sequence is completed accurately, with all the occlusal records taken at the same vertical dimension of occlusion, the technician will have an accurate three-dimensional plan for creating the definitive restorations.

This case was created using a refractory die technique. As the layers of ceramic were built and sintered, it was possible to return the articulated casts to the articulator to verify the position of the internal materials, such as the dentin layer, against the reference platform. The first layer of ceramic creates the translucency at the cervical and incisal margins and begins to develop the internal structure. Blending fluorescing, somewhat opaque materials at the incisal edge of the preparation will help control the value of the restoration.

After the dentin layer was built to the desired contours and checked against the reference platform on the articulator, it was sintered. This helped to control the ceramic shrinkage as the crown was brought to full contour with up to three thinner layers of ceramic. This also allowed adjustments to be made in color and translucency before the veneers were glazed and the refractory material blasted out. Additionally, firing the dentin layer provided a more stable platform to complete the incisal layering because the buildup can be unstable and break off or shift when the dies are removed to be placed in the furnace.

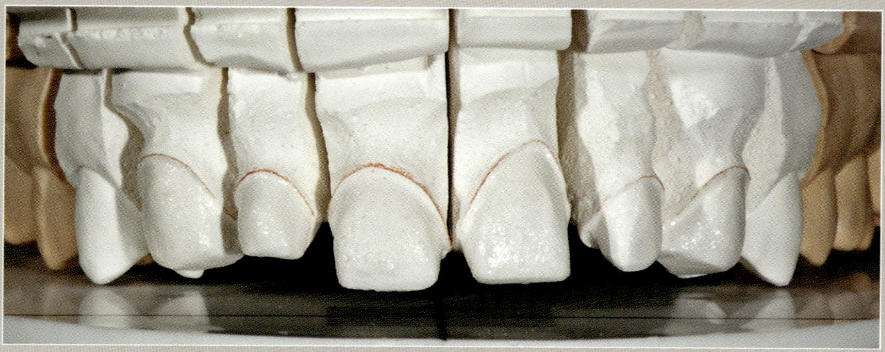

Refractory die showing the negative space to be augmented relative to the Dento-Facial Analyzer.

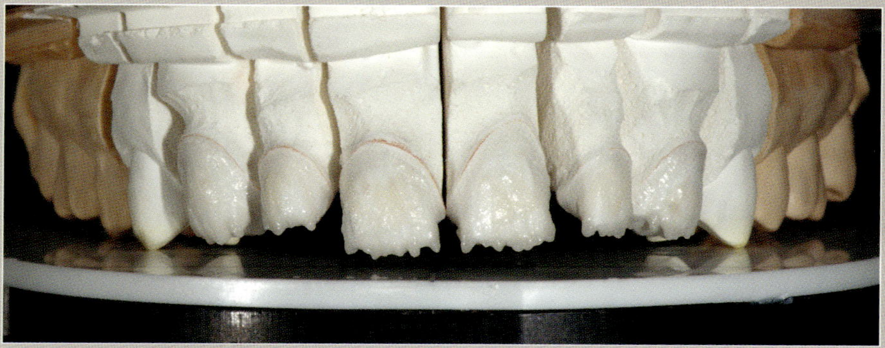

Refractory die with first layer of ceramic.

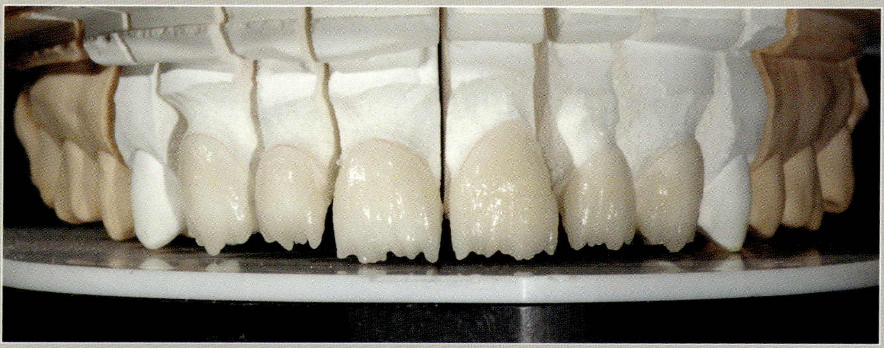

Addition of the dentin layer.

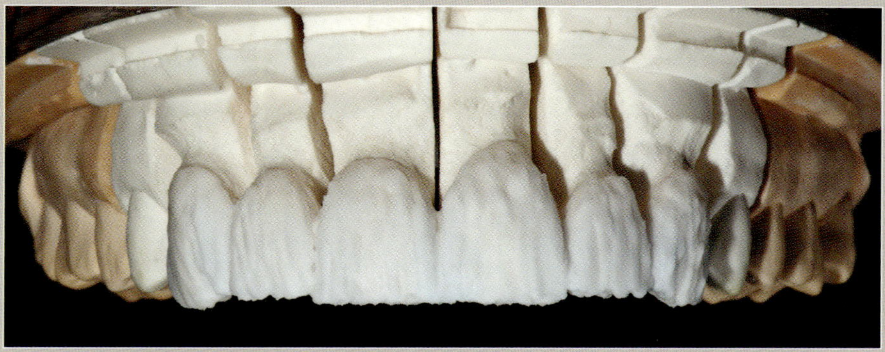

Incisal layering.

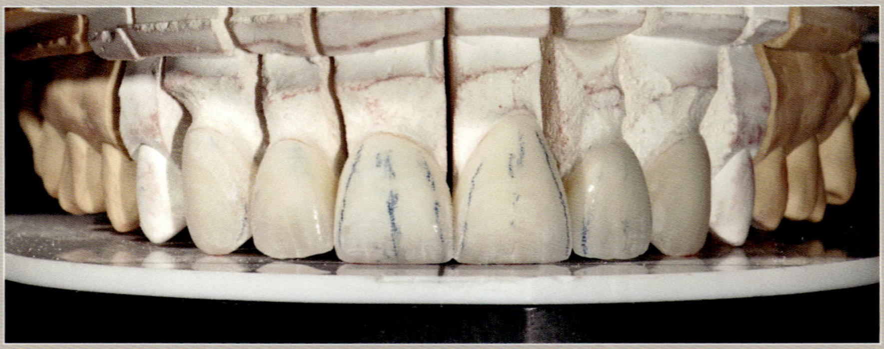

Contouring of the veneers.

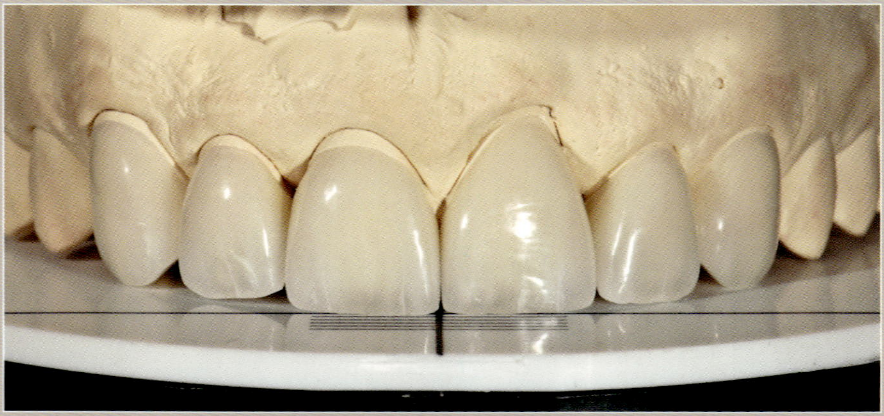

Definitive veneers seated on the working cast and verified facially to the platform and functionally to the guide table.

The first step in contouring the veneers was to establish the midline. To do this, either of the maxillary central incisors can be used. Once the veneer is placed in the cast on the articulator, the facial midline, which was transferred from the Dento-Facial Analyzer, is easily referenced on the index tray. The reference platform on the articulator was then used to determine the length and the facial position of the maxillary central incisors. The remaining teeth were added after adjusting their proximal contacts and altered for length on the reference platform. Using a custom incisal guide table, the lingual contours were formed to determine the appropriate functional parameters.

After the veneers were contoured, they were glazed, and the refractory material was removed using air abrasion with glass beads. The veneers were then fitted to a new stone die cast and the margins polished to follow the desired emergence profile. The proximal contacts were adjusted and verified on a solid stone cast, after which the length and facial position were checked in the articulator against the reference platform. The veneers were then etched using hydrofluoric acid, cleaned in distilled water in an ultrasonic bath, silanated (3M Primer, 3M ESPE), and thoroughly dried.

Veneer placement

Following try-in to verify fit and color, the veneers were cleaned by etching with 37% phosphoric rinse, silanated, and dried. The veneers were then luted using the following adhesive retention protocol: The teeth were microabraded with 27-μm aluminum oxide with a PrepStart air abrasion system (Danville) at 40 psi with a 0.015 tip. The teeth were etched using 37% phosphoric acid for 15 seconds, and 3 layers of an unfilled adhesive resin (One-Step, Bisco) was applied and light cured. All veneers were luted with a photo-activated resin (RelyX Veneer translucent cement, 3M ESPE) and cured with an LED light source. Following a minor occlusal adjustment, impressions were made for a maxillary occlusal nightguard, and the maxillary occlusal nightguard was seated and adjusted in a subsequent appointment.

Posttreatment

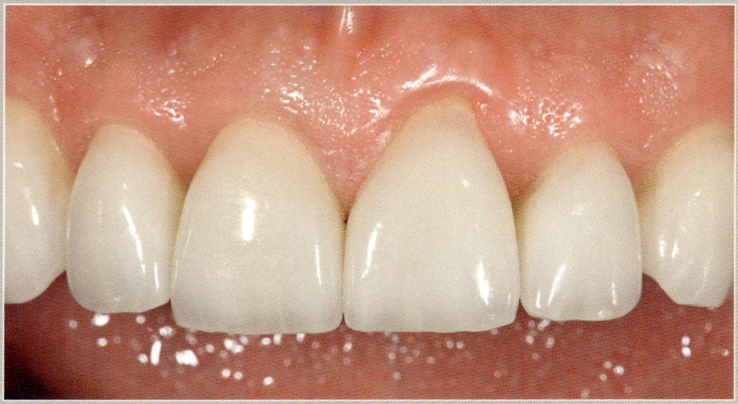

Definitive maxillary anterior veneers on teeth nos. 6 to 11.

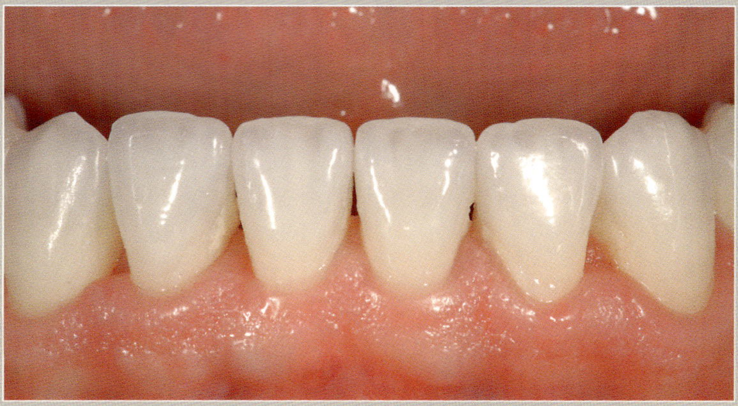

Definitive mandibular anterior veneers on teeth nos. 22 to 27.

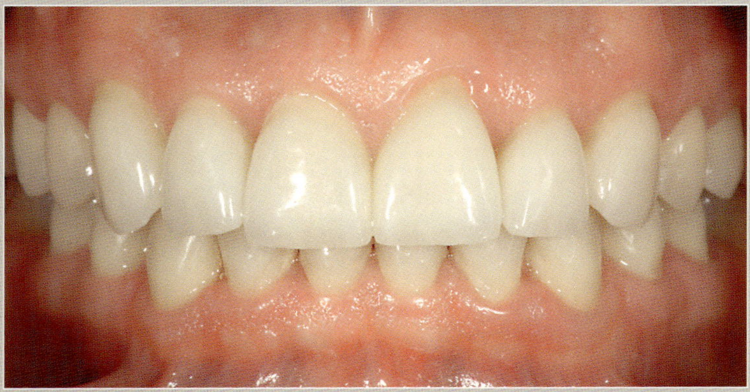

Frontal view.

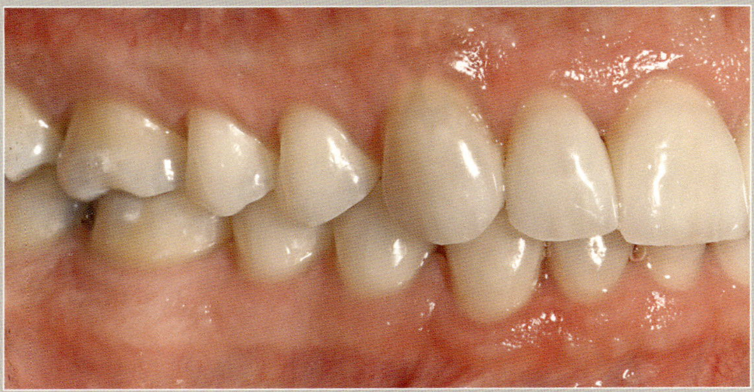

Right lateral view.

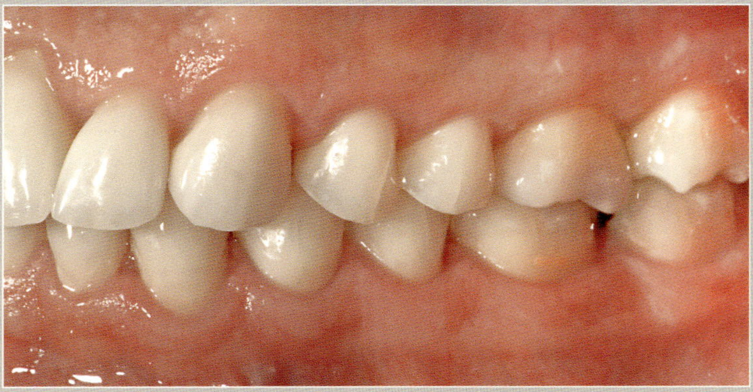

Left lateral view.

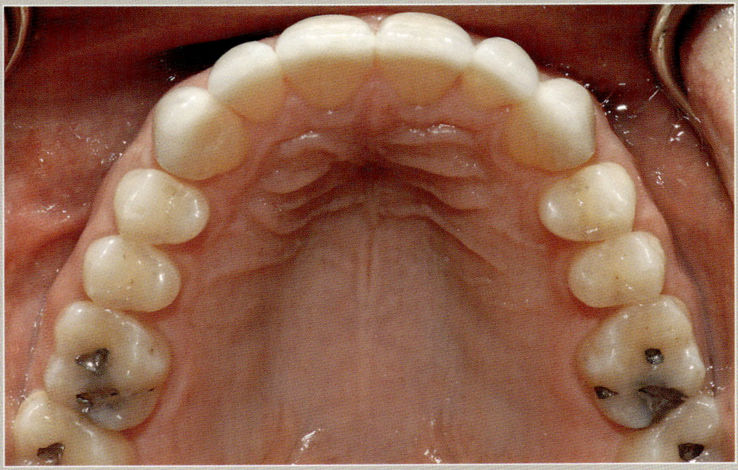

Maxillary occlusal view.

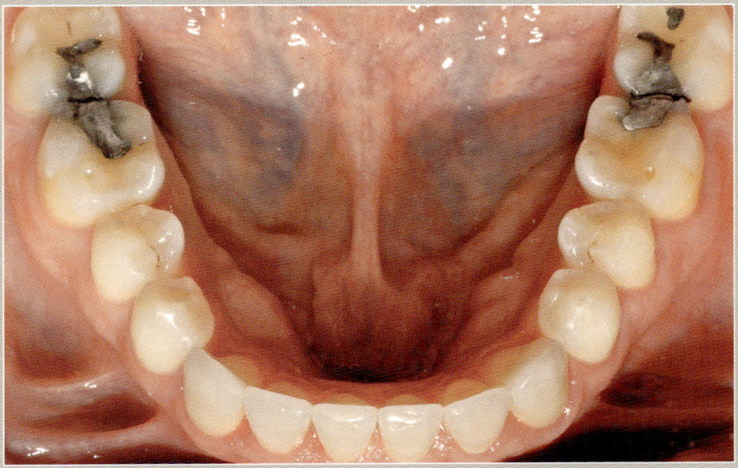

Mandibular occlusal view.

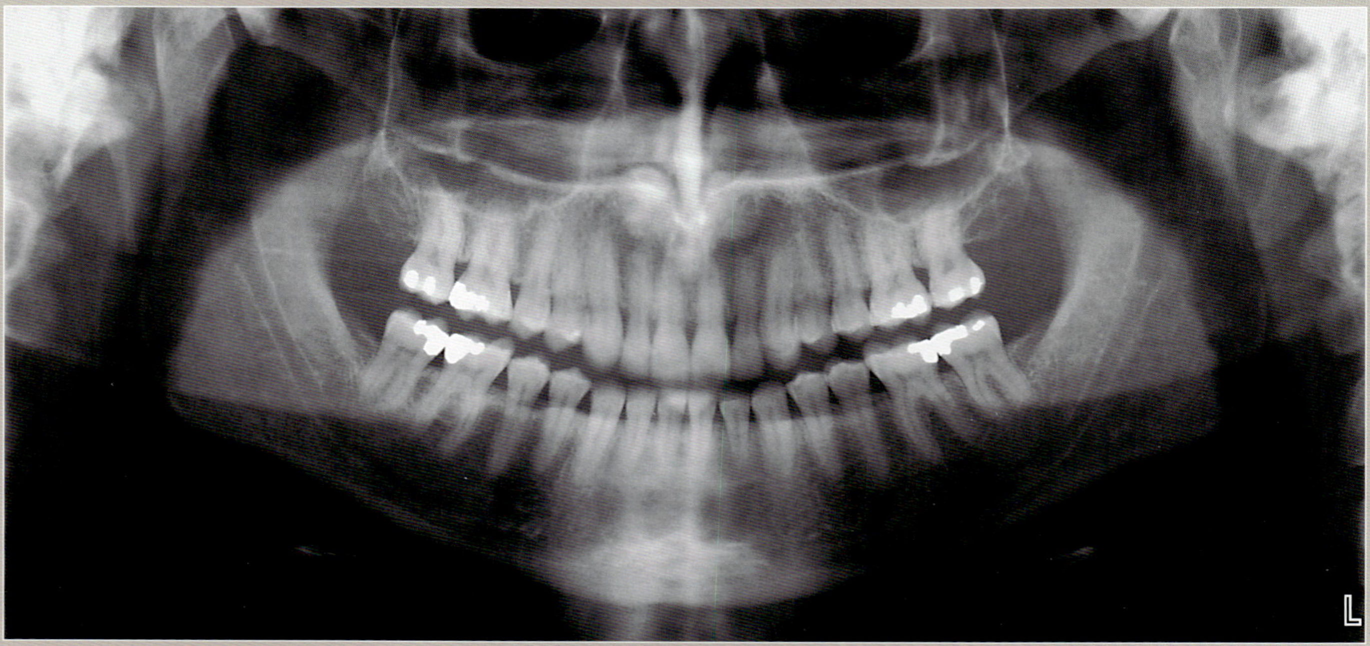

Panoramic radiograph.

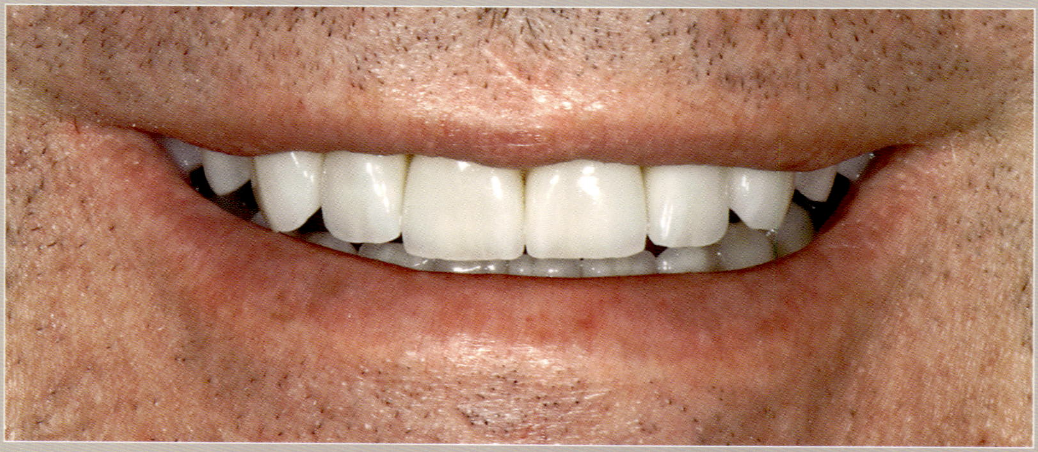

Close-up of full smile.

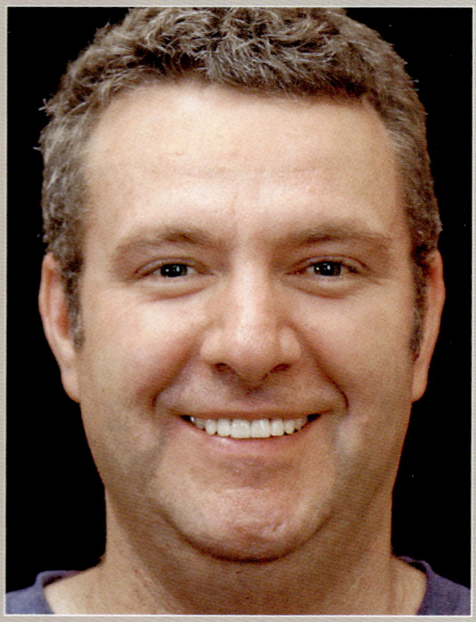

Facial view in MIP.

You may now place the corresponding posttreatment overlay found in the separate folder over the pretreatment periodontal chart on page 197.

Commentary

The final result exceeded the patient's expectations. Based on an understanding of the patient's individual risk factors, treatment was designed to reduce or minimize any additional risk to the entire dentition. Alternative treatment options to manage the occlusal concerns with orthodontics could have been accomplished by increasing the vertical dimension of occlusion. This would have created longer anterior teeth, which would have resulted in a less favorable esthetic result. Without orthodontics, increasing the vertical dimension of occlusion would have required complete-mouth rehabilitation. This would require restoring the posterior teeth, which would not otherwise be necessary and would have increased the biomechanical risk. Only the anterior teeth that were compromised by attrition and esthetically compromised required restoration. This is a classic case emphasizing the value of orthodontic treatment to address vertical changes in the posterior occlusion prior to initiating restorative care. The labial crown torque to maxillary incisors and intrusion of worn mandibular anterior teeth provides freedom from a constricted chewing environment and the proper emergence profile for conservative restorations.

All the necessary tooth preparation was restricted to the enamel, which further minimized biomechanical risks. Tooth preparation was also kept supragingival, which did not contribute to any periodontal risks. The occlusal management resolved all the TMD symptoms from the constricted chewing pattern and eliminated the concerns of friction contributing to ongoing tooth structure loss. The nightguard, however, is still required to protect the restorations from any episodes of nocturnal bruxism. The patient is also on a 6-month recall interval for maintenance. The only anticipated liability is the restorations (ie, chipped porcelain), not the remaining teeth. In conclusion, the patient's periodontal and biomechanical prognosis remains good. The dentofacial and functional prognosis was elevated from poor to good as long as the patient continues to wear the nightguard. By establishing a foundation that is in harmony with the surrounding musculature, the long-term prognosis of maintaining a beautiful smile and functionally balanced occlusion has greatly improved. At the 4-year follow-up interview, the patient reported an overall relaxation in both muscles of mastication and perioral musculature.

8

Biometric Determinants of Tooth and Gingival Esthetics

Stephen J. Chu, DMD, MSD, CDT
Dennis P. Tarnow, DDS

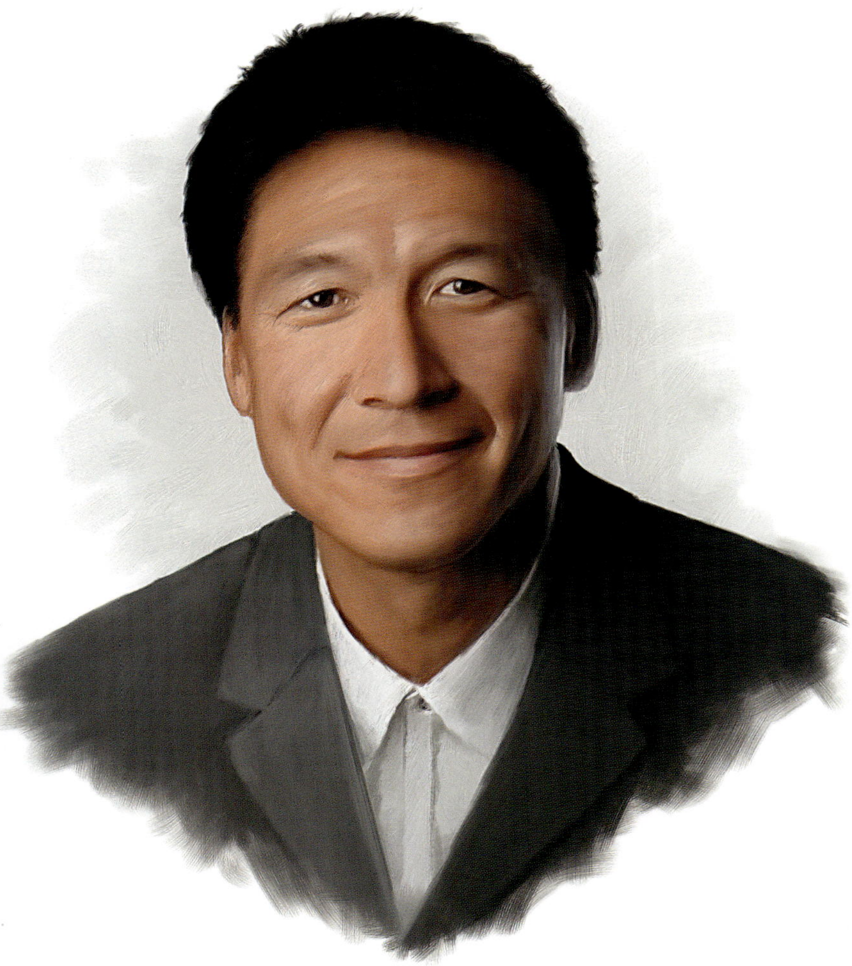

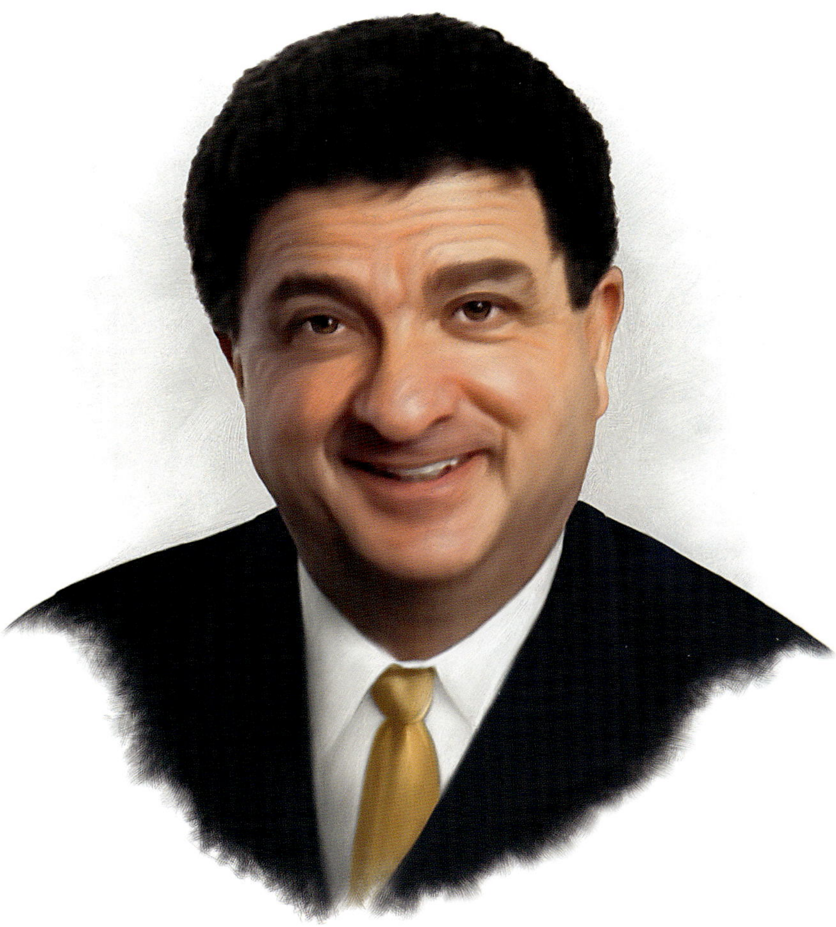

One of the goals in achieving esthetic enhancement is to determine the biometric and biologic endpoints that define and guide the course of therapy.

Philosophy and Background

Management of anterior tooth size and proportion as well as gingival architecture discrepancies is a thought-provoking and often ambitious diagnostic and treatment-planning endeavor in daily clinical practice. This is true whether the case involves natural teeth or dental implants. Over the past decade, while teaching advanced esthetic dentistry at the postgraduate level, I realized that what is needed is a common denominator that defines dental esthetics. I was not seeking subjective or descriptive parameters for esthetics but objective biometric (ie, quantitative) determinants that define tooth and gingival esthetics.

In all cases treated privately or at the university, whether the patient presented with excessive spacing or crowding of the dentition, once the correct incisal edge position within the proper vertical dimension of occlusion was established, treatment outcomes always focused on:

- Proper size and proportion of the teeth
- Establishment of a new arch form that met the biologic and esthetic requirements of the patient
- Achievement of occlusal stability

Several studies have been conducted to validate these concepts and to establish concrete determinants that practitioners can easily understand and integrate into their daily clinical practice.

The first study focused on tooth width.[1] The purpose of this investigation was to answer the question: How often do mean tooth width values apply to a given patient population? The answer was a surprisingly low 34% for the maxillary anterior dentition and 42% for the mandibular dentition.[2] This means that tooth width variation is the rule, not the exception.

The second question, addressed in another study,[2] was: Does tooth proportion vary commensurate with tooth size? Investigators determined that the answer was no; several authors[3,4] have shown that even though tooth size varies, the width-length proportion remains constant at about 80% for the maxillary anterior teeth and 60% to 65% for the mandibular teeth.

The final question taken in hand was: What is the correlation between the widths of the maxillary and mandibular anterior teeth? The most well-known correlation is based on the Bolton analysis,[5,6] which is commonly used in orthodontic therapy. Wayne Bolton was a University of Washington orthodontic graduate student in 1952. His master's thesis was a mathematic analysis of the maxillary anterior dentition in Angle Class I occlusion. He found that the sum of the widths of the mandibular anterior teeth was about 75% to 80% of the combined widths of the maxillary anterior teeth. If the summed widths were within this range, then there would be an absence of residual crowding or spacing. The only weakness in this analysis is that individual intra-arch tooth size discrepancies can be present without the finding of a Bolton discrepancy. The teeth will be aligned but may not appear esthetically pleasing if the individual tooth size discrepancy is not addressed.

Interestingly, if we know the width of the mandibular central incisor in a patient, we can determine, with relatively good predictability, the widths of all of the remaining anterior teeth. Research by Chu and Okubo[1,7] on tooth biometrics has shown that the size of the mandibular central incisor is the least variable of all 12 anterior teeth. Its width falls within a range of 5.0 to 5.5 mm about 90% of the time. The maxillary central incisor (Y) is about 3 mm wider than the mandibular central incisor (X), giving the equation Y = X + 3. Compared with the maxillary central incisor, the maxillary lateral incisor is about 2 mm narrower (Y – 2), and the canine is about 1 mm narrower (Y – 1). We call this the *Y – 2, Y – 1 rule* for the maxillary anterior arch. Compared with the mandibular central incisor, the mandibular lateral incisor is 0.5 mm greater in width (X + ½), and the canine is 1 mm greater in width, giving the *X + ½, X + 1 rule* for the mandibular anterior teeth.

Further studies have been conducted by our group and others on biometric gingival esthetic determinants, ie, gingival zeniths, gingival levels, and papillae heights.[8–10] These studies found that the range of the mesiodistal location of the gingival zenith in the maxillary anterior dentition is quite small: 0.5 to 1.0 mm distal of the vertical midline. The reported frequency of distal displacement of the zenith in maxillary canine teeth is fairly low (12%[8] and 60%[10]). Distal displacement of the zenith is more frequent and more pronounced in the maxillary central incisor than in the other maxillary anterior teeth.

Spear[11] and Kois[12] reported the height of the interdental papilla to be about 4.5 mm, measured from the gingival zenith. They evaluated 100 maxillary right central incisors to determine whether this mean value is applicable to all anterior teeth given that tooth size variation is the rule. Thorough investigation revealed that papillae height varies with tooth length: The interdental papillae height is about 40% of the clinical crown length no matter what size variation exists.[13] The clinically acceptable range is 30% to 50%, of which the lower end of the range is acceptable for a thick-flat gingival phenotype and the higher end for a thin-scalloped phenotype. In addition, the study[13] revealed that:

- There is no difference in the height of the mesial versus distal papillae.
- The most apical extent of the interdental contact area defines the height of the papillae.
- The most coronal extent of the interdental contact area defines the start of the incisal embrasure.

My colleagues and I find the following biometric deter-minants to be meaningful during diagnosis and treatment planning and in establishing esthetically pleasing tooth dimensions:

1. The ideal width of the maxillary central incisor (Y) is 3.0 mm greater than the width of the mandibular central incisor (X). The intra-arch rules for tooth width are the Y – 2, Y – 1 rule for the maxillary teeth and the X + ½, X + 1 rule for the mandibular teeth. This individual tooth size analysis conforms to the Bolton analysis but also provides information about individual tooth size discrepancies.
2. The distal displacement of the gingival zenith relative to the vertical midline of the tooth should be about 1.0 mm for the central incisor, 0 to 0.5 mm for the lateral incisor, and 0 mm for the canine.
3. The interdental papillae height should be about 40% of the length of the tooth measured from the gingival zenith, while 30% to 50% is an acceptable clinical range depending on the gingival phenotype.
4. The most coronal points of the interdental papillae should form a straight line.

The treatment described in the following case presentation is of particular interest because it encompasses all of the basic biometric and biologic determinants that define tooth and gingival esthetics. The reader should focus on the following list of concerns that the treating clinicians faced in treatment planning:

1. What are the appropriate tooth dimensions and proportions for this particular patient?
2. How can the vertical discrepancies in the positions of the interdental papillae be managed in a predictable manner?
3. How can the residual discrepancies in tooth length and midfacial soft tissue be managed on teeth previously prepared twice for full crown restorations with shoulder and deep chamfer finish lines?

Taking the time to familiarize yourself with the biometric esthetic determinants above will be helpful in treatment planning the following case and will also facilitate the pursuit of more satisfying esthetic results in practice.

—Stephen J. Chu

Case Presentation

Treating clinicians
Prosthetics/restorative dentistry: Stephen J. Chu, DMD, MSD, CDT
Adjunctive orthodontics: Mark N. Hochman, DDS
Periodontal plastic and implant surgery: Dennis P. Tarnow, DDS
Dental ceramics/laboratory work: Adam J. Mieleszko, CDT

Clinical Treatment Planning

Age at initial presentation: 43 years
Initial presentation: January 2005
Active treatment completed: December 2007

Introduction and background

This 43-year-old man presented with a history of multiple replacements of a maxillary anterior fixed dental prosthesis following the loss of his maxillary right central incisor as a result of a childhood sports accident. The resistance and retention form of the tooth preparations became compromised because of chronic problems with decementation and recurrent decay that required repeated treatment. The patient presented with full maxillary provisional restorations and ceramic laminate veneer restorations from mandibular first premolar to first premolar with a metal-ceramic crown on his mandibular right second premolar. He was a businessman with a very hectic schedule. Because of the patient's limited availability, it was necessary for tooth replacement to be accomplished over an extended period of time.

The patient complained that his teeth were too big and of different sizes and colors. He wanted his teeth lighter and more uniform in color. He stated, "I only show teeth when I smile; shouldn't I be showing some of my gums when I smile?" Food was becoming trapped around his maxillary left central incisor, which was quite bothersome to the patient. He had localized gingival recession around the mandibular veneer restorations and did not like the visibility of the restorative margins between the exposed roots and restorations. He wanted individual restorations so that he could clean and maintain them more easily.

Medical history

- Noncontributory

Diagnostic findings

Extraoral and facial findings

- Lack of facial symmetry

TMJ and mandibular range of motion

- Normal range of motion
- No joint pathology noted

Intraoral findings

Dental

- Acrylic provisional restorations on teeth nos. 2 to 15, 19, 20, 30, and 31
- Missing teeth nos. 1, 8, 16, 17, 18, and 32
- Dental implant in tooth no. 18 site with healing abutment attached
- Recurrent caries in teeth nos. 7, 9, 10, 11, 13, and 20
- Bonded ceramic veneer restorations on teeth nos. 21 to 28
- Metal-ceramic crown on tooth no. 29

Periodontal

- History of a gingival graft at edentulous site no. 8
- Generalized mild to moderate gingival recession of 1 to 3 mm with adequate zones of attachment
- Gingival recession of 4 to 5 mm at teeth nos. 7, 9, and 10
- Isolated 4-mm pocket at the mesiofacial aspect of tooth no. 9

Pretreatment

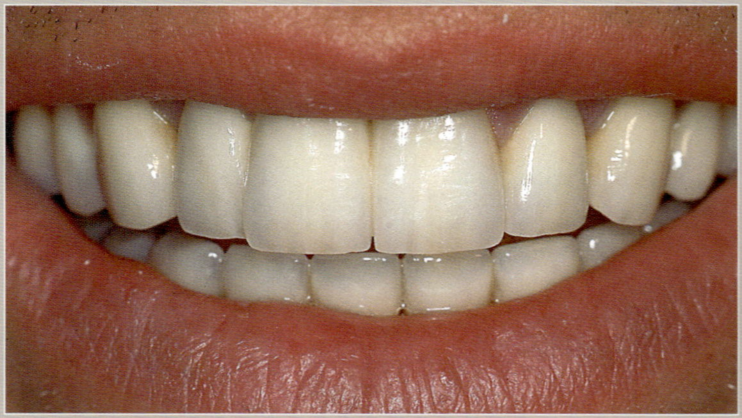

Smile.

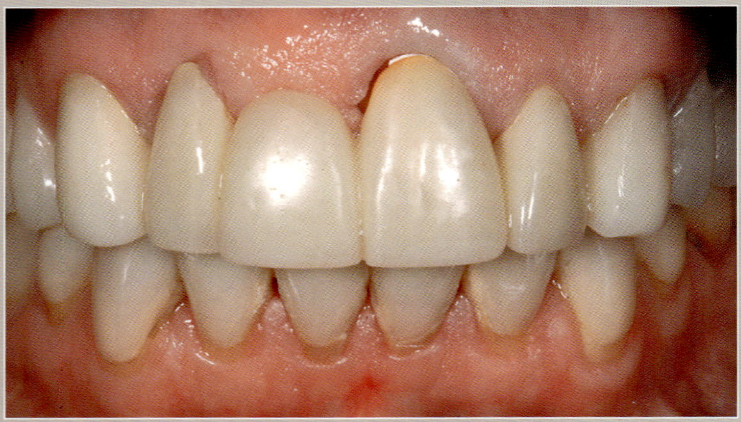

Intraoral frontal view.

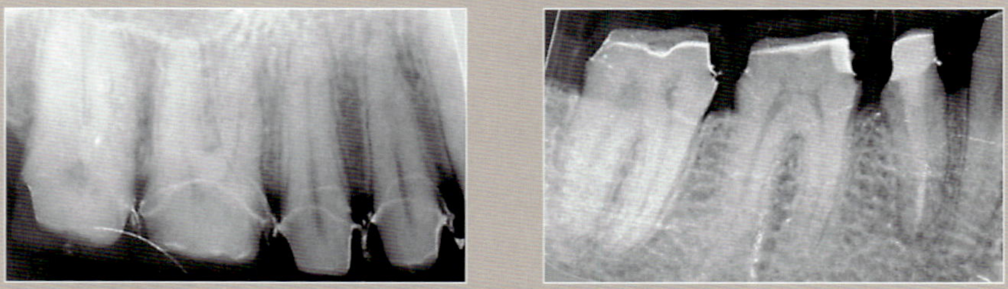

Periapical radiographs of right posterior area.

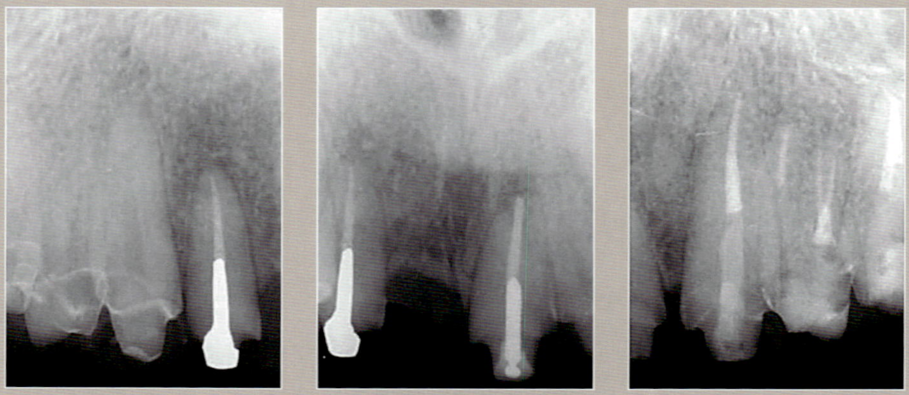

Periapical radiographs of maxillary anterior area.

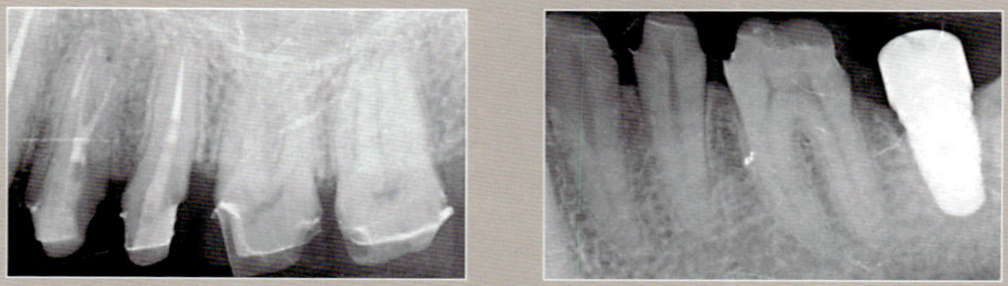

Periapical radiographs of left posterior area.

Occlusal notes

- Class II, division 1 malocclusion; Class II canine and molar relationships
- No discrepancy between centric relation (CR) and maximal intercuspal position (MIP)
- MIP with posterior tooth contacts and canine contacts
- Functional overbite of 1 mm and functional overjet of 0 mm
- Centric slide of 1 mm in protrusive movement to first point of contact
- Canine and first premolar contact in lateral excursions

Radiographic findings

- Maxillary and posterior mandibular provisional crown restorations
- Foundation restorations on teeth nos. 7, 9, and 11
- No evidence of caries
- Previous endodontic treatment in teeth nos. 7, 9, 11, 12, 13, and 29
- No horizontal or vertical bone defects noted

Biometric analysis

- Acceptable incisal edge position with regard to esthetics (smile line), phonetics (vermilion border), and occlusion (overbite/overjet)
- Disproportionate size of teeth nos. 7, 9, and 10
- Gingival zenith levels and interdental papillae heights not coincident with normative biometric values for teeth nos. 7, 9, and 10

Diagnosis and prognosis

- Healthy periodontium: AAP I; generalized gingival recession with advanced recession localized to the facial surfaces of the maxillary anterior teeth
- Excellent prognosis for all remaining teeth

Summary of concerns

1. How can we meet this patient's treatment expectations with:
   - Disproportionate tooth size?
   - Nonbiometric midfacial and interdental gingival architecture (disparate gingival levels)?
   - Zero functional overjet?
2. How can we establish long-term stability of the fixed dental prosthesis?
3. How can we create esthetic harmony between the implant restoration of tooth no. 8 and the adjacent teeth?
4. Can we re-establish solid foundation restorations with an adequate ferrule effect for teeth nos. 7, 9, and 10?

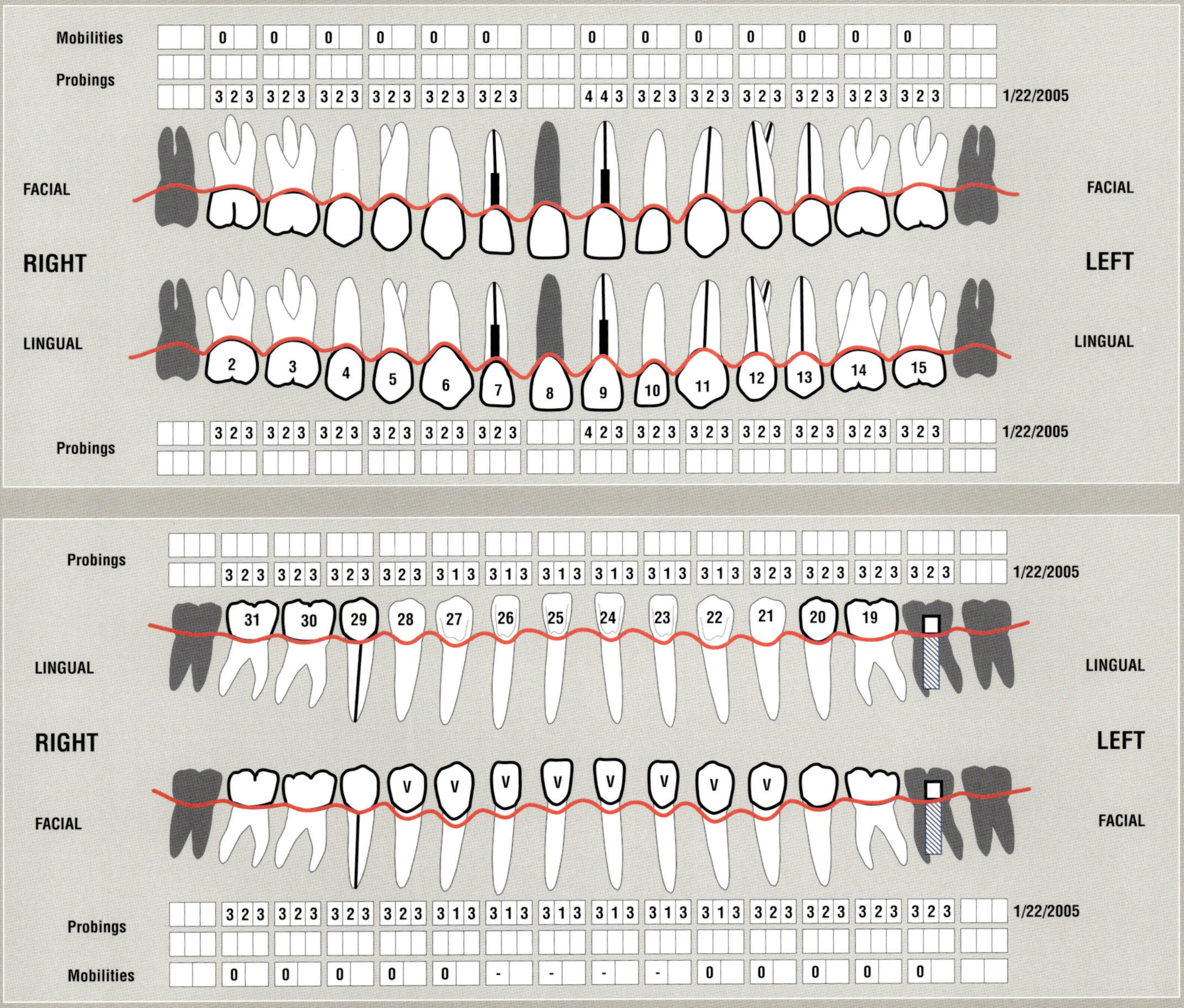

As a learning exercise, you may now outline goals/objectives of treatment and a treatment plan.

Proposed Treatment Plan

Goals/objectives of treatment

One of the goals in achieving esthetic enhancement is to determine the biometric and biologic endpoints that define and guide the course of therapy. Frequently, treatment is rendered without clear direction or a truly comprehensive perspective. This often results in a compromised treatment outcome. It is shortsighted to focus only on a restorative/prosthetic solution when a patient presents with a multitude of other problems. The treatment goals established for this patient were as follows:

- Establish the correct incisal edge position and then ascertain the proper tooth size and proportion of the anterior teeth.
- Determine relative position of associated gingival tissues, including the zone of keratinized attached gingiva, free gingival margin architecture, gingival zenith, and interdental papillae proportions.
- Use orthodontic alterations of vertical tooth positions to align the most coronal points of the contact areas and hence the interdental papillae from maxillary canine to canine.
- Correct the midfacial gingival architecture discrepancies through periodontal plastic surgery using coronally positioned flaps.

Phase I: Initial therapy

1. Comprehensive oral examination
2. Pretreatment digital photographs
3. Pretreatment radiographs
4. Diagnostic impressions
5. Prophylaxis and oral hygiene instruction
6. Fabrication of new acrylic provisional restorations

Phase II: Interdisciplinary treatment planning and sequencing

7. Referral to the periodontist for soft tissue evaluation
8. Referral to the orthodontist for evaluation
9. Patient consultation with the prosthodontist
10. Patient consultation with the dental technician

Phase III: Initial orthodontic therapy

11. Orthodontic treatment to extrude teeth nos. 7, 9, and 10 (ie, forced eruption), altering tooth position to level and align the interdental papillae of the maxillary anterior teeth

Phase IV: Implant therapy

12. Flapless procedure for placement of a single dental implant in the no. 8 site

Phase V: Initial periodontal plastic surgery

13. Coronally positioned flap to cover the roots of teeth nos. 9 and 10 and to decrease the clinical crown length

Phase VI: Final orthodontic therapy

14. Continued forced eruption of tooth no. 7 to favorably alter the position of its interdental papilla, with the implant at site no. 8 serving as additional anchorage

Phase VII: Second periodontal plastic surgery and second set of provisional restorations

15. Coronally positioned flap to cover the root of tooth no. 7 and to decrease the excessive clinical crown length
16. Chairside fabrication of a second set of provisional restorations to visualize the outcome following orthodontic and periodontal therapy

Phase VIII: Diagnostic wax-up and third set of provisional restorations

17. Facebow transfer for fabrication of a third set of provisional restorations for the maxillary anterior teeth
18. Use of the esthetic tooth proportion gauge for wax-up of the teeth based on a large tooth dimension
19. Creation of silicone matrices from the wax-up to fabricate an acrylic eggshell provisional for relining
20. Use of a silicone matrix as a guide for rebuilding the foundation restorations on teeth nos. 7, 9, and 10
21. Replacement of the posts in endodontically treated teeth nos. 7 and 9

Phase IX: Pickup impression

22. Try-in of the zirconia and metal-ceramic copings and pickup impression to remount the working casts

Phase X: Laboratory fabrication procedures

23. Fabrication of full crown restorations for the maxillary arch and mandibular posterior teeth
24. Fabrication of porcelain laminate veneers for the mandibular anterior teeth

Phase XI: Placement of definitive restorations

25. Try-in of definitive restorations and adjustment of occlusion
26. Bonding of mandibular anterior veneers
27. Six-month periodontal/restorative maintenance protocol

Active Clinical Treatment

Review of the goals/objectives of treatment

The key elements in the treatment plan and treatment sequence for this patient are as follows:

1. Establish the correct incisal edge position, and then ascertain the proper tooth size and proportion of the anterior dentition.
   - The proper tooth proportion is a width-length ratio of about 80% for the maxillary anterior teeth and 60% for the mandibular anterior teeth.
   - The maxillary anterior tooth size selected for this patient was large: 9.5 mm wide and 12 mm long.
   - This patient was to be restored in a Class II, division 1 occlusion with a long intercuspal contact area in MIP.
2. Orthodontically alter the anterior tooth position to align the coronal extents of the papillae from canine to canine.
   - The length of the papillae should be about 40% of the length of the tooth; the clinical range is 30% for thick-flat and 50% for thin-scalloped periodontal phenotypes, respectively.
3. Correct the midfacial gingival architecture discrepancies in the maxillary anterior teeth through periodontal plastic surgery using coronally positioned flaps.
   - The gingival zeniths should be 1 mm distal of the vertical midline for the maxillary central incisors and at the vertical midline for the maxillary lateral incisors and canines.

Phase I: Initial therapy

Treatment commenced with initial supportive periodontal therapy consisting of root planing, scaling, and oral hygiene instructions.

A soft tissue onlay graft had been previously placed to correct the proportions of the provisional pontic at site no. 8. The goal for proportion of the maxillary anterior teeth was an 80% width-length ratio (9.5-mm width and 12-mm length). New provisional restorations were placed in the maxillary arch to replace the existing provisional restorations.

Phase II: Interdisciplinary treatment planning and sequencing

The interdisciplinary treatment plan was re-evaluated after the existing provisional restorations were replaced. Orthodontic treatment was considered. The goal of orthodontic therapy was to extrude teeth nos. 7 and 9 to level and align the interdental papillae levels to be coincident and equal in height. The residual discrepancies in the midfacial tissue heights would be addressed surgically.

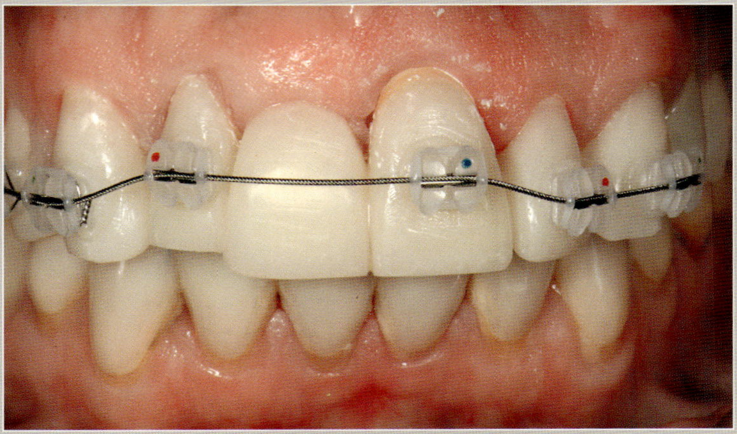
Orthodontic treatment (forced eruption) of teeth nos. 7 and 9.

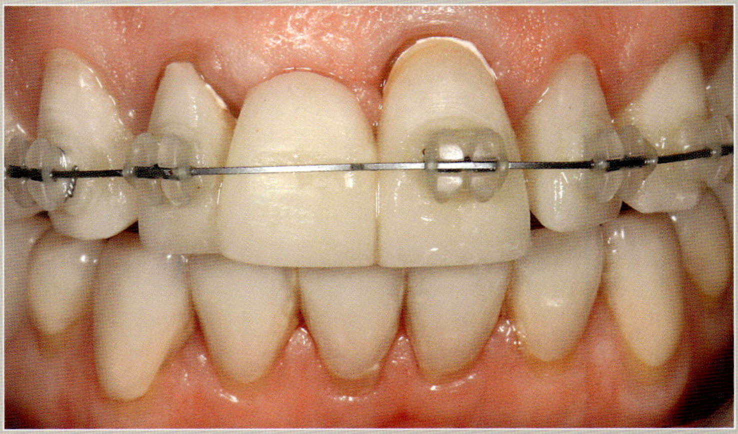
Frontal view after 6 weeks of orthodontic treatment.

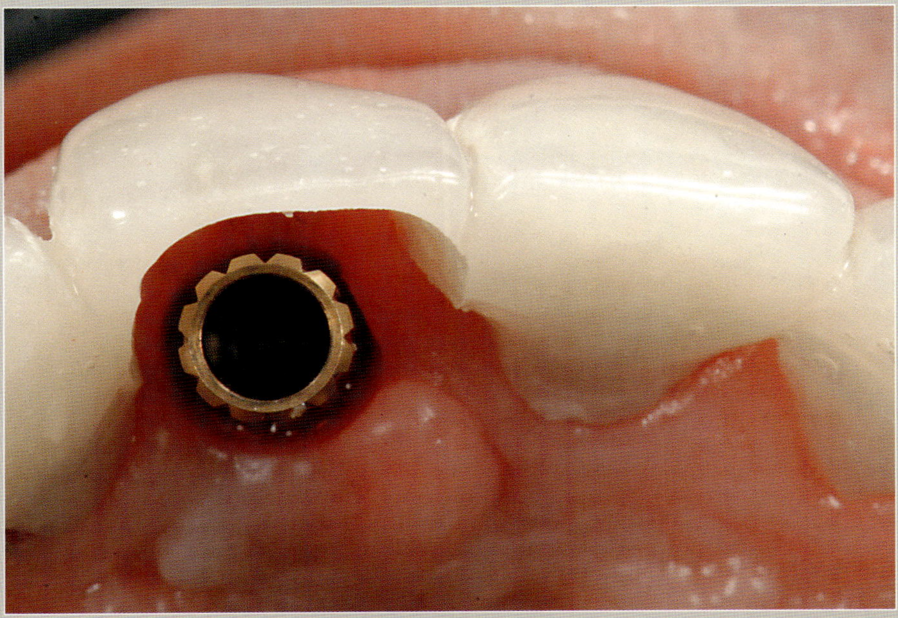
Occlusal view following implant placement with a flapless surgical approach in site no. 8.

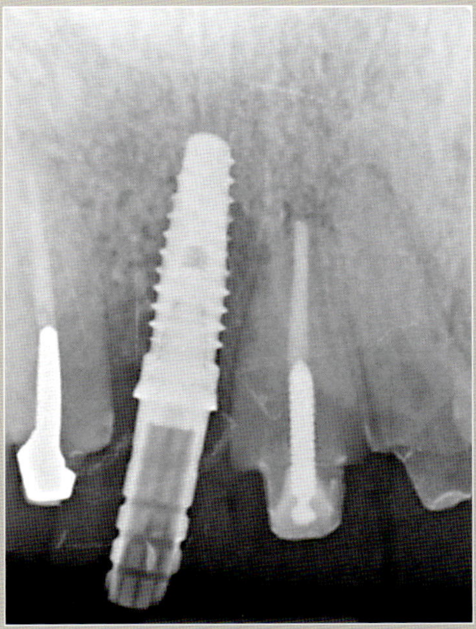
Digital radiograph verifying the seating of the provisional implant abutment.

Phase III: Initial orthodontic therapy

Ceramic orthodontic brackets with metal inserts were bonded with acrylic resin to the provisional restorations at teeth nos. 5 to 12. A coaxial 0.014 round wire was placed to initiate forced eruption. The anterior teeth nos. 7 to 9, including the provisional pontic at site no. 8, were forcibly erupted as a fixed unit. The provisional restorations were sectioned and separated at the mesial aspects of the maxillary right canine and left lateral incisor. The posterior provisional restorations were used as anchorage; the maxillary right provisional sextant was joined to tooth no. 6 with ligature wire tied to the brackets of teeth nos. 5 and 6.

The papilla on the mesial aspect of tooth no. 7 required further orthodontic extrusion, but the papilla of tooth no. 9 was corrected with this initial movement.

Phase IV: Implant therapy

An implant was placed in site no. 8 using a flapless surgical approach. A screw-retained temporary abutment was used to connect the provisional implant crown to the provisional splint.

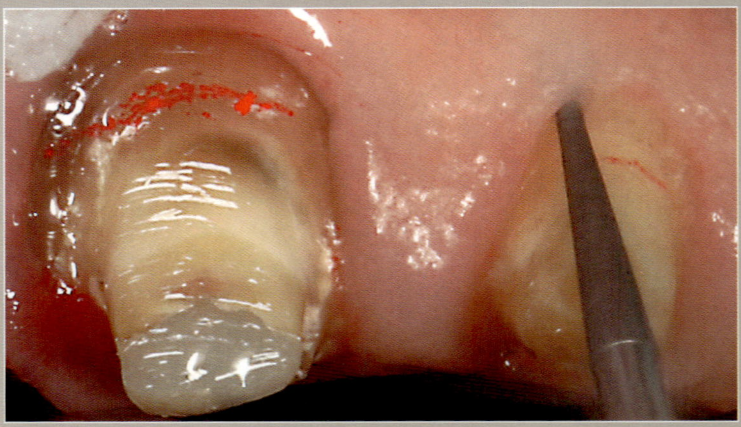

Reshaping and flattening of the shoulder of the crown preparations and root contours with a finishing diamond.

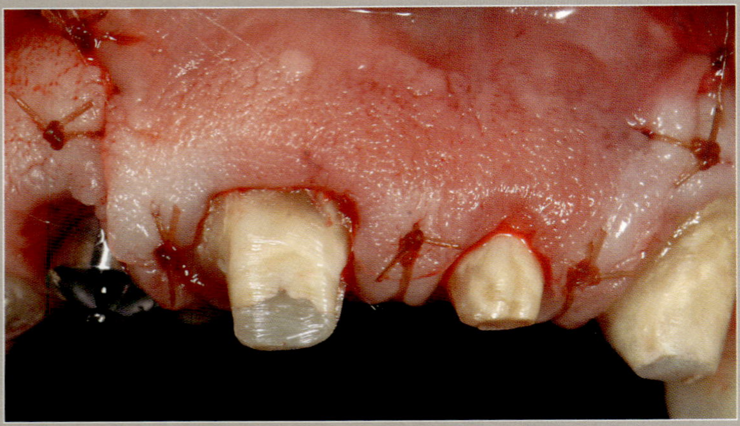

Coronally positioned flap.

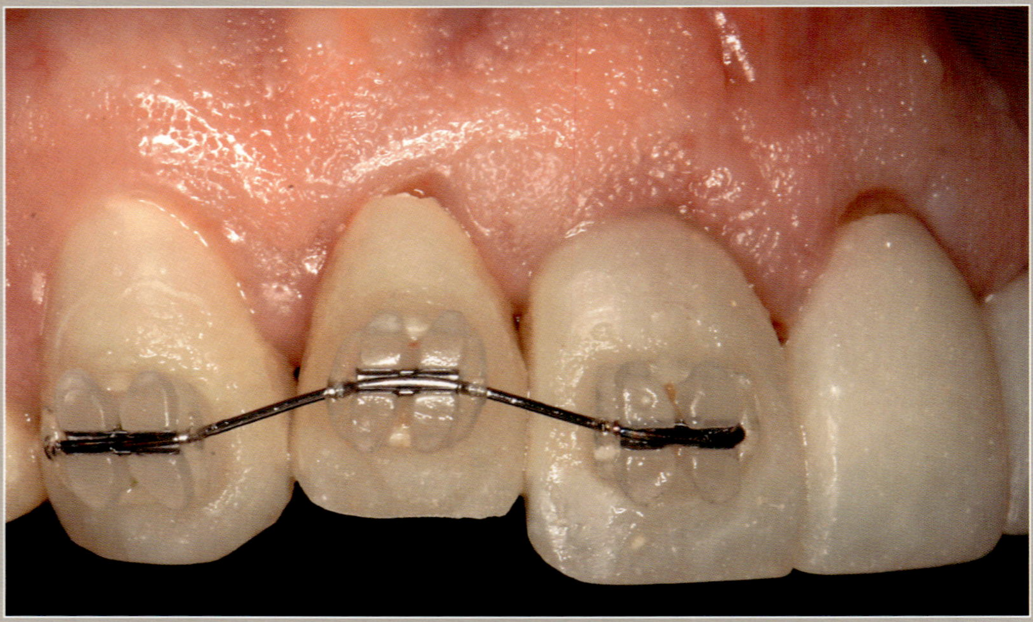

Continued forced eruption of tooth no. 7 using implant at site no. 8 as orthodontic anchorage.

Phase V: Initial periodontal plastic surgery

Because the teeth had been previously prepared for complete-coverage restorations, the finish line of the crown preparations had to be eliminated and flattened with a polishing diamond bur before periodontal plastic surgery was performed. After 2 weeks of healing, a coronally positioned flap procedure was performed to cover the prepared root surfaces of teeth nos. 9 and 10, decreasing the excessive crown length of these teeth. Vertical releasing incisions were made with a broad-based flap design to maintain maximum blood supply to the flap. The patient had a thick gingival phenotype, which was advantageous for this type of periodontal plastic surgery.

Phase VI: Final orthodontic therapy

Orthodontic forced eruption of tooth no. 7 was resumed, using the implant at site no. 8 as anchorage, until its papilla was aligned with those of tooth nos. 9 and 10.

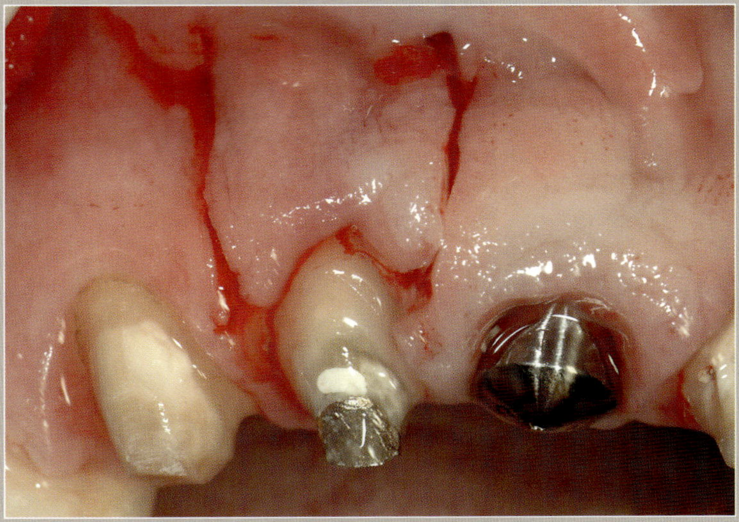

Split-thickness beveled incision used to preserve the interdental papillae around tooth no. 7.

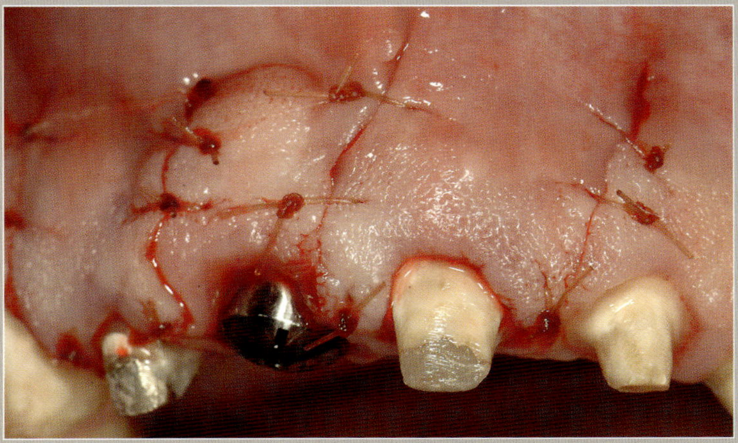

Coronally positioned flaps to correct gingival architecture of teeth nos. 7 and 9.

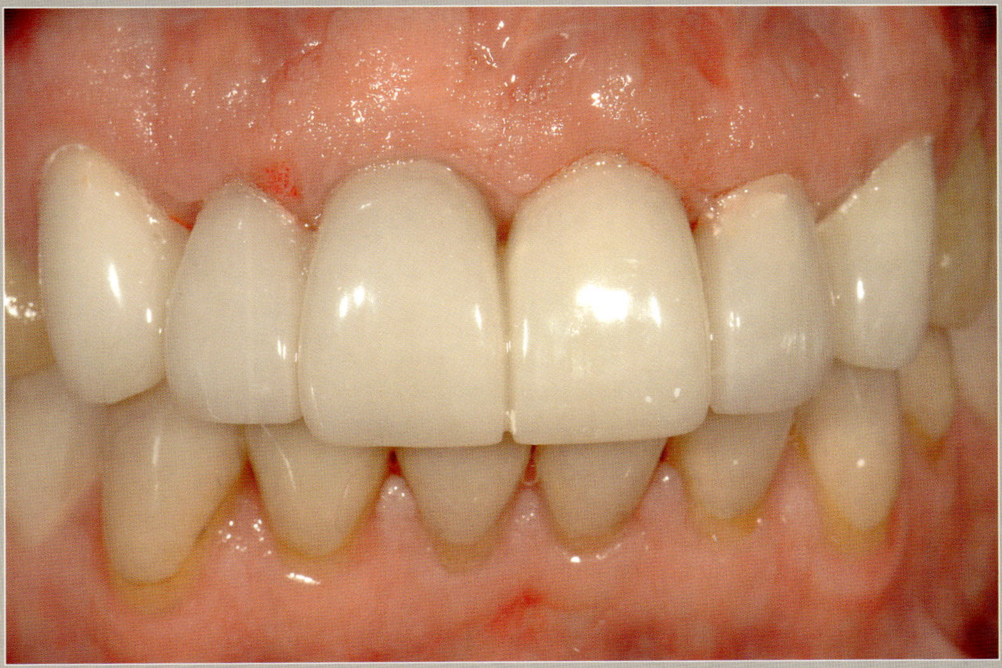

Provisional restorations placed 3 months after second periodontal plastic surgery.

Phase VII: Second periodontal plastic surgery and second set of provisional restorations

Six months after orthodontic therapy was completed, a coronally positioned flap procedure was performed on tooth no. 7. In addition, a second coronally positioned flap procedure was performed on tooth no. 9 because a slight additional gain of tissue was required to optimize the gingival architecture. After 3 months of healing, a second set of provisional restorations was fabricated chairside to allow visualization and re-evaluation of orthodontic and periodontal therapy.

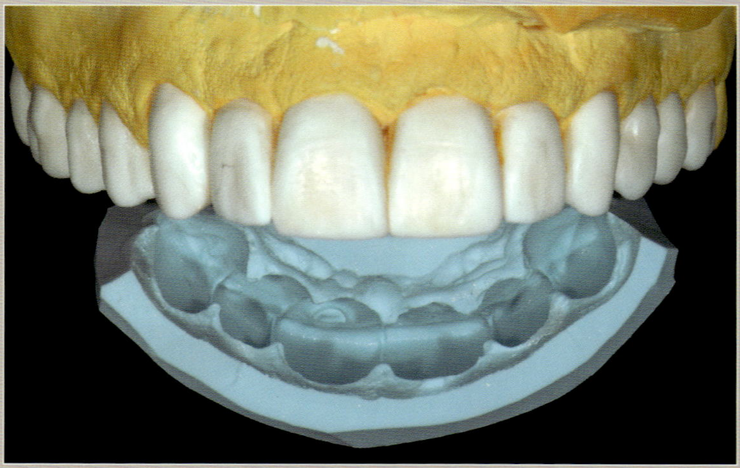

Wax-up with definitive tooth proportions and silicone preparation matrix.

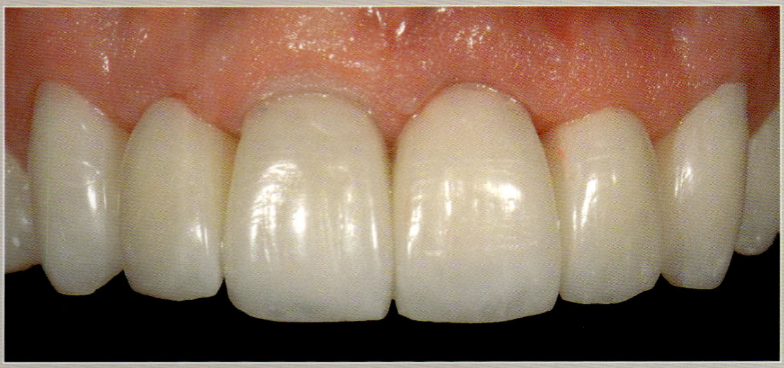

Acrylic eggshell provisional made from the anterior wax-up after intraoral relining, trimming, polishing, and cementation on teeth nos. 6 to 11.

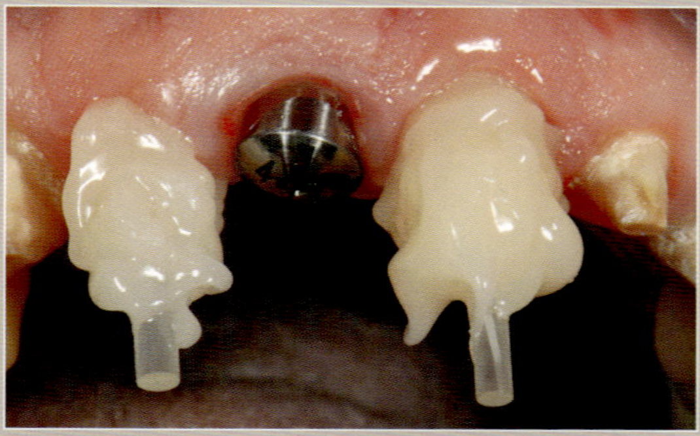

Foundation restorations fabricated on teeth nos. 7 and 9.

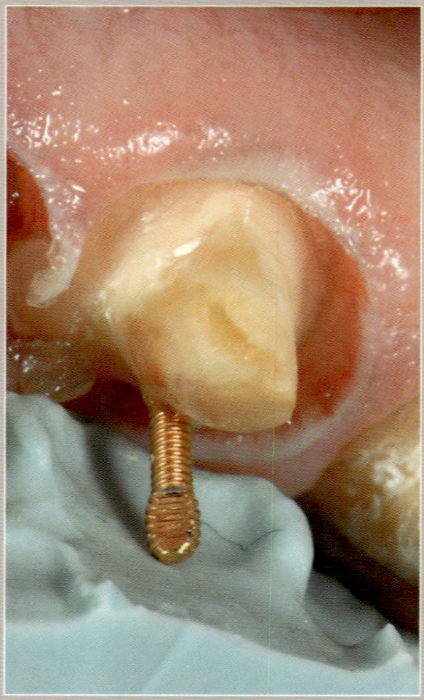

Gold pin placed in vital tooth no. 10.

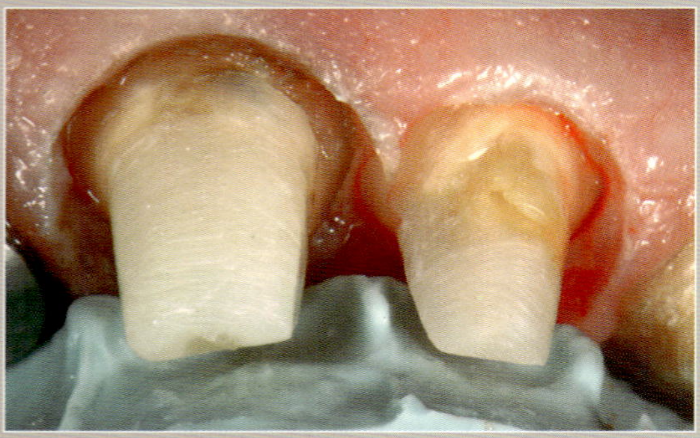

Definitive preparation of foundation restorations using a silicone preparation matrix.

Phase VIII: Diagnostic wax-up and third set of provisional restorations

After biometric correction of the tooth proportions and gingival architecture in the anterior dentition, a second set of diagnostic casts was made and mounted with a facebow transfer onto a semi-adjustable articulator. The details of the definitive tooth size, shape, and contour and occlusal scheme were defined in this final wax-up, which included the correction of the mandibular anterior teeth in regard to tooth position, size, shape, and contour in anticipation of new mandibular anterior veneer restorations. The wax-up was evaluated in centric occlusion as well as protrusive and lateral excursion of the mandible. The zero functional overjet discrepancy was corrected in the wax-up, establishing MIP in centric occlusion.

Silicone preparation matrices and a third set of provisional restorations were created using the new wax-up prior to final tooth preparation and impression taking.

Fiber-reinforced foundation restorations were placed in the endodontically treated teeth nos. 7 and 9. These dowels were bonded using resin cement and a core material with a modulus of elasticity similar to that of dentin. A pin-retained foundation restoration was placed on the vital tooth no. 10. The definitive preparations of these foundation restorations were made using a silicone preparation matrix fabricated from the laboratory wax-up.

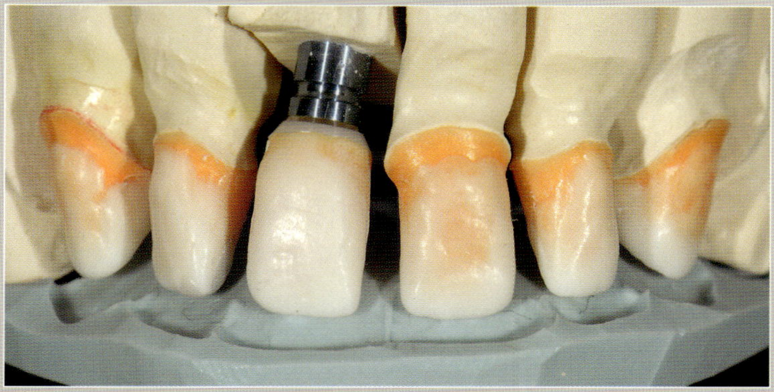

Stone die cast with wax-up of copings performed using a silicone preparation matrix.

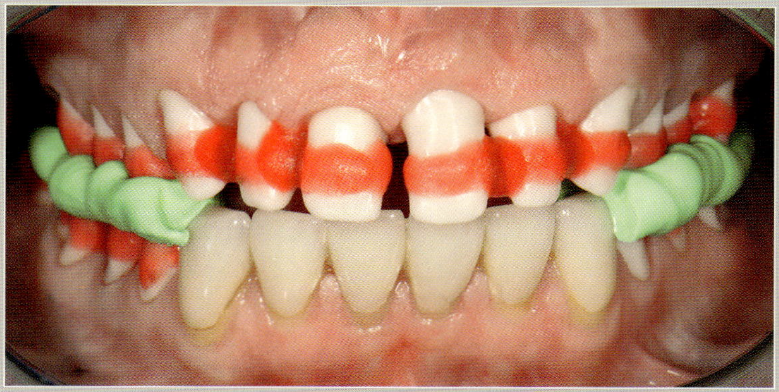

Maxillomandibular registration with zirconia copings seated on tooth preparations in the maxilla and mandibular posterior areas and joined with acrylic pattern resin.

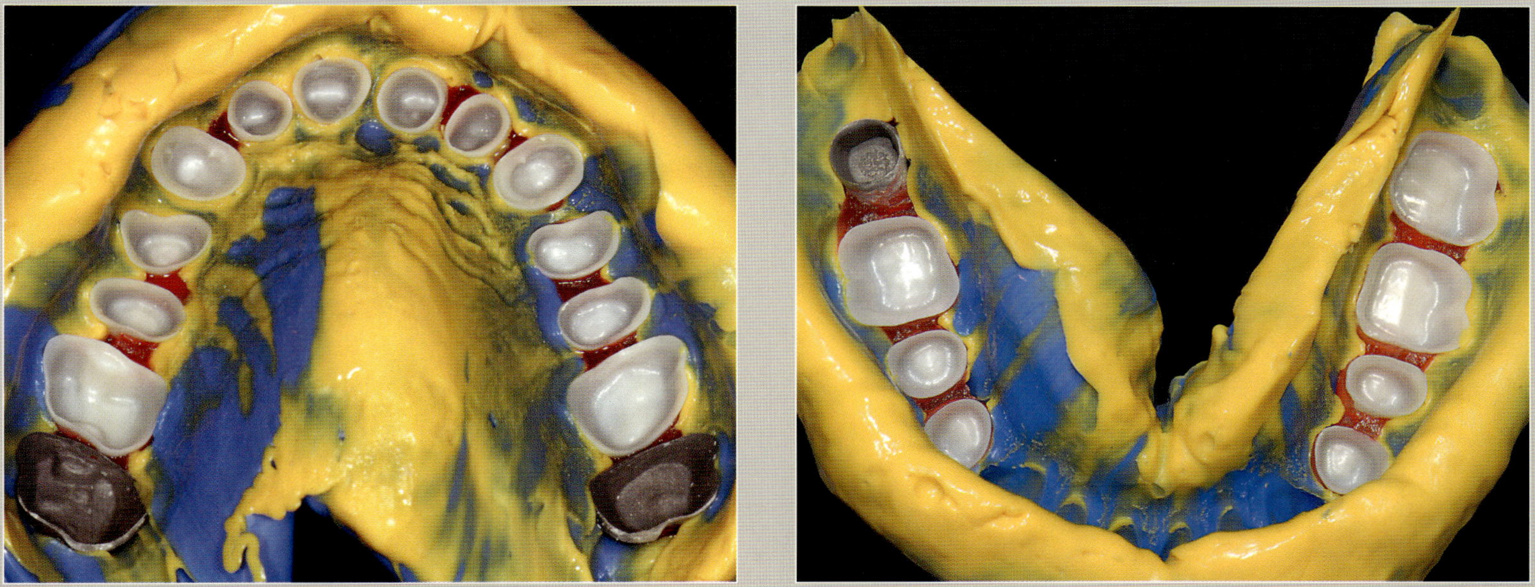

Maxillary and mandibular pickup impressions of the seated zirconia copings.

Phase IX: Pickup impression

Impressions were taken, stone die casts were fabricated, and working casts were mounted. Silicone preparation matrices were used to wax up and scan the patterns for zirconia copings. A stock zirconia abutment with a metal insert was placed on the implant in site no. 8 and prepared to receive a cement-retained restoration.

The zirconia copings for teeth nos. 3 to 14, 19 to 21, and 28 to 31 and three metal alloy copings for teeth nos. 2, 14, and 18 were tried in individually and evaluated with silicone paste to verify proper fit and seating of the copings. The zirconia copings were joined together intraorally with acrylic pattern resin. Maxillomandibular interocclusal records were made and cross-mounted with the working casts prior to the pickup impression with a polyvinyl siloxane material.

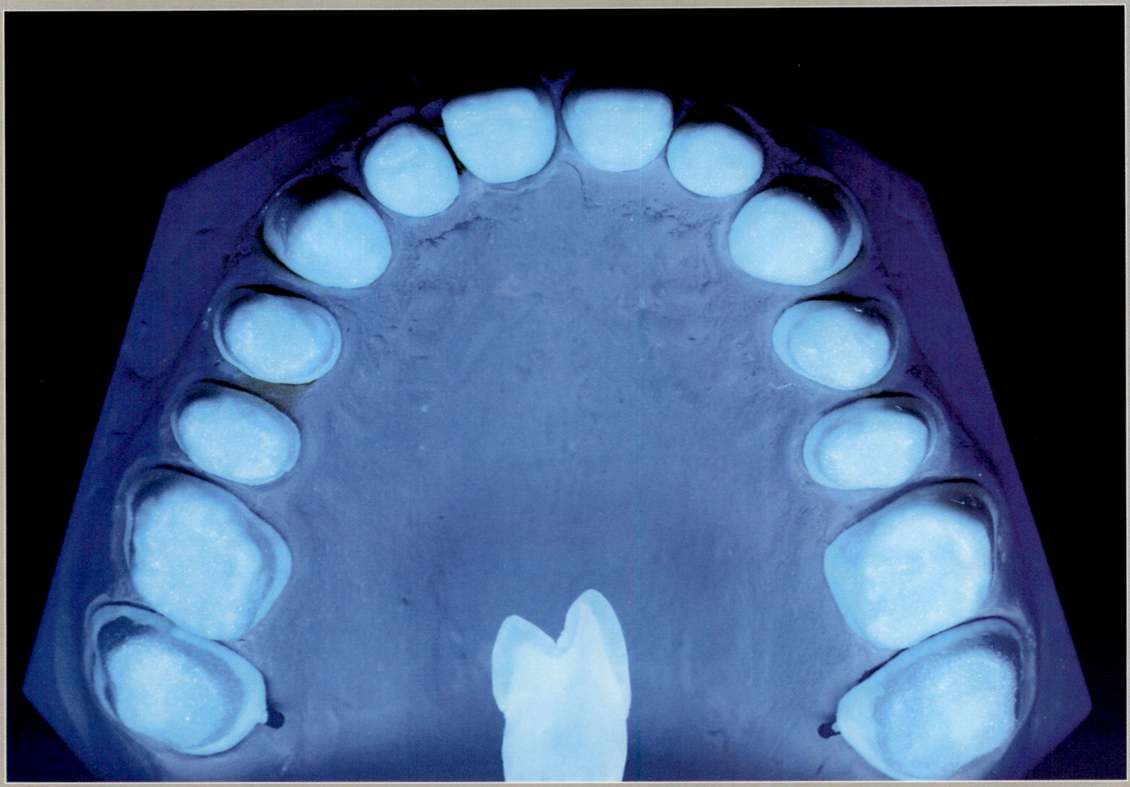

Ceramic bonding layer on zirconia copings and opaque porcelain on metal-ceramic restorations imparts fluorescence comparable with that of a natural tooth.

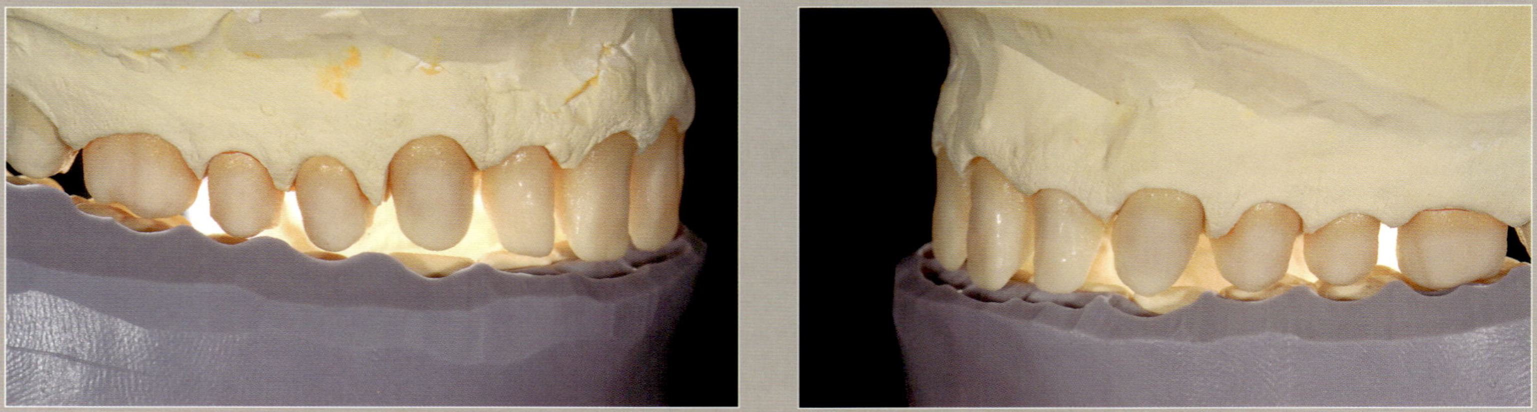

Polychromatic effect and increased chroma achieved using high-chroma dentin shoulder porcelain at the cervical area of the copings with silicone preparation matrix used as reference for anatomical shaping.

Phase X: Laboratory fabrication procedures

Working casts were fabricated and cross-mounted with the maxillomandibular interocclusal records. A bonding layer of high-fusing ceramic with fluorescence was applied to the zirconia copings prior to application of the veneering ceramic to ensure proper adhesion to the zirconia substructure. High-chroma ceramic shoulder material was applied and baked to increase the hue of the restorations at the gingival third, giving a polychromatic shading effect from the gingival to the incisal regions. The silicone matrices were used in the ceramic build-up process. The single crown restorations were contoured, finished, glazed, and polished. The occlusion was re-evaluated on the mounted casts in centric occlusion and lateral excursive movements.

A try-in of the definitive crowns was made; the shade, contours, and occlusion were evaluated and adjusted as necessary. The mandibular anterior teeth nos. 22 to 27 were prepared for veneer restorations, and the impression was taken with a polyvinyl siloxane material. Again, a silicone preparation matrix was used to guide the tooth preparation for the veneer restorations.

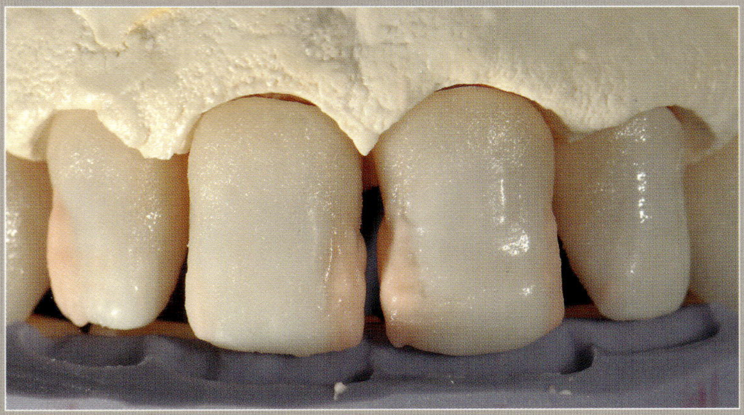

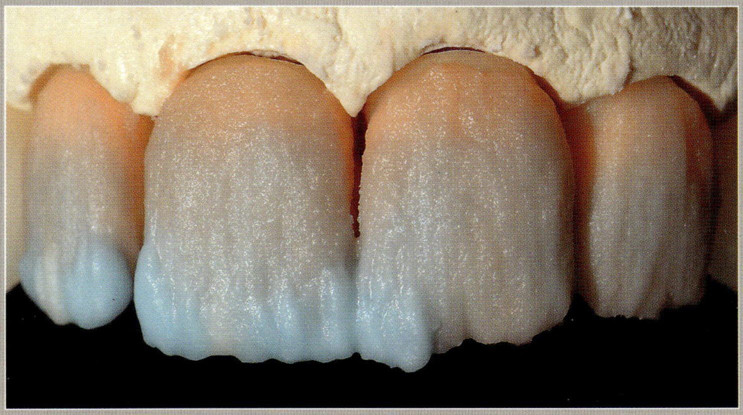

Silicone preparation matrix used in the dentin and enamel buildup.

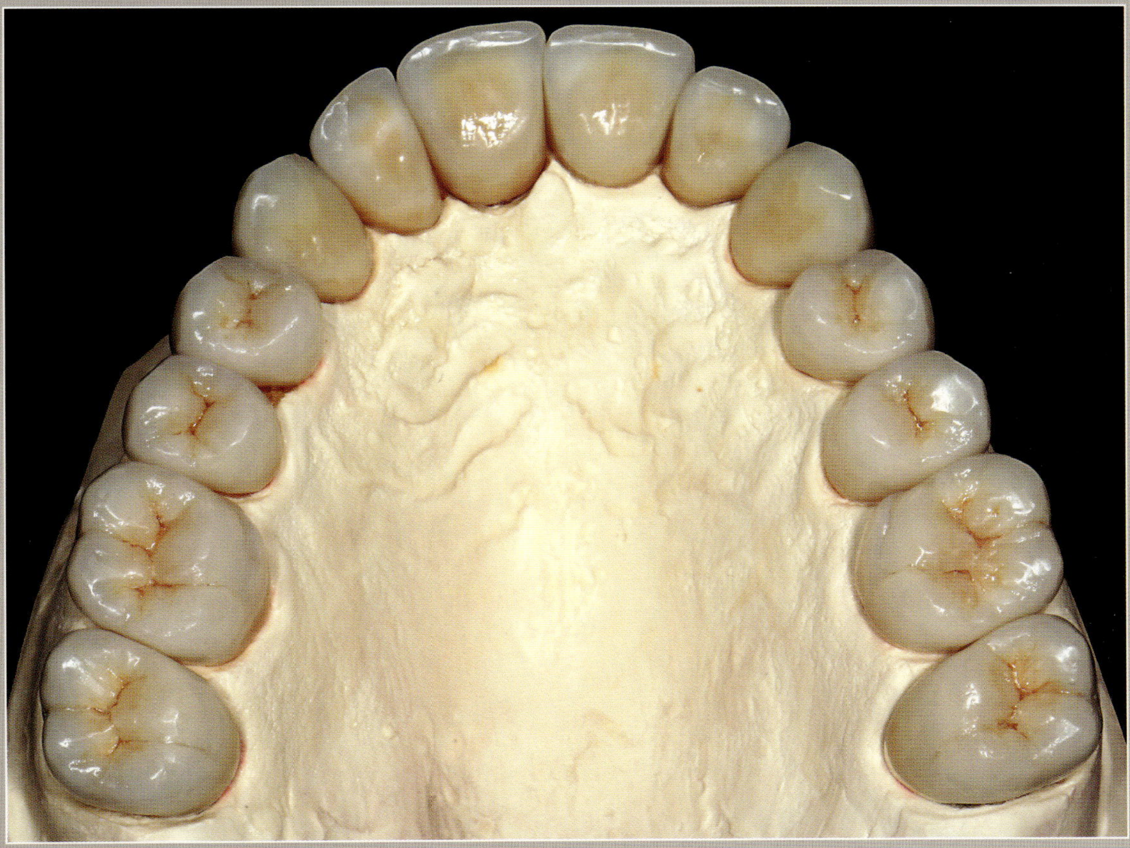

Definitive restorations glazed, polished, and assembled on the cast.

Phase XI: Placement of definitive restorations

The definitive restorations were temporarily seated with Temp-Bond NE (Kerr) for 6 months. The crowns were removed and definitive cementation was completed using Maxcem (Kerr). The provisional cement remained on the implant crown at site no. 8. The veneer restorations were bonded with transparent light-cured resin cement.

The patient's chief complaints were systematically addressed throughout therapy, and the goals of treatment were achieved. The size and proportion of the teeth as well as the gingival architecture were brought into harmony by planning treatment based on biometric goals and biologic principles. The smile reveals the anterior papillae, representing achievement of the goal of orthodontic therapy.

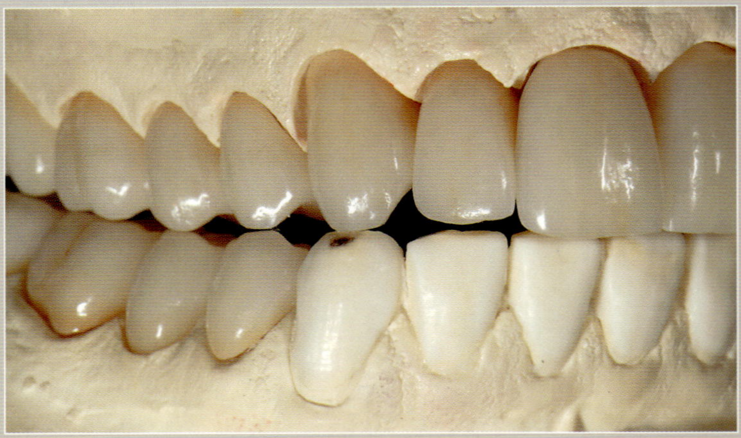
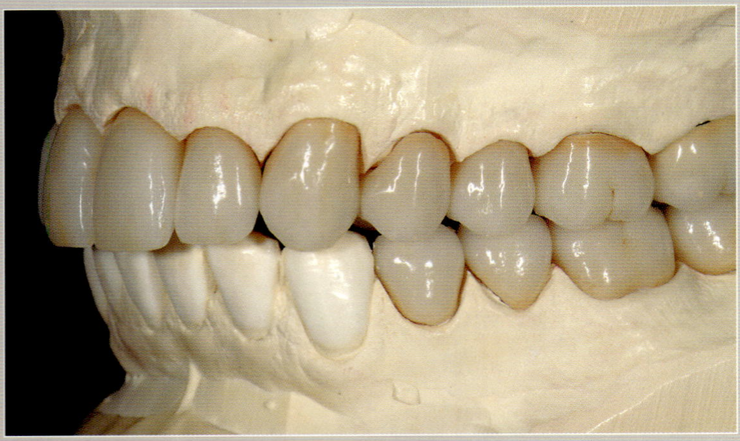

Mandibular posterior zirconia single crowns, a metal-ceramic implant crown for site no. 18, and the anterior teeth waxed up on the cast before replacement of the existing veneers.

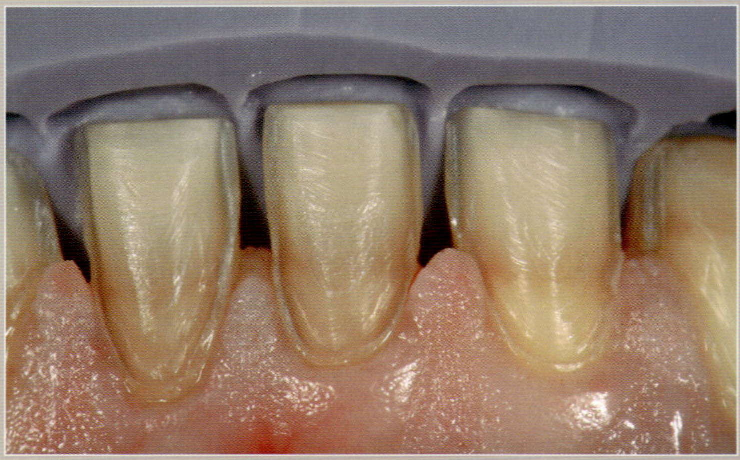

Preparation of mandibular anterior teeth for veneers verified using silicone preparation matrix.

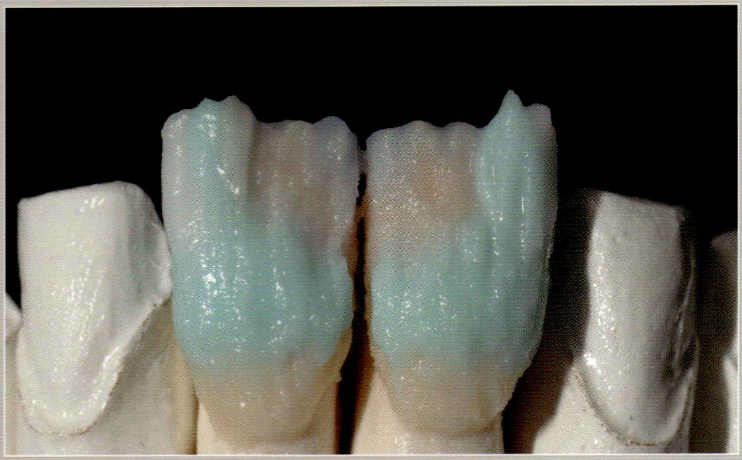

Ceramic powders mixed and layered on the refractory dies.

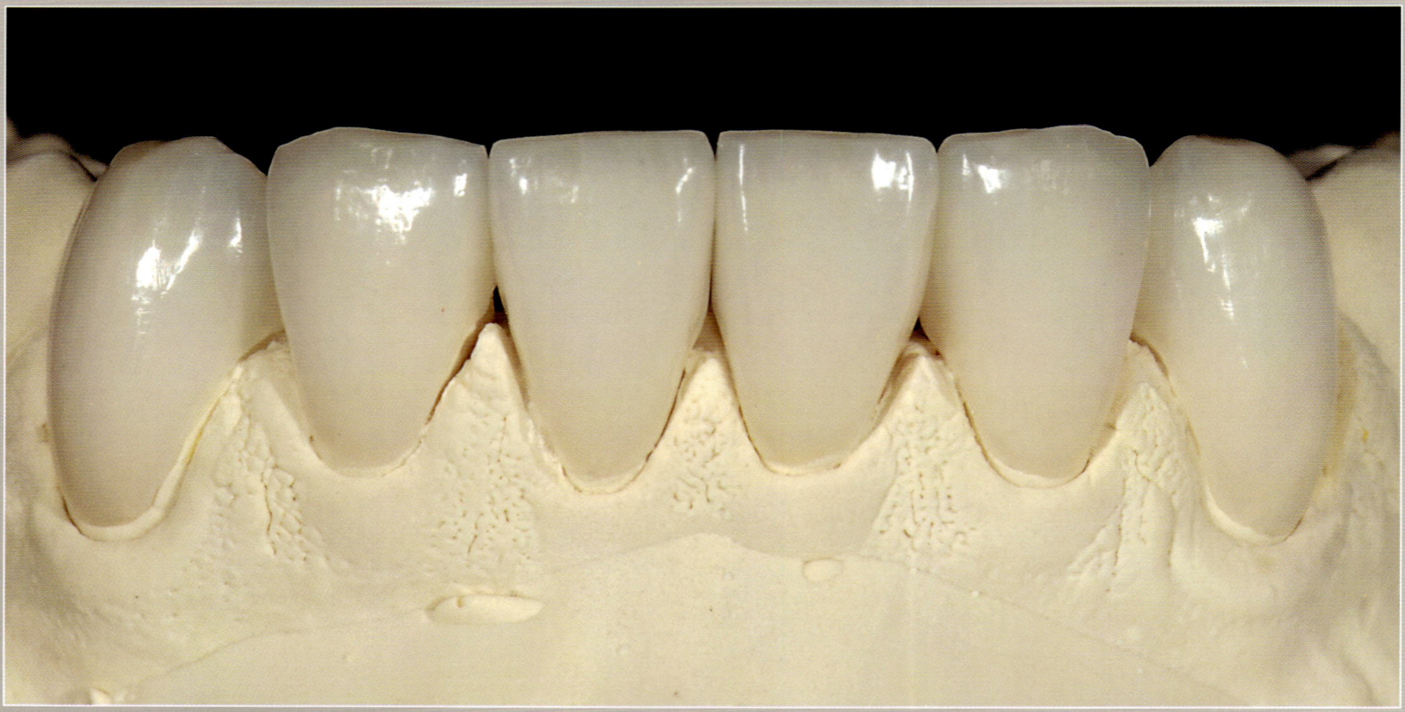

Mandibular anterior veneers following final contouring, shaping, glazing, and polishing.

Posttreatment

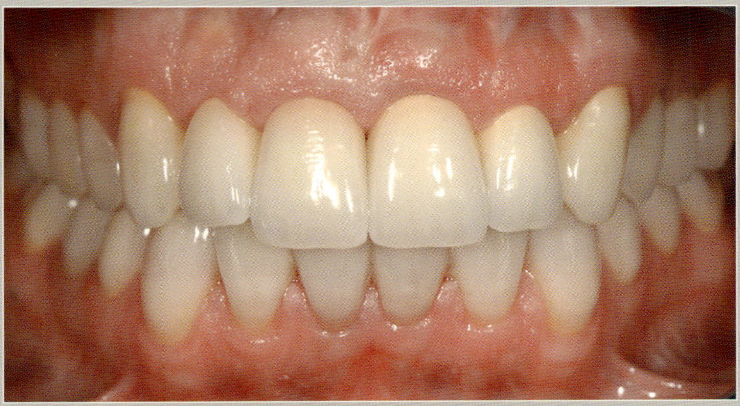

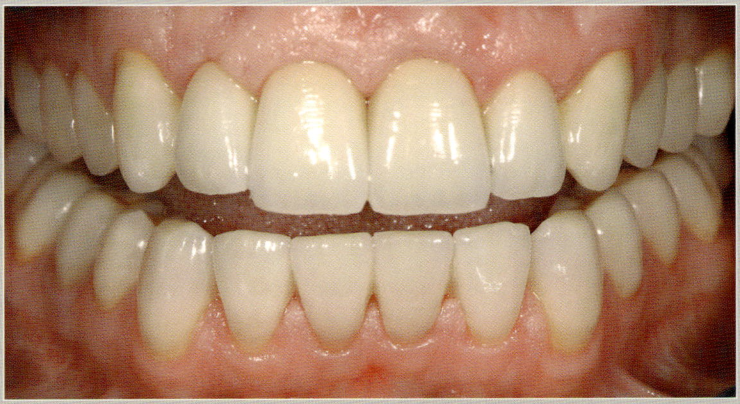

Intraoral frontal views of definitive restorations.

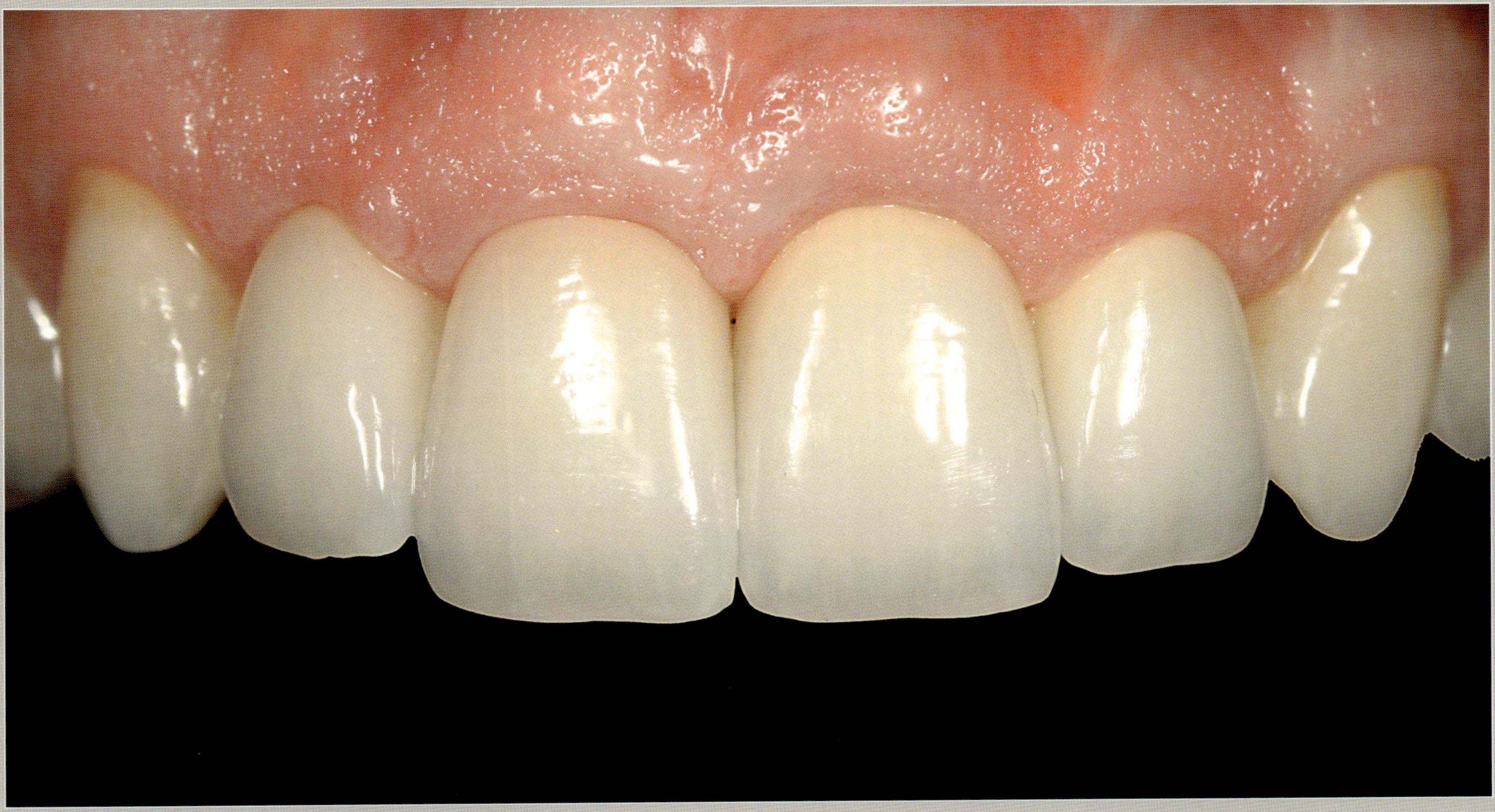

Esthetic integration of crowns on implant at site no. 8 and teeth nos. 6, 7, 9, 10, and 11.

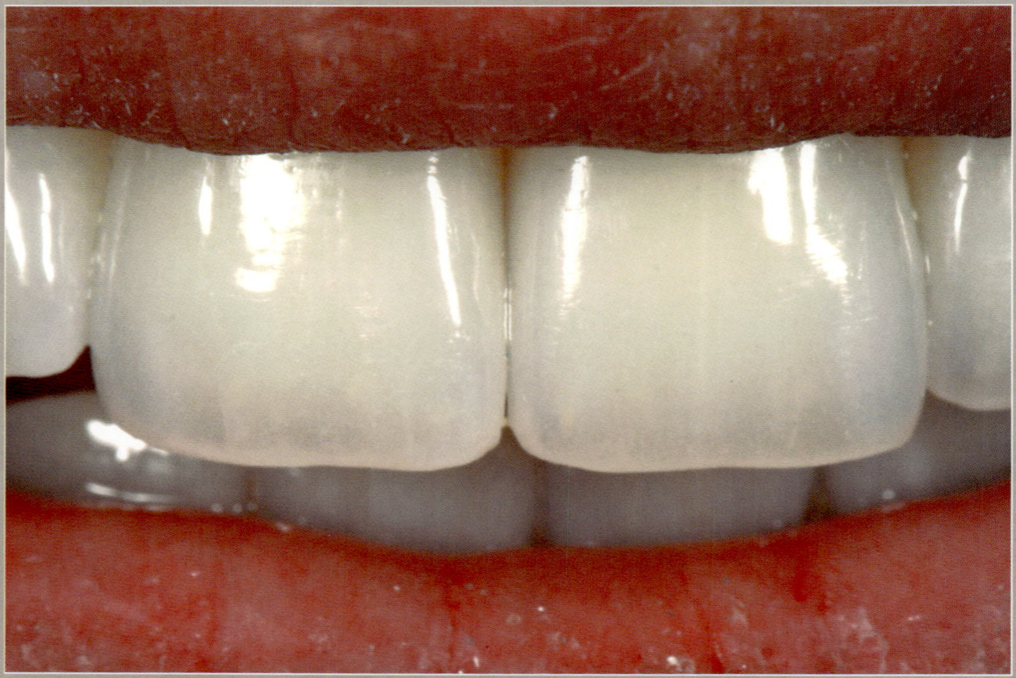

Integration of incisal translucency of crowns on implant at site no. 8 and tooth no. 9.

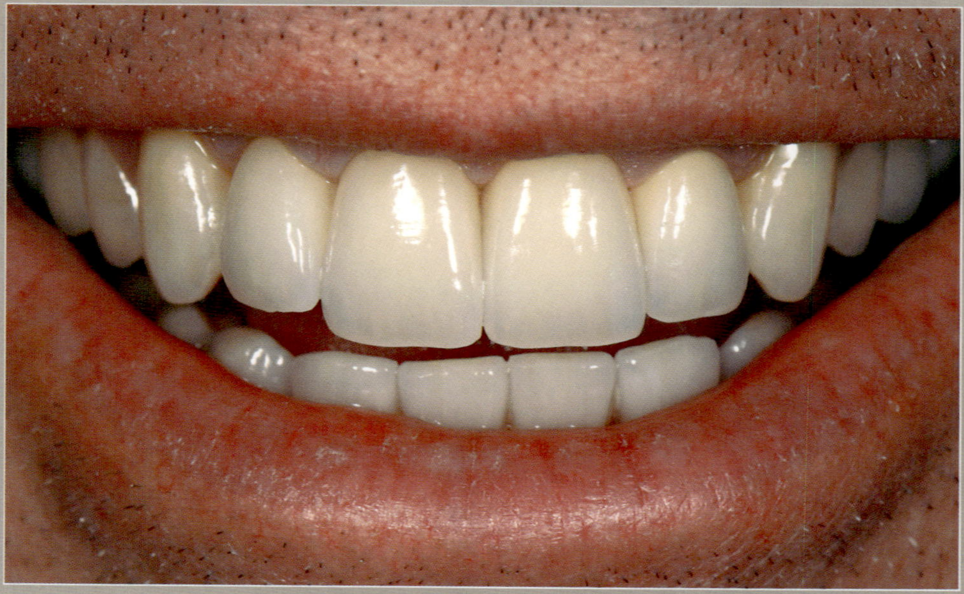

Smile.

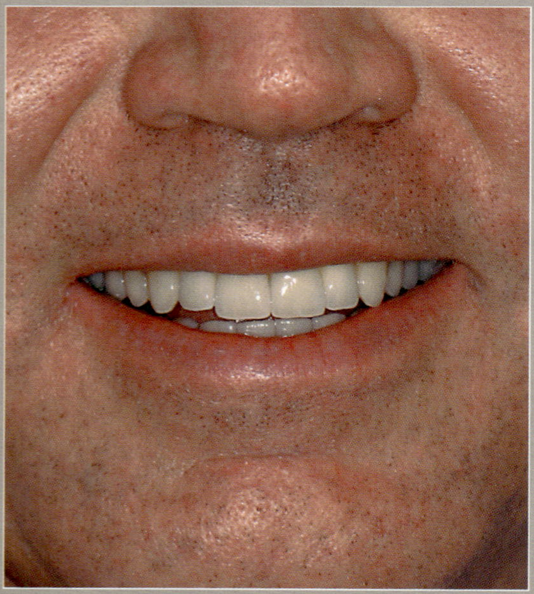

Facial view of smile.

You may now place the corresponding posttreatment overlay found in the separate folder over the pretreatment periodontal chart on page 217.

Commentary

Timing of implant placement

Implant placement was performed early in the treatment sequence to facilitate the orthodontic extrusion of tooth no. 7, for which anchorage was insufficient. The key is to envision the definitive esthetic outcome of the implant restoration prior to implant placement. Site development should have been completed before implant placement. If orthodontic anchorage had been sufficient, the implant would have been placed after completion of the orthodontic therapy.

Surgical root coverage therapy

Coronal positioning of the midfacial soft tissues has esthetic implications in regard to papillae length. The length of the papillae should be roughly 40% of the length of the tooth from free gingival margin to incisal edge. When the height of the gingival third of the tooth decreases (ie, root coverage), then the papillae proportion also decreases; conversely, an increase in the length of the midfacial gingival third of the tooth (ie, crown lengthening) leads to an increase in papillae proportion. Caution should be taken when midfacial crown lengthening is performed without papillae correction because this will result in excessively long papillae, probably exceeding 40% of clinical crown height (if the existing relationship was within the normative values).

Orthodontic therapy

In light of the fact that papillae height decreases with coronal positioning of the midfacial tissues, additional orthodontic extrusion of the teeth to increase the interdental papillae height could have been performed to overcompensate for this phenomenon. However, the most important part of orthodontic extrusion therapy was to bring the visually short papillae into view in the smile.

Smile line esthetics

The smile line is generally classified as low, average, or high based on the amount of midfacial tooth and gingival display. The amount of tooth and gingival display has been found to be greater in the dynamic (spontaneous) versus the static smile.[14] The exposure of interdental tissue is often overlooked in this analysis, but it has been shown to be a critical element in achieving smile line esthetics. Tjan et al[15] reported that papillae were evident in 100% of 454 photographs of randomly selected dental and dental hygiene students displaying a full smile, even though the amount of midfacial display varied. In a study the authors conducted with patients ranging in age from 30 to 90 years, the papillae were visible during smiling 91% of the time.[16] Because it is known that the length of the papilla should be 40% of the length of the tooth or about 4.5 mm measured from the gingival zenith, it makes sense that it would show during the smile, even if it is deficient and/or the smile line is low.

Therefore, the smile line should fit into one of the following four distinct categories:

1. High: 100% tooth and papillae display
2. Moderate: 75% to 100% tooth display and 100% papillae display
3. Low with papillae display: less than 75% tooth display with some papillae display
4. Low without papillae display: less than 75% tooth display with no papillae display

Identifying and managing the display of papillae in the smile line is critical in the complex esthetic case. It is an element that is often misunderstood and frequently overlooked when treating the esthetic-restorative patient presenting with vertical discrepancies of the hard and soft tissues within the esthetic zone.

Materials selection

Recently, zirconia has been the subject of controversy, with fracture problems being reported clinically. However, the high-strength ceramic industry has undergone a metamorphosis, improving the fracture resistance of second-generation materials. A recent study involving 702 zirconia restorations in 207 patients with 70% of the restorations in function for 3 to 5 years showed a failure (replacement) rate of only 2%.[17] The restorations provided to the patient shown in this case presentation have been in function for 4 years without any complications. Esthetically, zirconia offers high light-dynamic properties and white shades where gingival recession is likely and risk of margin exposure is high.

References

1. Chu SJ. Range and mean distribution frequency of individual tooth width of the maxillary anterior dentition. Pract Proced Aesthet Dent 2007;19:209–215.
2. Duarte S Jr, Schnider P, Lorezon AP. The importance of width/length ratios of maxillary anterior permanent teeth in aesthetic rehabilitation. Eur J Esthet Dent 2008;3:224–234.
3. Sterrett JD, Oliver T, Robinson F, et al. Width/length ratios of normal clinical crowns of the maxillary anterior dentition in man. J Clin Periodontol 1999;26:153–157.
4. Magne P, Gallucci GO, Belser UC. Anatomic crown width/length ratios of unworn and worn maxillary teeth in white subjects. J Prosthet Dent 2003;89:453–461.
5. Bolton WA. Disharmony in tooth size and its relation to the analysis and treatment of malocclusion. Angle Orthod 1958;28:113–130.
6. Bolton WA. The clinical application of tooth-size analysis. Am J Orthod 1962;48:504–529.
7. Chu SJ, Okubo, S. Range and mean discordance of individual tooth width of mandibular anterior dentition. Pract Proced Aesthet Dent 2008;20:313–320.
8. Mattos CM, Santana RB. A quantitative evaluation of the spatial displacement of the gingival zenith in the maxillary anterior dentition. J Periodontol 2008;79:1880–1885.
9. Chu SJ, Tan JH, Stappert CF, Tarnow DP. Gingival zenith positions and levels of the maxillary anterior dentition. J Esthet Restor Dent 2009;21:115–123.
10. Zagar M, Knezović Zlatarić D, Carek V. A quantitative evaluation of the distal displacement of the gingival zenith in the maxillary anterior teeth. Coll Antropol 2010;34(suppl 1):225–228.
11. Spear F. Maintenance of the interdental papilla following anterior tooth removal. Pract Periodontics Aesthet Dent 1999;11:21–28.
12. Kois JC. Altering gingival levels: The restorative connection. Part I: Biologic variables. J Esthet Dent 1994;6:3–9.
13. Chu SJ, Tarnow DP, Tan JH, Stappert CF. Papilla proportions in the maxillary anterior dentition. Int J Periodontics Restorative Dent 2009;29:385–393.
14. Van Der Geld P, Oosterveld P, Bergé SJ, Kuijpers-Jagtman AM. Tooth display and lip position during spontaneous and posed smiling in adults. Acta Odontol Scand 2008;66:207–213.
15. Tjan AH, Miller GD, The JG. Some aesthetic factors in a smile. J Prosthet Dent 1984;51:24–28.
16. Hochman MN, Chu SJ, Tarnow DP. Maxillary anterior papillae display during smiling: A clinical study of the interdental smile line. Int J Periodontics Restorative Dent (in press).
17. Nathanson D, Chu S, Yamamoto H, Stappert C. Performance of zirconia based crowns and FPDs in prosthodontic practice. Presented at the International Association of Dental Research General Session, Barcelona, 16 July 2010.

9

Endodontic Failure in the Esthetic Zone: Interdisciplinary Decision Making

John D. West, DDS, MSD

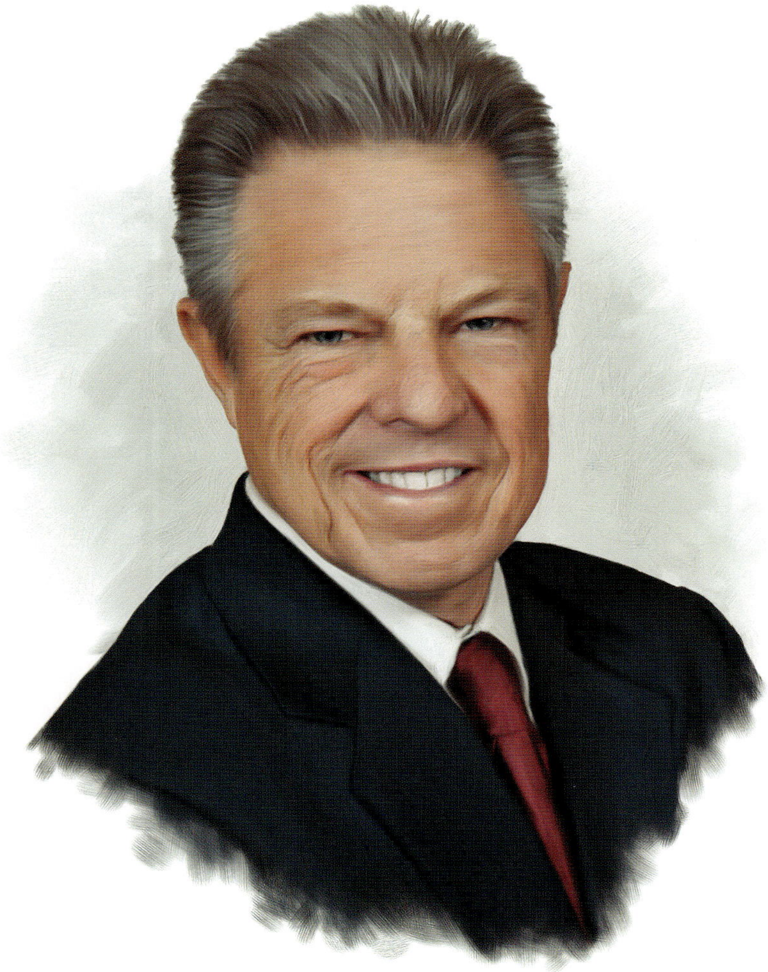

While the art of saving compromised teeth, particularly endodontically treated teeth, may seem to have been lost, in the proper hands it is alive and well.

Philosophy and Background

In this, the second decade of the 21st century, we are born out of the most humble biologic stance: that when the cause of a disease is removed, the disease is gone. Not only is the disease gone, but the results of the disease are no longer sustainable without a cause. It's that simple. We, as dentists, are the caretakers of this biologic tenant. And yet, we sometimes forget. We forget because it is easy. We forget because it is hard. We forget because we may be thinking of ourselves and not the patient. We forget for convenience. We forget because we fail to do the right thing.

I chose this highly predictable long-term case presentation as an example of doing the right thing. It may not have been the safest, the easiest, or the most dentally productive, but it was the right thing for the patient. Today, the trend is to "remove and replace" when in doubt. My goal is for this chapter to serve as a reminder that the "always" answer in treatment planning is easily found in the answer to the question, "What would I do if it were me?" I am convinced that upon reviewing this patient's options and considering that endodontists are truly skilled masters of preventing and curing lesions of endodontic origin, anyone would choose what this patient chose: the right thing. It is the right thing for the patient, for the dentist, and for dentistry. Making this choice, to me, is the hallmark of a true caregiver.

Case Presentation

Treating clinicians
Endodontist: John D. West, DDS, MSD
Restorative dentist: Randy McLeary, DDS

Clinical Treatment Planning

Age at initial presentation: 44 years
Initial presentation: January 1999
Active treatment completed: July 1999

Introduction and background

This 44-year-old man was referred by his family dentist for endodontic evaluation of his maxillary anterior fixed partial denture that had been placed in 1998. The patient had experienced pain in the maxillary anterior region a few months prior to recent slight swelling at the labial aspect of tooth no. 8. Tooth no. 9 had been lost during a car accident in 1975. Numerous provisional prostheses and unesthetic removable and fixed partial dentures had been placed over the years. When the patient was first examined in January 1999, he presented with a sinus tract labial to tooth no. 8, which was serving as a fixed partial denture abutment. He had experienced some pressure in the area for several months, but the sinus tract was first noticed only a few weeks prior.

A gutta-percha tracer cone led to the mesial aspect of the midroot of tooth no. 8. Probing in the gingival crevice was within normal limits, suggesting that the sinus tract was caused by a lesion of endodontic origin (LEO) rather than a lesion of periodontal origin and/or a vertical fracture. A periapical radiograph of tooth no. 10 suggested a necrotic pulp and an LEO.

This patient had undergone a great deal of treatment in this area and was becoming frustrated with the series of failures that had resulted in emergency appointments, significant chair time with each incident, and short-lived solutions with esthetic compromise. The latest partial denture was esthetically acceptable, and he felt that his best overall treatment option would be to save it and address the problem with a permanent solution in mind. The patient's desire was for the treatment to be as simple and minimally invasive as possible because he already was feeling weary of treatment.

Medical history

- Noncontributory

Diagnostic findings

Extraoral and facial findings

- Balanced facial profile and good facial symmetry
- Average lip mobility with low to average smile line

TMJ and mandibular range of motion

- No joint sounds with external palpation
- No joint or muscle pain with palpation, upon loading, or with movement
- Range of motion within normal limits
- Easy manipulation

Pretreatment

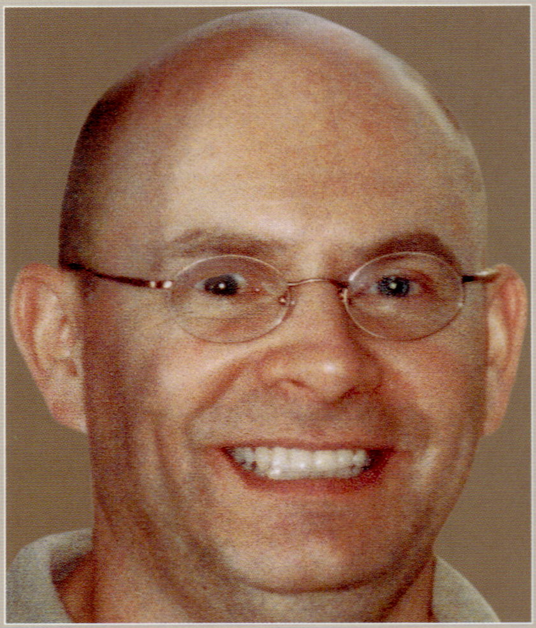

Frontal facial view in 1998, shortly after maxillary fixed partial denture placement.

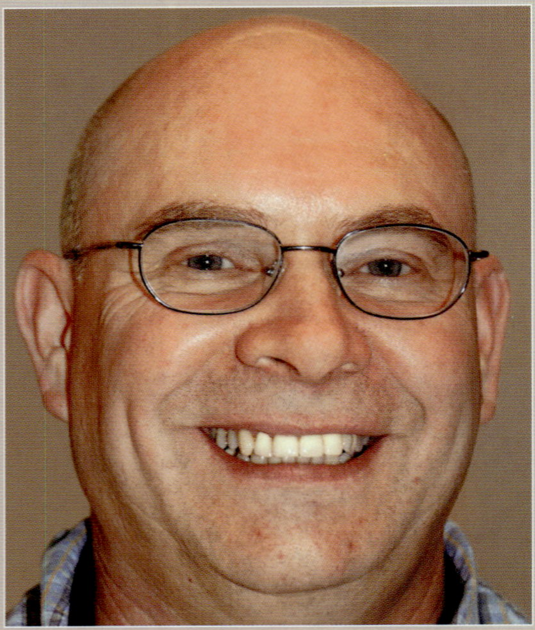

Frontal facial view at initial presentation (1999).

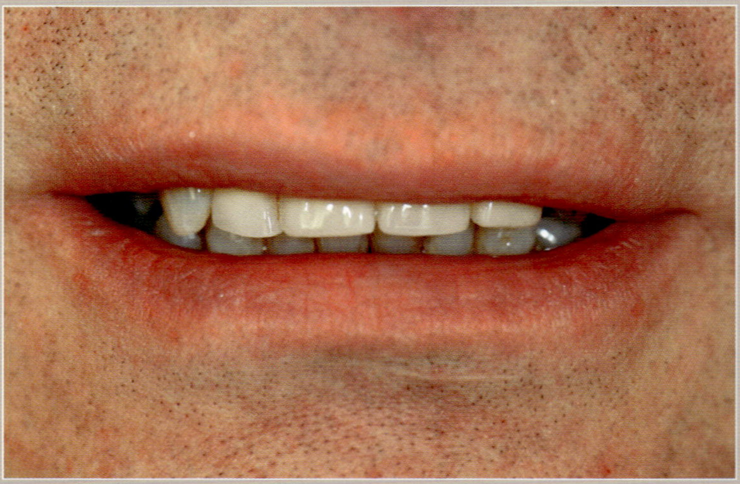

Lips in repose.

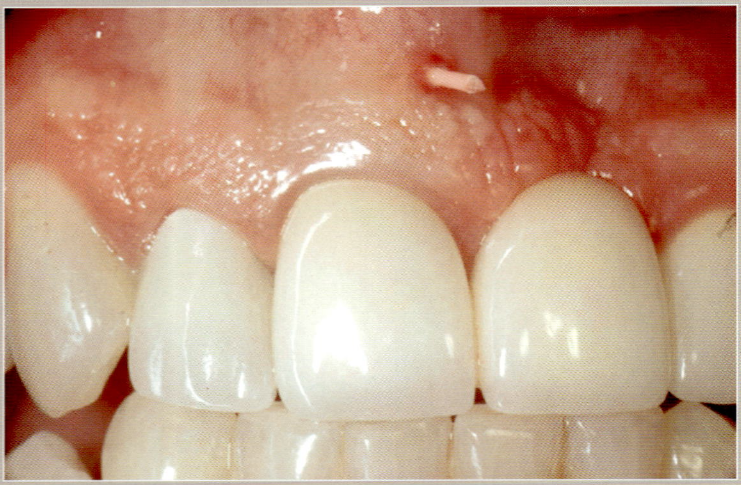

Gutta-percha cone tracing the labial sinus tract.

Intraoral findings

General

- Intraoral soft tissues within normal limits
- Negative cancer screen

Dental

- Maxillary gingival levels appropriate
- Pontic site of edentulous site no. 9 slightly concave
- Emergence profile of tooth no. 9, while prominent during lip retraction, does not have a negative esthetic affect due to low to medium smile line
- Intact dentition except for missing tooth no. 9

Periodontal

- Good plaque control and oral hygiene
- Healthy periodontium with generalized slight gingival inflammation
- Probing depths generally 3 mm or less
- Tooth mobility within normal limits

Endodontic

- Previous endodontic treatment of teeth nos. 7 and 11 appeared to be successful; both teeth were asymptomatic.
- The pulp of tooth no. 10 tested nonvital. Tooth no. 8 has an undersealed root canal system, lateral LEO, and draining sinus tract that can be traced to a probable mesial midroot lateral unfilled portal of exit (POE).

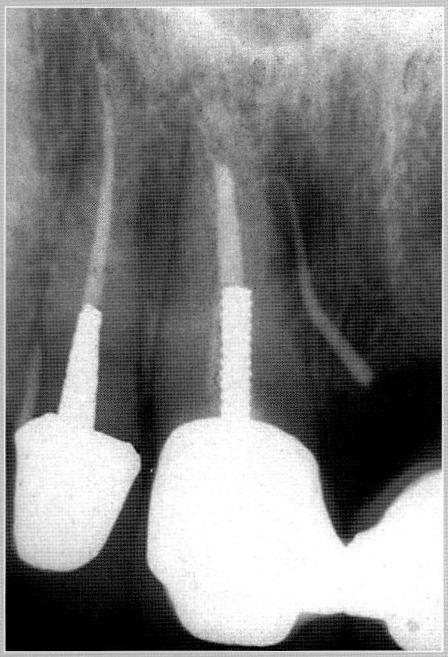

Periapical radiograph of tooth no. 8 with gutta-percha cone.

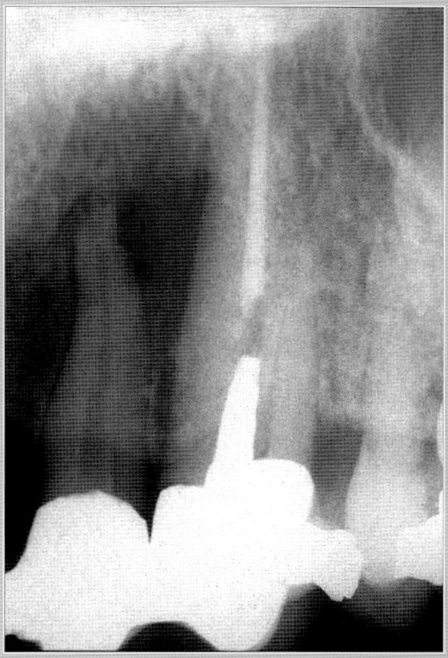

Periapical radiograph of tooth no. 10.

Occlusal notes

- Angle Class II molar and canine relationships
- Minimal overbite and overjet
- Mild incisal wear

Radiographic findings

- Acceptable anterior and posterior bone levels
- Presence of several anterior composite restorations
- Lateral radiolucency, diagnosed as an LEO, appearing on the mesial midroot surface of tooth no. 8, which had nonsurgical endodontic treatment 5 years previously; in addition to the presumed unfilled lateral POE, the apical portion of the root canal system was underfilled
- Apical radiolucency on tooth no. 10

Diagnosis

- Tooth no. 8 has an undersealed root canal system resulting in an LEO and draining sinus tract that can be traced to the mesial lateral border of tooth no. 8.
- The pulp of tooth no. 10 is nonvital.

Prognosis

- Tooth no. 7 prognosis is good because of healthy attachment apparatus, intact lamina dura, and asymptomatic status since previous endodontic treatment in 1992.
- Tooth no. 8 prognosis is excellent if endodontic seal can be achieved either nonsurgically or surgically.
- Tooth no. 10 prognosis is excellent because successful endodontic seal should be easily achieved if skillfully treated with nonsurgical endodontic re-treatment.
- Tooth no. 11 endodontic prognosis is good because of healthy lamina dura and asymptomatic status since endodontic treatment in 1991.

Summary of concerns

1. How long has the maxillary partial denture been in place?
2. Does the patient like the esthetics and function of the partial denture?
3. What material was used to cement the partial denture? (The answer to this question will influence how the area is treated.)
4. Can either or both of the abutment teeth nos. 8 and 10 be saved, or do extraction and tooth replacement comprise the most prudent approach?
5. If an attempt is made to save these teeth, is the best endodontic approach for predictable structural and esthetic success surgical or nonsurgical? If surgical correction of the endodontic seal is considered, what are the chances of finding the undersealed lateral POE? Could the POE be on the palatal side of the root, making it difficult or impossible to locate even with a microscopic approach? Will we be able to make a proper cavity preparation and seal? What if there is more than one lateral POE?
6. If tooth no. 8 is re-treated surgically, could or should the undersealed apical POE be treated?
7. If tooth no. 8 is re-treated surgically, what about necrotic tooth no. 10 with an LEO? Creating access through the fixed partial denture in order to treat tooth no. 10 nonsurgically may loosen the fixed partial denture, which would negate the consideration of fixed partial denture removal. Can the pulp of tooth no. 10 be reliably tested?
8. With surgical re-treatment, what is the possibility of creating an unesthetic black triangle?
9. If surgical re-treatment is chosen, what type of incision should be made and where should it be placed to maximize access and minimize an adverse gingival esthetic result?
10. If re-treatment is nonsurgical, should access be made through the partial denture or should it be removed? If it is removed, how will this be accomplished? What are the dangers of partial denture removal? What method produces the least risk of breaking the partial denture and/or the teeth?
11. If nonsurgical re-treatment is made through the partial denture, what problems does the post pose? Is the post part of a separate foundation or attached to the fixed partial denture abutment? What is the best way to remove a post if it previously was separately cemented? What measures must be taken to protect the integrity of the ferrule?
12. If nonsurgical re-treatment is used, how will the lateral POE(s) be discovered and cleaned? How then will the endodontic seal be produced?

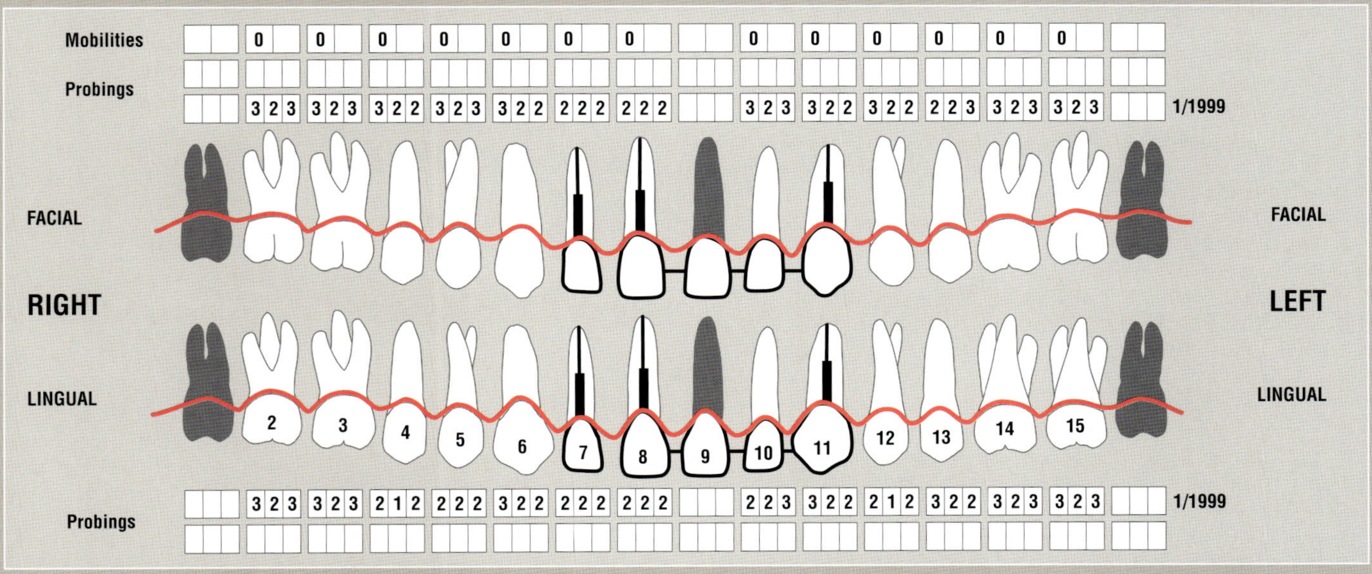

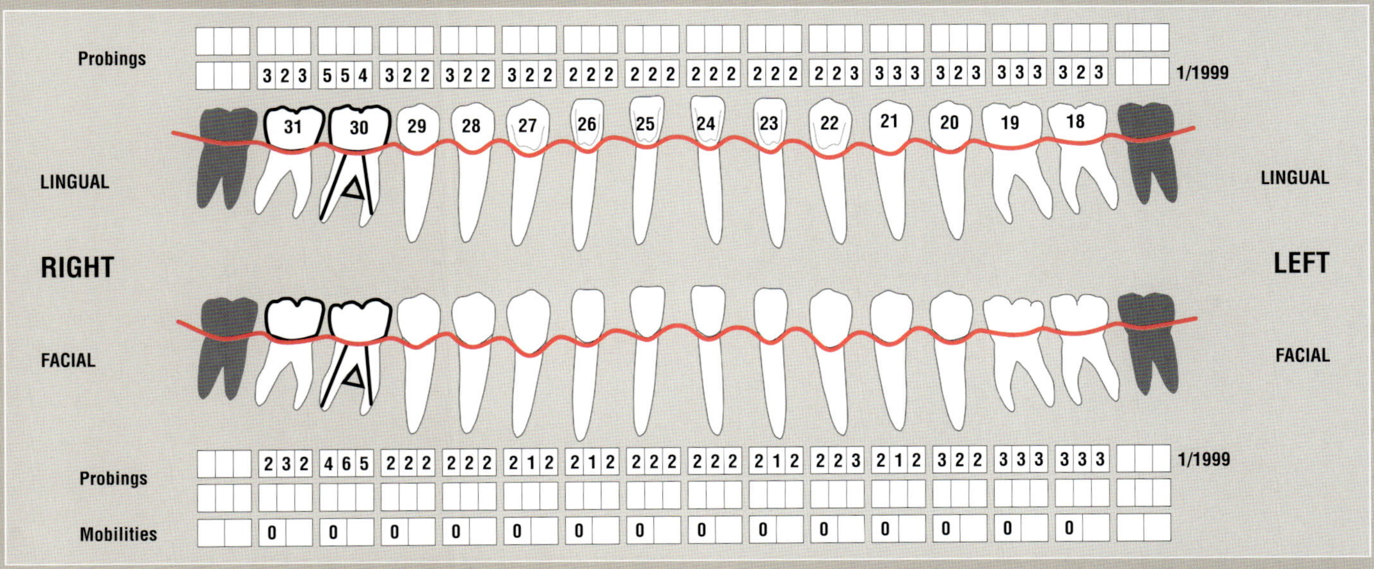

As a learning exercise, you may now outline goals/objectives of treatment and a treatment plan.

Proposed Treatment Plan

Goals/objectives of treatment

- Use a nonsurgical approach to resolve the LEOs on the fixed partial denture abutment teeth nos. 8 and 10.
- Successfully preserve the existing fixed partial denture and avoid periodontal, structural, and esthetic considerations of abutment teeth and/or partial denture damage that would require removal and replacement with a new and differently designed fixed partial denture or implant restorations.
- Find a long-term solution. This is of paramount importance because the patient has experienced frustration with the short-term nature of solutions in the past.
- Minimize cost without compromising the biologic, structural, functional, or esthetic result.
- Achieve periodontal stability.

Phase I: Data gathering

1. Comprehensive oral examination
2. Pretreatment photographic series

Phase II: Interdisciplinary planning and sequencing

3. Collaborative discussion with interdisciplinary treatment team members, including the restorative dentist, endodontist, and any other members who will be participating in treatment
4. Consultation with patient
5. Finalization of the treatment plan

Phase III: Fixed partial denture removal

6. Determination as to whether the fixed partial denture is cemented with bonded cement or zinc phosphate and, based on the answer, choice of appropriate method of removal
7. Discussion with patient about the risk of the fixed partial denture and/or teeth breaking (particularly crowns breaking off within the casting) during removal
8. Possible need for the restorative dentist to place a provisional restoration should the fixed partial denture be damaged

Phase IV: Endodontics

9. Determination of the pulpal health of tooth no. 10
10. Determination as to whether LEO is present surrounding previous endodontic treatment of tooth no. 11
11. Evaluation to see if teeth nos. 8, 10, and 11 are vertically fractured
12. Planning of disassembly strategy, sequence, and armamentarium for teeth nos. 8 and 10
13. If fixed partial denture removal and tooth no. 8 endodontic disassembly are successful, nonsurgical re-treatment of tooth no. 8 and nonsurgical treatment of tooth no. 10

Phase V: Definitive restorative treatment and endodontic follow-up

14. After 1 month, evaluation of closure of tooth no. 8 sinus tract and early radiographic healing of tooth no. 8 LEO and confirmation that the patient is asymptomatic, assessing that the LEO at tooth no. 10 is resolving and that the attachment apparatus surrounding endodontically treated teeth nos. 7 and 11 remains healthy
15. Reseating and cementation of the existing fixed partial denture
16. Routine periodontal maintenance every 6 months
17. Routine endodontic posttreatment follow-up for fixed partial denture abutments

Active Clinical Treatment

Review of the goals/objectives of treatment

This patient had been treated on numerous occasions for the problems associated with his maxillary anterior teeth. He was now faced with additional treatment, which would be expensive and related to teeth with very questionable long-term prognoses. The goals and objectives of the treatment team included:

- Finding a long-lasting solution
- Finding a simple and conservative approach that would accommodate the patient's desire for the least invasive treatment possible
- Successfully removing the existing fixed partial denture without having to destroy it and at the same time being able to keep the underlying teeth intact
- Successfully re-treating the endodontic failure on tooth no. 8 and nonvital root canal system of tooth no. 10
- Recementing and utilizing the existing fixed partial denture
- Accomplishing all of the above and not losing sight of the main goal, which is to make this patient happy, his dentition healthy, and his smile and teeth esthetically pleasing, while at the same time elevating his level of appreciation for our profession

Phase I: Data gathering

The patient's dentist confirmed that the fixed partial denture was cemented with zinc phosphate cement. The patient's records were presented to members of the Northwest Network for Dental Excellence for discussion and a consensus as to which treatment option would be best. His low smile line was advantageous because it hid the imperfect soft tissue–pontic interface due to prior loss of bone support on the edentulous ridge. In addition, the patient had several partial dentures placed in the past and finally was satisfied with the appearance of the present fixed partial denture, which he felt looked quite natural. All members of the Northwest Network agreed that, if the fixed partial denture could be successfully removed and an endodontic seal produced for teeth nos. 8 and 10, this approach would be in the patient's best interest because it was the most conservative and predictable from a biologic, structural, and esthetic standpoint.

Phase II: Interdisciplinary planning and sequencing

Both the patient and the dentist were optimistic that the proposed plan involving fixed partial denture removal, restorative disassembling, and endodontic nonsurgical re-treatment of tooth no. 8 and endodontic treatment of tooth no. 10, followed by recementation of the existing fixed partial denture, would provide the best possible outcome. If the fixed partial denture removal or endodontic treatment of either or both teeth nos. 8 and 10 were unsuccessful, the treating clinicians could always consider fabrication of a new fixed partial denture or the placement of implants.

Phase III: Fixed partial denture removal

Local anesthetic was administered in the maxillary anterior segment. Dental floss was ligated to the fixed partial denture to prevent it from being dropped or swallowed if it was abruptly dislodged during removal. After numerous failed attempts, the Coronaflex (Kavo) system was employed to uneventfully remove the partial denture. A tried and true, although potentially hazardous, instrument, this miniature pneumatic can be highly effective and does not require the creation of an access cavity through the existing crown or abutment. The porcelain of the partial denture was not damaged in any way because of the safe "saddles" in the Coronaflex system, and the abutments maintained complete structural integrity. The post remained in the fixed partial denture abutment casting.

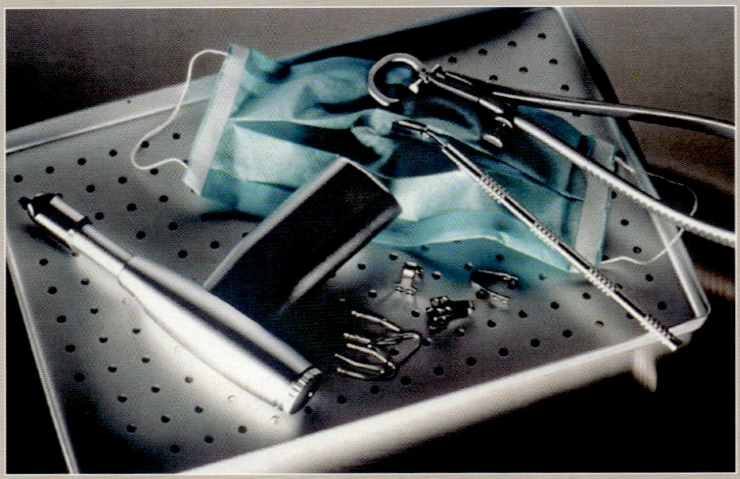

Coronaflex system used to remove the fixed partial denture.

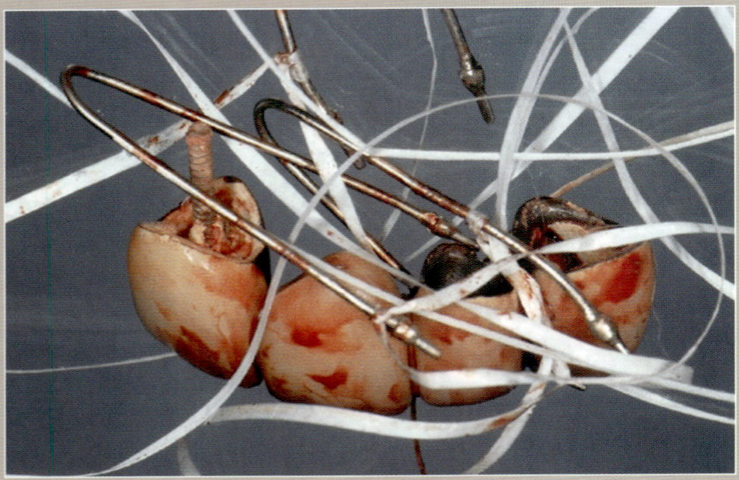

Fixed partial denture following removal.

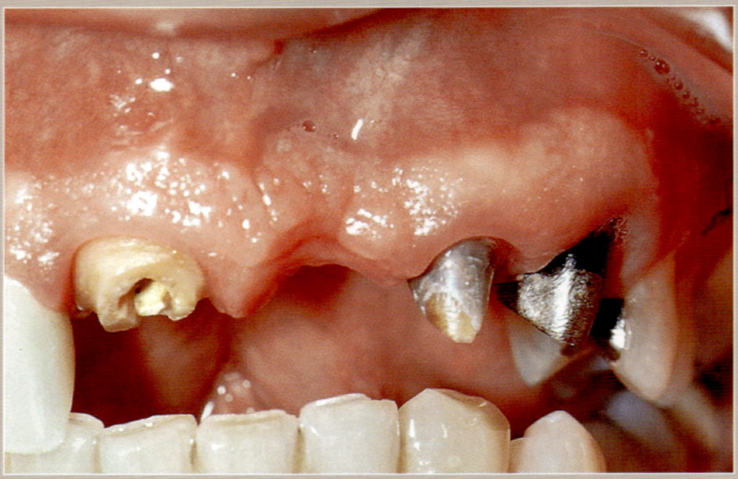

Intraoral view following removal of fixed partial denture.

Phase IV: Endodontics

Once the fixed partial denture was successfully removed, tooth no. 8 was isolated with rubber dam, and a proper access cavity was prepared by removing the previously unremoved remnant of triangle no. 1, which is essentially in enamel (and some dentin), and triangle no. 2, which is essentially in dentin.[1] After straight-line endodontic access was created, the endodontic disassembly continued by first removing the underfilled gutta-percha using heat (System B or Kerr Touch 'n Heat, SybronEndo). The key is to remove the gutta-percha and not change the landscape anatomy of the root canal system. The POE had been transported internally by one or a combination of the following three possible mechanical errors: *(1)* a block of dentinal debris during the cleaning and shaping attempt, *(2)* a dense pulpal collagen block when the pulp was vital, or *(3)* a ledge in the radicular preparation preventing apical patency. The treating clinician must discover which mechanical objective[2] has been violated without making the block or ledge worse. Therefore, the most apical gutta-percha needs to be carefully removed manually using commercially available gutta-percha solvents and delicate, precurved endodontic files.

Once an endodontic heat carrier has been used to remove the majority of gutta-percha, it is time to switch to the solvent and manual files. The operating microscope will reveal any remaining tags of gutta-percha that may not otherwise be evident on a radiograph or digital image. Rotary nickel-titanium files can be used to facilitate gutta-percha removal. Although not available at the time of treatment (1999), specially designed ProTaper Universal treatment and re-treatment endodontic files (Dentsply) are now available for nonsurgical endodontic retreatment. The final removal of remnant gutta-percha can be accomplished using paper-point wicking to absorb the gutta-percha–solvent mixture out of the root canal system. Also not available in 1999 but available today is an instrument that is highly useful for agitating root canal system irrigants—the EndoActivator (Dentsply). This instrument facilitates the flow of the endodontic solvent into the many fins, aberrations, and cul-de-sacs that make up the labyrinth that is the root canal system.

Once complete removal of the gutta-percha has been confirmed visually and radiographically, a series of additional irrigants are necessary to remove the gutta-percha solvent because it is not miscible in any single liquid. First, sodium hypochlorite is gently flushed and agitated into the root canal system, followed by ethylenediaminetetraacetic acid (EDTA) and then alcohol to desiccate the hollow root canal system prior to three-dimensional obturation.

At this point, the previous endodontic obturation material and solvents used to remove this obturation material are removed. The root canal system is then irrigated with copious amounts of sodium hypochlorite. There were two goals at this point in the endodontic cleaning and shaping. The first goal was to discover and then clean and shape the apical portion of the underfilled root canal system in order to create the proper shape for producing the apical endodontic seal. The second was to make a continuously tapering funnel shape (Schilder's mechanical objective no. 1) that would produce a resistance form that would result in lateral canal wall hydraulics.[3,4] This reflects Bernoulli's principle, which first described the *Venturi effect* (as it is referred to in engineering), and will often provide the conditions of restrictive fluid flow that enable the dentist to obturate biologically significant lateral POEs as were suspected in this patient. Gutta-percha and sealer are the fluid mediums in endodontic obturation. Because a probable underfilled lateral POE was blocked with dentinal debris or necrotic tissue, much irrigation with sodium hypochlorite was performed to digest the probable lateral POE contents.

Deblocking the apical portion of the root canal system was the next critical and essential step.[5,6] In order to accomplish this, the clinician must begin with the end in mind by imagining the endodontic file successfully reaching the radiographic terminus, which is always some distance from the physiologic terminus. The actual physiologic constriction position can be measured using an endodontic apex locator. A precurved no. 6 endodontic file is carefully followed to the blockage. Precurving is achieved by carefully stroking the no. 6 file's shaft with dental metal cotton pliers.[1] If the instrument easily slides into the patent apical canal, then cleaning and shaping can proceed. However, in this patient, the canal seemed blocked, and the first no. 6 file was followed to at least 3 mm from the desired apical POE. Patience, restraint, and delicacy are the watchwords when deblocking. After every file removal, the canal was thoroughly yet gently irrigated with sodium hypochlorite. The no. 6 file was precurved again, and the systematic and rhythmic process was continued until the apical plug was disrupted, and the no. 6 curved endodontic file slid to the default mechanical position—the radiographic terminus, which was easily verified with a radiograph.[7] The next step was to shape the canal inside the radiographic terminus at the level of the physiologic terminus, which was again identified using the apex locator.

Once the first instrument identified the radiographic terminus, the re-treatment canal was ready to clean and shape. In 1999, rotary endodontic shaping was in its infancy; therefore, manual shaping using files and reamers in the root canal system radicular body and Gates-Glidden drills were used for coronal third radicular shaping. Shaping was finished when the gutta-percha cone fit.[8]

After the cone had been fit, the root canal system was ready for vertical compaction of warm gutta-percha.[9] The objective of vertical endodontic compaction is to capture the maximum cushion of warmed gutta-percha and mold it apically and laterally. In this way, the gutta-percha–dentin interface is minimized by distorting the gutta-percha to better take on the shape of the asymmetric foramen. Endodontic sealer (Sybron Pulp Canal Sealer, SybronEndo) fills the interface but has, like all sealers, the potential of resorption; therefore, reliance on sealer needs to be reduced as much as possible.

A radiograph demonstrated apical movement into the apical preparation (ie, downpacking) as well as surplus sealer emanating from the apparent lateral POE and lateral LEO source. In this case, the hydraulic effect was significant enough to squeeze sealer through the lateral POE (which was too small to be seen in the radiograph), through the sinus tract, and out of the orifice of the clinical sinus tract.

After backpacking with the Obtura (Obtura Spartan), an access composite restoration (Revolution, Kerr) was placed as a protective seal over the gutta-percha to prevent possible future apical microleakage. The fixed partial denture was recemented with a temporary bonding agent until the sinus tract healed and endodontic treatment of tooth no. 10 was completed.

After 2 weeks, the sinus tract had completely closed, and the endodontic treatment on tooth no. 10 was completed.

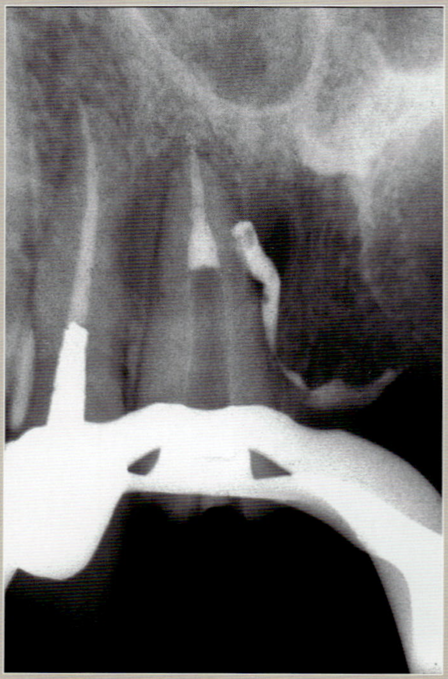

Periapical radiograph demonstrating downpacking.

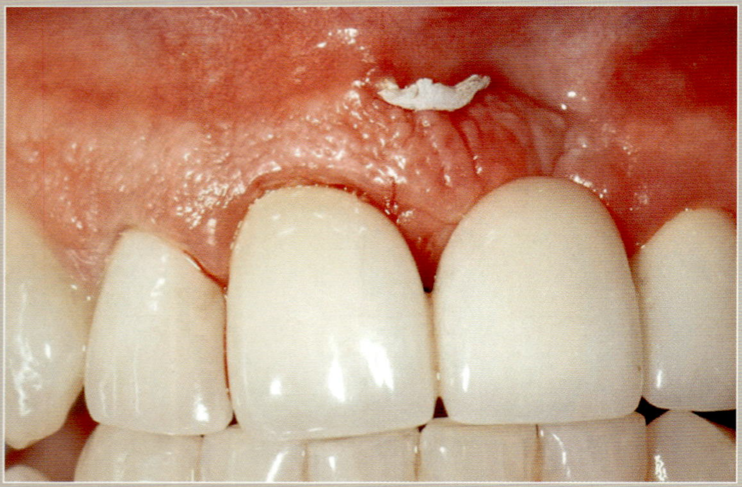

Intraoral view of surplus sealer emanating from sinus tract.

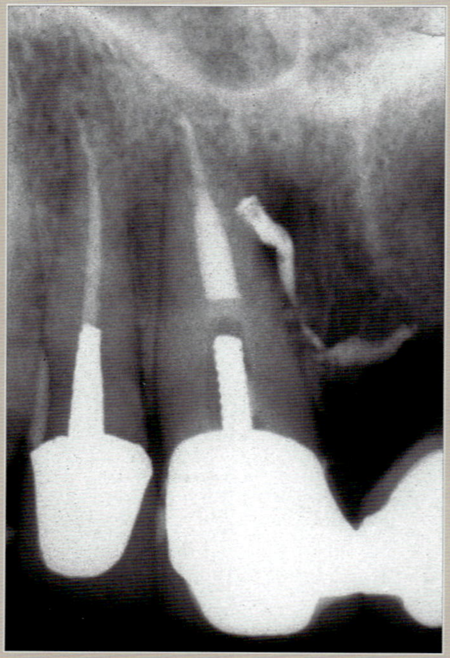

Completed nonsurgical re-treatment of tooth no. 8.

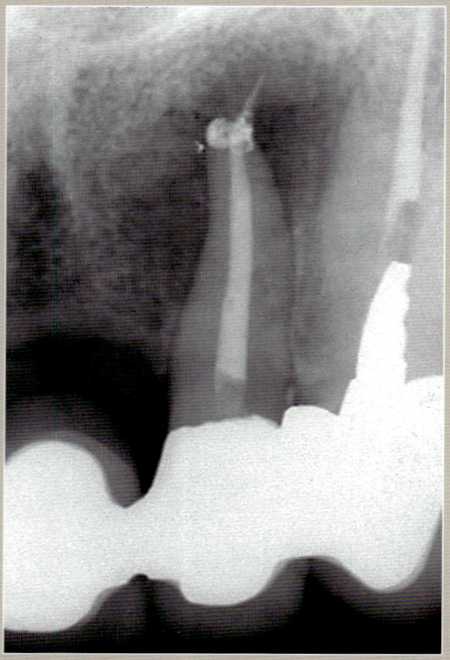

Completed nonsurgical re-treatment of tooth no. 10.

Phase V: Definitive restorative treatment and endodontic follow-up

The emphasis in treatment was directed toward solving the endodontic challenge in the maxillary anterior region. In addition, initial periodontal therapy was performed, including sessions of root planing and scaling with oral hygiene review. This was followed by periodontal surgery to reduce existing periodontal pocketing and to provide increased access for home care around tooth no. 30.

The fixed partial denture was permanently cemented, the LEO apical and lateral to tooth no. 8 and the apical LEO of tooth no. 10 completely healed, the sinus tract labial to tooth no. 8 healed, and the abutments became asymptomatic at the 6-month posttreatment recall. Periodontal pockets were well within normal levels (2 to 3 mm) at the 10- and 12-year follow-ups. The patient is now considering a new orthodontic evaluation to improve his biologic, structural, and esthetic appearance.

Posttreatment

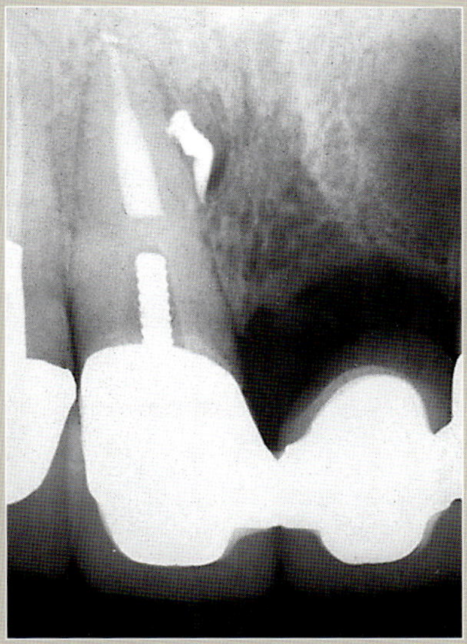

Radiograph of tooth no. 8 at
6 months posttreatment.

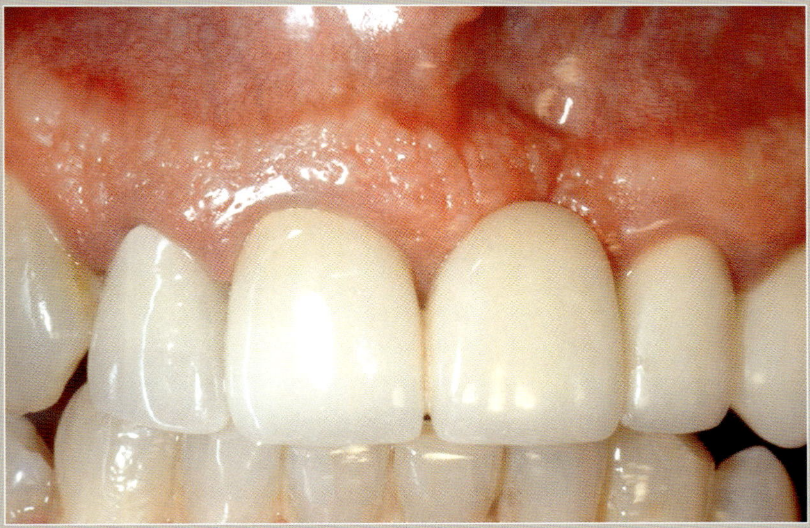

Intraoral view 6 months posttreatment.

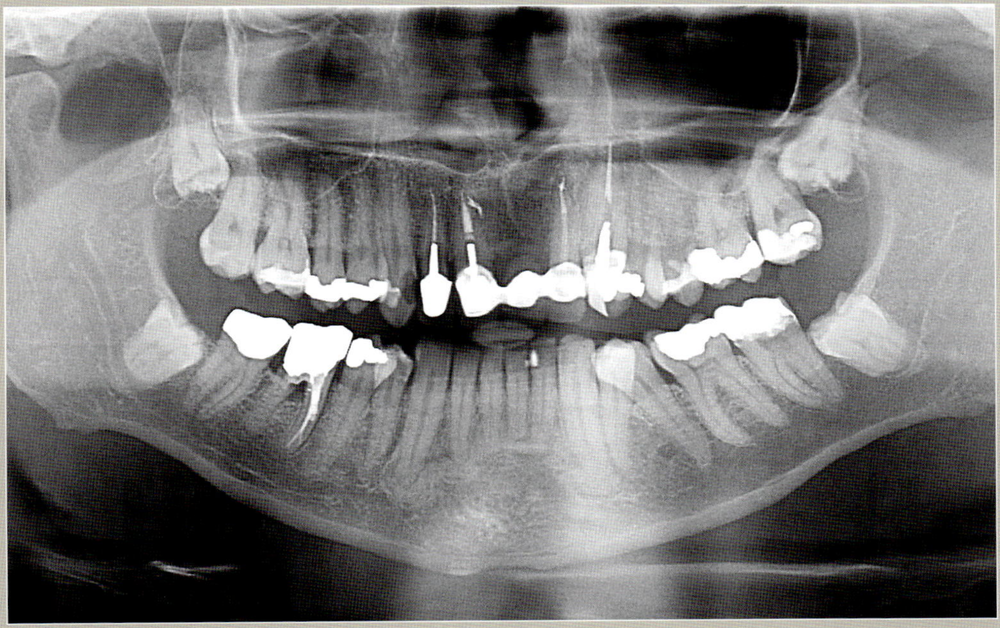

Panoramic radiograph 10 years posttreatment.

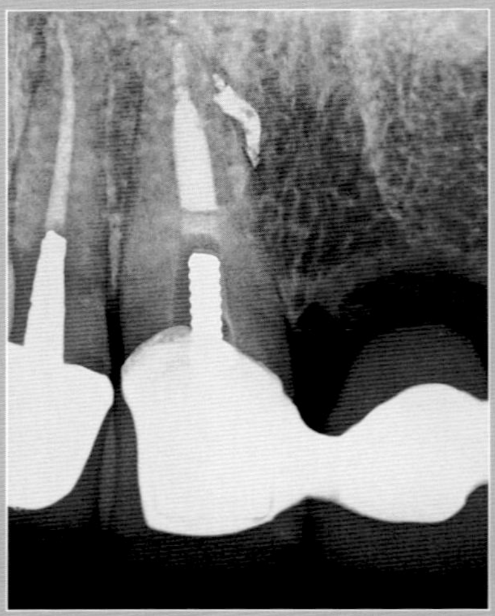

Periapical radiograph of tooth no. 8 at 10 years posttreatment.

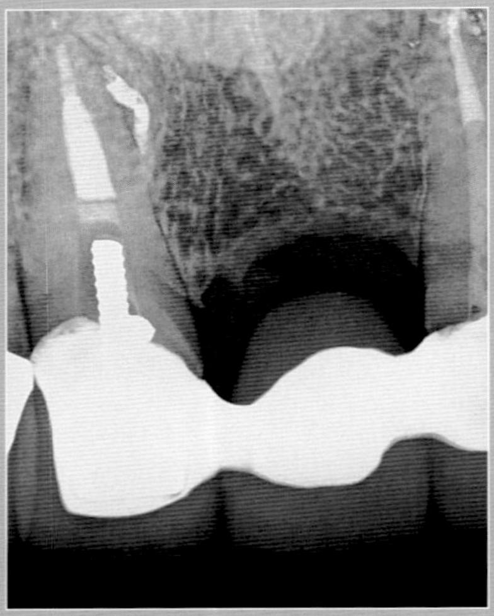

Periapical radiograph of pontic site no. 9 at 10 years posttreatment.

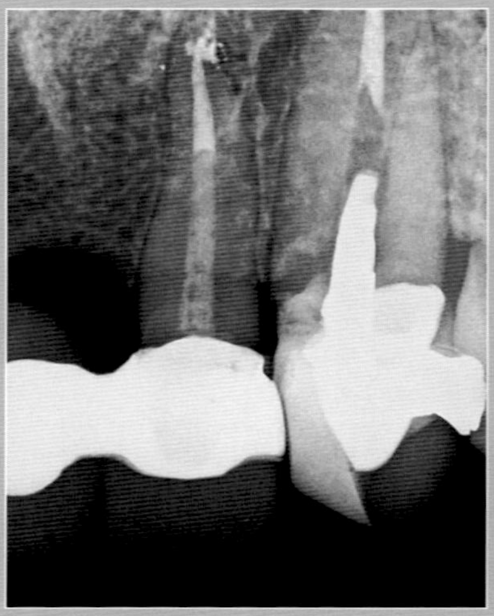

Periapical radiograph of tooth no. 10 at 10 years posttreatment.

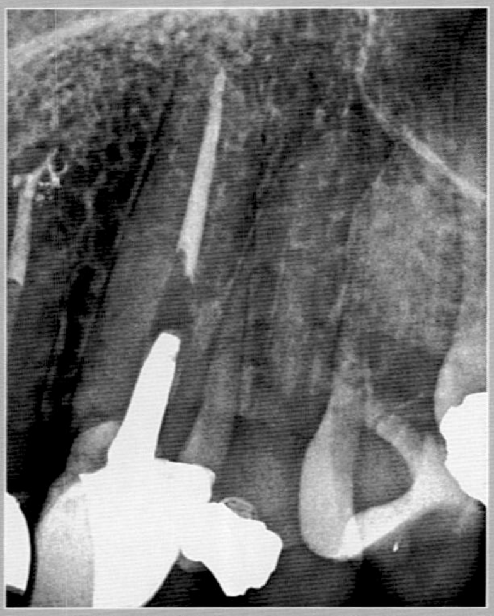

Periapical radiograph of tooth no. 11 at 10 years posttreatment.

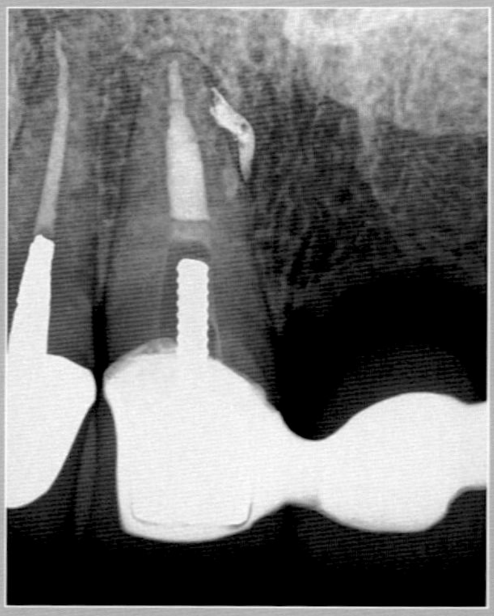

Periapical radiograph of tooth no. 8 at 12 years posttreatment.

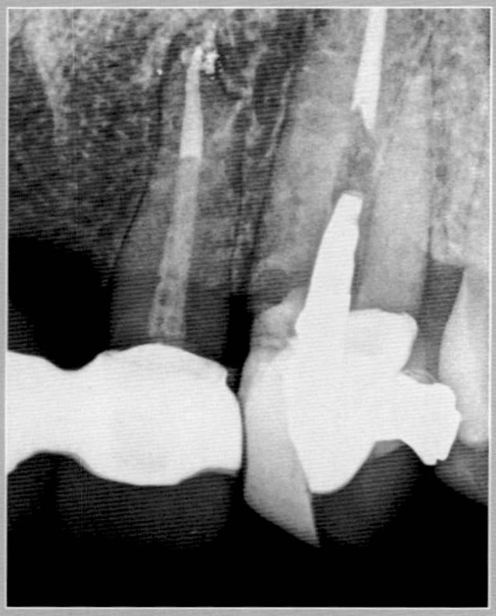

Periapical radiograph of tooth no. 10 at 12 years posttreatment.

You may now place the corresponding posttreatment overlay found in the separate folder over the pretreatment periodontal chart on page 239.

Commentary

Restore or remove?

When first diagnosing and treatment planning this patient, whether or not to save tooth no. 8 was the first consideration. While removal and replacement with a new and/or longer-span fixed partial denture or implants may have been the easy way out for the dentist, it would not necessarily have been the best option for the patient.[10] The treatment plan that was chosen instead:

- Afforded the least risk
- Resulted in the least biologic and structural sacrifice
- Presented the least esthetic risk
- Offered the least-expensive treatment option
- Provided the highest predictability as long as the nonsurgical endodontic re-treatment seal could be achieved

Safe fixed partial denture removal

This patient's entire treatment plan depended on the successful removal of his existing esthetic fixed partial denture. If the fixed partial denture fractured or if the underlying abutments were broken, the previously established backup plan could have been implemented almost immediately. This may have involved fabrication of a new and longer-span fixed partial denture or ridge preservation followed by ridge augmentation and the placement of dental implants.

Proper nonsurgical endodontic re-treatment mechanics

The purpose of endodontics is to heal or prevent LEOs. The real success of this patient's treatment lies in the belief that the capacity for endodontic healing is 100% when all significant POEs (foramina, iatrogenic perforations, or resorptions) are obturated either nonsurgically or surgically. The predictability of endodontic healing, therefore, is in direct relation to the clinician's success in achieving a three-dimensional endodontic seal.

The patient's decision to opt for this treatment plan was predicated on the confidence expressed by the endodontist that he could produce a nonsurgical endodontic seal for tooth no. 8. This confidence translated into taking the risk of fixed partial denture removal and honoring the endodontic mechanics that would allow the possibility of cleaning and obturating not only the apical POE but, more importantly, the offending LEO and sinus tract creating the lateral POE. Sufficient hydraulics was created, as evidenced by positive radiographic and clinical results during the 12-year post-treatment observation.

Would we choose this same treatment plan today?

The answer is *yes*. While the art of saving compromised teeth, particularly endodontically treated teeth, may seem to have been lost, in the proper hands it is alive and well. All that is required is the awareness that endodontists can either nonsurgically or surgically create the endodontic seal in virtually all teeth. The real question is whether or not the tooth is structurally restorable, periodontally sound or capable of being made so, and esthetically desirable.

In addition, knowing that endodontic re-treatment is a highly predictable option for dentist and patient, this gives both parties a chance to make the right choice. When doctor and patient have a number of viable choices and the patient truly understands the pros and cons of each, it is usually easier to find the right path on which to proceed. Then, and only then, are the dentist and the patient, in collaboration with the rest of the interdisciplinary team, able to design a dental future that they truly control.

The following quote by author M. H. McKee perhaps best summarizes the interdisciplinary lesson of this chapter: "Wisdom is knowing the right path to take . . . integrity is taking it."

References

1. West JD. The magic of mastering the glidepath: What every endodontist should know. Presented at the American Association of Endodontists Annual Session, San Diego, 16 April 2010.
2. Schilder H. Vertical compaction of warm gutta-percha. In: Gerstein H (ed). Techniques in Clinical Endodontics. Philadelphia: Saunders, 1983:84–90.
3. West JD. The Incidence of Underfilled Foramina in Endodontic Failures [thesis]. Boston: Henry M. Goldman School of Dental Medicine, 1975.
4. West JD. The cone fit: An essential step to creating exceptional endodontic obturation. Dent Today 2005;24(5):102–105.
5. West JD. Endodontic update 2006. J Esthet Restor Dent 2006;18:280–300.
6. West JD. Perforations, blocks, ledges, and transportations: Overcoming barriers to endodontic finishing. Dent Today 2005;24(1):68–73.
7. West JD. The endodontic Glidepath: "Secret to rotary safety". Dent Today 2010;29(9):86–93.
8. Schilder H. Cleaning and shaping the root canal. Dent Clin North Am 1974;18:269–296.
9. West JD. Finishing: The essence of exceptional endodontics. Dent Today 2001;20(3):36–41.
10. West JD. Endodontic predictability—"Restore or remove: How do I choose?" In: Cohen M (ed). Interdisciplinary Treatment Planning: Principles, Design, Implementation. Chicago: Quintessence, 2008:123–164.

10
Complex Full-Mouth Implant-Supported Reconstruction

Tal Morr, DMD, MSD

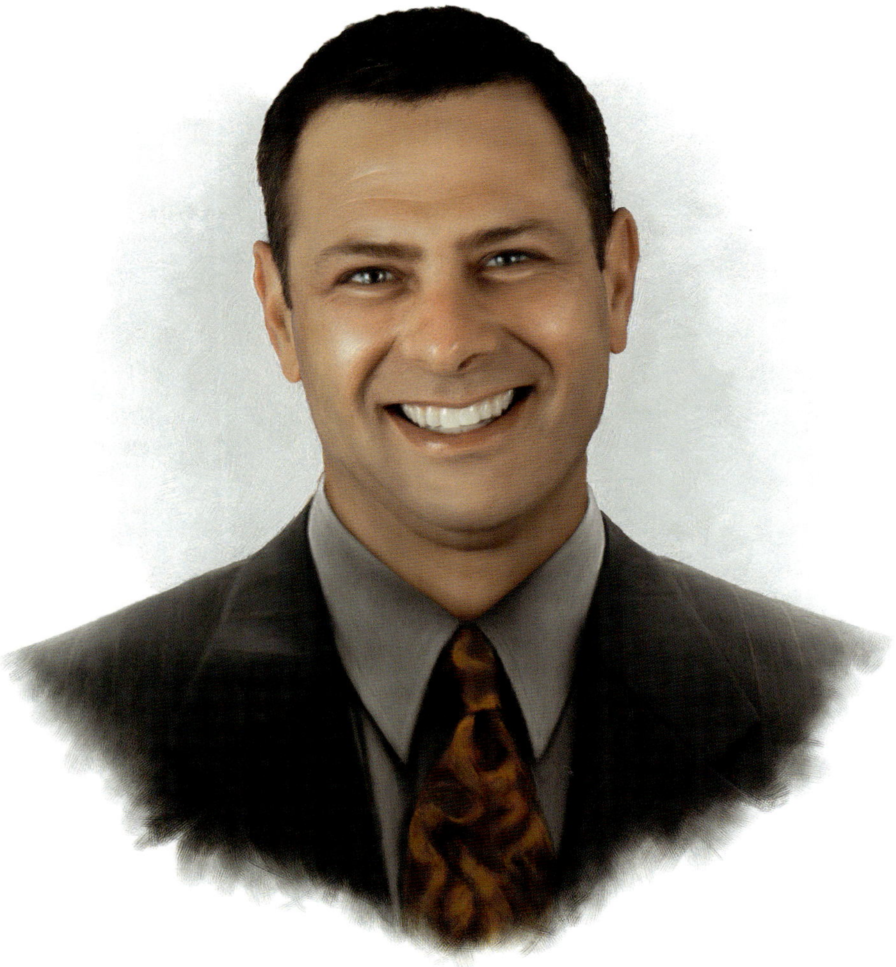

I always begin treatment planning cases by looking at the esthetic issues, starting with the patient's face and working my way inward.

Philosophy and Background

My treatment philosophy stems from my professional and personal association with some of the best dentists and technicians in the world. My passion for dentistry began at Tufts University School of Dental Medicine, where I was taken under the wing of Dr Hiroshi Hirayama, who is now the head of the prosthodontics program. Finishing my clinical requirements early gave me the opportunity to work on complex cases both in the clinic and in the laboratory. This experience sparked the initial passion for my present specialty. I will never forget when Dr Hirayama told me that I needed to become a prosthodontist and gave me a list of schools at which to interview for prosthodontics training. Alas, my adventure began.

I now look back at the path that I have taken, the people I have met on this journey, and the way they influenced me as a person and as a clinician, and I can honestly say that attending the graduate prosthodontics program at the University of Washington was the best decision I ever made. Having an extraordinary group of mentors gave me the passion and direction to strive for the highest standard of care while maintaining integrity, honesty, and the idealistic concept of doing what is best for the patient.

In our graduate program, the concept of interdisciplinary treatment was introduced and implemented on a daily basis. It was ingrained in each and every student through interaction with and treatment of patients, as well as in the interdisciplinary treatment-planning seminars with the other graduate specialty programs.

I began private practice with the mindset that I would treatment plan my patients from an idealistic point of view with the highest level of care. I began collaborating with the finest specialists in the area as well as some of the best technicians in the world. This interaction helped expand my knowledge base from an interdisciplinary as well as a technical standpoint and ultimately helped me become a more complete clinician.

I chose this particular clinical case because it is truly complex in nature and encompasses the full spectrum of variables, including esthetic, biologic, mechanical, structural, and functional problems. All of the variables are interrelated, making this case an interesting puzzle to solve. Readers may also discover some unfamiliar prosthetic techniques that I often use in daily practice with great success.

Case Presentation

Case Presentation

Treating clinicians
Prosthetic rehabilitation: Tal Morr, DMD, MSD
Periodontal and implant surgery: Isaac Garazi, DMD
Maxillary interim and final prosthesis: Onofrio Azzaretto, MDT
Mandibular final prosthesis: Harald Heindl, MDT, and Daniela Heindl, CDT

Clinical Treatment Planning

Age at initial presentation: 71 years
Initial presentation: August 2006
Active treatment completed: January 2008

Introduction and background

At the time of presentation, the patient was a retired widow living in Washington, DC. She was born in Sweden and had lived all over the world during her lifetime. Her son lived in Miami and had been a patient in our office for 3 years. During a visit with her son, she presented to our office with a feeling that her maxillary right fixed partial denture was "loose and about to fall out of her mouth." She was ready to address all of her dental needs after many years of living with patchwork dentistry. She wanted to begin with treatment in the maxillary arch and also desired a plan that would last long term.

Medical history

- History of high blood pressure, which was being treated with metoprolol
- History of sinus problems
- No other medical contraindications

Dental history

This patient had a long dental history but had a difficult time recalling past treatment dates. She was married, and because of her husband's occupation, they moved quite often, living in many foreign countries. Because she did not feel comfortable being treated comprehensively in a foreign country, she only sought treatment on an emergency basis. Around 1980, she went to see a dentist in Lebanon who suggested she have all her maxillary teeth prepared and a fixed partial denture made. She did not speak the language and was skeptical yet proceeded with treatment. A few years later, her dentition began to fall apart. The patient and her husband moved to Washington, DC, and she selected a family dentist who was not experienced in the discipline of implant dentistry. He told her that he had practiced on his staff and recommended implant placements on the mandibular right side due to failing teeth that exhibited advanced periodontal disease. Three implants were placed. A few years later, her dentist retired, and she went to see another dentist because she was experiencing discomfort in the mandibular left posterior area. He recommended extraction of the remaining teeth in that area and replacement with implants. A short while after having implants placed in the mandibular left posterior segment, the same dentist placed implants in the maxillary left posterior segment, and subsequently additional implants were inserted in the mandibular anterior region. The patient felt that her bite was never the same following the anterior implant placements and subsequent restoration. She was also concerned because she noticed some movement of her maxillary fixed partial denture. This was the impetus for her initial visit to our office.

Pretreatment

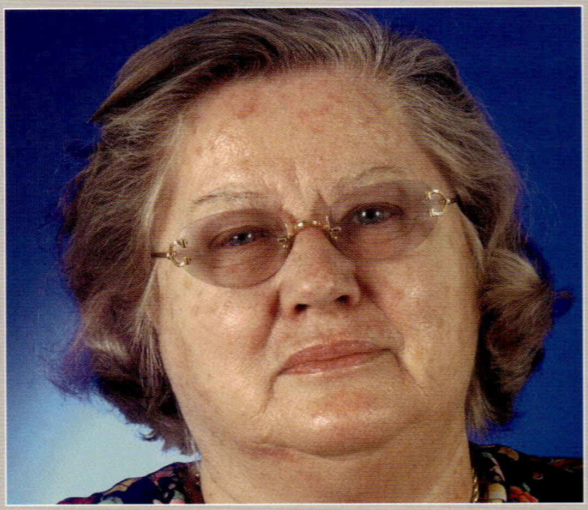

Facial view with lips together.

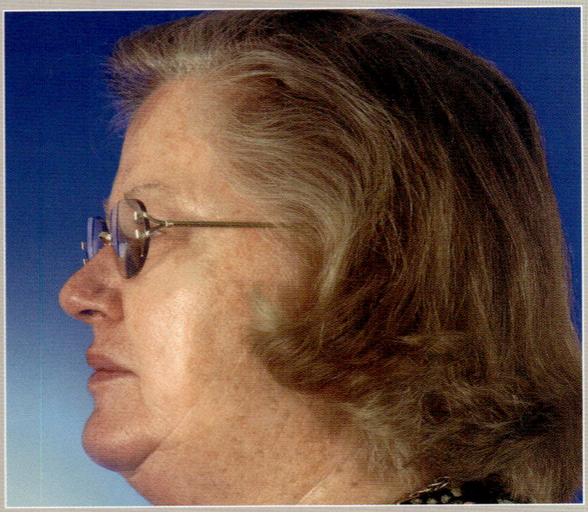

Profile view with lips together.

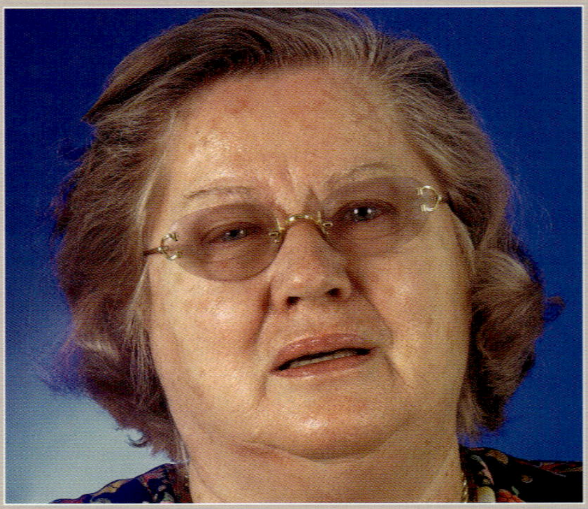

Facial view with lips at rest.

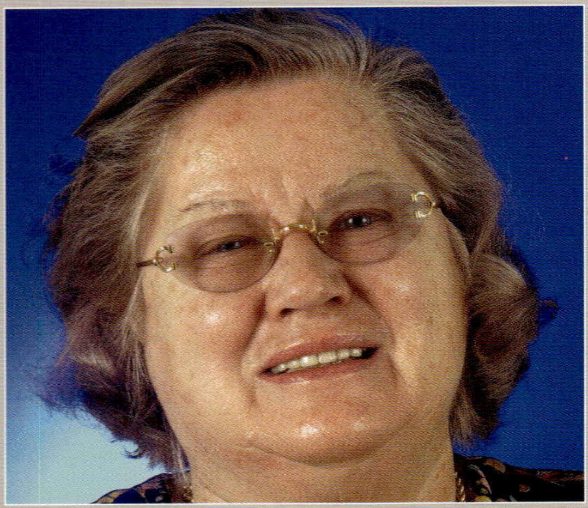

Facial view of smile.

Diagnostic findings

Extraoral and facial findings

- Slightly overclosed appearance with downturned commissure
- Large masseter muscles
- Flat to concave profile with deficiency localized to maxillary arch
- Maxillary teeth hidden at rest
- Low lip line during smiling
- Large negative space on left side when smiling
- Irregular maxillary occlusal plane due to deficiency in length of the maxillary left posterior teeth
- Irregular mandibular occlusal plane with a drop in the posterior occlusal plane distal to the canines and an irregular incisal plane

TMJ and mandibular range of motion

- TMJ within normal limits
- Mouth opening and range of motion within normal limits
- No muscle discomfort or tenderness to palpation

Intraoral findings

- Generalized bleeding on probing with plaque and calculus
- Missing teeth nos. 1, 5 to 7, 10, 12 to 16, 17 to 21, 24 to 26, and 28 to 32
- Implants in sites nos. 12 to 14, 19 to 21, 24, 26, and 28 to 30
- Maxillary right and anterior porcelain-fused-to-metal fixed partial denture from teeth nos. 2 to 11 with extreme mobility (Class III)

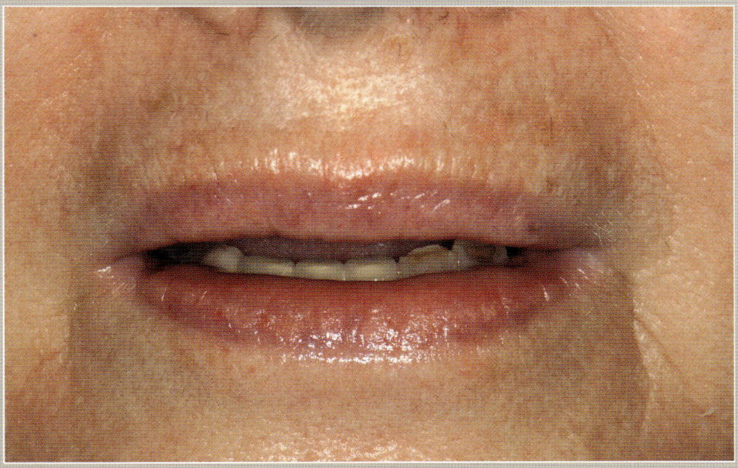

Lips at rest.

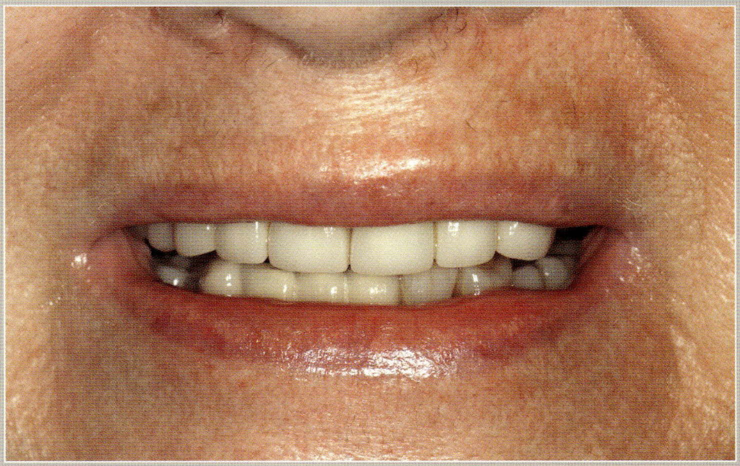

Smile.

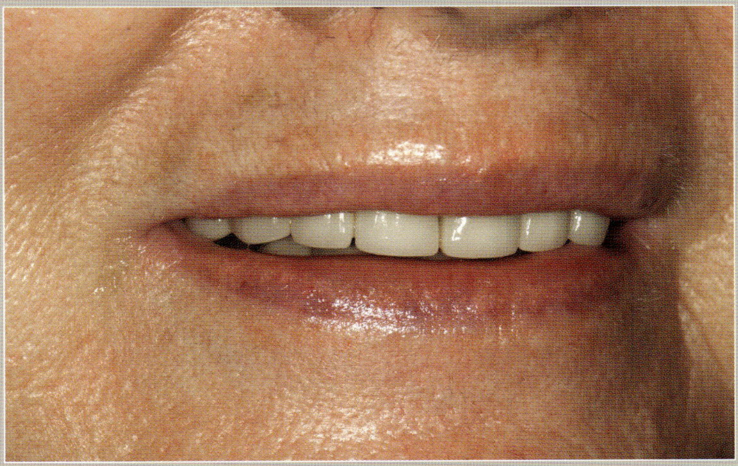

Right lateral view of smile.

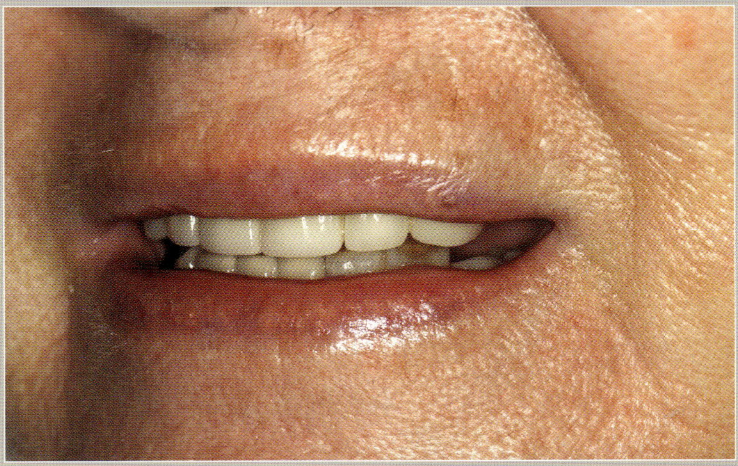

Left lateral view of smile.

- Fracture of metal frame between central incisors on existing fixed partial denture
- Maxillary and mandibular left implants are Bicon with friction-fit posts and composite crowns (single units)
- Mandibular anterior implants are Bicon with friction-fit posts and a porcelain-fused-to-metal fixed partial denture (splinted)
- Mandibular right implants have screwed-in abutments with a cemented fixed partial denture (splinted); records did not identify implant type
- Natural teeth nos. 22 and 23
- Porcelain-fused-to-metal crown on natural abutment of tooth no. 27
- Generalized gingival recession on all natural maxillary teeth
- Generalized horizontally deficient maxillary ridge with exaggerated defect at sites nos. 5 to 7
- Purulent exudate from mandibular anterior implant-supported fixed partial denture
- Very irregular gingival margin position in both arches with resultant disproportion of teeth
- Visual evidence of wear of the mandibular lateral incisors and left canine

Occlusal notes

- Centric relation (CR) not coincident with maximal intercuspal position; first point of contact in the anterior segment
- Deep vertical overlap with very steep anterior guidance
- Class II canine relationship on right and left sides
- Constricted envelope of function
- Patient reports clenching habit

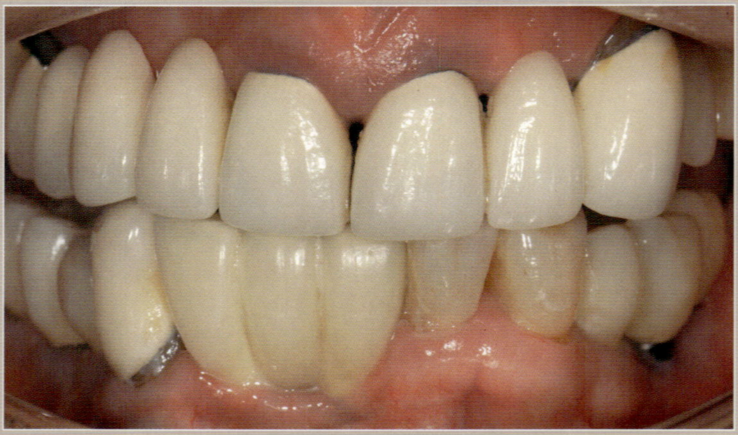

Intraoral frontal view.

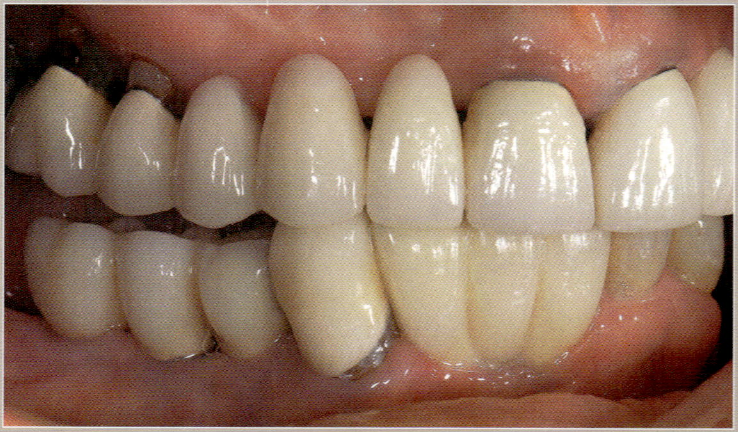

Intraoral right lateral view.

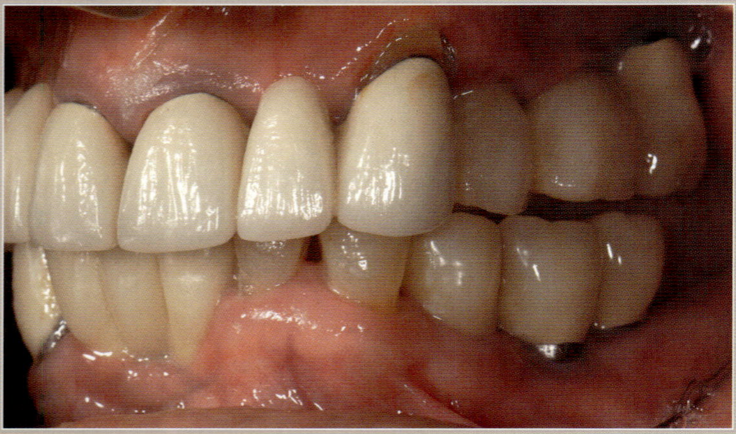

Intraoral left lateral view.

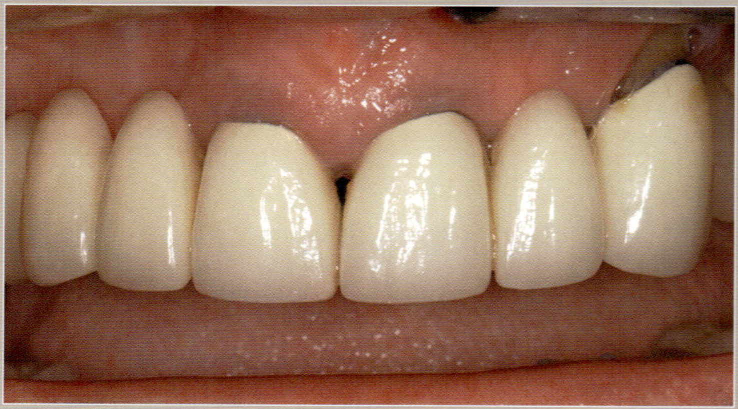

Maxillary anterior view.

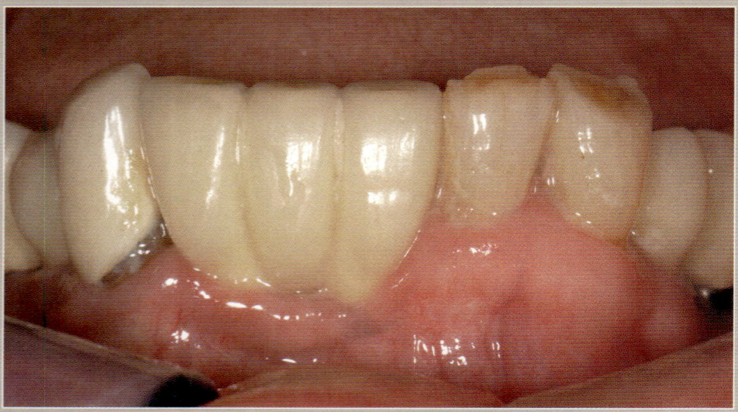

Mandibular anterior view.

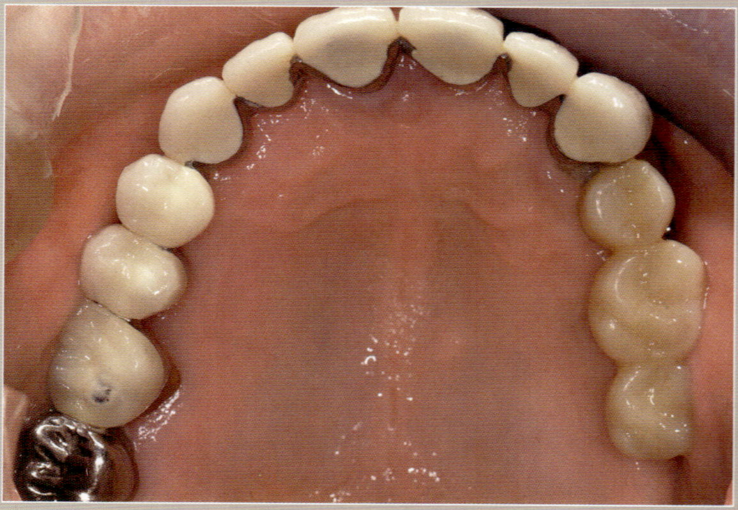

Maxillary occlusal view.

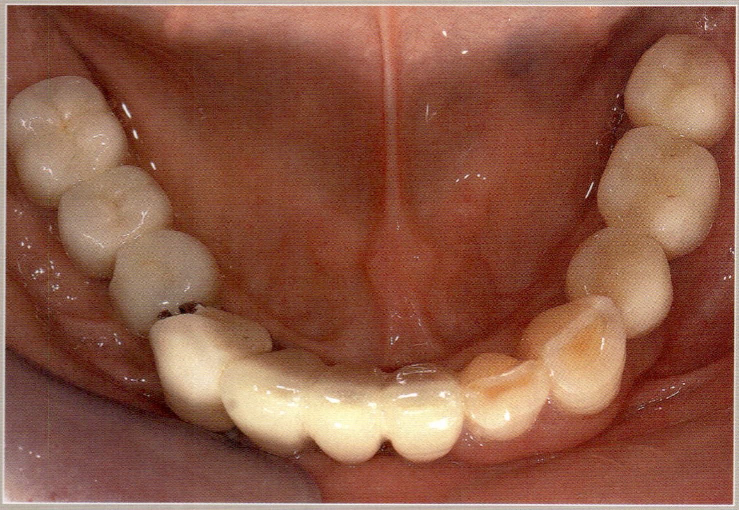

Mandibular occlusal view.

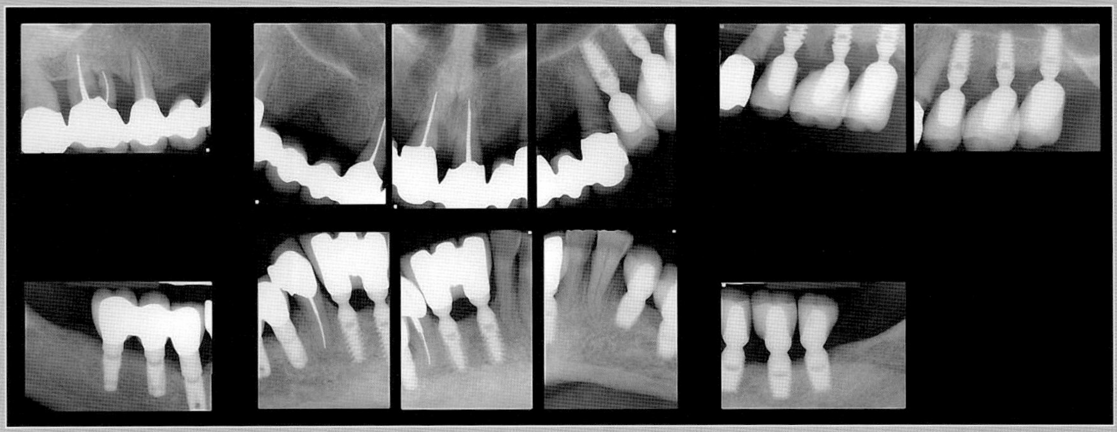

Complete full-mouth radiographs.

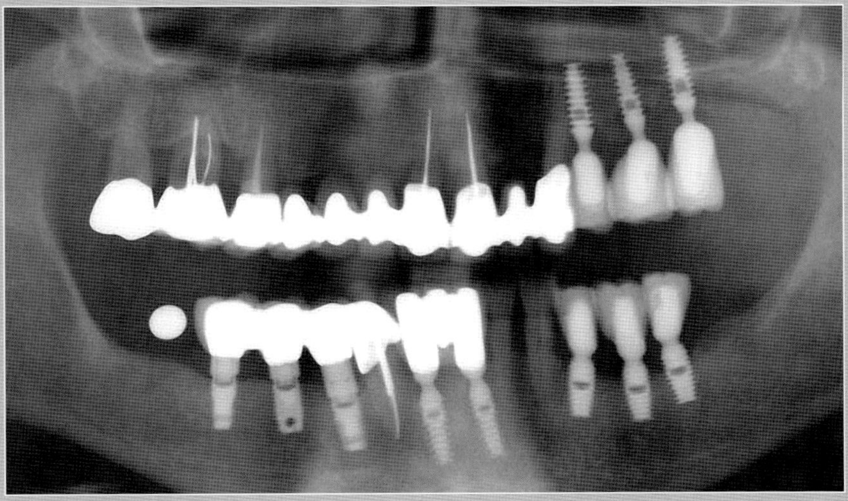

Panoramic radiograph.

Radiographic findings

- Advanced attachment loss on teeth nos. 2 to 4, 8, 9, and 11 with "well-like" defects on the maxillary teeth
- Bony defect on maxillary right ridge, sites nos. 5 to 7
- Exposure of one to two threads on all maxillary left implants with "well-like" bony defects present
- Exposure of two to three threads on all mandibular left implants, although bone loss is mostly horizontal
- Moderate to advanced bone loss on remaining mandibular teeth nos. 22, 23, and 27
- Fracture of tooth no. 11
- Class III furcation involvement of tooth no. 3 with root caries
- Caries noted on teeth nos. 2, 3, 8, 9, and 11

Oral hygiene habits

- Patient is afraid to brush her maxillary teeth due to mobility; she does swish with salt water.
- Patient brushes mandibular teeth two times per day.

Diagnosis

- Generalized moderate to advanced periodontitis
- Generalized early to moderate peri-implantitis with purulent discharge localized to mandibular anterior fixed partial denture
- Lack of attached tissue around the mandibular anterior implant-supported fixed partial denture, sites nos. 23 to 26
- Multiple missing teeth
- Failure of maxillary fixed partial denture at sites nos. 2 to 11
- Caries on teeth nos. 2, 3, 8, 9, 11, and 27
- Fracture of tooth no. 11
- Angle Class II canine relationship on right and left sides
- Constricted envelope of function

Prognosis

- General: good, with the assumption that all of the failing, periodontally involved teeth are extracted and a stable and supportive prosthesis is made with modification of the occlusal scheme and deep vertical overlap
- Teeth nos. 2, 3, 4, 8, 9, and 11: hopeless
- Teeth nos. 22, 23, and 27: questionable because of their lack of importance in overall treatment scheme
- Existing implants: fair to good, assuming establishment of plaque control, hygiene access, and controlled occlusal forces

Summary of concerns

1. How do we manage the patient's dental phobia due to negative past experiences?
2. How do we manage the patient's concern about undergoing extensive surgical treatment?
3. Are the patient's numerous existing implants, which have friction-fit, narrow abutments and compromised support, adequate?
4. When it comes to deciding which areas to address first, how will we reconcile the patient's priorities with those of the treatment team?
5. Can we help the patient improve her poor oral hygiene?
6. How do we manage the esthetic bony and soft tissue deficiencies and irregularities?
7. What type of maxillary prosthesis can we fabricate that will minimize surgery while providing rigidity and cross-arch stability and supporting the vertical dimension?
8. How do we manage the inability to remove the existing abutments and crowns from the implants?
9. How do we resolve the mandibular peri-implantitis?

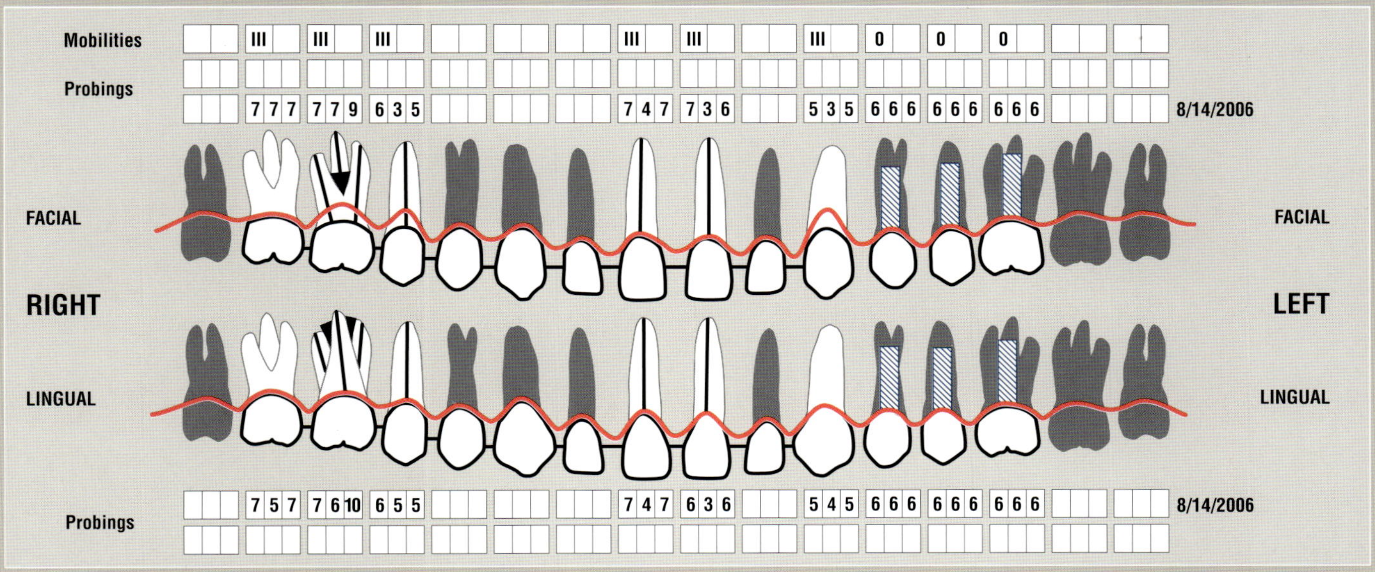

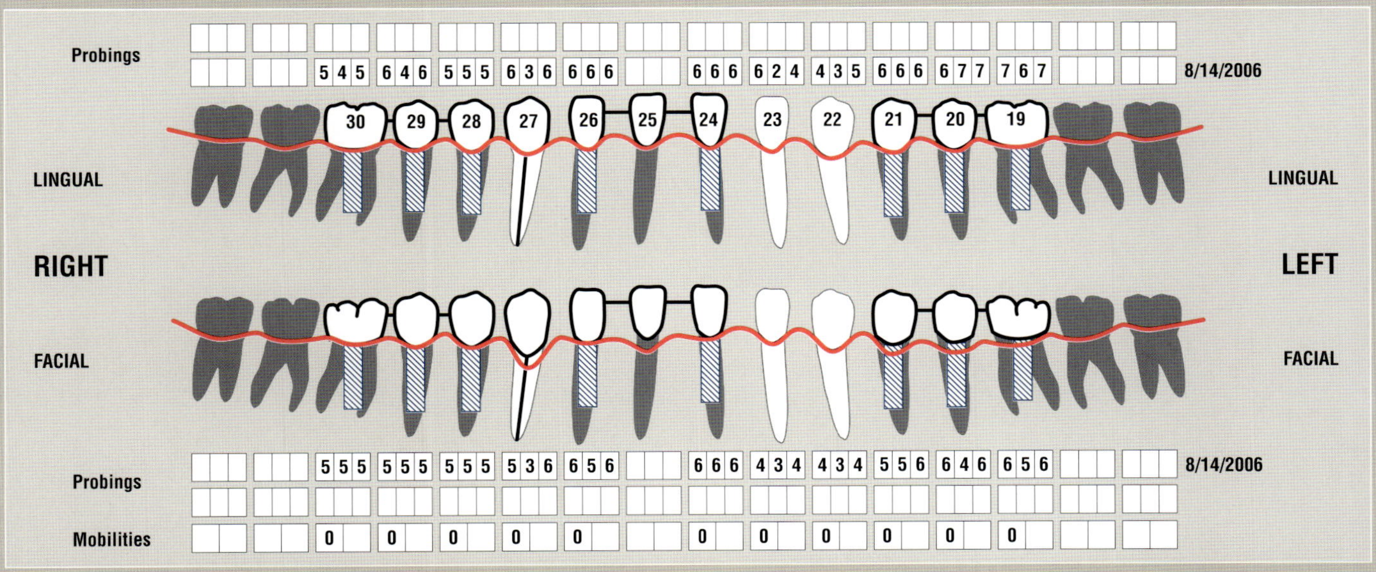

As a learning exercise, you may now outline goals/objectives of treatment and a treatment plan.

Proposed Treatment Plan

Goals/objectives of treatment

- Eliminate disease
- Improve esthetics
- Fabricate a full-mouth rehabilitation that is more functional, with cross-arch stability and support of the vertical dimension
- Establish an occlusal scheme that places less force on the future abutments

Phase I: Treatment planning

1. Radiographs
2. Extraoral evaluation
3. Intraoral evaluation
4. Photographs
5. Diagnostic casts
6. Occlusal plane guide to determine the correct occlusal plane
7. Mounting of the maxillary cast with the occlusal plane guide using the Kois Dento-Facial Analyzer (Panadent) mounting platform
8. Mounting of the maxillary and mandibular diagnostic casts using the Kois Dento-Facial Analyzer mounting platform on the Panadent semi-adjustable articulator

Phase II: Fabrication of maxillary provisional restorations and interim partial denture

9. Cutting of teeth nos. 3 to 11 off the cast and replacement with setup for interim partial denture
10. Waxing of teeth nos. 2 and 12 to 14 for provisional restorations
11. Fabrication of the maxillary interim partial denture and provisional shells by the laboratory using the Dento-Facial Analyzer platform to set the maxillary teeth

Phase III: Initial therapy

12. Scaling and root planing in maxillary left posterior segment and mandibular arch with placement of Arestin (OraPharma) around existing implants
13. Extraction of maxillary teeth nos. 3, 4, 8, 9, and 11 with debridement of sockets
14. Provisionalization of tooth no. 2
15. Preparation of composite crowns and reline with acrylic shell to fabricate implant provisional restorations on the maxillary left implants, sites nos. 12 to 14
16. Reline of the interim partial denture for sites nos. 3 to 11
17. Adjustment of mandibular anterior teeth with selective grinding to develop an appropriate incisal plane

Phase IV: Healing and surgical planning

18. Waiting period of 6 to 8 weeks for tissue to close over extraction sockets
19. Soft reline of the fixed partial denture
20. Duplication of the maxillary interim partial denture for surgical stent fabrication
21. Radiographic evaluation by the periodontist for appropriate implant placement in the maxillary arch using the surgical stent, a panoramic radiograph, and the diagnostic maxillary cast
22. Planning for the placement of two implants in the maxillary right posterior segment (sites nos. 3 and 4), two in the anterior region (sites nos. 8 and 9), and possibly two in the canine regions (if bone is available) for a friction-fit galvano prosthesis

Phase V: Surgery

23. Patient sent to periodontist for implant placements with surgical guide
24. Implants placed in sites nos. 3, 4, 8, and 9 with healing abutments
25. Soft reline of maxillary interim partial denture
26. Wait 3 months for integration of implants

Phase VI: Use of implants to stabilize maxillary interim partial denture

27. Placement of temporary abutments on implants and relining of the maxillary interim denture to add stability

Phase VII: Optimization of mandibular contour and occlusion

28. Alginate impressions of maxilla (with provisional restorations and partial denture) and mandible (as is)
29. Wax-up of mandibular arch to level and align the occlusal plane and idealize the bite relationship
30. Fabrication of provisional shell from the wax-up
31. Preparation of mandibular composite crowns on Bicon implants intraorally
32. Removal of porcelain-fused-to-metal fixed partial dentures from remaining implants without disturbing the existing abutments, if possible
33. Extraction of teeth nos. 22, 23, and 27 and reline of mandibular acrylic shell with acrylic
34. Optimization of contour and occlusion

Phase VIII: Free autogenous gingival graft at sites nos. 23 to 26

35. Patient referred to periodontist to perform a soft tissue graft in the area of sites nos. 23 to 26 to address lack of attached tissue

Phase IX: Maxillary final impression and CR record

36. Placement of impression transfers on implants and packing of cord on modified abutments in maxillary left area
37. Final impression in maxillary arch
38. CR record of maxillary to mandibular provisional using bite rim

Phase X: Finalization and delivery of maxillary prosthesis

39. Removal of healing abutments
40. Torquing down of telescopic abutments
41. Placement of galvano copings on telescopic abutments
42. Try-in of frame for passivity
43. Cementation of telescopic abutments to frame
44. Back to laboratory for processing of prosthesis
45. Delivery of prosthesis and modification of occlusion if necessary

Phase XI: Mandibular final impression and CR record

46. Removal of provisionals and packing of cord around implant abutments
47. Final impression and CR record of maxillary definitive prosthesis against mandibular implant abutments

Phase XII: Finalization and delivery of mandibular prosthesis

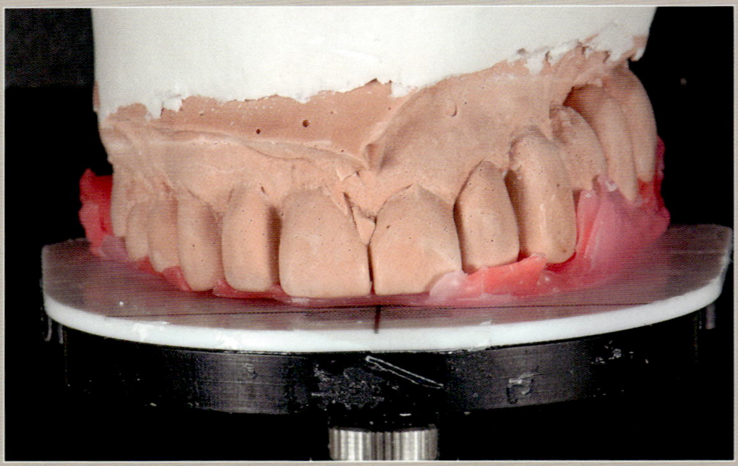

Occlusal plane guide on mounting plate.

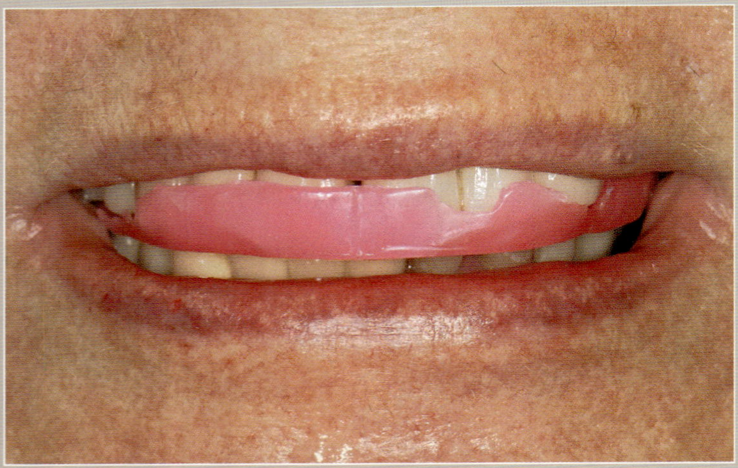

Occlusal plane guide try-in.

Review of the goals/objectives of treatment

- Eliminate disease
- Improve esthetics
- Fabricate a full-mouth rehabilitation that is more functional, with cross-arch stability and support of the vertical dimension
- Establish an occlusal scheme that places less force on the future abutments

Phase I: Treatment planning

At the initial examination, a full evaluation was performed on the patient, including esthetic, extraoral, and intraoral assessments, as well as taking radiographs, photographs, and alginate impressions for diagnostic casts. Taking the maxillary diagnostic impression involved blocking out the undercuts with wax and taking a maxillary alginate impression, being very careful not to remove the failing and loose maxillary fixed partial denture.

The patient was informed that due to the complexity of her case, a meeting would be necessary between the periodontist and prosthodontist in order to create a comprehensive and practical treatment plan. The patient was scheduled for a periodontal examination that day, and given the emergent nature of her disease and the importance of timely intervention, the treatment plan was completed the next day.

The patient returned a few days later, at which time the diagnosis, treatment plan, and fees were discussed with the patient, and she agreed to treatment. She emphasized that she wanted to start with the maxillary arch first because it was more of an emergency situation. We agreed to begin treatment in the maxillary arch; however, we also emphasized the importance of controlling the active exudate around the mandibular anterior teeth. The patient agreed to some initial periodontal therapy in the mandibular anterior segment, including prophylaxis and placement of Arestin (minocycline hydrochloride 1 mg) to control the exudate.

Given that the maxillary fixed partial denture (sites nos. 2 to 11) was failing and ready to completely dislodge from her mouth, time was of the essence. Treatment in a timely fashion would not only stabilize her occlusion and enable her to continue to function but also help build her self-esteem and improve her overall outlook regarding treatment. She had many past negative dental experiences, and the primary goal was to make her feel comfortable.

From an esthetic standpoint, we wanted to lengthen the teeth and bring them out labially; this critical information needed to be transferred to the laboratory. Three layers of pink baseplate wax (Allcezon Dental Wax, Mizzy) were folded, heated, and applied to the maxillary cast. The edges were rolled over the labial and lingual aspects. This was cooled and removed from the cast and tried in the mouth to evaluate the ideal tooth position and occlusal plane (in the same way that an occlusion rim is used for dentures).

The patient was asked to pronounce the letter *m* and to relax her jaw to evaluate the incisal edge position at rest. The patient was then asked to smile to evaluate the incisal and occlusal planes. The baseplate was removed and adjusted with a torch and a spatula until the ideal incisal edge position and occlusal planes were developed. A vertical line was made in the wax indicating the midline. The wax was then warmed in a hot water bath, and a CR record was taken using the occlusal plane guide[1] at an open vertical dimension to allow for decreasing the vertical overlap and lengthening the maxillary teeth.

The mandibular cast was marked with pencil in the anterior area to indicate the degree of incisal reduction necessary to establish an ideal incisal plane (ie, shortening teeth nos. 22, 23, and 27 to become level with the remaining incisors). The ideal incisal plane is based on the maxillary occlusal plane guide and the horizontal plane of the face. The objective was to shorten the teeth in the laboratory to the ideal position before fabricating a provisional restoration. Finally, VITA Physiodens denture teeth (Vita Zahnfabrik) were selected, and the patient was consulted for shade selection.

The maxillary cast was placed, with the wax occlusal plane guide, on the Kois Dento-Facial Analyzer mounting platform with the midline of the occlusal plane guide lined up with the midline on the platform and the facial aspect of the wax lined up with the horizontal line of the platform. This platform is made for use with a Panadent semi-adjustable articulator (Magna-Split II System). Aligning the cast on the plate places the maxillary anterior teeth 100 mm from the hinge axis of the articulator with the same horizontal relationship as the teeth have with the face. It has been shown in the literature[2–6] that 80% of the population falls within 1 standard deviation of the mean if the anterior teeth are placed 100 mm from the hinge axis of the articulator. Using this technique eliminates the need for an earbow or dentofacial analyzer to mount the maxillary cast because the wax allows the cast to be mounted relative to the correct horizontal plane of the face and the mounting plate allows the maxillary cast to be mounted the appropriate distance from the hinge axis by aligning it to the marks on the mounting plate.[1]

Once the casts were mounted in our office, the mandibular anterior teeth (nos. 22, 23, and 27) were shortened on the cast to the ideal length and horizontal plane (indicated by the pencil marks) based on the maxillary wax occlusal plane guide.

Phase II: Fabrication of maxillary provisional restorations and interim partial denture

The next step was to meet with the laboratory technician: Instructions were given to cut down teeth nos. 3 to 11 from the cast and fabricate a resin base. The technician was then directed to set the teeth following the contour of the wax. Once the teeth were ideally positioned, the remaining teeth on the cast (nos. 2 and 12 to 14) were waxed ideally to flow with the set teeth from an esthetic standpoint. Having the baseplate allowed the technician to remove the teeth from the cast so that the wax-up could be finished cleanly. The waxed-up cast, without the partial denture, was duplicated to allow fabrication of the provisional restorations on a separate cast. The final step was for the technician to bend clasps and process the interim partial denture.

Phase III: Initial therapy

The objective of initial therapy is always to eliminate disease. In this case, removing the remaining maxillary teeth would achieve our goal. Even though treatment was necessary in the mandibular arch, the patient was adamant about treating the maxillary arch first. She did agree to initial prophylaxis and insertion of Arestin around the anterior mandibular and maxillary left implants.

We also discussed with the patient the need to level and slightly shorten the mandibular anterior teeth with a bur to idealize the incisal plane and tooth length. She approved this measure, and we leveled the mandibular anterior teeth to mimic the original pencil marks drawn on the casts. The maxillary left implant crowns were then prepared with burs intraorally as if they were natural teeth, given that the existing crowns and abutments were one piece and friction-fit and therefore could not be removed. The next step was to anesthetize the patient. The maxillary right segment of the existing fixed partial denture was sectioned between teeth nos. 2 and 3. All of the existing maxillary teeth were extracted, the sockets were thoroughly debrided with various instruments, and a Gelfoam absorbable gelatin sponge (Pfizer) was inserted for hemorrhage control. Chromic gut sutures (Ethicon) were used to help hold the Gelfoam in place.

Given the amount of active infection, the periodontist wanted to allow the areas to heal without socket grafting.

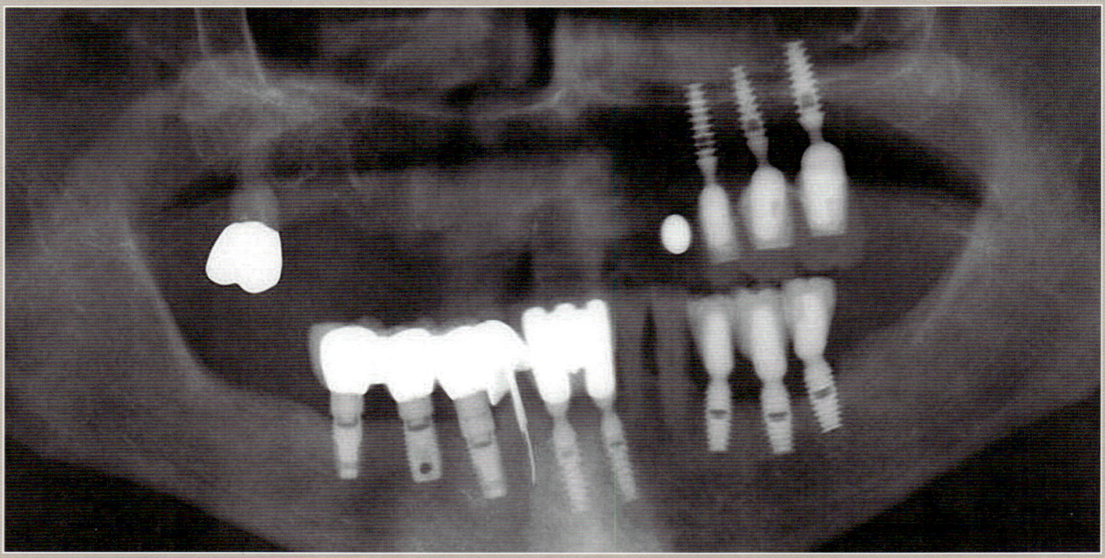

Radiograph after extraction of teeth and placement of provisional restorations.

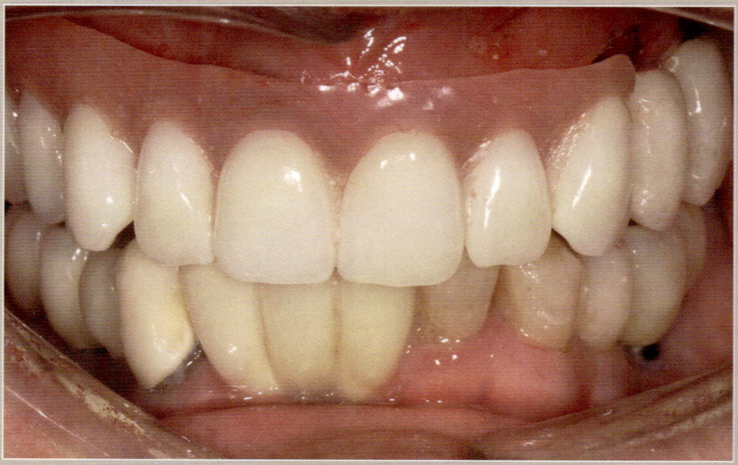

Maxillary interim partial with provisional on the day of extractions.

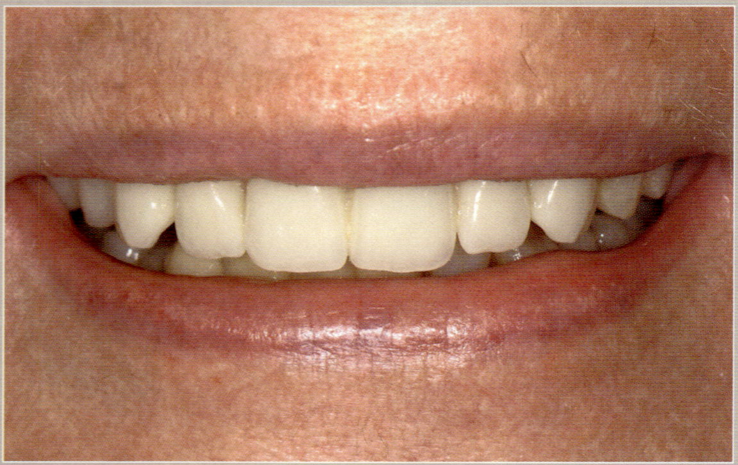

Smile view of maxillary provisional restoration at delivery.

The provisional shells were placed into the interim partial denture, and everything was tried in together. Adjustments were made until all the segments fit passively and properly at the same time. The interim partial denture was painted with petroleum jelly, and Alike acrylic (GC) was mixed and introduced into the provisional shell. The interim partial denture and provisional shells were placed into the mouth as one unit and pumped in and out until the provisional restorations were set. The provisional restorations were removed and trimmed. The next step was to grind the internal aspect of the interim partial denture and reline with PermaSoft denture liner (Denstply). Once set, the interim partial denture was removed and trimmed. The provisional restorations were polished on a lathe and cemented into place with Durelon carboxylate cement (3M ESPE). Final adjustments were made, and the patient was sent home with a prescription for antibiotics, pain medication, and a chlorhexidine rinse (Periogard, Colgate). Postoperative instructions were given to the patient.

Phase IV: Healing and surgical planning

The patient spent 6 weeks in Washington, DC, before returning for treatment. The interim partial denture was relined again with a soft reline material (PermaSoft) to stabilize the denture against the healing ridge. The interim partial denture was then removed and sent to the laboratory for duplication in clear acrylic for fabrication of a surgical stent. Once ready, the clear replica of the interim partial denture was tried in and verified for accurate fit. Drill slots were made to allow the duplicated denture to be used as a surgical guide for implant placement.

The patient was sent to the periodontist for radiographic evaluation with the surgical sent. The periodontist took a panoramic radiograph as his diagnostic tool. The plan was to place two implants in the maxillary right posterior area (in sites nos. 3 and 4). Two implants would be placed in the anterior region, in sites nos. 8 and 9, and possibly two additional implants would be placed in the maxillary canine

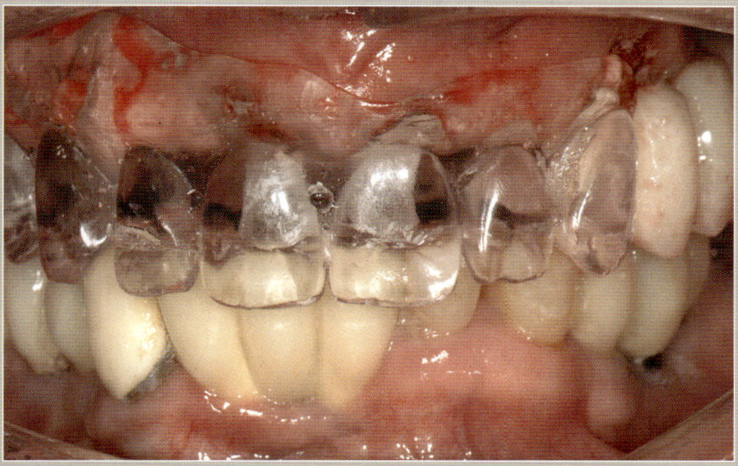

Clear acrylic duplicate of interim partial denture at try-in.

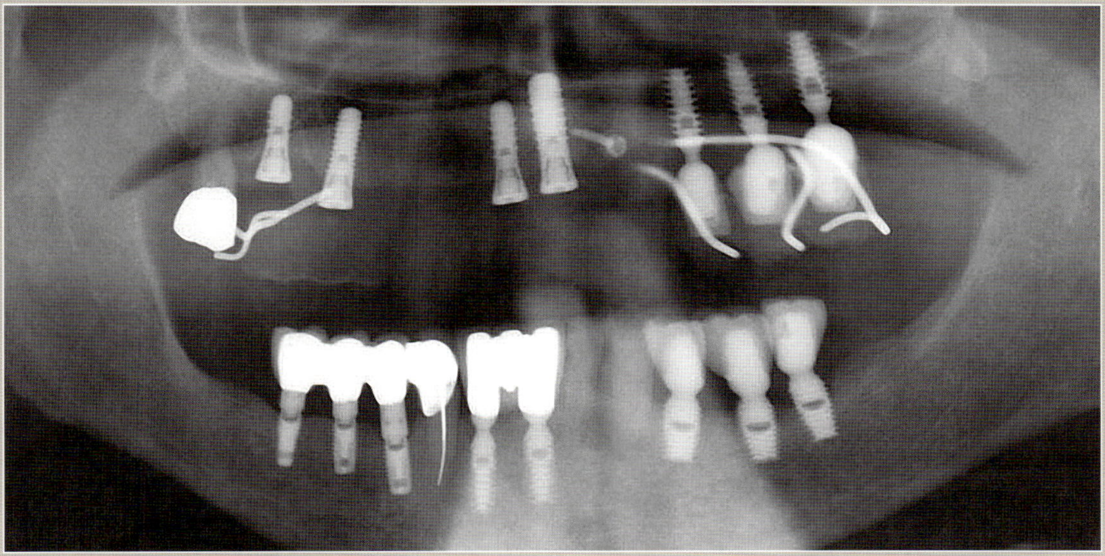

Panoramic radiograph after implant placement.

positions to obtain cross-arch stability and a large anteroposterior spread. However, the surgeon was not sure he could place implants in the canine positions because of the horizontal deficiencies in the ridge. Once the surgical implant planning was completed, surgical treatment was initiated.

Phase V: Surgery

The patient was now ready for implant placement in the maxillary arch. The objective was to gain cross-arch stability with the smallest number of implants to minimize the cost to the patient.

Upon reflecting the flap, the periodontist decided that the sites of teeth nos. 3, 4, 8, and 9 were best suited for implant placement. Due to the infection associated with the fractured tooth no. 11, there was a very large defect in that area. The surgeon chose to reconstruct the ridge in the area of sites nos. 9 to 11 with Regenaform (Exactech), a moldable allograft paste; an Ossix collagen membrane (OraPharma); and a tenting pin for possible future implant placement because the original plan was to possibly place implants in the canine regions. Although site no. 6 was not ideal for implant placement, a connective tissue graft procedure was performed to augment the ridge.

Four Straumann implants were inserted. The patient immediately returned to our office for seating of the interim partial denture and relining with a soft base material (PermaSoft). The patient was placed on antibiotic therapy, Periogard, and pain medications and given postoperative instructions. She was asked to return a week later for reevaluation. After uneventful healing was confirmed, she went home to Washington, DC.

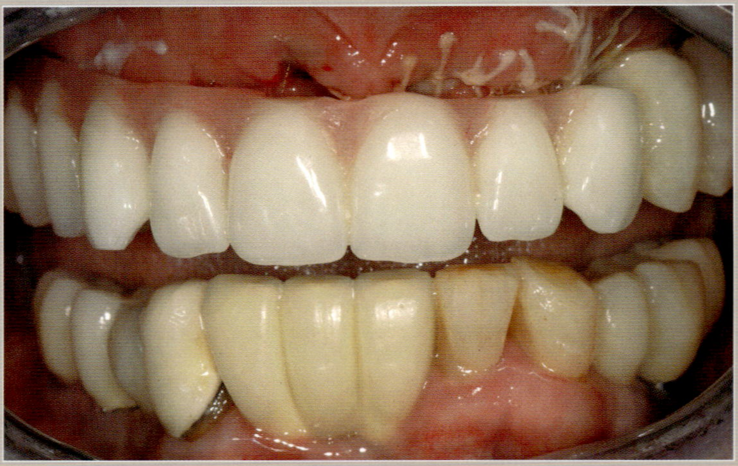

Maxillary interim partial denture after implant surgery and grafting.

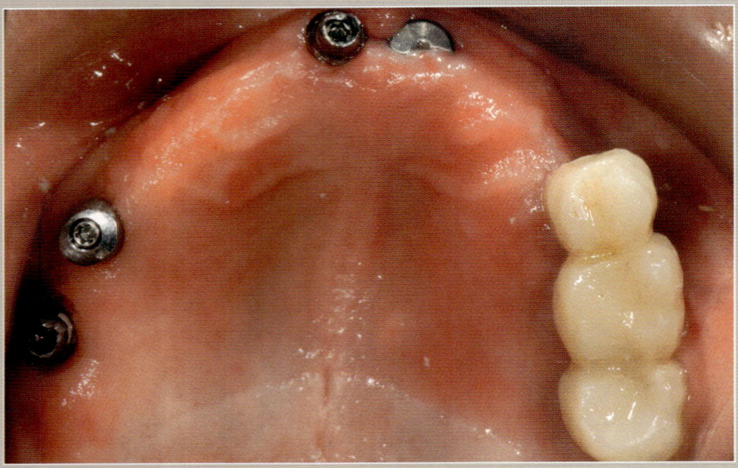

Maxillary occlusal view of temporary abutments.

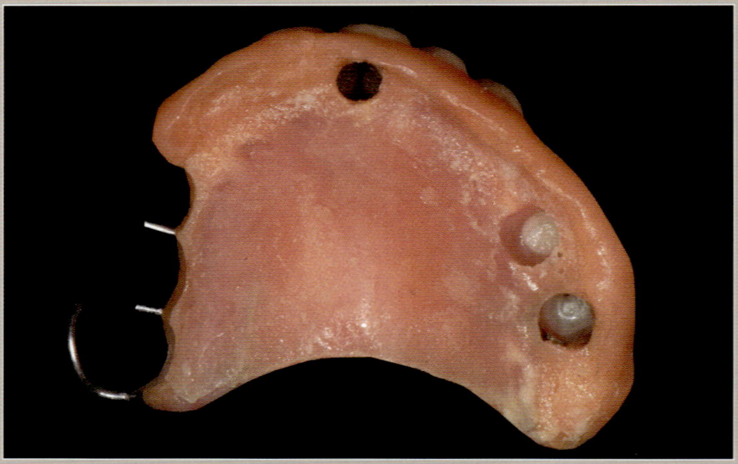

Maxillary interim partial denture hollowed out in areas of temporary abutments.

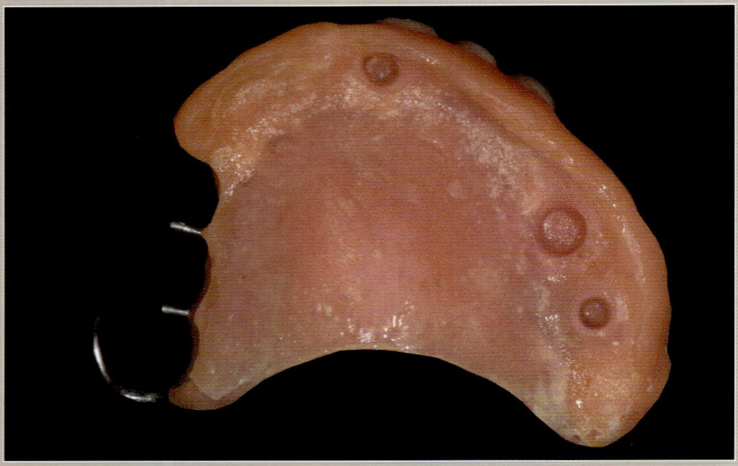

Relined maxillary provisional interim partial denture.

Phase VI: Use of implants to stabilize maxillary interim partial denture

The patient returned 3 months postoperatively. The implants were tested by the periodontist, who found they were all well integrated. Two temporary Straumann abutments were placed on implants nos. 3, 4, and 8 and marked with a black marker to indicate the path of draw relative to the existing prepared implants on the maxillary left side. The abutments were prepared at the laboratory and chairside and then placed back in the mouth, and minor adjustments were made so that they had the same path of draw as the prepared implants in the maxillary left quadrant.

The interim partial denture was hollowed out in the areas of the temporary abutments until it was completely seated without any interference. The whole inside of the interim partial denture was ground and relined so that the palatal aspect and the holes were filled with PermaSoft soft denture reline material to allow the maxillary interim partial denture to readapt to the healed ridge and to intimately fit around the temporary abutments and remaining healing caps. We again discussed with the patient the need to complete treatment in the mandible prior to completion of the maxillary prosthesis, based on the following considerations:

- The inability to perform adequate hygiene in the mandibular anterior segment
- The pseudo-hemiseptal defect in the anterior area
- The stepped mandibular occlusal plane

The patient agreed to proceed with provisionalization of the mandible.

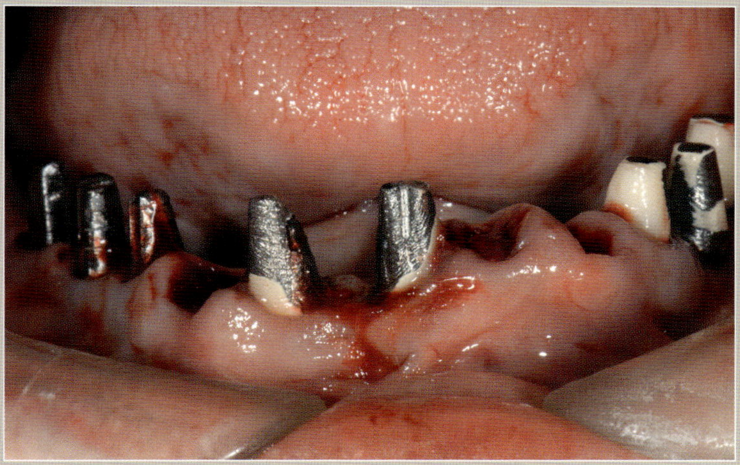

Following extraction of remaining mandibular teeth.

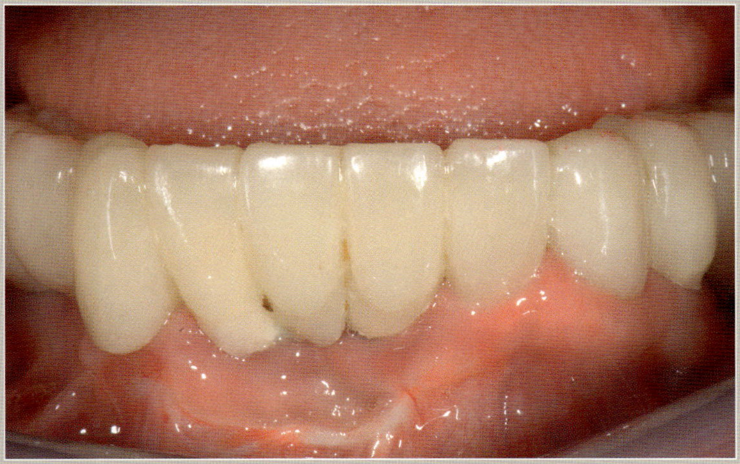

Mandibular provisional restoration following free gingival graft.

Phase VII: Optimization of mandibular contour and occlusion

Alginate impressions were taken of the maxillary provisional restorations and interim partial denture and the existing mandibular arch. These were poured and mounted on a semi-adjustable articulator (Magna-Split II). The mandibular arch was idealized in wax to level the plane and create a better occlusal relationship. Once the wax-up was completed, an acrylic shell was fabricated using a putty matrix of the wax-up and the "salt and pepper" technique with Alike acrylic. The mandibular left composite crowns were prepared with a bur in a fashion similar to that performed in the maxillary left quadrant. The remaining mandibular implant-supported fixed partial dentures were removed through preparation of the porcelain and the metal until the abutments were reached. We did not know if there were abutments underneath or if the fixed partial dentures were attached in one piece with the abutments. This was a long, painstaking process, but we managed to find abutments underneath the existing fixed partial dentures. All of the remaining mandibular teeth were extracted and the sockets debrided and filled with Gelfoam absorbable gelatin sponge. The provisional shell was filled with the same acrylic as the shell and relined in the mouth. It was trimmed, and the occlusion was idealized.

Phase VIII: Free autogenous gingival graft at sites nos. 23 to 26

Due to the lack of attached tissue in the area of sites nos. 23 to 26, the periodontist performed a free autogenous gingival graft procedure. Esthetics was not a concern in this area.

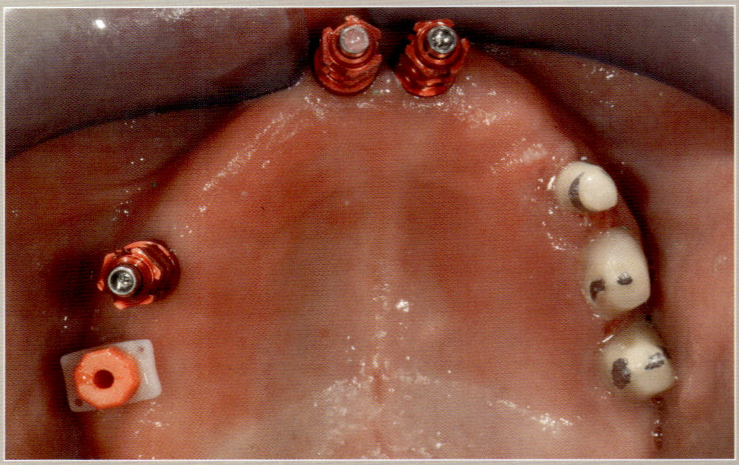

Transfer copings in the maxilla.

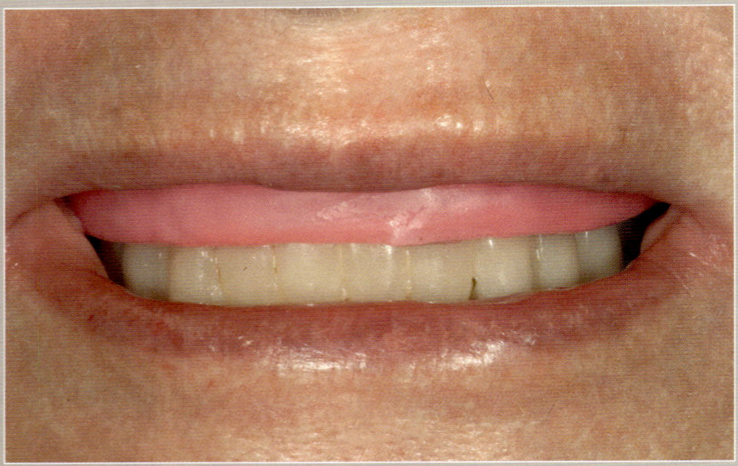

Maxillary occlusion rim try-in for mounting the maxillary definitive cast against the mandibular provisional cast.

Phase IX: Maxillary final impression and CR record

During the postoperative phase, we took final impressions in the maxillary arch. All of the healing abutments and the healing caps were removed, and transfer copings were placed on the implants. Cord was packed around the maxillary left prepared implants as would be done for a conventional fixed partial denture impression. A custom tray was used to capture the maxillary final impression. The provisional restorations were then reseated.

The impression was sent to the laboratory to pour and fabricate a maxillary occlusion rim. The patient returned, and the occlusion rim was modified to the ideal arch form, lip support, incisal plane, and occlusal plane, and a CR record was taken against the mandibular provisional restorations. A mandibular alginate impression was taken as well to allow mounting of the casts.

Phase X: Finalization and delivery of maxillary prosthesis

In the laboratory, the casts were mounted on the semi-adjustable articulator using the Kois Dento-Facial Analyzer mounting platform as described in the diagnostic section. The same denture teeth as in the interim partial denture were ordered by the technician and were set in the same relationship. This was sent back to our office for try-in. Once verified for accuracy in the mouth, a matrix was made of the teeth onto the cast, and the wax was boiled out. Using the teeth as a reference, UCLA-type Straumann abutments were trimmed, waxed, and milled to a 0- to 2-degree taper in the cervical 4 mm and a 4-degree taper for the remaining height. This was invested and cast in a precious high-gold alloy (Argedent Euro, Argen). Once cast, the abutments were polished and checked for ideal draw and taper.

For the maxillary left segment, copings were waxed and cast using the dyes fabricated from the final impression. Once milled and idealized on the final impression, a secondary galvano coping was fabricated directly on the primary abutments as described in the literature.[7] Basically, this type of fabrication is achieved by applying a thin layer of a silver conductor to the telescopic abutment and placing it in a galvano bath overnight. This process creates a galvano coping of about 3 mm in thickness with a friction fit. This coping is made of 99.9% pure gold and has been shown to allow a precise fit that is superior to that of conventional metal castings.[7-9] Once the abutments (ie, primary copings) and galvano copings (ie, secondary copings) are fabricated, the final impression with these two components is duplicated and poured in investment material (Bellavest SH, Bego). A chrome cobalt frame is waxed and cast in chrome cobalt alloy (Argeloy N.P. Partial, Argen).

Once the three components were ready, the primary copings were left on the cast, and a positioning jig was fabricated using Pattern Resin (GC). All of the abutments were screwed in the mouth, and the gold copings made for the maxillary left implants were cemented with a small amount of Freegenol temporary cement (GC). All of the galvano copings were placed on top of the abutments. The framework was tried in to ensure a passive fit of the frame with slight space between the frame and the galvano copings. The copings were then luted into the frame intraorally using a self-

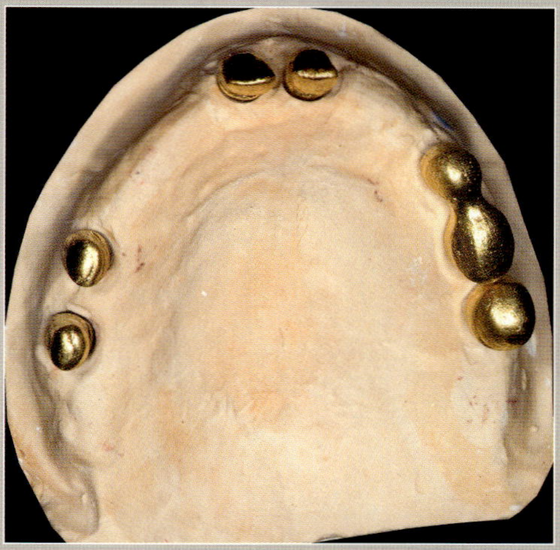

Galvano (secondary) copings placed on telescopic (primary) abutments.

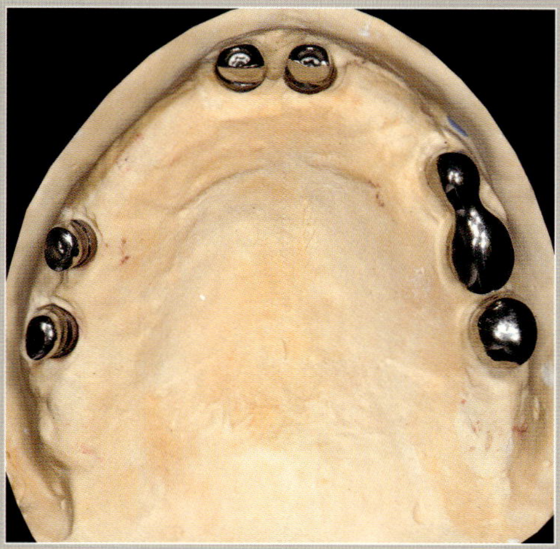

Telescopic (primary) abutments on the maxillary cast.

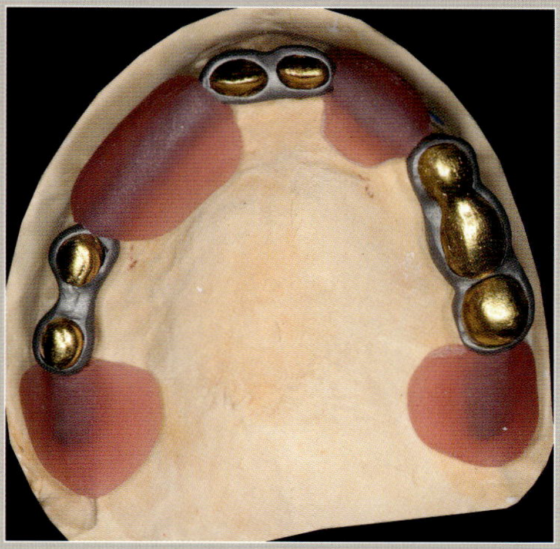

Chrome cobalt frame and resin positioning jig placed over the galvano copings.

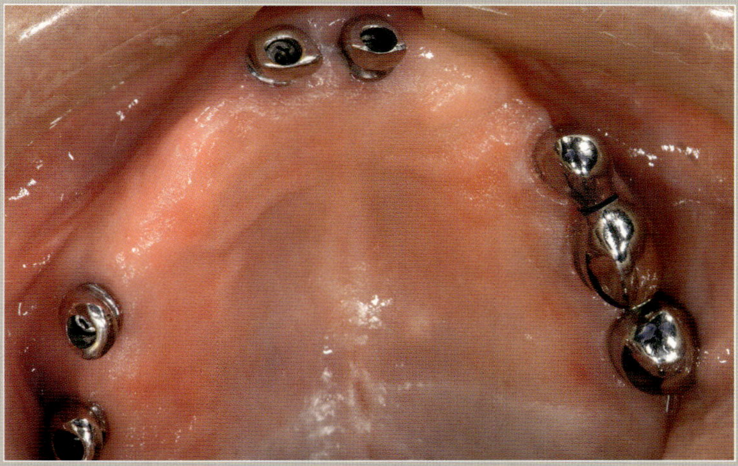

Maxillary occlusal view of telescopic (primary) abutments on the implants.

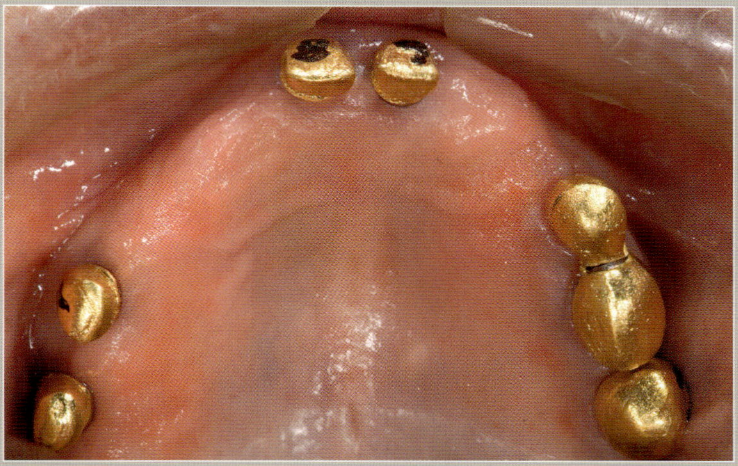

Maxillary occlusal view of galvano copings placed on telescopic abutments.

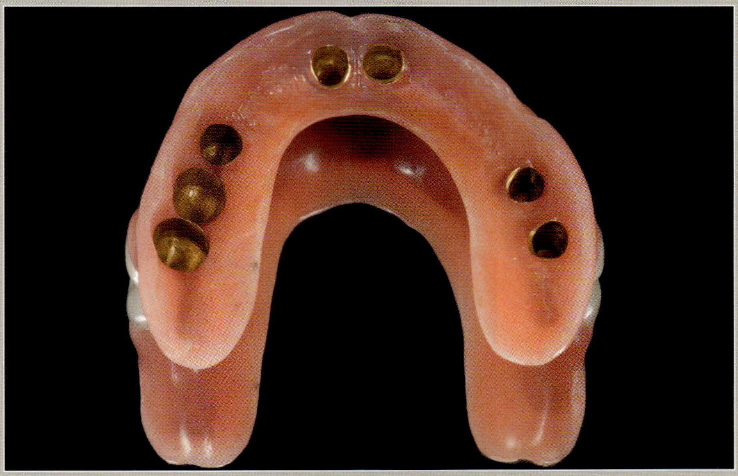

Occlusal view of maxillary definitive prosthesis.

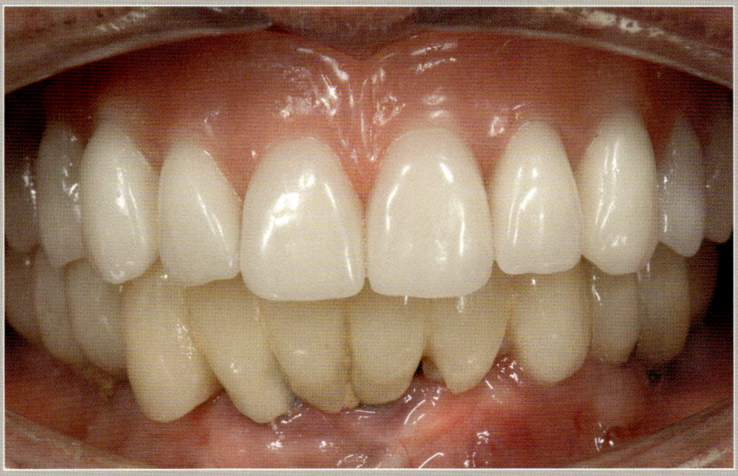

Maxillary definitive restoration and mandibular provisional restoration.

curing resin cement, Nimetic-Cem (3M ESPE), which is made specifically for this purpose.

The frame with the galvano copings was removed as one unit, and the abutments and copings were removed from the mouth. This was sent back to the lab to check the accuracy of the cast. Once the precision relative to the cast was confirmed, the teeth were waxed back to the frame using the matrix, and the wax-up was tried in the mouth. When the esthetics and occlusion were confirmed as appropriate, the prosthesis was finished in acrylic and delivered. All of the definitive abutments were torqued down to 35 Ncm, and the maxillary left gold copings were cemented with Panavia (Kuraray), using the definitive prosthesis to seat these copings during cementation to ensure proper positioning. Postoperative instructions, including those for care of the prosthesis, were given to the patient.

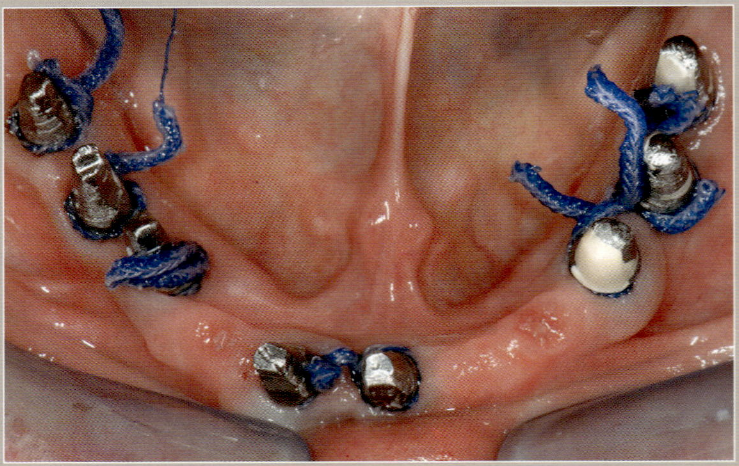

Cords in place for final mandibular impression.

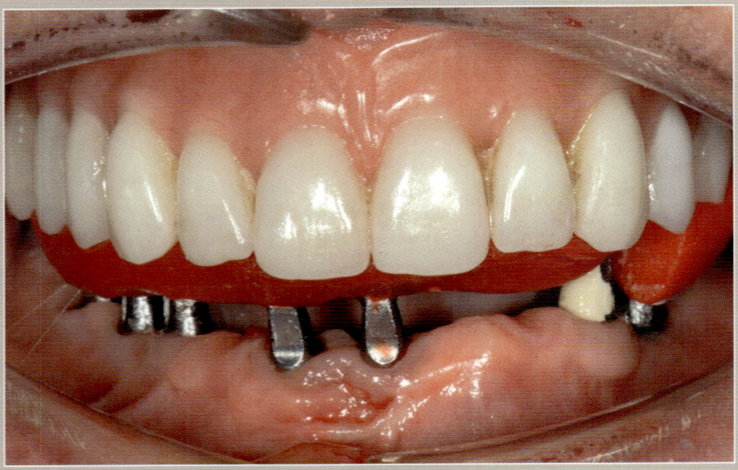

Registration of maxillary definitive prosthesis against mandibular implant abutments.

Phase XI: Mandibular final impression and CR record

By the time the maxillary prosthesis was delivered, the mandibular graft had healed. Exudate was no longer present around the implants, and the ridge and soft tissue had healed in the areas where the teeth had been extracted. Because we could not remove the mandibular left and anterior abutments from the implants, the mandible was treated with a conventional impression technique.

The patient was given anesthetic, and Ultrapak #1 cord (Ultradent) was dipped in ViscoStat Clear (Ultradent), a 25% aluminum chloride solution, and packed around the implant abutments. An impression was taken using a polyvinyl siloxane impression material (Imprint, 3M ESPE). The mandibular provisional restoration was sectioned in two pieces on the mesial of site no. 21, and the smaller segment was placed back onto the abutments. Pattern Resin was used as a registration material by mixing it, waiting until it reached the doughy stage, and placing it between the maxillary definitive prosthesis and the mandibular abutments. The patient was then guided into centric occlusion. Once the resin had set, the smaller segment of the provisional restoration was removed from the mouth, and more resin was mixed and placed in the mouth to capture the maxillomandibular relationship in the mandibular left quadrant. The Pattern Resin was then removed, and the provisional restoration was luted back together to form one piece using Alike acrylic. This mandibular provisional restoration was then cemented with Freegenol temporary cement.

Alginate impressions were taken of the maxillary definitive prosthesis and the mandibular provisional restorations to use for cross mounting.

Phase XII: Finalization and delivery of mandibular prosthesis

At the laboratory, all the casts were cross-mounted on the same Panadent articulator to allow them to be in the same three-dimensional position. Matrices were made from the provisional restorations, and the framework was fabricated in Pattern Resin. We had planned to fabricate the mandibular restorations with cross-arch stability, considering that the remaining implant abutments were delicate and because of the existing bone loss on the implants. However, casting a one-piece framework on a full arch of implants with accuracy and a passive fit is almost impossible. Therefore, the mandibular frameworks were cast in three pieces that connect via a telescopic extension of the posterior segments, allowing the anterior segment to sit on top and connect the three segments together. This is a casting technique that we have been using successfully for years in various case scenarios because it mimimizes the casting inaccuracies associated with a single, large, full-arch casting. Once the castings were finished, they were tried in and verified for passive fit. A maxillomandibular relationship record was taken and sent back to the lab. Porcelain

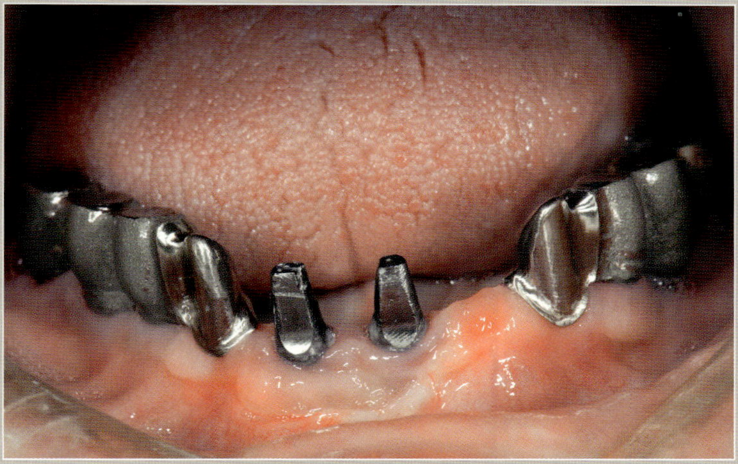

Try-in of mandibular posterior metal frameworks.

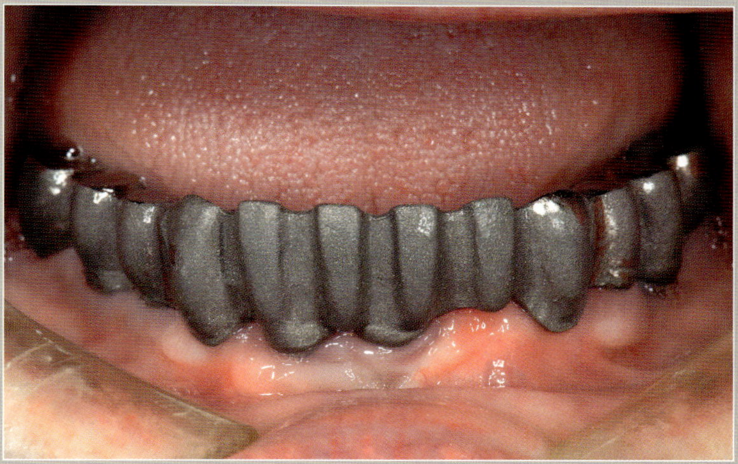

Try-in of all three mandibular metal frameworks.

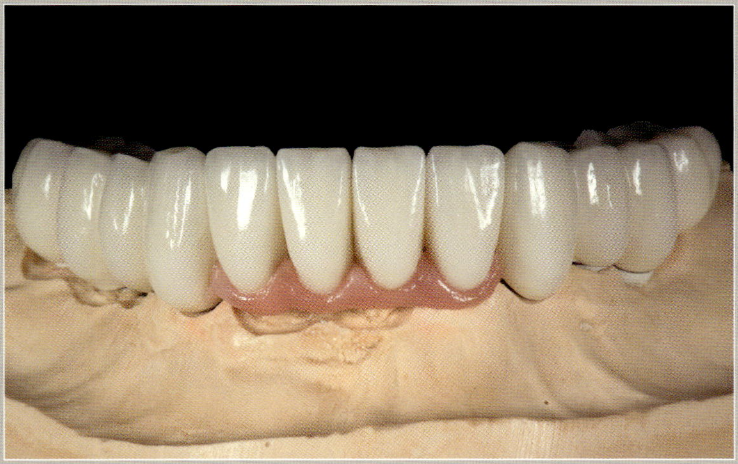

Definitive mandibular restorations on the cast.

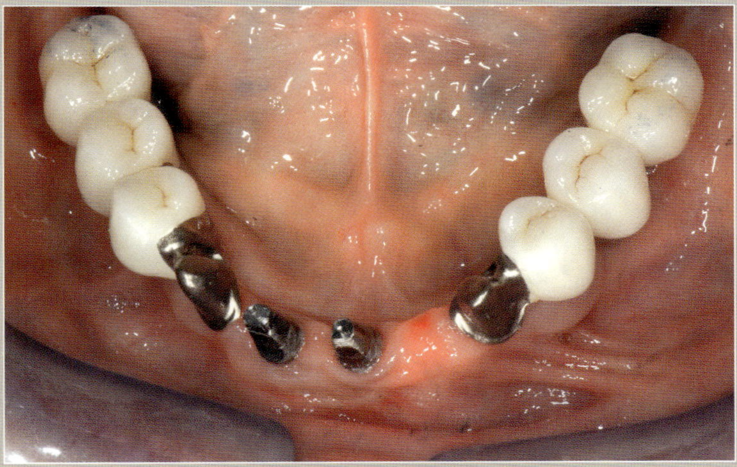

Mandibular occlusal view of definitive posterior restorations in place.

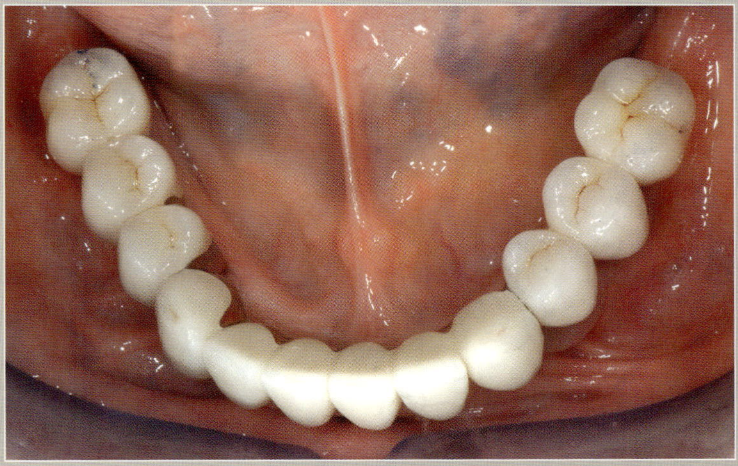

Mandibular occlusal view of all definitive restorations in place.

was applied to all segments, and pink ceramics was used in the mandibular anterior segment to create more ideal proportions for the mandibular anterior teeth.

When the patient presented for delivery, all of the frameworks with the porcelain were again tried in, and minor adjustments were made. The segments were then cemented with Freegenol cement to allow for retrievability. Alginate impressions were taken of the mandibular definitive prosthesis and the maxillary abutments and gold copings. Finally, a maxillary occlusal orthotic (short of the soft tissue) was fabricated to protect the mandibular ceramic from the metal abutments.

Posttreatment

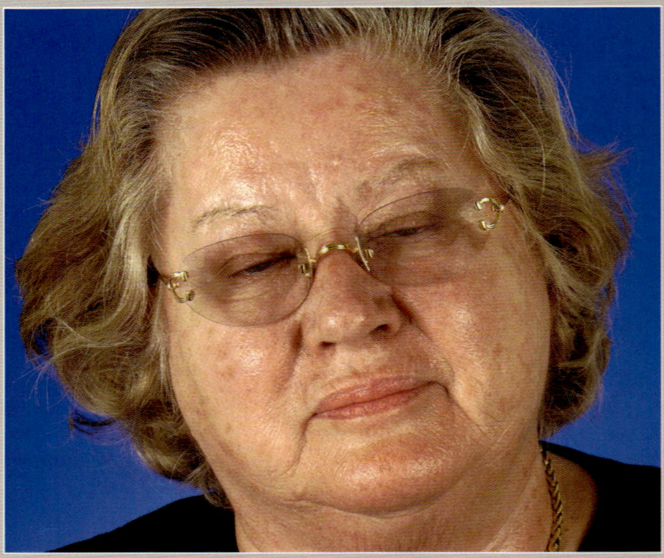

Facial view with lips together.

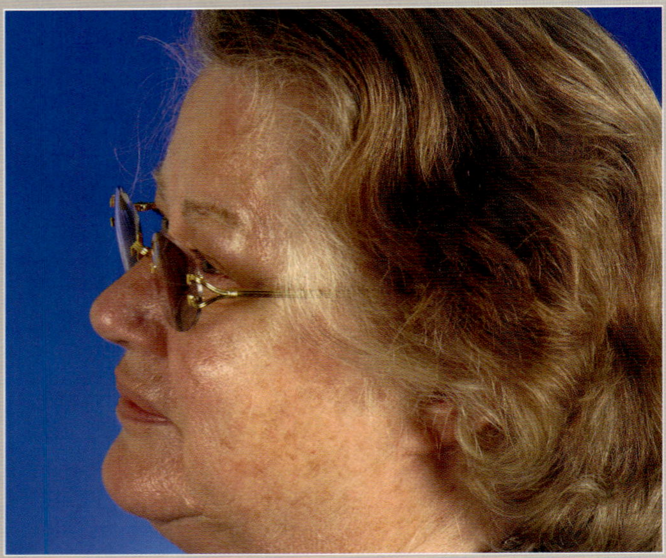

Profile view with lips together.

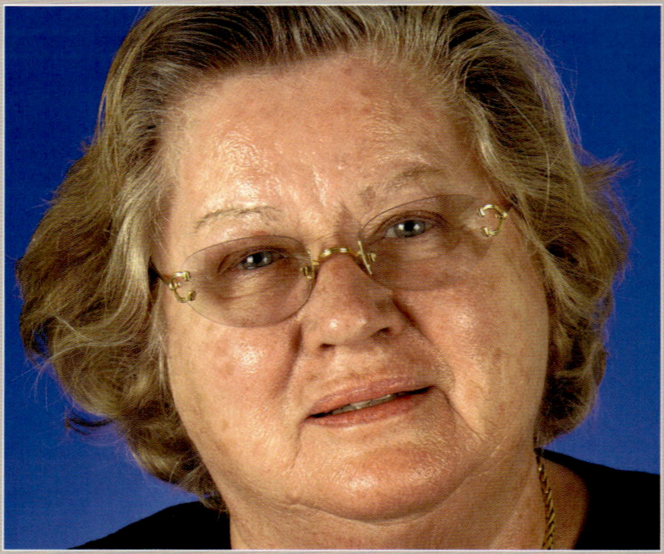

Facial view with lips at rest.

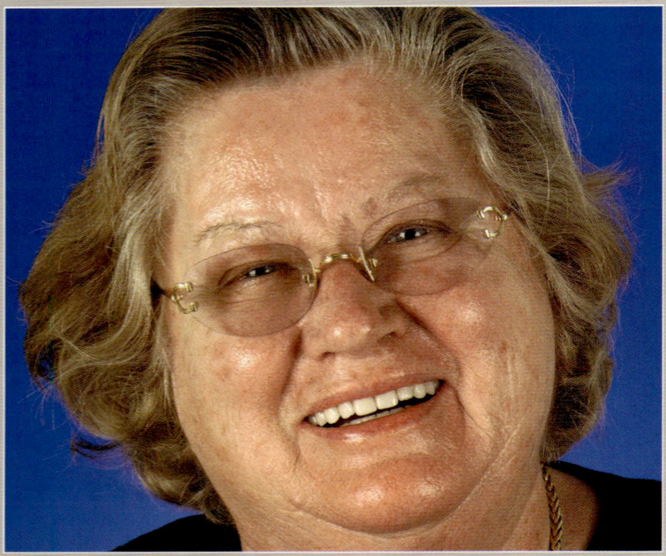

Facial view of smile.

Phase XIII: Recall/maintenance

Since the time of completion of active treatment, the patient has complied with a 3-month maintenance schedule, which gives her a chance to visit her son more often. During these sessions, we perform periodontal maintenance, including root planing and scaling and thorough examination. The wear of her maxillary prosthesis is evaluated very carefully to ensure support of her vertical dimension. She is comfortable and very happy and wears the occlusal orthotic (nightguard) religiously to protect the mandibular prosthesis from the maxillary metal abutments.

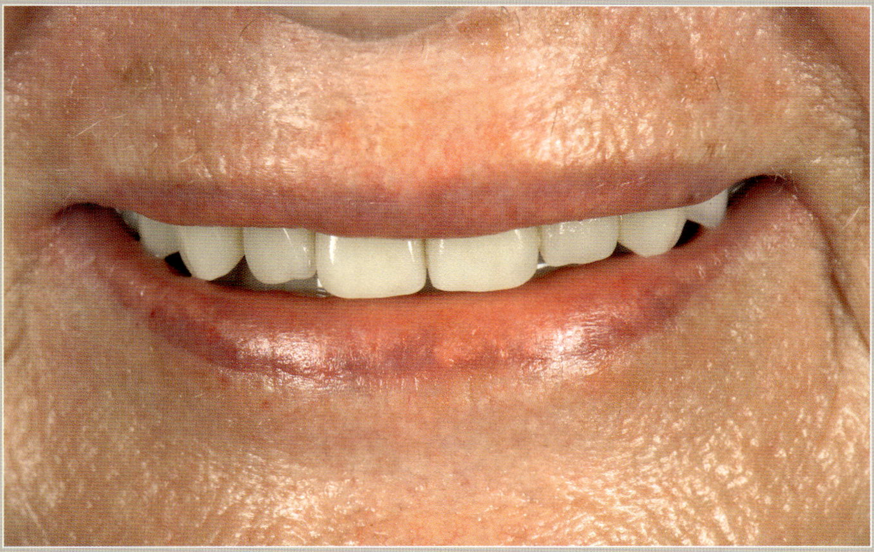

Frontal view of smile.

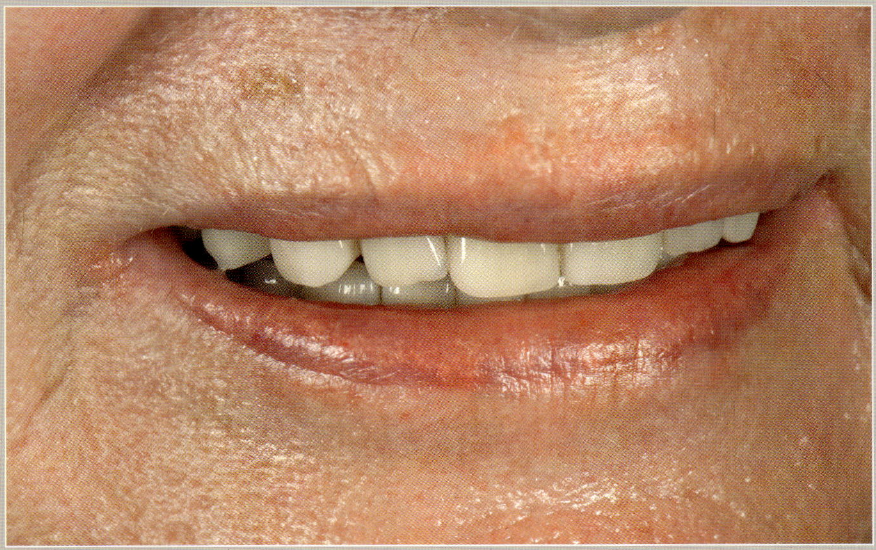

Right lateral view of smile.

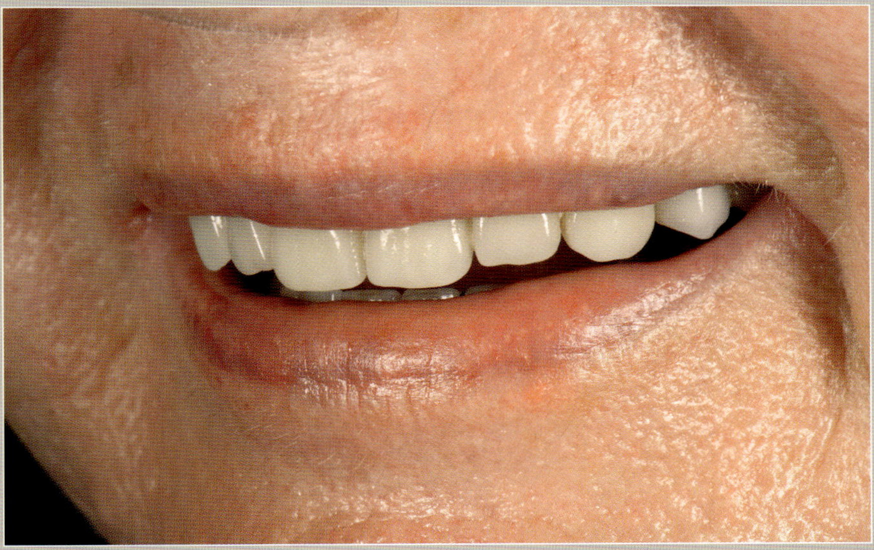

Left lateral view of smile.

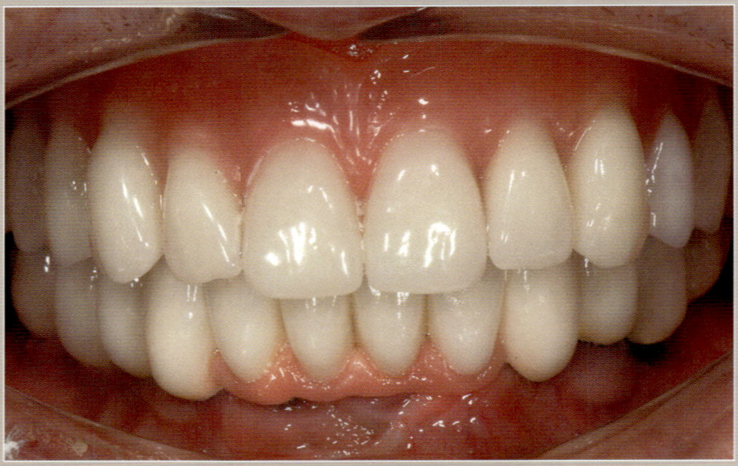

Intraoral frontal view.

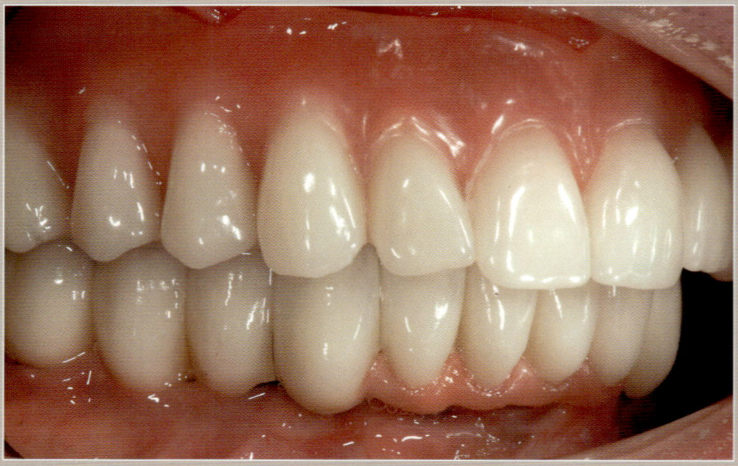

Intraoral right lateral view.

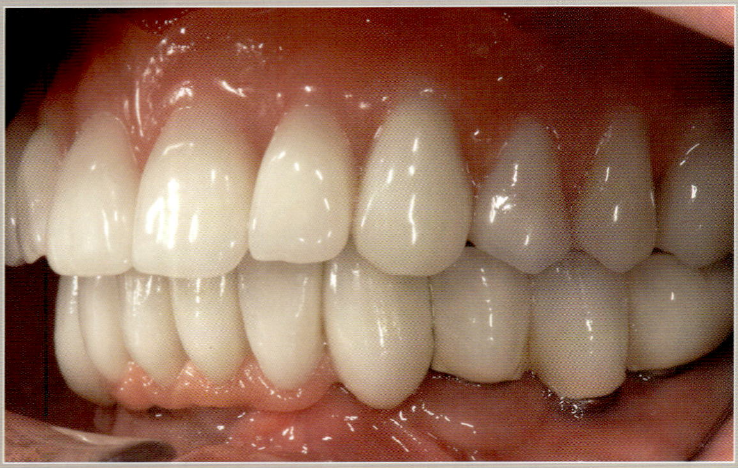

Intraoral left lateral view.

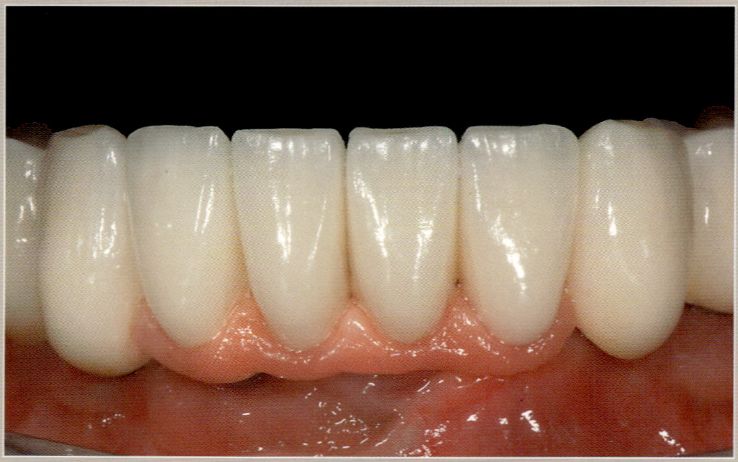

Mandibular anterior view.

You may now place the corresponding posttreatment overlay found in the separate folder over the pretreatment periodontal chart on page 257.

Commentary

All of the following types of issues were successfully addressed in this challenging case:

- Esthetic
- Biologic
- Functional
- Structural
- Biomechanical

It is clear that there was dramatic improvement in facial height, lip support, and tooth length. Although this case was quite complex, it was approached in an organized fashion by focusing on solutions in each of the above areas (Table 1), which led to the development of a manageable treatment plan and a gratifying outcome.

The following sections describe the thought process used in approaching this case. This case was very challenging due to the multitude of issues and considerations involved in treatment; therefore, each concern is addressed in a separate section. My aim is to share the thought process in selecting an appropriate treatment plan based on specific findings in complex cases.

I always begin treatment planning cases by looking at the esthetic issues, starting with the patient's face and working my way inward. With this philosophy, it is easier to integrate the esthetic changes you would like to make with all of the other issues that need to be addressed. Following is a discussion of each of these concerns, categorized by type, and the considerations involved in managing them.

Maxillary treatment

It is evident in all of the areas of concern that the most prudent treatment approach would be to extract the maxillary teeth. From an esthetic standpoint, the old restorations were too short and needed to be moved labially for improved lip support. The irregular soft tissues levels, which created disproportionate teeth, could not be resolved, even with augmentation. Based on the above considerations, a prosthesis with a gingival (pink) component would need to be fabricated.

All that would remain in the maxillary arch after extracting the teeth would be the implants in the left quadrant. These implants had friction-fit posts that could not be removed and very thin necks, which complicated the maxillary prosthetic choices.

Is a fixed maxillary prosthesis an option?

Considering that it was necessary to lengthen the maxillary teeth for esthetic purposes, the crown-root ratio would also increase on the remaining maxillary left implants. This would create a biomechanical issue with at least a 2:1 crown-root ratio. Considering the type of abutments on the implants, this would be a very risky choice. It would be necessary to add many more implants in the maxillary arch to stabilize a maxillary fixed partial denture, and we would still have a compromised maxillary left segment. This alone negated the choice of a fixed prosthesis. Considering the remaining anatomy of the maxillary ridge after extraction, adding the appropriate number of implants for a fixed partial denture (ie, approximately six additional implants), would necessitate major augmentation procedures as well as removal of the existing implants in the maxillary left quadrant and placement of new ones. This would be time-consuming, expensive, and traumatic for the patient, given her age and desire to do as little as possible to achieve the desired result. Although the surgeon chose to augment sites nos. 9 to 11 during the implant placement procedure for possible future implant placement, this was done in the event that the four new implants placed were not enough to support a removable prosthesis design. It was determined after the provisionalization that there was enough cross-arch support and stability with the number of implants placed for a removable prosthesis, and this was in line with the patient's desire to minimize cost and surgical procedures. The esthetic objectives from our evaluation indicated that we would like to increase support of the upper lip and create ideal proportion of the teeth. Using soft tissue (pink) prosthetics can solve both of these esthetic dilemmas. A fixed partial denture would involve pink ceramics and a ridge lap design and would have to be cemented into place. Hygiene and maintenance procedures for such a prosthesis would be much more difficult than for a removable prosthesis with pink acrylic. Given these considerations, a removable prosthesis would be the ideal choice in the maxilla.

Is a rigid or resilient system better for this case?

Given that the implants in the maxillary left quadrant represent a rigid system with abutments that cannot be removed, the remaining prosthesis also needs to be a rigid system to avoid overload of the maxillary left segment. Also, due to the crown-root ratio of the maxillary left segment once the teeth are lengthened, cross-arch stabilization is required to distribute the forces to all of the implants.

What type of rigid removable prosthesis should be used?

We chose a maxillary friction-fit telescopic abutment–galvano coping prosthesis. The use of telescopic crowns on natural teeth with a double-crown system is a treatment alternative that has been used successfully since the mid-1970s.[1,10–26]

(continued on p. 276)

TABLE 1 MANAGEMENT OF CONCERNS IN CHALLENGING CASES

Category		Concern	Considerations and solutions
Esthetic	*Extraoral*	· Flat or concave profile (deficient upper lip)	· Bring maxillary teeth labially to support lip (consider using pink ceramics)
		· No tooth exposure at rest and very little in smile	· Lengthen maxillary teeth
		· Large negative space in maxillary left buccal corridor due to short maxillary left restorative segment	· Lengthen maxillary left restorative segment to level occlusal plane
		· Mandibular incisal and posterior occlusal planes not level	· Shorten mandibular incisors and/or lengthen posterior teeth; in this case, better to shorten the incisors by 1 mm (subjective, based on lip relationship)
		· Short lower one-third of face	· Open vertical dimension
	Intraoral	· Irregular soft tissue margins and papillae in maxilla and mandible; disproportion of teeth	· If papillae involved or large discrepancy, as in this case, consider pink ceramics or acrylic; sufficient regeneration impossible due to biologic limitations
Biologic		· Severe periodontitis on all maxillary teeth	· Consider extraction
		· Fractured maxillary left canine	· Consider extraction
		· Decay on all remaining maxillary teeth	· Consider extraction due to the combination of severe periodontal attachment loss and stuctural compromise
		· Early to moderate peri-implantitis with purulent exudate on mandibular anterior fixed partial denture	· In this case, it is a soft tissue problem: No attached tissue, no embrasure form in area to allow thorough debridement; treat area locally with antimicrobials, scaling, and root planing, and change contour of teeth to make cleansable; consider grafting to create attached tissue
		· Soft tissue between tooth no. 23 and implant no. 24 not level (pseudo pocket); difficult to clean	· Importance of teeth in overall treatment plan: In this case, patient has enough support from implants to plan for a full mandibular implant-supported fixed rehabilitation; the teeth create a problem in maintenance and health of adjacent implants; consider extraction; however, if teeth were important, consider crown lengthening

TABLE 1 *(cont)*

Category	Concern	Considerations and solutions
Functional	· Irregular occlusal planes in maxillary and mandibular arches	· In this case, all maxillary teeth need to be lengthened for esthetics, especially in the left quadrant; need to determine the correct mandibular incisal position and level plane to that point—from a subjective point of view, the best incisal position relative to the lower lip was slightly (1 mm) lower than at presentation; therefore, shorten the mandibular incisors slightly and lengthen the posterior teeth to open the bite, which decreases the overbite and lessens the stress on the anterior teeth
	· Loss of vertical support and stability due to failing maxillary tooth-supported fixed partial denture	· Consider implants and a rigid prosthesis that will have cross-arch stability and support the vertical dimension
	· Deep overbite and Class II canine relationship	· Consider opening the vertical dimension and using a prosthesis for which you can choose the width of the teeth and that does not need to emerge directly from the implants, allowing manipulation of the position of the teeth to compensate for the ridge deficiency, lip support, and occlusal relationship; rigid removable prosthesis for maxilla
	· History of parafunction	· Consider ways to lessen stress; in this case, consider a maxillary removable appliance with acrylic teeth to help reduce the force and minimize ceramic fracture; also consider a nightguard once finished with the rehabilitation
Structural	· All remaining maxillary teeth have severe cement washout and decay	· Consider extraction
	· Abutments on implants have a very narrow neck width; posts are all tapped into place with a friction fit and cannot be removed	· Consider a way to lessen the stress on the implants; consider rigid cross-arch splinting
Biomechanical	· Ideal cusp tip or incisal edge position relative to implant head in maxilla (especially on left side) creates an unfavorable crown-root ratio	· Consider cross-arch splinting and a removable prosthesis with acrylic teeth to dampen stress with a rigid splinting effect when in place
	· No cross-arch stability in maxilla due to failing maxillary teeth	· Consider distributing more implants throughout the arch with a large anteroposterior spread and rigid cross-arch splinting
	· Maxillary anterior fixed partial denture fractured at midline	· Patient has constricted bite; consider increasing maxillary dental protrusion

(*continued from p. 273*)

Although the literature regarding implant-supported telescopic prostheses is limited, the results so far indicate that this treatment modality can lead to good long-term treatment outcomes.[27-30] In my office, I have been successfully using telescopic prostheses for more than 10 years on both teeth and implants.

What are the advantages of this type of prosthesis?

- *Passive fit:* We know that a misfit of an implant framework can transfer stress to the implants.[29,31-34] Although there is no evidence-based numeric formula for acceptable implant prosthesis fit, we strive to make the fit of our frameworks as passive as possible.[35] In this case, any aberrant stress, such as a misfit casting, can exaggerate the stress on the already compromised maxillary left implants. This type of prosthesis allows us the ability to create a totally passive fit by intraorally luting the electroformed copings directly to the framework.[30]
- *Oral hygiene:* Individual abutments and copings are much easier to clean than a fixed partial denture or a prosthesis with a metal bar or framework connecting the implants.
- *Cross-arch stability and stress distribution:* This type of prosthesis has a cast metal frame. Once the prosthesis is seated, all of the abutments and copings become splinted, thereby creating cross-arch stability and stress distribution.
- *Repairability:* If a removable prosthesis with acrylic denture teeth needs repair, it is simple to remove and replace the denture teeth, whereas if the porcelain fractures on a fixed partial denture, all of the ceramic must be removed. Moreover, if an implant fails, the chosen prosthesis is still functional and is likely to remain functional even if more than one implant fails. If it is necessary to place a new implant, it is easy to make a new abutment and galvano coping, which can be picked up in the prosthesis.

What are the advantages particular to this case?

In this case, the patient had enough support for a fixed implant prosthesis in the mandibular arch. This was to be fabricated with porcelain-fused-to-metal fixed partial dentures. There have been high incidences of porcelain fracture in implant-supported prostheses reported in the literature,[36,37] and the full-arch prosthesis has the highest rate of veneer chipping.[38]

My clinicial experience supports this data, especially when implants with fixed restorations involving ceramics are used in both arches. We know that natural teeth have periodontal mechanoreceptors that provide feedback regarding the magnitude, direction, and rate of occlusal load for sensory perception and motor function.[39,40] The loss of teeth and their replacement with implants affects the proprioceptive response. Patients with implants do not feel touch sensation until greater force is applied compared with patients with natural teeth. This passive tactile threshold has been shown to be 3.47 times higher with implants than with natural teeth.[41] Some researchers have shown it to be 100 times higher with implants than with natural teeth.[42-44] Active threshold, which is determined by the patient's interocclusal detection of the thickness and shape of various objects, was found to be six times higher for implants than for teeth.[45]

The difference between active and passive discrimination is that passive discrimination depends on periodontal and/or intrabony mechanoreception and is activated by the application of a controlled force to a tooth or implant. Active discrimination is based on objects placed between the teeth or implants and involves a number of mechanoreceptor inputs such as the teeth, periodontium, gingiva, jaw muscles, and the TMJ.[40,45,46]

Either way, this can lead to overload of the implant or prosthesis.[40] This can be dangerous when the restorations in both arches are supported by implants and involve ceramics. Because of this, one arch should be developed as the weak link in the system. This can be accomplished by the use of acrylic restorations in one arch, as was done in this case. Acrylic materials have a dampening effect on the force delivered to the implants. If acrylic restorations are planned in one of the arches, the acrylic will wear before the opposing porcelain fractures. Moreover, acrylic restorations are easily replaceable. Unfortunately, not all patients will accept having one arch restored in acrylic and the other in ceramic, but all patients must be informed of the risks prior to fabrication of full-arch, fixed, implant-supported ceramic restorations in the maxilla and mandible.

One last important consideration is the need to use similar materials in the same arch. If the decision is made to use acrylic restorations, the whole arch should be restored using the same material to allow for even wear, thus minimizing the risk of overload. If one segment of an arch is restored using a different material, the most rigid segment would eventually be overloaded as a result of the weaker material wearing more quickly.

Mandibular treatment

Although the implants in the mandibular left quadrant had some horizontal bone loss, we believed that eight implants would provide sufficient support for a mandibular fixed implant prosthesis. My decision in this case, considering the bone loss in the mandibular left segment and the type of abutments in the Bicon system, was to splint the mandible for the purpose of creating cross-arch support, stability, and transfer of forces throughout the arch. Casting a full-arch frame on implants and having a passive fit is virtually impossible given the inevitable distortion that occurs throughout the process of taking impressions, fabricating casts, and casting the frameworks.[29,31,47–49] It appears that these inaccuracies may be proportionate to the framework length.[49,50] In order to compensate for the distortion associated with casting a full arch, a special frame design that we have been using for years was used. This design allows fabrication of the frame in three smaller segments, making it easier to cast with greater accuracy. The distal segments were cast with a cantilevered telescopic extension anteriorly, and the anterior segment was overlaid and connected to these extensions. Once they are connected, they function as one unit. There have been numerous articles that describe flexure of the mandible upon opening[51–53] as a contraindication to a full-arch framework in the mandible. Medial mandibular flexure is a deformation of the mandible characterized by a decrease in arch width during jaw opening and protrusion movements because of the contraction of the lateral pterygoid muscles, causing strain in the symphysis region.[54–56] Although these findings should not be wholly discounted, Fischman[57] found that flexure was reduced with all types of splints, although none of the splints totally inhibited flexure of the mandible. Moreover, dentists have been fabricating implant-supported prostheses that cross the symphyseal region for many years without any problems. In my practice, I have been using this framework design for at least 10 years and have had no evidence of loosening, breakage of components, or any problem as a result of this flexure. It is possible that the cement layer between the segments helps to relieve some of this reported stress. All of the mandibular segments were cemented with a temporary cement (Freegenol) that allowed for retrievability in case something needed to be repaired or replaced.

Aspects of this treatment plan that could be challenged

Type of maxillary prosthesis

Another very good rigid removable prosthesis that would have worked for the maxillary arch is a spark erosion prosthesis.[58] This type of prosthesis employs the use of electrical discharge machining to allow very precise framework design and very rigid prosthesis fabrication. In this case, however, there are three negatives to this type of prosthesis compared with the telescopic abutment–electroformed coping prosthesis. One is the difference in cleansability between the two prostheses, which is important considering the age of the patient and her poor oral hygiene history. It is much easier to clean single-unit telescopic abutments than it is to clean under a bar. The second advantage of the telescopic prosthesis is the ease in creating a passive fit by picking up all of the galvano copings in the mouth within the frame. A spark erosion prosthesis is made with precision on a cast. If one were to fabricate a spark erosion prosthesis for the maxillary arch, it would become complicated with regard to the maxillary left segment, in which the abutments cannot be removed from the implants. An intricate and complex prosthesis, which may or may not splint the whole arch, would need to be fabricated. The last advantage is in long-term maintenance. It is much easier to repair or replace a galvano coping in the prosthesis than to have to replace the entire maxillary prosthesis should the maxillary left implants fail in the future.

Retention of existing implants

Although the remaining implants were compromised both biologically and mechanically, they were well integrated. Removing the old implants would have caused extensive bone loss and would necessitate grafting. Considering the complications that could arise from removing the old implants, as well as the time and cost involved, it was not a good option. Moreover, if the maxillary implants were to fail, the maxillary prosthesis would not be lost, and if the mandibular implants were to fail, only a small segment of the prosthesis would require attention.

Lack of medial segmentation of the mandibular prosthesis

Considering the suboptimal implant type, it was felt that bilateral segments extending from the distal implants and sectioned at the midline would result in a span that was excessively long. To expect a friction-fit post as a terminal abutment to support this span is risky. In addition, the bilateral anteroposterior implant positions were fairly straight. This creates greater lateral forces, which could be better managed by a full-arch prosthesis with cross-arch support and stability.

Acknowledgments

I would like to thank my mentors, who have changed my life at both a personal and professional level, and without whom I would not be the person I am today. These include Drs Hiroshi Hirayama, Ralph Youdelis, John Kois, Frank Spear, Ward Smalley, and Warren Libman, as well as the countless graduate students, local specialists, and amazing technicians I have met on my journey.

I would also like to acknowledge all those who helped in the treatment of this case. These include Dr Isaac Garazi, a fine periodontist in Aventura, Florida, who is not only a great clinician but also a great friend.

We cannot treat these complex cases without the help of our laboratory technicians, who work meticulously to create the beautiful outcomes we achieve. Onofrio Azzaretto is a fine technician from Germany with great skill in fabricating removable telescopic prostheses. We have made many of these restorations over many years with much success, thanks to his fine work. Harald Heindl and I have been working together for the last 10 years. He is one of the finest technicians in the world, with amazing precision and esthetics. We have been fabricating this type of interdigitating prosthesis on implants for many years with many cases and have had wonderful success thanks to his and Daniela Heindl's abilities.

References

1. Morr T. Transfer of information for esthetic and functional predictability in the severe wear case. Quintessence Dent Technol 2007;30:55–65.
2. Kois JC, Kois D. Simplified facebow rationale and technique (in press).
3. Bonwill WGA. The scientific articulation of the human teeth as founded on geometrical, mathematical, and mechanical laws. Dent Items Interest 1899;21:617–643.
4. Weinberg LA. An evaluation of basic articulators and their concepts. Part I: Basic concepts. J Prosthet Dent 1963;13:622–644.
5. Weinberg LA. An evaluation of basic articulators and their concepts. Part II: Arbitrary, positional, semiadjustable articulators. J Prosthet Dent 1963;13:645–663.
6. Monson GS. Occlusion as applied to crown and bridge work. J Am Dent Assoc 1920;7:399–413.
7. Wirz J, Hoffmann A. Electroforming in Restorative Dentistry: New Dimensions in Biologically Based Prostheses. Chicago: Quintessence, 2000:132–161,238–267.
8. Dolger J, Gadau C, Rathmer R. Treatment behavior and complete mouth rehabilitation using AGC crowns: A case report. Int J Periodontics Restorative Dent 2001;21:373–379.
9. Setz J, Diehl J, Weber H. The marginal fit of cemented galvanoceramic crowns. Int J Prosthodont 1989;2:61–64.

10. Englehardt JP. Telescopic crowns and attachments in partial dentures (II). Quintessence Dent Technol 1976;1:31–47.
11. Reitemeier B, Retemeier G. Experiences with the use of the double crown system. 1. Telescoping partial denture [in German]. Stomatol DDR 1976;26:538–544.
12. Reitemeier VB, Reitemeier G. Experiences in the use of the double crown system. 3. Removable bridge prosthesis [in German]. Stomatol DDR 1976;26:669–674.
13. Langer A. Telescope retainers and their clinical application. J Prosthet Dent 1980;44:516–522.
14. Langer A. Telescope retainers for removable partial dentures. J Prosthet Dent 1981;45:337–343.
15. Diedrichs G. Is the telescope system still reasonable? [in German]. ZWR 1990;99:78–92.
16. Ericson A, Nilsson B, Bergman B. Clinical results in patients provided with conical crown retained dentures. Int J Prosthodont 1990;3:513–521.
17. Johnke G. Investigations on the incorporation of telescopic crown-partial dentures in comparison with bridgework and total dentures [in German]. Dtsch Stomatol 1991;41:362–368.
18. Molin M, Bergman B, Ericson A. A clinical evaluation of conical crown retained dentures. J Prosthet Dent 1993;70:251–256.
19. Sethi A, Sochor P. Restoration of the maxillary arch using implants, natural teeth and the Konus crown: A cast study. Dent Update 1994;21:52–55.
20. Hou GL, Tsai CC, Weisgold AS. Periodontal and prosthetic therapy in severely advanced periodontitis by the use of the crown sleeve coping telescopic denture. A longitudinal case report. Aust Dent J 1997;42:169–174.
21. Igarashi Y, Goto T. Ten year follow-up study of conical crown-retained dentures. Int J Prosthodont 1997;10:149–155.
22. Wenz HJ, Lehmann KM. A telescopic crown concept for the restoration of the partially edentulous arch: The Marburg double crown system. Int J Prosthodont 1998;11:541–550.
23. Wenz HJ, Hertrampf K, Lehmann KM. Clinical longevity of removable partial dentures retained by telescopic crowns: Outcome of the double crown with clearance fit. Int J Prothodont 2001;14:207–213.
24. Behr M, Hofmann E, Rosentritt M, Lang R, Handel G. Technical failure rates of double crown-retained removable partial dentures. Clin Oral Investig 2000;4:87–90.
25. Eisenburger M, Gray G, Tschernitschek H. Long-term results of telescopic crown retained dentures—A retrospective study. Eur J Prosthodont Restor Dent 2000;8(3):87–91.
26. Beschnidt SM, Chitmongkolsuk S, Prull R. Telescopic crown-retained removable partial dentures: Review and case report. Compend Contin Educ Dent 2001;22:927–932.
27. Weischer T, Mohr C. Implant-supported mandibular telescopic prostheses in oral cancer patients: An up to 9-year retrospective study. Int J Prosthodont 2001;14:329–334.
28. Heckman SM, Winter W, Meyer M, Weber HP, Wichmann MG. Overdenture attachment selection and the loading of implant and denture-bearing area. Part 2: A methodical study using five types of attachment. Clin Oral Implants Res 2001;12:640–647.
29. Heckmann SM, Karl M, Wichmann MG, Winter W, Graef F, Taylor TD. Cement fixation and screw retention: Parameters of passive fit. An in vitro study of three-unit implant-supported fixed partial dentures. Clin Oral Implants Res 2004;15:466–473.
30. Greven B, Luepke M, von Dorsche SH. Telescoping implant prostheses with intraorally luted galvano mesostructures to improve passive fit. J Prosthet Dent 2007;98:239–244.
31. Jemt T. Three-dimensional distortion of gold alloy castings and welded titanium frameworks. Measurements of the precision of fit between completed implant prostheses and the master casts in routine edentulous situations. J Oral Rehabil 1995;22:557–564.
32. Karl M, Rosch S, Graef F, Taylor TD, Heckmann SM. Static implant loading caused by as-cast metal and ceramic-veneered superstructures. J Prosthet Dent 2005;93:324–330.
33. Pietrabissa R, Gionso L, Quaglini V, Di Martino E, Simion M. An in vitro study on compensation of mismatch of screw- versus cement-retained implant supported fixed prostheses. Clin Oral Implants Res 2000;11:448–457.
34. Setz J, Kramer A, Benzing U, Weber H. Completed dentures fixed on dental implants: Chewing patterns and implant stress. Int J Oral Maxillofac Implants 1989;4:107–111.
35. Kan JY, Rungcharassaeng K, Bohsali K, Goodacre CJ, Land BR. Clinical methods for evaluating implant framework fit. J Prosthet Dent 1999;81:7–13.
36. Pjetursson BE, Tan K, Lang NP, Bragger U, Egger M, Zwahlen M. A systematic review of the survival and complication rates of fixed partial dentured (FPDs) after an observation period of at least 5 years. Clin Oral Implants Res 2004;15:625–642.

37. Sharma P. Implant supported fixed partial dentures survival rate high, but biological and technical complications common. Evid Based Dent 2005;6:72–73.
38. Linkevicius T, Vladimirovas E, Grybauskas S, Puisys A, Rutkunas V. Veneer fracture in implant-supported metal-ceramic restorations. Part 1: Overall success rate and impact of occlusal guidance. Stomatologija 2008;10:133–139.
39. Hoshino K, Miura H, Morikawa O, Kato H, Okada D, Shinki T. Influence of occlusal height for an implant prosthesis on the periodontal tissues of the antagonist. J Med Dent Sci 2004;51:87–196.
40. Klineberg I, Murray G. Osseoperception: Sensory function and proprioception. Adv Dent Res 1999;13:120–129.
41. Grieznis L, Apse P, Blumfelds L. Passive tactile sensibility of teeth and osseointegrated dental implants in the maxilla. Stomatologija 2010;12:80–86.
42. Hämmerle CH, Wagner D, Brägger U, et al. Threshold of tactile sensitivity perceived with dental endosseous implants and natural teeth. Clin Oral Implants Res 1995;6:83–90.
43. Muhlbradt L, Ulrich R, Mohlmann H, Schmid H. Mechanoperception of natural teeth versus endosseous implants revealed by magnitude estimation. Int J Oral Maxillofac Implants 1989;4:125–130.
44. Mericske-Stern R, Hofmann J, Wedig A, Geering AH. In vivo measurements of maximal occlusal force and minimal pressure threshold on overdentures supported by implants or natural roots: A comparative study, Part I. Int J Oral Maxillofac Implants 1993;8:641–649.
45. Jacobs R, van Steenberghe D. From osseoperception to implant-mediated sensory-motor interactions and related clinical implications. J Oral Rehabil 2006;33:282–292.
46. Jacobs R, van Steenberghe D. Comparative evaluation of the oral tactile function of teeth or implant-suppported prostheses. Clin Oral Implants Res 1991;2:75–80.
47. Jemt T, Lie A. Accuracy of implant-supported prostheses in the edentulous jaw: Analysis of precision of fit between cast gold-alloy frameworks and master casts by means of three-dimensional photogrammetric technique. Clin Oral Implants Res 1995;6:172–180.
48. Tan KB, Rubenstein JE, Nicholls JI, Youdelis RA. Three-dimensional analysis of the casting accuracy of one-piece, osseointegrated implant-retained prostheses. Int J Prosthodont 1993;6:346–363.
49. Safarti E, Harter JC. Comparative accuracy of fixed partial dentures made as one-piece castings or joined by solder. Int J Prosthodont 1992;13;275–281.
50. Huling JS, Clark RE. Comparative distortion in three-unit fixed prostheses joined by laser welding, conventional soldering, or casting in one piece. J Dent Res 1977;56:128–134.
51. Burch JG, Borchers G. Method for study of mandibular arch width change. J Dent Res 1970;49:463.
52. De Marco TL, Paine S. Mandibular dimensional change. J Prosthet Dent 1974;31:482–485.
53. Goodkind RJ, Heringlake CB. Mandibular flexure in opening and closing movements. J Prosthet Dent 1973;30:134–138.
54. Gates GN, Nicholls JI. Evaluation of mandibular arch width change. J Prosthet Dent 1981;46:385–392.
55. Hylander WL. Stress and strain in the mandibular symphysis of primates: A test of competing hypotheses. Am J Phys Anthropol 1984;64:1–46.
56. Hobkirk JA, Schwab J. Mandibular deformation in subjects with osseointegrated implants. Int J Oral Maxillofac Implants 1991;6:319–328.
57. Fischman BM. The influence of fixed splints on mandibular flexure. J Prosthet Dent 1990;64:483–485.
58. Van Roeke NB. Prosthesis fabrication using electrical discharge machining. Int J Oral Maxillofac Implants 1992;7:56–61.

11

Digital Image Morphing for Collaborative Treatment Planning

Glenn D. Krieger, DDS

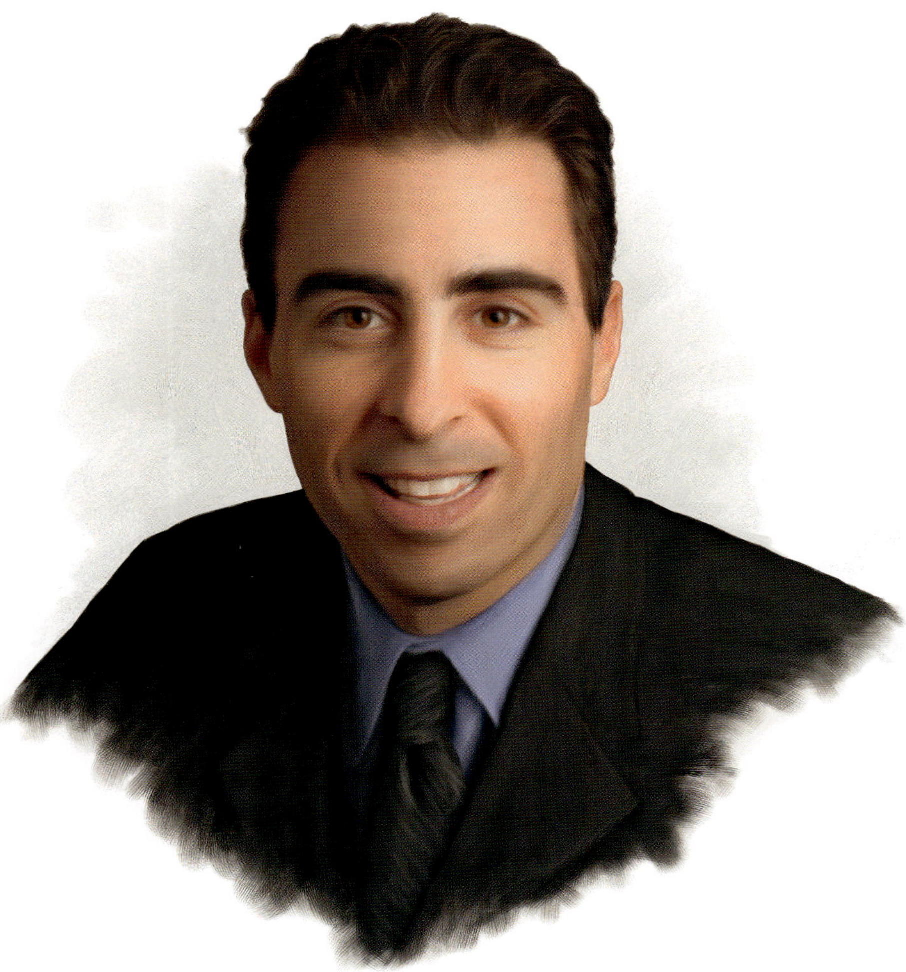

One of the least recognized truisms in dentistry is that it is as easy to be fooled in the simplest of cases as it is in the most complex.

Philosophy and Background

One of the least recognized truisms in dentistry is that it is as easy to be fooled in the simplest of cases as it is in the most complex. In reality, very few of the cases that we treat are truly straightforward and simple. The more a clinician is willing to carefully investigate and thoroughly examine a case, the more likely the complexities will be uncovered and an accurate diagnosis achieved. In many of these assiduously approached cases, the practitioner will ultimately realize that a comprehensive line of attack is required, usually resulting in a more favorable outcome. It was with this in mind that this particular case was chosen for review.

When evaluating this case, it can be easily dismissed as undemanding and trouble-free. However, when one scrutinizes the existing soft tissue display and its relationship to the overall harmony of facial esthetics, it becomes clear that several clinical management challenges exist.

Successful management of this case requires the clinician to first focus on establishing an accurate diagnosis. Once this is in hand, there are many treatment options possible depending on the specific needs and wants of the patient. Important mitigating factors are the patient's past dental treatment and experiences. This patient had already been treated for exactly the same chief complaint without success. It was essential for us to avoid a repeat performance.

While treatment planning this case, it was important to keep in mind the overall relationship of the teeth, gingiva, and face to one another. The normal parameters related to tooth size, shape, and display that are generally regarded as esthetically pleasing had to be considered, and the factors that must be addressed and managed in the treatment plan to provide an outcome that will meet or exceed this patient's expectations had to be uncovered.

The diagnosis was of paramount importance in this case. The proper place to begin was to ask why this patient did not like her smile rather than how it should be corrected. The failure to do so was, in part, why the patient presented for treatment. Once the proper diagnosis is achieved, we can begin to visualize the final treatment outcome. What should it look like? What are potential obstacles that may stand in the way during treatment? What is the simplest, most direct path to achieve our treatment goals? By first visualizing the desired outcome, this path becomes far more predictable.

This case could easily be viewed as a "simple" anterior esthetic dilemma, although doing so would be a mistake. By slowing down and evaluating all of the information, new challenges will become evident. Each answer will lead to other potentially complicating questions. Most clinicians have treated many anterior cases involving esthetic challenges, but this case can best be characterized as deceptive.

While evaluating the clinical data, take into consideration ways in which the soft tissue "gumminess" can be corrected, while keeping in mind the morphology and length of the roots of the anterior teeth. Creating even more difficulty is the fact that the anterior teeth, the very center of this case's challenge, have been restored for many years, leaving no information about the patient's original tooth shape and size. Determining the proper size of the proposed "new" outcome and its relationship to the arch should be considered. Again, you will find that the answer to one question may create another question.

While looking at ways to improve the anterior esthetics, consider the effect that such treatment would have on the posterior teeth, which are also visible when the patient smiles. Creating a harmonious esthetic outcome without unduly compromising posterior support might be a potential challenge in this case. Preparing a considerable number of teeth to "harmonize" proposed restorations also brings about a number of long-term biologic considerations.

This case isn't about simply doing as much dentistry as possible to make the smile look better. On the contrary, it is about solving the patient's esthetic concerns as simply and predictably as possible, keeping in mind the liability an extremely high smile line brings with it.

If a stepwise approach is followed, this case offers many pearls of wisdom that can assist clinicians in daily clinical practice. The issues presented in terms of the relationship between teeth and the periodontium allow a deeper understanding of a majority of cases that we treat on a daily basis.

Case Presentation

Treating clinicians
Restorative dentist: Glenn D. Krieger, DDS
Periodontist: Lloyd M. Tucker, DMD, MSD

Clinical Treatment Planning

Age at initial presentation: 37 years
Initial presentation: August 2006
Active treatment completed: September 2008

Introduction and background

This patient presented with a chief complaint of unhappiness with her gummy smile and a general dissatisfaction with the shorter length of her teeth. Furthermore, she did not like the color of her teeth, which did not look natural to her.

The patient reported that 3 years earlier she had four crowns placed on her anterior teeth with an outcome that did not meet her expectations. She also stated that immediately after placement, the crowns were longer than they currently are, but were adjusted because she felt that they were too long. As a result, the patient was not only unhappy with the outcome of her previous treatment but was also exasperated with the dental profession as a whole. Her previous experience left her feeling confused about why a reasonable outcome could not be achieved.

Her desire was to gain a more appealing smile with teeth that appear more natural and a smile that shows less gingiva, if possible.

Medical history

- Noncontributory
- Codeine allergy
- No current medications
- Nonsmoker

Diagnostic findings

Extraoral and facial findings

- Flat to slightly convex facial profile
- Slightly obtuse nasolabial angle
- Excessive gingival display during smiling
- Mandible and chin deviated 3 to 4 mm to right
- Excessive lip mobility
- Size and form of lips symmetric during smile and repose
- Asymmetric midface, particularly around nose
- Appearance suggestive of vertical maxillary excess

Smile analysis

- Excessive maxillary tooth display at repose (6 to 7 mm of central incisors)
- Maxillary midline approximately 2 mm to left of facial midline
- Excessive gingival display (6 to 7 mm) with broad smile
- Maxillary central incisors display excessive width-height ratio
- Wide buccal corridor
- Anterior four maxillary teeth appear too monochromatic and too high in value
- Slight cant of incisors to patient's right from gingival to incisal
- Descending gingival zenith heights from teeth nos. 6 to 10, leading to inappropriate gingival relationships among the six anterior teeth
- Maxillary lateral incisors are different sizes and shapes with considerable variation in gingival zeniths
- Diastema of 1 mm between teeth nos. 7 and 8
- Mandibular midline deviation 1 to 2 mm to right visible in broad smile

Pretreatment

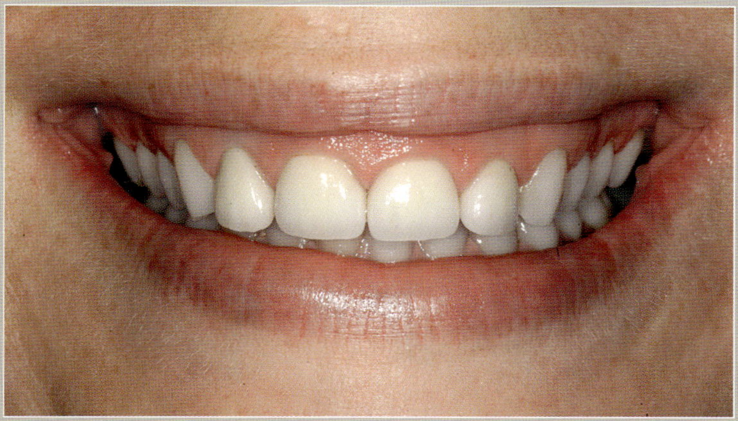

Close-up of smile

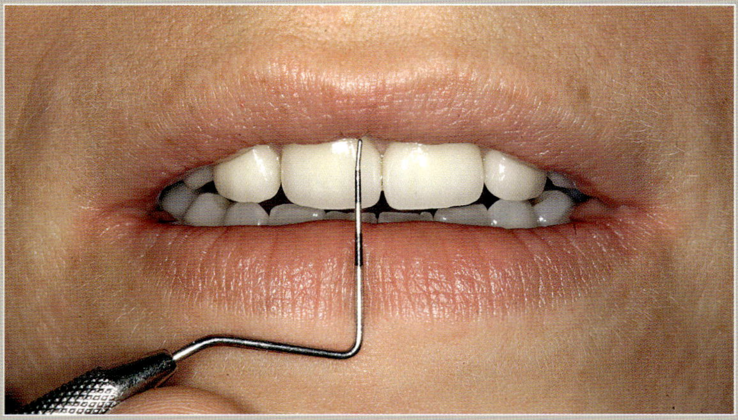

Approximately 6.5 mm of incisal edge visible in repose.

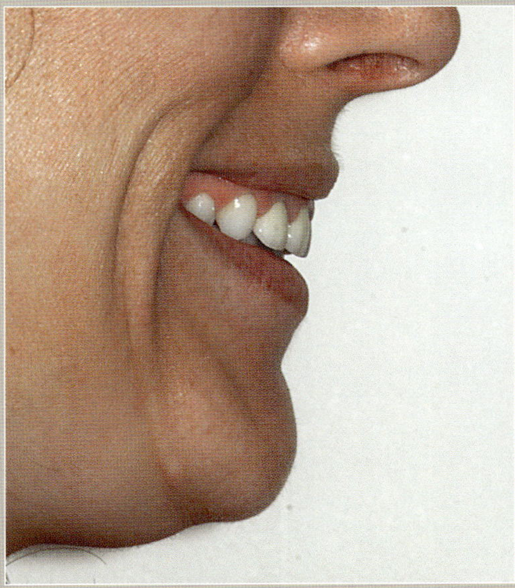

Profile view of smile.

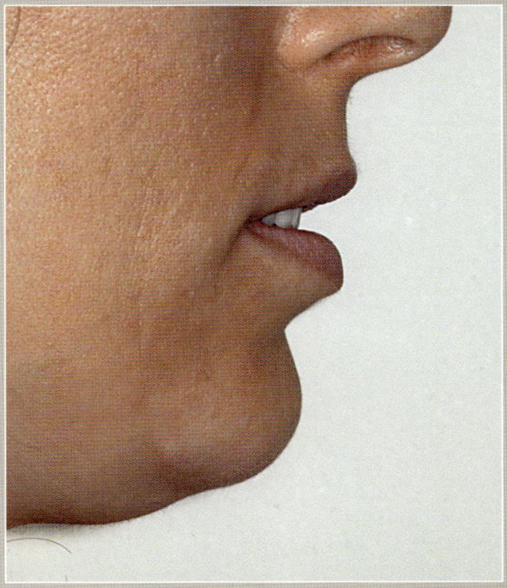

Profile view in repose.

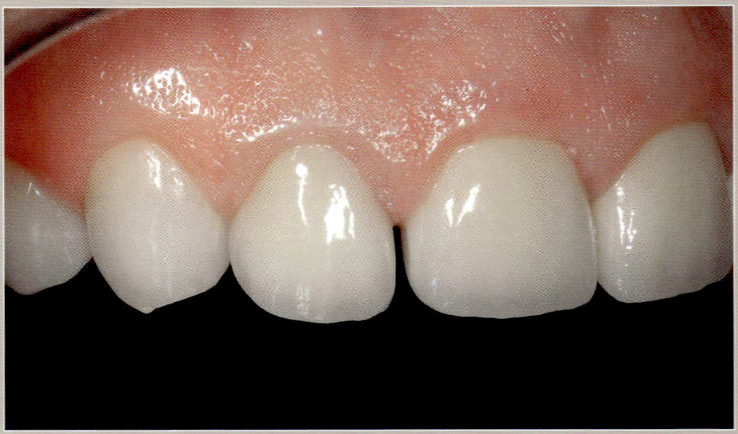

Intraoral view of right maxilla.

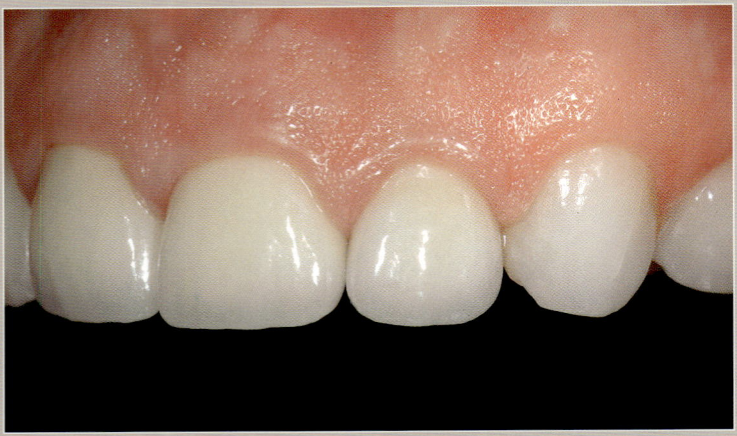

Intraoral view of left maxilla.

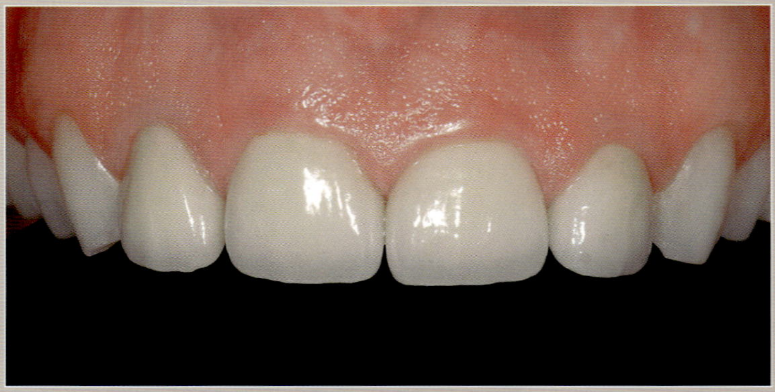

Intraoral view of anterior maxilla.

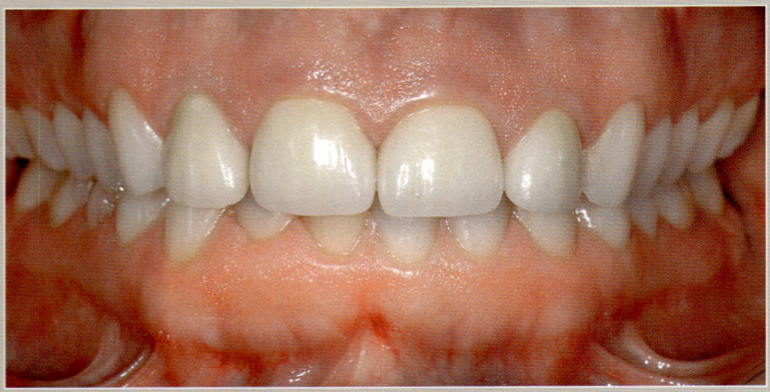

Intraoral frontal view.

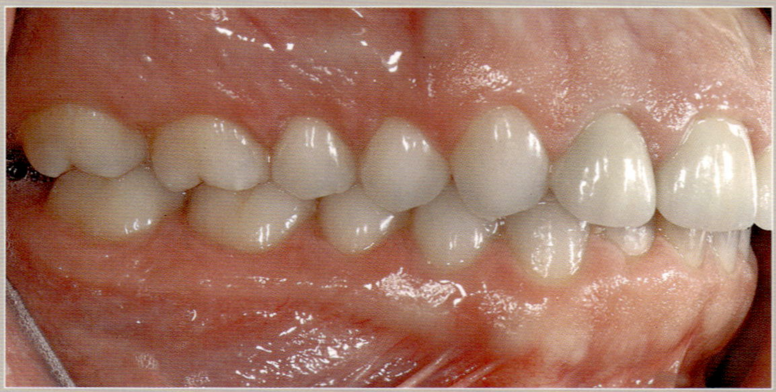

Intraoral right lateral view.

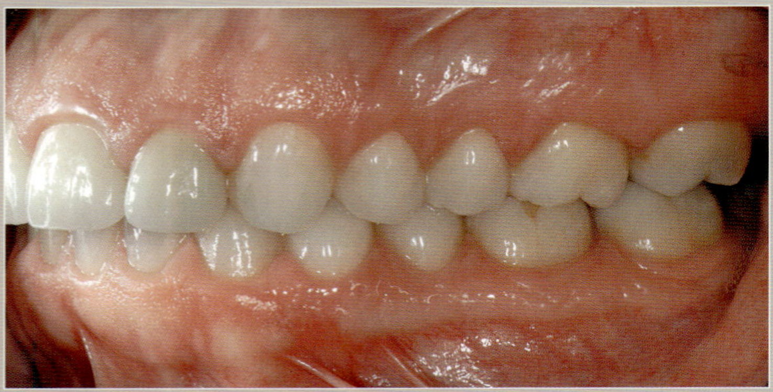

Intraoral left lateral view.

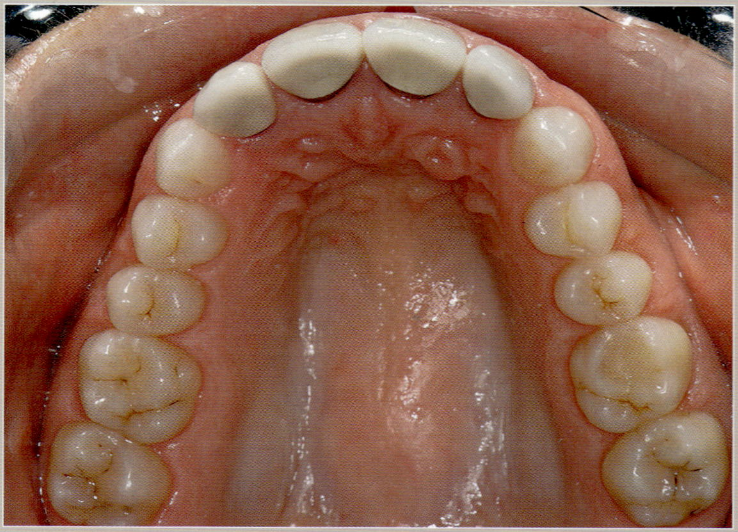

Occlusal maxillary view.

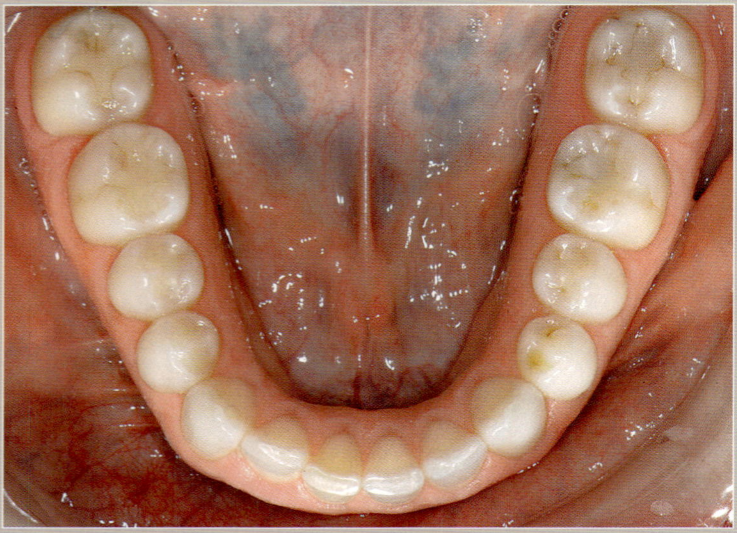

Occlusal mandibular view.

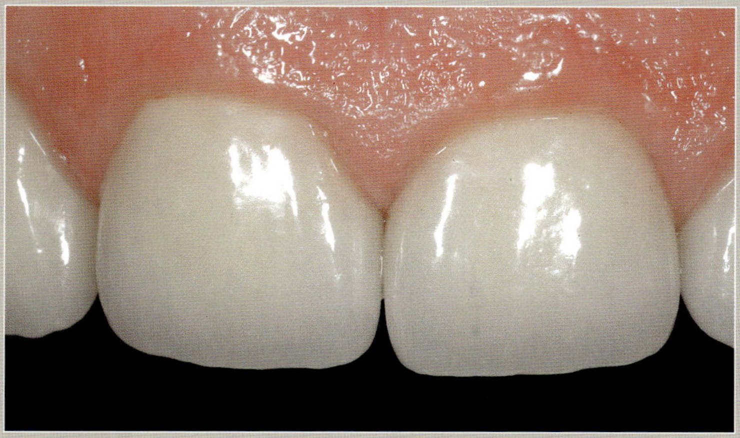

Close-up view of existing crowns on teeth nos. 8 and 9.

TMJ and mandibular range of motion

- Deviation of mandible 2 mm to left upon initial opening with midlines in alignment at full opening
- Full range of motion
- No pain or discomfort upon loading in centric relation (CR)
- No evident clicking or popping in the joint areas
- No pain or discomfort upon opening/closing

Intraoral findings

Dental

- Missing teeth nos. 1, 16, 17, and 32
- Slight to moderate attrition/wear of mandibular anterior teeth
- Slight wear of teeth nos. 6, 11, 13, 20, 22, and 27
- Adequate marginal adaptation of crowns on teeth nos. 7 to 10
- Caries around restoration on tooth no. 15

Periodontal

- Generally healthy periodontium with cyanotic tissue around crowns of teeth nos. 7 to 10
- Adequate zone of attached gingiva throughout
- Thick, flat, fibrous gingival phenotype
- Moderate gingival scalloping
- Excessive gingival stippling in anterior region
- Disparate gingival levels in maxillary anterior region
- Cementoenamel junctions (CEJs) of teeth nos. 7 to 10 palpable roughly 1 to 2 mm subgingivally
- Excellent oral hygiene with minimal plaque

Occlusal notes

- Angle Class I occlusion
- Horizontal overlap (overjet): 3 mm
- Vertical overlap (overbite): 4 mm (50%)
- Retroclined teeth nos. 7 to 10
- CR coincident with maximal intercuspal position
- Canine guidance in right lateral excursion
- Early contact between teeth nos. 13 and 20 gives way to canine guidance in left lateral excursion
- Anterior disocclusion of the posterior teeth during protrusion
- Appropriate mandibular and maxillary curves of Spee
- Appropriate curve of Wilson
- Maxillary arch displays slight concavity in premolar regions bilaterally
- Teeth nos. 4, 5, 12, 13, 21, and 28 rotated between 5 and 15 degrees

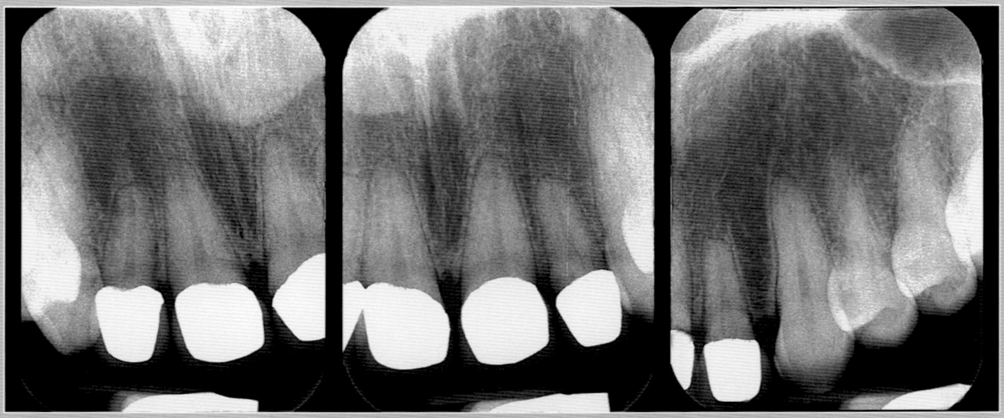

Radiographs of maxillary anterior teeth.

Radiographic findings

- Shortened and blunted roots on teeth nos. 7 to 10 and 29
- Calcified pulp space in tooth no. 24
- Multiple radiopacities below apex of tooth no. 29, not attached to root (ultimately diagnosed as osteosclerosis)

Diagnosis and prognosis

- Altered passive eruption and vertical maxillary excess
- Prognosis: excellent for all teeth

Summary of concerns

1. How can we determine if the patient's complaint that her teeth are "too short" is technically true or simply her perception?
2. Can we meet or exceed her treatment expectations?
3. How will the excessive gingival display be addressed?
4. How can we overcome the anatomical and biologic concerns that may be barriers to achieving the proposed ideal outcome?
5. Knowing this patient's past treatment experience, how can the restorative dentist best communicate to the interdisciplinary team the emotional circumstances surrounding treatment, a clear picture of the intended treatment outcome, and the importance of effective communication throughout the entire treatment process?

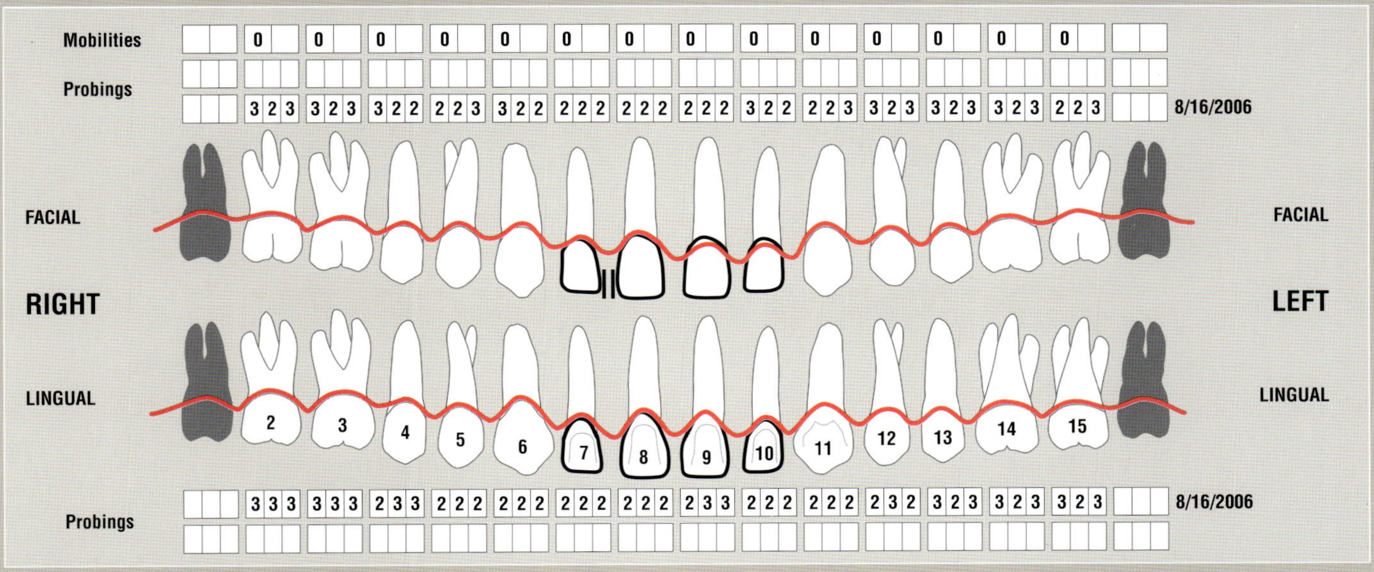

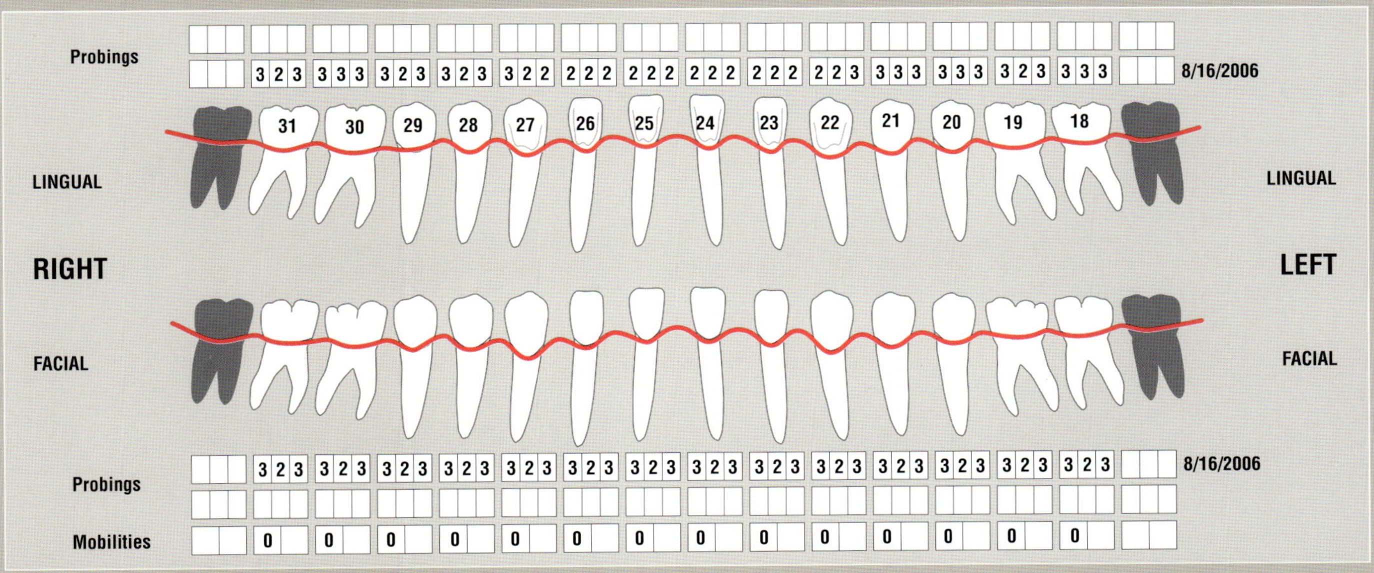

As a learning exercise, you may now outline goals/objectives of treatment and a treatment plan.

Proposed Treatment Plan

Note: While treatment planning this case, it is important to keep in mind that although the patient was referred for both orthodontic and orthognathic evaluations, she chose not to follow through with the orthognathic component of the treatment plan. Nonetheless, the proposed treatment plan for this case will include the appropriate referrals as part of the diagnostic phase, as the information garnered by the patient during the referral process was a key component of her decision to decline orthognathic surgery.

Goals/objectives of treatment

- Create a less gummy smile that the patient finds more pleasing
- Move the incisal edge superior to its current position so that the patient does not perceive that her maxillary anterior teeth are too "low" (not long)
- Close the diastema between teeth nos. 7 and 8
- Develop more pleasing proportions for teeth nos. 7 to 10
- Establish a mutually protected articulation
- Maintain gingival health
- Protect the dentition from parafunctional habits for long-term stability
- Restore the patient's confidence in the dental profession as a whole

Phase I: Diagnostic evaluation

1. Obtain initial records (including maxillary and mandibular casts, intraoral images, facebow transfer, CR record).
2. Perform digital codiagnosis to create initial awareness and discussion of broader dental issues as they relate to potential outcomes.
3. Refer the patient to an orthodontist for consultation.
4. Refer the patient to an oral and maxillofacial surgeon for orthognathic evaluation.
5. Refer the patient to a periodontist for evaluation of soft tissue.
6. Consult with the interdisciplinary team to discuss and determine possible treatment options.
7. Consult with the patient to present initial treatment-planning options (including digital morphing of current smile to determine an esthetic outcome that the patient finds pleasing).
8. Using the final morphed image, communicate with the lab to produce a diagnostic wax-up of the proposed periodontal/restorative outcome.
9. Consult with the patient to review diagnostic wax-ups.

Phase II: Periodontal surgery and provisional restorations

10. Fabricate a surgical guide for the periodontist to perform esthetic crown lengthening.
11. Remove existing porcelain-fused-to-metal crowns nos. 7 to 10 immediately prior to gingival surgery.
12. Perform esthetic crown lengthening on teeth nos. 3 to 14 with the objectives of achieving:
    - Less visible gingiva during smile
    - More pleasing proportions of the anterior teeth
    - Harmonious gingival margins throughout the entire maxillary arch
    - The ability to establish more superior incisal edges of the anterior teeth
13. Prepare teeth for provisional restorations, keeping in mind anticipated final gingival margins.
14. Place a splinted provisional restoration in the sites of teeth nos. 7 to 10 immediately following surgery.
15. Allow for appropriate healing before moving to phase III.

Phase III: Definitive restorations

16. Modify the provisional restorations, if necessary, to aid in determination of the definitive restoration's contours and to assist soft tissue healing and maturation.
17. Perform definitive preparations on teeth nos. 7 to 10 for all-ceramic full-crown restorations.
18. Fabricate and cement all-ceramic restorations.
19. Fabricate maxillary occlusal appliance (nightguard).

Active Clinical Treatment

Review of the goals/objectives of treatment

The main treatment goal expressed by the patient was to reduce the "gumminess" of her smile and to create a more harmonious relationship between the anterior crowns and the rest of the dentition. The treatment objectives established for this patient are as follows:

- Remove the existing unesthetic restorations on teeth nos. 7 to 10
- Alter the soft tissue heights in such a way as to allow less gingival display in the anterior region
- Place definitive restorations that provide the patient with a natural and esthetically pleasing smile
- Restore the patient's faith in the dental profession as a whole

Phase I: Diagnostic evaluation

Diagnostic casts and images were obtained to determine the best course of action for all subsequent steps. The records included diagnostic casts of the maxillary and mandibular arches, facebow transfer, CR record, and a standard set of digital photographic images.

All of this was performed prior to referring the patient to the specialist. It was at this time that all of the images were brought together in a digital case presentation, during which there was much discussion that focused on broader dental issues and helped the patient understand potential solutions and possible barriers to treatment. The importance of the digital case presentation prior to referral cannot be overstated. Using a process called *digital codiagnosis*, patients are educated regarding their current state of dental health. They are not shown potential solutions until they agree that there is a problem to be solved and show a desire for resolution. By allowing the patients to visualize and, most importantly, fully understand their current dental condition, they not only become more of an active participant in the development of their treatment plan but also better understand the importance of a specialty referral. Engaged patients who own their particular dental problems are more likely to accept treatment recommendations and to fully understand the benefits and risks of proposed treatment.

After the orthodontic consultation, the patient declined orthodontics and orthognathic surgery. Her decision not to pursue this potential treatment was one that every member of the team accepted. The interdisciplinary team met to discuss potential options, and because the orthodontic/orthognathic surgery option was no longer viable, the treatment plan was developed by the periodontist and restorative dentist.

The information gained during the process of initial records, digital codiagnosis, and team collaboration allowed for the fabrication of a diagnostic wax-up to exact specifications. By accurately diagnosing the case, developing a hypothesis of possible treatment options, and testing the hypothesis using digitally morphed images before creating a diagnostic wax-up and provisional restorations, the patient, laboratory, and treating clinicians moved into the next phase of treatment with as little left to chance as possible.

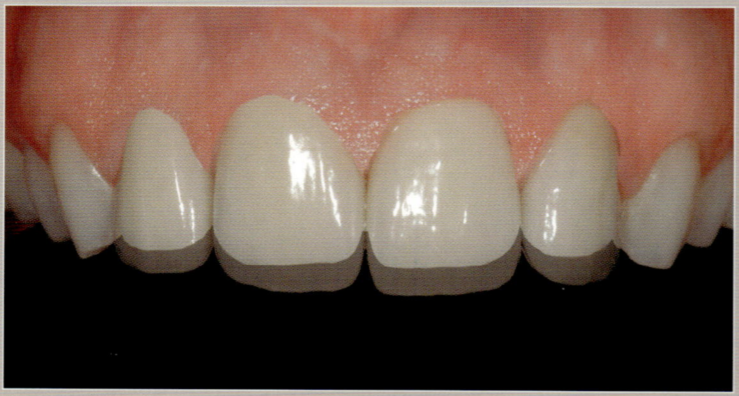

Digital morphing demonstrating approximately 3.5 mm of crown lengthening on teeth nos. 7 to 10 and superior placement of the incisal edge.

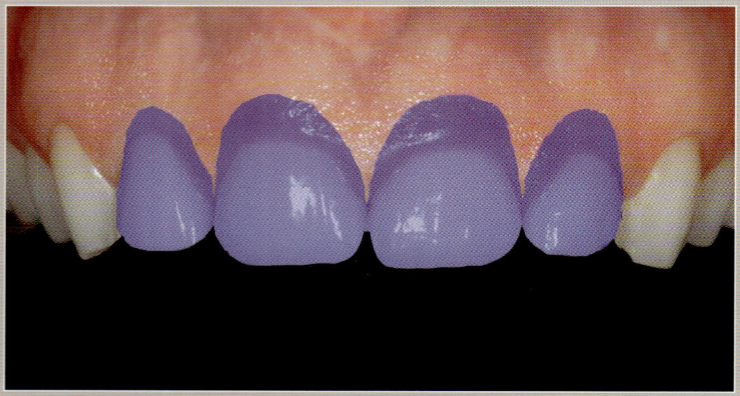

Digital morphing showing proposed shapes of new crowns in purple and volume of tissue to be removed.

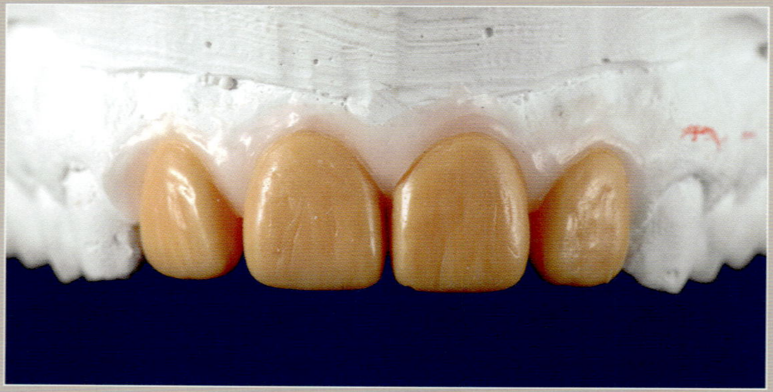

Wax-up produced using morphed images as a guide.

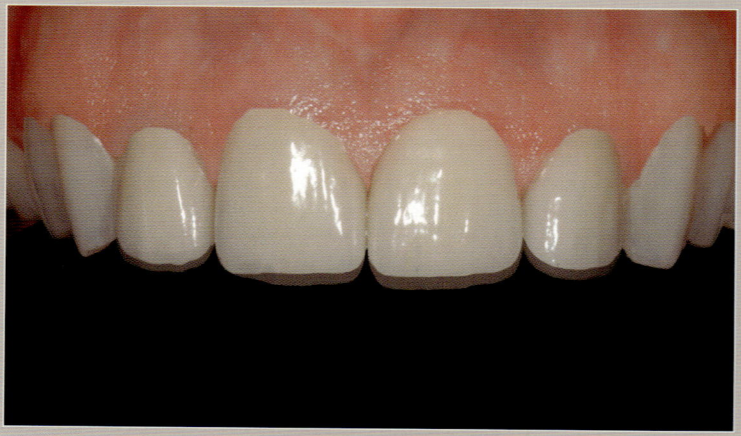

Digitally altered image demonstrating an alternative treatment option that included crown lengthening teeth nos. 4 to 13 and superior placement of the incisal edge.

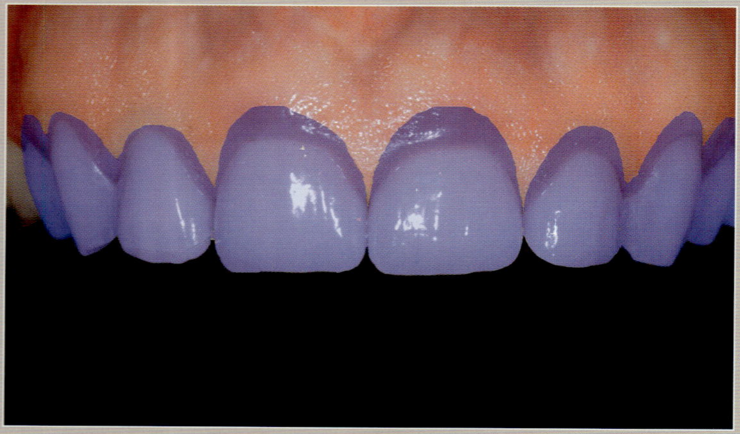

Image demonstrating proposed new crown shapes and smaller volume of tissue to be removed in the alternative treatment plan.

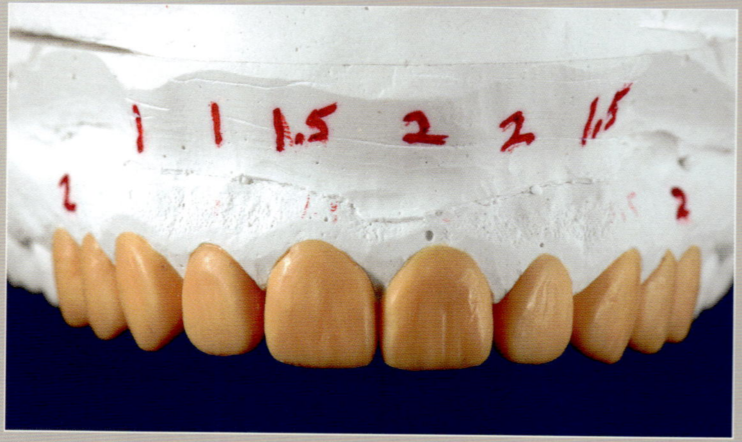

Wax-up of the alternative treatment plan produced using the morphed images.

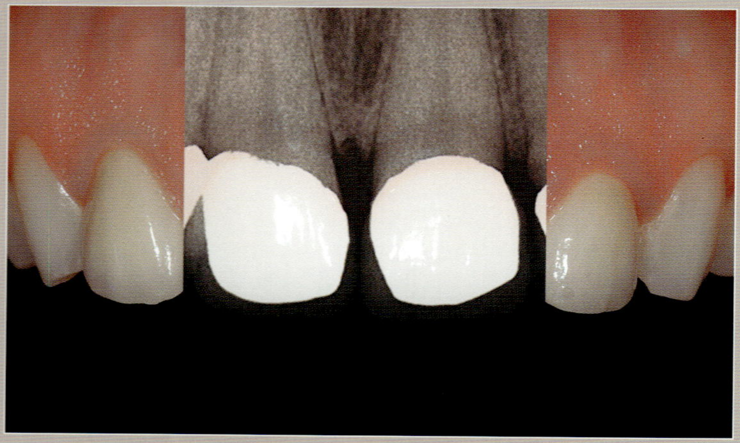

Superimposition of the radiograph on the image of the maxillary teeth.

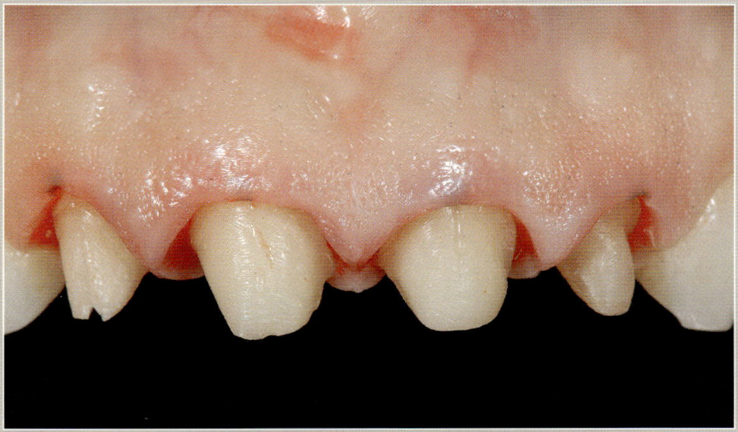

Existing crowns removed prior to crown lengthening.

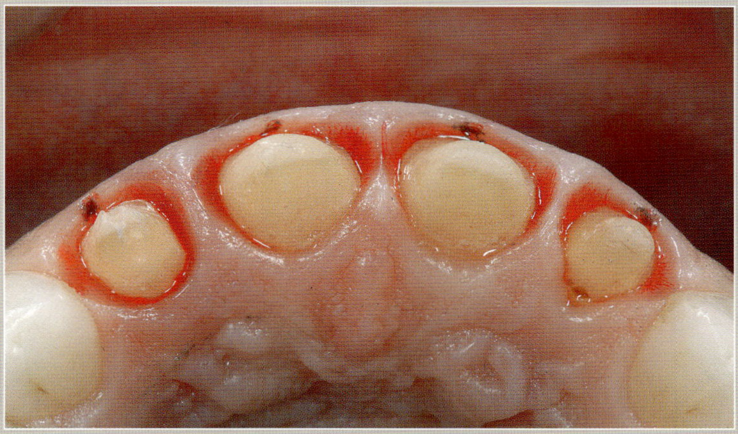

Occlusal view with existing crowns removed.

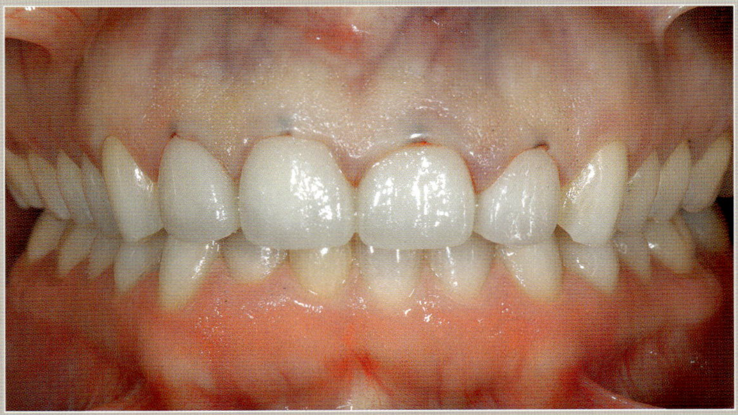

Presurgical try-in of provisional restorations on teeth nos. 7 to 10. (Note: Margins are considerably subgingival here.)

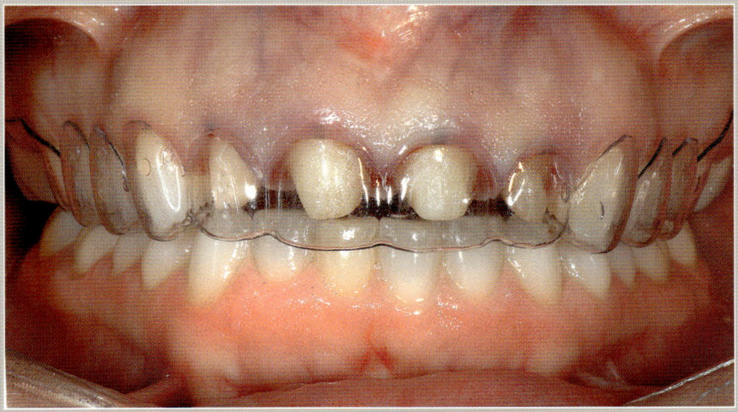

Presurgical view of surgical stent in place.

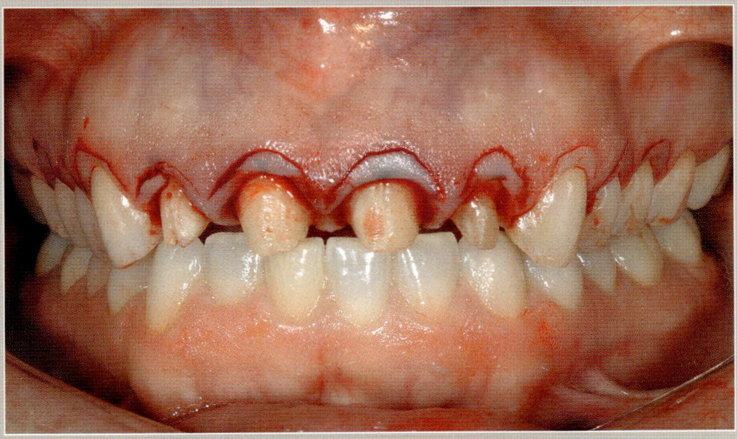

Initial incision.

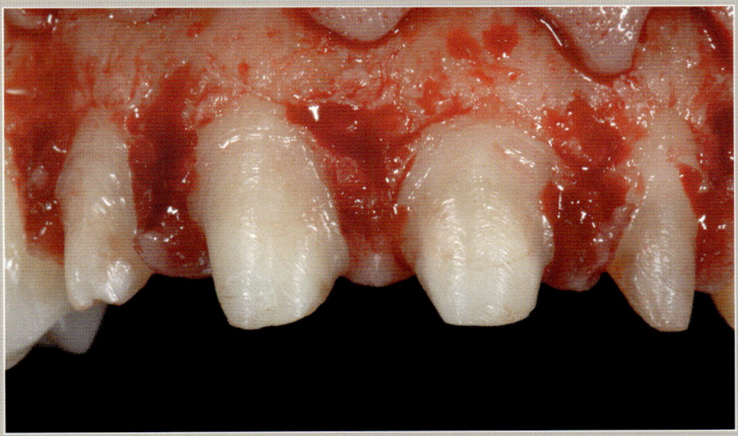

Initial retraction of surgical flap.

Phase II: Periodontal surgery and provisional restorations

The existing crowns on teeth nos. 7 to 10 were removed, and the provisional crowns were tried in to ensure that the incisal edges were in the most ideal position. At this time, because a large part of the provisional restoration was subgingival, it was impossible to fully visualize its appearance; however, when the clear surgical guide was placed, one could, for the first time, begin to appreciate the proposed esthetic outcome. In the periodontist's office, using the clear plastic matrix as a guide, the surgeon removed excess tissue around teeth nos. 3 to 14. Once this was completed, a full-thickness buccal flap was elevated around all the maxillary teeth, with great caution taken

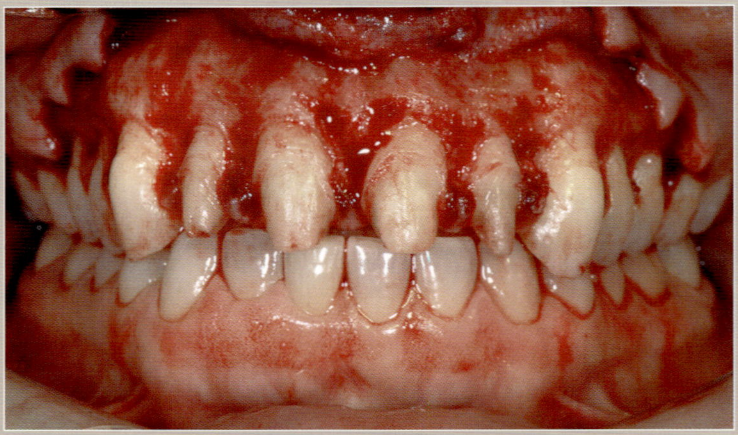

Altered bone contours resulting from crown lengthening.

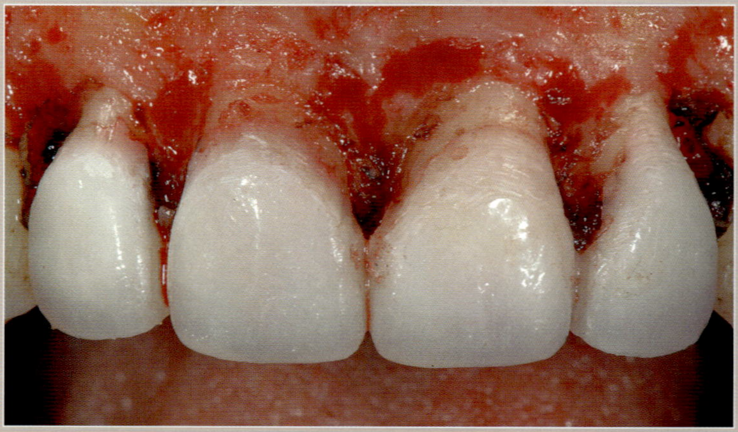

Provisional restorations finished and cemented prior to flap closure.

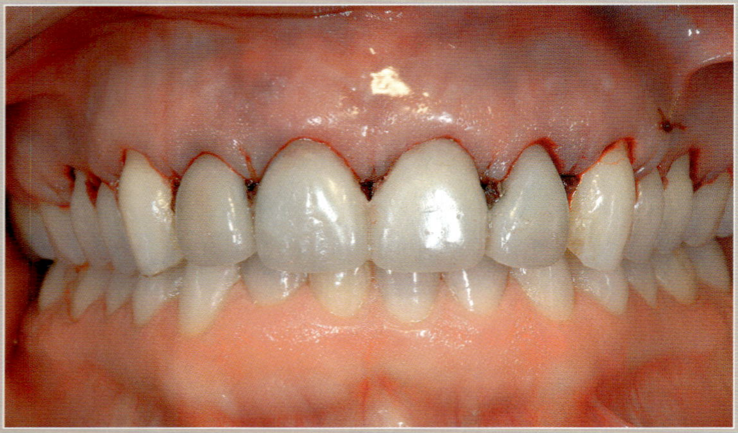

Surgical flap replaced and sutured around the provisional restorations.

to preserve the interdental papillae. The CEJs of the anterior teeth were exposed, and bone was removed to a height of 2 mm from the CEJ. With appropriate healing, this would allow the zeniths of the anterior teeth to be in a more appropriate coronal position compared with their preoperative position.

Note that, because the patient turned down the orthodontic/orthognathic option, a significant amount of time was spent determining where the tissue should be placed using esthetic crown lengthening alone. The preoperative crown-root ratio was already less than ideal, and the thought of removing considerable bone was not appealing to either treating clinician. Additionally, because all-porcelain restorations were going to be used, bonding to enamel was far more propitious than bonding to cementum. The final concern was that the more apically the tissue was placed on the root surface, the less ideal the emergence profiles of the crowns would be. The decision to remove 2 mm of bone apical to the CEJ was made after taking all of these factors into consideration.

Once the appropriate amount of bone was removed and the remaining bony architecture recontoured (with the flap still elevated), the restorative dentist relined, finished, and cemented the provisional restorations with TempBond Clear (Kerr). This allowed unimpeded access to the margins for ideal adaptation and cement removal. However, during surgery and for some time afterwards, the patient demonstrated an unusual amount of bleeding, which was extremely difficult to control. As a result, small amounts of blood were inadvertently incorporated into the provisional restorations, later leading to considerable discoloration of the acrylic. Approximately 1 month later, which was still too early for definitive restorations, a new set of provisional restorations was fabricated to replace the discolored first set.

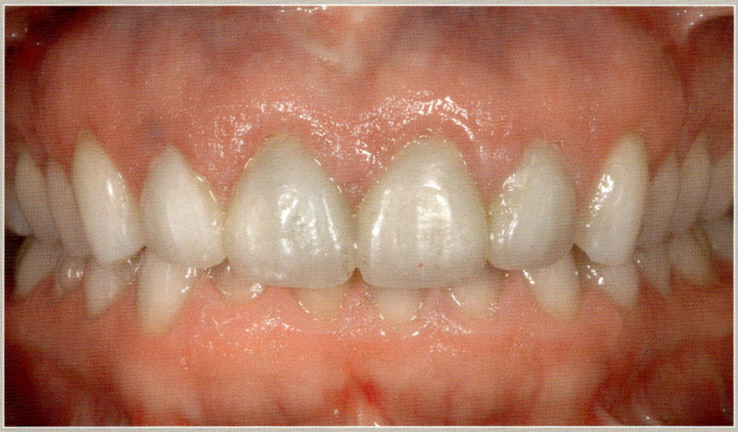

Intraoral frontal view of provisional restorations 9 months after surgery.

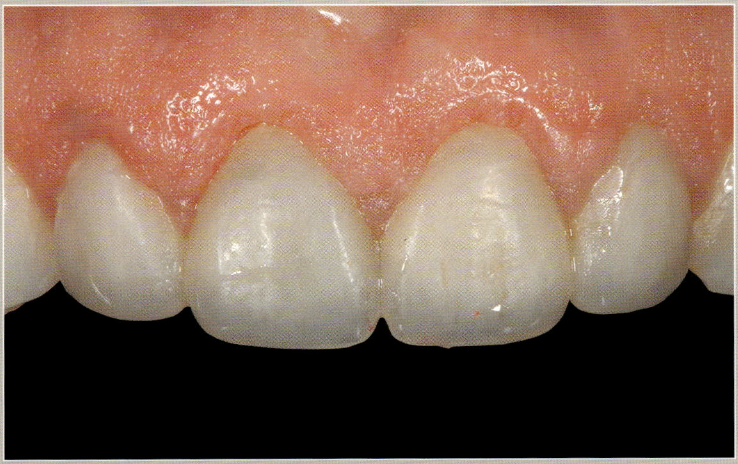

Close-up of provisional restorations 9 months after surgery.

Phase III: Definitive restorations

After approximately 9 months had passed and a palpable gingival sulcus had formed, the decision was made to replace the provisional restorations with the definitive crown restorations.

The provisional restorations were removed, impressions were made, and the definitive restorations were fabricated. The patient was pleased with the shape, size, and contours of the provisional crowns; therefore, they were used as a guide for fabrication of the definitive restorations. The patient went to the dental laboratory to meet with the technician, and they discussed details of the definitive crowns, such as surface texture, incisal translucency, halo, color, and contour.

Empress Esthetic crowns (Ivoclar Vivadent) were fabricated for teeth nos. 7 to 10. The definitive restorations were cemented using Variolink II (yellow shade; Ivoclar Vivadent). A maxillary acrylic nightguard was fabricated to prevent breakage due to her nighttime bruxing and clenching habit. The nightguard was delivered and adjusted in CR and excursive movements. The patient was placed on a 6-month recall schedule.

Posttreatment

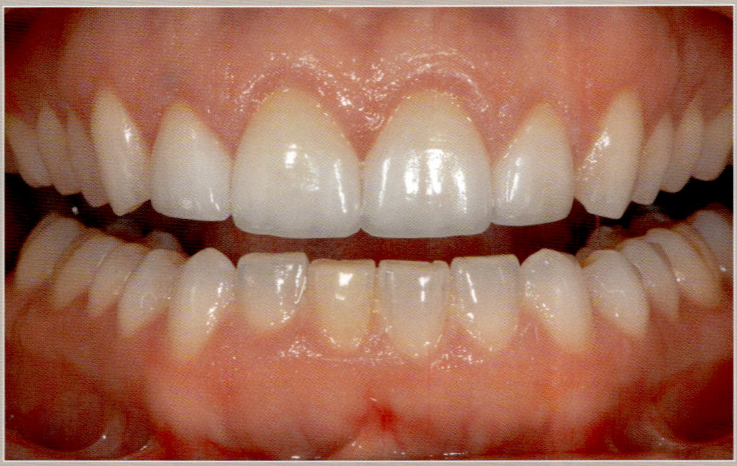

Intraoral frontal view.

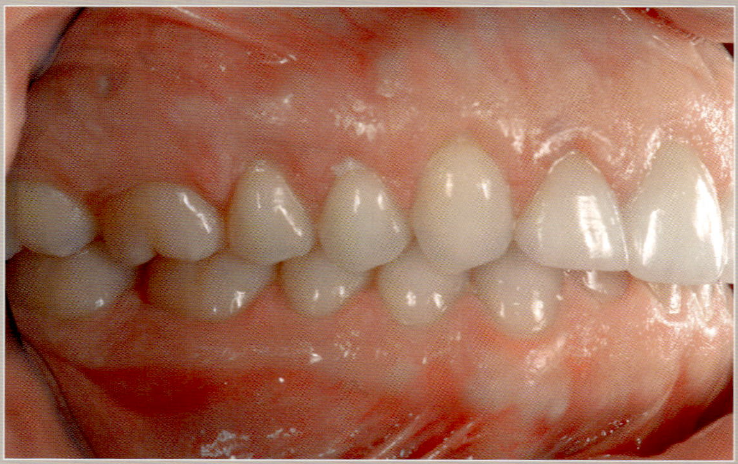

Intraoral right lateral view.

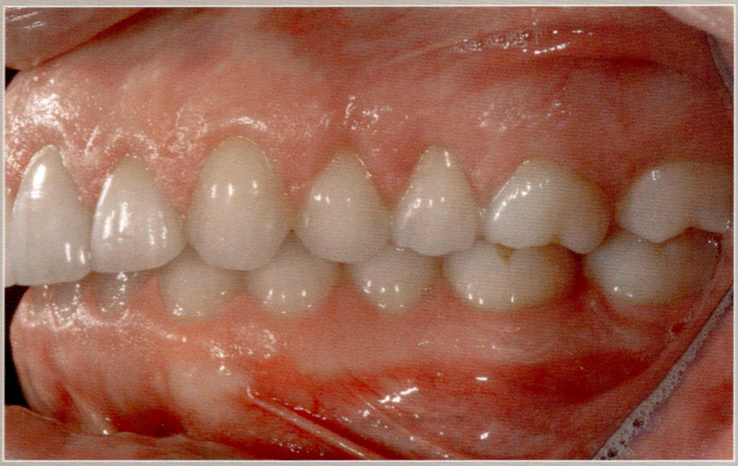

Intraoral left lateral view.

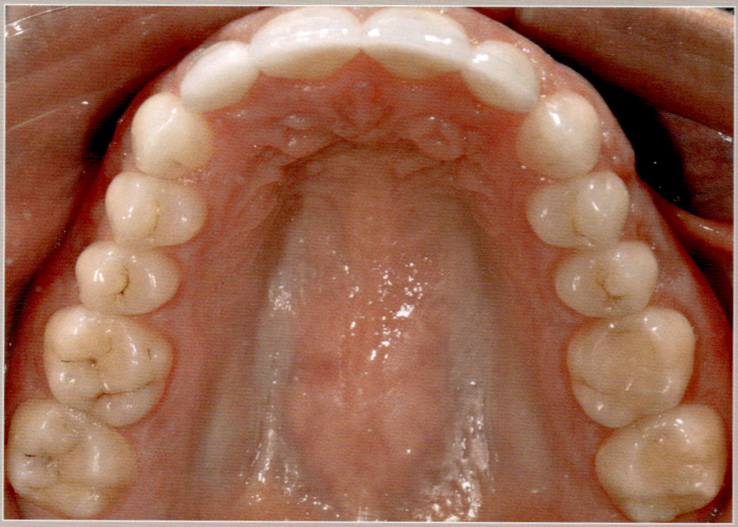

Maxillary occlusal view.

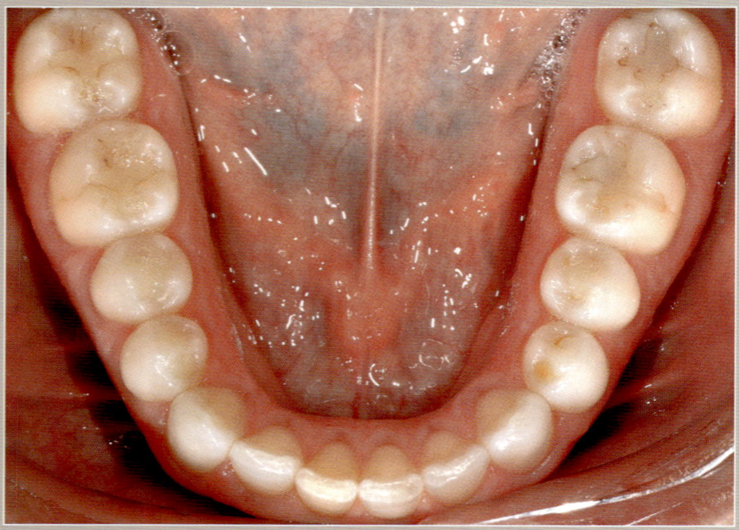

Mandibular occlusal view.

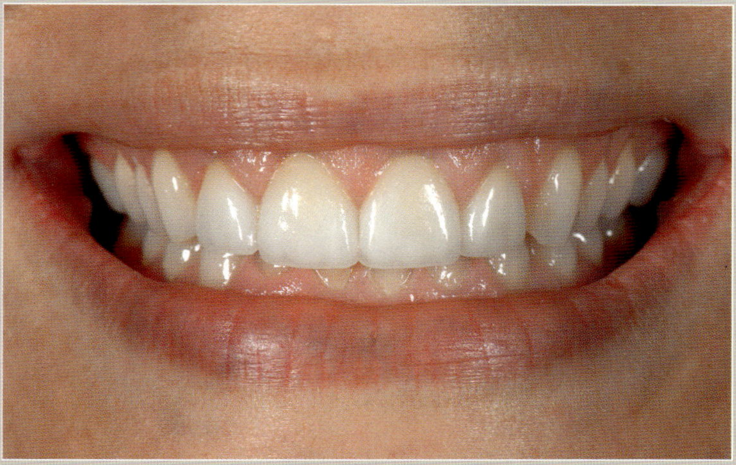

Close-up of smile.

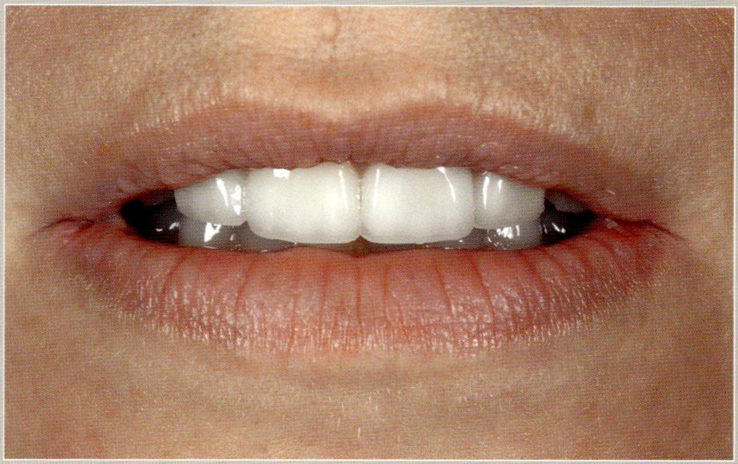

Close-up of mouth in repose.

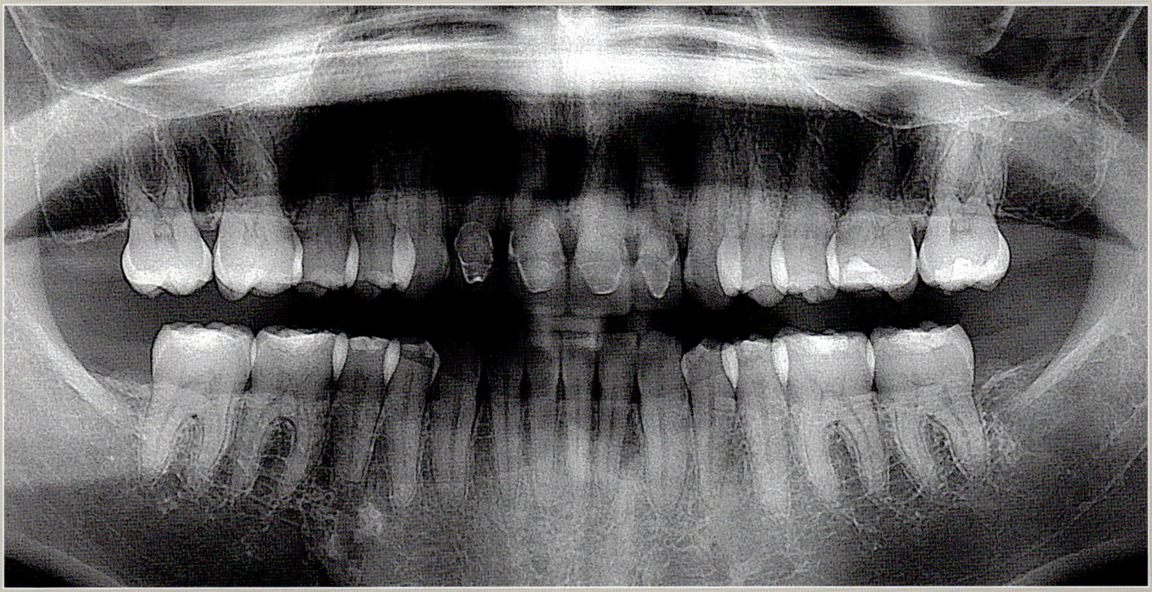

Panoramic radiograph.

You may now place the corresponding posttreatment overlay found in the separate folder over the pretreatment periodontal chart on page 289.

Commentary

Virtually every practitioner has seen this type of case at some point in his or her career. Its difficulty presented in the recognition of subtle challenges lurking below the surface rather than complexity in restorative or surgical treatment. Many clinicians recognize complex interdisciplinary implant or restorative cases as being beyond their ability and either treat or refer them based on comfort level. However, this case was insidious in that most clinicians would look upon it as being an "easy" crown replacement or crown lengthening only to find a nightmare of complexity during the stages of active treatment had the challenges been overlooked or missed.

This case was an excellent example of how attention to detail in the diagnostic stages pays significant dividends during treatment. Although this seemed like a simple case of replacement of four anterior crowns, complete records were nonetheless procured. The patient's decision not to undergo orthodontic therapy and orthognathic surgery complicated matters; however, by remaining vigilant in the comprehensive diagnosis of the case before proceeding, the clinicians were able to adapt to the changes in the parameters of the case. The digital mock-up with patient participation allowed us to approach every step—from diagnostic wax-up to definitive restorations—by beginning with the end in mind.

The challenges of this case were numerous because every answer led to another potential challenge. For instance, once esthetic crown lengthening of the anterior teeth was chosen, would that have caused an unacceptable undermining of the osseous structure? While viewing the preoperative radiographs, one can see that the roots of the anterior teeth were neither long nor morphologically advantageous. There was a great deal of concern that crown lengthening around such short roots gave the surgeon very little latitude in which to balance correction of the altered passive eruption with proper osseous support. By utilizing the digital mock-up and diagnostic wax-up, a lot more predictability for the proper balance was achieved.

When the decision was made to perform surgical crown lengthening in the maxillary arch, a number of new questions arose. How far back in the arch should the lengthening extend? If the cementum of posterior teeth is exposed while harmonizing the tissue, how should that be handled? Surely, placing esthetic restorations on teeth nos. 3 through 14 would create a beautiful smile, but is that necessary? Less is certainly better, but how little is enough? By trying to be conservative, it actually made the case far more challenging.

Furthermore, the existing restorations were too wide compared to many of the other teeth in the arch, and yet the patient did not want to involve any other teeth. Nonetheless, her current Class I relationship did not allow any orthodontic space closure to assist in providing "smaller" teeth. Had the arch been able to be reduced by retroclining of the roots, it would have produced advantageous results. The concern was not simply the width of the teeth but the emergence profiles created by having to close up spaces that were simply too large relative to the rest of the arch. Crown lengthening would further exacerbate this.

As previously mentioned, had one approached this case as being "straightforward," problems would have been encountered at later stages of treatment with no ability for correction. There were issues related to bone support, arch space, and soft tissue treatment planning that, although seen individually in many cases, rarely combine in a "simple" four crown anterior case. Thankfully, by our commitment to a process of diagnostic records and a team approach, these issues were recognized prior to active treatment and subsequently became a part of the treatment-planning process.

As this case illustrates, diagnostic records would not be complete without an excellent set of clinical images. In many respects, clinical images can be as important as diagnostic casts, particularly for this patient, who was able to use visual tools to better communicate her esthetic expectations.

Well-composed images allowed the interdisciplinary team to test certain esthetic outcomes during the diagnostic phase using digital morphing. It was through the use of this technology that all team members and the patient were able to evaluate treatment-planning options before creating a diagnostic wax-up. Through digital technology, we demonstrated *(1)* the option of crown lengthening only teeth nos. 7 to 10 and superior placement of the incisal edge and *(2)* the alternative option of crown lengthening teeth nos. 4 to 13 with subsequent alteration of the incisal edges in the anterior region. We then produced the final wax-ups that resulted from each respective option's digital "hypothesis." One can imagine how easy it is to discuss the pros and cons of each treatment plan using these morphed images. Without highly diagnostic images, however, even this technology has significant limitations.

The treating dentist can also combine easy-to-understand images with the clinical data. For instance, we demonstrated to the patient the effect that esthetic crown lengthening has on the crown-to-root ratio by superimposing the radiograph over an image of the proposed final outcome. This effect is something that must be kept in mind, particularly in a case such as this where shorter roots and a less-than-ideal crown-to-root ratio already exists.

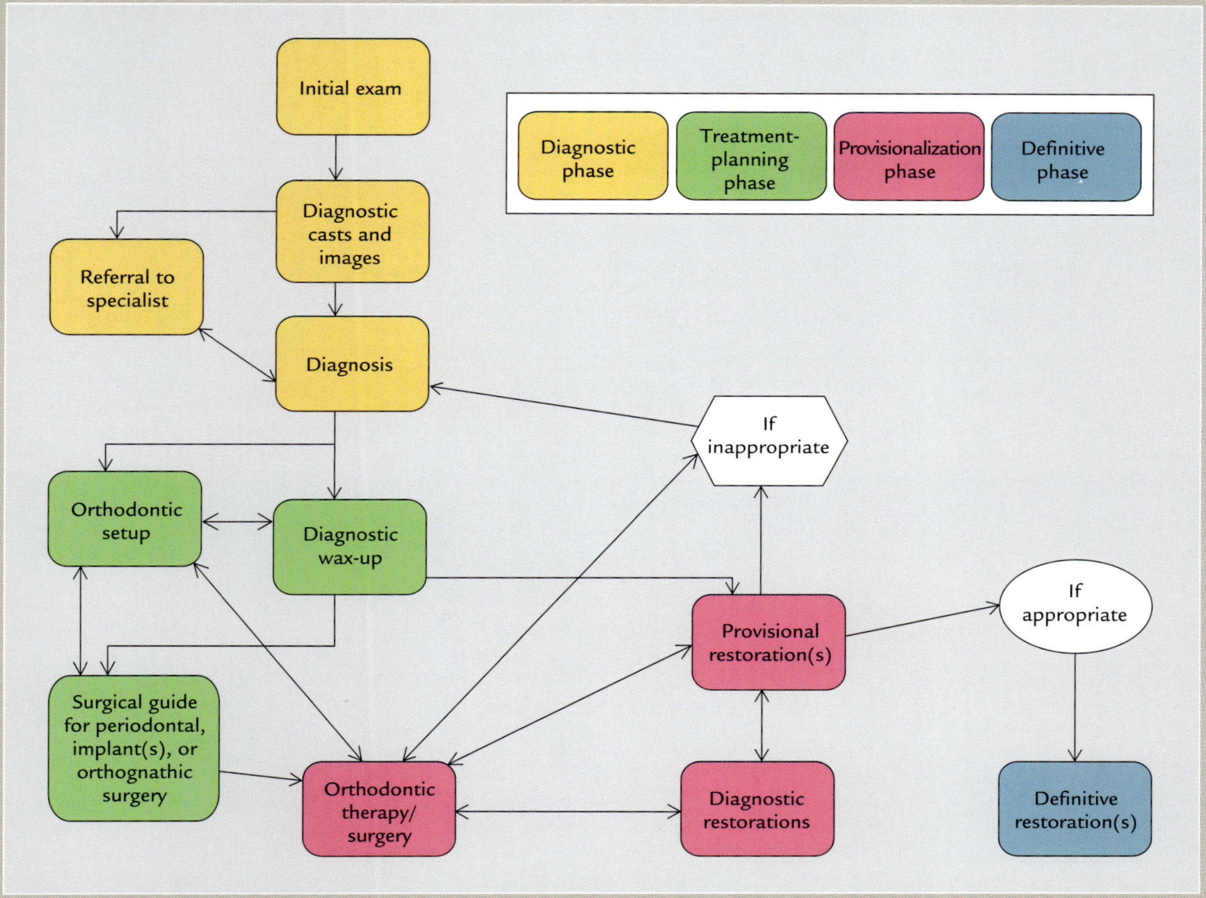

Interdisciplinary treatment algorithm.

Interdisciplinary treatment algorithm

Analyzing and integrating the clinical data into a meaningful comprehensive treatment plan takes time to master. However, if one creates a decision tree that relates to the underlying clinical decision-making pathway, this entire process can be repeated again and again with consistent results, regardless of the intricacies of the case being treated. To this end, we created an interdisciplinary diagnostic treatment algorithm that demonstrates a series of potential treatment pathways from start to finish. There are four distinct phases: *(1)* diagnostic, *(2)* treatment planning, *(3)* provisionalization, and *(4)* definitive restoration.

Diagnostic phase

The diagnostic phase commences when the dentist meets the patient and begins discussing the chief concern. A comprehensive exam, radiographs, mounted casts, and well-composed clinical images are essential components of this phase. It is at this point that specialist referral and team collaboration become essential. The final goal of the diagnostic phase is to develop a comprehensive treatment plan that addresses all concerns related to the patient's dental needs and overall expectations.

The diagnosis was of paramount importance to this case because it was the previous failure to properly diagnose that led the patient to her current chief complaint. By determining the exact causes for the patient's unhappiness with her smile, namely vertical maxillary excess and altered passive eruption, we were able to address them directly. Asking *why* assisted in arriving at a diagnosis: Why are the gingival levels in their present position? Why is there an excess of gingiva displayed? Why did the previous treatment not solve the problem?

Treatment-planning phase

Once a proper diagnosis was established, we could begin to visualize how the outcome of treatment should look and use this information to formulate the final plan. Questions that arose during treatment planning centered on what to do and how to do it: What will the definitive restorations look like? How will the case be provisionalized? How will the definitive incisal edge position be determined?

The clinical images were important in helping the treating clinicians gain answers to all of the *why, what,* and *how* questions. Because it has been shown that dentists and patients have different acceptable standards for many esthetic components[1] and there are unique patterns of communication between patients and clinicians,[2,3] morphing proposed outcomes with the patient's assistance fosters more congruency between expectations and the final results. In this case, it was essential that the patient understand the esthetic possibilities and differences in outcome for each treatment plan. Once the patient and clinician agreed on the final esthetics, the images were given to the laboratory to develop a wax-up to see if the outcome was feasible from an occlusal perspective.

There are, unfortunately, numerous cases where digital mock-ups demonstrate that a desired esthetic outcome is not possible within the parameters outlined by the patient. Although such a finding is disheartening, it is better to find out at this stage than to end up with an unacceptable outcome, such as the one this patient presented with, solely because the diagnostic phase was never effectively completed.

During the treatment-planning phase, a surgical guide and provisional restorations were created from the diagnostic wax-up. Had the patient accepted the orthodontic/orthognathic option, an orthodontic setup might also have been included.

The defining characteristic of the treatment-planning phase is the determination, through a well-defined treatment plan, that the factors associated with the diagnosis can be solved with an orthodontic, surgical, restorative, or combined approach.

Provisionalization phase

If the diagnostic phase is where one develops a hypothesis regarding the final outcome, the provisionalization phase is where it is tested. It is far better to see the inadequacies of a proposed treatment plan in the provisionalization phase than when definitive restorations begin failing. The cost, time, and emotional investment of fixing a problem in definitive restorations makes the provisional stage of critical importance. If there are any questions related to the viability of the treatment plan, this is where they should be answered. One should think of the provisionalization stage as a process and not as a means to an end. This is where details regarding the occlusal scheme are worked out and final soft tissue forms contoured through orthodontics and the judicious use of provisional restorations.

During this phase, one must ultimately decide whether or not the patient is ready for definitive treatment. If there is any degree of uncertainty regarding the provisional restorations or if orthodontic therapy is not progressing as desired, the treatment team should return to the diagnostic phase. New casts should be made, images taken, and a new treatment plan developed to address the shortfalls in the first approach.

The provisionalization phase is considered complete only when the patient and treating clinician(s) agree that the biologic, functional, and esthetic considerations of the case have been properly addressed and the case is ready to enter the definitive phase of treatment.

Definitive phase

If the diagnostic and provisionalization phases have been properly managed, the definitive phase may be nothing more than swapping out provisional restorations for definitive ones. Moreover, the provisional restorations may act as a useful aid in fabricating the definitive restorations.[4,5]

In this case, because the patient liked the appearance of the provisional restorations, the laboratory had an easy time transitioning to definitive crowns, and allowing time for the gingival tissue to mature[6–8] was not a problem. The patient was thrilled with the definitive treatment result.

The myriad treatment options currently available to clinicians provide the opportunity to offer patients an unprecedented level of care. It is vital that the treating clinician and patient understand the benefits and risks of each plan under consideration. The opportunity to do this lies within the clinician's ability to bridge the gap between clinical knowledge and patient understanding. With the use of high-quality clinical images and the digital codiagnostic process, a treatment plan can be created that is born out of the combination of the clinician's knowledge and the patient's desires. Treatment options are chosen through educated reasoning rather than simple, visceral emotional responses. It is by way of this partnership that clinicians can most predictably serve the needs of the patient in a way that goes far beyond simply fixing teeth.

References

1. Kokich VO, Kokich VG, Kiyak HA. Perceptions of dental professionals and laypersons to altered dental esthetics: Asymmetric and symmetric situations. Am J Orthod Dentofacial Orthop 2006;130:141–151.
2. Sondell K, Söderfeldt B, Palmqvist S, Adell A. Communication during prosthodontic treatment—Dentist, patient, and dental nurse. Int J Prosthodont 2000;13:506–512.
3. Sondell K, Söderfeldt B, Palmqvist S. Dentist-patient communication and patient satisfaction in prosthetic dentistry. Int J Prosthodont 2002;15:28–37.
4. Nemcovsky CE, Gross MD. Transferring provisional restorations to final master casts. J Oral Rehabil 1994;21:157–163.
5. Nemcovsky CE. Transferring the occlusal and esthetic anatomy of the provisional to the final restoration in full-arch oral rehabilitations. Compend Contin Educ Dent 1996;17:72–80.
6. Pontoriero R, Carnevale G. Surgical crown lengthening: A 12-month clinical wound healing study. J Periodontol 2001;72:841–848.
7. Deas DE, Moritz AJ, McDonnell HT, Powell CA, Mealey BL. Osseous surgery for crown lengthening: A 6-month clinical study. J Periodontol 2004;75:1288–1294.
8. Perez JR, Smukler H, Nunn ME. Clinical evaluation of the supraosseous gingivae before and after crown lengthening. J Periodontol 2007;78:1023–1030.

12

Management of Patients with Missing/Abnormally Proportioned Teeth, Part II*

Ward M. Smalley, DDS, MSD

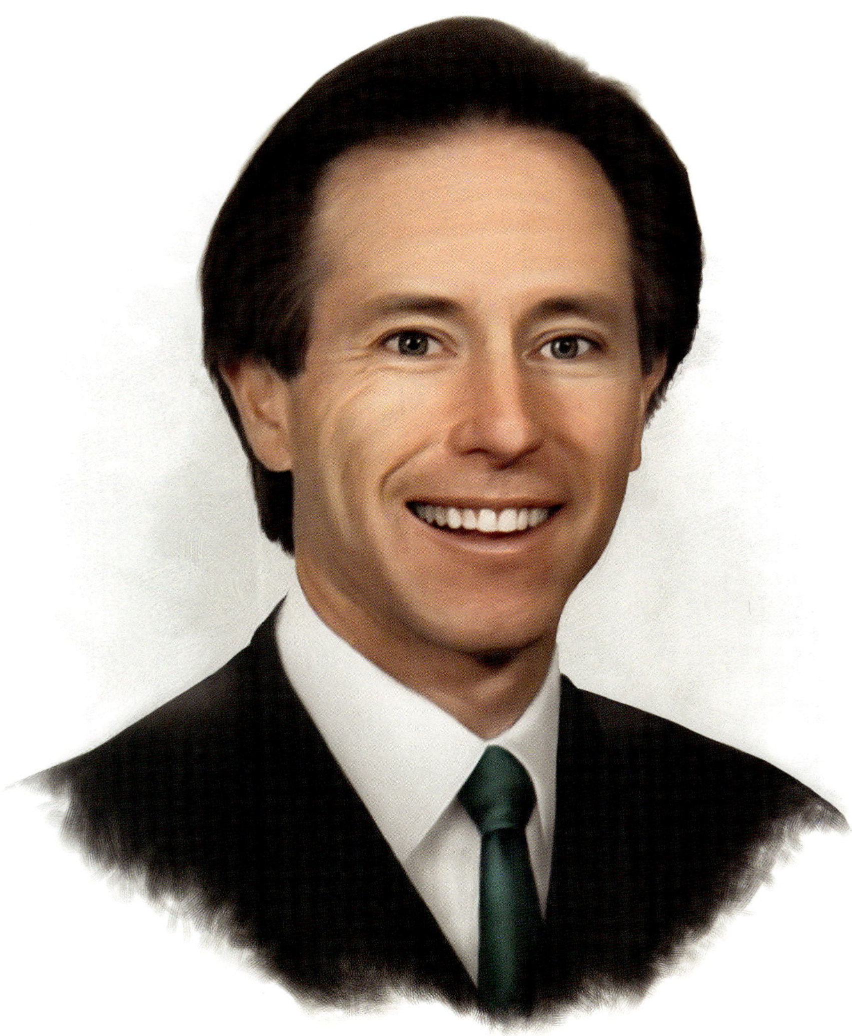

When it comes to appropriating space for tooth replacement,

the only parameter of real importance is actual tooth width.

*To read Part I ("Comprehensive interdisciplinary management of patients with missing and/or abnormally proportioned teeth"), see *Interdisciplinary Treatment Planning*, ed M. Cohen (Quintessence, 2008):343–382.

PHILOSOPHY AND BACKGROUND

There are two reasons why the following case presentation was selected for this chapter. The first is that the patient's dentition manifested considerable spatial concerns related to tooth position induced by a congenital anomaly, amelogenesis imperfecta, which is a disorder of tooth development characterized by abnormal enamel formation. There are four main types of amelogenesis imperfecta based on enamel effects: hypoplastic (type I), hypomaturation (type II), hypocalcified (type III), and hypomaturation/hypoplasia/taurodontism (type IV). Fourteen subtypes have also been identified based on clinical appearance and mode of inheritance. The disorder may be inherited as an X-linked, autosomal dominant, or autosomal recessive genetic trait, depending on the type.

All of this patient's permanent teeth developed with abnormally thin, pitted enamel. As a result, the clinical crowns of her teeth had atypical morphology and were deficient in all dimensions. The spaces between many of her teeth had been compromised by the absence of normal proximal contours and compensatory tooth movement that resulted in root proximity and insufficient space proximally and vertically to manage restoration of normal coronal dimensions and morphology.

Furthermore, her teeth were very unattractive. In addition to the enamel deficiency and pitted surfaces, her teeth appeared brownish-yellow in color from the intense, saturated color of the underlying dentin that was visible through the thin enamel. The lack of enamel and other structural deficiencies also led to accelerated wear, compromised occlusal function, and increased sensitivity of her teeth. To address some of these problems, her pediatric dentist placed stainless steel crowns on her posterior teeth.

The second reason for choosing this case presentation is that the patient has an earnest desire to help others afflicted with the same or similar dental anomalies. She has actively shared the successful resolution of her problems through a variety of modalities. This patient's unselfish efforts to help others in this regard is admirable. It is my hope that the publication of her treatment will increase the level of awareness of the anomaly within the profession and demonstrate what can be done to correct such problems, improving the quality of life for other patients suffering from amelogenesis imperfecta and similar disorders.

Space appropriation

I suggest that when planning treatment for this or any other patient with similar dental problems, the reader should focus primarily on the requirements for optimal space appropriation in all three planes of space. All of her teeth are in need of restoration to establish normal contours for appearance (undoubtedly the patient's primary goal), function, and protection from accelerated breakdown (eg, wear, caries, sensitivity, inflammation). To facilitate this, one needs to know the average dimensions and morphology of all the crowns of the teeth, including the mesiodistal, buccolingual, and occluso-/incisogingival dimensions as well as the ratios of clinical coronal width to height[1–13] (Figs 1 and 2).

With these dimensions in mind, the arch length deficiencies that exist as a result of compensation for the coronal insufficiencies can be determined and managed to achieve an optimal treatment result. The positions of the teeth can then be altered by orthodontic treatment to resolve the deficiencies and establish ideal spacing to facilitate definitive restoration of the teeth.

Use of the golden proportion or percentage to determine the size of spaces needed to either restore or replace maxillary anterior teeth is inappropriate because it only relates to an optical perspective of aligned teeth from a frontal view and not the actual sizes of teeth. Levin[14] clearly

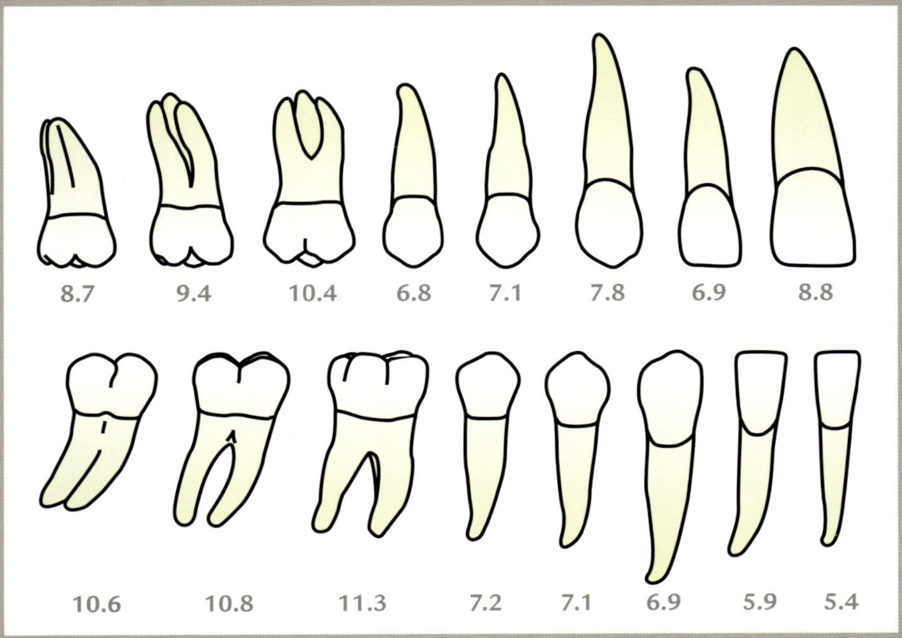

Fig 1 Average mesiodistal crown dimensions (mm) of natural teeth compiled from several sources.[1–13]

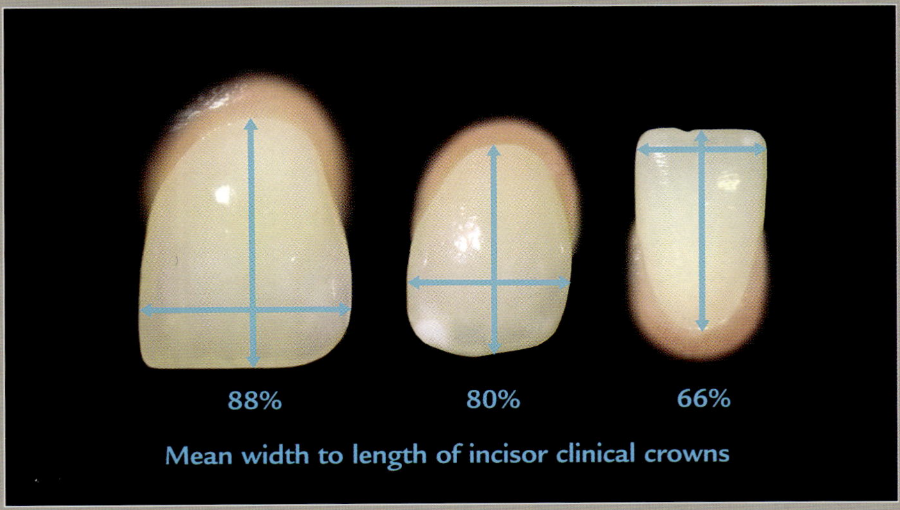

Fig 2 Width-to-length proportions of maxillary central incisors (range, 84% to 91%; mean, 88%), maxillary lateral incisors (range, 76% to 84%; mean, 80%), and mandibular incisors (range, 62.5% to 71%; mean, 66%), compiled from several sources.[5,6,8–10]

stated that "the widths of the incisors are in golden proportion to each other as seen from the front." Lombardi,[15] who was the first to discuss the golden proportion relative to teeth, stated that the ratio "is too strong for dental use." Magne et al[11] concurred and reported that use of the golden proportion applied to teeth would lead to the development of relatively narrow arches. Gillen et al[9] and Preston[16] also showed a poor correlation between actual tooth dimensions and the golden proportion. Furthermore, Preston found that, even from a perceived perspective, the golden proportion was relevant in only 17% of the population. Based on this relatively low incidence and the absence of any correlation between the golden proportion and actual tooth dimensions, it is clear that the golden proportion is of little or no value in restorative or prosthetic dentistry. Moreover, from a purely esthetic standpoint, the perceived widths of teeth can easily be changed by altering their facial contours to change the amount of light reflected off a tooth's labial surface, effectively making a tooth appear narrower or wider as desired without changing the actual width of a tooth. However, when it comes to appropriating space for tooth replacement, the only parameter of real importance is actual tooth width. The perceived width is of no value in this regard.

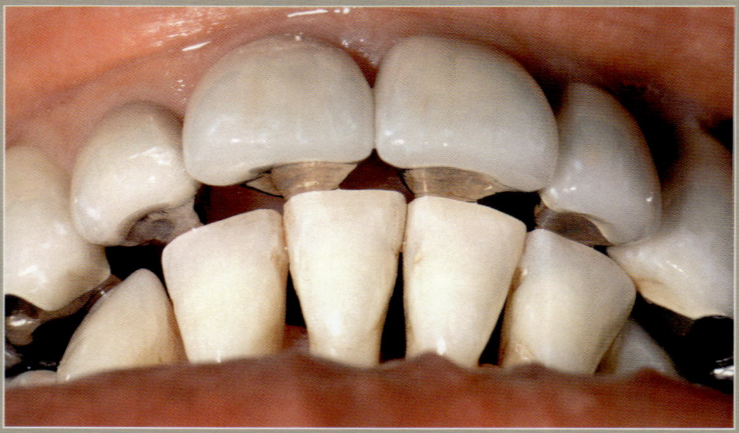

Fig 3 Restored maxillary teeth with increased labiolingual dimensions and pronounced cingulum to establish occlusal contact with mandibular anterior teeth in MIP (with MIP coincident with centric occlusion and centric relation) to compensate for increased horizontal overlap (overjet) caused by a unilateral Class II relationship.

Occlusal relationship

To achieve optimal appearance and occlusion of the teeth, it also is essential to have the anterior teeth aligned in a Class I relationship, a topic I discussed briefly in the first volume of this series (Interdisciplinary Treatment Planning, Quintessence, 2008). A Class I anterior relationship of the teeth allows a normal vertical and horizontal overlap of the teeth (2 to 4 mm) to be established, as well as the most desirable proclination of the incisors with the teeth in maximal intercuspal position (MIP). From a functional perspective, having the anterior teeth in a Class I relationship promotes the most favorable guidance of the teeth in and out of MIP.

Without having or establishing an anterior Class I relationship, a number of compromises are inevitable regarding orientation and/or size of the anterior teeth. In Class II situations or tendencies, any one or more of the following will occur:

- Horizontal and/or vertical overlap (ie, overjet and overbite, respectively) of the incisors becomes compromised (to establish contact in MIP). Horizontal overlap of the incisors usually decreases as the maxillary incisors become more upright, and vertical overlap of the incisors increases as both the maxillary and mandibular incisors overerupt.
- The incisors become unfavorably inclined, usually with the maxillary incisors relatively upright and the mandibular incisors excessively proclined, by attempting to achieve contact of the incisors orthodontically without a Class I relationship.
- The width of the maxillary incisors may be reduced, often to the point of being too narrow to be esthetically pleasing, and/or the mandibular incisors may be made wider. Both are performed in an effort to reduce horizontal overlap of the incisors.
- Crowding or overlapping of the maxillary incisors—in lieu of making the incisors narrower—is accomplished in an effort to reduce horizontal overlap of the incisors and achieve occlusal contact of the anterior teeth in MIP.
- The curve of Spee becomes exaggerated on the mandibular arch and reversed on the maxillary arch.

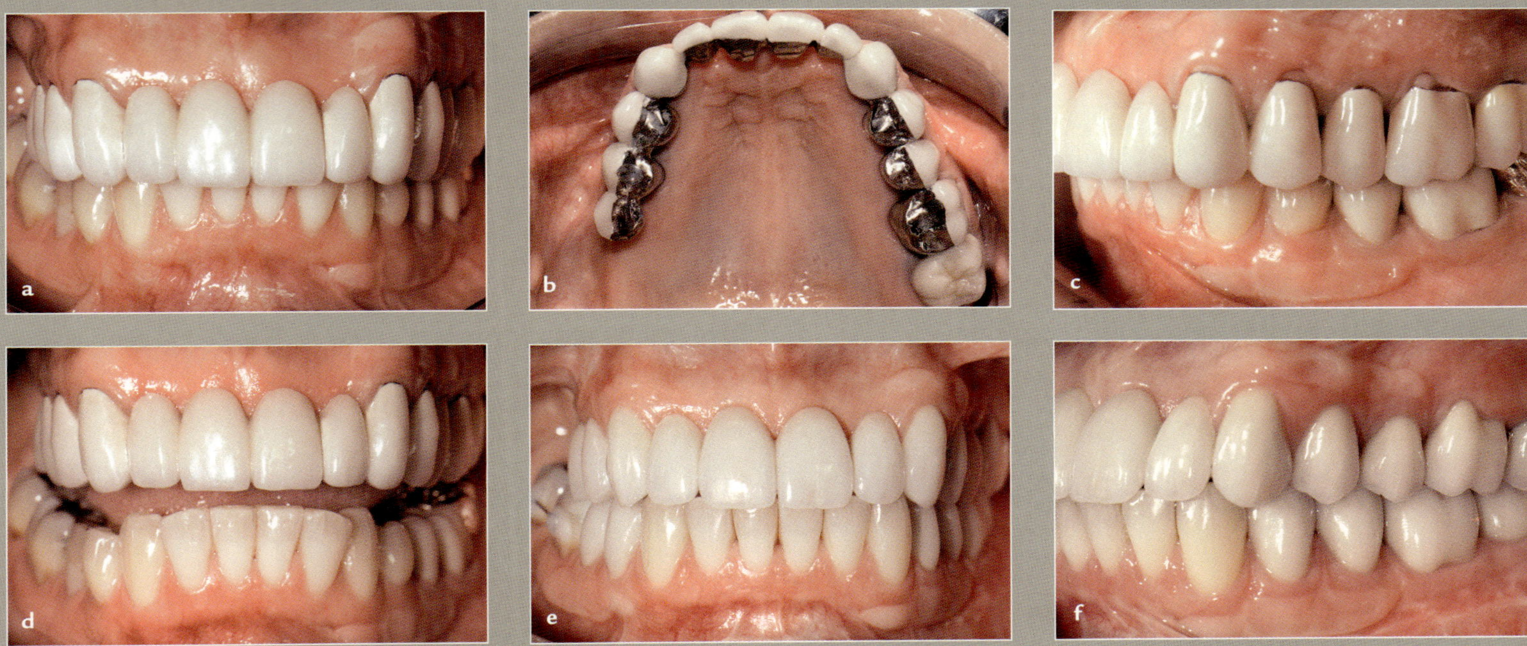

Fig 4 *(a)* Frontal view of unesthetic prosthetic replacement of maxillary incisors with pontics that are too narrow for their length in a misdirected effort to reduce excessive horizontal overlap of the anterior teeth caused by a Class II relationship. *(b)* Occlusal view of pontics reveals exaggerated cingula on the central incisors that proved to be insufficient to provide stable occlusal contact with the mandibular incisors in MIP. *(c)* Left lateral view showing Class II relationship. Note that the horizontal overlap of incisors is less than the normal 8 mm associated with Class II, division 1 relationships having aligned incisors. *(d)* Frontal view showing overeruption of mandibular incisors as a result of the unstable occlusal relationship that occurred after prosthetic reconstruction of the maxillary teeth. *(e and f)* Frontal and left lateral views after establishment of anterior Class I relationship and replacement of previous restorations. Note normal size and proportions of the incisors (and other teeth) and the normal vertical and horizontal overlap of the anterior teeth.

With the anterior teeth in a Class II relationship or tendency, it is impossible to have anterior teeth of a normal width, ideally aligned and level, and contacting in MIP with the mandibular condyles in centric relation (CR). The greater the magnitude of the Class II relationship, the greater the horizontal overlap of the incisors. In Class III situations, the opposite is true, ie, the horizontal overlap of the incisors decreases with increasing magnitude of the Class III relationship and may even become nonexistent or negative.

From a restorative perspective, having the anterior teeth in any relationship other than Class I usually leads to additional compromises resulting from an effort to compensate for the lack of normal incisor contact. To manage the excessive horizontal overlap of the incisors that is inevitable in Class II relationships or tendencies with relatively aligned and level teeth, the labiolingual dimension of restorations placed on maxillary incisors is often increased, and the height of the cingulum area is moved incisally to establish occlusal contact of the maxillary and mandibular incisors in MIP and, hopefully, stability of incisor position (Fig 3). This often increases the thickness of the crowns on the maxillary incisors well beyond that of normal contours. The amount of contour change is dependent on the amount of horizontal and vertical overlap that exists, which again is dependent on the magnitude of the Class II relationship. Patients often find this restorative solution to the problem less than desirable because the teeth feel too thick and unnatural. Moreover, the stability of such an incisor position can be unreliable over time because minimal contact of the incisors in MIP exists in these situations. The usual and undesirable result of any instability is compensatory eruption of the incisors with increased vertical overlap of the teeth. In an effort to reduce the increased horizontal overlap of the incisors, the maxillary anterior teeth, especially the incisors, are often made narrower to retract and position them closer to the mandibular incisors (Fig 4).

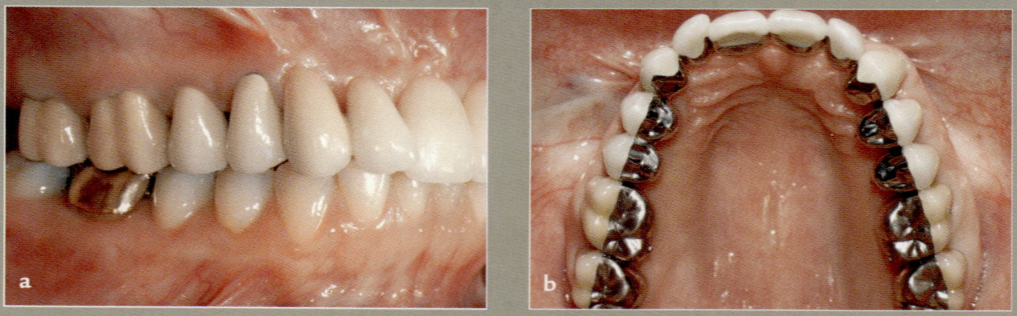

Fig 5 Class II relationship with prosthetic replacement of incisors. Maxillary lateral incisors overlap the central incisors to maintain a normal width of teeth while reducing the inherent horizontal overlap associated with a Class II relationship. The resulting compromise is crowded incisors. Note that the vertical overlap of maxillary and mandibular incisors is also increased, which is typical of a Class II, division 2 relationship. *(a)* Lateral view. *(b)* Occlusal view.

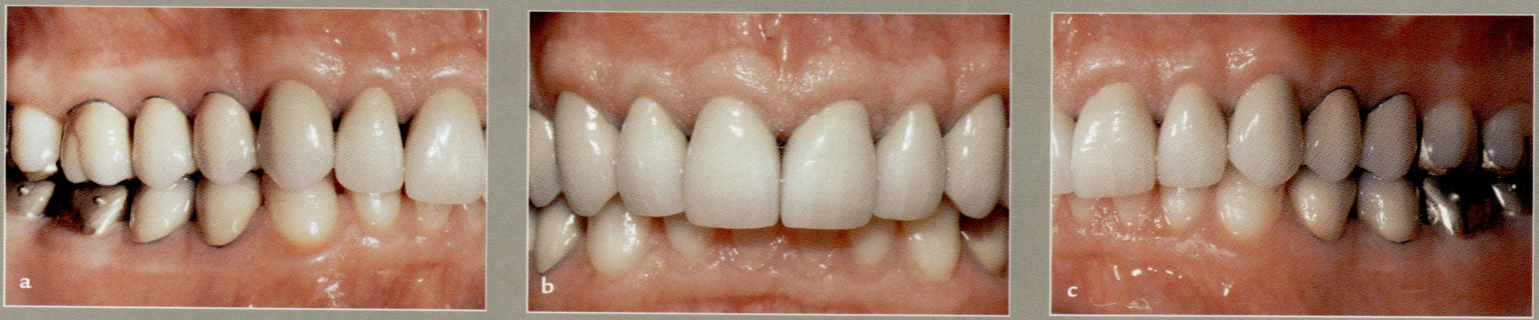

Fig 6 Restored Class II malocclusion with multiple compromises to establish incisor occlusal contact in MIP and reduce horizontal overlap of incisors: upright maxillary incisors, excessive vertical overlap of incisors, steep anterior guidance, reverse maxillary curve of Spee, and exaggerated mandibular curve of Spee. *(a)* Right lateral view. *(b)* Frontal view. *(c)* Left lateral view.

Unfortunately, as the incisors are made narrower they also become more upright, which together leads to an unesthetic appearance of the teeth. As an alternative to making incisors narrower to reduce the excessive horizontal overlap inherent in Class II, division 1 relationships, the incisors may be overlapped, which establishes a crowded appearance of the anterior teeth (Fig 5). This arrangement of teeth is consistent with that of Class II, division 2 relationships. Most patients, however, prefer to have relatively straight teeth. Decreasing horizontal overlap of the anterior teeth in Class II relationships also usually leads to increased vertical overlap of the incisors, which often results in a reverse maxillary curve of Spee and an exaggerated mandibular curve of Spee (Fig 6).

In short, having a Class I anterior relationship of the teeth negates any of these compromises and facilitates the development of an attractive smile with normal-sized teeth and a more stable, functional relationship.

Additional considerations

The next consideration in managing this patient's problems should be the requirements for resistance and retention form to adequately retain complete-coverage restorations on a long-term basis. Retention of artificial crowns on prepared teeth requires sufficient length and appropriate taper to prevent dislodgement of the crowns as a result of occlusal forces.

The patient's skeletal relationships need to be considered as well to achieve an optimal result of treatment with respect to the patient's maxillary teeth relative to her mandibular teeth, her teeth relative to her face, and her facial proportions relative to norms. The patient's facial appearance can be impacted by changes in the position, orientation, and shape of her teeth as well as the size, position, and orientation of her jaws. It is important to be aware of these dentofacial relationships to avoid compromising an individual's facial appearance while managing the care of his or her teeth. Facial proportions and balance should either be maintained or improved during the management of dental care, but not negatively impacted. If one thinks about managing a patient's dental care from the overall perspective that includes the face relative to the teeth, a more optimal result can be achieved in terms of appearance, function, and stability. In fact, the best way to evaluate a patient is from the face to the teeth. This is not always easy, especially considering that the dental education most of us received focused primarily on the teeth almost to the exclusion of the face, except, perhaps, in managing a patient for dentures. Also, considering most dentists graduated from dental school essentially as reparative dentists, it is not surprising we often neglect to evaluate the structures that surround the teeth and instead focus our treatment on the patient's restorative needs.

Developing a treatment plan

The key parameter to consider when planning treatment for this patient—or any patient—is to establish very specific goals or objectives for every problem the patient presents. This is assuming, of course, that the treating clinicians recognize all of the problems that exist. Any individual clinician may not know how to correct a specific problem but should be able to recognize the problem or deformity that exists and the possible need for change.

The purpose of interdisciplinary care is to address the how-to element of comprehensive care and compensate for any deficiency in an individual clinician's knowledge base with regard to a specific disease, dysfunction, or deformity as well as any lack of the technical expertise necessary to provide treatment, should it be desired. With the patient presented in this chapter, it is readily apparent that her teeth need to be restored. However, to achieve this goal in an optimal manner, a number of other problems need to be recognized and managed as well. Some of these have been delineated in the aspects of care mentioned above.

What I hope the reader learns from this chapter is how to better plan the overall treatment for any patient. This is perhaps the greatest deficiency in the dental education of most dentists, myself included. The best way to improve one's ability to plan treatment for any patient is having sufficient diagnostic information to facilitate recognition of the problems presented by the patient. This would include a comprehensive examination comprising a dental and periodontal charting of the teeth and supporting structures, intraoral and extraoral photographs, articulated casts of the teeth, panoramic and periapical radiographs of the teeth with vertical bitewings, and a lateral cephalometric radiograph. A cone beam computerized tomogram (CBCT) also may be indicated depending on the problem the patient presents with or treatment planned (eg, bony defects, impacted teeth, replacement of missing teeth with implants). Without the information these records provide, it would be impossible to assess a patient's problems sufficiently, let alone establish acceptable goals and a plan for treatment that would be capable of managing any patient's problems beyond perhaps restoring individual teeth.

Three benefits come to mind for those planning treatment for the patient presented in this chapter. First and foremost is the opportunity to learn to plan treatment according to the specific goals or objectives of treatment established before considering any particular modality of treatment. This allows one to focus only on treatment that is actually pertinent to treating the patient. The second benefit is understanding how to manage treatment of a patient's dentition relative to the face and not limit one's focus to only the teeth. Finally, this case presents the opportunity to learn how to develop appropriate spacing between the teeth to facilitate the placement of definitive restorations with normal proportions for optimal appearance and function.

Case Presentation

Treating clinicians
Prosthodontist: Thomas Junge, DDS, MSD
Orthodontist: Ward M. Smalley, DDS, MSD
Periodontist: Ralph Yuodelis, DDS, MSD
Oral and maxillofacial surgeon: Roger West, DDS
Oral and maxillofacial surgeon: Dale Bloomquist, DDS
Laboratory technicians: Harald Heindl, MDT, and Daniela Heindl, CDT

Clinical Treatment Planning

Age at initial presentation: 13 years
Initial presentation: January 1995
Active treatment completed: October 2006

Introduction and background

The patient was referred by Dr Doug Ramsey at the University of Washington Dental School, and she presented for examination with her mother. They expressed concern about the appearance and sensitivity of her teeth, her difficulty eating, and her "narrow" oral cavity. The patient was diagnosed with amelogenesis imperfecta type I (ie, associated with enamel hypoplasia). She had been a patient in the Department of Pediatric Dentistry at the University of Washington for a number of years and received treatment consisting of plaque control and provisional restoration of some involved teeth with composite resin or stainless steel crowns. The patient had a family history of amelogenesis imperfecta on her father's side. Her father was treated for the same disorder at the University of Washington Graduate Prosthodontics Program in the early 1980s.

Medical history

- Severe enamel hypoplasia
- Family history of amelogenesis imperfecta
- Hypersensitivity to hydrocodone

Diagnostic findings

Extraoral and facial findings

- Convex facial profile
- Increased lower facial height
- Slight lip incompetence with strain during closure
- Retrognathic mandible
- Steep mandibular plane
- Deficient chin
- Relatively symmetric face
- Maxillary incisor to upper lip within normal limits
- Excessive display of mandibular incisors

TMJ and mandibular range of motion

- Within normal limits
- Opens to 55 mm

Intraoral findings

Dental

- Enamel hypoplasia of all teeth
- Tooth sensitivity
- Stainless steel crowns on teeth nos. 3 to 5, 12 to 14, 19 to 21, 28, and 30
- Delayed eruption of teeth nos. 2, 6, 8, 11, 18, and 31
- Retained primary teeth C and H
- Class I malocclusion

Periodontal

- Generalized mild to moderate gingival inflammation
- Bleeding on probing
- Short clinical crowns
- Disproportionate levels of marginal gingiva

PRETREATMENT

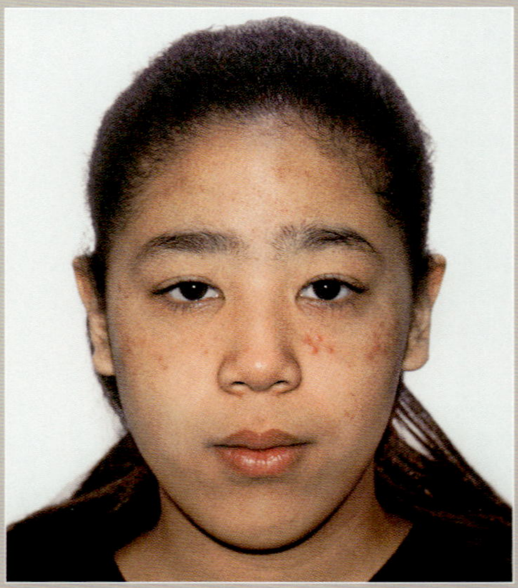

Facial view at rest.

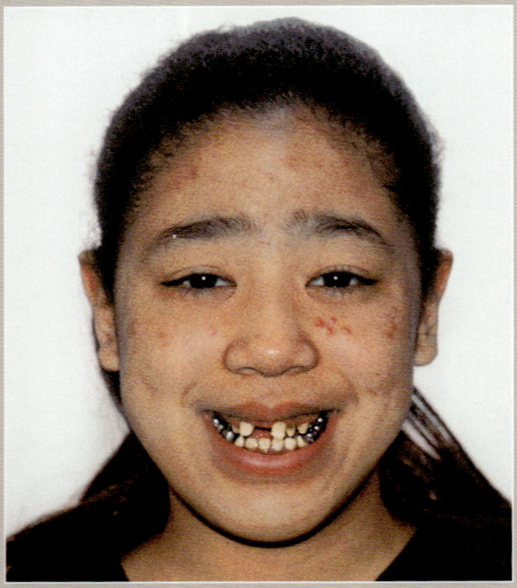

Facial view of smile.

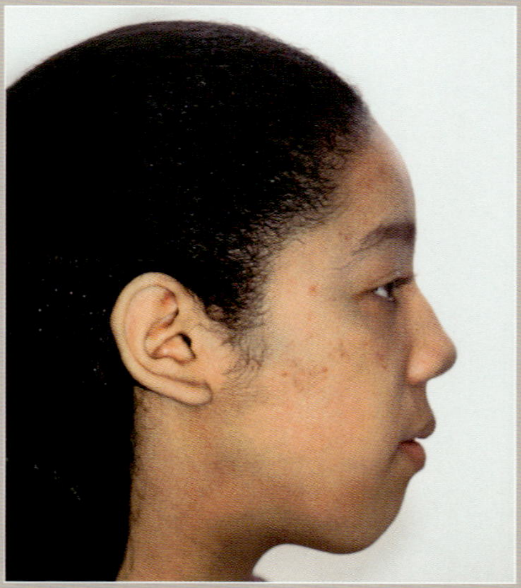

Lateral facial view.

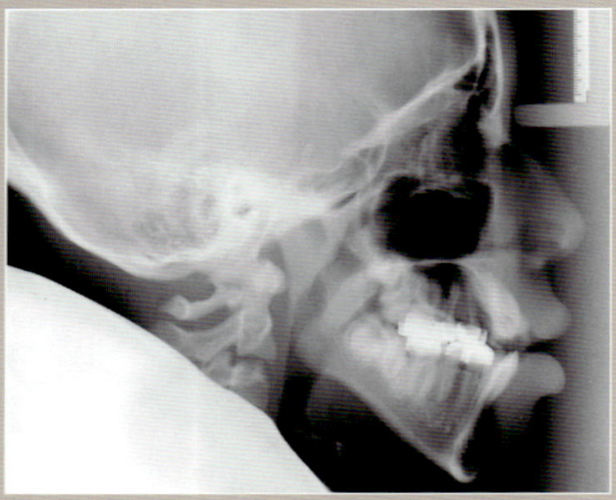

Lateral cephalometric radiograph.

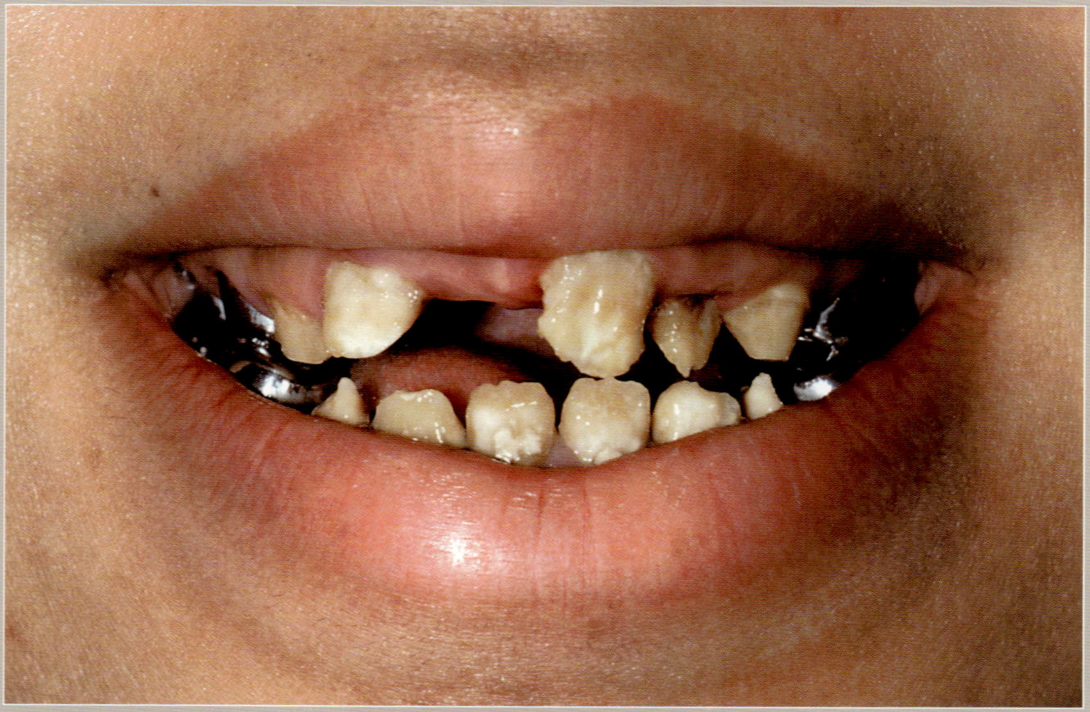

Close-up of smile.

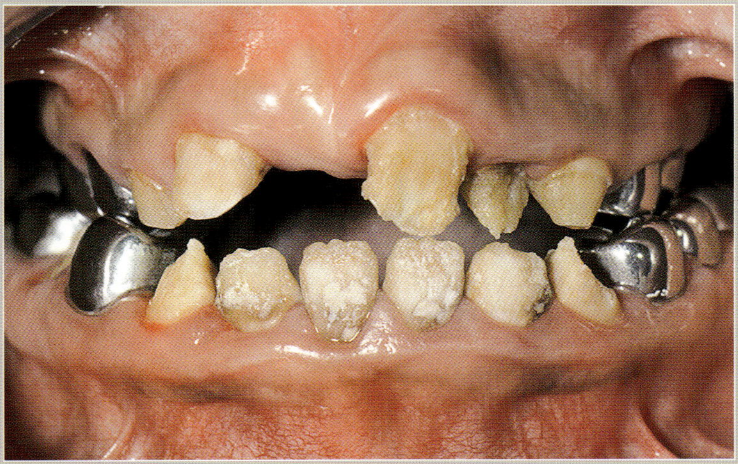

Frontal view.

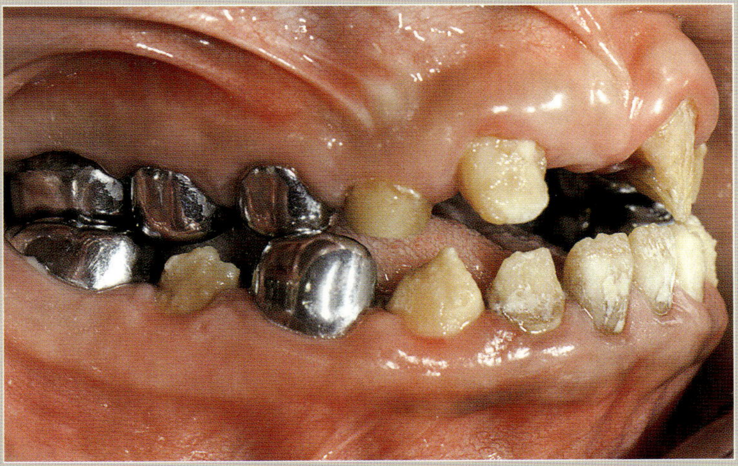

Right lateral view.

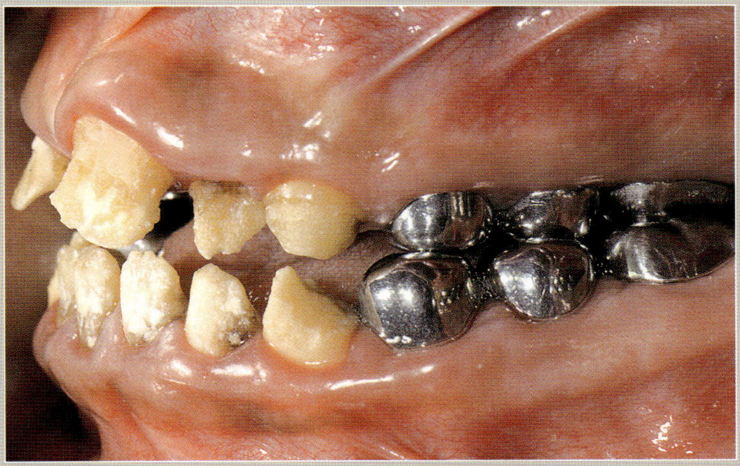

Left lateral view.

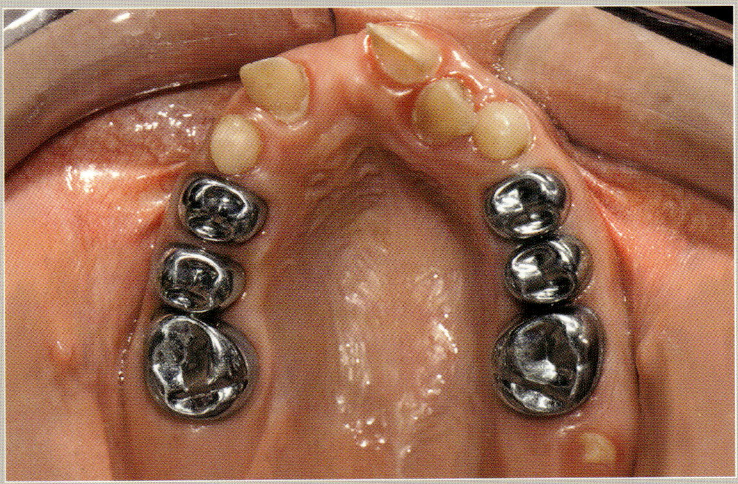

Maxillary occlusal view.

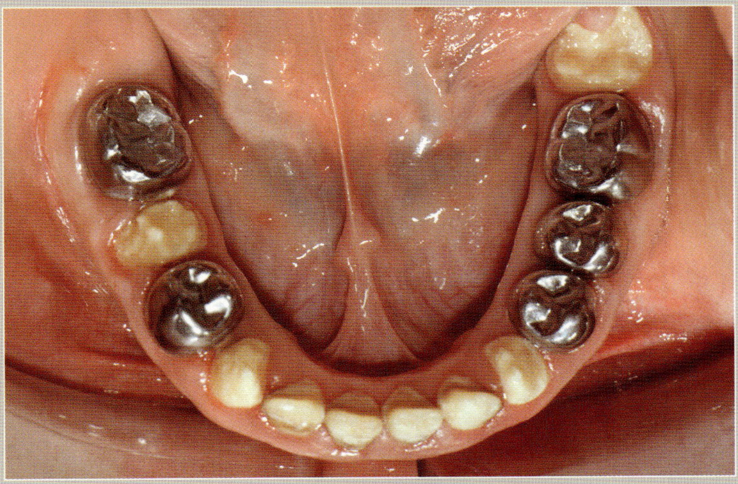

Mandibular occlusal view.

Occlusal notes

- Class I relationship (left canines end-on Class II)
- Horizontal overlap (overjet): 5 mm
- Anterior reverse articulation (crossbite) of teeth C and no. 27, nos. 10 and 23, and H and no. 22
- Mandibular dental midline deviated about 2 mm to the left
- Constricted maxillary arch with associated bilateral posterior reverse articulation
- Anterior open occlusal relationship; no anterior guidance
- Maxillary and mandibular arch length deficiencies of 2 to 4 mm anteriorly with root proximity and insufficient space to restore involved teeth
- Rotated teeth
- Proclined tooth no. 7
- Centric occlusion (CO) = MIP (with condyles in centric relation [CR])

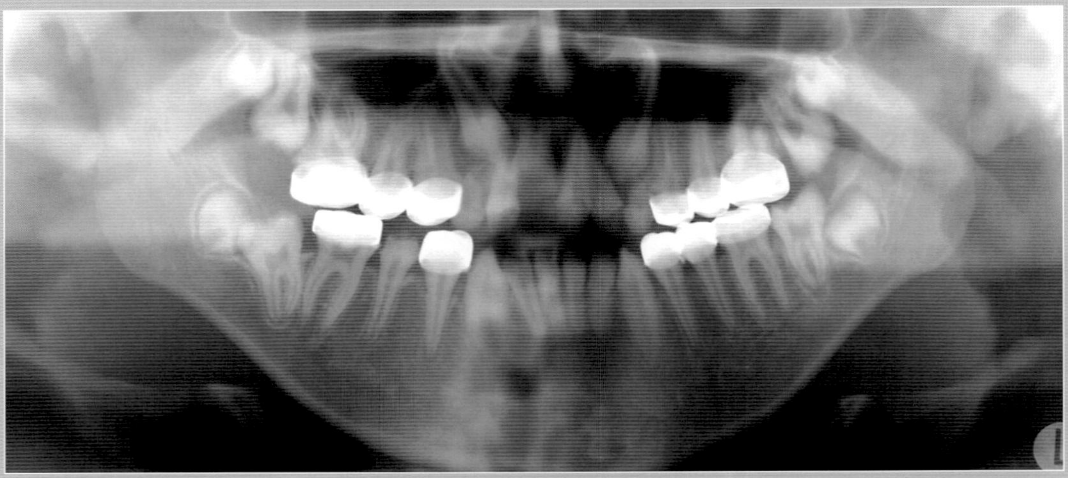

Panoramic radiograph.

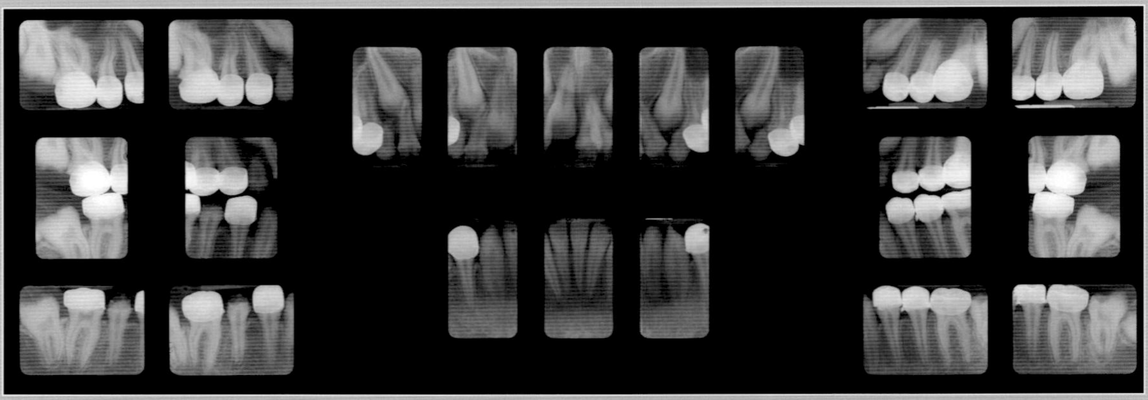

Periapical radiographic survey with bitewings.

Radiographic findings

- Root proximity of incisors
- Poor fit of existing stainless steel crowns with overhanging margins and areas of excess cement
- Close proximity of unerupted maxillary canines relative to roots of lateral incisors
- Dilaceration of maxillary canine roots at apices

Oral hygiene habits

- The patient brushed her teeth twice a day with a manual toothbrush.
- Moderate amounts of plaque and calculus present.

Diagnosis

- Amelogenesis imperfecta type I (characterized by enamel hypoplasia)
- AAP Type I
- Class I malocclusion with constricted maxilla
- Inadequate restorations on posterior teeth

Etiology

- Dentition: genetics (inherited disorder from father, related to a mutation of ENAM gene inherited in an autosomal-dominant pattern)
- Skeletal: genetics

Prognosis

- Periodontal: good
- Biomechanical: good
- Functional: good
- Esthetic: good

Summary of concerns

1. How will we address the delayed eruption of teeth with possible ankylosis and proximity to adjacent teeth?
2. How will we manage the sensitivity of the patient's teeth?
3. What effect will the root morphology of teeth nos. 6 and 11 have on active or passive eruption of teeth?
4. How will we manage the patient's orthodontic problems considering the existing tooth morphology; specifically, how will we attach the orthodontic appliances to the teeth and address the current esthetic concerns of the patient?
5. Can the patient's dentition be restored predictably with a stable and esthetic result?
6. What will be the financial cost of treatment?
7. What will be the length of treatment, especially if orthodontics is started before teeth have erupted?
8. What will be the psychologic impact of treatment on the patient, especially if treatment is delayed or protracted?

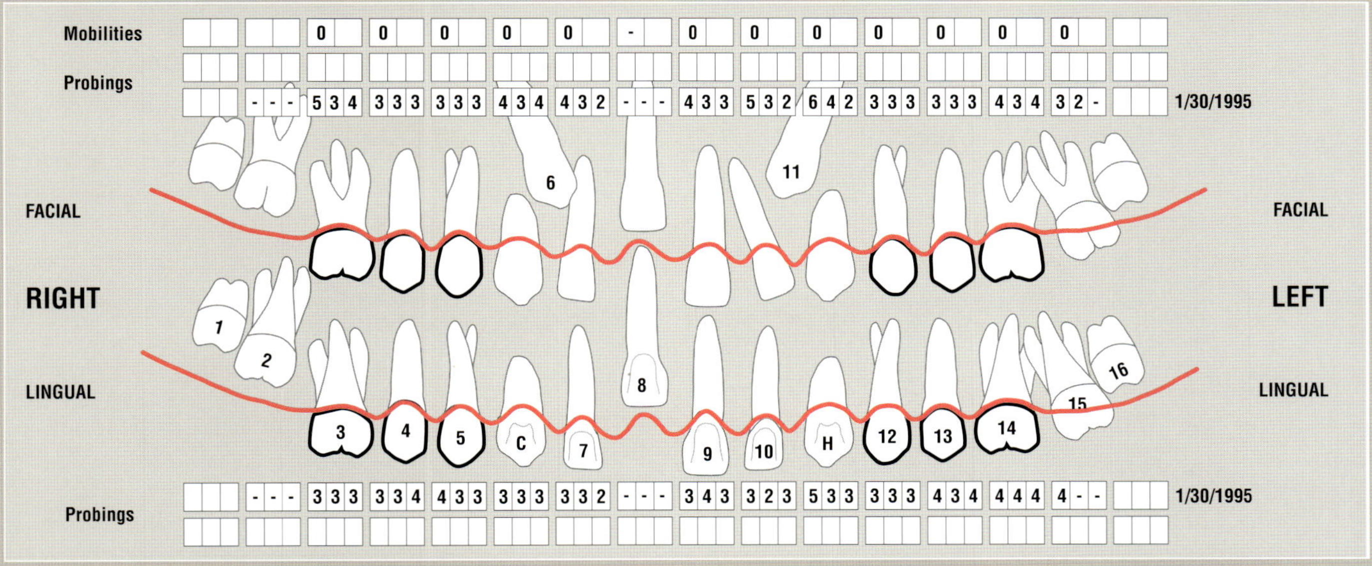

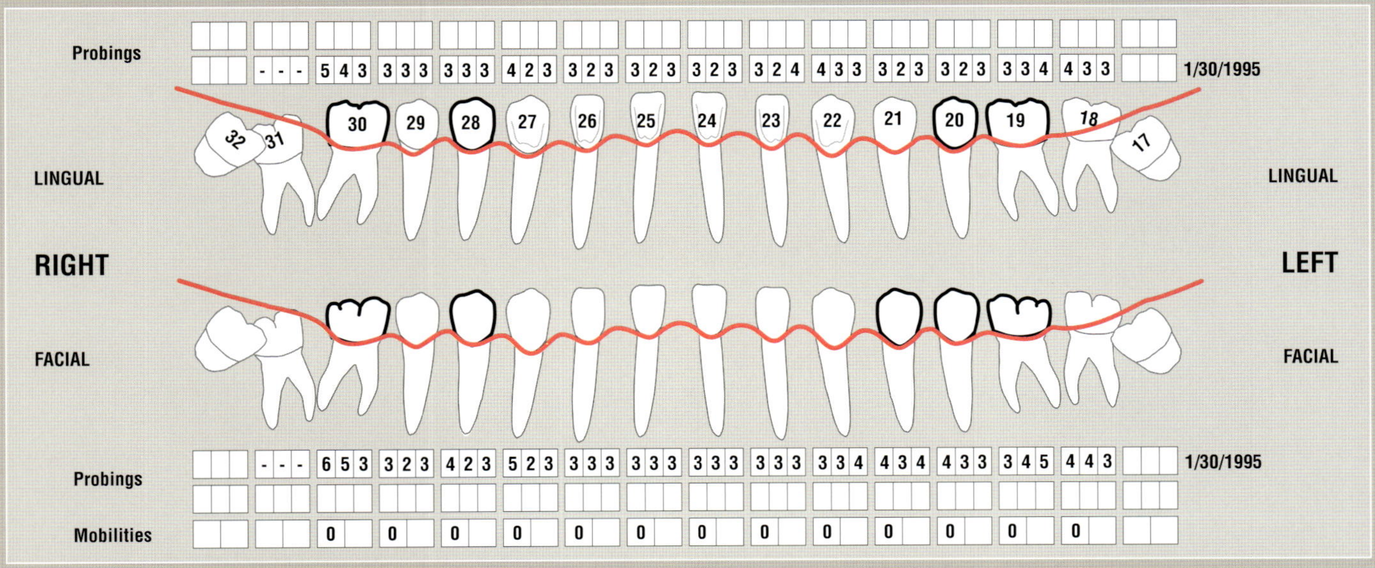

As a learning exercise, you may now outline goals/objectives of treatment and a treatment plan.

Proposed Treatment Plan

Goals/objectives of treatment

Face

- Improve facial balance/profile—reduce convexity
- Reduce lower facial height
- Increase prominence of chin
- Eliminate slight lip incompetence and muscle strain during closure

Smile

- Improve appearance of teeth with respect to shape, size, color, and position
- Balance levels of maxillary marginal gingiva
- Improve alignment of teeth
- Manage apparent absence (relative lack of eruption) of maxillary anterior teeth

Dentition

- Eliminate stainless steel crowns
- Balance levels of maxillary and mandibular marginal gingiva
- Establish normal morphology of clinical crowns with appropriate dimensions
- Establish adequate tooth length to facilitate retention of restorations and resistance to displacement
- Eliminate caries lesions
- Correct malocclusion of teeth and associated dental and skeletal findings (in conjunction with restoration of teeth)
- Align teeth and correct rotations
- Maintain/establish Class I relationship, at least anteriorly
- Facilitate eruption of unerupted teeth
- Establish optimal horizontal and vertical overlap of teeth—eliminate anterior open bite relationship
- Level occlusal and incisal planes
- Eliminate constriction of maxilla and associated posterior reverse articulation
- Establish symmetric dental arches
- Eliminate arch length deficiencies and associated crowding of teeth
- Establish appropriate spacing for optimal restoration of teeth
- Coordinate dental arches
- Restore affected teeth to improve occlusion, function, appearance, stability of tooth position, and ability of patient to maintain health of teeth and supporting structures

Overall

- Monitor/promote health of TMJ, dentition, and periodontium throughout treatment

Phase I: Diagnostic evaluation

1. Diagnostic records (complete dental and periodontal charting, facial and intraoral photographs, articulated casts of teeth, and radiographs—cephalometric, panoramic, and complete periapical/bitewing surveys)
2. Periodontal evaluation for clinical crown lengthening and exposure of unerupted anterior teeth
3. Orthodontic evaluation
4. Restorative evaluation
5. Referral to oral and maxillofacial surgeon for orthognathic surgical evaluation
6. Consultation with interdisciplinary team members to establish goals, plan, and sequence of treatment
7. Consultation with patient by participating clinicians regarding goals, proposed plan, alternatives, estimated time, and financial commitment required of treatment

Phase II: Initial treatment

8. Removal of existing stainless steel crowns
9. Surgical clinical crown lengthening of all teeth and exposure of unerupted anterior teeth
10. Articulated diagnostic casts for evaluation
11. Diagnostic wax-up of teeth to establish normal size and morphology of clinical crowns
12. Fabrication of initial provisional restorations
13. Preparation of all erupted teeth for complete-coverage restorations, impressions, and placement of initial provisional restorations
14. Definitive wax-up of prepared teeth for long-term provisional restorations
15. Fabrication of heat-cured provisional restorations
16. Placement of long-term provisional restorations

Phase III: Orthodontic treatment

17. New diagnostic records and re-evaluation/confirmation of treatment plan
18. Another referral for surgical evaluation to address skeletal disparities
19. Placement of fixed orthodontic appliances including palatal expander
20. Regular hygiene recall to monitor and manage patient's overall dental health

Phase IV: Orthognathic surgery (initial phase)

21. Maxillary osteotomies and midline split to facilitate progressive expansion of maxilla
22. Removal of third molars

Phase V: Orthodontic progress

23. Continuance of fixed appliance treatment after expansion of maxilla and healing to:
    - Facilitate eruption of unerupted teeth
    - Align and level teeth
    - Eliminate arch length deficiencies and establish appropriate spaces to facilitate optimal restoration of teeth
    - Align dental and facial midlines
    - Coordinate dental arches

Phase VI: Orthognathic surgery (second phase)

24. Surgical advancement of chin via horizontal osteotomy and correction of any skeletal disparities that remain or become apparent

Phase VII: Orthodontic treatment (postsurgical/finishing)

25. Continuance of fixed appliance treatment after surgery and healing to:
    - Establish a solid Class I relationship bilaterally
    - Establish appropriate horizontal and vertical overlap of teeth
    - Establish stable, functional occlusion with CO = MIP, anterior guidance, and no posterior excursive occlusal interferences
    - Fabricate and place retainers
26. Referral back to the restorative dentist during orthodontic treatment to provisionally restore newly erupted teeth and add to existing restorations that are deficient in size as appropriate space to do so is established

Phase VIII: Definitive restorative treatment

27. Removal of existing provisional restorations
28. Definitive preparation of all teeth
29. Placement of provisional restorations
30. Evaluation of provisional restorations with regard to resistance and retention, occlusion, function, and appearance
31. Determination of definitive restorations depending on patient's desires, habits, appearance, and existing/remaining tooth structure
32. Impressions, facebow, and maxillomandibular relationship record for definitive restorations
33. Fabrication of definitive restorations
34. Placement of definitive restorations
35. Fabrication and placement of maxillary occlusal appliance (nightguard)

Phase IX: Documentation of treatment result

Phase X: Recall

Active Clinical Treatment

Phase I: Diagnostic evaluation

Following an initial examination, diagnostic records were obtained initially for a comprehensive evaluation of the patient's dental needs. These included complete dental and periodontal charting of teeth; facial and intraoral photographs; articulated casts of the teeth; and cephalometric, panoramic, periapical, and bitewing radiographs. Once evaluation was complete, a consultation was held with the patient and her father to review her diagnostic findings, goals of treatment, and anticipated plan and sequence of treatment. The patient was subsequently referred to the University of Washington Graduate Fixed Prosthodontics Program for evaluation and management of her restorative dental needs, to a periodontist for evaluation and management of her short clinical crowns and unerupted anterior teeth, and to an oral and maxillofacial surgeon for evaluation and management of her skeletal disparities. After the patient was seen and evaluated by the interdisciplinary treatment team, a meeting was held between the participating clinicians to finalize the goals/objectives of treatment consistent with those desired by the patient as well as the plan and sequence of treatment that would meet the established goals. Finally, the participating clinicians met with the patient and her mother and/or father to review the desired goals/objectives of treatment, plan of treatment, treatment alternatives that would be acceptable but may not achieve all of the treatment goals desired, estimated time of treatment, and the financial commitment treatment would involve.

Phase II: Initial treatment/disease control

The patient's stainless steel crowns were removed to more easily evaluate the involved teeth and to determine whether or not there was adequate crown length. The patient's teeth were cleaned via oral prophylaxis, and oral hygiene was reviewed. Peridex (3M ESPE) was prescribed in preparation for periodontal surgery.

Phase III: Surgical crown lengthening

The clinical crowns of all the patient's teeth were surgically lengthened in three separate appointments. The objective was to establish sufficient clinical crown height for adequate retention and resistance to displacement of the planned coronal restorations. The maxillary arch and mandibular right posterior teeth were completed first, followed by the mandibular anterior and left posterior teeth about 1 month later. Healing progressed well with no complications.

Phase IV: Diagnostic phase for provisional restorations

Diagnostic records were obtained to evaluate planned provisional restoration of the patient's teeth in preparation for comprehensive orthodontic treatment. These included impressions and photographs of the teeth, facebow registration, and a maxillomandibular relationship record with the patient's condyles in CR.

A preliminary diagnostic wax-up of the teeth with normal crown contours and dimensions was then completed on articulated casts of the teeth. It is important to note that the teeth were and should be provisionally restored without any compensation or correction for rotated and/or tipped teeth to facilitate orthodontic correction of any malposed teeth that exist. After completion of the diagnostic wax-up, provisional restoration shells were fabricated out of polymethyl methacrylate (PMMA) resin in preparation for placement on the teeth. The patient's teeth were then prepared and curetted as needed for complete-coverage restorations in a series of appointments in conjunction with the placement and cementation of provisional restorations. Each tooth was etched with 37% phosphoric acid followed by the application of a preparation disinfectant to reduce sensitivity.

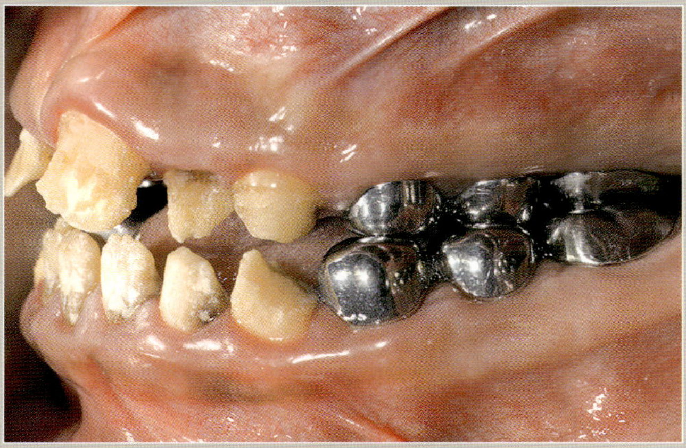
Left lateral view before crown lengthening.

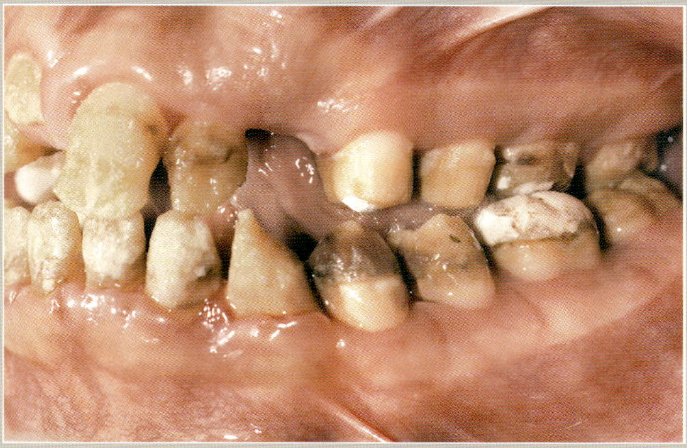
Left lateral view after crown lengthening.

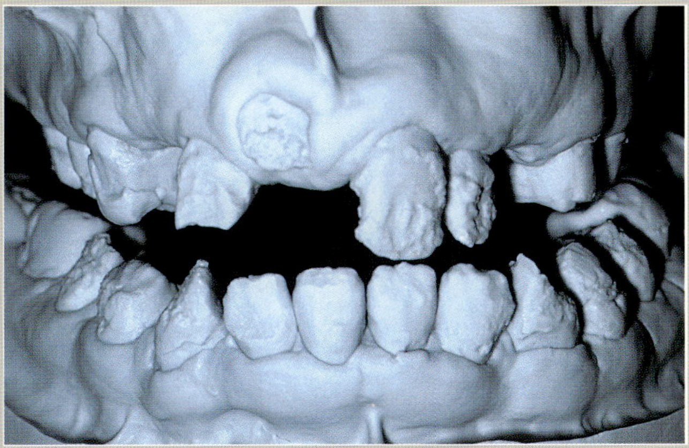
Articulated casts after crown lengthening.

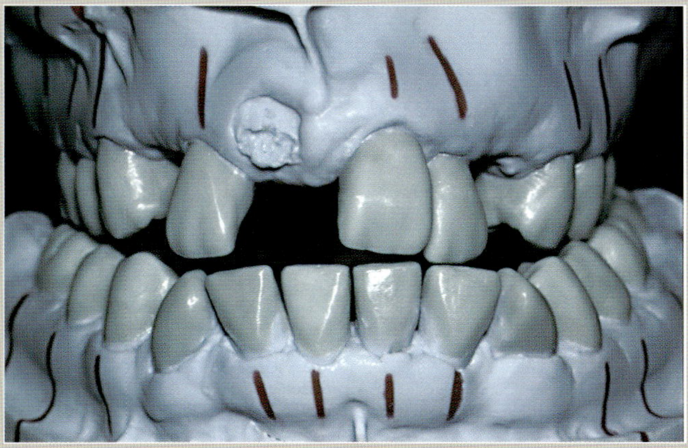
Preliminary diagnostic wax-up.

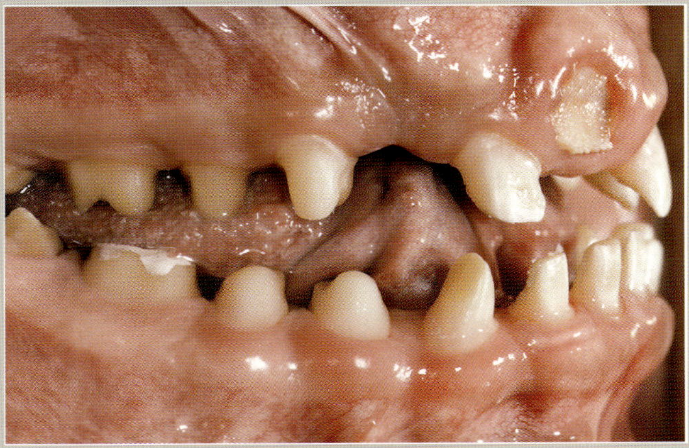
Right lateral view of prepared teeth.

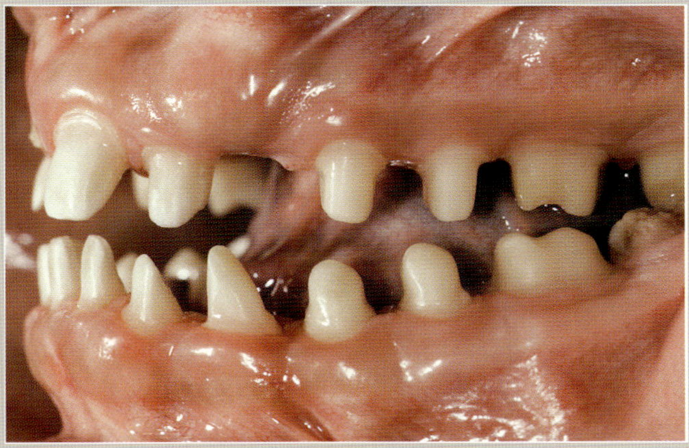
Left lateral view of prepared teeth.

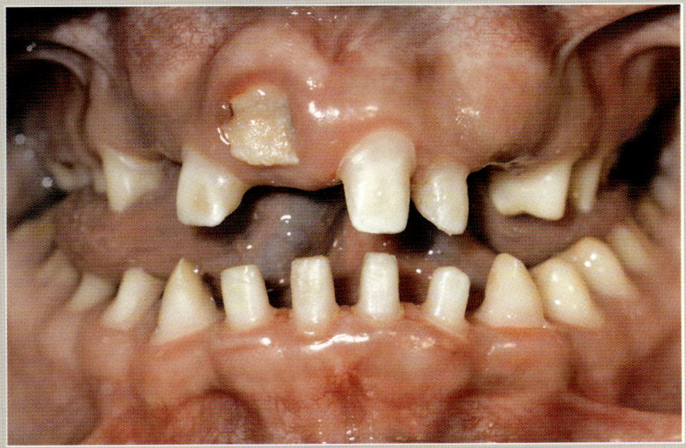
Frontal view of prepared teeth.

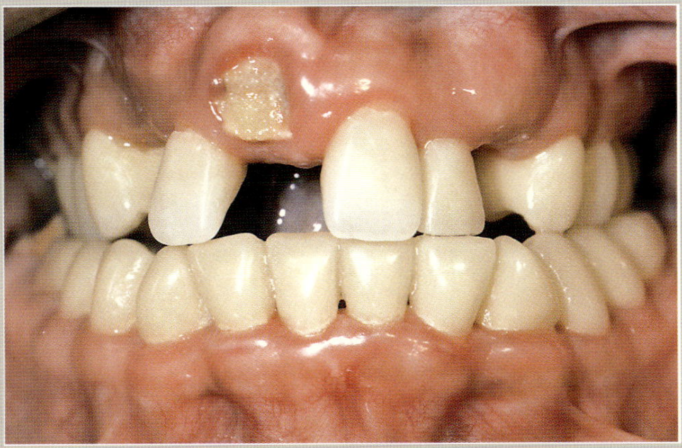
Frontal view of initial provisional restorations.

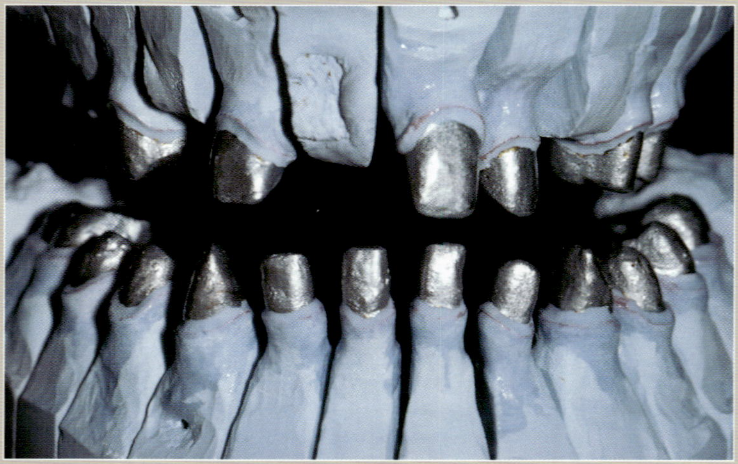

Articulated casts of prepared teeth.

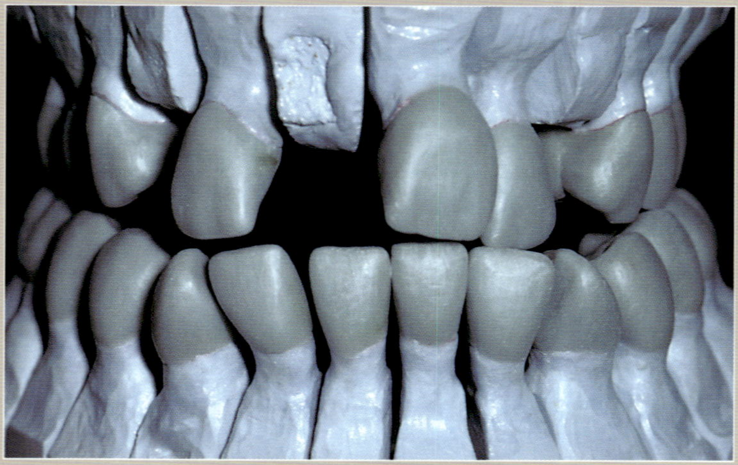

Articulated casts with diagnostic wax-up.

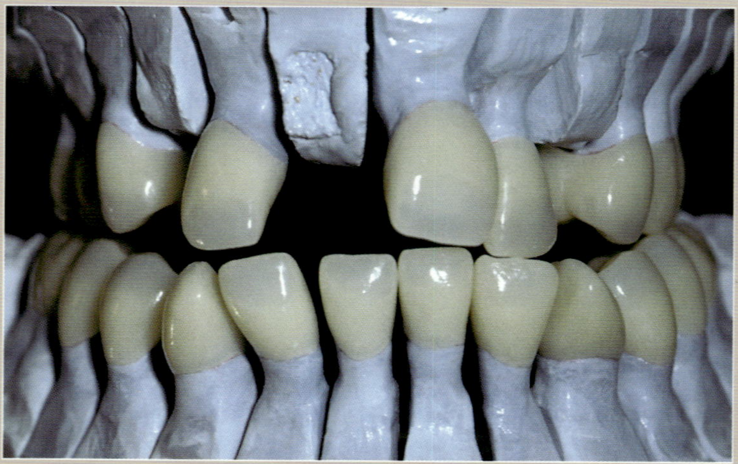

Articulated casts with long-term provisional restorations.

Following the completion of tooth preparations and placement of the initial provisional restorations, the restorations were removed, and full-arch impressions of the prepared teeth were taken. A facebow transfer and a maxillomandibular relationship record of the prepared teeth were then obtained. The resultant casts were articulated for definitive wax-up of the teeth for fabrication of long-term provisional restorations. Each tooth was again waxed to nor-

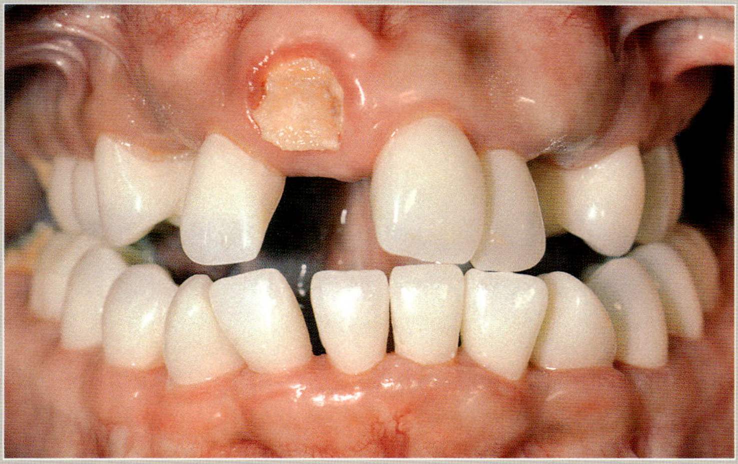

Frontal view of long-term provisional restorations.

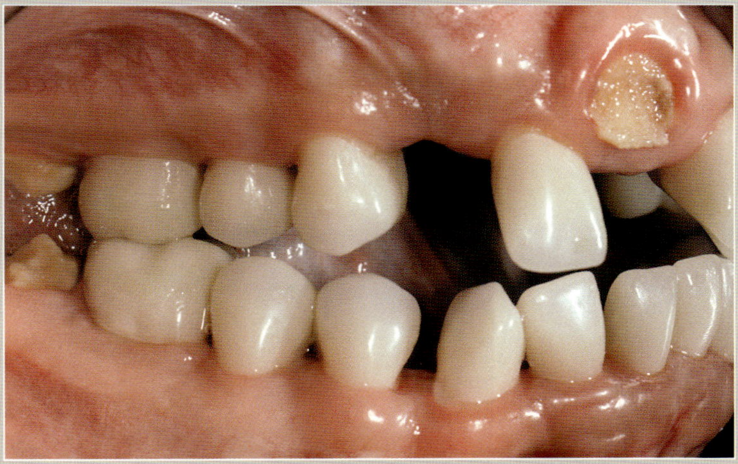

Right lateral view of long-term provisional restorations.

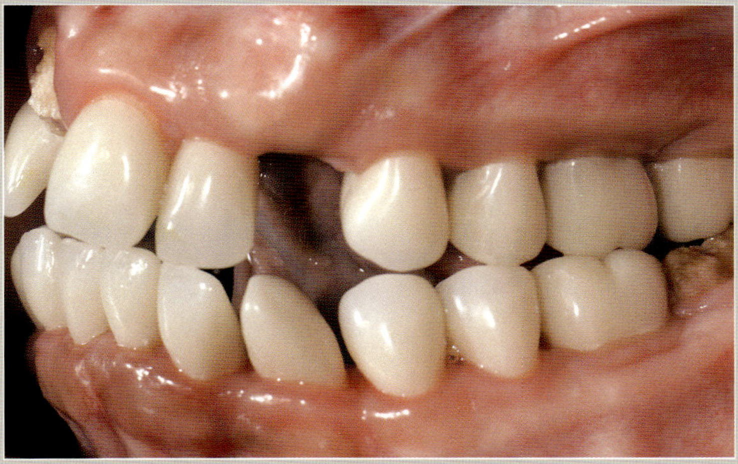

Left lateral view of long-term provisional restorations.

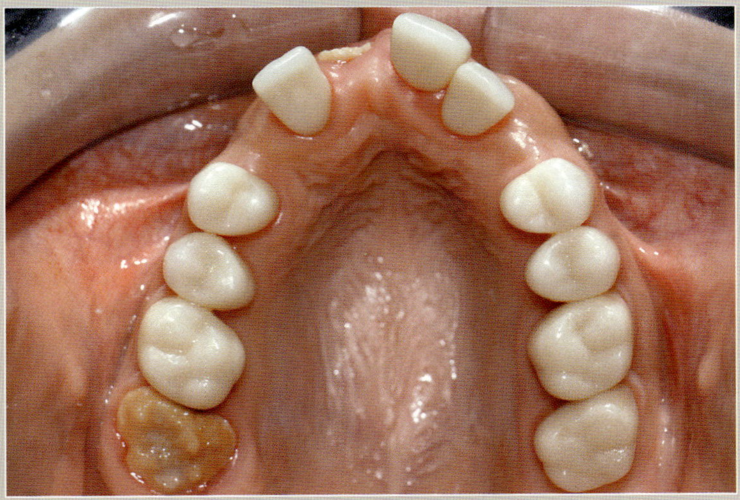

Maxillary occlusal view of long-term provisional restorations.

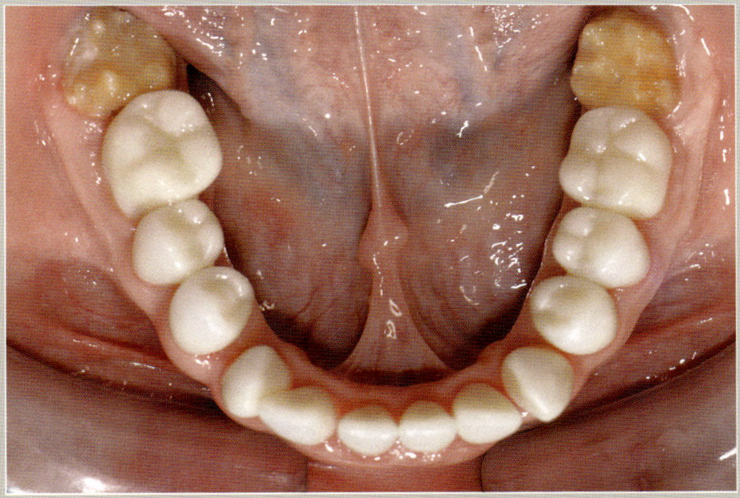

Mandibular occlusal view of long-term provisional restorations.

mal contours and dimensions, as existing root orientation and space permitted. The waxed teeth were then flasked to produce heat-cured acrylic resin restorations made of Biolon (Dentsply), which is capable of maintaining long-term dimensional stability (note that no appropriate microhybrid composite resin restorative veneering material existed at that time). The provisional heat-cured resin restorations were then placed on the prepared teeth and cemented with Vitremer (3M ESPE) cement.

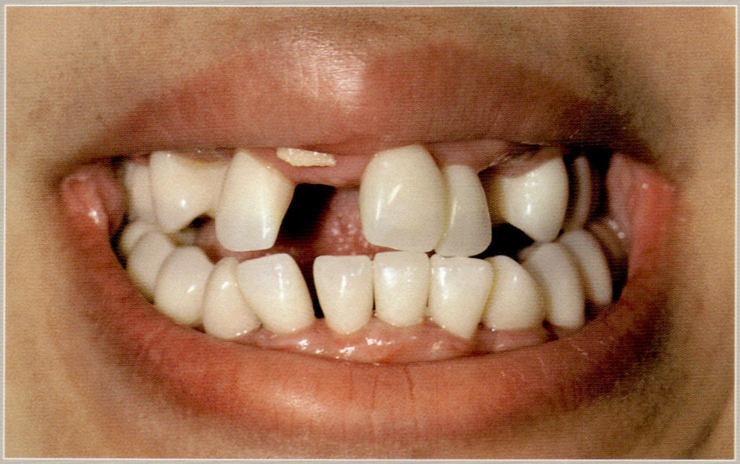

Close-up of smile with long-term provisional restorations.

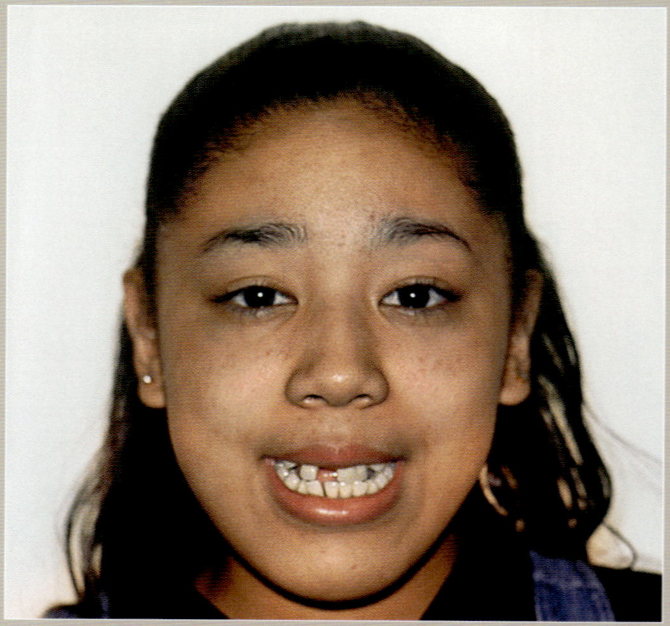

Facial view of smile with long-term provisional restorations.

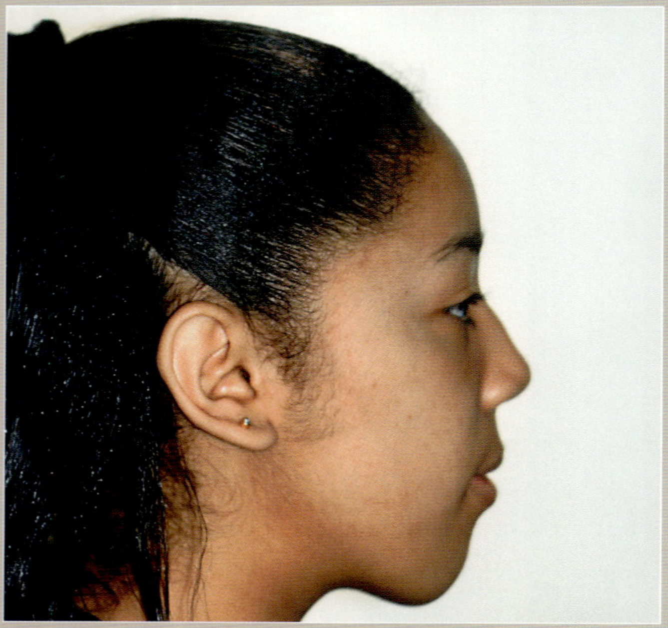

Lateral facial view with long-term provisional restorations.

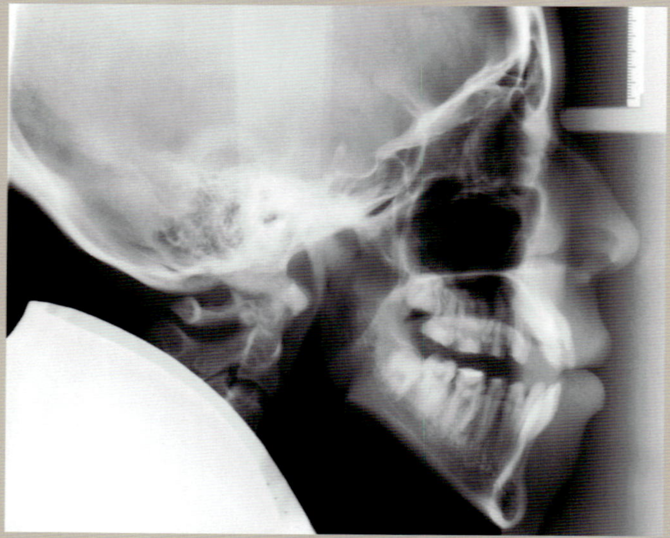

Lateral cephalometric radiograph with long-term provisional restorations.

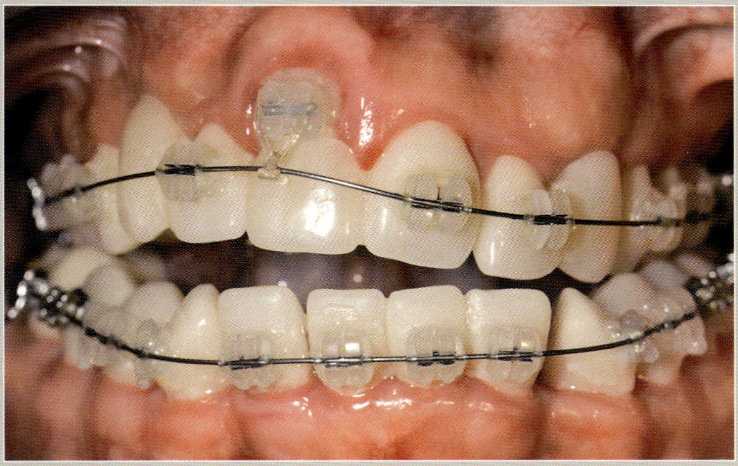

Frontal view at start of orthodontic treatment.

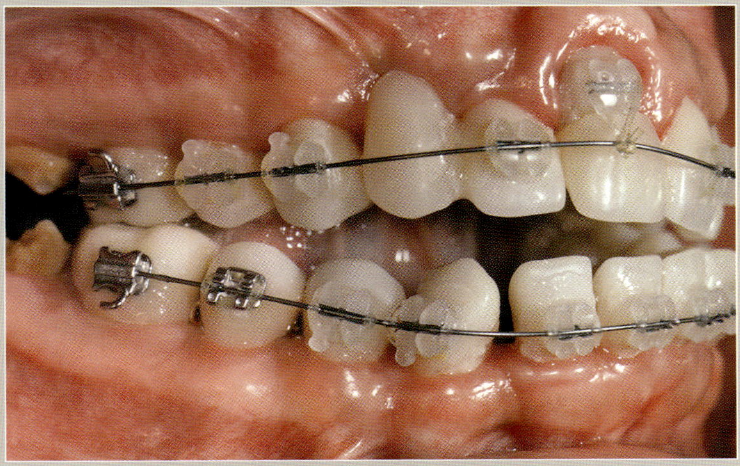

Right lateral view at start of orthodontic treatment.

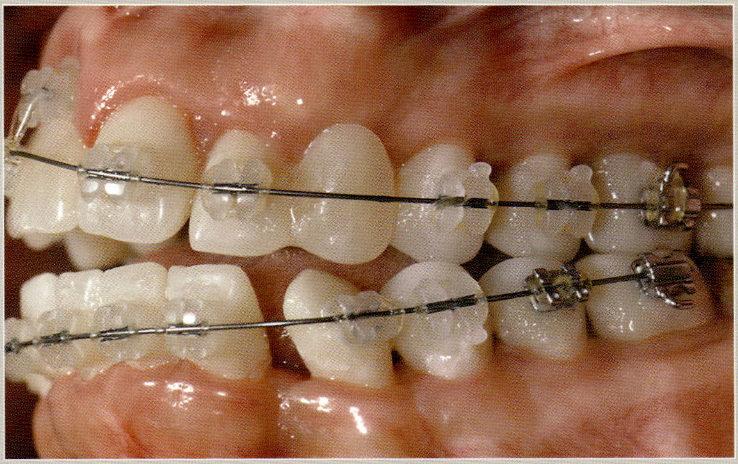

Left lateral view at start of orthodontic treatment.

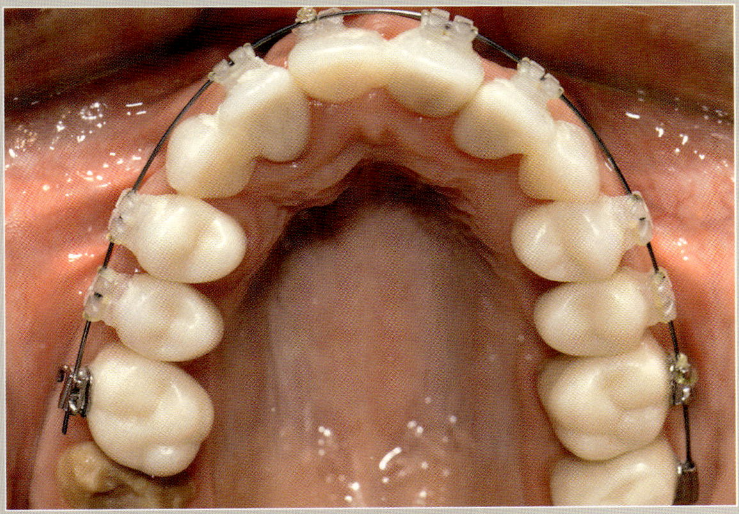

Maxillary occlusal view at start of orthodontic treatment.

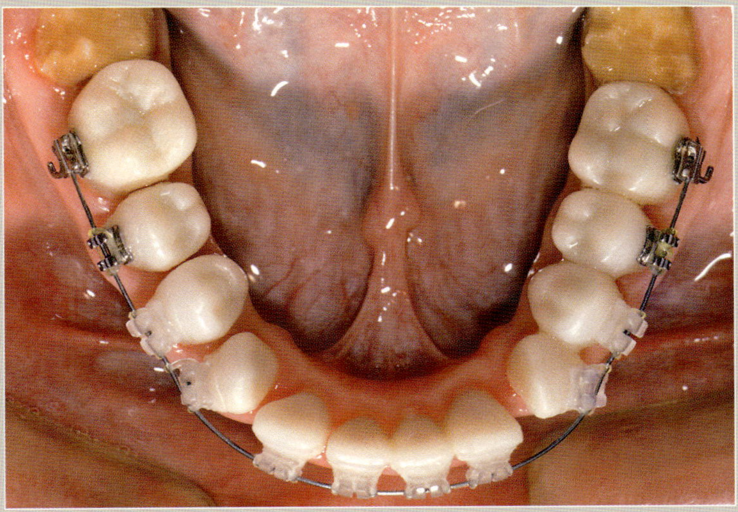

Mandibular occlusal view at start of orthodontic treatment.

Phase V: Orthodontic treatment and initial orthognathic surgery

Orthodontic diagnostic records were obtained to review the plan of treatment. Fixed orthodontic appliances were placed on all erupted teeth, including a jackscrew (Hyrax type) palatal expander. The patient was referred to the oral and maxillofacial surgeon for appropriate osteotomies to facilitate surgically assisted expansion of the patient's maxilla and for removal of her third molars. This procedure was favored over a Le Fort I

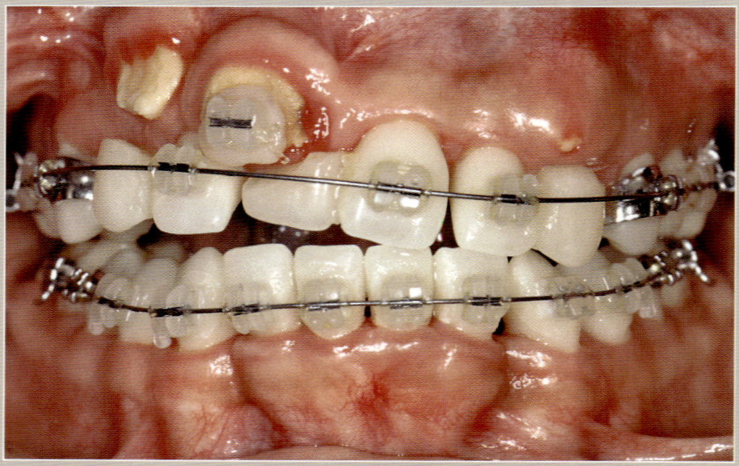

Frontal view at completion of maxillary expansion.

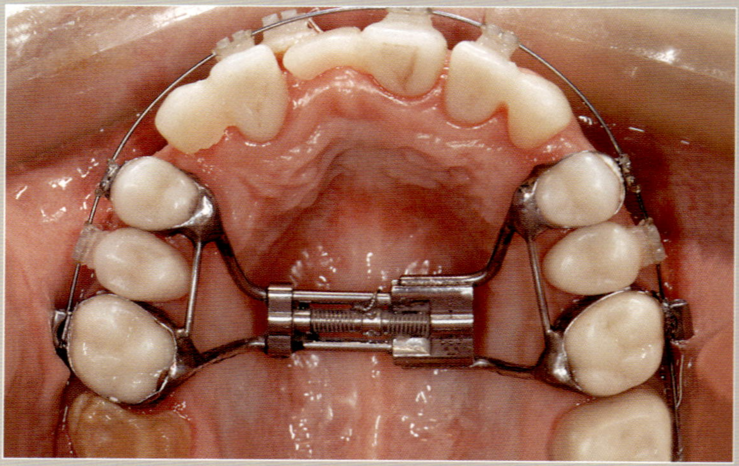

Maxillary occlusal view at completion of maxillary expansion.

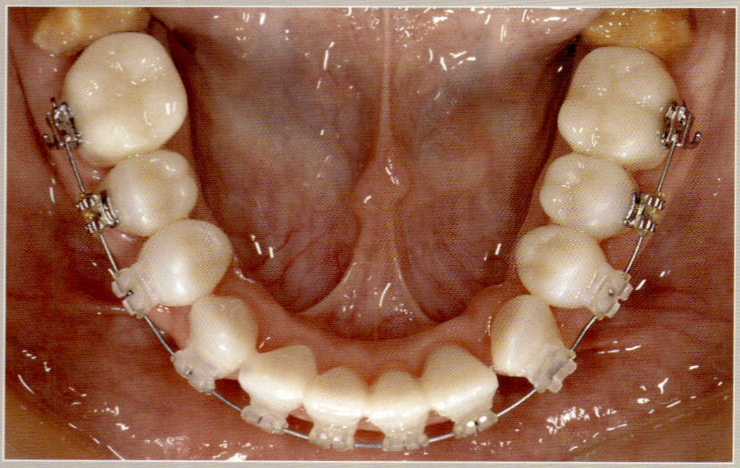

Mandibular occlusal view of orthodontic progress.

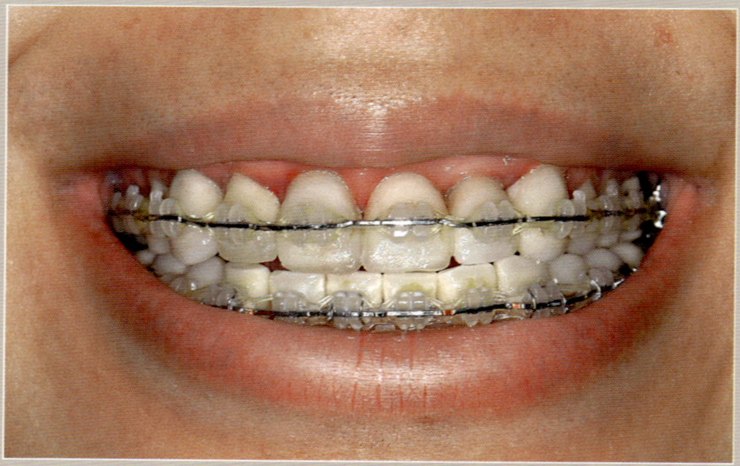

Close-up view of smile at completion of presurgical orthodontics.

osteotomy to achieve the desired amount of expansion anteriorly as well as posteriorly. In addition, the unerupted maxillary right canine was further exposed during the surgery with apical positioning of the overlying soft tissue. After about 10 mm of expansion was achieved, the expander was secured for several months to allow for complete healing of the osteotomy sites and stabilization of the expansion that had taken place.

Following expansion of the patient's maxilla, the teeth were aligned and leveled. As the unerupted maxillary anterior teeth erupted, brackets were attached to facilitate further

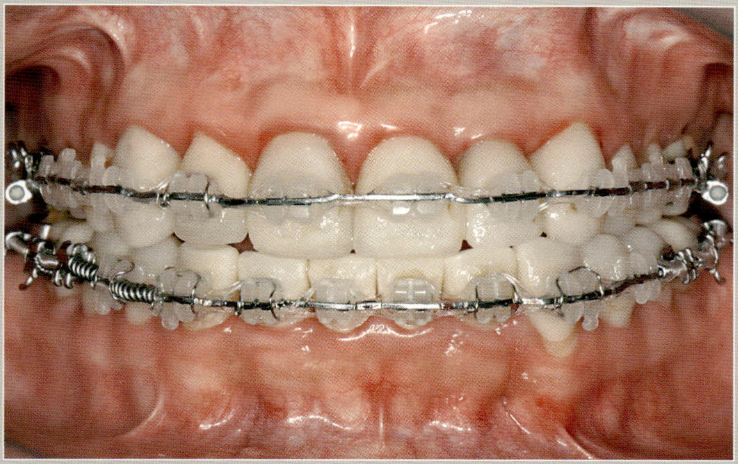

Frontal view at completion of presurgical orthodontics.

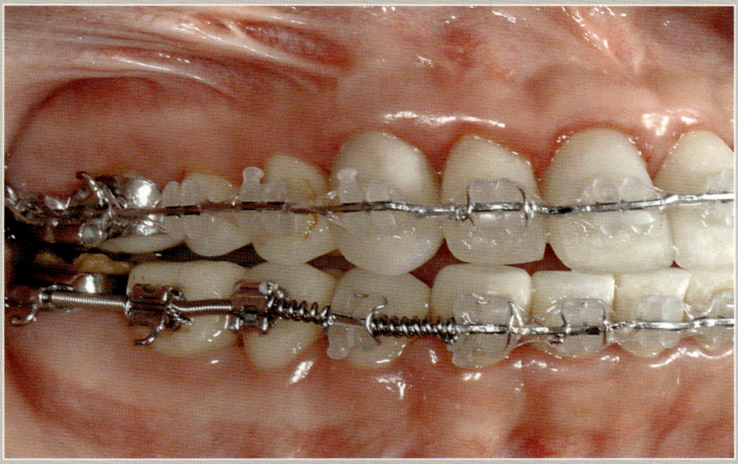

Right lateral view at completion of presurgical orthodontics.

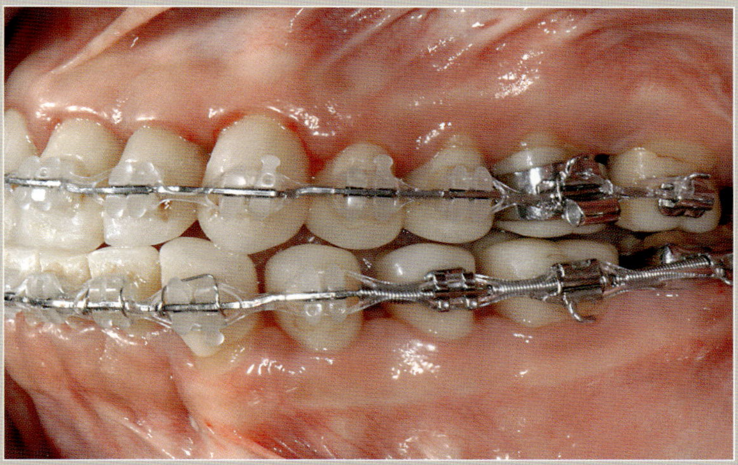

Left lateral view at completion of presurgical orthodontics.

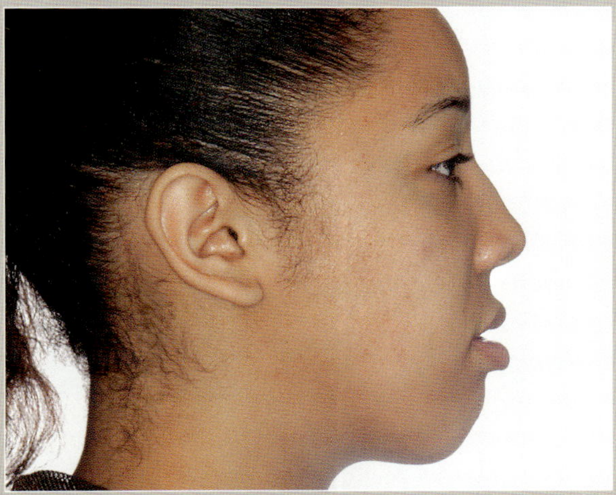

Lateral facial view at completion of presurgical orthodontics.

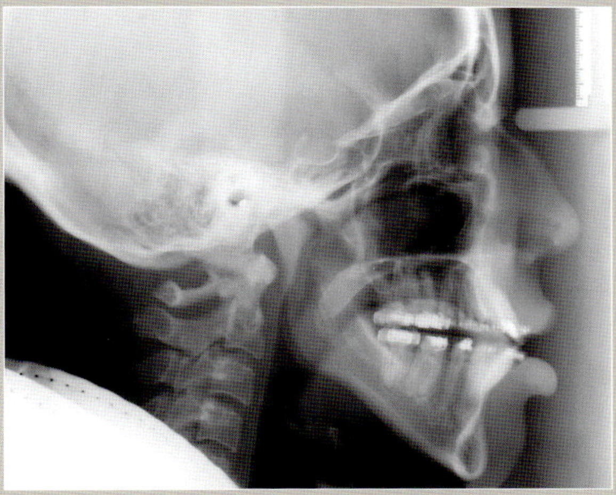

Lateral cephalometric radiograph at completion of presurgical orthodontics.

eruption until adequate tooth structure became exposed to facilitate placement of provisional restorations. The patient was then referred back to her restorative dentist to prepare the erupted anterior teeth and place long-term provisional restorations. Orthodontic brackets were placed on the newly restored teeth, and bands were placed on the newly erupted second molars to facilitate further alignment and leveling of the teeth with closure of the patient's existing open bite. Appropriate spaces were opened mesiodistally between teeth as needed to facilitate the establishment of optimal clinical crown size and contour for each tooth.

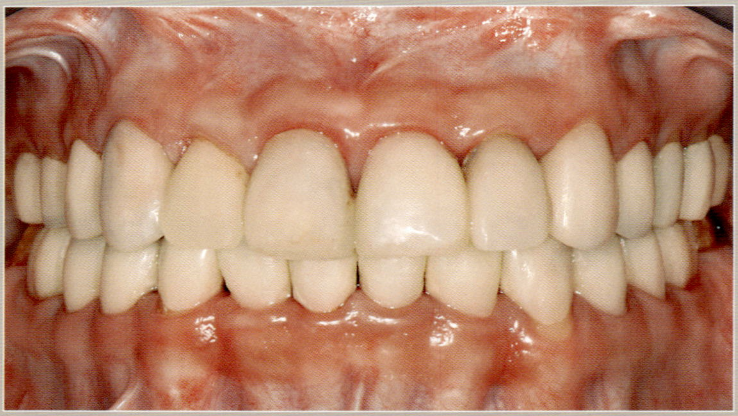

Frontal view after completion of orthognathic surgery and postsurgical orthodontics.

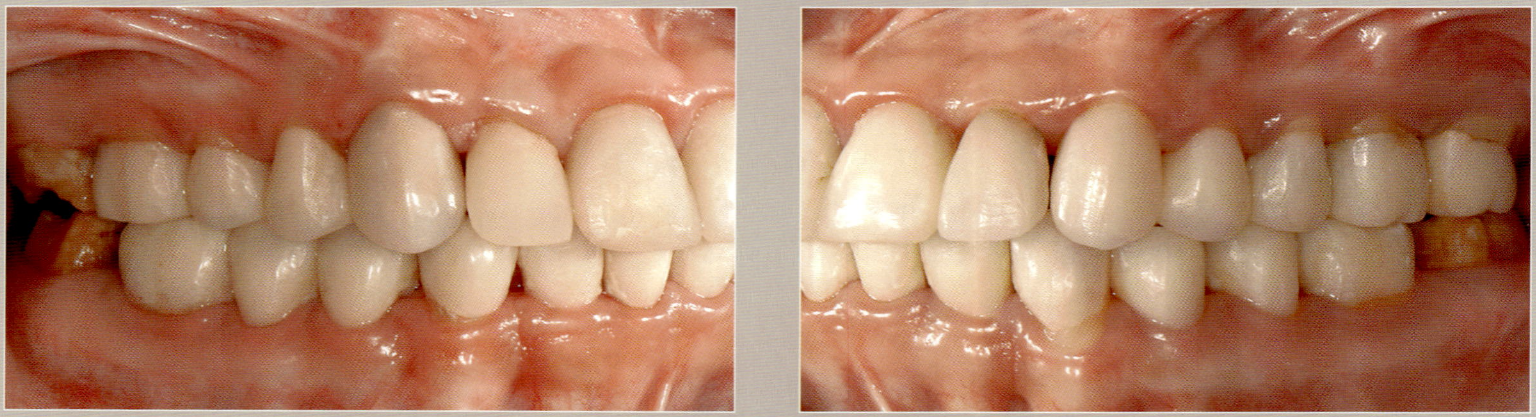

Lateral views of Class I relationship and appropriate intercuspation of teeth in MIP.

As orthodontic treatment progressed, it became apparent that an asymmetry had developed, with rotation of the patient's maxillary arch to the right. As a result, her maxillary dental midline also shifted to the right, a Class III relationship of the teeth developed on the right side, and essentially no horizontal or vertical overlap existed on the left side or anteriorly. To correct the asymmetry and establish an acceptable, esthetically pleasing, and functional occlusal relationship, the patient's maxilla needed to be advanced and rotated to the left. Because a second phase of orthognathic surgery was planned to advance the patient's chin, movement of her maxilla was included in the surgical plan.

Phase VI: Orthognathic surgery (second phase)

A Le Fort I osteotomy and palatal split of the patient's maxilla was completed to advance her maxilla and rotate it to the left. A horizontal osteotomy of the patient's bony chin at the symphysis also was completed, with removal of a 5-mm tapered section of bone and advancement of the symphyseal fragment to improve her facial profile and reduce her anterior lower facial height. Rigid fixation was used to stabilize the bony fragments during healing.

Phase VII: Orthodontic treatment (postsurgical/finishing)

Orthodontic treatment was resumed after healing of the osteotomy sites was complete. Detailing and final tooth position was established with good parallelism of the tooth roots. The orthodontic treatment goals/objectives established initially were essentially met. These included a solid Class I relationship bilaterally, relatively level curves of Spee and Wilson, appropriate vertical and horizontal overlap of the anterior teeth for anterior guidance, relatively balanced levels of marginal gingiva, appropriate spacing between the teeth for optimal restoration for normal tooth dimensions and contours, dental and facial midlines aligned, and a stable, functional occlusion at CR = CO = MIP that was free of any posterior occlusal interferences.

Maxillary and mandibular removable retainers were placed to maintain the tooth positions established during orthodontic treatment. Orthodontic records of the completed treatment were obtained. These included facial and intraoral photographs, casts of the teeth, and cephalometric, panoramic, periapical, and bitewing radiographs. The patient was referred back to her restorative dentist for definitive restoration of her teeth.

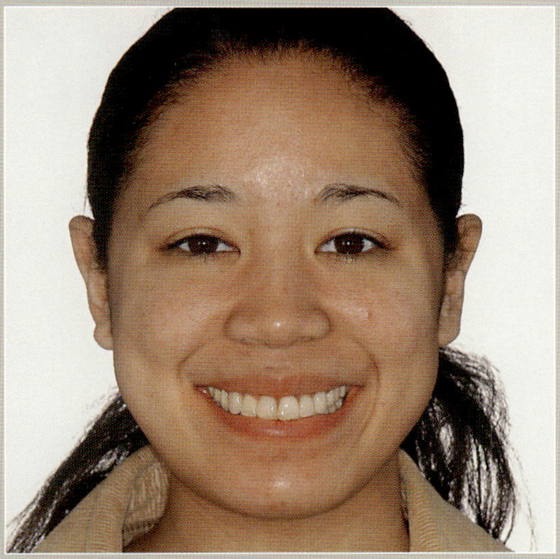

Facial view of smile with decreased lower facial height.

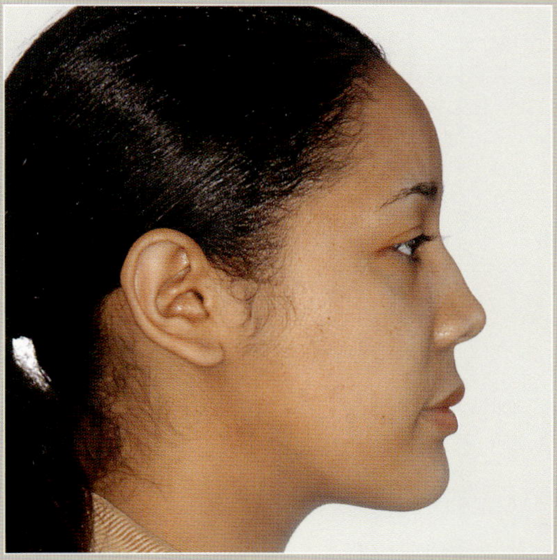

Lateral facial view with decreased lower facial height and establishment of lip competence.

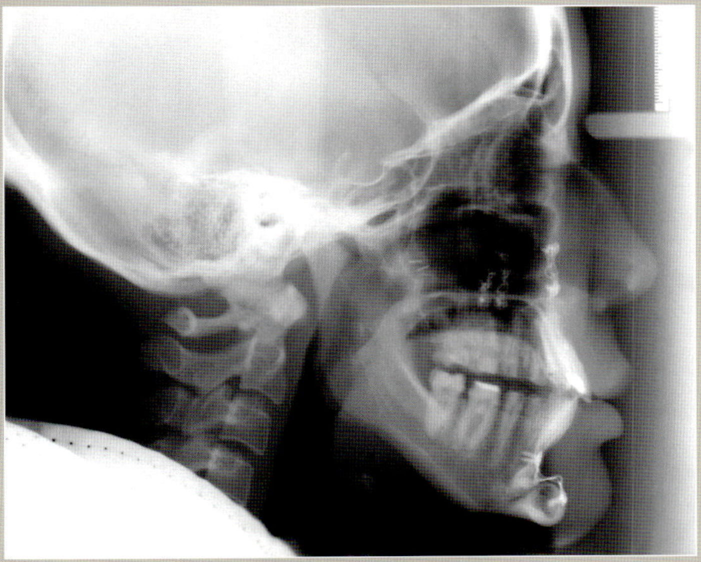

Lateral cephalometric radiograph after completion of orthognathic surgery and postsurgical orthodontic treatment.

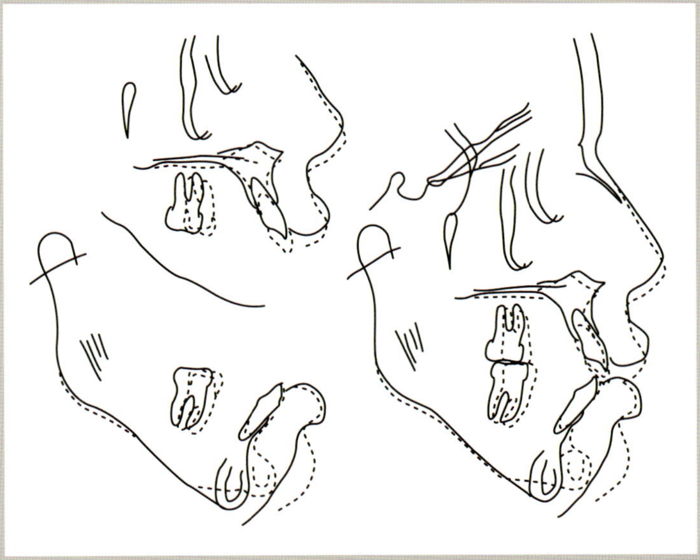

Composite tracings of cephalometric radiographs: *(solid line)* pretreatment; *(dashed line)* posttreatment.

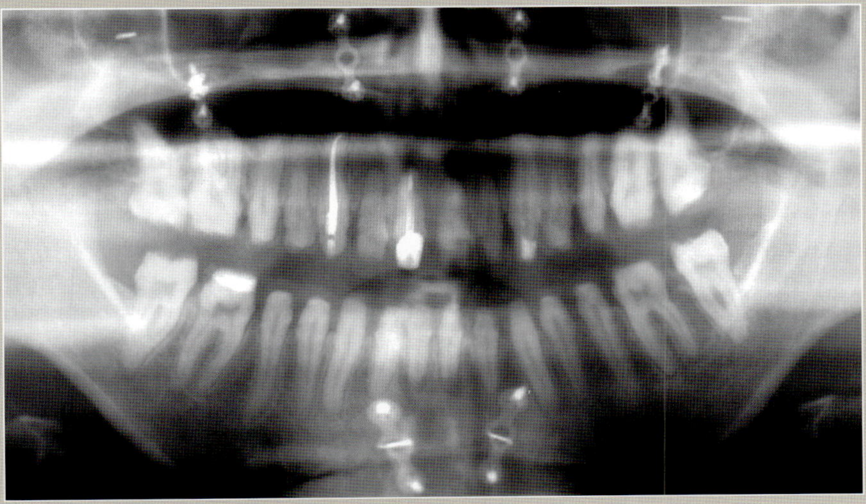

Panoramic radiograph after completion of orthognathic surgery and postsurgical orthodontics.

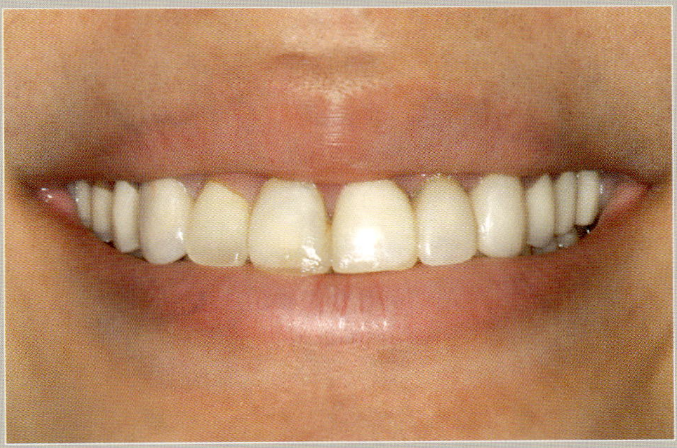

Close-up view of smile with coincident maxillary dental midline and facial midline.

Posttreatment

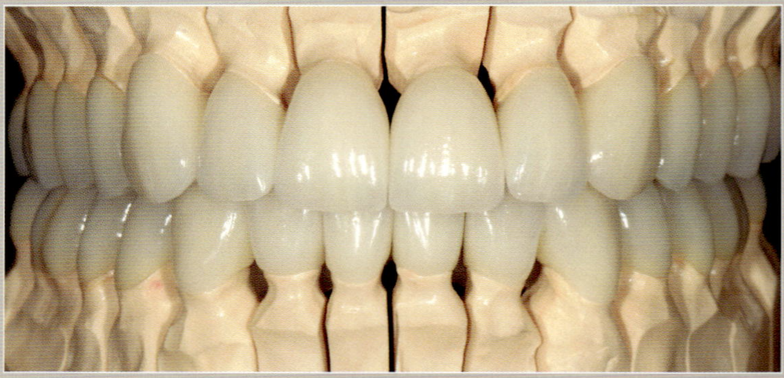

Laboratory view of completed definitive restorations.

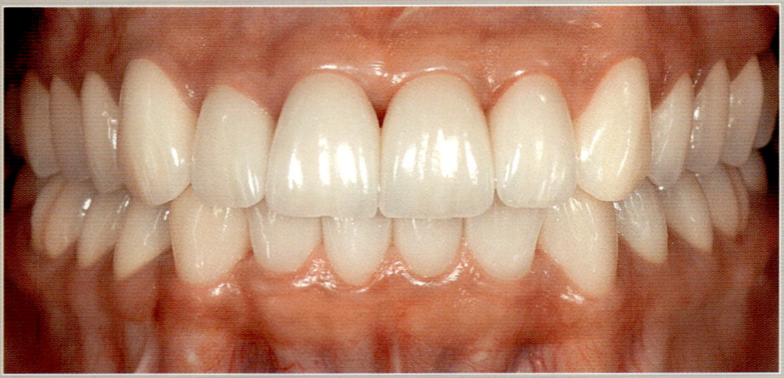

Frontal view of definitive restorations.

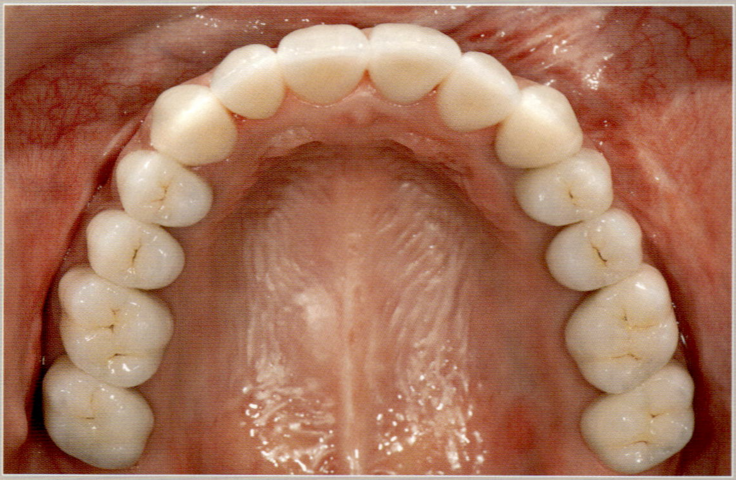

Maxillary occlusal view.

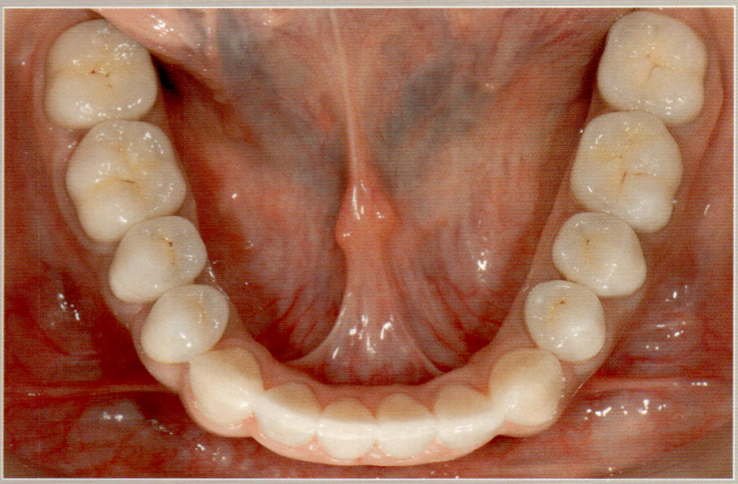

Mandibular occlusal view.

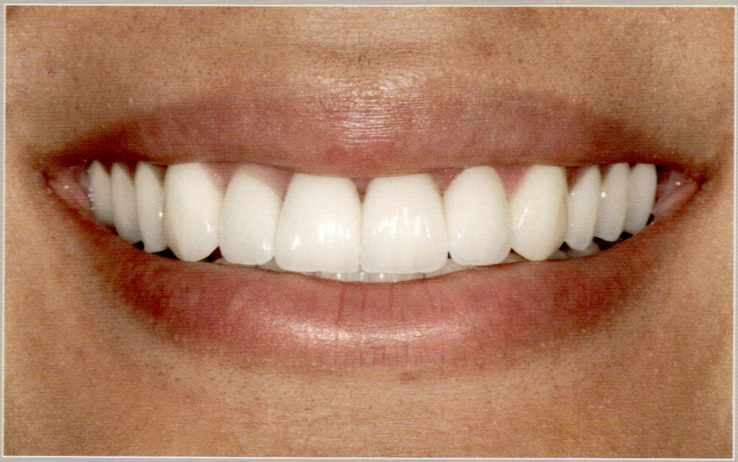

Close-up view of smile.

Phase VIII: Definitive restorative treatment

A diagnostic wax-up was completed on articulated casts of the patient's teeth, and provisional restorations were fabricated from the wax-up in preparation for removal of the long-term restorations used throughout orthodontic treatment. Next, the long-term provisional restorations were removed, the teeth reprepared as needed, and new provisional restorations placed. After an appropriate period of evaluation to assess the patient's occlusion, function, appearance, hygiene, and stability, definitive impressions of the prepared teeth were obtained, and definitive restorations were fabricated and placed on the teeth. Complete-coverage metal-ceramic crowns—design feldspathic porcelain (Ivoclar)—were placed on all posterior teeth, and complete-coverage ceramic crowns—Procera alumina copings (Nobel Biocare) with VM7 feldspathic porcelain (Vita)—were placed on the anterior teeth. Finally, a maxillary occlusal nightguard was fabricated, adjusted, and delivered.

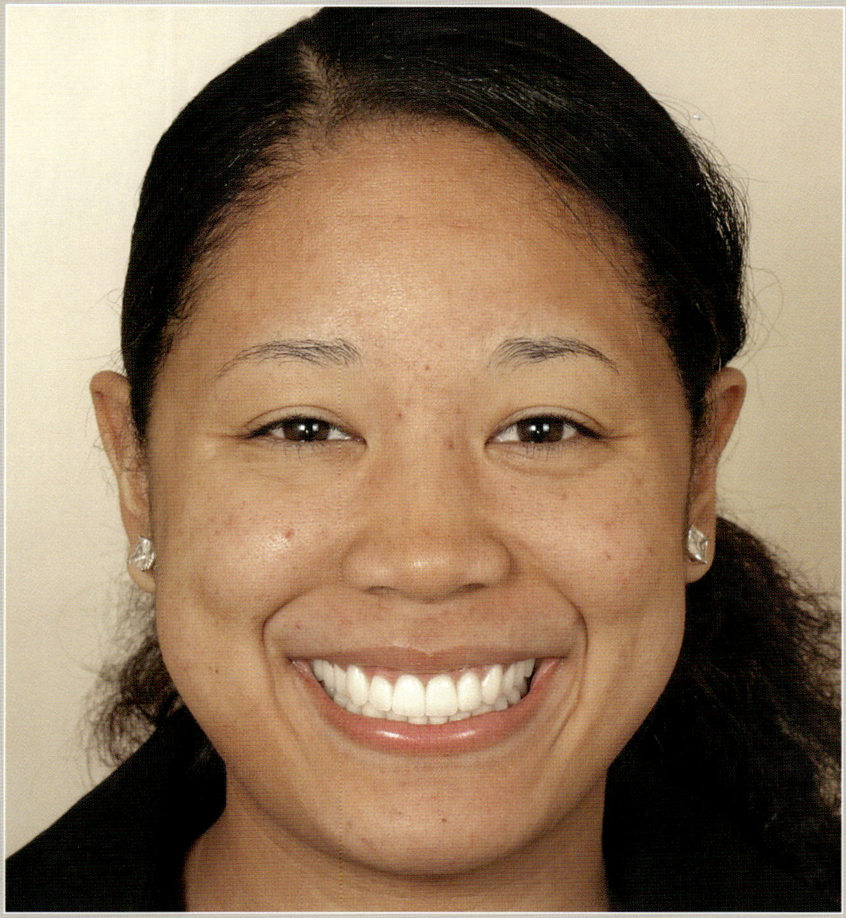

Facial view of smile.

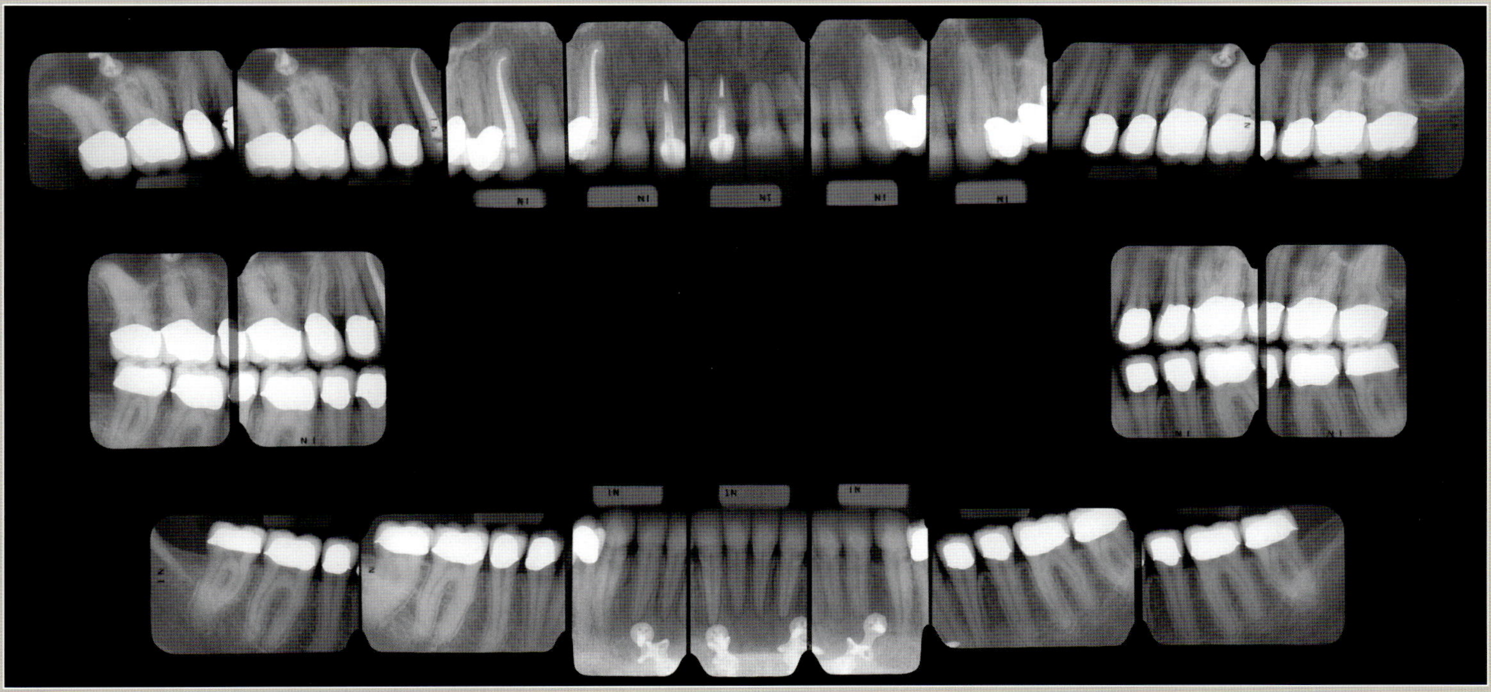

Complete periapical radiographic survey with bitewings.

You may now place the corresponding posttreatment overlay found in the separate folder over the pretreatment periodontal chart on page 315.

Commentary

This case illustrates the ultimate restorative challenge with regard to tooth size and proportional relationships of the teeth. No frame of reference existed because of the absence of normal crown contours due to the substantial deficiency of enamel on every tooth. As a result, her teeth had considerably compromised her appearance, occlusion, function, psychologic development, and general well-being. In addition, the patient had a skeletal disharmony that had negatively affected her facial balance and appearance.

The two principles related to diagnosis and treatment planning discussed in my chapter in the first volume in this series and expanded upon in this chapter (ie, space appropriation and a Class I relationship of the anterior teeth) were essential to treatment success in this case. Optimal space appropriation in the vertical and transverse planes of space achieved through surgical crown lengthening of the teeth, surgical expansion of the maxilla, orthodontics, and the placement of provisional restorations of normal size and shape facilitated the placement of definitive restorations that resemble natural teeth in size and proportion. This, in turn, facilitated the establishment of optimal appearance and occlusal relationships of the teeth. The establishment of a Class I relationship of the teeth achieved through the combination of orthodontics, provisionally restored teeth of normal size and shape, and orthognathic surgery to reposition the patient's maxilla facilitated optimal intercuspation of her teeth in MIP and appropriate horizontal and vertical overlap of her teeth with relatively normal proclination of her incisors.

The combination of achieving optimal space appropriation and a Class I relationship of the teeth allowed the dentition to be definitively restored in an optimal manner with an excellent result in terms of occlusion, appearance, function, hygiene, and stability. If an interdisciplinary team approach and these key principles were not implemented, treatment results would have fallen far short of what was ultimately achieved. Restorative dentistry alone would certainly not have provided a favorable result. Orthodontic treatment without first provisionally restoring the patient's teeth to normal size and shape would have made it nearly impossible to establish optimal tooth position to facilitate optimal definitive restoration of the teeth. In addition, by establishing goals/objectives of treatment that addressed the patient's facial considerations as well as her teeth, we were able to improve her facial profile, balance, and appearance as well.

Prior to the placement of definitive restorations, it was noted that the marginal gingiva labial to tooth no. 7 was more coronal than desired. The patient declined esthetic enhancement in this area.

Acknowledgments

First and foremost, I thank my Lord and Savior, Jesus Christ, and my family for the opportunities in life that have allowed me to participate in the dental education of others, including the contribution I have made to this book. Hopefully, my efforts in this regard will help those who engage in the process of planning treatment for their patients and specifically those who become involved with patients that have problems similar to those of the young lady presented in this chapter.

I also want to thank the clinicians who participated with me in the management of this patient's complex dental needs. They are all friends of mine and excellent clinicians. They have certainly blessed my life and the lives of the patients I have had the honor of treating with them as interdisciplinary team members. Dr Ralph Yuodelis, a periodontist and fixed prosthodontist, provided his surgical expertise in lengthening the clinical crowns of the patient's teeth and exposure of the central incisor. In addition, he is one of the outstanding leaders in the discipline of prosthodontics and was instrumental in my dental education during my graduate training at the University of Washington. Dr Thomas Junge, one of the best prosthodontists I know, completed all of the restorative procedures, initially as a graduate student and, after the orthodontic and orthognathic treatment was completed, while in private practice. Dr Dale Bloomquist, an oral and maxillofacial surgeon, provided his surgical expertise to facilitate initial expansion of the patient's maxilla, removal of her third molars, and soft tissue exposure of her right unerupted canine. Dr Roger West, an oral and maxillofacial surgeon, also provided his surgical expertise to correct the patient's asymmetric maxilla and advance her chin. His treatment significantly improved her overall facial balance and appearance. Mr Harald Heindl, MDT, and his daughter, Daniela Heindl, CDT, dental technicians extraordinaire and true artists, provided the technical and artistic expertise involved in the fabrication of the beautiful restorations placed by Dr Junge. Finally, I thank Dr Robert Faucher, a mentor of mine and many others, for contributing a number of pictures to illustrate problems associated with restoring teeth in patients without anterior Class I relationships, which we both prefer not to do. He is also one of the best and one of the most knowledgeable prosthodontists I know.

References

1. Black GV. Descriptive Anatomy of the Human Teeth, ed 4. Philadelphia: S. S. White, 1902:17,18.
2. Ballard ML. Asymmetry in tooth size: A factor in the etiology, diagnosis and treatment of malocclusion. Angle Orthod 1944;14:67–71.
3. Bolton WA. Disharmony in Tooth Size and Its Relation to the Analysis and Treatment of Malocclusion [thesis]. Seattle: University of Washington, 1952:12.
4. Garn SM, Lewis AB, Walenga AJ. Maximum confidence values for the human mesiodistal crown dimension of human teeth. Arch Oral Biol 1968;13:841–844.
5. Shillingburg HT, Kaplan MJ, Grace SC. Tooth dimensions—A comparative study. J South Calif Dent Assoc 1972;40:830–839.
6. Bjorndal AM, Henderson WG, Skidmore AE, Kellner FH. Anatomic measurements of human teeth extracted from males between the ages of 17 and 21 years. Oral Surg Oral Med Oral Pathol 1974;38:791–803.
7. Richardson ER, Malhotra SK. Mesiodistal crown dimension of the permanent dentition of American Negroes. Am J Orthod 1975;68:157–164.
8. Wheeler RC. Wheeler's Atlas of Tooth Form. Philadelphia: Saunders, 1984.
9. Gillen RJ, Schwartz RS, Hilton TJ, Evans DB. An analysis of selected normative tooth proportions. Int J Prosthodont 1994;7:410–417.
10. Sterrett JD, Oliver T, Robinson F, Fortson W, Knaak B, Russell CM. Width/length ratios of normal clinical crowns of the maxillary anterior dentition in man. J Clin Periodontol 1999;26:153–157.
11. Magne P, Gallucci GO, Belser UC. Anatomic crown width/length ratios of unworn and worn maxillary teeth in white subjects. J Prosthet Dent 2003;89:453–461.
12. Chu SJ. Range and mean distribution frequency of individual tooth width of the maxillary anterior dentition. Pract Proced Aesthet Dent 2007;14:209–215.
13. Chu SJ. Range and mean discordance of individual tooth width of the mandibular anterior dentition. Pract Proced Aesthet Dent 2008;20:313–320.
14. Levin EI. Dental esthetics and the golden proportion. J Prosthet Dent 1978;40:244–252.
15. Lombardi RE. The principles of visual perception and their clinical application to denture esthetics. J Prosthet Dent 1973;29:358–382.
16. Preston JD. The golden proportion revisited. J Esthet Dent 1993;5:247–251.

13

Designing the Fixed Implant-Supported Reconstruction for the Fully Edentulous Patient

Ricardo Mitrani, DDS, MSD

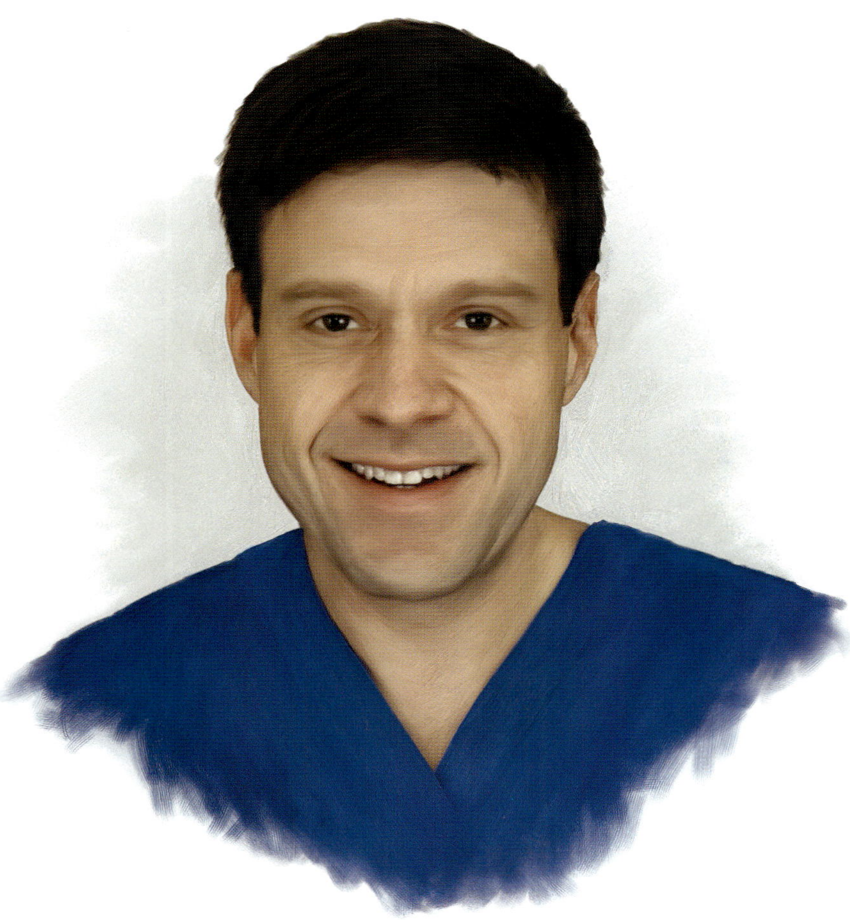

It is when we automatically default to what has worked best in the past

that we are most likely to encounter failure.

Philosophy and Background

Since I adopted the concept of interdisciplinary dentistry in my practice and began working in a collaborative environment with a group of very talented clinicians, dentistry has become far more satisfying and enjoyable. As the restorative dentist on our team, more often than not, I have been accountable for tailoring and then delivering the definitive restoration to our patients. This responsibility has involved being able to outline a clear and detailed treatment path for all participants on our interdisciplinary team. It has required strong leadership skills, one of the most important being the ability to keep all the lines of communication open and active.

Treatment success is directly dependent on the effectiveness of team members in communicating their varying treatment ideas, thoughts on the cost-benefit ratio, updates on the progress of treatment, and changes in expectations for treatment outcome. It calls to mind the *Medici effect*, which is named after a prominent family in Florence, Italy, who promoted intimate interaction among individuals from various disciplines, such as painters, philosophers, architects, and writers. By doing so, they sparked innovative ideas and concepts that are said to have been instrumental in precipitating the Renaissance era. One can only imagine the creative strategies that can be generated and ultimately implemented by a group of individuals willing to meet and share their thoughts and ideas throughout treatment, and this is why I am committed to an interdisciplinary approach to treatment. Ultimately, the patient is the beneficiary.

One modality of treatment that epitomizes the necessity for an interdisciplinary approach is the implant rehabilitation of patients who present with hopeless dentitions or total edentulism. The fixed implant-supported reconstruction for the fully edentulous patient represents one of the most fascinating challenges in contemporary dentistry. As a prosthodontist, I find that being able to re-establish form and function when it has been radically lost (ie, the edentulous state) challenges my creative threshold both technically and technologically. Designing and implementing the treatment approach involves numerous fundamental aspects that cannot be overlooked. With today's diagnostic tools, virtual treatment can be explored, but it is only through a systematic and comprehensive approach that we can achieve predictable long-term success.

Among the aspects that make treating these types of cases so fascinating is the fact that no clinical situation presents in exactly the same way. Every patient presents with his or her own unique set of circumstances, clinical conditions, and personal desires. Each new case must be approached as if it is the first patient the clinician has ever treated. It is when we automatically default to what has worked best in the past that we are most likely to encounter failure. Past triumphs do not necessarily guarantee future success.

This case was chosen more for the journey than the destination of treatment. Numerous questions come to mind when considering the path of treatment to be taken:

- How do we set the stage for long-term success both functionally and esthetically in a complete-mouth, fixed, implant-supported case?
- How does the introduction of multiple implant placements in severely compromised edentulous ridges potentially complicate overall treatment?
- Why is an interdisciplinary team approach beneficial when planning for fabrication of a complete-mouth, fixed, implant-supported reconstruction?
- How is the sequencing, which is very important in ensuring successful treatment outcomes in these types of cases, determined?
- How can new technologies be used to help guide and facilitate treatment in more advanced and complex cases?

When it comes to implant therapy, there are several myths that should be dispelled, such as the idea that implant-supported restorations last forever. While there is a plethora of evidence-based literature that substantiates the long-term success of osseointegrated implants, realistic expectations dictate that these restorations may suffer eventual biomechanical breakdown that will require repair.[1] This is especially true for the fully edentulous patient who not only has lost his or her dentition but also has impaired proprioception, which is an essential protective mechanism for natural teeth or artificial replacements.

All features pertaining to restorative design must be well thought out prior to implant placement because some of these features will dictate how sensitive the precise three-dimensional (3D) placement of the implants will be. For instance, if the restorative plan requires screw-retained restorations, the buccolingual placement and angulation play a crucial role because it would be quite cumbersome to correct if the implants were angled toward the buccal aspect of the anticipated restoration.

The biomechanical principles associated with implant-supported restorations dictate the number, diameter, length, and distribution of the implants. When considering the optimal number of implants, one must also think about two important aspects: *(1)* the splinting scheme and *(2)* the opposing arch. Common sense plays an important role in this regard. We should recognize that placing too many implants is as inefficient as not placing enough implants, and both can negatively affect the overall outcome. Placing as many implants as possible does not necessarily produce a better result because implants that are placed too close together can lead to interimplant bone loss and make access for oral hygiene maintenance difficult or impossible. Placing too few implants, on the other hand, can result in mechanical failure.

When assessing anteroposterior spread, we should not only consider the distal cantilever but also the buccal and vertical cantilevers as well. All of these contribute to increased stress concentration at the implant-abutment interface,[2] and if implants are placed at odd angles,[3] care must be taken to ensure that retrievability is considered to allow easy management of future failures.

Planning for complete dentures is difficult even without the introduction of implant treatment into the overall scheme. This underscores the importance of thorough initial planning, effective interdisciplinary team case management, and diligent monitoring during the posttreatment phase of therapy.

Case Presentation

Treating clinicians
Prosthodontist: Ricardo Mitrani, DDS, MSD
Oral and maxillofacial surgeon: Ignacio Calleja, DDS
Ceramist: Joel Lopez, CDT

Clinical Treatment Planning

Age at initial presentation: 68 years
Initial presentation: July 2008
Active treatment completed: March 2009

Introduction and background

This 68-year-old woman was seeking fixed treatment because she was weary of using removable appliances. She stated that she was willing to invest the time required and had sufficient financial resources but admitted being anxious about potential surgeries.

She had been wearing a maxillary complete denture for the last 20 years and had ill-fitting mandibular bilateral distal extension removable partial dentures (Kennedy Class I). The mandibular anterior teeth had advanced periodontal involvement.

Medical history

- Noncontributory
- No known allergies
- No contraindications to dental treatment

Diagnostic findings

Extraoral and facial findings

- Relatively flat facial profile
- Good frontal symmetry
- Low lip mobility

TMJ and mandibular range of motion

- Within normal limits
- Maximum opening: 48 mm
- No history of muscle pain

Intraoral findings

Dental

- Incisal wear of maxillary denture teeth

Periodontal

- Mandibular anterior teeth exhibit advanced periodontitis.

Occlusal notes

- Vertical dimension of occlusion appears to be adequate.

Pretreatment

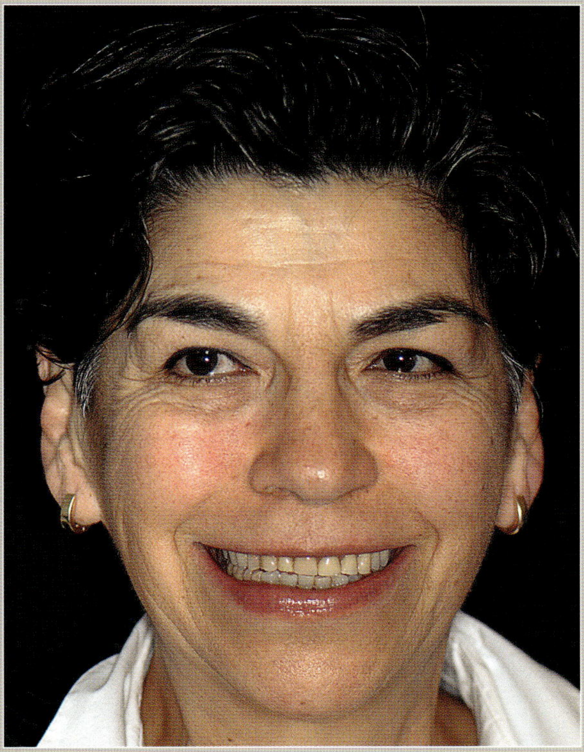

Facial view of smile.

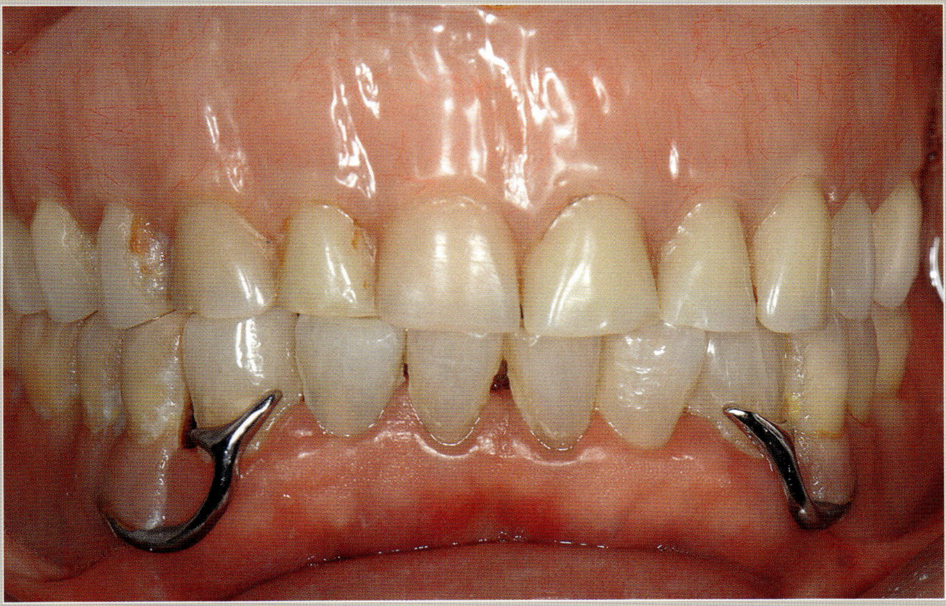

Intraoral frontal view.

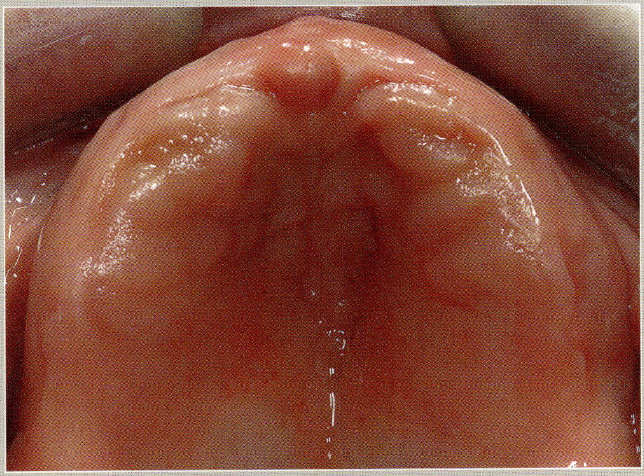

Maxillary occlusal view.

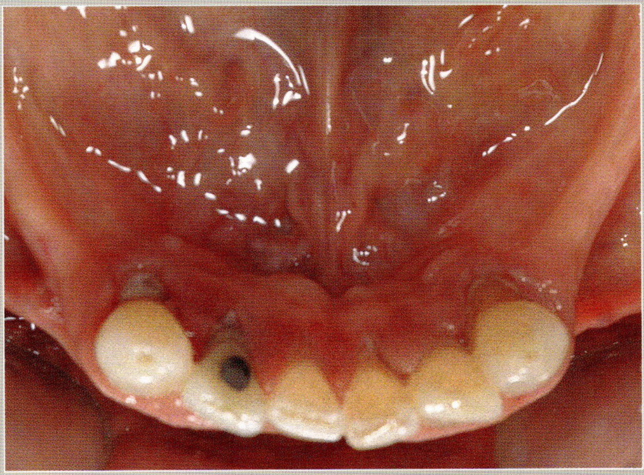

Mandibular occlusal view.

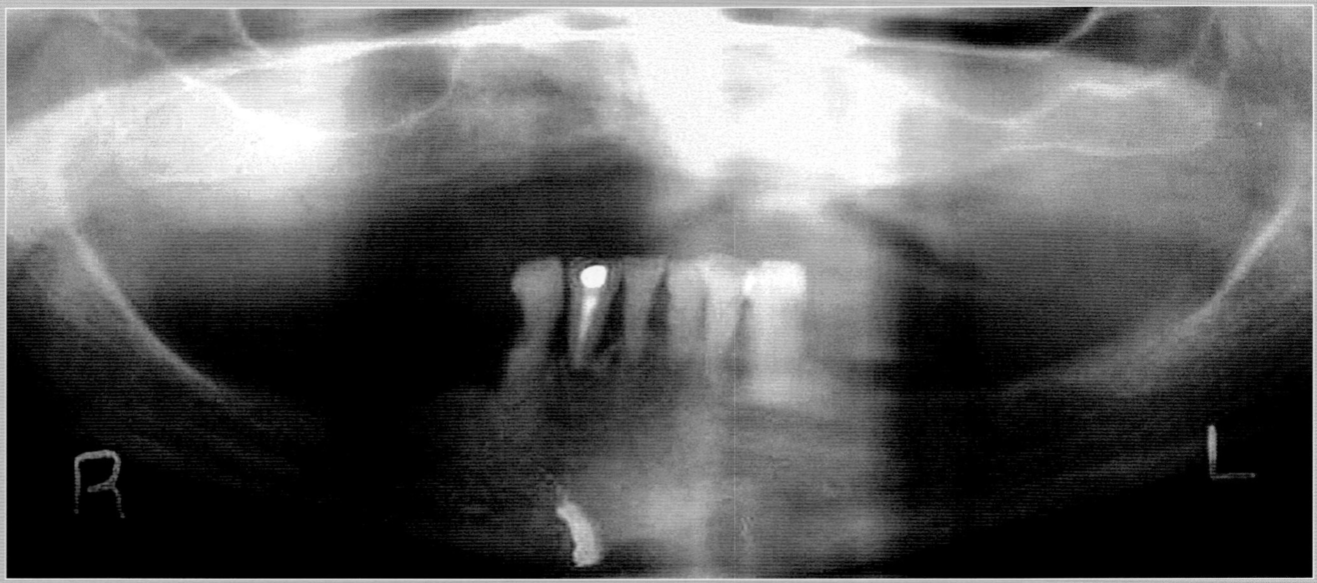

Panoramic radiograph.

Radiographic findings

- Panoramic radiograph depicts slight pneumatization of the maxillary sinuses and what appears to be sufficient bone for implant placement.
- In the mandible, the regions distal to the mental foramina seem rather atrophic, and significant bone loss was noted in the anterior sextant.
- Tooth no. 26 has been endodontically treated.

Oral hygiene habits

- The patient brushed her teeth twice a day with a manual toothbrush.
- Moderate amounts of plaque and calculus present.

Diagnosis

- Total maxillary edentulism
- Partial mandibular edentulism
- AAP Type IV
- Parafunctional habits

Prognosis

- Periodontal: hopeless for the remaining dentition
- Biomechanical, functional, and esthetic: poor without treatment; very good with treatment

Summary of concerns

1. How can we satisfy the patient's esthetic and functional concerns?
2. Can we consider immediate implant loading for this patient?
3. Considering the resorption pattern in the anterior maxilla, should we graft the area first or work with the existing structure?
4. Ridge configuration of the mandible: Considering the limited anteroposterior spread for the mandibular arch,[4–6] should we consider grafting the posterior mandible or lateralize the mental nerve in order to be able to place at least one implant distal to the mental foramen and avoid lengthy cantilevers?
5. Should we consider fabrication of a mandibular implant-supported overdenture with tissue support as an alternative?
6. What materials should be used for the definitive restorations?
7. Should we plan for cement- or screw-retained restorations?
8. Can we use computer-aided design/computer-assisted manufacture (CAD/CAM) to generate a surgical stent for implant placement in an area where extensive osteoplasty needs to be done?
9. Can we perform CAD/CAM-guided surgery and sinus elevation procedures at the same time?
10. Can we restore this patient with long-term predictability?
11. Can we protect our restorations from potential parafunctional damage?

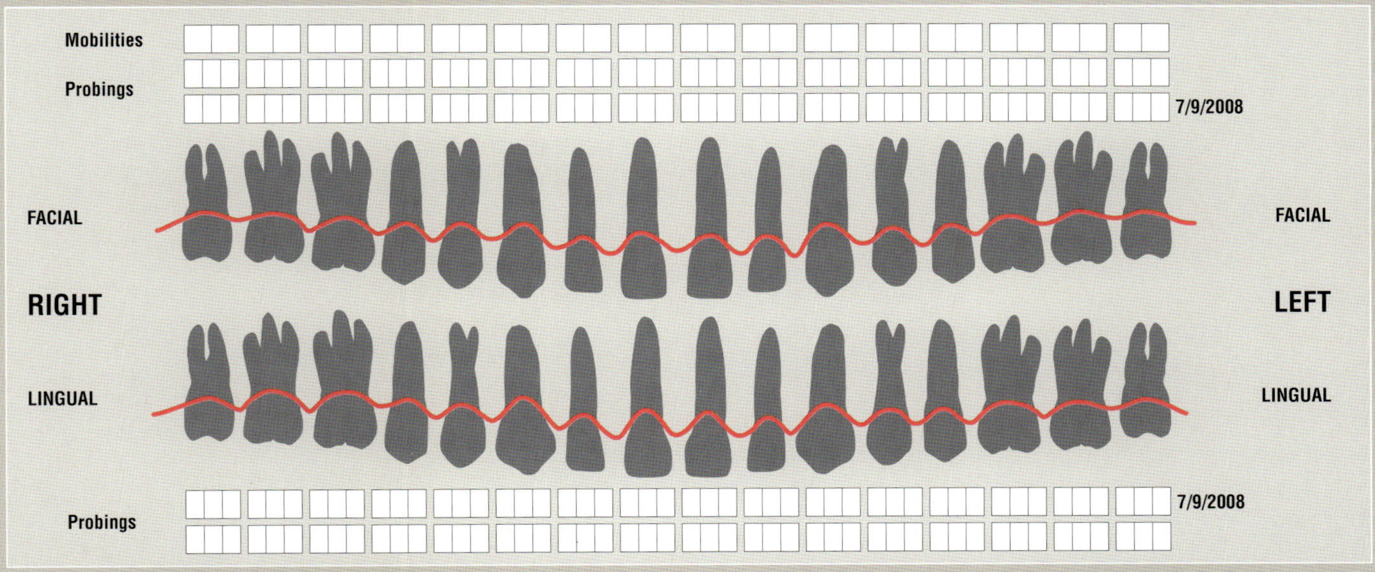

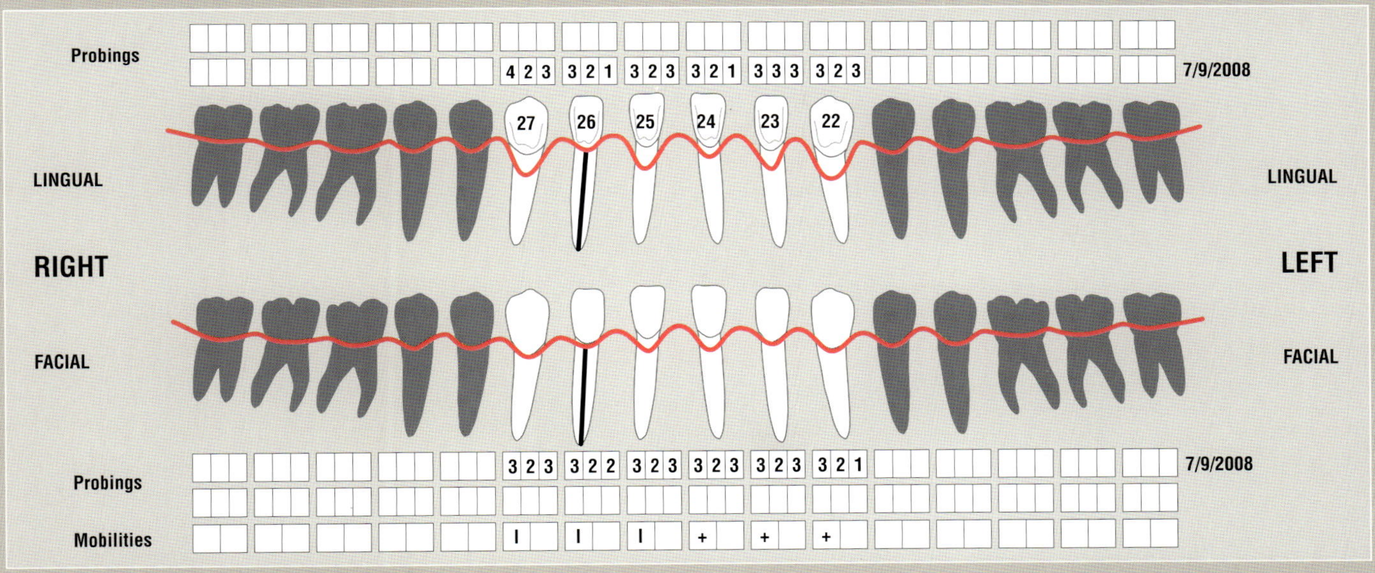

As a learning exercise, you may now outline goals/objectives of treatment and a treatment plan.

Proposed Treatment Plan

Goals/objectives of treatment

- Improve overall esthetics
- Maximize function with full-denture occlusion
- Provide fixed implant-supported restorations
- Provide a reconstruction with a built-in contingency plan that will allow easy, low-cost repair when needed

Phase I: Initial extractions and provisional interim denture

1. Extraction of the hopeless mandibular anterior teeth and delivery of an immediate provisional conventional denture, which will facilitate gathering all the diagnostic data and defining the prosthetic design

Phase II: Diagnostics

2. Fabrication of a trial denture to communicate to the patient the most ideal esthetic outcome
3. Computed tomography (CT) scans using software that will allow us to closely relate the anatomical structures and any bone deficiencies to the ultimate implant/crown positions
4. Fabrication of surgical templates and provisional restorations

Phase III: Maxillary implant placements and immediate provisional restorations

5. Implant placements in the maxillary arch concomitant with bilateral sinus grafts
6. Delivery of fixed, screw-retained, immediate provisional restorations[7]

Phase IV: Mandibular implant placements

Phase V: Provisionalization of the mandibular implants

Phase VI: Impressions, records, and fabrication of provisional and definitive restorations

Phase VII: Try-in and delivery of the definitive reconstruction

Phase VIII: Recall program

7. Six-month recall maintenance program

Active Clinical Treatment

Review of the goals/objectives of treatment

- Improve overall esthetics
- Maximize function with full-denture occlusion
- Provide fixed implant-supported restorations
- Provide a reconstruction with a built-in contingency plan that will allow easy, low-cost repair when needed

Phase I: Initial extractions and provisional interim denture

The treating clinicians decided that it would be best to extract the periodontally compromised mandibular anterior teeth and give the patient a provisional interim denture in the mandible, which would allow appropriate healing of the area and provide a better, more controlled diagnostic work-up for the definitive treatment.

Phase II: Diagnostics

The treatment team sought the patient's approval by presenting a mock-up of the proposed esthetic outcome by means of a trial denture. Impressions were taken, and conventional complete denture procedures were carried out.

Once the impressions were made, baseplates and wax rims were fabricated in order to establish an appropriate vertical dimension, which usually is arbitrarily obtained by assessing esthetics. Other parameters such as freeway space may also be considered, but at this stage we generally adhere to the idea that if it looks right, it usually is right.[8]

Using a facebow transfer, the casts were then mounted on a semi-adjustable articulator, and a trial denture was fabricated. At the waxing stage, the trial denture was tried in, and the patient was asked to provide input regarding esthetics because this would be used as the ultimate reference for fabrication of the definitive prosthesis.

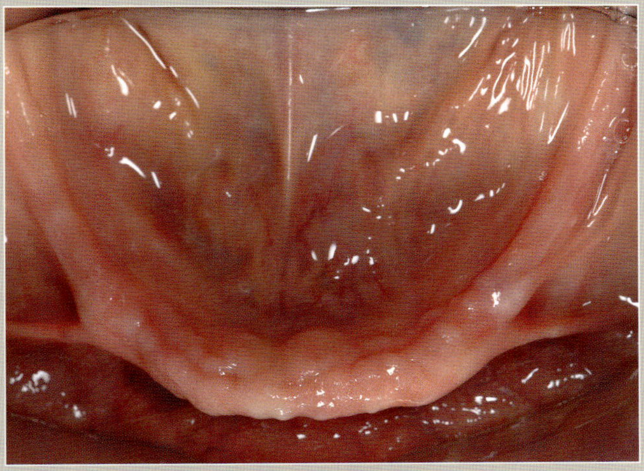

Mandibular occlusal view following extractions and healing.

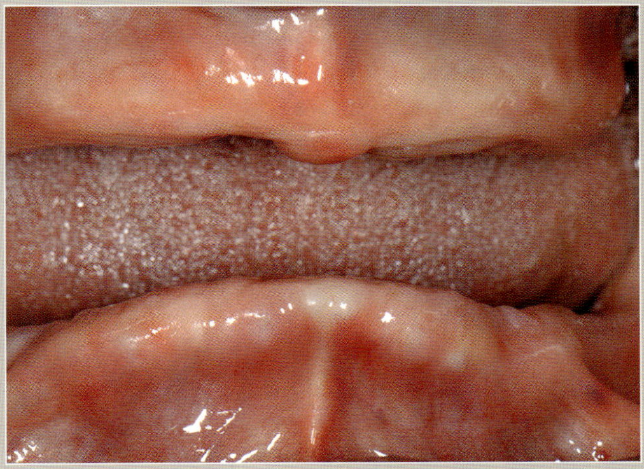

Intraoral frontal view.

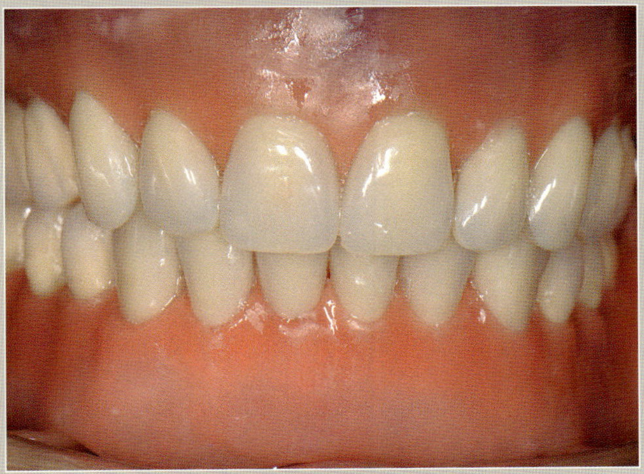

Intraoral view of trial denture try-in.

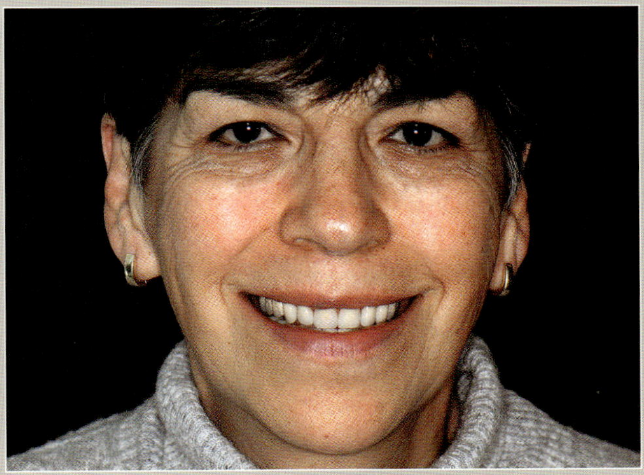

Extraoral view of trial denture try-in.

Because implant placement is prosthetically driven,[9] this was the time for any modifications in 3D tooth position to be made and discussed with the patient. We would not move forward until we were certain that she was completely comfortable with the proposed esthetic outcome. Once this first step was accomplished, the trial denture was duplicated with clear acrylic using a denture duplicator flask (Lang Dental).

Ten radiographic markers of approximately 2-mm diameter were randomly distributed throughout the duplicated denture. Using a round fissure bur on a slow-speed handpiece, 1-mm-deep indentations were drilled and then filled with warm gutta-percha.

Markers on the radiographic guide are essential during the double-scan procedure because they create a perfect match between the high-resolution scan of the radiographic guide and the patient's 3D dataset. This software allows the clinician to navigate the entire area of interest without losing the reference of the ultimate implant/crown positions.

With the double-scan protocol, both the patient's anatomy and the radiographic guide were digitized. In this way, anatomical data, as well as prosthetic targets, were visualized. Planning in 3D provides the closest representation of the actual patient situation and allows for precise diagnostics and treatment implementation.[10]

With the relatively small installation base of cone beam CT (CBCT) scanners, CT imaging has become an increasingly accessible technology with excellent accuracy.[11-15] These scanners deliver low radiation doses and are becoming more affordable. It is surprising how often their accuracy and zooming ability allow us to find measurable space to place implants. This may also enable the insertion of implants in areas of thin bone, thereby avoiding surgical augmentation.

Another key feature of the software is the ability to micrometrically change the 3D position and angulation of the implants, which may become a critical factor because we need the implant position to optimally match the restorative design.

Initially, the plan was to place implants bilaterally in the maxillary canine regions. Clinically it seemed quite feasible, but the CT and the planning software proved otherwise. In both the canine and lateral incisor regions, the amount of bone resorption and remaining bone topography made it impossible to consider the placement of fixtures with conventional diameters. However, the central incisor region, although also resorbed, allowed the placement of two fixtures. While perhaps an ideal approach would have been to graft the areas of the canines first and then place the implants in a subsequent procedure, this was not consistent with the patient's desire to limit the number of surgeries.

Another interesting feature of this case was that the posterior areas required sinus elevation[16-18] in order to accommodate implants. It was therefore important to determine if adjunctive grafting of the sinus could be carried out simultaneously with the placement of the implants using a CAD/CAM-generated surgical stent.

Because there was more than 5 mm of native bone at the floor of the sinus, it was decided that it was possible to graft and place the implants at the same time.[19-21] In order to allow lateral access for the sinus elevation procedures, the surgical stent was modified slightly. Using a slow-speed, pear-shaped carbide bur, approximately 6 mm was removed from the surgical template's flange.

Treatment in the mandibular arch presented three important challenges:

1. Severe atrophy distal to the mental foramina
2. Square configuration of the ridge
3. A knife-edge ridge in the anterior mandible

This, in turn, meant that:

- All implants had to be placed anterior to the mental foramina.
- The anteroposterior spread was unfavorable, especially considering that the prosthesis potentially could be negatively affected by three different cantilever forces (distal, buccal, and vertical).[2,5,6]
- In order to accommodate the implants buccolingually without ending up with an unsuitable fenestration, an 8-mm ostectomy was required to level the ridge prior to implant placement.

Because of the required ostectomy, it was not possible to use a CAD/CAM-generated stent similar to the one used for the placement of the implants in the maxilla, so it was decided to fabricate a conventional surgical stent–supported reconstruction consisting of a screw-retained, CAD/CAM-generated, zirconium oxide framework veneered with dissimilar materials (ie, ceramic in the maxilla and acrylic resin in the mandible).

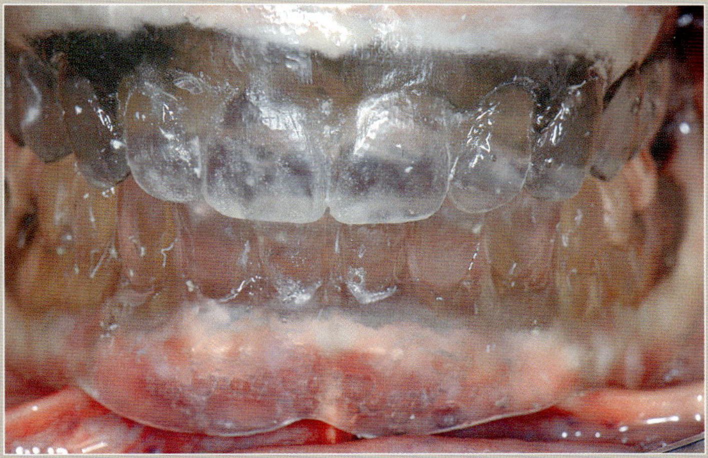

Try-in of the clear acrylic duplicate of the trial denture.

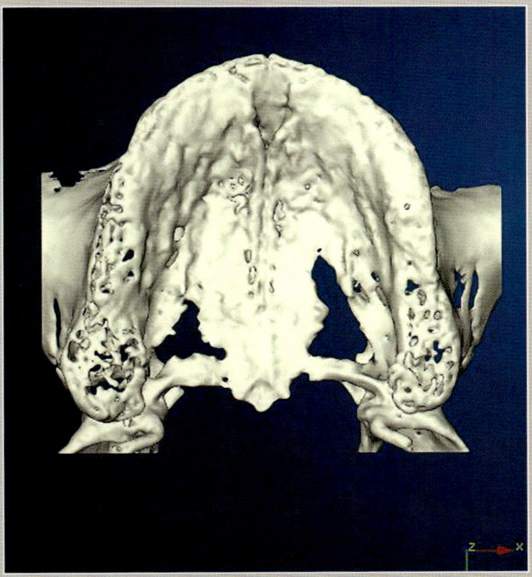

Occlusal view of the maxillary CT.

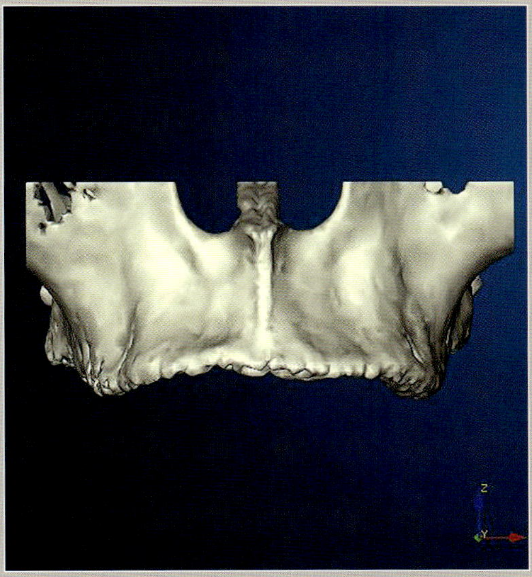

Frontal view of the maxillary CT.

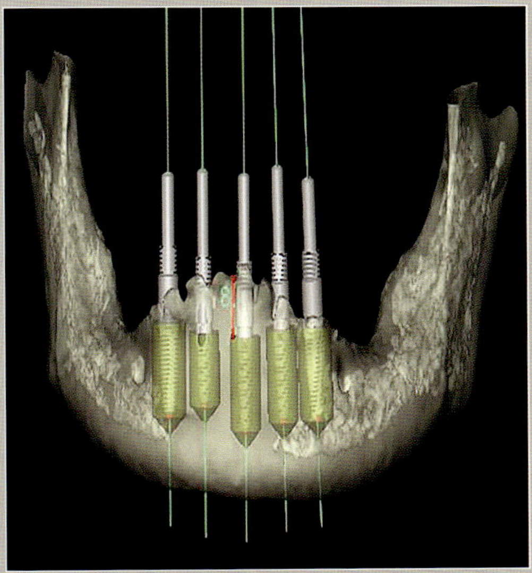

Frontal view of the mandibular CT showing implant placement.

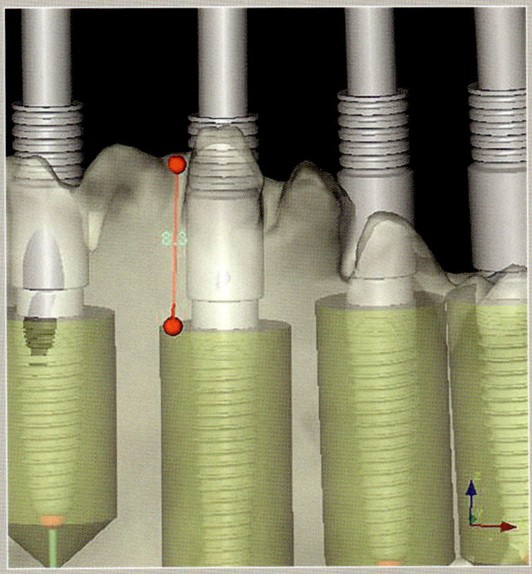

Amount of ostectomy needed.

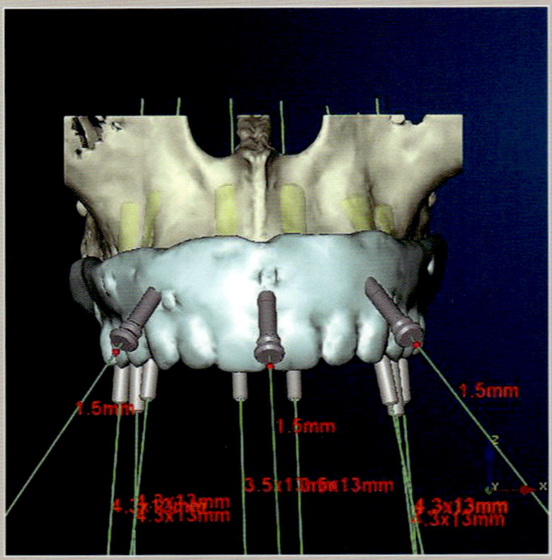

Frontal view of approved implant planning in the maxilla.

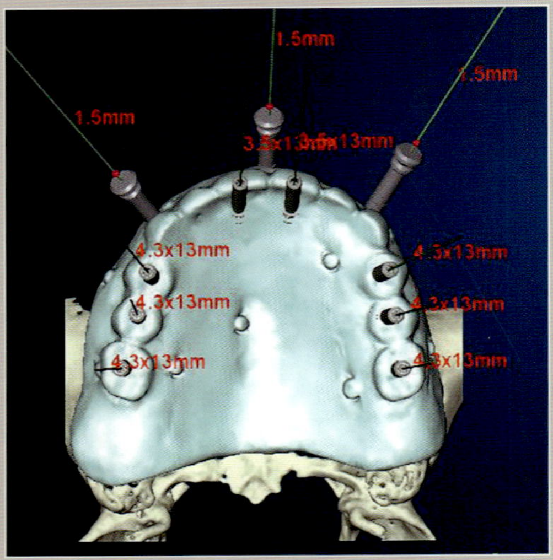

Occlusal view of implant planning in the maxilla, showing the implant angulation for a screw-retained design.

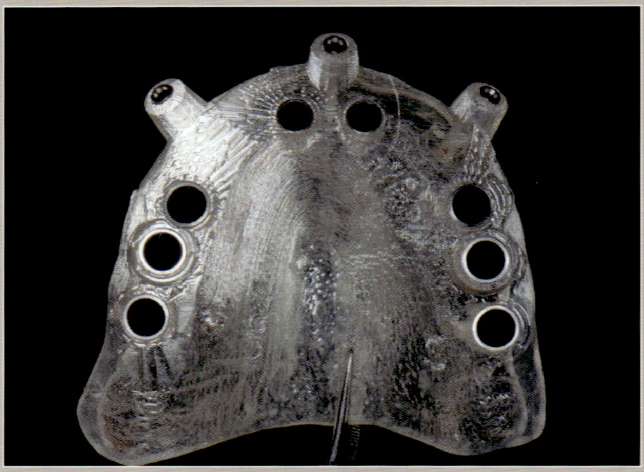

Occlusal view of CAD/CAM-generated surgical template.

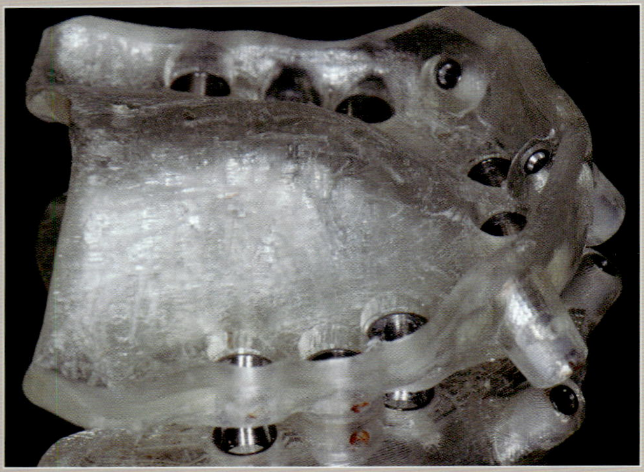

Lateral view of the modified CAD/CAM-generated surgical template.

Phase III: Maxillary implant placements and immediate provisional restorations

This phase of treatment involved placing implants in the maxillary arch. Sinus elevation procedures[16-21] were performed at the same time.

The CAD/CAM-generated surgical stent was tried in and then fixed using the anchor pins. The osteotomies were carried out through the washers embedded in the surgical template.

Once all the osteotomies were completed, the sinus elevation procedures were performed. Starting with the lateral windows, the sinus membrane was carefully detached, and the sinus was grafted using a mix of the autogenous bone collected from the osteotomies and demineralized freeze-dried bone.

Once the medial aspect was fully filled with bone, the implants were placed, and then the remainder of the cavity was filled with bone. This process ensured that the implants would have grafted bone circumferentially. There was a little more than 5 mm of native bone beyond the floor of the sinus, which ensured primary stability and the ability to place the implants concomitantly with the elevation procedures.

Once all implants were placed, healing abutments were secured, sinus sites sutured, and the pre-existing complete denture relined.

The patient had an appointment 24 hours later to receive the fixed immediate provisional restoration. The armamentarium for this prosthesis consisted of the processed trial denture and nonengaging titanium temporary abutments. Perforations in the processed trial denture were made at the estimated sites of implant placement. Because the angulation of the implants was well planned and the restricted surgical template replicated this plan very precisely, the abutments were easily located.

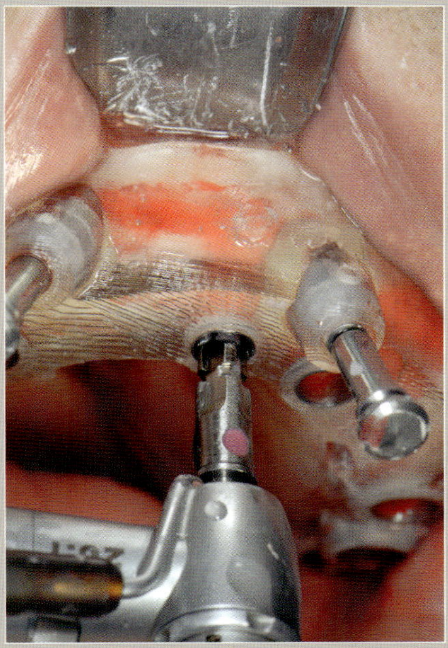

Osteotomies carried out through the surgical stent.

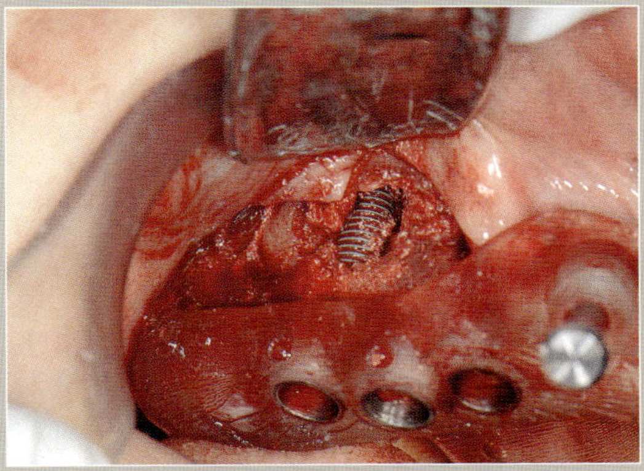

Maxillary sinus grafting and implant placement.

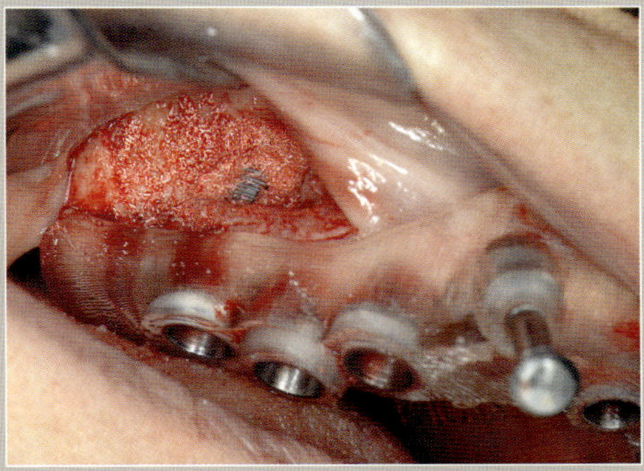

Placement of additional grafting material before suturing.

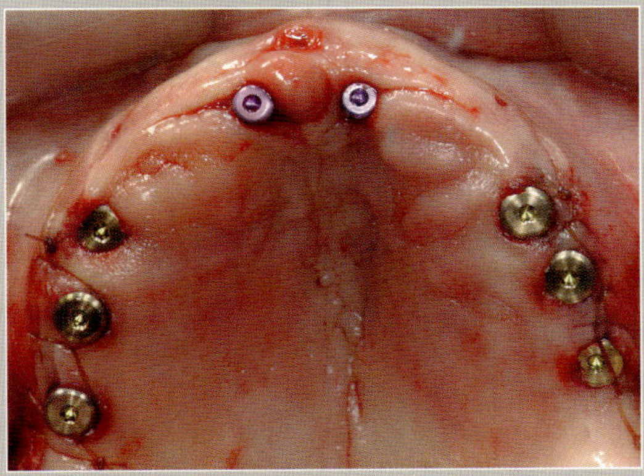

Following stent removal and securing the temporary abutments.

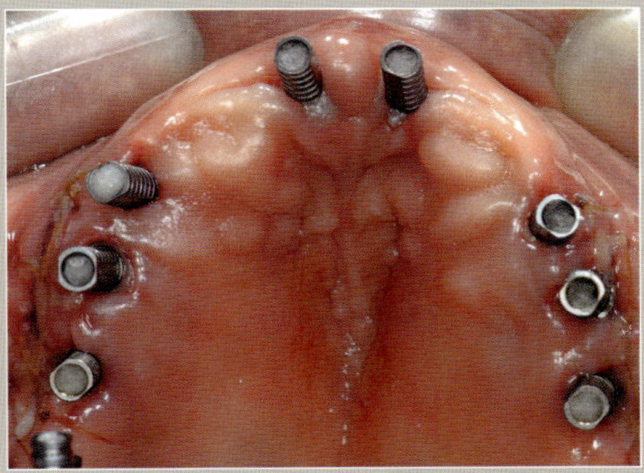

Nonengaging titanium temporary abutments screwed in place with cotton pellets placed in the screw access holes.

The healing abutments were removed, and titanium nonengaging temporary abutments were secured, with radiographic validation of their seating.[22] Care was taken to ensure that their length was customized so that they did not bypass the occlusal surfaces of the denture teeth, causing an occlusal interference.

Verifying full seating of the denture, mainly using the palate as a reference, was essential during the pickup process; each temporary abutment was picked up individually with autopolymerizing acrylic resin using the salt and pepper technique. The screw access holes were filled with a cotton pellet or orthodontic white wax, which was important to prevent the acrylic resin from flowing into the temporary abutments.

Once the last temporary abutment was picked up, we allowed an additional 10 minutes for completion of the polymerization process,[23] ensuring that there would not be

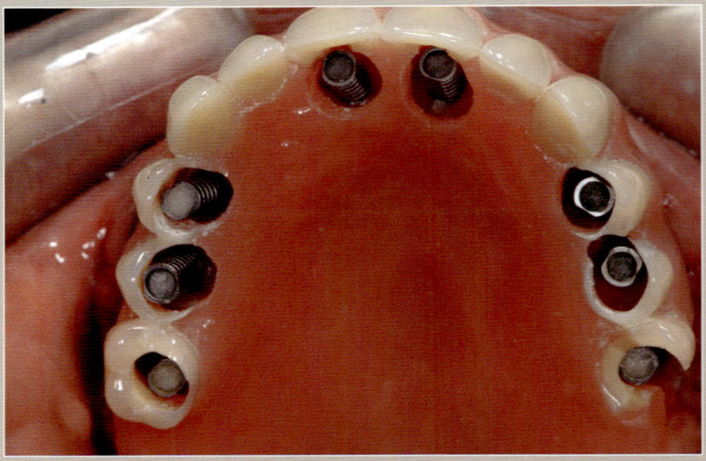

Perforated denture is seated in place in order to do the pickup of the temporary abutments.

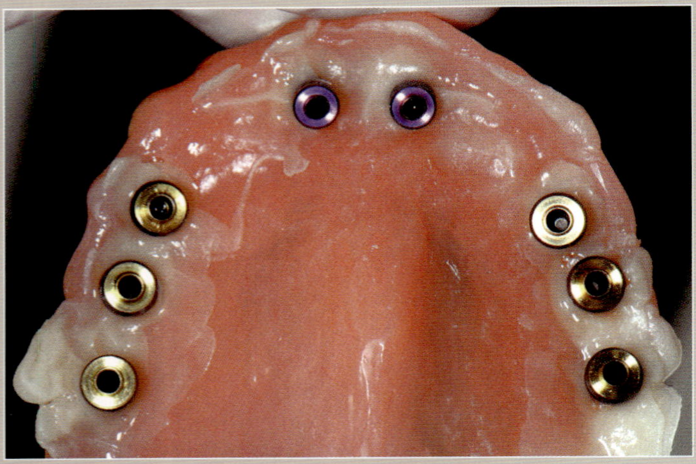

Intaglio surface of the trial denture with the picked up temporary abutments.

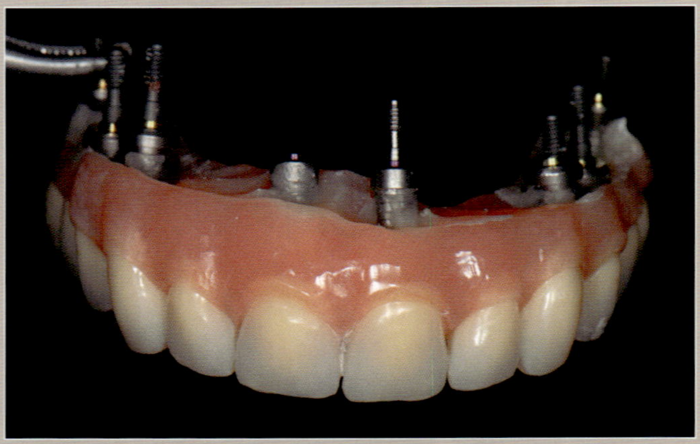

Frontal view of the modified provisional restoration.

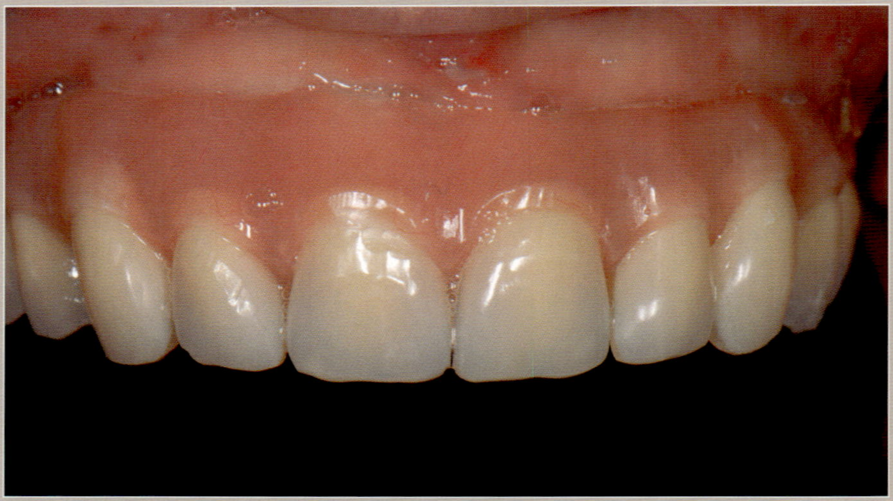

Intraoral view of the seated provisional restoration.

additional contraction of the resin. The denture was then removed for recontouring of the provisional restoration. This recontouring consisted of removing the palatal coverage as well as the buccal flanges. Because it was now going to become a fixed, screw-retained provisional restoration, it was important to eliminate unnecessary flanges that could contribute to food entrapment.

Once the acrylic was removed using slow-speed carbide burs, the provisional restoration was smoothed and polished with a rag wheel and pumice powder. It was then screwed in place, and the access holes were obliterated using cotton pellets and light-activated temporary restorative material.

We instructed the patient that it was important to refrain from chewing hard food and to limit herself to a relatively soft diet for the next 6 to 7 weeks.

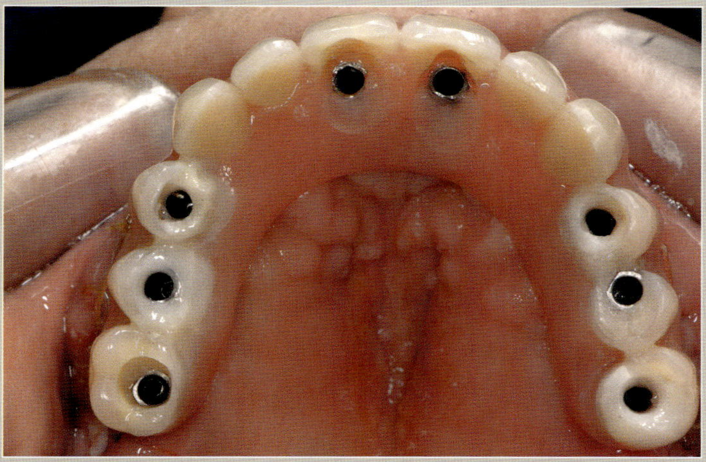

Occlusal aspect of the screw-retained provisional restoration.

Phase IV: Mandibular implant placements

The CAD/CAM-generated surgical stent was rendered inapplicable due to the extensive (8-mm) ostectomy required to allow the anterior mandible to accommodate the implants without risk of fenestration. Instead, the radiographic template (a clear acrylic resin duplicate of the trial denture) was used as the surgical template, leaving the buccal contour of the teeth portion intact to ensure that the angulation of the implants would be confined to the lingual aspect, thus favoring a screw-retained prosthesis.

The ostectomy was performed, and five 4.3 × 13-mm implants were inserted. Healing abutments were secured, and the area was sutured.

Phase V: Provisionalization of the mandibular implants

The same protocol described for the provisionalization of the maxillary arch was carried out for the mandible; the pre-existing immediate complete interim denture was modified and converted into a screw-retained implant-supported prosthesis.

Phase VI: Impressions, records, and fabrication of provisional and definitive restorations

After the 3-month osseointegration period, the patient was recalled in order to take the final impressions and transfer the records to the laboratory, where the prototypes of the definitive restorations would be fabricated and the frameworks for the reconstruction designed.

The impression procedure was significantly simplified because care was taken during the preliminary provisionalization steps to do individual pickups of each temporary abutment. All that was required was to make a simple alginate impression of the maxillary arch with the provisional restoration in place. In order to ensure accurate transfer of the gingival topography to the master cast, caution was exercised to ensure that the intaglio surface of the preliminary provisional was in intimate contact with the residual ridge.

A facebow transfer was obtained using the Panadent system. The provisional restoration was unscrewed and removed, and the laboratory analogs were carefully secured in each of the temporary abutments. The provisional restoration was carefully repositioned inside the alginate impression.

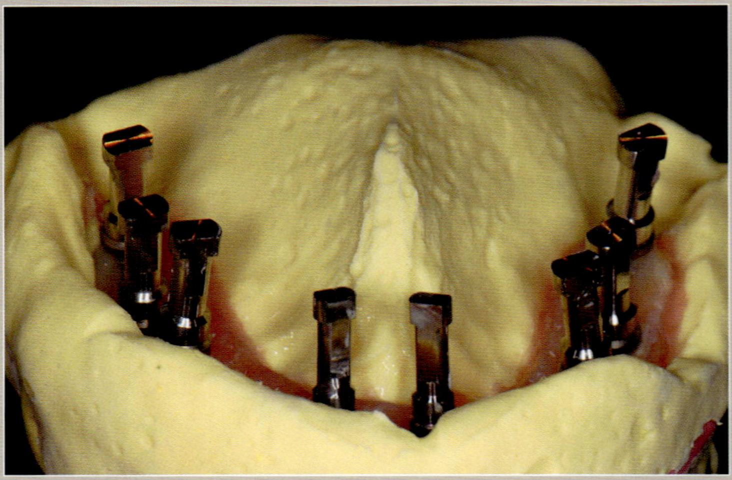

Frontal aspect of the alginate pickup impression.

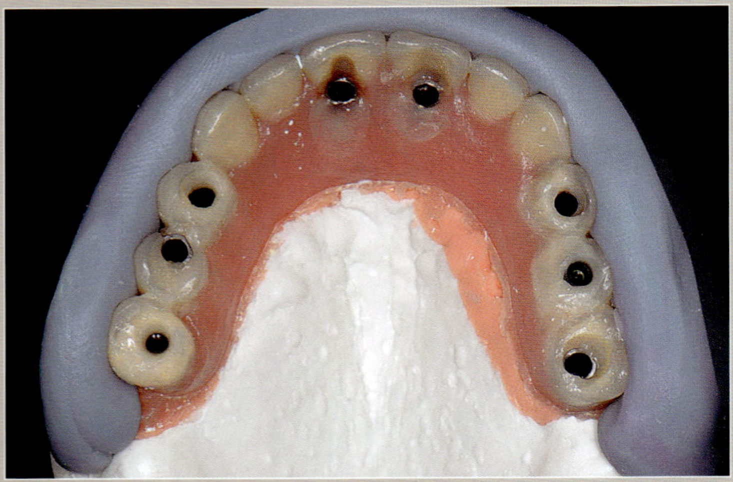

Fabrication of a maxillary silicone matrix.

A thin coat of separating medium (petroleum jelly) was applied at the intaglio surface of the provisional restoration. Soft tissue polyvinyl siloxane impression material was injected to lightly cover the temporary abutment-analog interface, followed by pouring of the impression using class IV stone.

We allowed 45 minutes for the setting of the stone. A master cast was then obtained, and, using the facebow transfer, the cast was immediately mounted on a semi-adjustable articulator.

Silicone matrices of the buccal and lingual contours of the provisional restorations in the cast were fabricated in order to preserve those references for the fabrication of the prototype restorations and the framework design.

Once the impression was made for the mandibular arch, the master cast was obtained and mounted against the maxillary master cast.

Using a new set of temporary abutments, and aided by the silicone matrices as a tooth position reference, the technician completed a new trial denture, verifying that the implant position could adequately accommodate a screw-retained definitive prosthesis.

Once tried in, the trial denture was processed and reinforced using bent wires, and this became the prototype for the definitive reconstruction.

The prototype not only would allow the patient to test the anticipated esthetic result and function but also would eventually become the spare denture in case the definitive prosthesis required repair. The security of having this backup, especially in complex cases, is invaluable. If there is ever a need to reveneer or repair the definitive prosthesis, it is as simple as unscrewing it and immediately screwing in the prototype while the laboratory performs the repair. This retrievability is an enormous advantage of the screw-retained design.

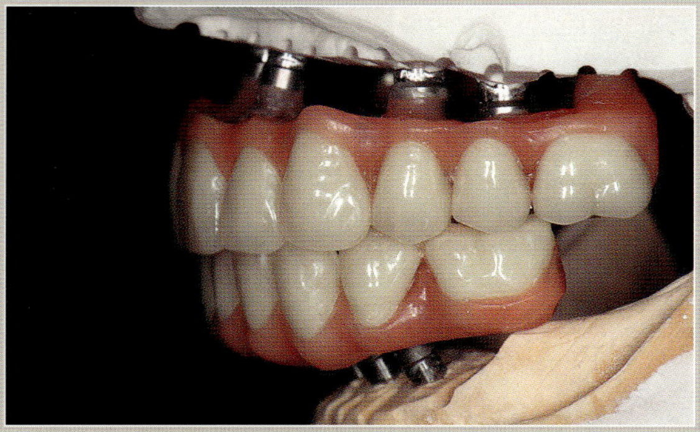

Lateral view of the new trial denture in a semi-adjustable articulator.

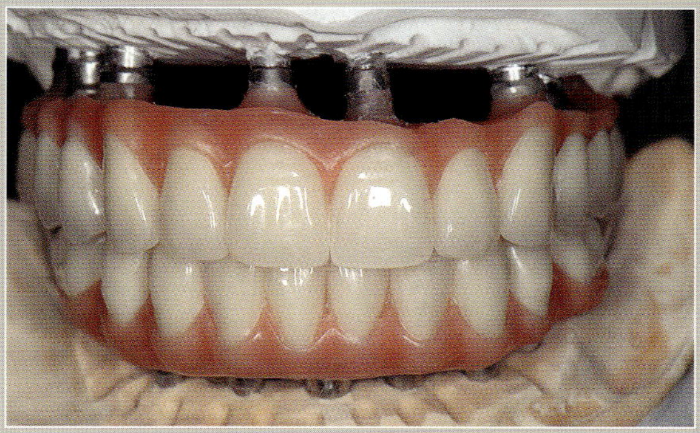

Frontal view of the new trial denture in a semi-adjustable articulator.

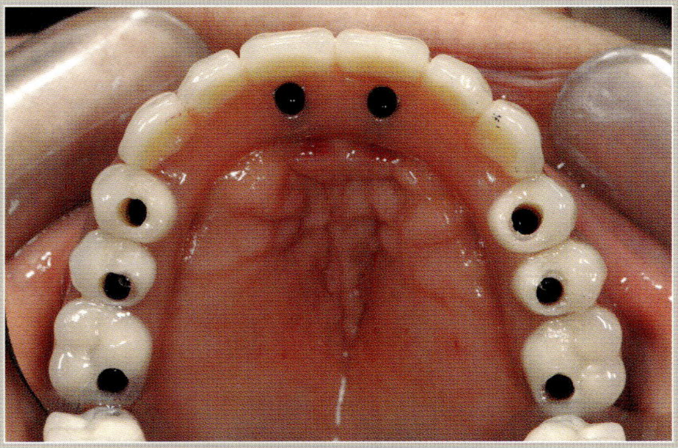

Occlusal view of the maxillary prototype restoration.

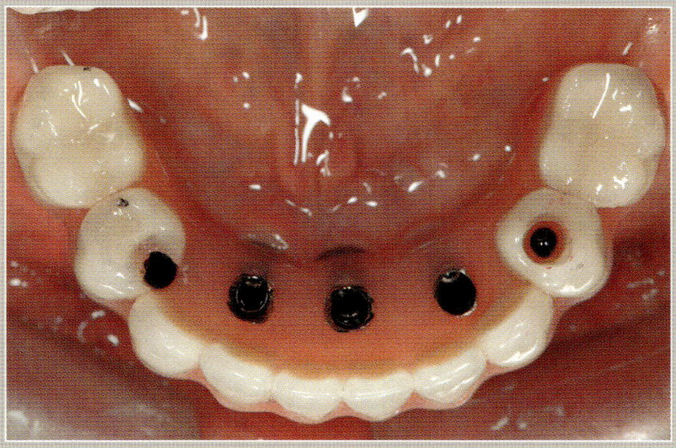

Occlusal view of the mandibular prototype restoration.

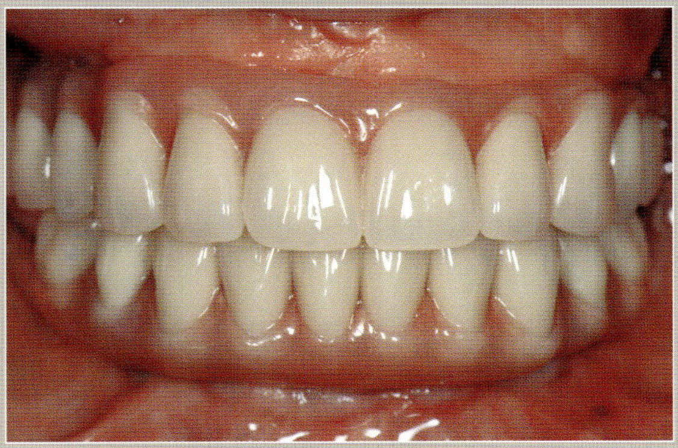

Intraoral view of the prototype restorations.

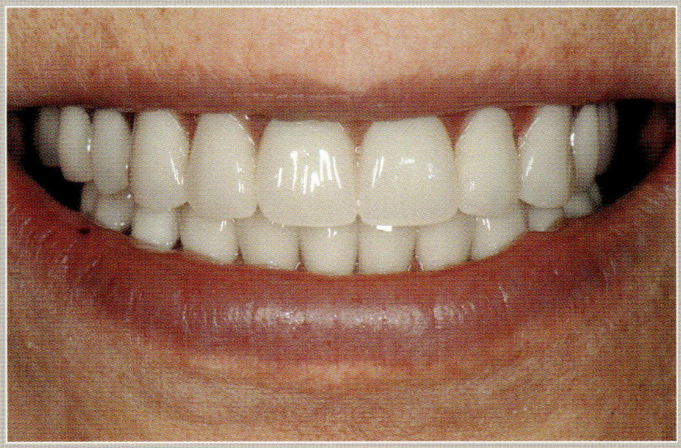

Smile view of the prototype restorations.

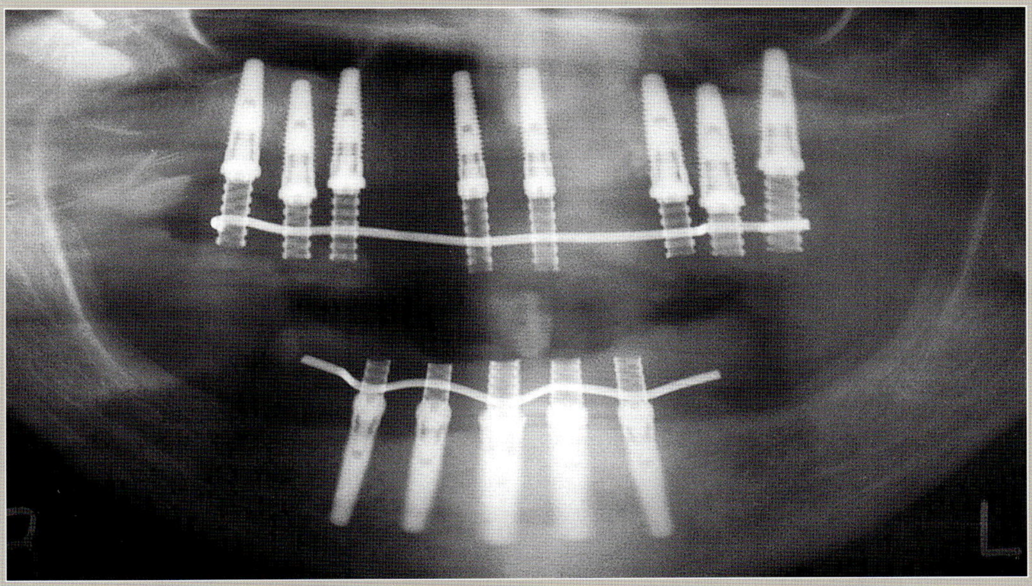

Panoramic radiograph of the prototype restorations.

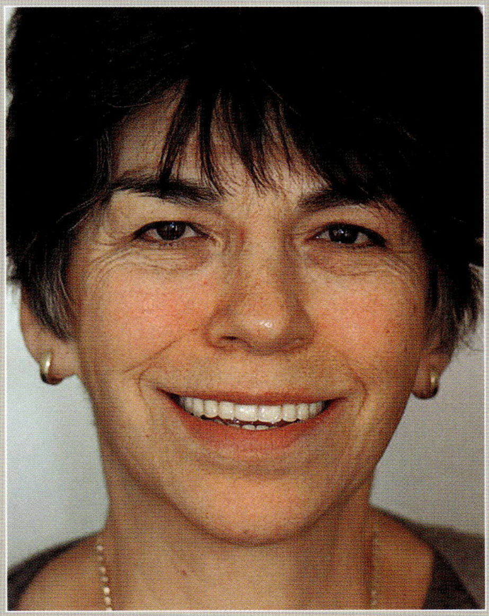

Facial view of the smile with the prototype restorations.

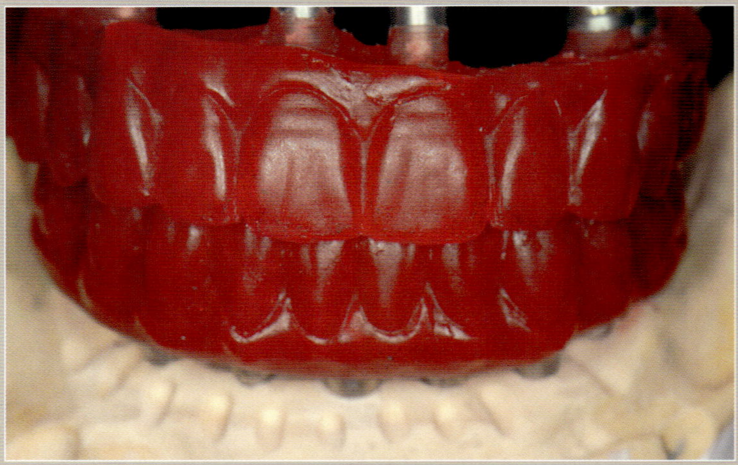

Full-contour setup in pattern resin.

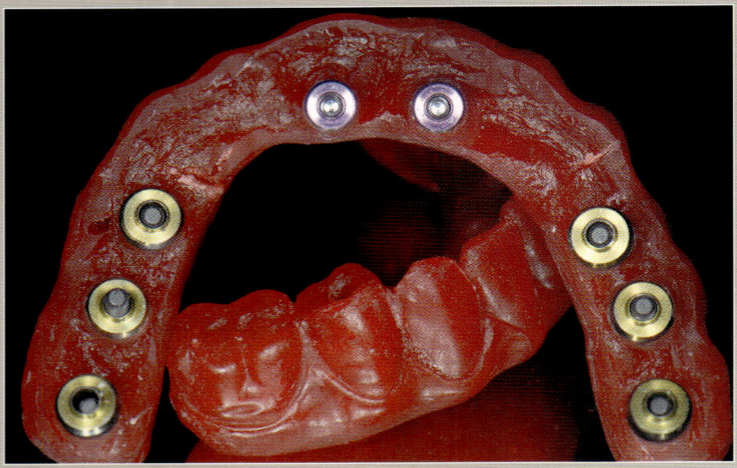

Intaglio view of the full-contour pattern resin setup.

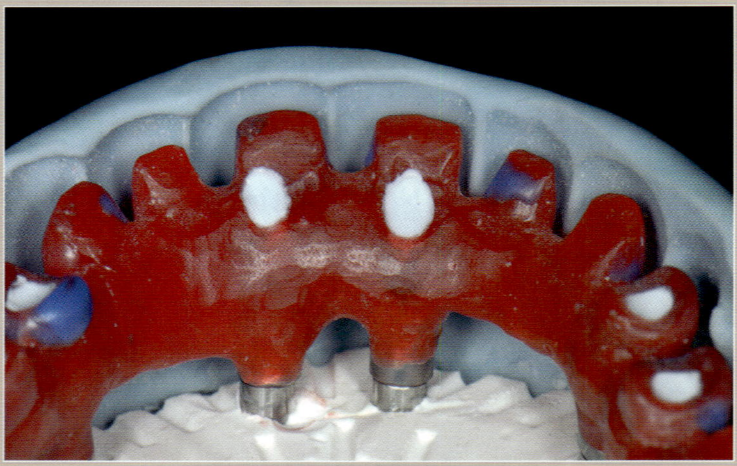

Cutback of the pattern resin setup using the silicone matrix.

Before the prototypes were delivered, silicone matrices were made from their buccal and palatal contours as a reference for the fabrication of the frameworks. Using a new set of nonengaging temporary abutments, a full-contour setup in pattern resin was made. Aided by the silicone matrices, a cutback was made in order to have an even thickness of the veneering material.

The cutback resin pattern setups were then scanned, and the prototype frameworks generated in zirconium oxide using CAD/CAM. The veneering material of choice in this case was ceramics for the maxillary arch and acrylic resin for the mandibular arch. The rationale for the use of dissimilar materials was simple: "Any mechanical system will be as strong as its weakest link."[24] In a patient with impaired propioception and potential parafunctional activity, the risk of chipping and fracturing the veneering ceramics, if this was the material of choice for both arches, would be considerably high, making the repairs both costly and cumbersome.

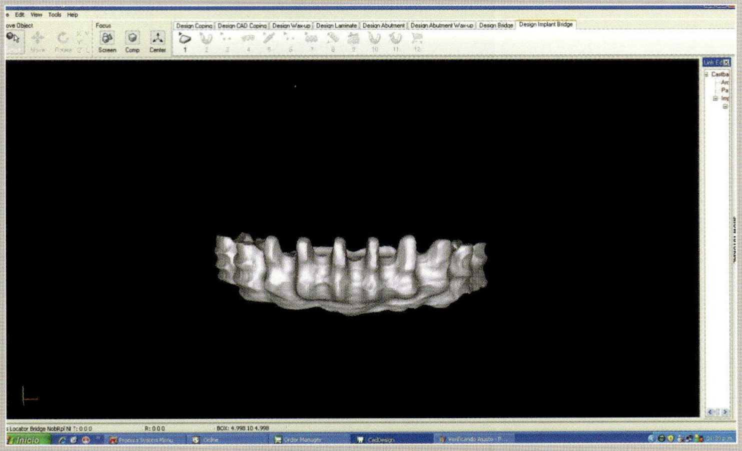

Scanning of the mandibular framework.

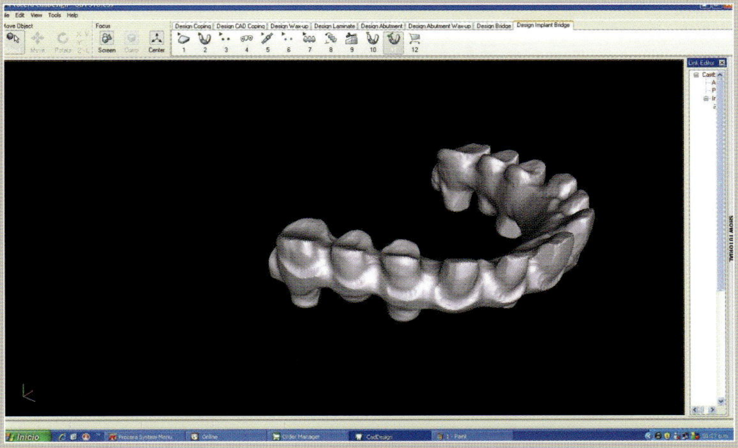

Virtual view of the scanned maxillary framework.

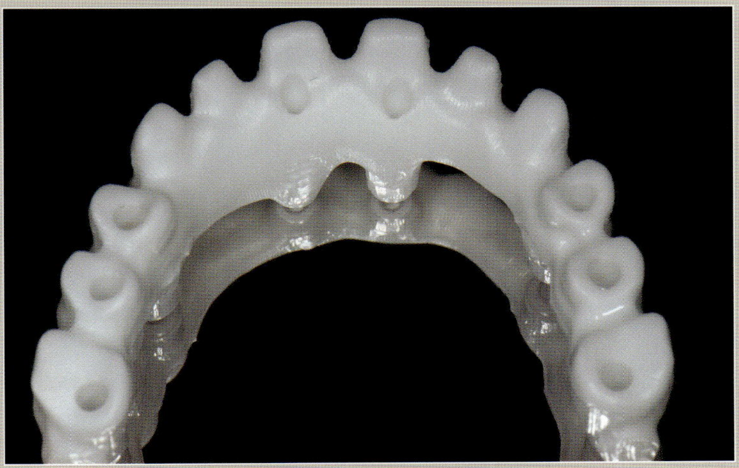

Occlusal view of the zirconium oxide CAD/CAM-generated maxillary framework.

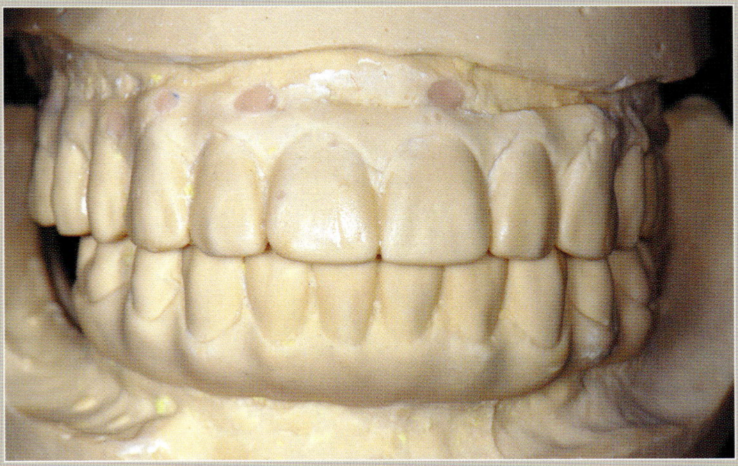

Mounted casts of the approved prototype provisional restoration.

Instead, the acrylic resin used in the mandible would become the weak link and would be much simpler and inexpensive to repair when needed (eg, after extensive wear). Furthermore, because of the potential deleterious effect of the cantilevers (distal, buccal, and vertical), which increase stress concentration at the implant restoration level,[3] veneering the framework with acrylic resin acts like a fuse in the system.

It should also be noted that with a mounted duplicate of the prototype provisional and a secondary mounting plate,[25] the ceramist was able to reproduce the exact orientation of the incisal/occlusal plane of the prototype provisionals with the ceramic reconstruction.

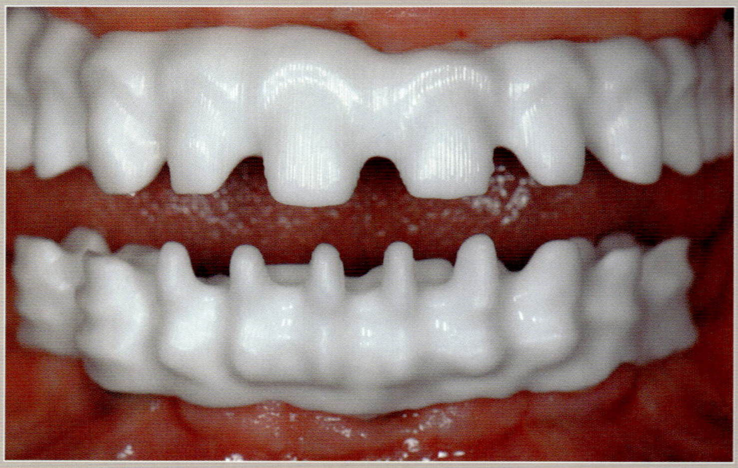

Maxillary and mandibular zirconium oxide frameworks at try-in.

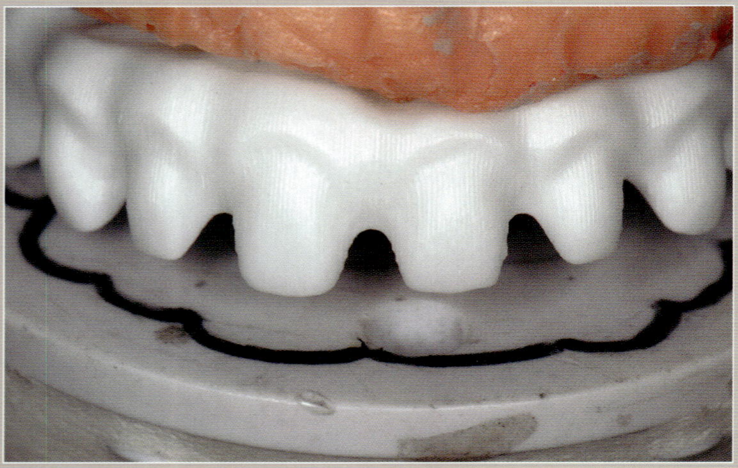

Use of the secondary mounting plate for incisal/occlusal reference.

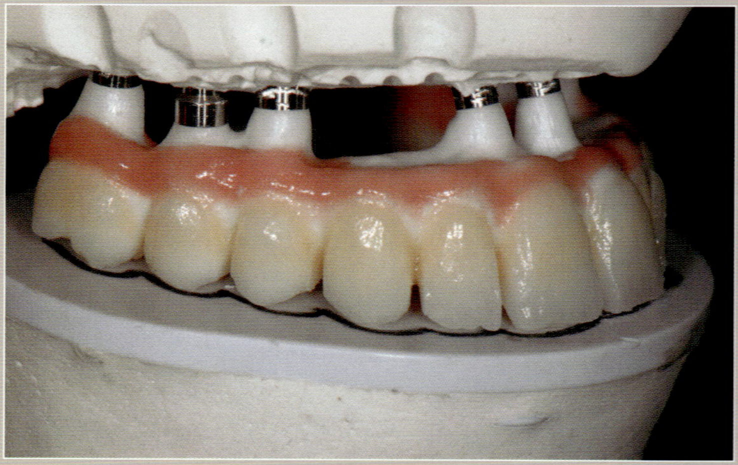

Maxillary framework ready for ceramic layering using the secondary mounting plate.

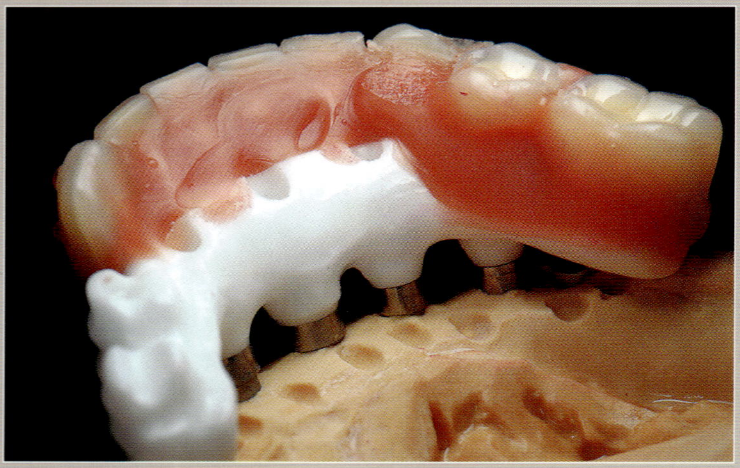

Lateral view of first bake on secondary mounting plate.

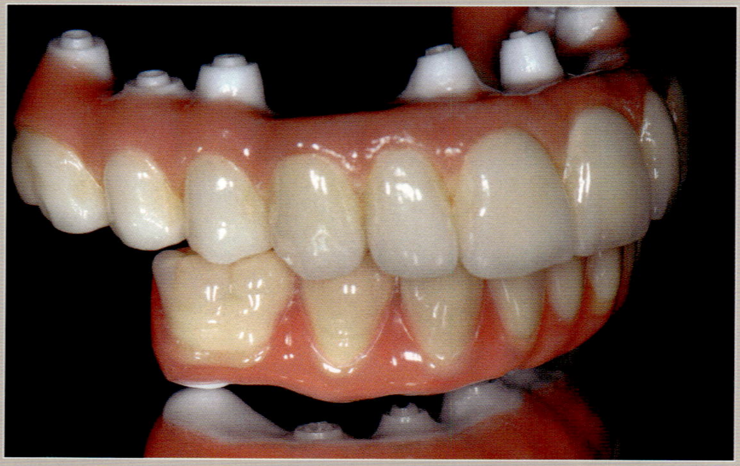

Veneering of acrylic resin on the mandibular zirconium oxide framework.

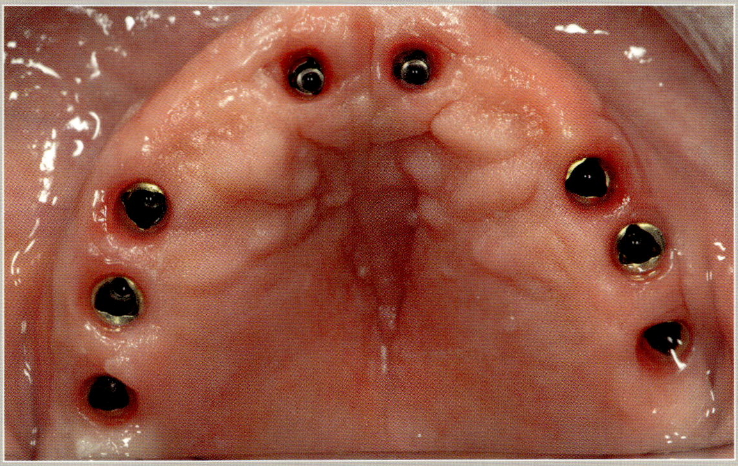
Occlusal view of the healed maxilla.

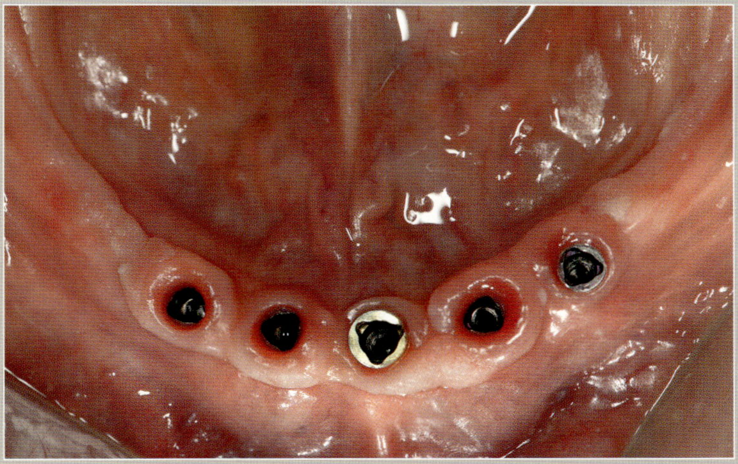
Occlusal view of the healed mandible.

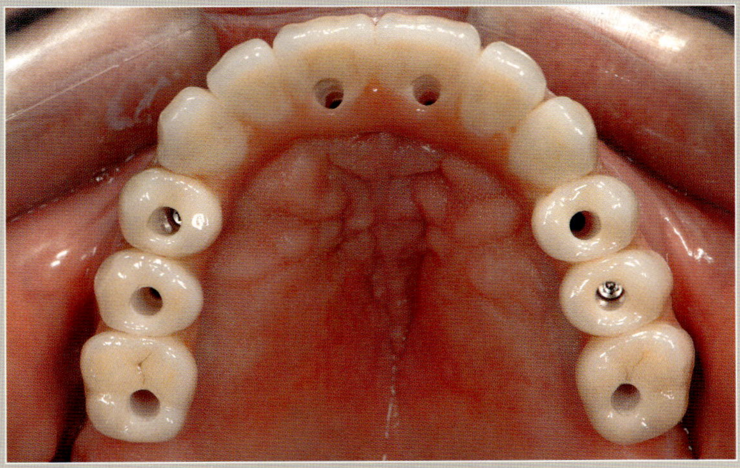
Definitive maxillary reconstruction in place.

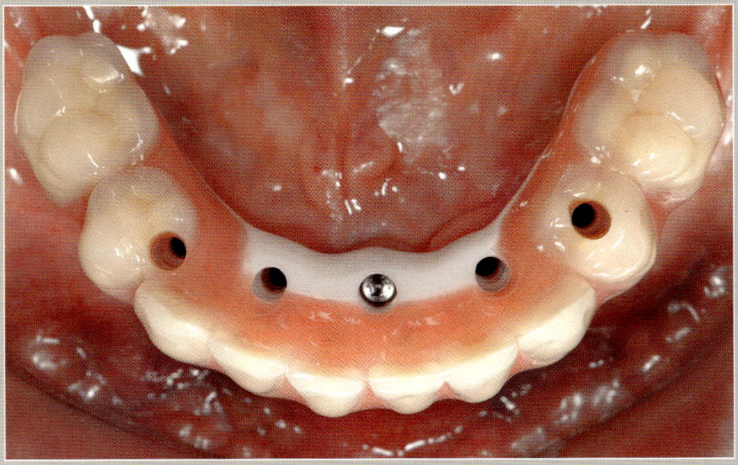
Definitive mandibular reconstruction in place.

Phase VII: Try-in and delivery of the definitive reconstruction

When using dissimilar materials, adjusting the occlusion becomes a much simpler task, and normally if there is any adjustment necessary, this will be carried out in the mandible, where the veneering material is acrylic. Once evenly distributed homogenous bilateral occlusal contacts[26-28] were verified using shim stock articulating paper, the screws were torqued with a calibrated torque wrench in order to ensure optimal torque values.[29-32]

The screw access holes were then obliterated using cotton pellets and a light-activated temporary obturation material.

Phase VIII: Recall program

The patient was placed on a 6-month maintenance program.

Posttreatment

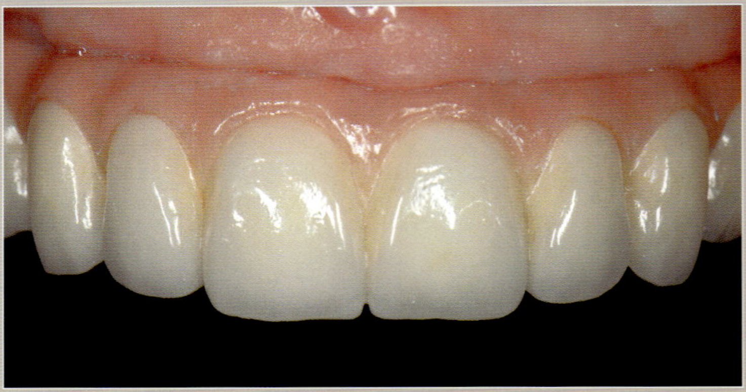

Intraoral frontal view of the maxillary reconstruction.

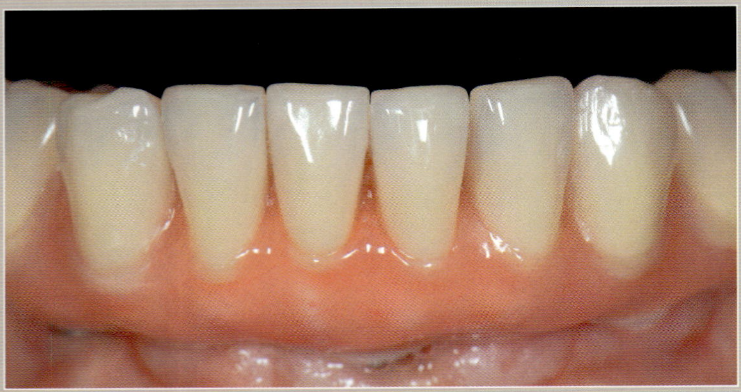

Intraoral frontal view of the mandibular reconstruction.

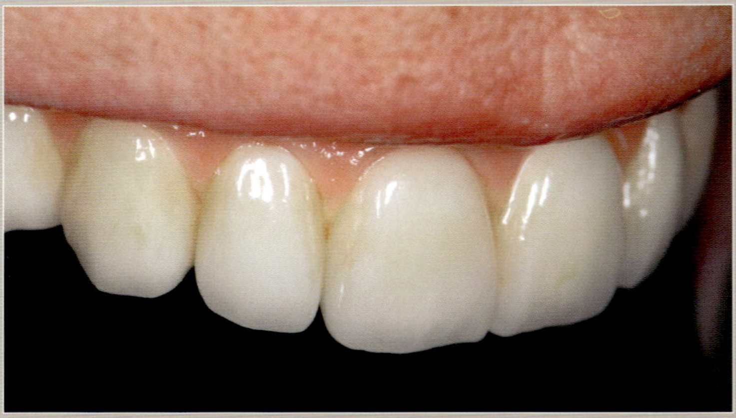

Oblique view showing that the lips hide the interface of the prosthetic gingival component with the gingiva.

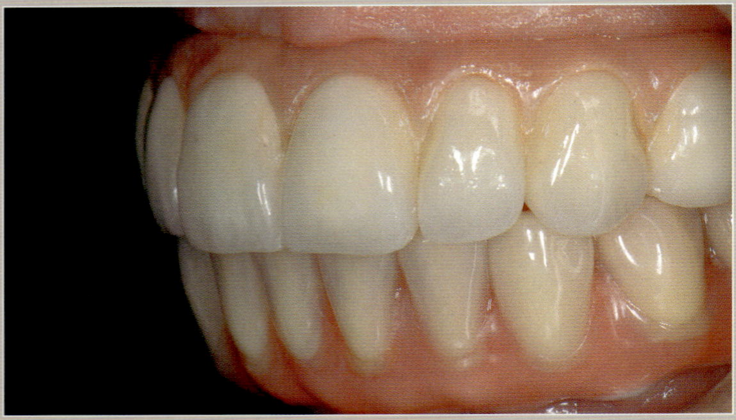

Intraoral lateral view.

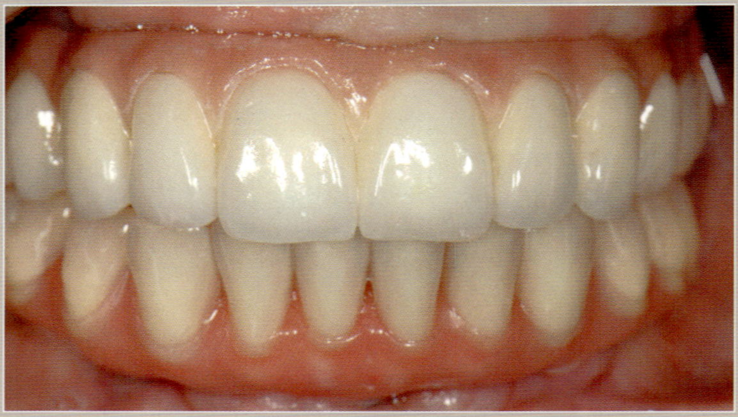

Intraoral frontal view.

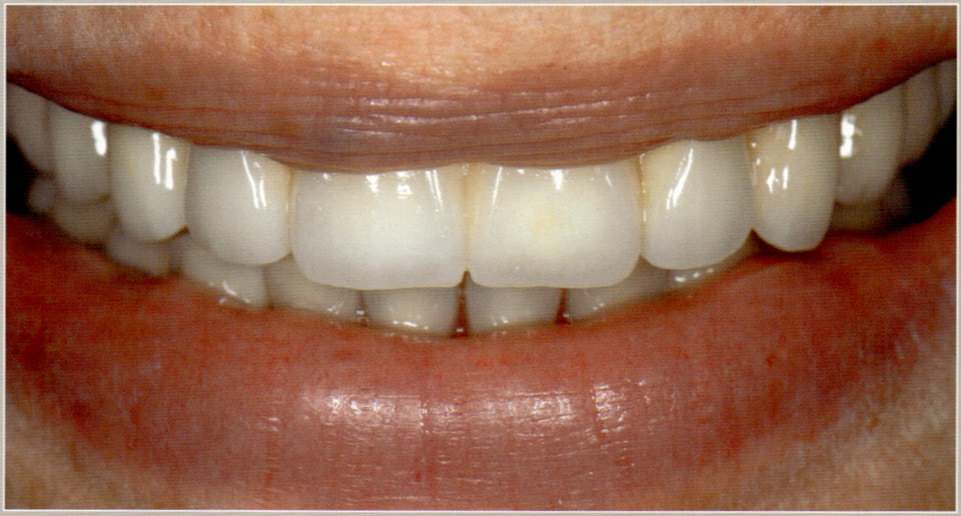

Smile view.

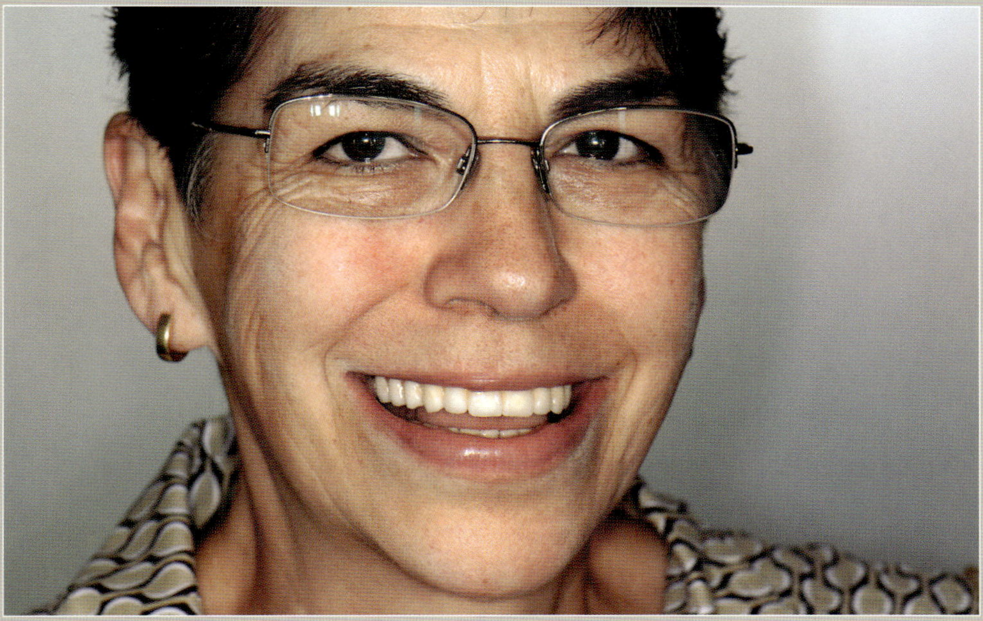

Facial view of smile.

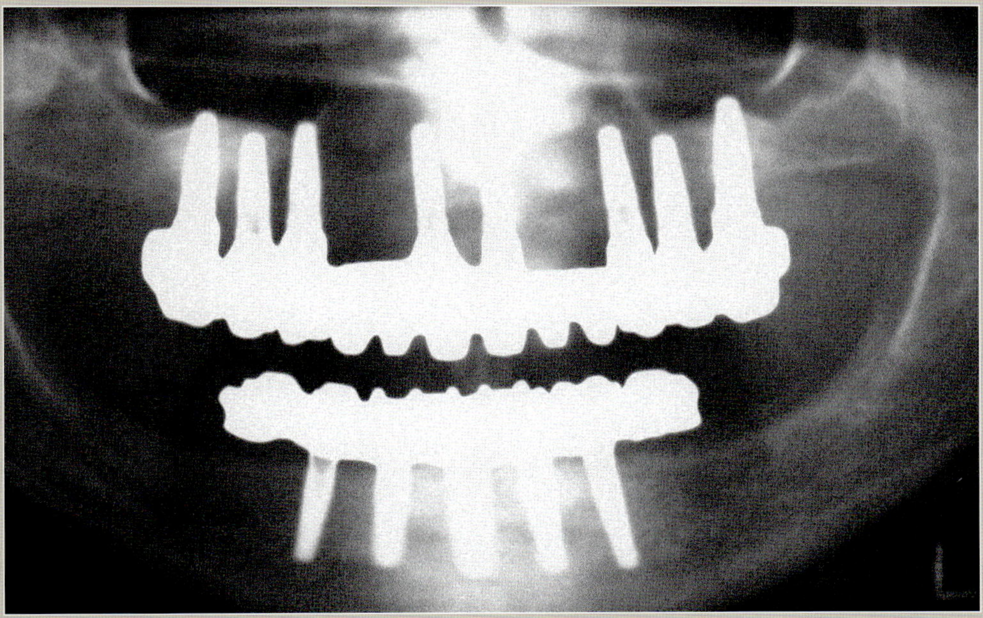

Panoramic radiograph.

You may now place the corresponding posttreatment overlay found in the separate folder over the pretreatment periodontal chart on page 339.

Commentary

Treating the fully edentulous patient with fixed implant-supported restorations is both fascinating and challenging.

With today's available technology, virtual treatment can be explored, and the interdisciplinary team can have precise CAD/CAM-generated surgical templates[11] as well as CAD/CAM-generated frameworks,[33] enabling them to perform with unprecedented proficiency.[34] However, it should be emphasized that in spite of such remarkable tools, the mind and the hands behind the machine can make a vast difference.

As far as operating the diagnostic software, it should be noted that as in any other field, there is a learning curve, and time is needed to understand how to handle each feature of the system. Nevertheless, there is no question that being able to navigate through software that provides the complete picture (eg, 3D ultimate implant/crown positions, available bone, anatomical landmarks, potential anatomical interferences) makes working through the initial challenges worthwhile. Having the ability to direct the orientation of each implant with unparalleled predictability makes the planning process both pleasurable and exciting.

Treatment planning requires a comprehensive vision that entails not only designing and sequencing the procedures but also the foresight to develop a plausible contingency plan should things not work as well as planned. For example, in this case, the surgery carried out in the mandible required an altered approach. Although all of the presurgical planning was carried out via a CAD/CAM-generated stent, a more conventional flap procedure was ultimately used because of the extent of the ostectomy required to level the ridge for implant placements.

Furthermore, as a prosthodontist, I have tried numerous prosthetic designs in the rehabilitation of my fully edentulous patients and all have their advantages and shortcomings.[33,35-38] This inevitably underscores the need to fully understand the implications of each design in order to select the most appropriate option for each clinical situation.[39-43]

As stated by Professor P. I. Branemark, "A passive and impeccable fit is essential in order to avoid the accumulation of adverse stress concentration in one or more implants."[44] Therefore, an essential goal in the fabrication of an implant-supported reconstruction is overcoming distortion.

Distortion as a concept in dentistry was defined in 1977 by Dr Jack Nicholls as "the relative movement of one point or a group of points far from a previously established reference, in such a way that there is a permanent deformation."[45-48] There is the potential for some amount of inherent distortion in every single step or procedure in the fabrication of a prosthesis (eg, impression, pouring of the cast, waxing, investing, casting, soldering, firing ceramics, and even polishing).[49-57]

Selecting the type of retention (cement- versus screw-retained) for a fixed implant-supported reconstruction can be regarded as a controversial and even emotional decision. There are clearly different groups of thought, each with reasonable rationale.[58-66] Perhaps the choice of prosthetic design should be determined in each case by considering the relative ease of fabrication, versatility, esthetics, cost, and retrievability.

The nature of the cement-retained design is more forgiving,[58] which has been considered to compensate for the framework´s potential lack of passive fit because it reduces the stress induced at the implant-abutment interface. On the other hand, studies have shown that, when comparing the fit discrepancies of cast versus CAD/CAM-generated frameworks, the CAD/CAM frameworks have significantly greater accuracy.[67,68] Considering such an improvement in the now available CAD/CAM-generated screw-retained substructures, these are unquestionably a viable alternative.

As stated in the introduction to the chapter, among the aspects that make this modality of treatment so fascinating is the fact that no clinical situation presents in exactly the same way. Every patient will present with his or her own unique set of circumstances, different clinical conditions, and diverse personal desires. I chose the design described for this case (ie, CAD/CAM-generated, screw-retained zirconium oxide frameworks using dissimilar veneering materials) because I believe it provides a system with extraordinary fit, adequate esthetics, simple retrievability, and the ability to repair at low cost when needed.

Acknowledgments

The treating clinicians would like to thank Dr Alejandro Asz for referring the patient and for his clinical involvement during treatment.

References

1. Goodacre CJ, Bernal G, Rungcharassaeng K, Kan JY. Clinical complications with implants and implant prostheses. J Prosthet Dent 2003;90:121–132.
2. Weinberg LA, Kruger B. Comparison of implant/prosthesis loading with four clinical variables. Int J Prosthodont 1995;8:421–433.
3. Brosh T, Pilo R, Sudai D. The influence of abutment angulation on strains and stresses along implant/bone interface: Comparison between two experimental techniques. J Prosthet Dent 1998;79:328–334.
4. McAlarney ME, Stavropoulos DN. Determination of cantilever length-anterior-posterior spread ratio assuming failure criteria to be the compromise of the prosthesis retaining screw-prosthesis joint. Int J Oral Maxillofac Implants 1996;11:331–339.
5. English CE. Critical A-P spread. Implant Soc 1990;1(1):2–3.
6. Kim Y, Oh TJ, Misch CE, Wang HL. Occlusal considerations in implant therapy: Clinical guidelines with biomechanical rationale. Clin Oral Implants Res 2005;16:26–35.
7. Suarez-Feito JM, Sicilia A, Angulo J, Banerji S, Cuesta I, Millar B. Clinical performance of provisional screw-retained metal-free acrylic restorations in an immediate loading implant protocol: A 242 consecutive patients' report. Clin Oral Implants Res 2010;21:1360–1369.
8. Kois JC, Phillips KM. Occlusal vertical dimension: Alteration concerns. Compend Contin Educ Dent 1997;18:1169–1177.
9. Katsoulis J, Pazera P, Mericske-Stern R. Prosthetically driven, computer-guided implant planning for the edentulous maxilla: A model study. Clin Implant Dent Relat Res 2009;11:238–245.
10. van Steenberghe D, Ericsson I, Van Cleynenbreugel J, Schutyser F, Brajnovic I, Andersson M. High precision planning for oral implants based on 3-D CT scanning. A new surgical technique for immediate and delayed loading. Appl Osseointegration Res 2004;4:27–31.
11. van Steenberghe D, Glauser R, Blombäck U, et al. A computed tomographic scan-derived customized surgical template and fixed prosthesis for flapless surgery and immediate loading of implants in fully edentulous maxillae: A prospective multicenter study. Clin Implant Dent Relat Res 2005;7(suppl 1):111–120.
12. Marchack CB. An immediately loaded CAD/CAM-guided definitive prosthesis: A clinical report. J Prosthet Dent 2005;93:8–12.
13. Balshi SF, Wolfinger GJ, Balshi TJ. Surgical planning and prosthesis construction using computed tomography, CAD/CAM technology, and the Internet for immediate loading of dental implants. J Esthet Restor Dent 2006;18:312–325.
14. Balshi SF, Wolfinger GJ, Balshi TJ. Surgical planning and prosthesis construction using computer technology and medical imaging for immediate loading of implants in the pterygomaxillary region. Int J Periodontics Restorative Dent 2006;26:239–247.

15. Kupeyan HK, Shaffner M, Armstrong J. Definitive CAD/CAM-guided prosthesis for immediate loading of bone-grafted maxilla: A case report. Clin Implant Dent Relat Res 2006;8:161–167.
16. Esposito M, Grusovin MG, Rees J, et al. Effectiveness of sinus lift procedures for dental implant rehabilitation: A Cochrane systematic review. Eur J Oral Implantol 2010;3:7–26.
17. Tong DC, Rioux K, Drangsholt M, Beirne OR. A review of survival rates for implants placed in grafted maxillary sinuses using meta-analysis. Int J Oral Maxillofac Implants 1998;13:175–182.
18. Wallace SS, Froum SJ. Effect of maxillary sinus augmentation on the survival of endosseous dental implants. A systematic review. Ann Periodontol 2003;8:328–343.
19. Summers RB. A new concept in maxillary implant surgery: The osteotome technique. Compendium 1994;15:152,154–156,158.
20. Summers RB. Sinus floor elevation with osteotomes. J Esthet Dent 1998;10:164–171.
21. Rosen PS, Summers R, Mellado JR, et al. The bone-added osteotome sinus floor elevation technique: Multicenter retrospective report of consecutively treated patients. Int J Oral Maxillofac Implants 1999;14:853–858.
22. Ercoli C, Romano PR, Al Mardini M, Cordaro L. Restoration of immediately placed implants in 3 appointments: From surgical placement to definitive prostheses. J Prosthet Dent 2006;96:212–218.
23. Mojon P, Oberholzer JP, Meyer JM, Belser UC. Polymerization shrinkage of index and pattern acrylic resins. J Prosthet Dent 1990;64:684–688.
24. Bickford JH. An Introduction to the Design and Behavior of Bolted Joints, ed 3. New York: Decker, 1995:74–77.
25. Phillips K, Morgan R. The acrylic occlusal plane guide: A tool for esthetic occlusal reconstruction. Compend Contin Educ Dent 2001;22:302–304,306.
26. Wiskott HW, Belser UC. A rationale for a simplified occlusal design in restorative dentistry: Historical review and clinical guidelines. J Prosthet Dent 1995;73:169–183.
27. Hobo S, Ichida E, García LT. Osseointegration and Occlusal Rehabilitation. Chicago: Quintessence, 1989.
28. Phillips KM, Mitrani R. Implant management in comprehensive occlusal reconstruction. Compend Cont Educ Dent 2001;22:235–245.
29. Binon PP. The role of screws in implant systems. Int J Oral Maxillofac Implants 1994;9(suppl):48–63.
30. Haack JE, Sakaguchi RL, Sun T, Coffey JP. Elongation and preload stress in dental implant abutment screws. Int J Oral Maxillofac Implants 1995;10:529–536.
31. Gutierrez JJ, Nicholls JI, Libman WJ, Butson TJ. Accuracy of the implants torque wrench following time in clinical service. Int J Prosthodont 1997;17:562–567.
32. Mitrani R, Nicholls JI, Phillips KM, Ma T. Accuracy of the electronic implant torque controllers following time in clinical service. Int J Oral Maxillofac Implants 2001;16:394–399.
33. Mitrani R, Vasilic M, Bruguera A. Fabrication of an implant-supported reconstruction utilizing CAD/CAM technology. Pract Proced Aesthet Dent 2005;17:71–78.
34. Riedy SJ, Lang BR, Lang BE. Fit of implant frameworks fabricated by different techniques. J Prosthet Dent 1997;78:596–604.
35. Mitrani R, Phillips K, Escudero F. Prototype provisional restorations for implant-supported, full-mouth, metal-ceramic reconstructions: The hybrid technique. Pract Proced Aesthet Dent 2003;15:807–814.
36. Mitrani R, Phillips K, Escudero F. A simplified approach in the fabrication of an implant-supported, full-mouth, fixed metal-ceramic restoration. Pract Proced Aesthet Dent 2004;16:125–127.
37. Mitrani R, Beerli M. Full rehabilitation of teeth and osseointegrated implants. Quintessence Dent Technol 2007;30:113–125.
38. Hofstede TM, Ercoli C, Hagan ME. Alternative complete-arch cement-retained implant-supported fixed partial denture. J Prosthet Dent 1999;82:94–99.
39. Zitzmann NU, Marinello CP. Clinical and technical aspects of implant-supported restorations in the edentulous maxilla: The fixed partial denture design. Int J Prosthodont 1999;12:307–312.
40. Sadowsky SJ. The implant-supported prosthesis for the edentulous arch: Design considerations. J Prosthet Dent 1997;78:28–33.
41. Zitzmann NU, Marinello CP. Fixed or removable implant-supported restorations in the edentulous maxilla: Literature review. Pract Periodontics Aesthet Dent 2000;12:599–608.
42. Desjardins RP. Implants for the edentulous patient. Dent Clin North Am 1996;40:195–215.
43. Grossmann Y, Finger IM, Block MS. Indications for splinting implant restorations. J Oral Maxillofac Surg 2005;63:1642–1652.
44. Bränemark P-I, Zarb GA, Albrektsson T. Tissue-Integrated Prostheses: Osseointegration in Clinical Dentistry. Chicago: Quintessence, 1985:303.

45. Nicholls JI. The measurement of distortion: Theoretical considerations. J Prosthet Dent 1977;37:578–586.
46. Nicholls JI. The measurement of distortion: Mathematical considerations. J Prosthet Dent 1978;39:339–343.
47. Nicholls JI. The measurement of distortion: Concluding remarks. J Prosthet Dent 1980;43:218–223.
48. Tan KB. The clinical significance of distortion in implant prosthodontics: Is there such a thing as passive fit? Ann Acad Med Singapore 1995;24:138–157.
49. Kaiser DA, Nicholls JI. A study of distortion and surface hardness of improved artificial stone casts. J Prosthet Dent 1976;36:373–381.
50. Harper RJ, Nicholls JI. Distortions in indexing methods and investing media for soldering and remount procedures. J Prosthet Dent 1979;42:172–179.
51. Bryant RA, Nicholls JI. Measurement of distortions in fixed partial dentures resulting from degassing. J Prosthet Dent 1979;42:515–520.
52. Willis LM, Nicholls JI. Distortion in dental soldering as affected by gap distance. J Prosthet Dent 1980;43:272–278.
53. Faucher RR, Nicholls JI. Distortion related to margin design in porcelain-fused-to-metal restorations. J Prosthet Dent 1980;43:149–155.
54. Bridger DV, Nicholls JI. Distortion of ceramometal fixed partial dentures during the firing cycle. J Prosthet Dent 1981;45:507–514.
55. Linke BA, Nicholls JI, Faucher RR. Distortion analysis of stone casts made from impression materials. J Prosthet Dent 1985;54:794–802.
56. Jasim FA, Brudvik JS, Nicholls JI. Impression distortion from abutment tooth inclination in removable partial dentures. J Prosthet Dent 1985;54:532–538.
57. Tan KB, Rubenstein JE, Nicholls JI, Yuodelis RA. Three-dimensional analysis of the casting accuracy of one-piece, osseointegrated implant-retained prostheses. Int J Prosthodont 1993;6:346–363.
58. Guichet DL, Caputo AA, Choi H, Sorensen JA. Passivity of fit and marginal opening in screw- or cement-retained implant fixed partial denture designs. Int J Oral Maxillofac Implants 2000;15:239–246.
59. Cicciu M, Beretta M, Risitano G, Maiorana C. Cemented-retained vs screw-retained implant restorations: An investigation on 1939 dental implants. Minerva Stomatol 2008;57:167–179.
60. Assenza B, Scarano A, Leghissa G, et al. Screw- vs cement-implant-retained restorations: An experimental study in the Beagle. Part 1. Screw and abutment loosening. J Oral Implantol 2005;31:242–246.
62. Assenza B, Artese L, Scarano A, et al. Screw vs cement-implant-retained restorations: An experimental study in the beagle. Part 2. Immunohistochemical evaluation of the peri-implant tissues. J Oral Implantol 2006;32:1–7.
63. Smith RB. Cemented vs screw-retained implant prostheses: The controversy continues. Alpha Omegan 1997;90(2):58–63.
64. Sherif S, Susarla SM, Hwang JW, Weber HP, Wright RF. Clinician- and patient-reported long-term evaluation of screw- and cement-retained implant restorations: A 5-year prospective study. Clin Oral Investig 2010 Sept 1 [epub ahead of print].
65. Lee A, Okayasu K, Wang HL. Screw- versus cement-retained implant restorations: Current concepts. Implant Dent 2010;19:8–15.
66. Al-Omari WM, Shadid R, Abu-Naba'a L, El Masoud B. Porcelain fracture resistance of screw-retained, cement-retained, and screw-cement-retained implant-supported metal ceramic posterior crowns. J Prosthodont 2010;19:263–273.
67. Jemt T, Lie A. Accuracy of implant-supported prostheses in the edentulous jaw: Analysis of precision of fit between cast gold-alloy frameworks and master casts by means of a three-dimensional photogrammetric technique. Clin Oral Implants Res 1995;6:172–180.
68. Riedy SJ, Lang BR, Lang BE. Fit of implant frameworks fabricated by different techniques. J Prosthet Dent 1997;78:596–604.

14

Minimizing the Liability of Re-entry: A Clinician's Projection of Risk

Henry I. Nichols, DDS

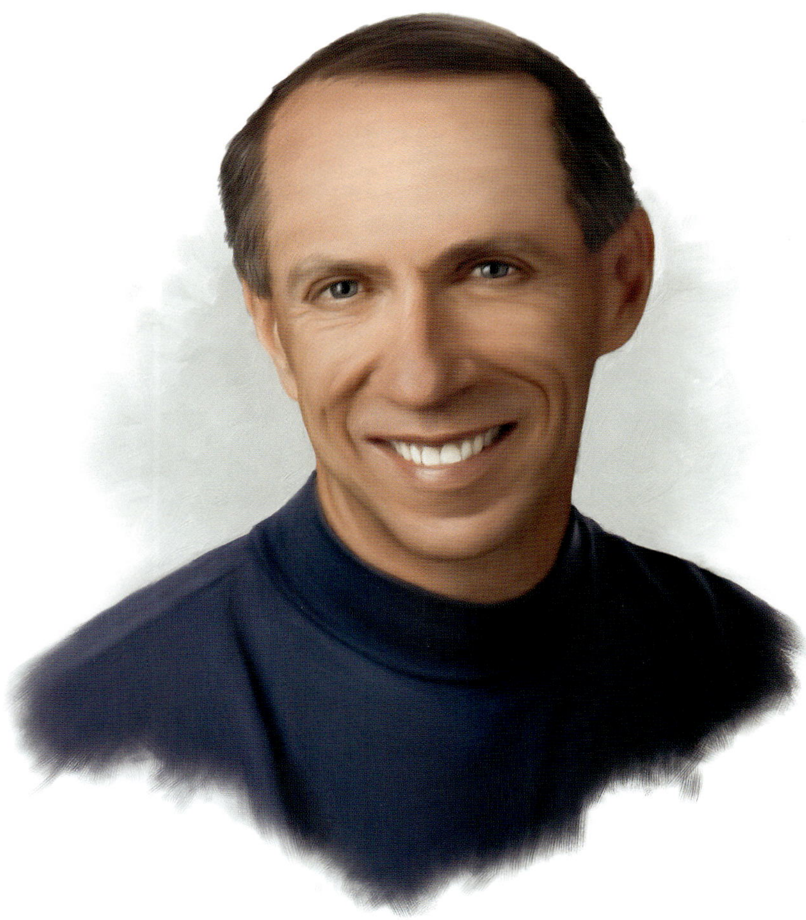

When treatment planning, it is imperative to make provision for future failure and to minimize the impact of its consequences.

Philosophy and Background

When dramatic change occurs, it takes those who are entrenched in the current culture time to adapt. Dentistry is no different, and those involved in it may be slow to accept change because of the conservative nature of its evidence-based roots and the dogmas that have historically pervaded the profession. To best serve our patients in the current dental culture, it is imperative to balance adaptation to rapidly changing technology with methodical evidence-based science.

A *dogma* is an established belief or opinion put forth as authoritative without adequate grounds or evidence. A few of our current dogmas include: always splint implants, never put implants adjacent to each other in the anterior maxilla, and fixed partial dentures are more cost-effective than implants. It is my hope that, through reading this chapter and completing the treatment-planning exercise, the reader will consider the impact these dogmas have on our patients and an adaptive change will occur.

In my chapter in the first volume of *Interdisciplinary Treatment Planning*,[1] I discussed three guiding principles needed to comprehensively treatment plan cases for predictable long-term treatment success:

1. Individualize restorations and minimize the liability of re-entry.
2. Design anterior guidance in harmony with the neuromuscular envelope of function.
3. Create adequate posterior support.

I apply these fundamental principles to the vast majority of patients I treat. When adopted by the clinician and applied to even the most challenging of cases, they help to demystify the treatment-planning process.

For this chapter, I have chosen a case that is challenging with regard to biologic, structural, and functional risk factors. By applying a systematic approach to diagnosis, treatment planning, and sequencing, clinicians can create a favorable treatment outcome that minimizes and/or better manages these risk factors. All three of the above guiding principles must be taken into consideration in treatment planning this case. However, I would like to focus on the first one—minimizing the liability of re-entry—because this will be most important for arriving at a favorable case solution.

It is fairly well accepted that restorative materials, no matter their design, fabrication, or patient delivery technique, are predisposed to potential failure.[2] Any restorative material is subject to failure due to a variety of mechanisms. Some of these include:

1. Biologic
2. Structural (from cyclic stress—mechanical, thermal, and/or chemical)
3. Technique limitations
4. Trauma (occlusal or external)

In short, our materials are not sufficiently biomimetic, our techniques are inherently flawed, and our engineering is inadequate to restore teeth to the full functionality of the intact natural dentition. Moreover, intervention occurs when the dentition has already been compromised by pathology and/or trauma. These limitations become magnified when treating a high-risk, debilitated dentition such as the one presented in this chapter.

When treatment planning, it is imperative to make provision for future failure and to minimize the impact of its consequences. Minimizing the liability of re-entry is a way to accomplish this. Minimizing the liability of re-entry is the clinician's projection of risk assessment as it pertains to the proposed treatment plan. The type, location, probability, and magnitude of failure are important risk assessment considerations as a treatment plan is developed. These risk assessment variables must be combined with the patient's unique inherent risk factors (eg, biologic, biomechanical, functional, and esthetic), which are determined during diagnosis, for the clinician to create and predict successful treatment. A simple example would be comparing the probability of failure of a ceramic crown restoration to a gold crown restoration on a second molar (the potential treatment plan) on a patient with significant parafunction (the diagnostic risk factor). The probability of failure of the gold crown in terms of fracture potential would be significantly less and thus a better treatment choice.

Minimizing the liability of re-entry has broad application when used as a treatment-planning objective. Individualization of restorations, minimally invasive and proper preparation design, and appropriate material choices are a few ways that this can be accomplished. For the treatment-planning exercise, it is important to focus on individualizing restorations to minimize the liability of re-entry for this patient.

When reading through the initial documentation, focus on the diagnostic findings and the risk factors they disclose. What are the etiologies of these diagnostic findings, and how should they be managed? What available treatment options will create the most favorable outcome? Be sure to use the three treatment-planning principles described above to help manage the risk factors.

The objective with this case is not only to create a treatment plan but also to visualize and create a treatment sequence that will facilitate the implementation of this plan in an efficient and effective manner. The ultimate goal is to develop a treatment plan that will minimize the risk and magnitude of future failure for this very discouraged patient.

Case Presentation

Treating clinicians
Restorative dentist: Henry I. Nichols, DDS
Periodontist: Stig Osterberg, DDS, MSD
Laboratory technician: Joseph Choy

Clinical Treatment Planning

Age at intial presentation: 66 years
Initial presentation: June 2006
Active treatment completed: December 2007

Introduction and background

The patient, a 66-year-old man, was referred by a general practitioner who was concerned about his ability to manage the complexity of treatment required. The patient complained of occasional pain in the mandibular right posterior segment and was not able to adequately chew on that side. He stated that he had his first dental reconstruction 15 years prior to the initial appointment. That reconstruction failed after 10 years, at which time he was provided with a second reconstruction. He now realized that the current dental reconstruction was failing after only 5 years. This patient was frustrated by his situation and wondered what could be done to restore and maintain his dental health. He did not want any removable appliances. He complained about two front crowns (teeth nos. 7 and 8) that had fractured multiple times and required recementation as well as other chipped and fractured teeth.

Medical history

- Colon cancer in 1995
- Hypertension, controlled with medication

Dental history

- Two previous reconstructions 5 and 15 years prior to initial examination

Diagnostic findings

Extraoral and facial findings

- Facial anatomy relatively symmetric
- Maxillary midline and facial midline coincidental
- Low smile dynamics (ie, gingiva does not show)
- Flat smile line (ie, teeth do not follow lip curvature)

TMJ and mandibular range of motion

- Mandibular range of motion: approximately 35-mm interincisal opening
- No pain on loading and no history of pain
- Bilateral crepitus/no deviation

Intraoral findings

- Negative cancer screen
- Extensively restored dentition
- Missing teeth nos. 1, 2, 5, 15, 16, 17, 18, 31, and 32
- Multiple exostoses
- Many failing restorations
- Recurrent caries on teeth nos. 3, 6, 19, 20, 21, 28, 29, and 30
- Previous nonsurgical endodontic treatment on teeth nos. 8, 10, 11, 12, and 19
- Fractured fixed partial denture on teeth nos. 4 to 6 with previous composite repair
- Square, short anterior teeth with long contact areas

Periodontal

- Flat, thick gingival morphology
- Poor plaque control
- Posterior pocket depths ranging from 3 to 10+ mm

Pretreatment

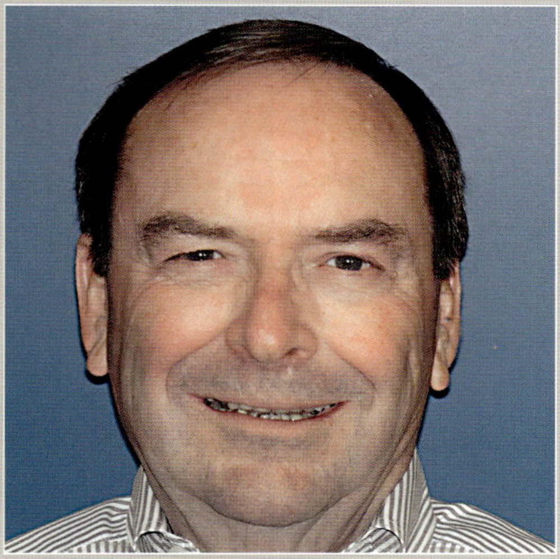

Full face with smile.

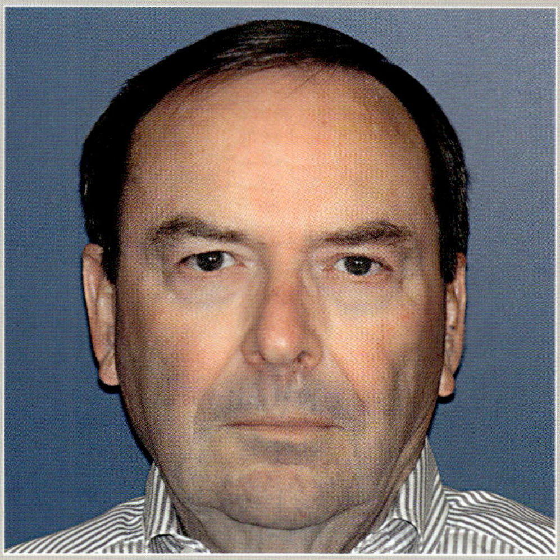

Full face in repose.

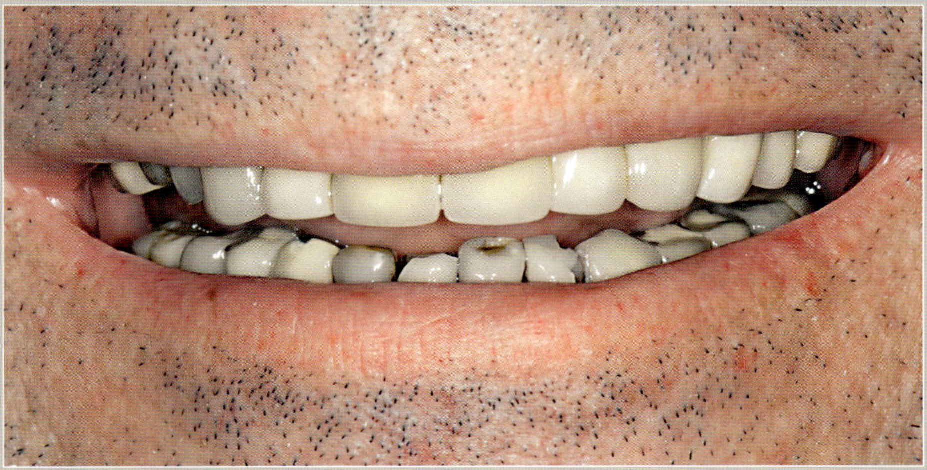

Smile.

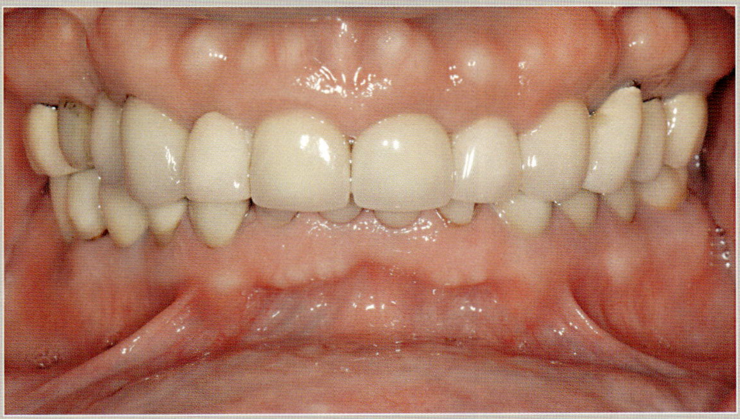

Intraoral frontal view of MIP.

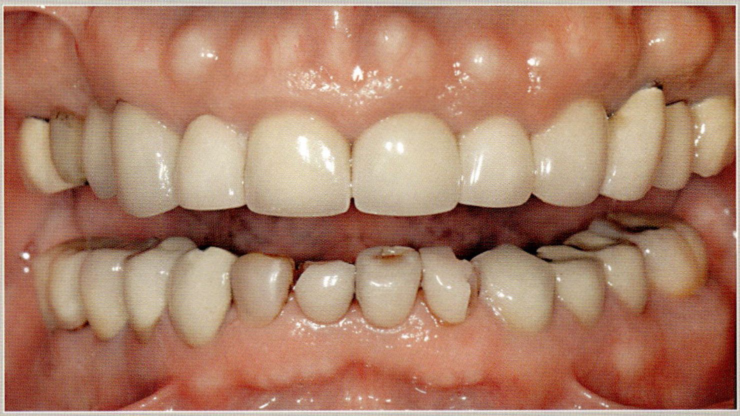

Intraoral frontal view with teeth apart.

- No significant tooth mobilities except teeth nos. 12 and 30
- Generalized favorable crown-root ratios
- Isolated narrow, deep probing (7 mm) associated with tooth no. 12 (possible vertical root fracture)

Occlusal notes

- Right side: Angle Class I; left side: Angle Class II
- Deep overbite
- Steep anterior guidance
- Adequate arch form
- Irregular occlusal plane
- Centric relation (CR) not coincident with maximal intercuspal position (MIP); approximately 1-mm translatory movement
- Suspected parafunction
- Dyskinesia related to mandibular movements
- Neuromuscular envelope of function not in harmony with the dental envelope

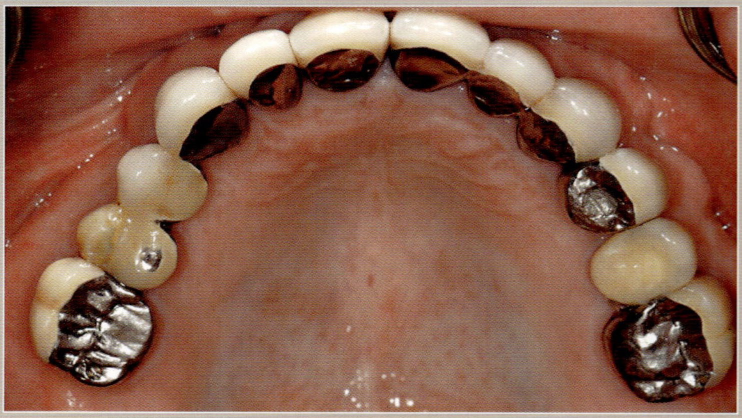

Maxillary occlusal view.

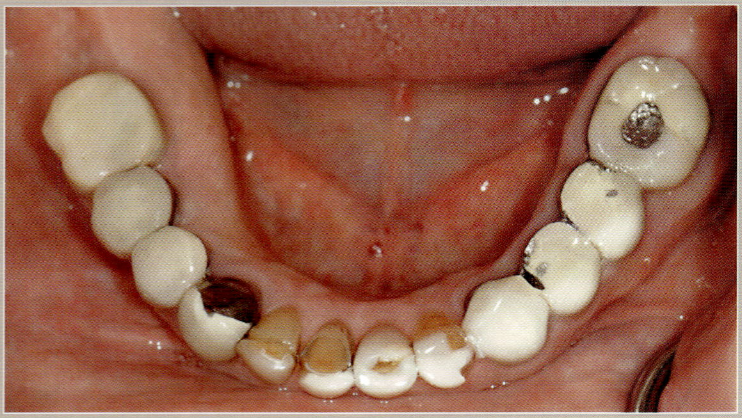

Mandibular occlusal view.

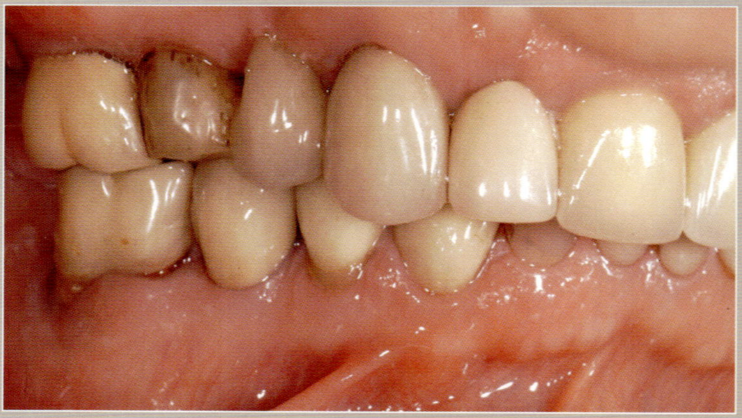

Right lateral view with teeth in MIP.

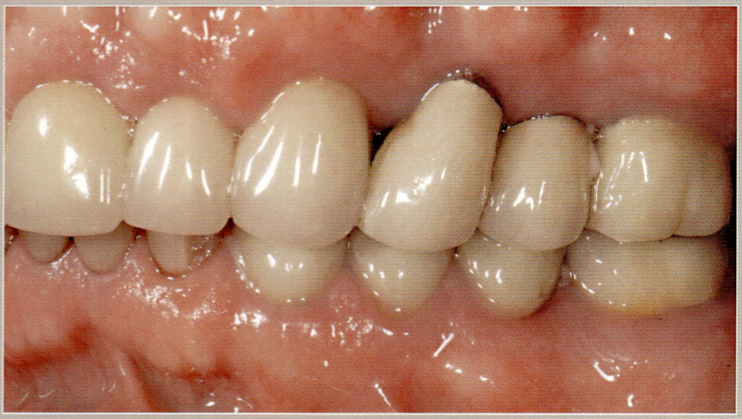

Left lateral view with teeth in MIP.

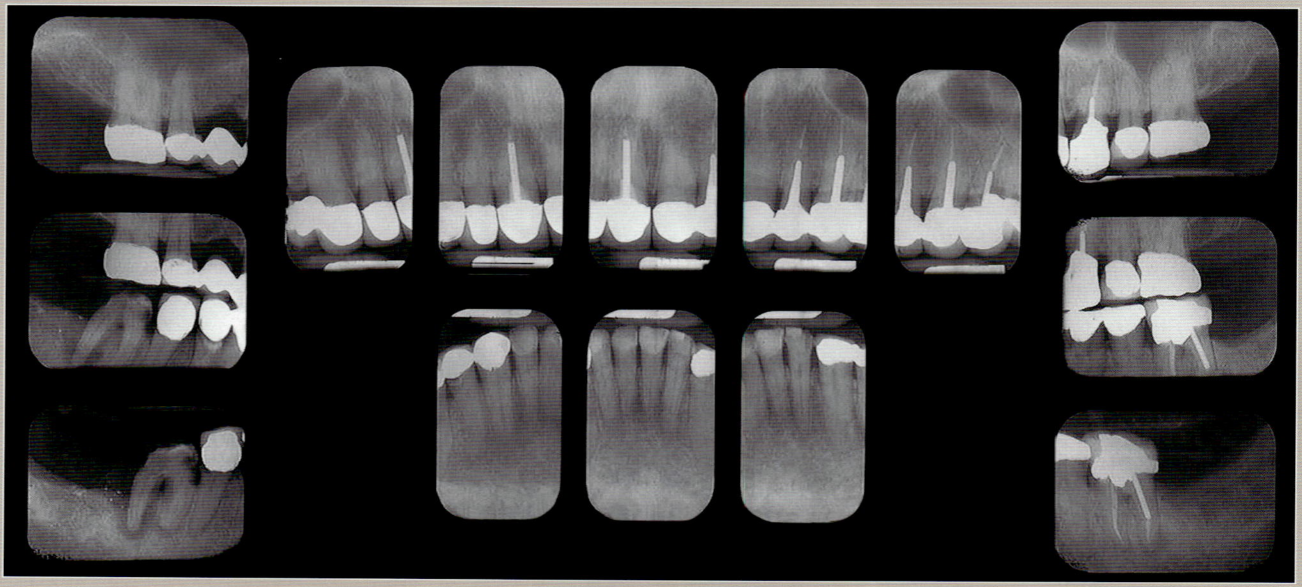

Complete-mouth radiographs.

Radiographic findings

- Periradicular radiolucencies associated with teeth nos. 19 and 30
- Poor crown-root ratio associated with tooth no. 12
- Previous nonsurgical endodontic treatment and posts in teeth nos. 8, 10, 11, 12, and 19
- Extensive caries associated with teeth nos. 19, 28, 29, and 30

Diagnosis

- AAP Type III: moderate to moderately advanced periodontitis with localized areas displaying more advanced bone loss

Prognosis

- General: poor
- Hopeless: teeth nos. 19 and 30
- Guarded: teeth nos. 7, 8 (previously fractured off), 12, 28, and 29
- Poor: teeth nos. 10 and 11

Risk assessment

- Biologic: high risk
- Structural: high risk
- Functional: high risk

Summary of concerns

1. How can we establish trust with this patient, who has already had two failed dental reconstructions?
2. What options are available to this patient to create a more favorable and stable occlusion?
3. What are the associated risks regarding these options?
4. How can we visualize and test the proposed occlusion in this high-risk patient?
5. What are the best treatment options for minimizing the liability of re-entry?
6. How can we decide which teeth have favorable prognoses and which teeth need to be removed?

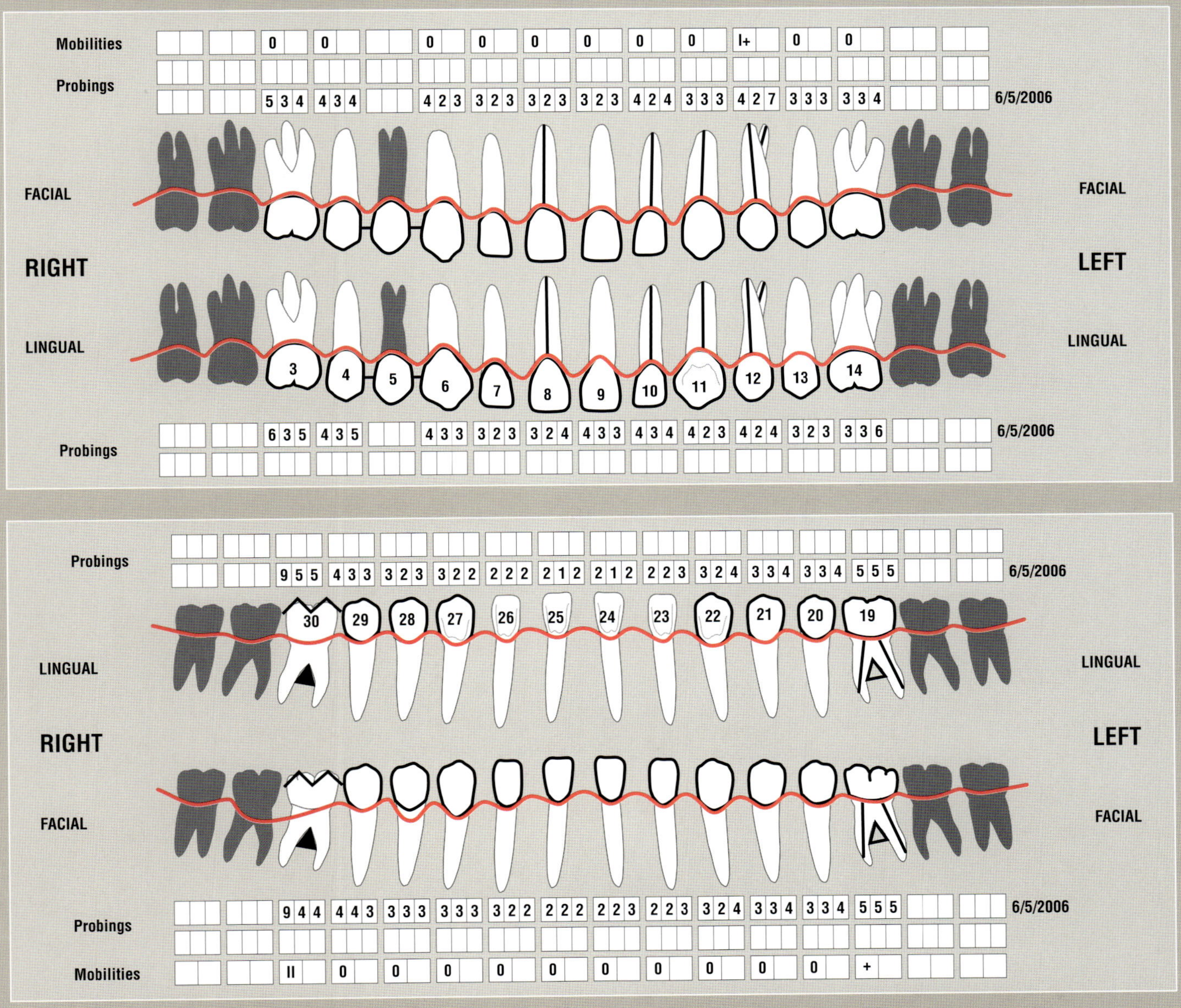

As a learning exercise, you may now outline goals/objectives of treatment and a treatment plan.

Proposed Treatment Plan

Goals/objectives of treatment

- Re-establish trust with the patient regarding dental treatment and risk management
- Create a more favorable and stable occlusion
- Enlist patient cooperation to manage caries, periodontitis, parafunction, and dyskinesia
- Improve esthetics
- Minimize the liability of re-entry (ie, impact of future failure)
- Create a result that meets or exceeds the patient's expectations

Phase I: Initial therapy

1. Oral examination and complete-mouth radiographs
2. Removal of hopeless teeth nos. 19 and 30
3. Gross periodontal debridement followed by complete-mouth scaling and root planing
4. Oral hygiene and nutritional instruction
5. Periodontal re-evaluation
6. Caries control/evaluation of prognoses for teeth nos. 28 and 29

Phase II: Diagnostic work-up

7. Records: two sets of casts mounted in CR on a semi-adjustable articulator using a facebow transfer and a full set of photographs
8. Patient consultation
9. Orthodontic/surgical consultation

Phase III: Initial surgical phase

10. Removal of teeth nos. 12, 28, and 29
11. Implant placement in sites nos. 5, 12, 19, 28, 29, and 30

Phase IV: Initial provisionalization

12. Provisional fixed partial dentures on teeth nos. 4 to 6 and 11 to 13 (patient did not want to be edentulous in these areas during treatment)
13. Re-evaluation and consultation with patient

Phase V: Diagnostic work-up

14. New diagnostic records (casts mounted in CR using a facebow transfer, photographs)
15. Diagnostic wax-up

Phase VI: Second provisionalization

16. Provisionalization of maxillary arch using a segmented restoration: teeth/sites nos. 3 to 4, 5 to 12, and 13 to 14
17. Provisionalization of mandibular arch using a segmented restoration: teeth/sites nos. 19 to 21, 22 to 27, and 28 to 30

Phase VII: Re-evaluation

18. Re-evaluation of provisional parameters: function, esthetics, and phonetics
19. Patient consultation, discussing prognoses and treatment options for teeth nos. 7, 8, 10, and 11

Phase VIII: Second surgical phase

20. Extraction of teeth nos. 7, 8, 10, and 11 and immediately place implants in these sites
21. Waiting period for osseointegration to take place

Phase IX: Re-evaluation

22. Complete-mouth radiographs
23. Re-evaluation of function, esthetics, phonetics, and biologic parameters
24. Patient consultation

Phase X: Definitive restoration

25. Refining of preparations and final impression taking for fabrication of definitive restorations for teeth nos. 6 and 9 as well as implant sites nos. 5, 7, 8, 10, 11, and 12
26. CR record and facebow transfer
27. Communication with the laboratory technician regarding definitive restoration fabrication using mounted casts with provisional restorations and photographs; discussion with patient and laboratory technician regarding shade and characterization parameters
28. Delivery of definitive restorations for teeth nos. 6 and 9 as well as implant sites nos. 5, 7, 8, 10, 11, and 12 with standard abutments in sites nos. 5 and 12 and custom abutments in sites nos. 7, 8, 10, and 11
29. Final impression for definitive restoration fabrication on teeth nos. 3, 4, 13, and 14
30. CR record and facebow transfer
31. Delivery of definitive crown restorations for teeth nos. 3, 4, 13, and 14
32. Final impression for definitive restoration fabrication for teeth nos. 22 to 27
33. Delivery of definitive crown restorations for teeth nos. 22 to 27
34. Final impression for fabrication of definitive restorations for teeth nos. 20 and 21 and implant sites nos. 19, 28, 29, and 30
35. Delivery of definitive restorations for teeth nos. 20 and 21 and implant sites nos. 19, 28, 29, and 30 using standard abutments

Phase XI: Re-evaluation and maintenance

36. Fabrication and delivery of a maxillary occlusal splint
37. Posttreatment evaluation and consultation
38. Follow-up photographs and complete-mouth radiographs
39. Four-month periodontal and occlusal recall

Active Clinical Treatment

Review of the goals/objectives of treatment

This patient presented with extremely difficult challenges: a debilitated dentition, two previously failed reconstructions, and a distrust of dentistry. Once time was spent with the patient to help him understand the causes of the failures and associated risks he presented, his trust increased. He became motivated to restore his dentition based on his desire to function at a high level without removable appliances and to improve his esthetics. He agreed to proceed with a third reconstruction once he understood the following concepts:

- We could mitigate his extreme biomechanical and functional risk but not eliminate it.
- He needed to be an integral part of the solution by managing his periodontal and caries risk and by cooperating with strict occlusal appliance (nightguard) wear.

He understood that, given the inherent risk associated with his parafunction and dyskinesia, he may have failures in the future. However, by individualizing his restorations and barring any major trauma, future failures would likely be limited to repairing or replacing single teeth. Once this patient's trust was gained, he became an ideal treatment partner. His treatment progressed as proposed.

Phase I: Initial therapy

Initial therapy commenced with a thorough orofacial examination, including a medical and dental history and complete-mouth radiographs. A periodontal referral was initiated, followed by scaling and root planing and extraction of hopeless teeth nos. 19 and 30. Caries control progressed through this phase of treatment. After caries removal, teeth nos. 28 and 29 had unfavorable prognoses, and extraction was recommended.

Phase II: Diagnostic work-up

The restorative dentist acquired two sets of casts mounted in CR on a semi-adjustable articulator and diagnostic photographs. Using this information, the interdisciplinary team met to discuss diagnostic findings and treatment options. The patient was then evaluated by the orthodontist. Due to his age, parafunction, and dyskinesia, it was determined that the risks were too great to pursue orthodontic treatment with or without mandibular advancement. A consultation with the patient followed, and a tentative treatment plan was agreed upon.

Phase III: Initial surgical phase

Teeth nos. 12, 28, and 29 were removed, and implants were placed in sites nos. 5, 12, 19, 28, 29, and 30 using a delayed approach.

Phase IV: Initial provisionalization

The patient did not want to be without teeth in sites nos. 5 and 12 during implant integration. Therefore, two provisional fixed partial dentures (teeth nos. 4 to 6 and 11 to 13) were provided to satisfy the patient's esthetic concerns.

Phase V: Diagnostic work-up

Once the implants had integrated, new diagnostic records were gathered, and a diagnostic wax-up was created. The vertical dimension of occlusion (VDO) was increased to facilitate a more favorable anterior relationship. This created less vertical and more horizontal overlap, providing the space needed to decrease the incisal guidance angle and comply with the second principle (creating anterior guidance in harmony with the patient's neuromuscular envelope of function). The parameters used to determine this were visualized when starting the diagnostic wax-up with the anterior teeth. Normal tooth sizes, preferred incisal guidance angle, and coupling of the anterior teeth all play a role. In this patient's situation, the Class II skeletal relationship necessitated some compromises. As we increased the VDO, the Class II relationship became more pronounced. A change in anterior tooth angulation was needed to maintain anterior coupling. In this way, the occlusal goals were met in the diagnostic wax-up: CR coincidental with MIP, anterior guidance in harmony with the neuromuscular envelope of function, and adequate posterior support.[1,3]

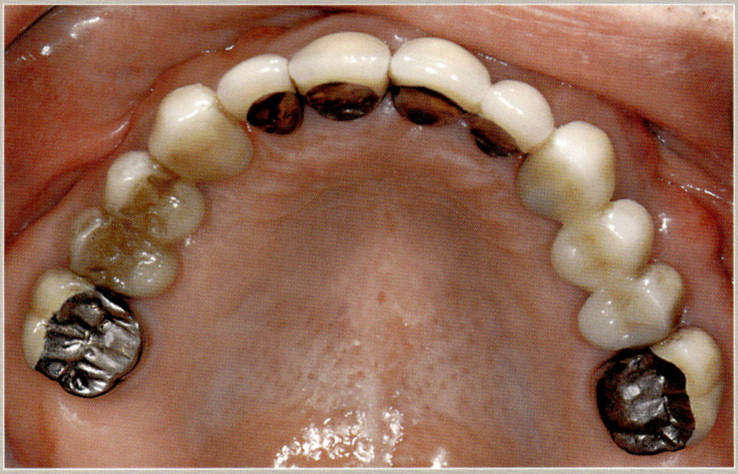

Provisional fixed partial dentures following implant placement in sites nos. 5 and 12.

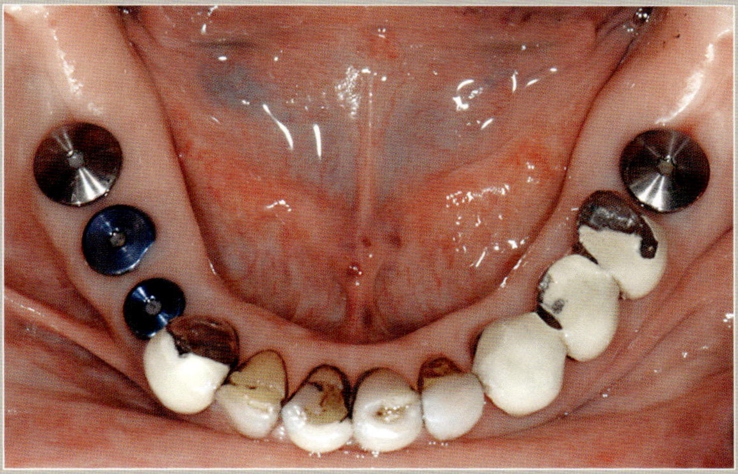

Implants in sites nos. 19, 28, 29, and 30.

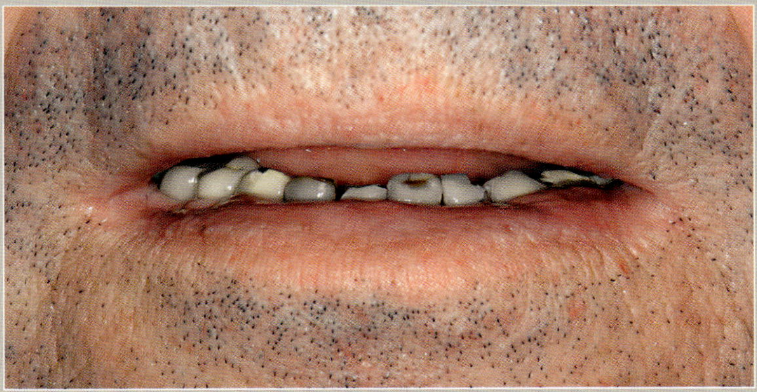

Lips in relaxed position.

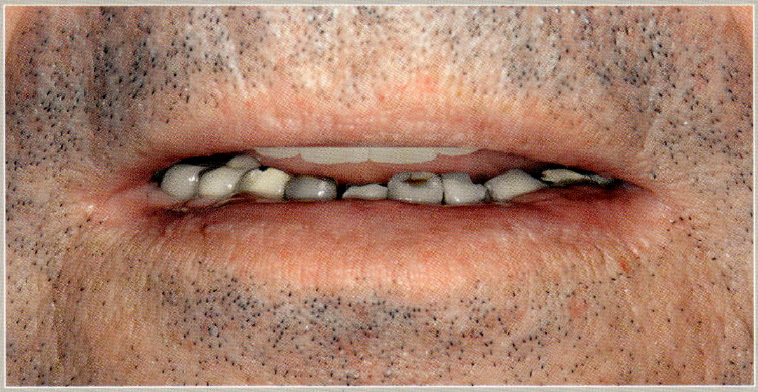

A hypothetical mock-up addition (approximately 2 mm) to the maxillary incisors to demonstrate the proposed incisal edge position.

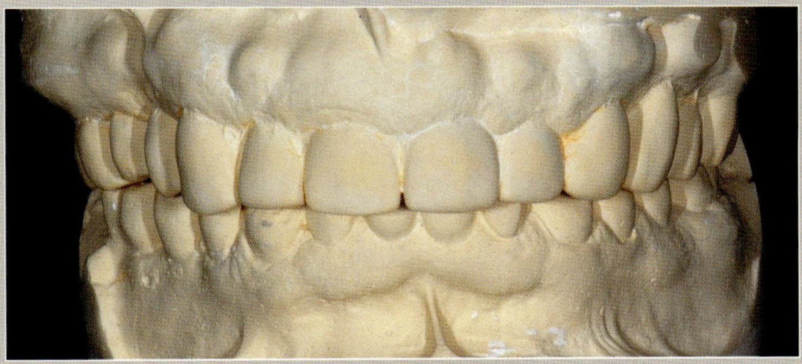

Articulated casts showing short teeth and deep overbite.

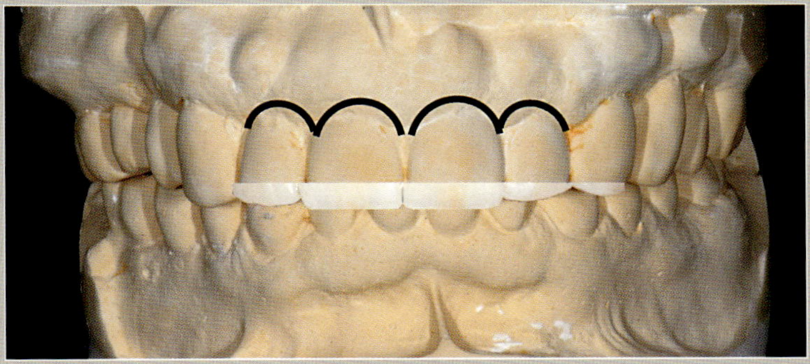

Casts showing transfer of additional tooth length (approximately 2 mm to central incisors) and proposed gingival crown lengthening (approximately 1 mm) to create proper tooth position, size, and proportion.

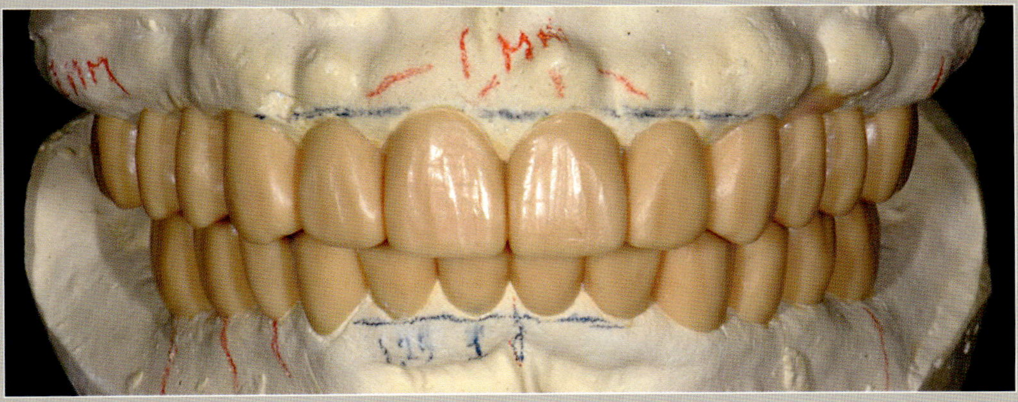

Diagnostic wax-up demonstrating the transfer of the proposed added maxillary incisal edge and gingival crown length.

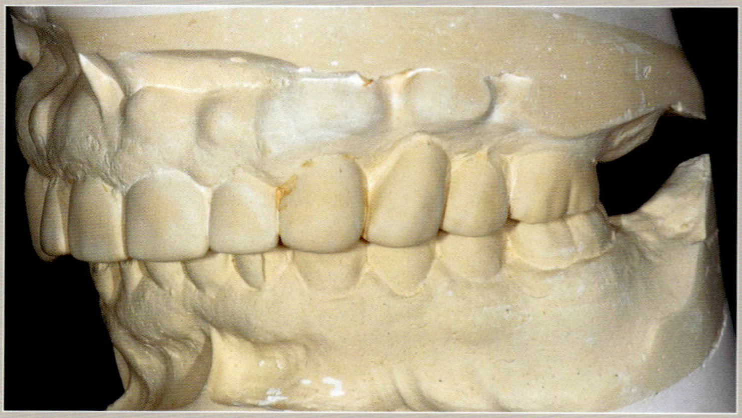

Left lateral view of mounted casts.

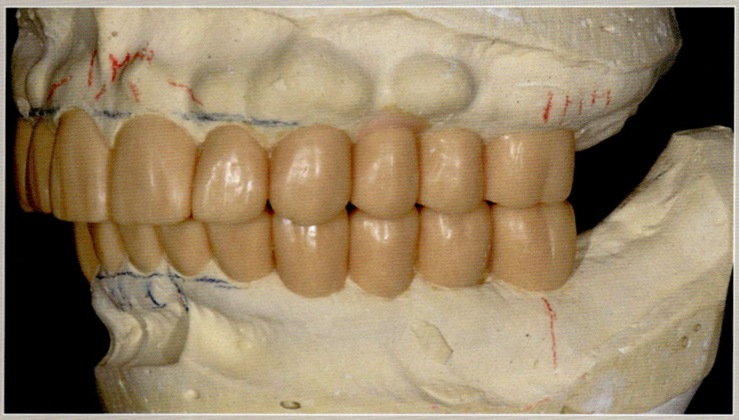

Lateral view of the diagnostic wax-up demonstrating an increase in the VDO creating less vertical overlap and a decrease in the incisal guidance angle.

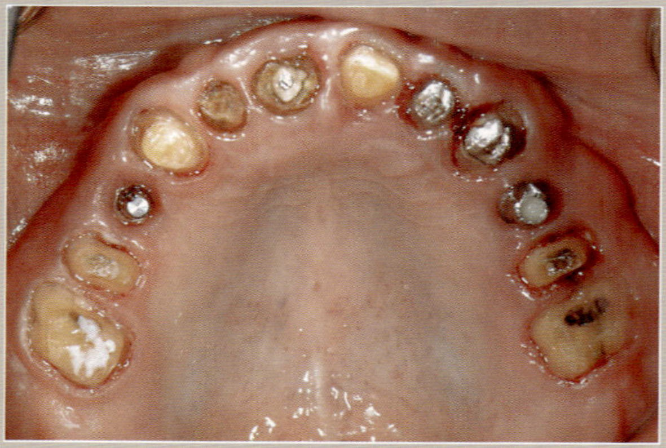

Maxillary occlusal view after removal of existing restorations.

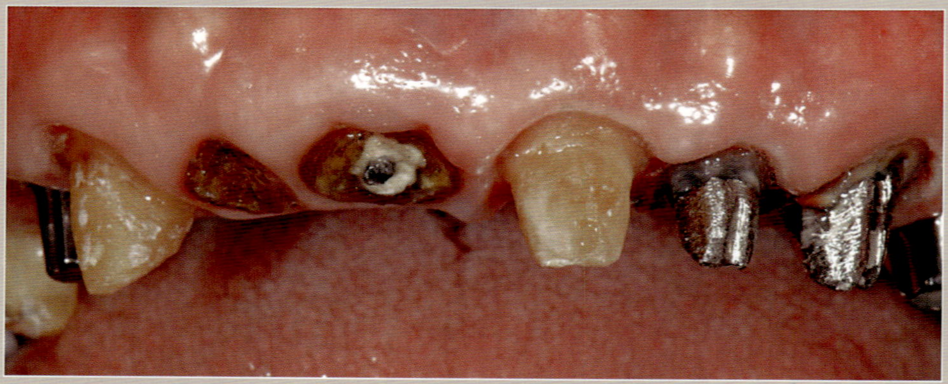

Frontal view of maxilla after removal of existing restorations.

Phase VI: Second provisionalization

From the diagnostic wax-up, shell provisional restorations were fabricated and delivered. The provisional was segmented in the maxilla (teeth/sites nos. 3 and 4, 5 to 12, 13 and 14) and in the mandible (teeth/sites nos. 19 to 21, 22 to 27, 28 to 30). This approach used the newly integrated implants (sites nos. 5, 12, 19, 28, 29, 30) and allowed for a controlled transition in case teeth with unfavorable prognoses (nos. 7, 8, 10, 11) would require removal. The provisional stage was critically important. It allowed for a structural evaluation of the remaining dentition. The restorative dentist and the patient were able to evaluate function, phonetics, and esthetics over a significant time period. This allowed the patient time to adapt to the changes. Any necessary alterations could be made and evaluated until the patient and the restorative dentist were satisfied.

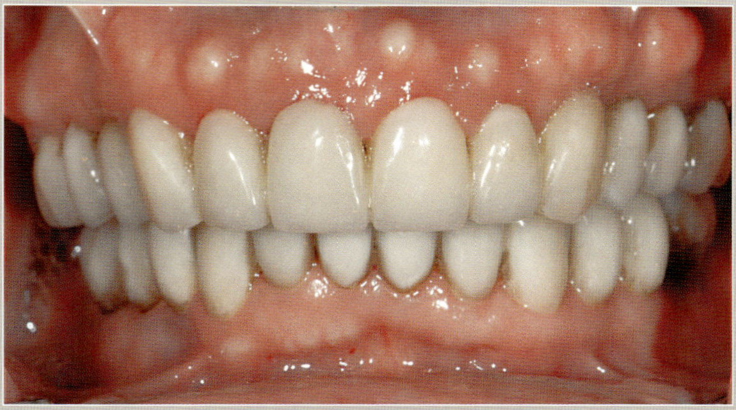

Provisional restorations in MIP.

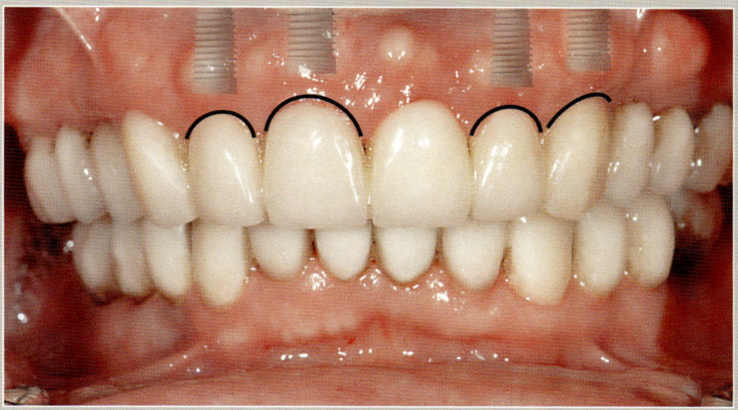

Provisional restorations demonstrate the proposed gingival position, thereby serving as a surgical guide for proper implant placement.

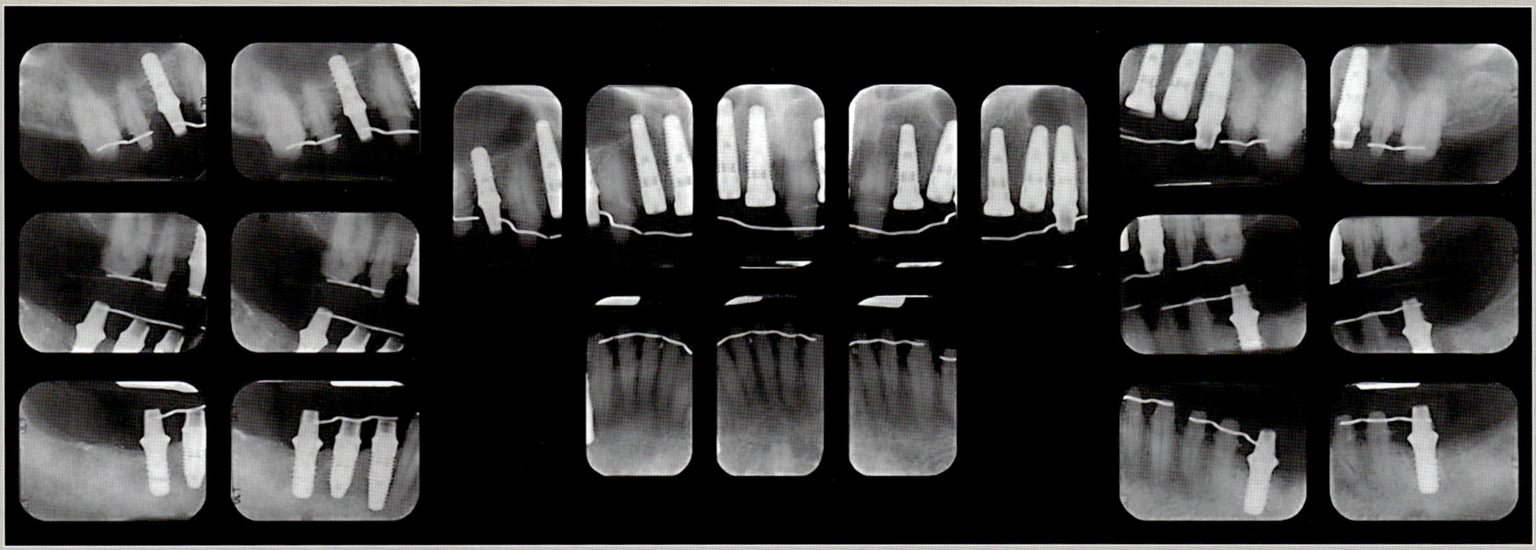

Complete-mouth interim radiographs.

Phase VII: Re-evaluation

After provisionalization, a consultation was initiated to discuss the prognosis and treatment options. Teeth nos. 7 and 8 had previously fractured to the gingival line, and only the roots remained. Teeth nos. 10 and 11 had endodontic therapy, large posts, and minimal remaining tooth structure. All the other teeth had favorable prognoses. After a discussion regarding treatment options and prognoses, the patient accepted a plan involving extraction of teeth nos. 7, 8, 10, and 11, followed by immediate placement of implants into these sites.

Phase VIII: Second surgical phase

The provisional restoration was removed. Teeth nos. 7, 8, 10, and 11 were extracted, and immediate implants were placed in these sites. The provisional restoration contained the definitive cementoenamel junction position and served as a surgical guide, allowing the surgeon to place the implants in the correct vertical, mesiodistal, and buccolingual positions. Thoughtful segmenting of the provisional restorations facilitated the transition from tooth-supported to implant-supported restorations. Early in the diagnostic phase, the prognoses for teeth nos. 7, 8, 10, and 11 were identified as guarded; in the event that all of these teeth were lost, the provisional restoration in the anterior maxilla would be supported by the integrated implants in site nos. 5 and 12 and the teeth in positions nos. 6 and 9. This allowed for a smooth transition during the integration of implants in sites nos. 7, 8, 10, and 11 and a seamless adaptation by the patient, who was able to use the same provisional restoration throughout this phase.

Phase IX: Re-evaluation

After implant integration, complete-mouth radiographs were obtained. The radiographs demonstrated a favorable prognosis for the remaining teeth and implants. An ongoing evaluation of function, esthetics, and phonetics was performed. The patient had adapted well to the new occlusion and approved of the overall tooth sizes and positions. A discussion with the patient was initiated to determine desired shade and characterization of the definitive restorations.

Posttreatment

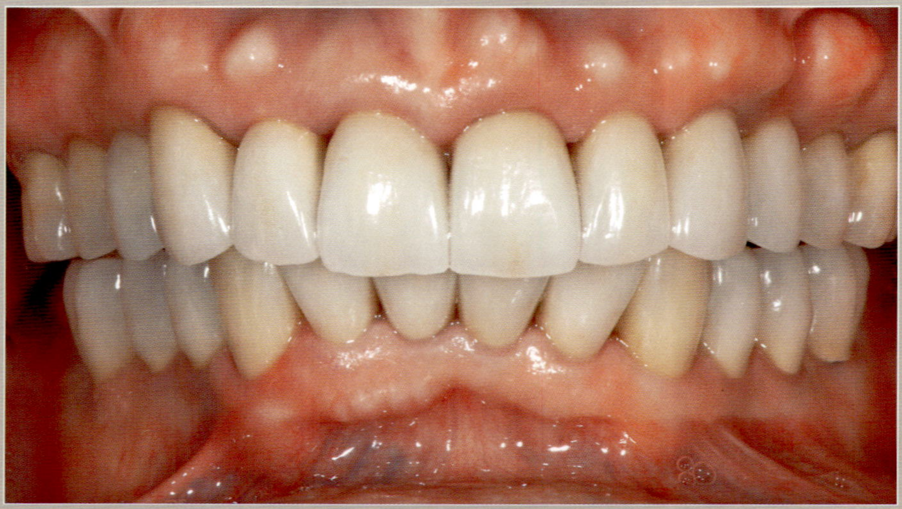

Intraoral frontal view of MIP.

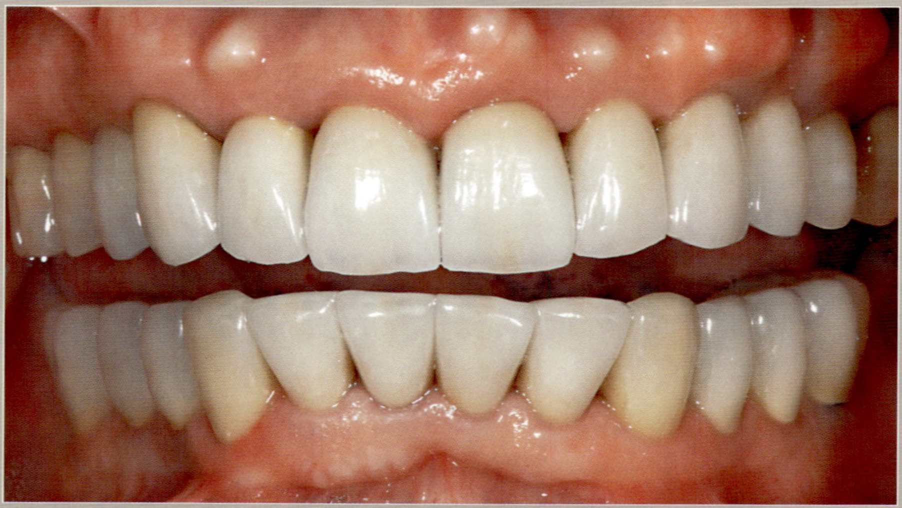

Intraoral frontal view with teeth apart.

Phase X: Definitive restoration

A staged approach was used for definitive restoration. A final impression was obtained for teeth nos. 6 and 9 and implant sites nos. 5, 7, 8, 10, 11, and 12. The segmented provisional restorations were left in place on teeth nos. 3, 4, 13, and 14. This facilitated an accurate CR record at the correct vertical dimension as well as an easily obtained and accurate final impression. Models of all provisional restorations along with a CR record, facebow transfer, and photographs were provided to the laboratory technician. Specific instructions were provided to the technician regarding the shade and characterization desired by the patient in the definitive restorations. The technician fabricated custom abutments for implants in sites nos. 7, 8, 10, and 11. Standard abutments were used on implants in sites nos. 5 to 12. Metal-ceramic crowns were fabricated and delivered. This staged approach was repeated for teeth nos. 3, 4, 13, and 14; then for teeth nos. 22 to 27; and finally for implant sites nos. 19, 28, 29, and 30 and teeth nos. 20 and 21. Standard abutments were used for all posterior implants, and metal-ceramic crowns were used throughout.

Phase XI: Re-evaluation and maintenance

A maxillary occlusal splint was fabricated and delivered for nighttime wear. A posttreatment consultation was held to determine patient satisfaction and to discuss ongoing maintenance. Follow-up photographs and radiographs were taken.

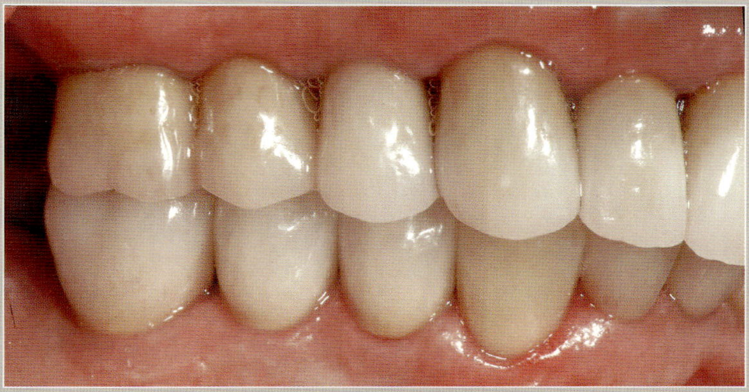

Right lateral view of MIP.

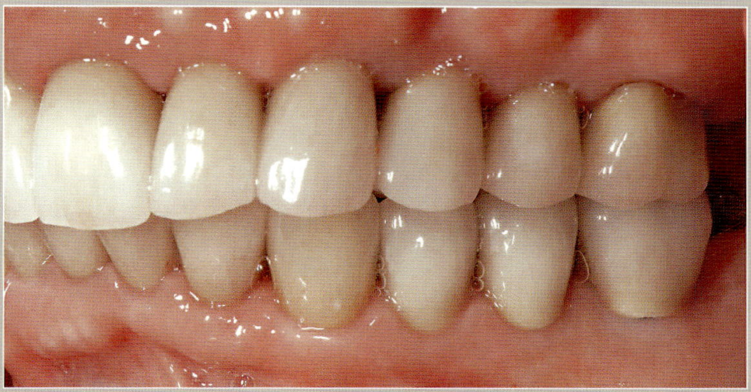

Left lateral view of MIP.

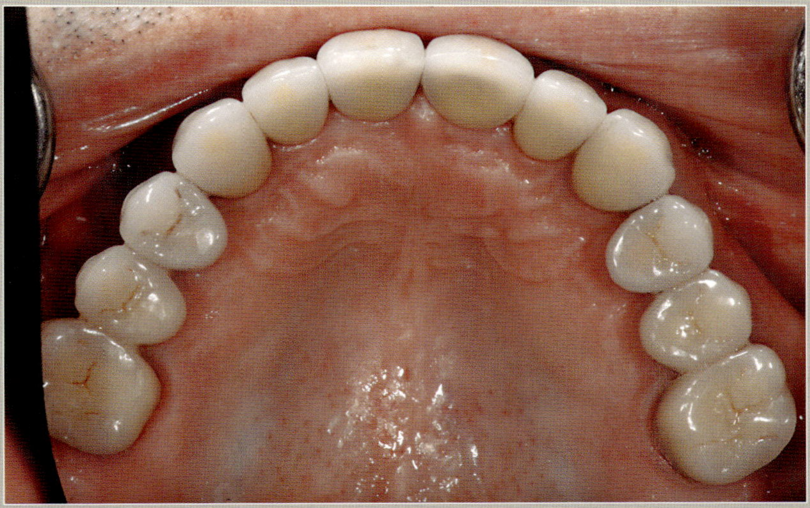

Maxillary occlusal view.

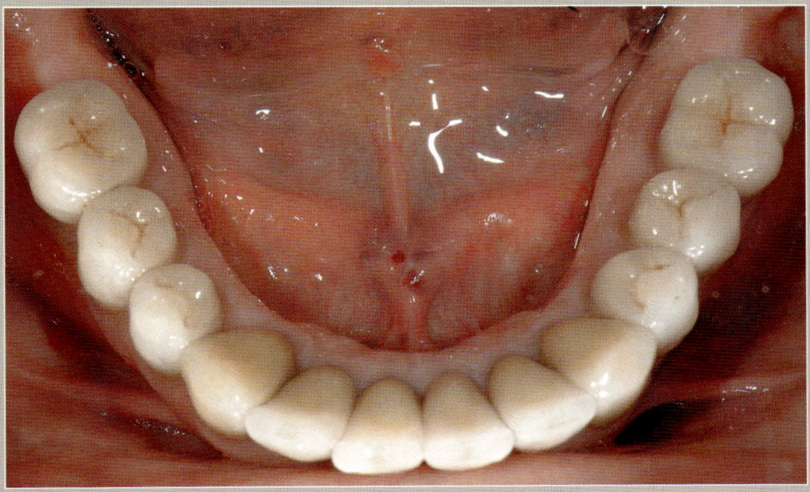

Mandibular occlusal view.

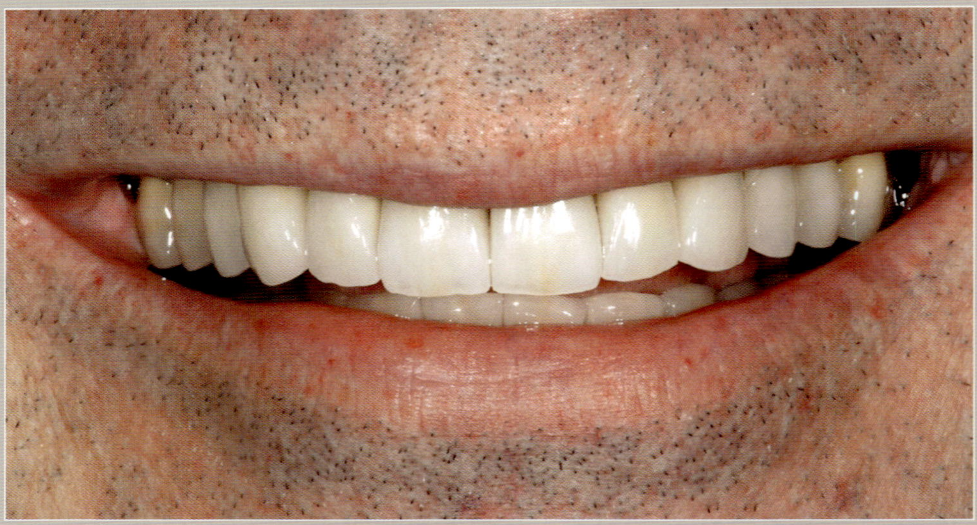

Smile.

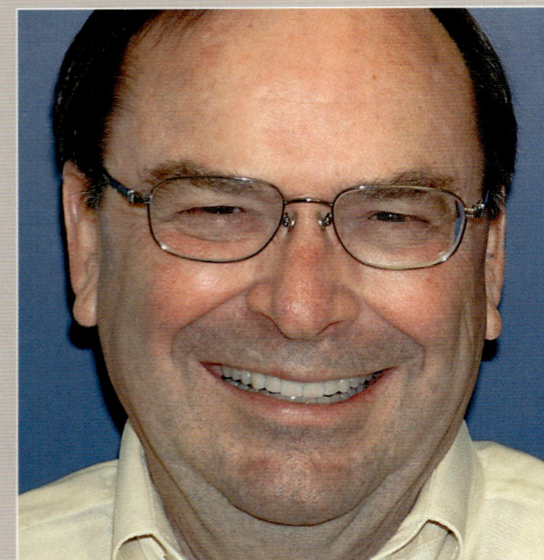

Full face with smile.

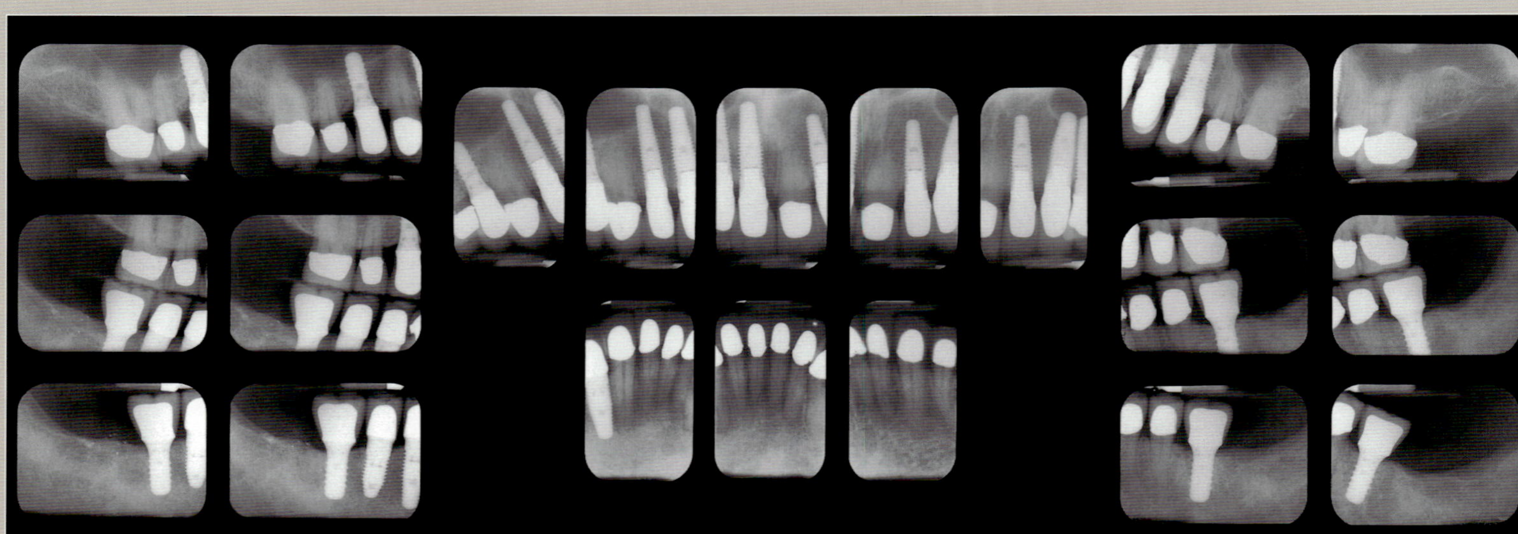

Complete-mouth radiographs 6 months after completion of treatment.

You may now place the corresponding posttreatment overlay found in the separate folder over the pretreatment periodontal chart on page 367.

Commentary

Treatment planning requires careful identification of the diagnostic risk factors combined with an application of the three fundamental treatment-planning principles in a creative, conceptual process that leads from hypothetical to definitive treatment. Minimizing the liability of re-entry is always an important consideration when treatment planning. The application of this principle was particularly critical for this patient, given his history of treatment failures. Minimizing the liability of re-entry primarily required removing teeth with poor prognoses, creating a favorable and stable occlusion, managing parafunction with a maxillary occlusal splint, and individualizing the restorations.

At a fundamental level, individualizing restorations as a treatment objective invites a direct comparison between restoring a single edentulous site with a fixed partial denture or with an implant-supported crown restoration. There are circumstances that necessitate restoration with a fixed partial denture, but it is my assertion that this may not be optimal treatment for the patient. The ramifications and consequences of this course of therapy must be considered and may include increased risk of failure and complexity of re-treatment should anything go wrong. While the literature is not conclusive when directly comparing the long-term survival of three-unit fixed partial dentures with a single implant-supported crown, there is strong evidence to support my hypothesis.[4-7] The mean survival of the three-unit fixed partial dentures we provide for our patients is 10 years or less,[8-16] although there is a false perception that they last much longer. The abutment teeth of fixed partial dentures may be at risk as well; reports show that 30% require extraction after 14 years.[17,18]

When forced to re-treat these failures, the clinician must consider the following issues:

- Would it be wise to place another fixed prosthesis with a longer span and associated higher risk of failure?[13]
- Will the edentulous area have to be restored with a removable partial denture with the associated risk factors this treatment option carries?[19-23]
- Will the age, health, and economic status of the patient at the time of failure become liabilities in providing optimum care?
- Will a potentially resorbed alveolar ridge become an additional obstacle to achieving more ideal results if dental implants are considered?[24-27]
- What are the psychosocial and economic impacts of these failures on our patients?

The answers to these questions would be academic if the teeth (restorations) were individualized in the original treatment. Even if the survival rates of a fixed partial denture and an individually restored implant were the same, it is clear that re-treating a failure on one unit is far preferable to having to re-treat three units.

When a patient is faced with the extraction of a tooth, the most likely etiologies are caries, periodontal disease, and/or trauma from occlusion or an external source. Given this diagnostic history, it does not seem reasonable to restore this newly edentulous site with a fixed partial denture, which increases the risk and magnitude of the future failure that the diagnostic history predicts. It is also clear that when a tooth is lost, a significant amount of associated alveolar bone is lost as well. We have a window of opportunity to prevent most of this resorption and thus limit future liability by planning for the placement of an implant.[28,29] With the high-risk debilitated-dentition patient such as the one in this treatment-planning exercise, it is imperative that we decrease risk factors and minimize the likelihood and magnitude of future failure.

In contrast to fixed partial dentures, single implant-supported crowns have demonstrated excellent success rates and do not impact the adjacent teeth.[30-39] Because efficacious treatment is of primary importance, the single implant-supported crown creates an opportunity to minimize the liability of re-entry by individualizing restorations.

Clinical experience has provided me the opportunity to live with my own failures. Through anecdotal evidence, literature review, and with invaluable mentoring, I have come to the conclusion that we must plan for and understand the impact of our potential and realized treatment failures. By doing so, we can become more effective and more complete clinicians. Only through critical re-evaluation that includes thorough examination as well as follow-up radiographs and photographs can we determine the degree of treatment success or failure.

As an example of fixed partial denture failure, Fig 1a shows complete-mouth radiographs of a patient restored with multiple fixed partial dentures, and Fig 1b shows complete-mouth radiographs of the same patient 9 years later, after failure of several of the fixed partial dentures. Some of the failed fixed partial dentures were replaced with individual implant- and tooth-supported restorations.

When we can restore the debilitated dentition of a patient with individualized restorations, we have given that patient

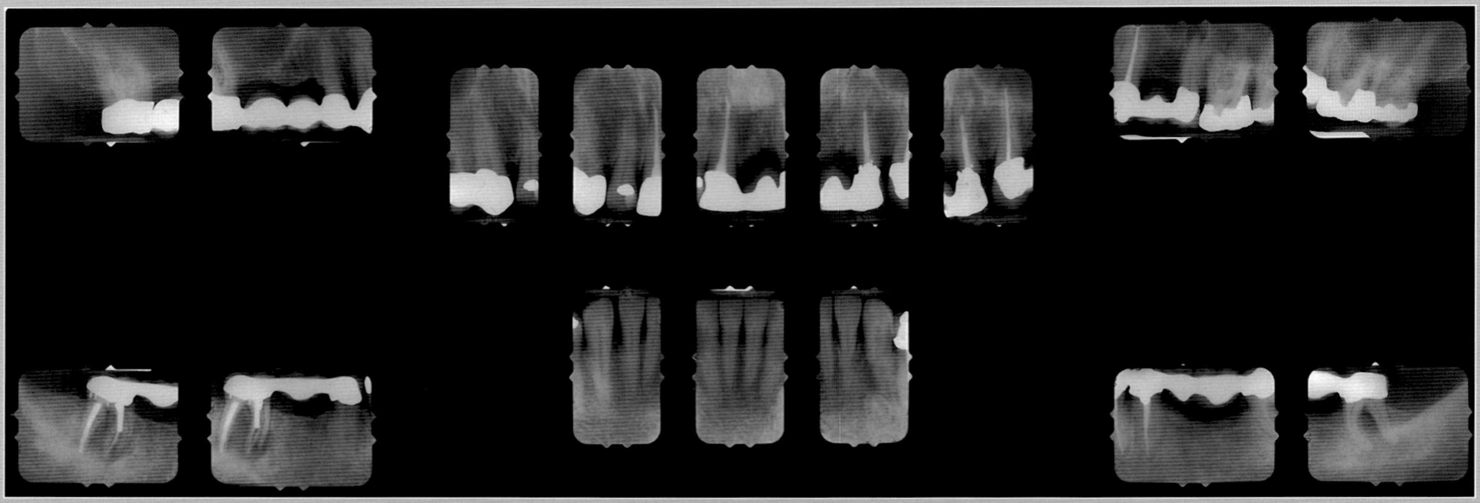

Fig 1a Complete-mouth radiographs of a patient with multiple fixed partial dentures.

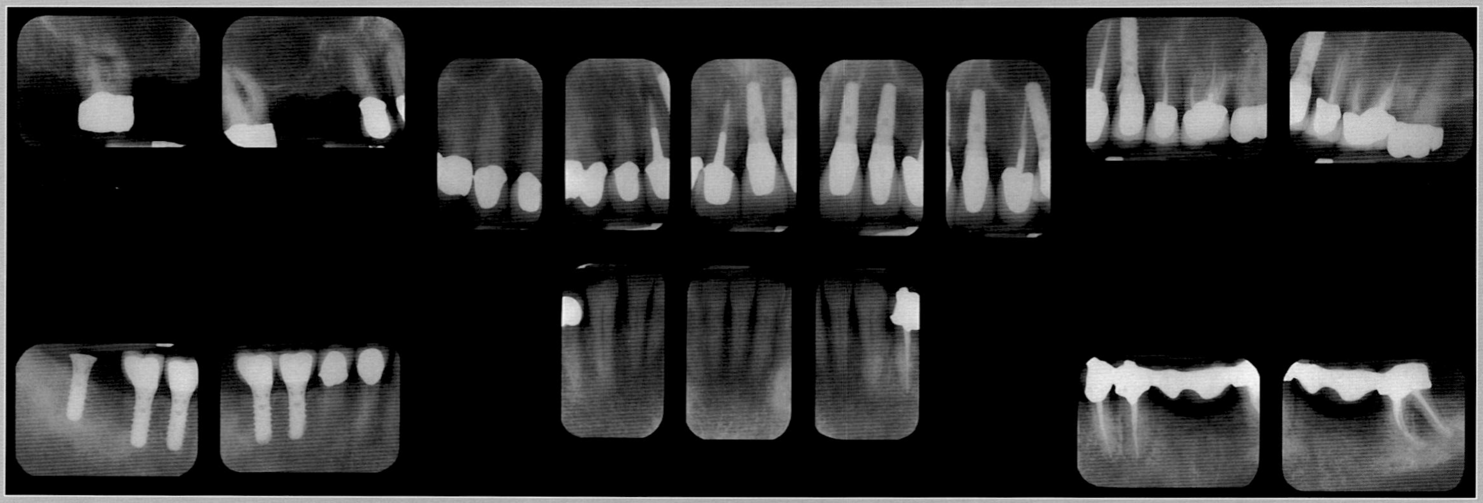

Fig 1b Complete-mouth radiographs of the same patient 9 years later after multiple fixed partial denture failures and placement of new restorations.

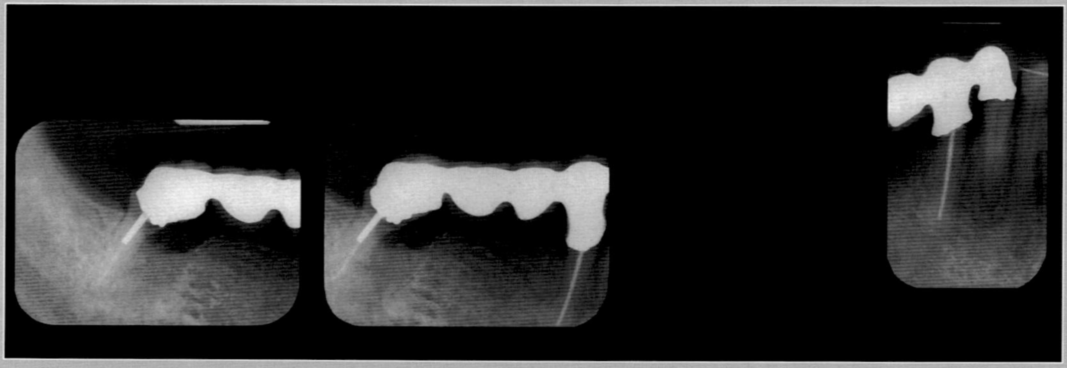

Fig 2a Radiographs demonstrating failure of a five-unit fixed partial denture that was less than 2 years old.

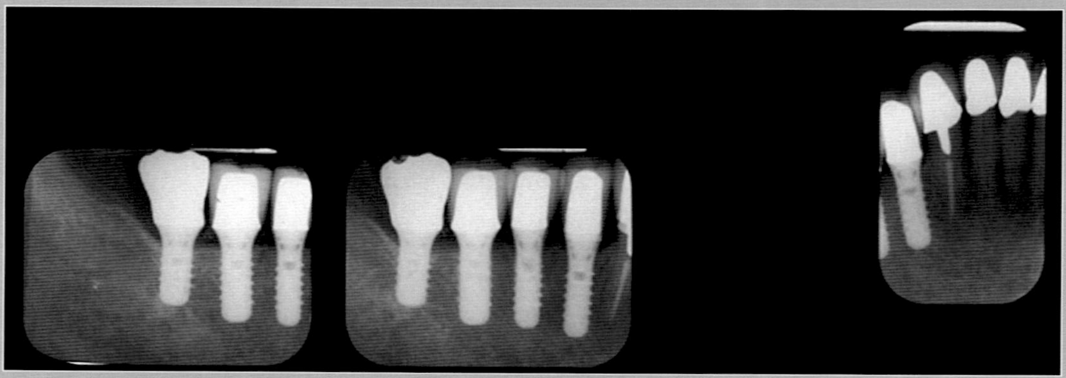

Fig 2b Radiographs of the same patient with individually restored implants and teeth. Two of the original abutment teeth were lost.

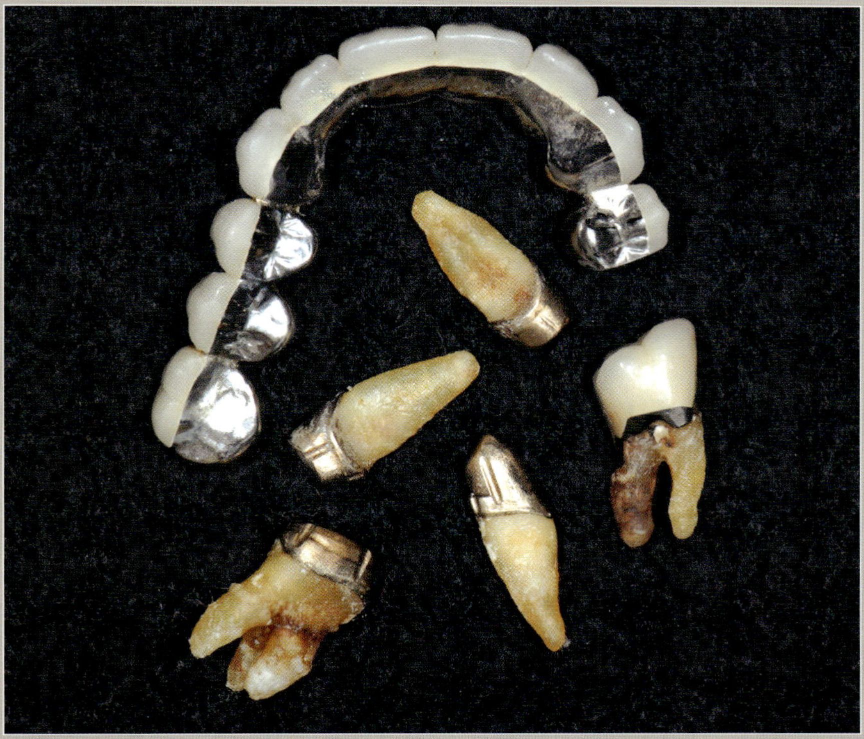

Fig 3 Periodontal prosthetic reconstruction after catastrophic failure.

optimum treatment. While we cannot promise these high-risk patients a future without failure, solutions to any problems that may arise will likely entail straightforward single-tooth replacement. Patients ultimately realize the benefits of this approach, even though initial treatment costs might be higher, and the duration of treatment may be longer.

Figure 2a shows a failed fixed partial denture that was less than 2 years old, and Fig 2b shows the quadrant after restoration with implants and individual restorations. While there may be extenuating circumstances that would justify treatment planning for short-span fixed partial dentures on sound abutments, it is clear that the increased risk and magnitude of failure associated with long-span fixed partial dentures and unsound abutments should be avoided.

Figure 3 shows an example of a periodontal prosthesis failure. While periodontal prosthetic reconstructions have historically demonstrated reasonable longevity, catastrophic failure can occur when key abutments are lost. This patient's age, health, and financial concerns precluded any re-treatment option other than a maxillary removable complete denture. The psychosocial and functional impact on this patient was significant. While we cannot predict when a failure will occur, we can anticipate the magnitude of the failure based on our treatment plan.

I am not suggesting we abandon fixed partial dentures or splinting as treatment options, but we must be acutely aware of their limitations.[40] As our dental techniques and materials evolve, so should our understanding of minimizing the liability of re-entry and how we can apply this concept. While individualizing restorations is an ideal treatment goal, this is not always possible or practical. The following examples demonstrate treatment plans where the principle of individualizing restorations was not the ideal strategy.

Figure 4 shows adjacent implants and individualized restorations that created significant problems as a result of inadequate spacing and lack of keratinized tissue. Proper space appropriation and interimplant distance are important treatment-planning considerations for successful implant therapy, especially when contemplating adjacent implants.[41,42]

Figures 5a and 5b show pretreatment and posttreatment radiographs. Judiciously placed implant-supported fixed partial dentures were used in the mandible.[43] Space requirements in the anterior mandible, financial limitations, and the occlusion opposing a maxillary implant-supported overdenture were important considerations in the design of this treatment plan. These practical concerns and treatment-planning compromises are part of everyday practice. However, a potentially greater re-entry liability exists in the probability, magnitude, and complexity of re-treatment should any of these fixed partial dentures and splinted restorations fail in the future.

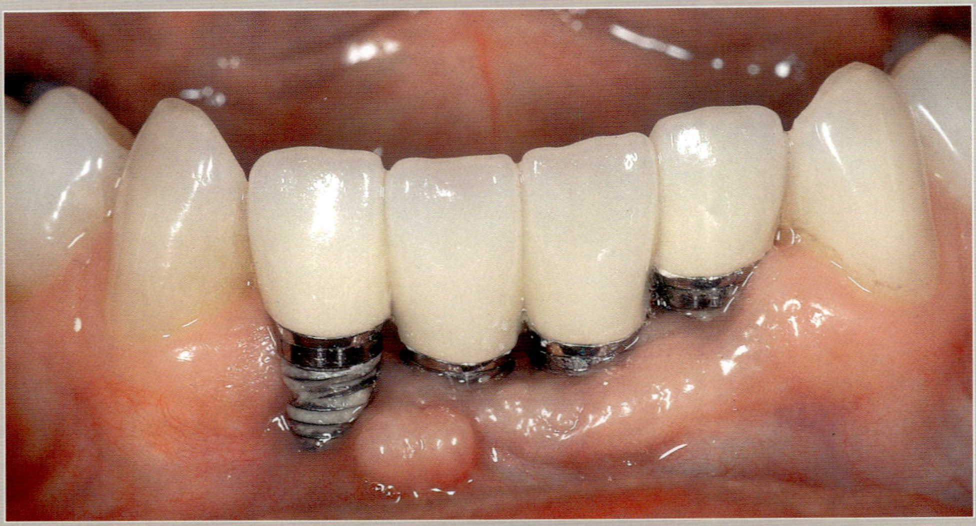

Fig 4 Failing implant-supported restorations of the mandibular incisors due to inadequate interimplant distance.

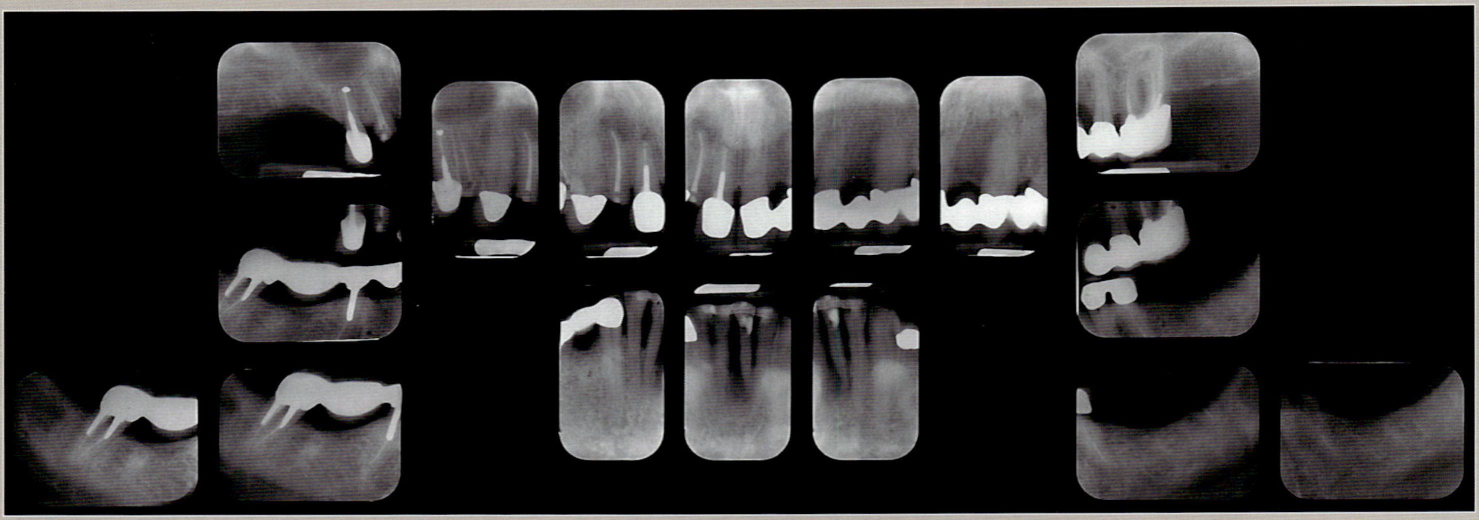

Fig 5a Pretreatment radiographs of a failing dentition.

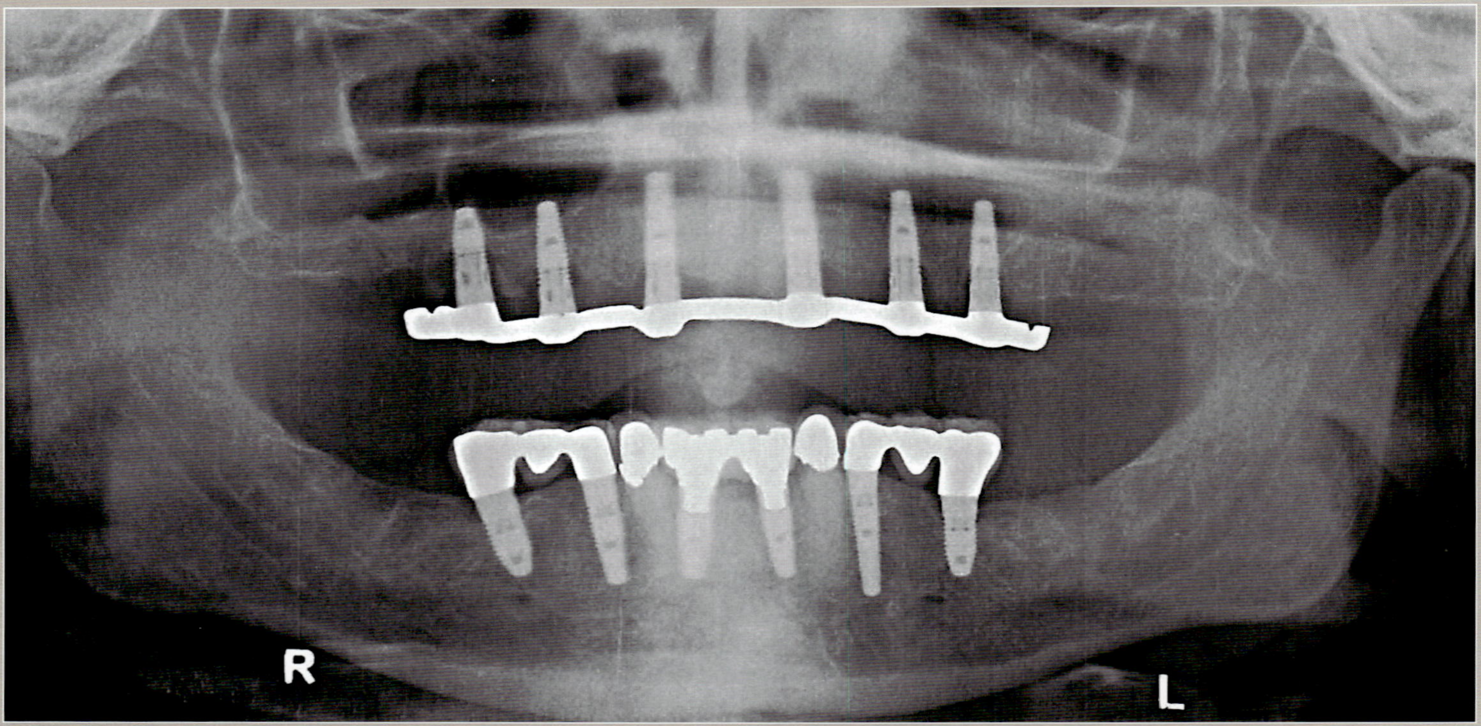

Fig 5b Posttreatment panoramic radiograph of the same patient, demonstrating judicious use of implant-supported fixed partial dentures in the mandible and a bar-supported overdenture in the maxilla.

An unspoken and uncomfortable aspect of compromised treatment plans is who is responsible for remediation of a failure when it occurs. The patient and clinician may accept a compromised treatment plan for economic or practical reasons, only to have to re-enter a few years later. The stress and lost trust associated with this situation is potentially avoidable when the clinician identifies and discusses the patient's intrinsic risk factors. This helps the patient understand the limitations of the materials and techniques available and, by individualizing restorations, minimizes the magnitude of potential failure. Patients appreciate this type of frank discussion, which allows them to participate in and take ownership of their unique treatment plan. It also facilitates shared responsibility, especially when they choose a compromised plan.

As a clinician who has practiced in the same location for more than 32 years, my empirical observations have led me to the conclusion that patients are best served by having individualized restorations where possible. This minimizes the liability of re-entry and the psychologic, functional, and financial impact should failure occur. We can diagnose historical and current risk factors, but we have difficulty forecasting and controlling future risk factors and the failure they predict. Minimizing the liability of re-entry appears to be a valuable tool for managing risk and predicting treatment success.

I began this chapter by asking the reader to consider some common dogmas that pervade our profession: always splint implants, never place implants adjacent to each other in the anterior maxilla, and fixed partial dentures are more cost-effective than implants. Imagine if the patient in the treatment-planning exercise had been treated with fixed partial dentures in order to reduce initial treatment costs or to try to achieve "ideal" esthetics. What would have been the impact of splinting the implants?[44] Something as simple and likely as a porcelain fracture on this functionally high-risk patient could have profound consequences. For this patient, the diagnostic findings of low lip dynamics, thick and flat tissue architecture, adequate bone quality and volume, and ideal interimplant distances allowed us to place and restore adjacent implants. For other patients, there are alternative diagnostic findings that may not have led to that treatment decision. The key is that the diagnostic information unique to every individual must drive our treatment decisions. In this case, minimizing the liability of re-entry by individualizing the restorations far outweighed any questionable esthetic or economic gain.

The old dogmas no longer apply. As available technology and our treatment options evolve, our cognitive treatment-planning skills must adapt as well. Failure is a reality we must consider in terms of probability and magnitude when we treatment plan. By minimizing the liability of re-entry, we have the opportunity to provide treatment plans that predict a successful outcome not only at completion but throughout the lives of our patients.

ACKNOWLEDGMENTS

I would like to recognize and thank Dr Stig Osterberg and Mr Joseph Choy for their talent and skill in helping to create a favorable treatment outcome for this patient and for their many years of friendship and teamwork. I have immense gratitude for Dr Michael Cohen's vision and commitment to a university without walls, which I have had the good fortune to attend; for Dr Gerrard Schultz and his teaching and dedication to excellence; and for my wife, Karen, who makes it all possible.

REFERENCES

1. Nichols HI. Fundamental treatment planning: Application of three basic principles. In: Cohen M (ed). Interdisciplinary Treatment Planning: Principles, Design, Implementation. Chicago: Quintessence, 2008:283–311.
2. Magne P, Belser U. Understanding the intact tooth and the biomimetic principle. In: Bonded Porcelain Restorations in the Anterior Dentition: A Biomimetic Approach. Chicago: Quintessence, 2002:23–56.
3. Spear F, Kinzer G. Approaches to vertical dimension. In: Cohen M (ed). Interdisciplinary Treatment Planning: Principles, Design, Implementation. Chicago: Quintessence, 2008:249–281.
4. Balevi B. Root canal therapy, fixed partial dentures and implant-supported crowns, have similar short term survival rates. Evid Based Dent 2008;9:15–17.
5. Salinas TJ, Eckert SE. In patients requiring single-tooth replacement, what are the outcomes of implant- as compared to tooth-supported restorations? Int J Oral Maxillofac Implants 2007;22(suppl):71–95.
6. Pjetursson BE, Lang NP. Prosthetic treatment planning on the basis of scientific evidence. J Oral Rehabil 2008;35(suppl 1):72–79.
7. Anusavice KJ, Kakar K, Feree N. Which mechanical and physical testing methods are relevant for predicting the clinical performance of ceramic-based dental prostheses? Clin Oral Implants Res 2007;18(suppl 3):218–231.
8. Schwartz NL, Whitsett LD, Berry TG. Unserviceable crowns and fixed partial dentures: Life span and causes for loss of serviceability. J Am Dent Assoc 1970;81:1395–1401.
9. Walton JN, Gardner FM, Agar JR. A survey of crown and fixed partial denture failures: Length of service and reasons for replacement. J Prosthet Dent 1986;56:416–421.
10. Torabinejad M, Anderson P, Bader J, et al. Outcomes of root canal treatment and restoration, implant-supported single crowns, fixed partial dentures, and extraction without replacement: A systematic review. J Prosthet Dent 2007;98:285–311.
11. Kinsel RP, Lin D. Retrospective analysis of porcelain failures of metal ceramic crowns and fixed partial dentures supported by 729 implants in 152 patients: Patient-specific and implant specific predictors of ceramic failure. J Prosthet Dent 2009;101:388–394.
12. Sailer I, Pjetursson BE, Zwahlen M, Hammerle CH. A systematic review of the survival and complication rate of ceramic and metal-ceramic reconstructions after an observation period of at least 3 years. Part II: Fixed dental prostheses. Clin Oral Implants Res 2007;18(suppl 3):86–96.
13. De Backer H, Van Maele G, De Moor N, Van den Berghe L. Long-term results of short-span versus long-span fixed dental prostheses: An up to 20-year retrospective study. Int J Prosthodont 2008;21:75–85.
14. Pjetursson BE, Tan K, Lang NP, Brägger U, Egger M, Zwahlen M. A systematic review of the survival and complication rates of fixed partial dentures (FPDs) after an observation period of at least 5 years. Clin Oral Implants Res 2004;16:624–642.
15. De Backer H, Van Maele G, De Moor N, Van den Berghe L. Single-tooth replacement: Is a 3-unit fixed partial denture still an option? A 20-year retrospective study. Int J Prosthodont 2006;19:567–573.

16. Pjetursson BE, Brägger U, Lang NP, Zwahlen M. Comparison of survival and complication rates of tooth-supported fixed dental prostheses (FDPs) and implant-supported FDPs and single crowns (SCs). Clin Oral Implants Res 2007;18(suppl 3):97–113 [erratum 2008;19:326–328].
17. Shugars DA, Bader JD, White BA, Scurria MS, Hayden WJ Jr, Garcia RI. Survival rates of teeth adjacent to treated and untreated posterior bounded edentulous spaces. J Am Dent Assoc 1998;129:1089–1095.
18. Aquilino SA, Shugars DA, Bader JD, White BA. Ten-year survival rates of teeth adjacent to treated and untreated posterior bounded edentulous spaces. J Prosthet Dent 2001;85:455–460.
19. Wetherell J, Smales R. Partial dentures failure: A long-term clinical survey. J Dent 1980;8:333–340.
20. Wilding R, Reddy J. Periodontal disease in partial denture wearers: A biologic index. J Oral Rehabil 1987;14:111–124.
21. Vermeulen AH, Keltjens HM, van't Hof MA, Kayser AF. Ten-year evaluation of removable partial dentures: Survival rates based on retreatment, not wearing and replacement. J Prosthet Dent 1996;76:267–272.
22. Roberts BW. A survey of chrome-cobalt partial dentures. N Z Dent J 1978;74:203–209.
23. Hummel SK, Wilson MA, Marker VA, Nunn ME. Quality of removable partial dentures worn by adult U.S. population. J Prosthet Dent 2002;88:37–43
24. Van der Weijden F, Dell'Acqua F, Slot DE. Alveolar bone dimensional changes of post extraction sockets in humans: A systematic review. J Clin Periodontol 2009;36:1048–1058.
25. Araujo MG, Lindhe J. Dimensional ridge alterations following tooth extraction. An experimental study in the dog. J Clin Periodontol 2005;32:212–218.
26. Kingsmill VJ. Post-extraction remodeling of the adult mandible. Crit Rev Oral Biol Med 1999;10:384–404.
27. Schropp L, Wenzel A, Kostopoulos L, Karring T. Bone healing and soft tissue contour changes following single-tooth extraction: A clinical and radiographic 12-month prospective study. Int J Periodontics Restorative Dent 2003;23:313–323.
28. Kline R, Hoar JE, Beck GH, Hazen R, Resnik RR, Crawford EA. A prospective multicenter clinical investigation of a bone quality-based dental system. Implant Dent 2002;11:224–234.
29. Norton MR. Biologic and mechanical stability of single-tooth implants: 4- to 7-year follow-up. Clin Implant Dent Relat Res 2001;3:214–220.
30. Schmitt A, Zarb GA. The longitudinal clinical effectiveness of osseointegrated dental implants for single tooth replacement. Int J Prosthodont 1993;6:187–202.
31. Ekfeldt A, Carlsson GE, Borjesson G. Clinical evaluation of single tooth restorations supported by osseointegrated implants: A retrospective study. Int J Oral Maxillofac Implants 1994;9:179–183.
32. Haas R, Mensdorff-Pouilly N, Mailath G, Watzek G. Brånemark Single tooth implants: A preliminary report of 76 implants. J Prosthet Dent 1995;73:274–279.
33. Jemt T, Laney WR, Harris D, et al. Osseointegrated implants for single tooth replacement: A 1-year report from a multicenter prospective study. Int J Oral Maxillofac Implants 1991;6:29–36.
34. Laney WR, Jemt T, Harris D, et al. Osseointegrated implants for single-tooth replacement: Progress report from a multicenter prospective study after 3 years. Int J Oral Maxillofac Implants 1994;9:49–54.
35. Henry PH, Laney WR, Jemt T, et al. Osseointegrated implants for single-tooth replacement: A prospective 5-year multicenter study. Int J Oral Maxillofac Implants 1996;11:450–455.
36. Misch CE, Poitras Y, Dietsh-Misch F. Endosteal implants in the edentulous posterior maxilla: Rationale and clinical report. Oral Health 2000;90(8):7–16.
37. Misch CE, Misch-Dietsh F, Silc J, Barboza E, Cianciola LJ, Kazor C. Posterior implant single-tooth replacement and status of adjacent teeth during a 10-year period: A retrospective report. J Periodontol 2008;79:2378–2382.
38. Priest G. Single-tooth implants and their role in preserving remaining teeth: A 10-year survival study. Int J Oral Maxillofac Implants 1999;14:181–188.
39. Jung RE, Pjetursson BE, Glauser R, Zembic A, Zwahlen M, Lang NP. A systematic review of the 5-year survival and complication rates of implant-supported single crowns. Clin Oral Implants Res 2008;19:119–130.
40. Baruch H, Ehrlich J, Yaffe A. Splinting—A review of the literature [in Hebrew]. Refuat Hapeh Vehashinayim 2001;18:29–40,76.
41. Rodriguez-Ciurana X, Vela-Nebot X, Segala-Torres M, et al. The effect of interimplant distance on the height of the interimplant bone crest when using platform-switched implants. Int J Periodontics Restorative Dent 2009;29:141–151.
42. Tarnow DP, Cho SC, Wallace SS. The effect of inter-implant distance on the height of inter-implant bone crest. J Periodontol 2000;71:546–549.
43. Abt E. Growing body of evidence on survival rates of implant-supported fixed prostheses. Evid Based Dent 2008;9:51–52.
44. Grossman Y, Finger IM, Block MS. Indications for splinting implant restorations. J Oral Maxillofac Surg 2005;63:642–652.

15

Management of an Esthetic Implant Complication

Anthony G. Sclar, DMD

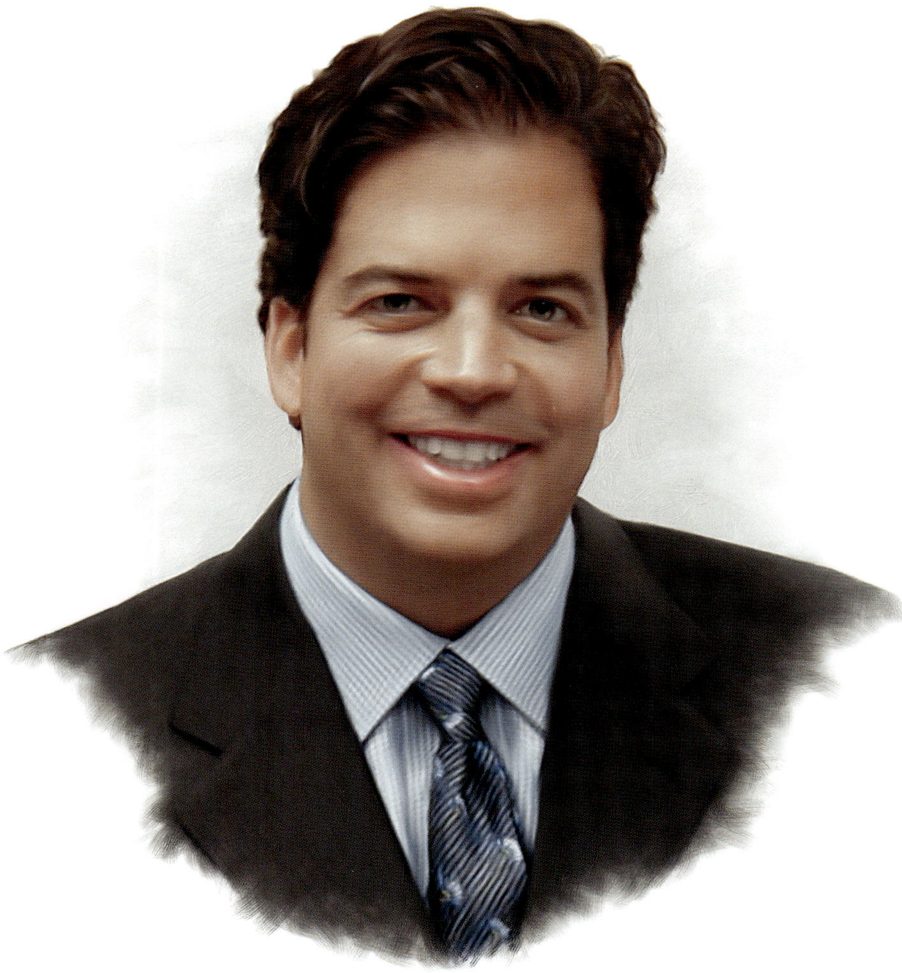

The management of this case exemplifies how interdisciplinary treatment planning and precise execution of biologically acceptable prosthetic and surgical protocols are essential to avoid and manage complications in esthetic implant therapy.

Philosophy and Background

In simple terms, an *esthetic implant complication* is defined as the failure to deliver an inconspicuous restoration in an area of high esthetic concern. This may arise in the eyes of the patient and/or significant others who have influence on the patient's perception of and expectations for the treatment outcome.[1]

Although the protocol for delivering an implant restoration in an area of high esthetic concern may seem straightforward, it is recognized that esthetic implant therapy is a complex treatment modality requiring interdisciplinary treatment planning and precise execution of the indicated treatment sequence by clinicians with advanced training and experience.[2–7] Prerequisites for the treatment team include:

- A keen and progressive diagnostic acumen
- A firm grasp of smile esthetic principles
- The ability to identify the diagnostic factors associated with esthetic complications and failures
- Excellent patient education and risk management skills
- In-depth knowledge of biologic mechanisms that impact long-term esthetic outcomes
- The ability to properly select, sequence, and precisely execute prosthetic and surgical treatment protocols
- A sense of artistry not typically required when providing dental implant therapy in areas of low esthetic concern[2,4–12]

Evolution of predictable implant esthetics

During the late 1980s and early 1990s—the developmental and growth period of esthetic implant therapy—a lack of scientific validation and clinical consensus concerning treatment protocols for achieving natural esthetic outcomes with dental implant therapy contributed to the occurrence of the majority of esthetic complications. Many clinicians erroneously applied the principles and treatment protocols designed to provide functional outcomes without regard for esthetics.

During this developmental and growth period, we experienced great success with esthetic implant therapy, but we also experienced a significant incidence of unexpected and disheartening complications and failures. It became evident that the decision to employ a particular treatment protocol had to be based on a clear understanding of the patient's objectives for treatment outcome, clinical findings from a systematic patient evaluation, and the determinations of esthetic risk for individual patients based on their unique clinical case presentation. Critical analysis of our esthetic outcomes on a case-by-case basis allowed us to identify numerous factors that were associated with esthetic implant complications as well as specific anatomical limitations and special treatment-planning considerations that precluded successful esthetic implant outcomes.[6,7]

We also learned that the ability to achieve initial esthetic success did not ensure the maintenance of a satisfactory long-term result despite ideal implant placement and use of a biologically acceptable prosthetic treatment protocol. In a significant number of our early cases in which implants were placed at healed sites, despite proper planning and execution of our treatment plan, we subsequently observed peri-implant soft tissue recession. This often resulted in disharmonious proportions of the implant restoration and progressive darkening of the peri-implant tissues. In the absence of other risk factors, the observed esthetic deterioration was correlated with the loss of crestal bone detected on follow-up radiographs and attributed to the biologic width phenomenon. Conversely, we observed that the deterioration of esthetics over time was virtually eliminated when preemptive soft tissue augmentation was performed at healed sites prior to or at the time of implant placement.

In an attempt to better understand and quantify our clinical observations, we measured the tissue thickness (labiopalatal dimension) of the peri-implant soft tissues at 20 esthetic implant sites in 16 consecutive patients who presented 3 years posttreatment for evaluation. The peri-implant soft tissue thickness was measured at points 2, 5, and 8 mm apical to the midfacial gingival margin of each implant restoration. The mean orofacial soft tissue dimension was determined for two individual groups based upon whether the esthetic outcome had deteriorated (group 1 = 6 sites) or had been maintained (group 2 = 14 sites) over time. The mean orofacial soft tissue dimension for the 6 sites that had experienced a deterioration of esthetics over time was 1.3 mm, and the mean orofacial soft tissue dimension for the 14 sites that maintained a natural esthetic outcome over the same time period was 2.5 mm. Interestingly enough, preemptive soft tissue augmentation was performed in 13 of 14 sites that had maintained pleasing soft tissue esthetics 3 years after completion of active treatment.

As a result of this translational approach of combining our clinical observations over time with labiopalatal peri-implant soft tissue measurements, we concluded that when implant placement is planned in an area of high esthetic concern, peri-implant soft tissue augmentation is indicated in almost all cases in order to satisfy the lateral biologic width requirement of the site and to mask the underlying metal implant components, which contribute to unesthetic discoloration of peri-implant soft tissues. Eventually, evidence-based information and clinical consensus regarding esthetic risk factors and biologically acceptable treatment protocols for esthetic implant therapy became available.[2,9,11–26]

Based on our clinical experience and the quantitative information gained from measurements performed at patient recall examinations, we subsequently developed a clinical guideline of 2.5 to 3.0 mm as the desired labiopalatal dimensions of peri-implant soft tissues in areas of high esthetic concern.[6,7,27,28] Through ongoing critical analysis of the outcomes that we were or were not able to achieve for our esthetic implant patients, we furthered our understanding of how peri-implant soft tissue architecture and esthetics depended on adequate underlying vertical and horizontal bony support. From a clinical perspective, it became evident that a minimal labial bone wall thickness of approximately 2.0 mm or greater was required at esthetic anterior maxillary and mandibular implant sites compared with earlier recommendations of approximately 1.0 mm for the minimum bone wall thickness surrounding implants placed at nonesthetic sites.[29,30] From a biologic perspective, we attributed this observation to the propensity of the alveolar ridge in these areas to experience significantly greater negative dimensional changes following tooth loss compared with posterior sites.[14,15,17]

This information, combined with our ongoing clinical observations, led us to develop a series of treatment algorithms for esthetic implant therapy that reliably provided natural esthetic outcomes while minimizing risk for patients who presented with what had emerged as commonly occurring clinical case scenarios.[7]

As a result of the above, in the mid-1990s, we entered the period of predictability in esthetic implant therapy based on our improved understanding of:

· Key biologic principles
· Anatomical and patient-related factors associated with esthetic implant complications
· Clinical concepts that defined ideal restoration-driven implant placement
· Dimensional requirements for hard and soft tissues at esthetic sites
· The importance of interdisciplinary treatment planning and precise execution
· Sequencing of biologically acceptable treatment protocols by clinicians with advanced levels of training, experience, and clinical skills

As a result of following the treatment-planning principles and treatment algorithms for esthetic implant therapy, we experienced a high level of predictability and very few esthetic implant complications. A consensus among experienced implant clinicians gradually developed, and our early clinical observations and those of other experienced clinicians eventually became supported by clinically oriented evidence-based information.[2,5–35] With the introduction of improved biomaterials and regenerative technologies related to hard and soft tissue implant site development, treatment protocols for esthetic implant therapy evolved and improved.

In subsequent years, despite the emergence of worldwide clinical consensus and evidence-based information in the area of esthetic implant therapy, an increasing percentage of my referral practice revolved around providing consultations, opinions, and care for patients seeking help after experiencing esthetic implant complications. The successful management of these patients was based on the same diagnostic planning and treatment principles that we used to achieve good esthetic outcomes for our new implant patients. However, the psychologic management of these patients differed greatly. Patients who have experienced significant esthetic implant complications have almost invariably suffered some level of emotional distress and financial harm, making it more difficult to establish the level of trust and cooperation required for successful management of their unfortunate situations. This was especially true for the many patients we treated who had already experienced numerous attempts to correct their problems that only resulted in further clinical deterioration. In these cases, clinical and psychologic management can be extremely challenging. Nevertheless, the issues of trust and confidence can be handled in the patient interview process by eliciting the details of the previous treatment experience, acknowledging the patient's misfortune, clearly identifying and educating the patient about the pre-existing risk factors, and establishing realistic treatment expectations.

Unfortunately, detailed case analysis of the many patients who presented with esthetic implant complications indicated that the majority of these complications were preventable and most often associated with a lack of requisite knowledge, diagnostic acumen, and/or clinical experience of the treatment team resulting in an error, omission, or failure to achieve the desired objective in one or more of the following critical phases of patient care in esthetic implant therapy:

1. Patient interview and consultation: Discover the patient's desires and objective(s) for treatment and establish realistic expectations for the clinical process and the treatment outcome.
2. Systematic patient evaluation and esthetic risk assessment: Identify the individual case factors that favor, detract from, or preclude the ability to achieve the desired esthetic outcome. Use appropriate diagnostic aids.

3. Interdisciplinary treatment planning: Formulate treatment options using a comprehensive approach that includes the patient, restorative dentist or prosthodontist, implant surgeon, other specialists, and the dental technician(s). Choose appropriate biomaterials that are strongly supported by evidence-based information and an established record of reliable clinical success.
4. Case presentation: Discuss the details of the potential treatment options, including the number of procedures required, choice and origin of biomaterials, options for provisional restorations, treatment time, relative risk of complications, worst-case scenario, and patient responsibilities. Establish realistic expectations for the treatment outcome, and strongly recommend the treatment approach with the least risk to the patient, avoiding treatment approaches that potentially exceed the healing potential of the site(s).
5. Properly sequence and precisely execute biologically acceptable prosthetic, surgical, and technical procedures: Soft and hard tissue implant site development; precise restoration-driven implant placement; use of provisional restorations to develop esthetic peri-implant soft tissue architecture; and use of individualized impression procedures and digital photography to communicate the desired emergence profile, optical parameters, and surface characterization of the definitive restoration with the dental technician.
6. Completion of the restorative phase of treatment: Following verification of precise contours and fit of abutment(s) and restoration(s), deliver the definitive restoration. Accessible margins are required for cement-retained restorations to avoid devastating biologic complications.
7. Assess the biologic response as it relates to the definitive restoration at recall visits: Closely monitor the clinical and radiographic appearance of the restoration during the first year following delivery and intervene if unexpected tissue recession or progressive bone loss occurs. After the first year, annual recall visits should be performed for a minimum of 2 additional years.

Rationale for case selection

In the following case study, a young female patient presented with a preventable and somewhat devastating esthetic implant complication. She was quite distraught with the results of previous treatment that involved the replacement of her failing maxillary central incisors with implant restorations. This case study demonstrates that treating clinicians must possess the requisite knowledge, experience, patient communication skills, clinical skills, and sense of artistry to provide implant restorations in areas of high esthetic concern. In addition, the importance of using a dental implant system and biomaterials that are compatible with the proposed indication and buttressed by strong evidence-based information is underscored. Finally, the key diagnostic determinants used to decide whether reparative implant site development procedures should be performed versus removal, submergence, or repositioning of a poorly placed and esthetically compromised implant are brought to light by the management of this particular esthetic complication.

Based on the background information provided above and the diagnostic information provided below, readers should focus on developing conventional and implant treatment-planning options for management of this esthetic complication. The key element to consider in this case is whether the desired esthetic outcome can be predictably achieved using the existing implants or an alternative treatment approach is likely to result in a more natural-appearing restoration. This exercise should reinforce the principles for achieving predictable outcomes as well as avoiding and managing complications in esthetic implant therapy.

Case Presentation

Treating clinicians
Surgeon: Anthony G. Sclar, DMD
Prosthodontist: Nuria Otero, DDS, CAGS, MSc
Laboratory technician: Stefano Inglese, RDT

Clinical Treatment Planning

Age at initial presentation: 30 years
Initial presentation: January 2009
Active treatment completed: August 2009

Introduction and background

This 30-year-old female patient presented with a chief complaint of feeling self-conscious about her smile and unhappy with her implant restorations. She was very concerned about the artificial appearance of the "false gums and white porcelain restorations and the purple-black discoloration of the gum tissues" around her maxillary central incisor implant restorations. She stated that she had learned to limit the elevation of her upper lip when she smiled and that this resulted in an awkward appearance in photographs. Her singular objective for seeking treatment was to be able to recapture her natural, unrestricted smile and lost social confidence.

Medical history

- Healthy nonsmoker
- No known allergies
- Not taking any medications or supplements

Dental history

- Traumatic avulsion of teeth nos. 8 and 9 at age 7 years with immediate reimplantation and short-term stabilization followed by endodontic therapy.
- Orthodontic therapy initiated in her late teen years and completed at age 22 years.
- Following initial orthodontic retention, teeth nos. 8 and 9 developed mobility and were removed.
  —Interdisciplinary treatment-planning process was not initiated.
  —Orthodontic extrusion was not considered.
  —Ridge preservation was not performed.
- Lateral ridge augmentation was performed using a guided bone regeneration procedure with particulate allograft bone approximately 1 year after tooth removal.
- Six months after hard tissue site development, endosseous implants were placed at nos. 8 and 9.
  —Peri-implant soft tissue augmentation was not performed.
  —Provisional implant restorations were not used for esthetic soft tissue conditioning.
- Definitive restoration was delivered 6 months after implant placement with an obvious esthetic compromise.
- Esthetic appearance of the restoration continued to deteriorate over the next 3 years with progressive darkening and shrinkage of the peri-implant tissues.

Diagnostic findings

Extraoral and facial findings

- Facial symmetry from the frontal perspective
- Patient smile was restricted for fear of embarrassment
- Exposure of the gingival embrasures and interdental papilla of the maxillary anterior dentition were evident using the phonetic method
- Coincidence of facial, dental, and chin midlines
- Incisal plane parallel to level interpupillary line
- Head and neck examination was negative for pathology

Pretreatment

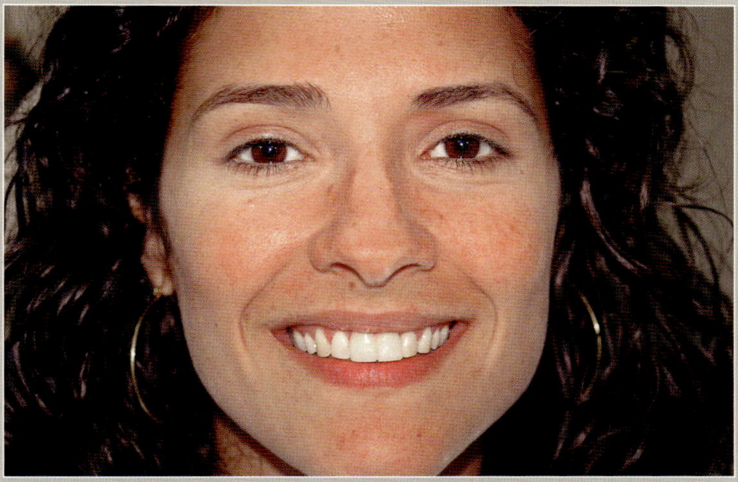

Smile.

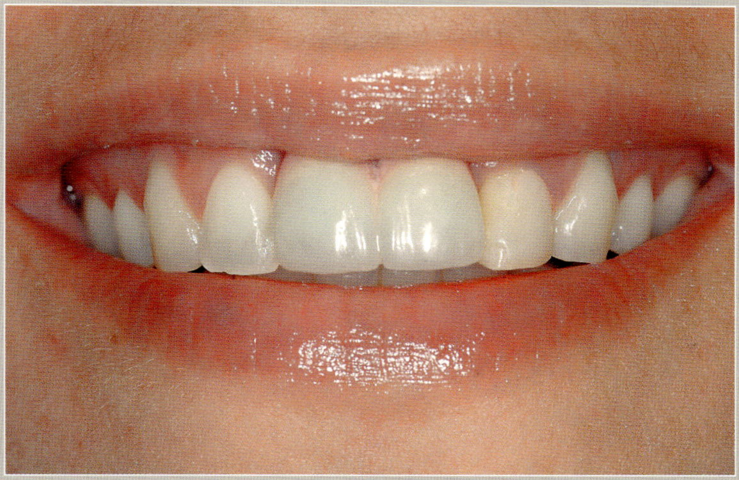

Close-up view of smile.

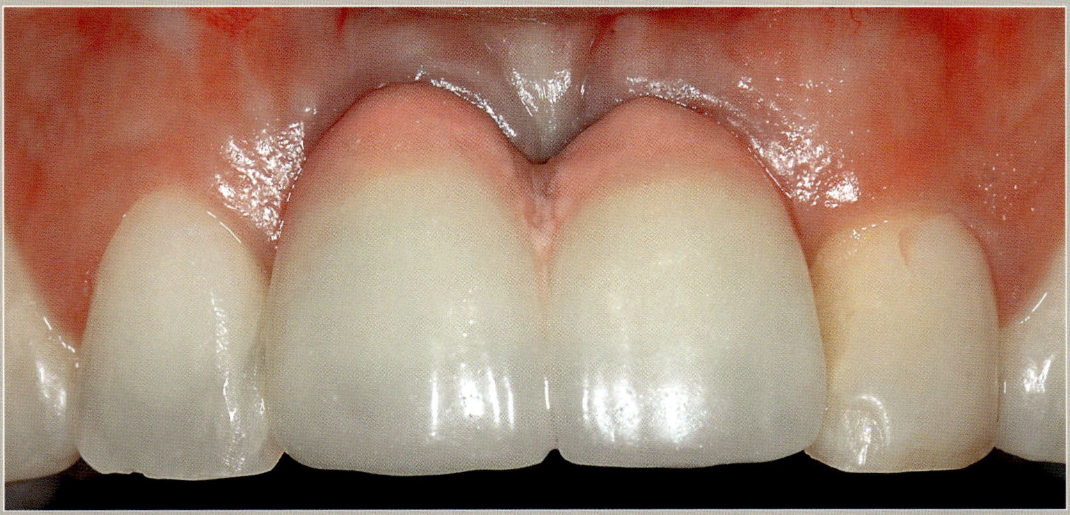

Intraoral frontal view.

TMJ and mandibular range of motion

- Negative for muscle hypertonicity, clinical signs of intracapsular joint pathology, or internal derangement.
- Vertical and excursive jaw motions were normal without evidence of discoordinate movements normally associated with parafunction.

Intraoral findings

- Intraoral examination was unremarkable for oral pathology.
- Periodontal status was very good: probing depths between 2 to 3 mm throughout the mouth except for 5- and 6-mm midfacial probing depths at sites nos. 8 and 9, raising suspicion of potential dehiscence defects in the facial bone. Home care was excellent with low plaque levels.
- Small-volume combination hard and soft tissue esthetic ridge defect evident at implant sites nos. 8 and 9.
- Severe discoloration of peri-implant soft tissue at sites nos. 8 and 9.
- No signs of fibrotic wound healing at sites nos. 8 and 9.
- Suboptimal facial implant positions and axial inclinations.
- Acceptable mesiodistal and apicocoronal implant positions.
- Unesthetic axial inclination (distal tipping) of teeth nos. 7 and 10.
- Moderate deficiency of the mesial papillae of teeth nos. 7 and 10.
- Severe deficiency of the papilla between the implants.

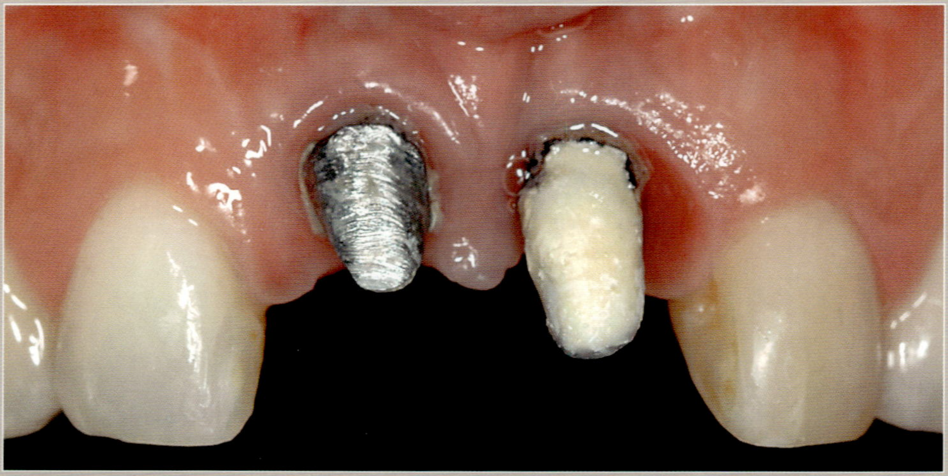

Frontal view of implant abutments.

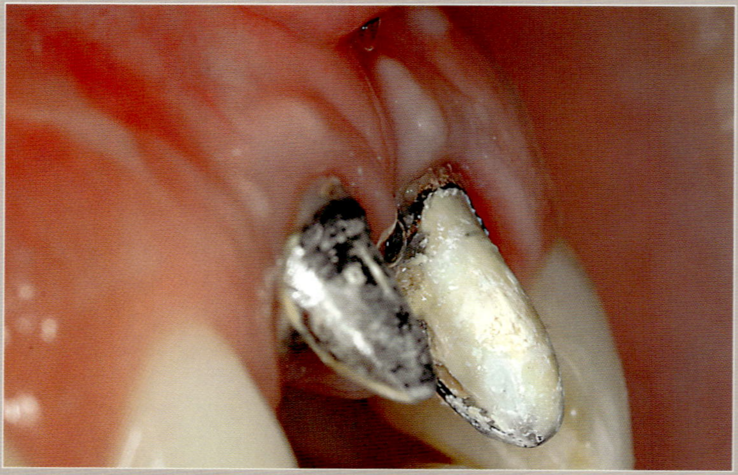

Lateral view of implant abutments.

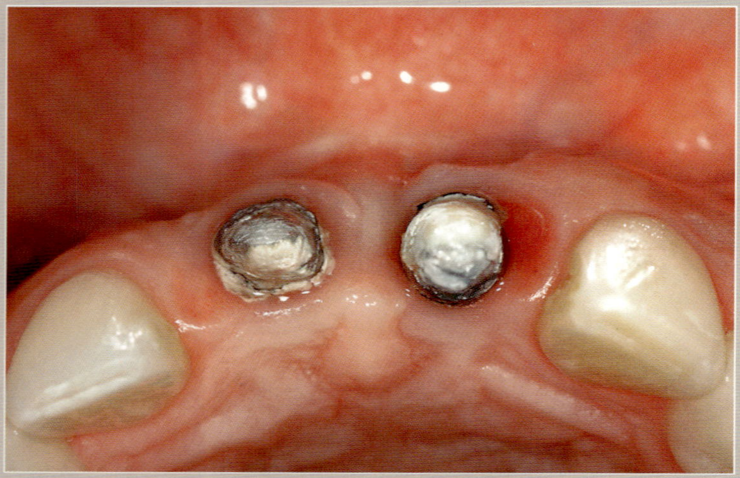

Occlusal view of implant abutments.

- Unesthetic intrinsic proportions of teeth nos. 8 and 9 (width-height ratio: 60%).
- Unfavorable tooth-to-tooth proportions and relationships among the maxillary anterior teeth.
- Bone sounding under local anesthesia using specialized instrumentation revealed that the labiopalatal peri-implant soft tissue dimension at sites nos. 8 and 9 was between 1.0 and 1.25 mm when measured at points 2, 5, and 8 mm apical to the midpoint of the marginal gingiva.

Occlusal notes

- Angle Class I occlusion
- 3-mm overjet and slight anterior open bite
- Group function in lateral excursions with canine-premolar guidance
- Absence of lateral or protrusive contacts on teeth nos. 7, 8, 9, and 10

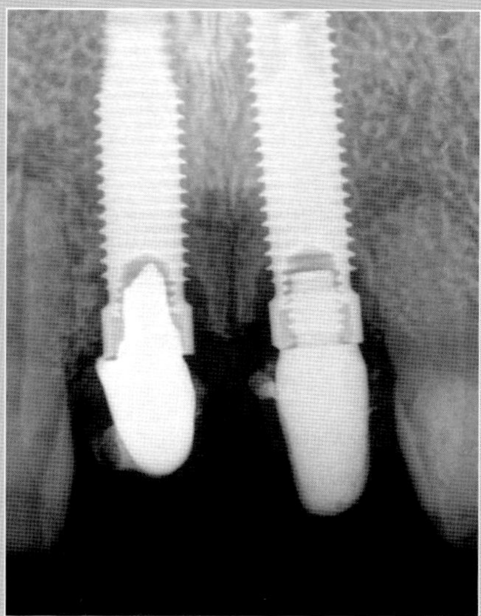

Radiograph of implants.

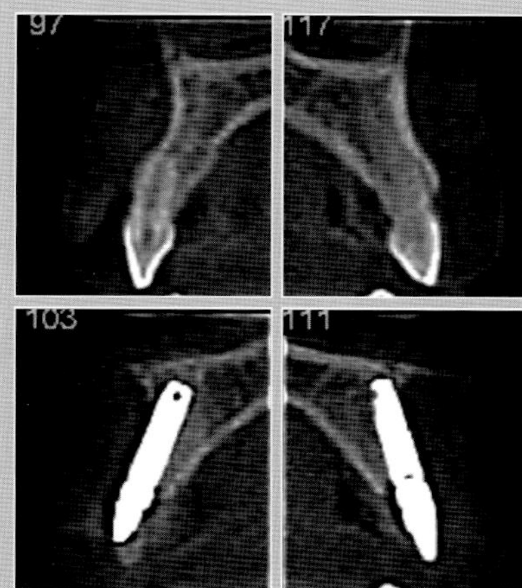

CT imaging.

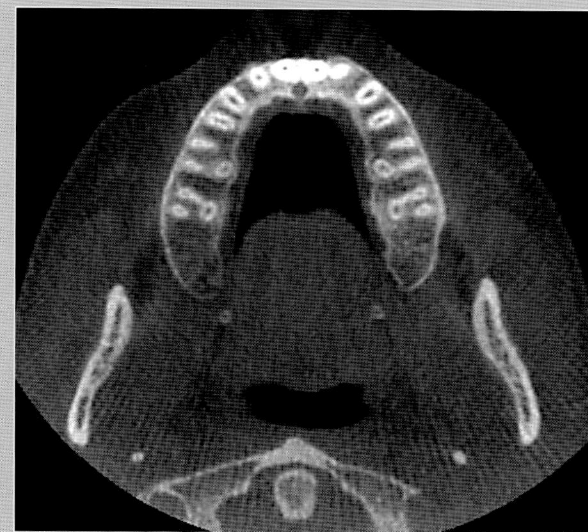

CT imaging.

Radiographic findings

- Implants appear well integrated with excellent density and apposition of peri-implant bone viewed on periapical radiographs.
- Implants in acceptable mesiodistal positions with approximately 1.5 mm between the implants and the lateral incisors and approximately 4.5-mm interimplant distance as measured on periapical radiographs and cone beam computed tomography (CT) images.
- Implants in acceptable apicocoronal positions: about 3 mm apical to an ideal facial gingival margin position, allowing for normal central incisor height of 10 to 11 mm as measured on periapical radiographs and cone beam CT images.
- Implants are positioned facially with suboptimal facial inclinations as viewed on cone beam CT images.
- Cone beam CT images show either bony dehiscences on the facial aspect of the implants at sites nos. 8 and 9 or beam-hardening artifacts.
- Shortened roots of teeth nos. 7 and 10 with unfavorable distal axial inclination.
- Compromised interimplant bone crests and adjacent lateral incisor bone crests.
- Calcified endodontic canal in tooth no. 10.

Diagnosis

Periodontal

- AAP Type I
- Healthy periodontium with generalized periodontal pocketing of 2 to 3 mm

Orthodontic

- Class I occlusion with group function in lateral excursions; anterior open bite with absence of lateral or protrusive contacts on the central incisor implant restorations and adjacent lateral incisors
- Shortened roots of teeth nos. 7 and 10 with unfavorable (distal) axial inclination
- Suboptimal facial position and inclination of implants
- Small-volume combination hard and soft tissue esthetic ridge defects at implant sites
- Severe purple-black discoloration of peri-implant soft tissue at sites nos. 8 and 9
- Compromised interimplant and peri-implant bone crests and papillae
- Intermediate smile pattern with exposure of interdental papillae via the phonetic method (exaggerated *e* sounds)

Prognosis

- Guarded: teeth nos. 7 and 10. Although currently stable without evidence of endodontic or periodontal compromise, teeth nos. 7 and 10 have an uncertain prognosis. Postorthodontic root resorption makes these teeth questionable abutments to support a fixed partial denture.
- Guarded: implants at sites nos. 8 and 9. Although the implants are well integrated and do not demonstrate signs of a biologic or biomechanical compromise, the current esthetic compromise gives them a guarded prognosis.
- Guarded: opportunity to provide esthetically pleasing restorations in the maxillary anterior region.
- Good: all remaining teeth.

Summary of concerns

1. Are the patient's expectations for the treatment outcomes realistic? Does the patient fully comprehend the risks, worst-case scenario, and long-term implications of the individual treatment options?
2. How do we determine whether to remove the existing implants or perform reparative implant site development procedure(s)? What are the restorative and surgical determinants that influence our decision making?
3. If a decision is made to proceed with reparative implant site development procedures, should the implant restorations be removed so as to temporarily submerge the implants or should the restorations be modified or replaced with provisional restorations designed to facilitate the grafting procedures? What are the restorative and surgical determinants that influence our decision making?
4. If a decision is made to proceed with a conventional fixed partial denture, should the lateral incisors be used as abutments or removed? Should the existing implants be removed or submerged? What are the restorative, surgical, and technical determinants that will influence our decision making?
5. The compromise of the interimplant and adjacent lateral incisor bone crests in this case are known risk factors to achieving an esthetically pleasing implant restoration with a natural-appearing scalloped soft tissue architecture. This esthetic risk is greatly magnified with adjacent multi-unit implant restorations. How can we mitigate the negative esthetic effect of this anatomical limitation in this case?
6. Which treatment option will best satisfy the patient's esthetic concerns?
7. Which treatment option is likely to yield the best long-term functional and esthetic outcome for the patient?

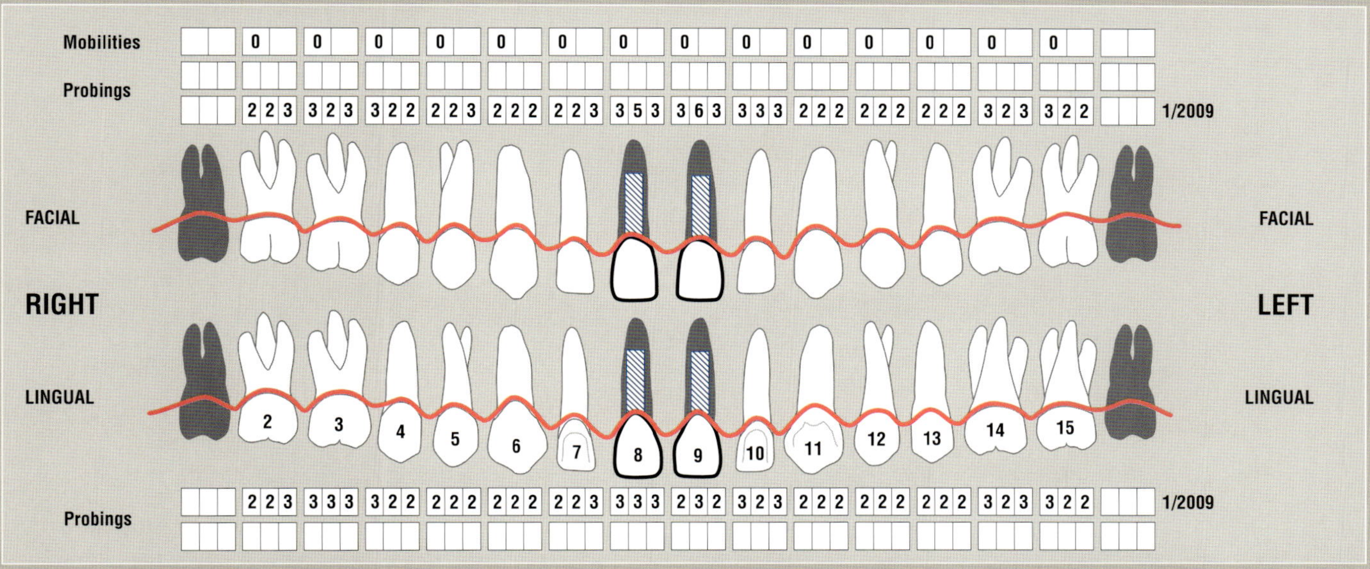

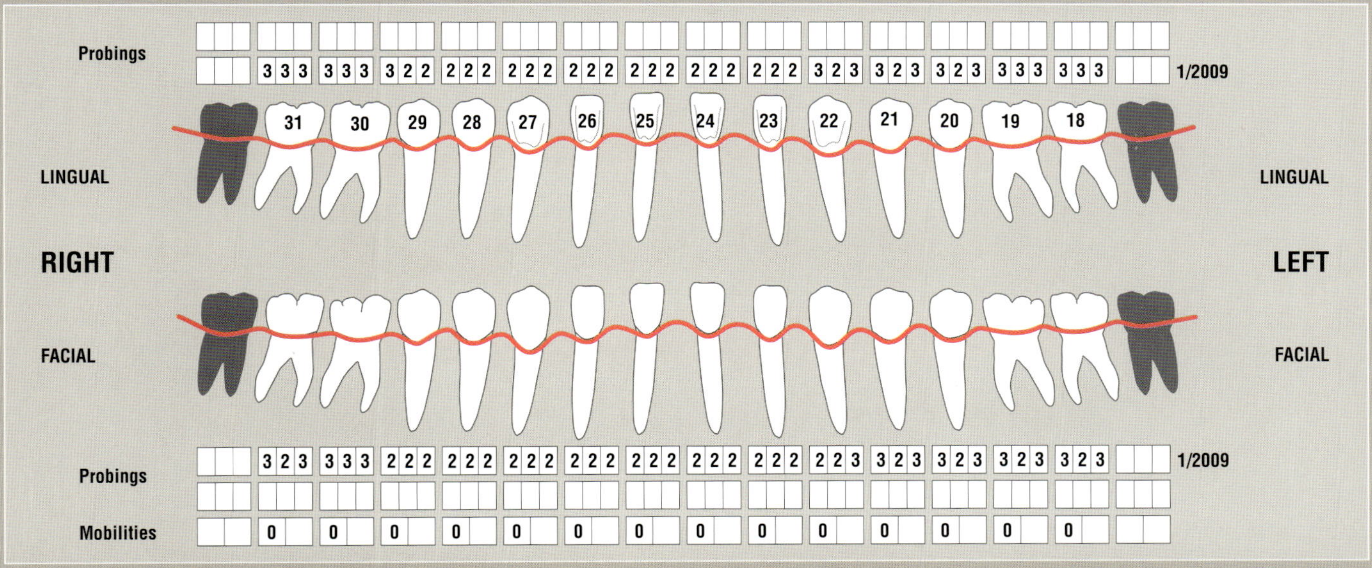

As a learning exercise, you may now outline goals/objectives of treatment and a treatment plan.

Proposed Treatment Plan

Treatment options

Following an interdisciplinary approach to diagnosis and treatment planning that included the prosthodontist, surgeon, laboratory technician, and the patient's stated objectives for treatment, four treatment options were presented to the patient.

Treatment option 1: We would perform necessary surgical implant site development procedures to restore natural labial and interproximal soft tissue esthetic appearance at sites nos. 8 and 9. Following an estimated 3-month healing period, we would employ prosthetic soft tissue conditioning and stabilization using provisional implant restorations to gain some degree of scalloped soft tissue architecture. This would take place over an additional 3-month period. We would then re-evaluate for possible surgical follow-up procedures such as scar revision, additional augmentation procedures, or soft tissue surgical sculpting. Treatment would be completed with custom abutments and individual ceramic implant restorations and porcelain laminate restorations for the lateral incisors to harmonize esthetic tooth-to-tooth proportions and facilitate prosthetic compensation of deficient papillae as needed. Fixed provisional implant restorations would be used at all stages of treatment.

Treatment option 2: We would perform minimally traumatic removal of the maxillary lateral incisors with ridge preservation and perform surgical implant and pontic site development procedures at sites nos. 7, 8, 9, and 10. After a 3-month period for healing, we would follow the prosthetic soft tissue conditioning treatment sequence as outlined in option 1 and complete treatment with two individual fixed implant restorations with cantilevered lateral incisor pontics. Fixed provisional implant restorations would be employed at all stages of treatment.

Treatment option 3: We would begin with the minimally traumatic removal of the maxillary lateral incisors and the central incisor implants with ridge preservation and surgical implant site development procedures at sites nos. 7, 8, 9, and 10. After a 3- to 6-month healing period, we would place smaller-diameter implants at sites 7, 8, 9, and 10 with additional site development procedures as needed. We would follow the prosthetic soft tissue conditioning treatment sequence as outlined in option 1 and complete treatment with four individual fixed esthetic implant restorations. Options for interim provisional restorations would include removable tooth- or tissue-borne restorations or a fixed provisional restoration supported by prepared maxillary canine abutments.

Treatment option 4: We would begin with minimally traumatic removal of the maxillary lateral incisors and the central incisor implants with ridge preservation and surgical and prosthetic pontic site development procedures at sites nos. 7, 8, 9, and 10. After a 3- to 6-month healing period, treatment would be finalized with a six-unit conventional fixed partial denture. Options for interim provisional restorations would be the same as those outlined for option 3.

After comparative discussion of the treatment process, relative benefits, risks, and long-term implications of the four treatment options outlined above, the patient expressed her desire to "avoid a dental or implant bridge" and to "maintain her maxillary lateral incisors as is" and agreed to cosmetic porcelain laminate restorations. Based on the patient's goals and objectives for treatment and our diagnostic findings, we made a strong recommendation for treatment option 1. The patient accepted our recommendation but qualified her decision by expressing an absolute expectation for individual implant restorations without "false gums." This made it clear that the patient did not fully understand the worst-case scenarios for the implant treatment options that were discussed during the case presentation. The treatment team re-educated her about the potential limitations of treatment based largely on our inability to predict the wound healing response of the site. As a result of this discussion, the patient understood, acknowledged, and accepted these possible limitations and consequences. She acknowledged that there was a possibility that a conventional or implant-supported fixed partial denture with artificial gingival tissue would turn out to be the best option for esthetic reconstruction of the area in question should there be further deterioration of her condition following any of the proposed surgical or prosthetic procedures.

Goals/objectives of treatment

- To provide a restorative solution that is as straightforward and minimally invasive as possible based on the patient's previous negative dental experience and her desire to preserve her remaining dentition
- To achieve an esthetically pleasing outcome in the midst of pre-existing suboptimal implant positions and compromised hard and soft tissue architecture
- To maintain focus on well-founded biologic principles in developing the final treatment plan in a compromised and very challenging clinical situation
- To ensure that all members of the interdisciplinary treatment team are well informed and on the same page throughout every step in treatment

Although all of the treatment options discussed during the case presentation had the potential to successfully address the patient's initially stated chief concern, the interdisciplinary approach to treatment planning that included the patient, prosthodontist, surgeon, and technician led to the selection of treatment option 1. This option was viewed as the least invasive approach involving the application of biologically acceptable prosthetic and surgical treatment protocols used to reliably achieve a pleasing esthetic outcome based on our diagnostic findings. Although the implants were located in a suboptimal labial position and inclination, the location of the crestal implant emergence was the key diagnostic determinant that influenced our decision to perform reparative procedures rather than remove, submerge, or reposition the implants. Despite the less-than-ideal labial position and inclination, the labial crestal emergence of the central incisor implants was approximately 1.5 to 2.0 mm palatal to the labial emergence of the adjacent lateral incisors at the level of the gingival margin, thereby satisfying the surgical requirements that the implants must be located within the alveolar housing in order to achieve success with reparative peri-implant soft and hard tissue procedures.[36-41]

Had the degree of labial malposition or inclination of the implants resulted in a crestal emergence 0 to 1.0 mm palatal to the labial emergence of the adjacent lateral incisors, consideration would have been given to temporarily submerging the implants by removing the restorations and placing cover screws in preparation for performing the reparative implant site development procedures after an appropriate healing period. If the crestal emergence of the implants had been labial to the emergence of the adjacent teeth at the gingival level or if there had been a concomitant apicocoronal and mesiodistal implant malposition, consideration would have been given to *(1)* permanently submerging the implant in preparation for a conventional restoration, *(2)* removing the implant in preparation for subsequent replacement in an acceptable anatomical position, or *(3)* repositioning the implant via an osteotomy procedure.

Because it had been a number of years since the implants were placed, there was a question as to whether suitable restorative components would be available to customize the provisional and definitive restorations. After some investigation, the prosthodontist and dental technician confirmed that they could fabricate custom components that would meet the case requirements, and we proceeded to formulate potential treatment options for the patient. Based on our past experience with esthetic complications and compromise, we believed that treatment option 1 would pose a low level of esthetic risk while meeting or exceeding the patient's treatment expectations.

Furthermore, it was understood by the patient and the treatment team that should a failure in the course of treatment result in further loss of peri-implant hard and soft tissues, we would then have to consider one of the other more invasive and complex treatment options.

The discussion of the relative risks of each treatment option during the critical case presentation phase helped the patient make an informed decision to proceed. After further discussion, she was able to understand and accept the worst-case scenarios that she might experience during treatment. The patient's expectations were set at a realistic level by following the same patient education and risk management process that we use with new esthetic implant patients.

The long-term implications of any selected treatment option must also be understood by the patient and treating clinicians. For treatment option 1, this included the need for close monitoring of the maxillary lateral incisors, which, because of their shortened roots, had a guarded prognosis even in the absence of an occlusal biomechanical risk. Although orthodontic extrusion of the lateral incisors was considered to improve the height of the bone crests adjacent to the existing implants, thereby improving support for the papillae, the compromised root lengths precluded this option. This also conflicted with the patient's desire to "maintain her lateral incisors for as long as possible and avoid any type of fixed partial denture." However, the patient also understood that if the lateral incisors subsequently began to fail, orthodontic extrusion could be considered to improve vertical bone and soft tissue heights prior to extraction of these teeth. This would ultimately improve the peri-implant papillae and the overall esthetic result.

Phase I: Prosthetic preparation for implant site development procedures

1. Delivery of customized provisional restorations on implants at sites nos. 8 and 9 in preparation for implant site development procedures
2. Monitoring of biologic response of peri-implant hard and soft tissues prior to surgery

Phase II: Implant site development procedures

3. Simultaneous hard and soft tissue implant site development
4. Close monitoring of biologic response with postoperative clinical and radiographic evaluation at 10 days, 6 weeks, and 3 months
5. Reinforcement of oral hygiene and dietary instructions at each follow-up visit
6. At 3-month follow-up visit, clinical and radiographic evaluation to determine whether the implant site development procedures were successful in restoring appropriate soft tissue bulk and levels for prosthetic soft tissue conditioning

Phase III: Prosthetic soft tissue conditioning

7. Delivery of second set of provisional restorations to support adjacent papilla, determine the final gingival margin positions, and develop the gingival zeniths
8. Monitoring of tissue response over the first 7 to 10 days and modification of cervical contours as needed to refine the soft tissue architecture
9. Allowance of approximately 3 months for tissue maturation, stabilization of marginal tissues, and maturation of the peri-implant sulcus

Phase IV: Definitive restoration

10. Final impression procedure using a custom impression technique designed to register implant position and capture the cervical contours and esthetic soft tissue architecture at the sites
11. Try-in and modification of definitive abutments as needed
12. Delivery of definitive restorations

Phase V: Assessment of the biologic response to the definitive restorations

13. Clinical and radiographic examinations performed at 2 weeks, 3 months, 7 months, 1 year, and 2 years following delivery of the definitive restorations in order to monitor the biologic response of the hard and soft tissues
14. Additional recall visits planned for 3 and 5 years after delivery of the definitive restoration to verify long-term stability of the esthetic outcome and monitor the status of the adjacent dentition

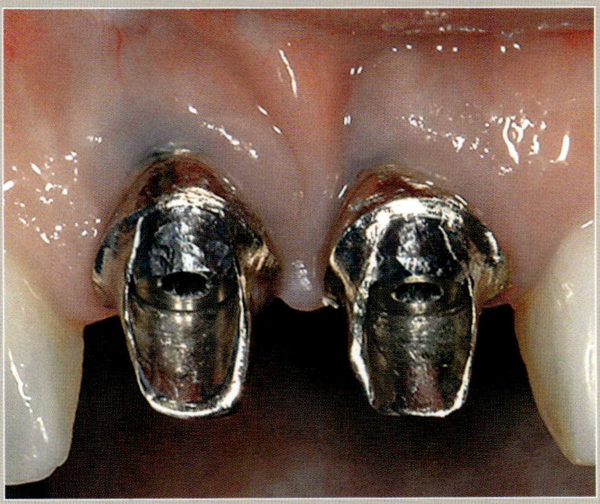

Custom abutments with concave gingival design.

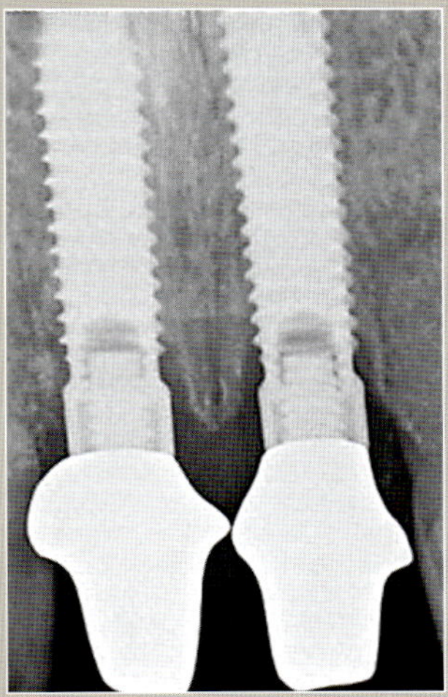

Radiograph of provisional abutments.

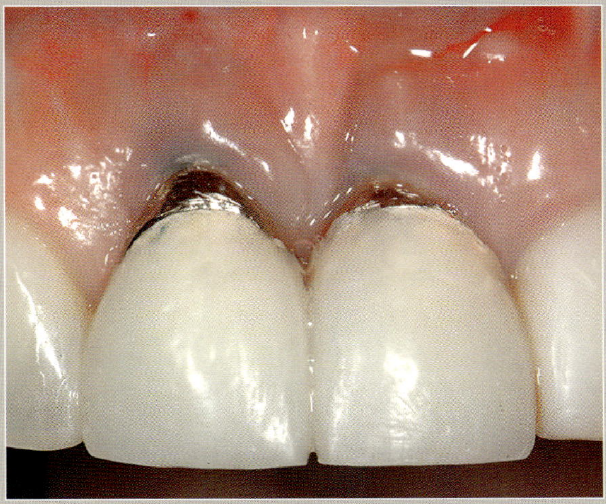

First set of provisional restorations.

Phase I: Prosthetic preparation for implant site development

After clinical and radiographic examinations confirmed that the crestal emergence of the implants was within the alveolar housing and thereby amenable to surgical repair, a request was made for the fabrication and delivery of custom abutments and provisional restorations. These were designed to compensate for the labial inclination and malposition of the central incisor implants and to optimize the initial healing and subsequent maturation of the hard and soft tissue grafts. In this case, manufacturer-discontinued implants and parts (Nobel Biocare) limited the prosthetic options available to address the existing problem. The sole remaining option was to fabricate a gold custom abutment (UCLA). Each abutment incorporated a highly polished concave gingival design with a coronally positioned supragingival finish line. Provisional restorations (Luxatemp, DMG) were fabricated for cementation over the provisional abutments.

Commentary

When grafting procedures are contemplated around esthetic implants with suboptimal labial position and inclination, prosthetic correction is required to decrease the prominence of the emerging implant components, providing room for hard or soft tissue grafts. This process is analogous to the mechanical preparation of an exposed root surface when there is a Miller Class III recession defect in order to convert it to Miller Class I or II, thereby mitigating the negative effect of root prominence and improving the potential to achieve full root coverage via the bridging phenomenon.[36,37,40]

Should the crestal emergence of an esthetic implant be labial to the point of emergence of the adjacent natural teeth, reparative implant site development procedures may be futile because the coronal portion of the implant is outside the alveolar housing. Implants malpositioned to this extent are analogous to excessively prominent natural teeth with Miller Class IV recession defects. The anatomical characteristics of an excessively prominent implant limit the level of success that can be achieved with reparative implant site development procedures.[6,28] In these situations, it is best to consider removal or submergence of the implant(s). Under certain circumstances, a repositioning osteotomy to relocate and reorient the implant into a biologically acceptable three-dimensional position can be performed.[42]

Reducing the prominence of the implant abutments by incorporating a concave design reduces tension on the margins of the coronally advanced cover flaps at the time of the reparative surgery, thereby reducing the risk of compromising circulation to the flap margin.[6,43–45] The concave gingival portion of the abutment also functions as a guide for tissue growth after hard and soft tissue augmentation surgery.[4,6–9,13,16,17,24,25]

In this case, supragingival finish lines, coronal to the concave gingival portion of the abutment, were planned for the surgery to allow for maximal coronal positioning of the grafts and cover flaps. This also aided in avoiding the potential negative effect of microbial contaminants on the development of a healthy and stable peri-implant sulcus before implementing dynamic tissue shaping with subsequent provisional restorations.[46]

Although the treatment team would have preferred to use one-piece screw-retained provisional implant restorations, the less-than-ideal labial position and inclination of the central incisor implants precluded their use in this case.

Phase II: Implant site development procedures

Simultaneous hard and soft tissue peri-implant augmentation was performed using a guided bone regeneration procedure and thick connective tissue grafts harvested from maxillary tuberosity areas. The standard operating room aseptic technique was used with sterile draping. The exposed implant surfaces were thoroughly scrubbed with chlorhexidine-soaked gauze sponges and chemically prepared with 24% ethylenediaminetetraacetic acid (EDTA) root surface conditioner (PrefGel, Straumann) followed by copious lavage with sterile saline solution.

A full-thickness–partial-thickness papilla-sparing curvilinear incision was used to gain access to the site with vertical releasing incisions camouflaged in the interdental space between the canine and first premolar. This provided ample access for debridement of the defect area to remove all soft tissue remnants and decontamination of the dehisced implant surfaces using a CO_2 laser with saline irrigation.

The hard tissue recipient site was prepared with multiple cortical bone perforations and grafted with a combination of autogenous bone harvested from the local area and cancellous bovine bone mineral (Bio-Oss, Geistlich). Platelet-rich plasma (PRP) was used to improve the workability of the graft complex, allowing restoration of the natural arch of the alveolar ridge in the defect area. The graft was isolated with two layers of a resorbable collagen barrier membrane (Bio-Gide, Geistlich).

The connective tissue grafts were intimately adapted over the facial aspect of the concave portion of the provisional abutments and stabilized with sutures anchored to the deepithelialized papillae and to the adjacent prepared connective tissue beds.

The cover flap was coronally advanced to ensure complete coverage of the hard and soft tissue grafts and passively secured with periodontal sling sutures around the neck of the abutments. This resulted in an appropriate vertical soft tissue level and soft tissue augmentation of the papillae in the area. The releasing incisions were closed with simple interrupted sutures.

Commentary

When the bone-loading surface of an implant is exposed to the oral cavity, the surface must be decontaminated if reintegration is to occur in that area. Although no one method has proven superior, mechanical and chemical preparation of contaminated surfaces is recommended, and the use of laser technology has shown promise in animal studies, where it has allowed reintegration of implant surfaces that have been exposed and contaminated as a result of peri-implantitis.[47–49] In this particular case, a portion of the facial implant surfaces was exposed and contaminated as a result of labial wall dehiscence defects. There was no evidence of peri-implant inflammation or infection. Nevertheless, the decision to follow the steps required to decontaminate the implant surfaces seemed prudent and was a matter of clinical judgment and experience.

The decision to use a coronally repositioned, curvilinear, papilla-sparing flap was based on the superiority of this approach for simultaneous hard and soft tissue augmentations and the avoidance of further compromise of the interimplant and adjacent interdental bone crests, which can occur following the use of papilla elevation flaps.[50–56] In addition, this surgical approach provided the opportunity to simultaneously enhance the compromised papillae, ultimately leading to a better esthetic result in this difficult case.[6,28,57,58]

The decision to use a slow substitution rate bovine bone mineral graft (Bio-Oss) and a resorbable collagen membrane (Bio-Gide) to isolate the graft was based on the success of these materials for contour grafting over implants in esthetic areas.[59–62] In this case, autogenous bone was first grafted directly to the implant surface and stabilized with PRP, after which the contour bovine mineral graft was applied. The decision to use the PRP was based on the tremendous technical advantage that it provides for delivering, molding, and stabilizing particulate bone grafts and barrier membranes during surgery. It also has the added benefits provided by the cellular adhesion molecules and growth factors contained within, which may potentiate enhanced early wound healing and reintegration of the exposed implant surfaces.[63–69]

The decision to use subepithelial connective tissue grafts harvested from the maxillary tuberosity areas was based on the increased volume of good quality connective tissue typically available from these donor sites. Compared with donor tissue harvested from the palate, these grafts provide greater contour augmentation and superior masking of underlying metal implant components.[5,70,71]

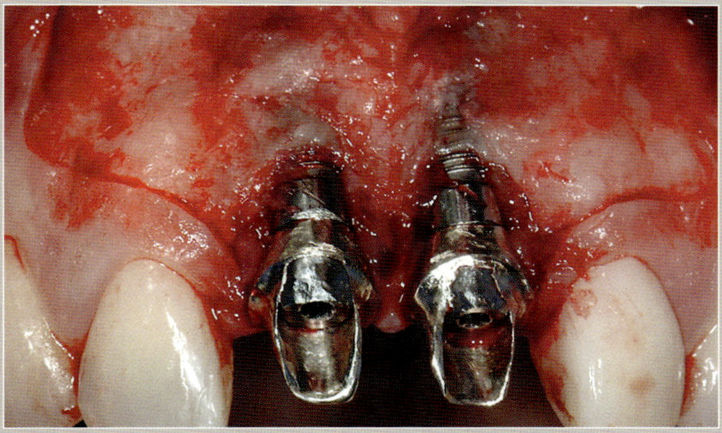

Incision to gain access to the augmentation site.

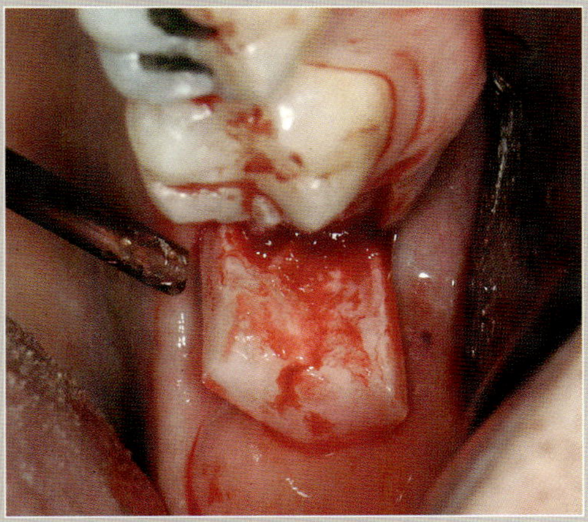

Graft harvest.

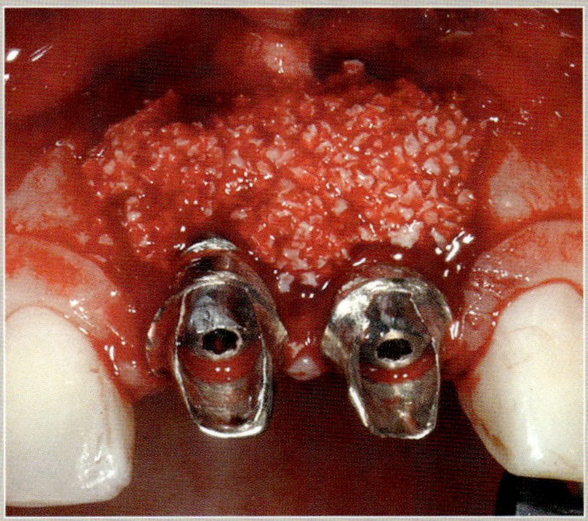

Placement of bone graft material.

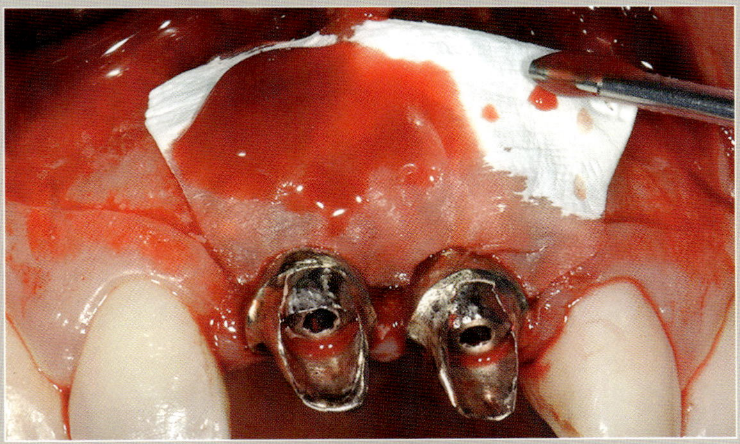

Placement of Bio-Gide membrane.

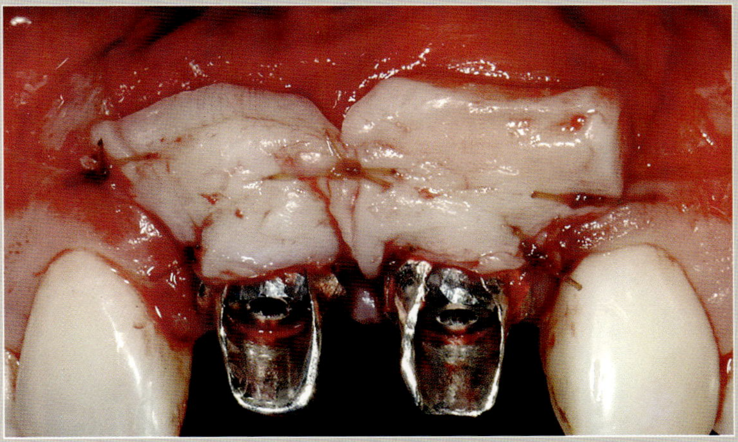

Sutured connective tissue grafts.

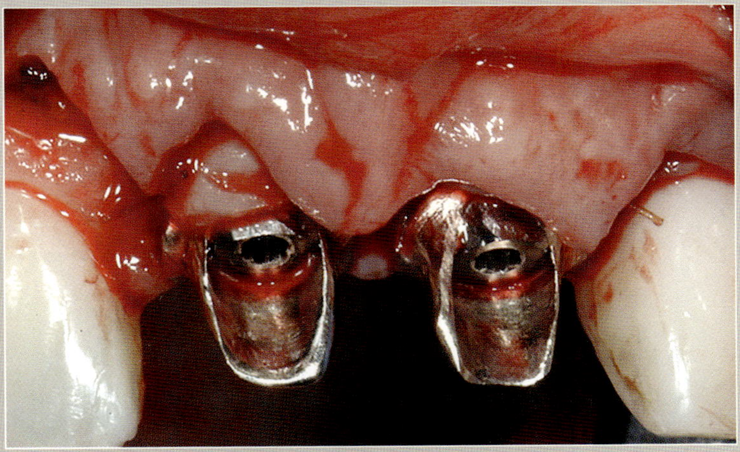

Passive coronal advancement of the cover flap.

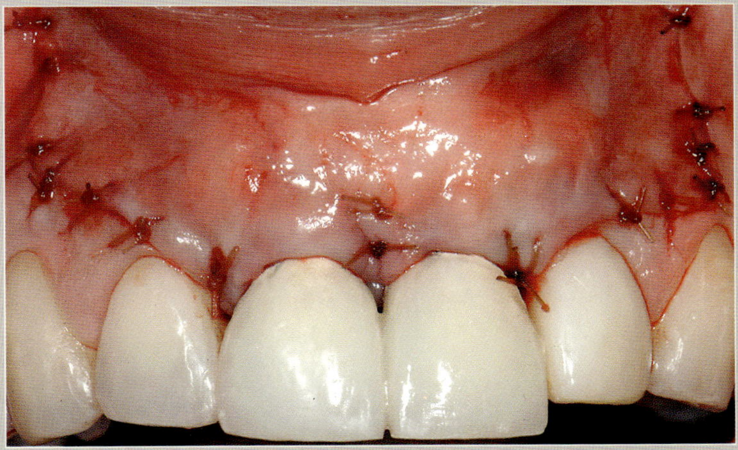

Frontal view following hard and soft tissue peri-implant augmentation.

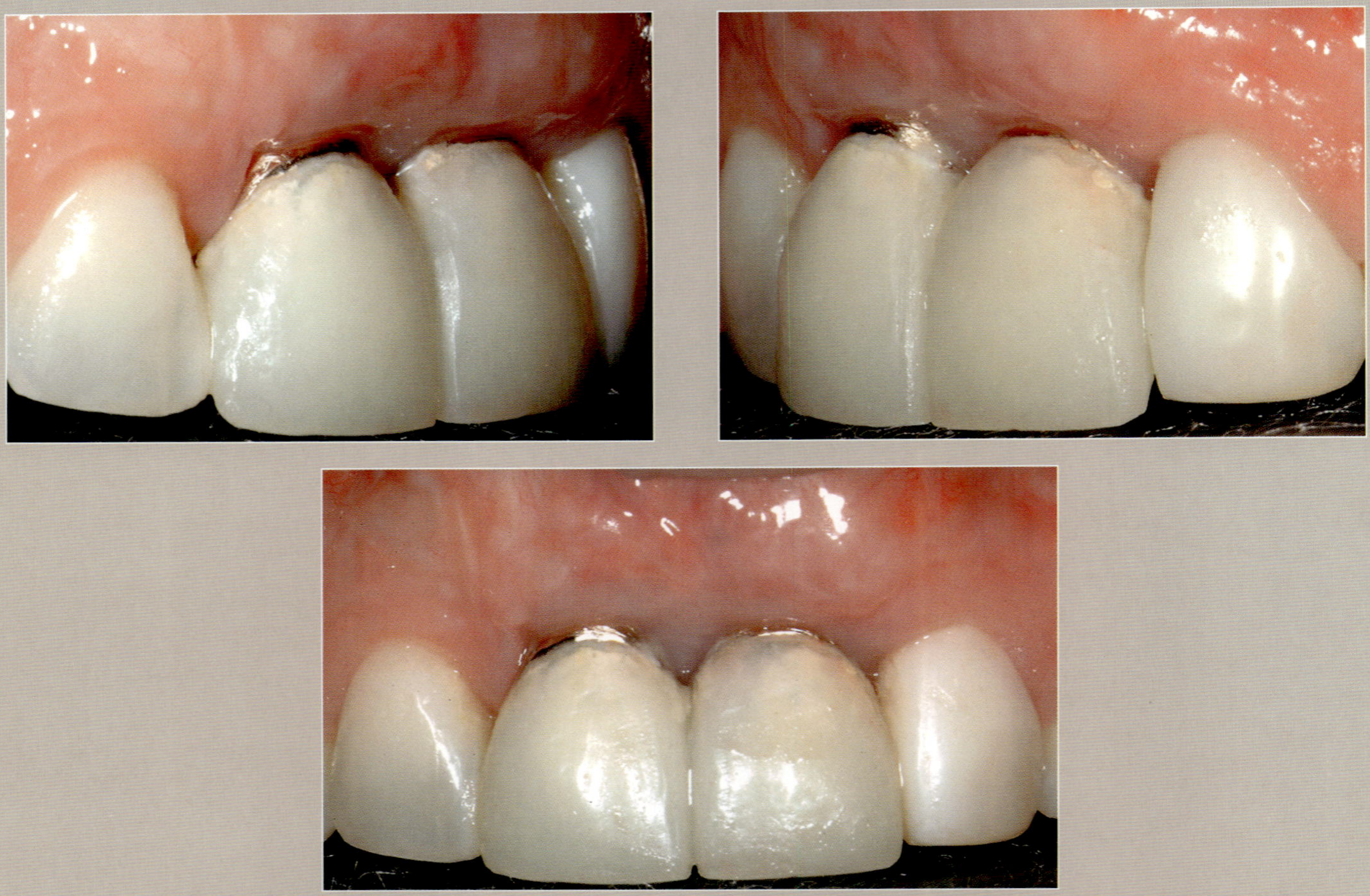

Lateral and frontal views after healing of grafts.

Phase III: Prosthetic soft tissue conditioning

After allowing 3 months for maturation of the hard and soft tissue grafts, a second set of provisional restorations was delivered using an aseptic technique. The new provisional restorations were designed for dynamic soft tissue shaping with appropriate cervical contours to support adjacent papillae and to precisely determine the labial gingival margin position. Accessible intrasulcular finish lines were located approximately 1.0 to 1.5 mm within the sulcus. Although sequential modifications of the contours are typically required to establish the desired gingival margin position and define the gingival zenith, none were required in this case. Another 3-month period was allowed for tissue maturation and stabilization of marginal tissues and the peri-implant sulcus before proceeding with the definitive restoration.[45–47,72]

Commentary

Whenever an abutment is removed and reconnected or replaced, an aseptic and minimally traumatic approach should be used because it has been documented that this seemingly innocuous procedure can reset the biologic width, causing apical migration of the crestal bone and soft tissue attachments.[73] Evidence-based information indicates that this process is typified by damage to the peri-implant soft tissue and bacterial contamination arising from the implant-abutment junction.[74–80]

A common sense practice when changing abutments is to use an aseptic technique and disinfect the area by irrigating with 0.12% chlorhexidine solution or applying a chlorhexidine gel. Furthermore, abutment changes should be accomplished quickly, thereby avoiding soft tissue collapse and subsequent tissue trauma caused by an attempt to seat an abutment over collapsed peri-implant soft tissues.

Another important concept related to the seating of abutments or delivery of esthetic provisional restorations is the need to monitor tissue blanching, which should resolve within 5 to 10 minutes, to avoid tissue necrosis and loss of the peri-implant soft tissue volume that can lead to esthetic deformities. In this particular case, no additional contour modifications were required after delivery of the second set of provisional restorations. Nevertheless, it is always important to closely monitor the tissue response for the first 7 to 10 days following the delivery of an esthetic implant-supported provisional restoration and to modify the cervical contours as needed to perfect and preserve the soft tissue architecture.[6,7,24,45,81–85]

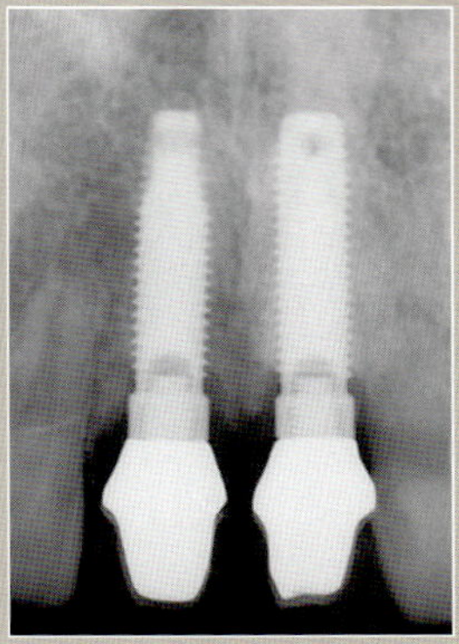

Radiograph following graft healing.

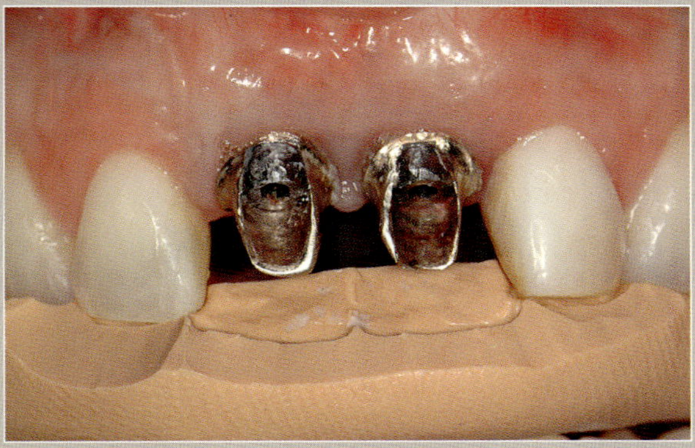

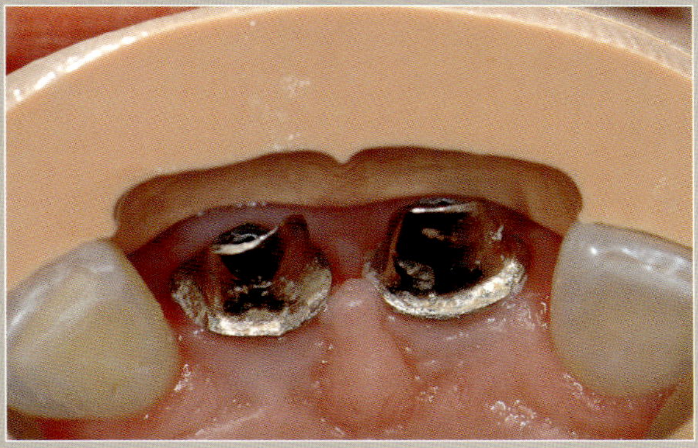

Modification of abutments for the second set of provisional restorations verified with silicone matrices.

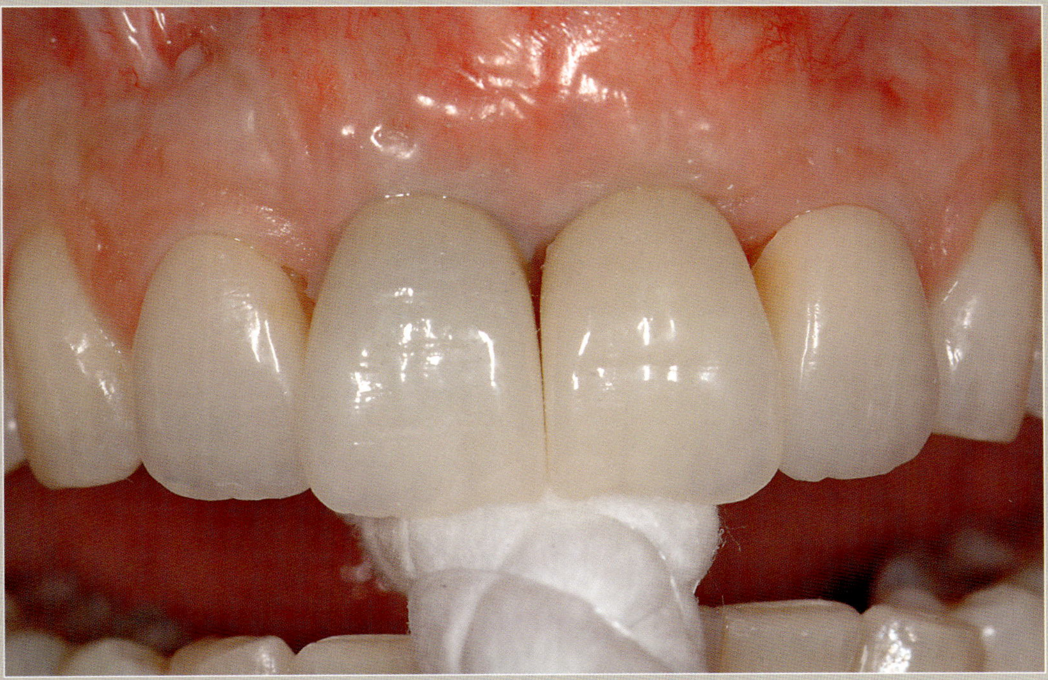

Intraoral view of second set of provisional restorations.

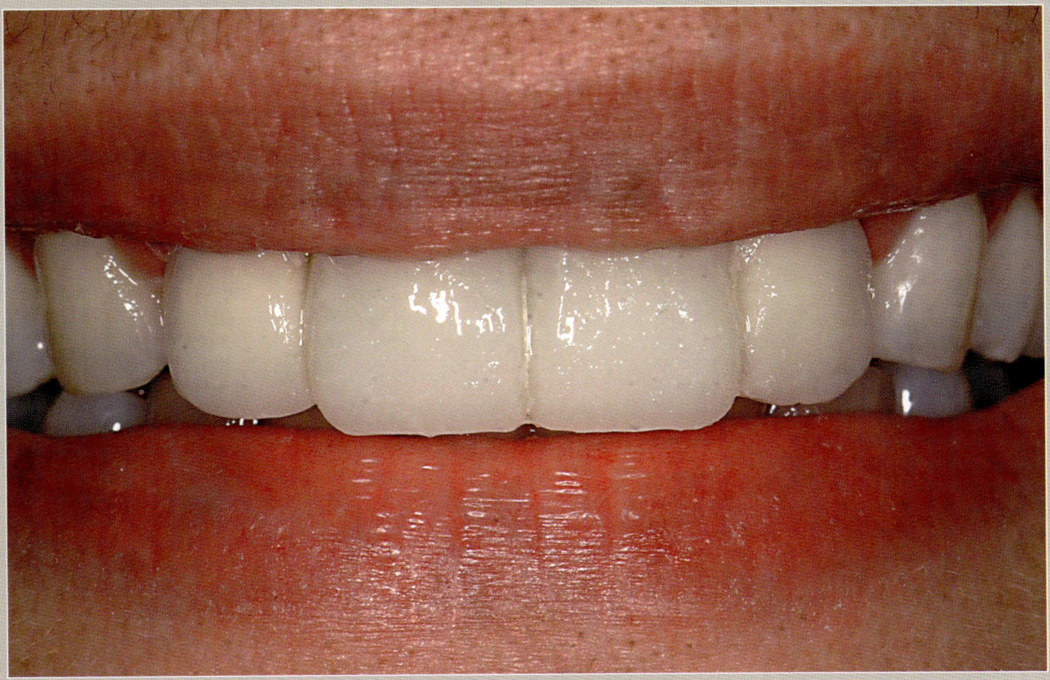

Close-up of smile with second set of provisional restorations.

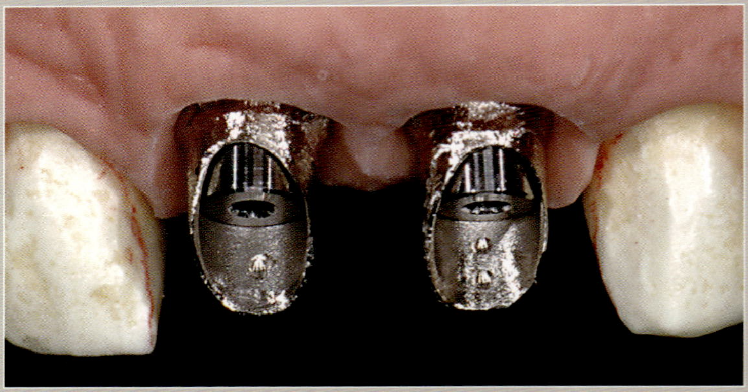

Gold casting of definitive custom abutments.

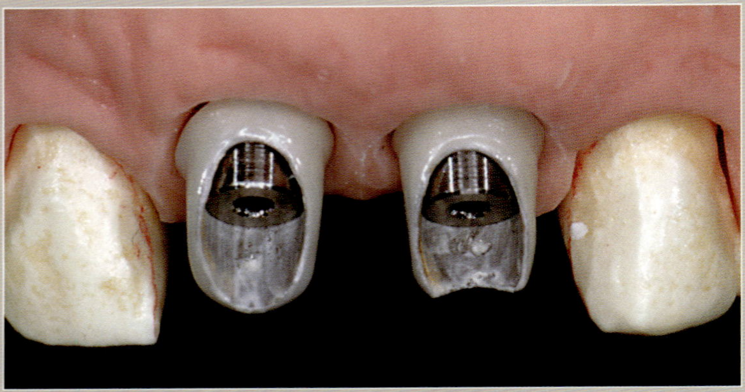

Ceramic covering on definitive abutments.

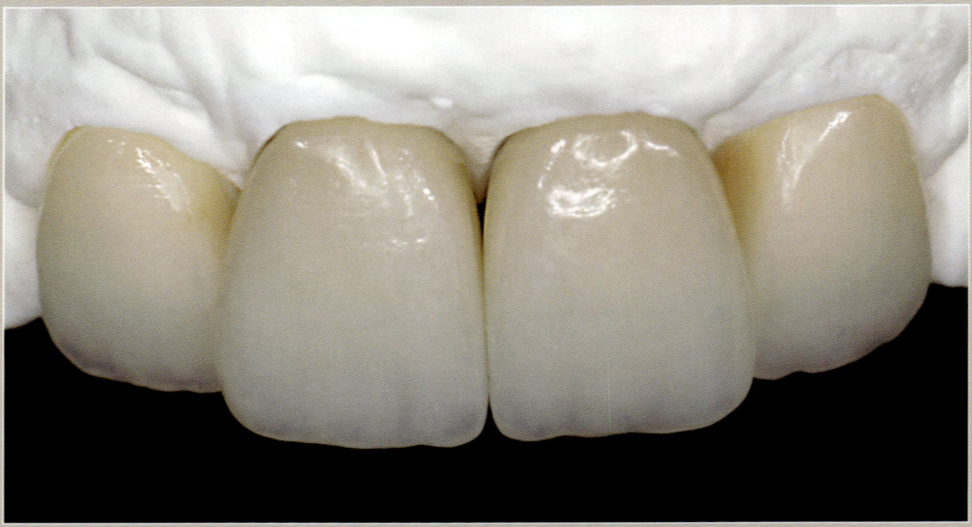

Definitive restorations on master cast.

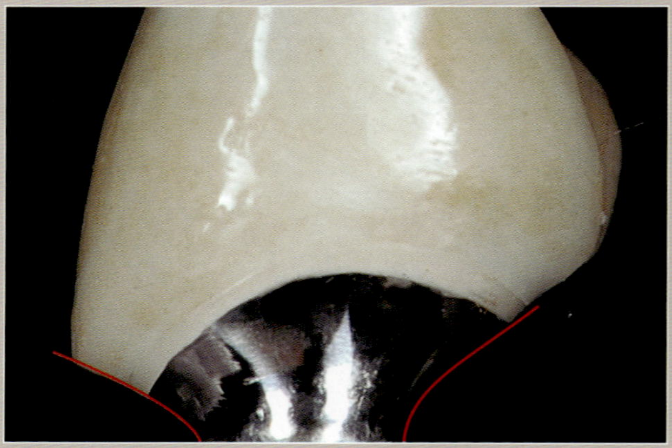

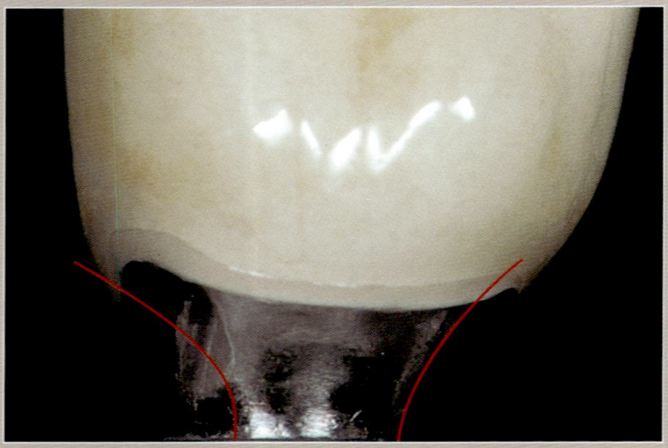

Emergence profiles of definitive restorations.

Phase IV: Definitive restoration

Once stability of the reconstructed esthetic soft tissue architecture surrounding the central incisor implants had been achieved (6 months postoperatively), final impressions were taken using a closed-tray customized impression procedure with polyvinyl siloxane material (Exaflex, GC). The impression procedure registered the implant positions and captured the cervical contours and labial gingival margin position developed by the second set of implant provisional restorations.

The definitive custom abutments (UCLA) were fabricated to duplicate the cervical contours and emergence profile developed by the second set of provisional restorations. The abutments were cast with a high-quality gold casting material to prevent porosity and covered with opaque and translucent ceramic to achieve a more natural-appearing implant

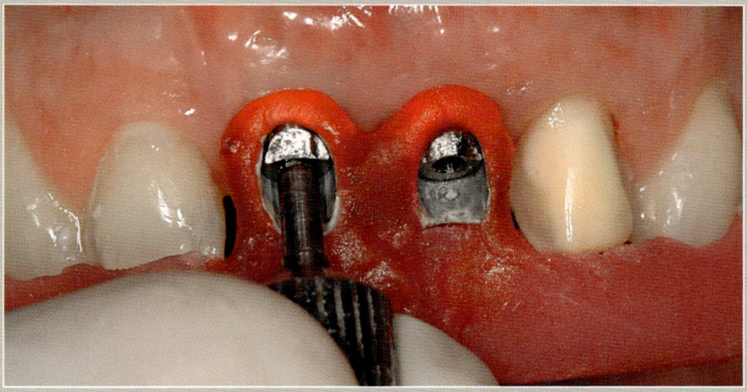

Try-in of abutments.

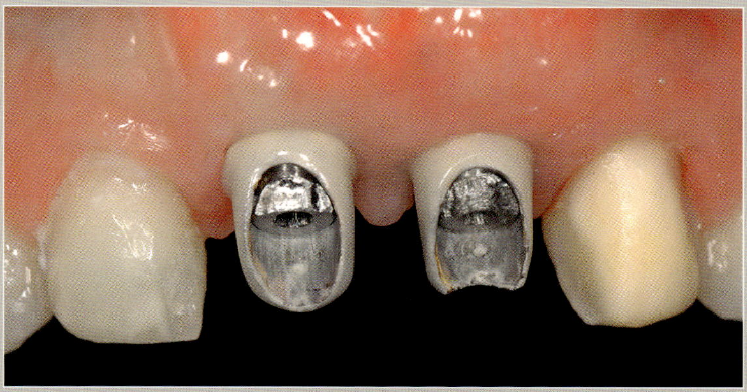

Definitive custom abutments in place.

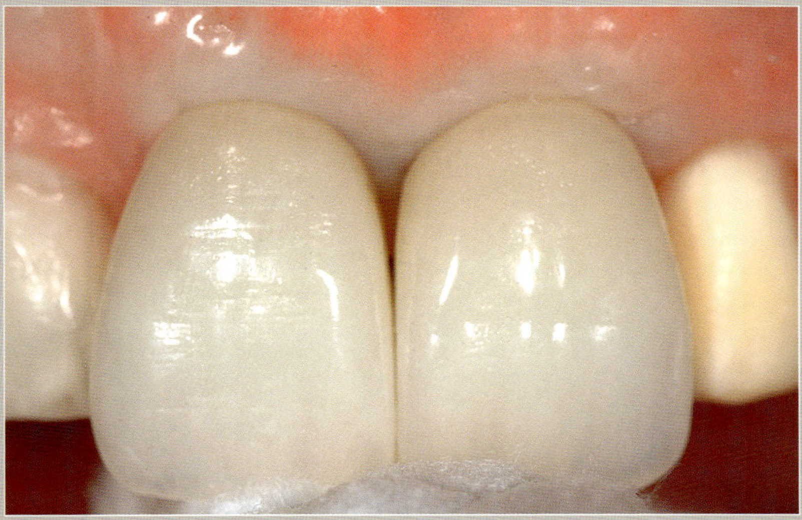

Definitive restorations in place.

restoration. Abutment try-in procedures were performed to verify the position and accessibility of the finish lines.

Because parts were no longer being manufactured for the existing implants, a positioning jig fabricated from Duralay pattern resin (Reliance) was required to properly orient the custom abutments. Crowns (e.max Press LT, Ivoclar Vivadent) were fabricated for the central incisor implants, and porcelain laminate veneers of the same material were fabricated for the maxillary lateral incisors in order to achieve harmonious tooth-to-tooth proportions and to establish the appearance of progressive mesial tipping of the maxillary anterior teeth for a better overall esthetic outcome.

Commentary

The definitive restorations were delivered 7 months after the reparative implant site development procedures were performed. This extended period of time was required to allow for maturation of the grafts, subsequent prosthetic tissue conditioning, and stabilization of the esthetic peri-implant soft tissue architecture.[86–89] Once this has been achieved, a customized impression procedure that captures the cervical contours of the provisional restorations should be performed so that the laboratory technician can replicate these contours in the definitive restoration, thus avoiding unwanted changes in the esthetic soft tissue architecture following delivery of the definitive prosthesis.[82,83] The prosthetic tissue conditioning protocol and customized impression procedures are critical to achieving and maintaining successful esthetic implant outcomes. This process requires clinical skill, experience, and a sense of artistry on behalf of the restorative team. Failure to perform these procedures with precision and respect for the biologic processes can result in loss of peri-implant tissues and is a serious omission that predictably results in esthetic compromise, complication, or failure.

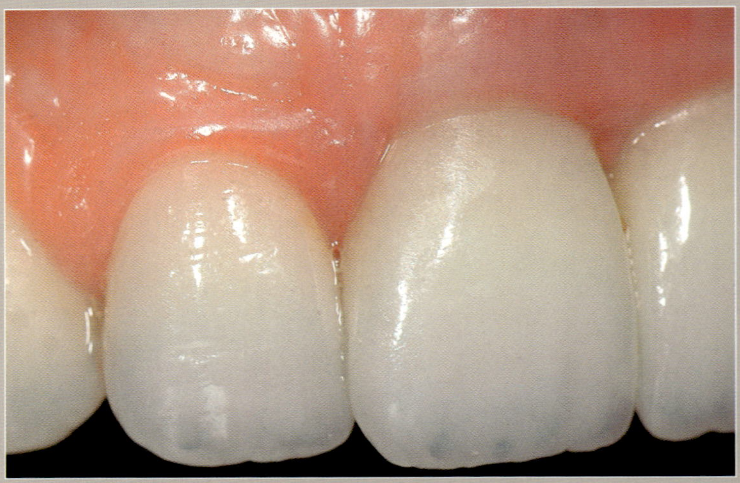

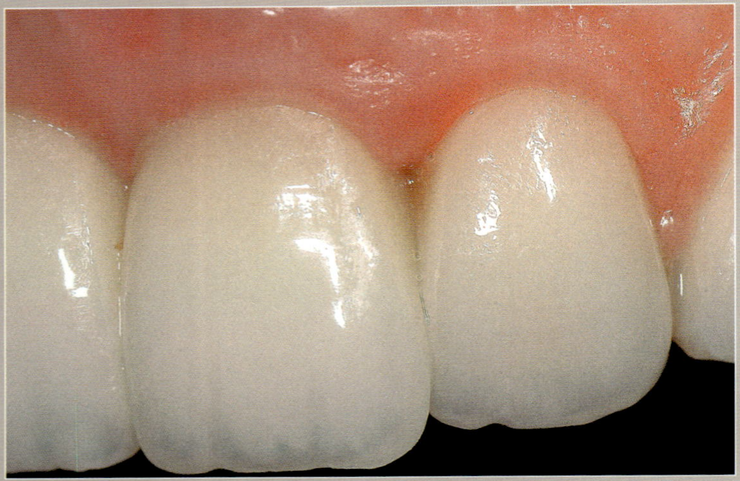

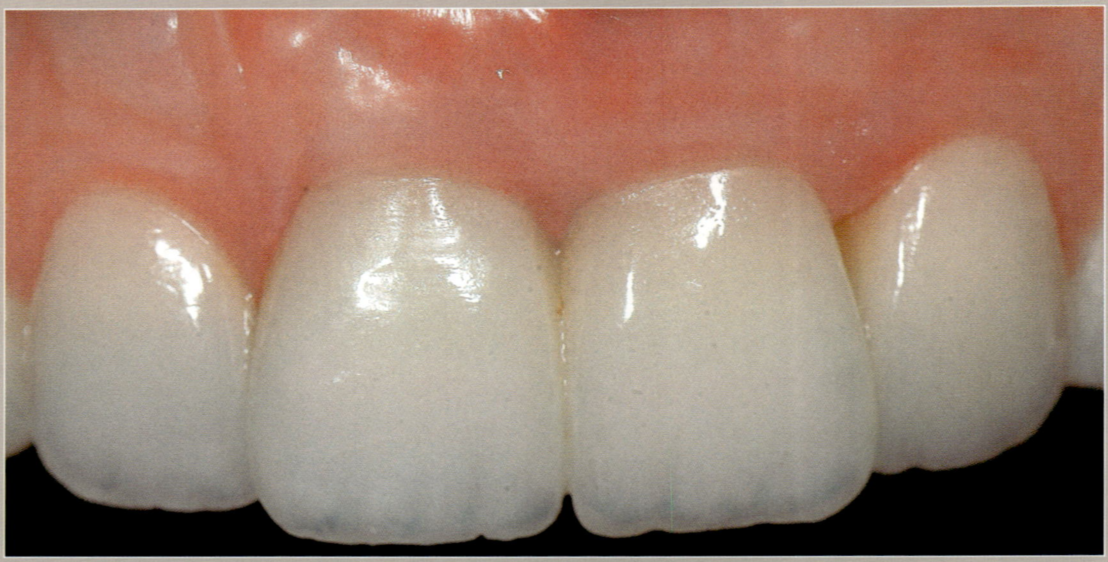

Close-up intraoral views of definitive restorations.

Phase V: Assessment of the biologic response to the definitive restorations

Clinical and radiographic examinations performed at 2 weeks, 3 months, 7 months, 1 year, and 2 years following delivery of the definitive restorations demonstrated a pleasing esthetic outcome with stability of the reconstructed peri-implant hard and soft tissues. There was no evidence of peri-implant inflammation or infection. The patient's oral hygiene was excellent, and probing depths remained between 2 to 3 mm at all sites. Additional recall visits are planned for 3 and 5 years after delivery of the definitive restorations to verify long-term stability of the esthetic outcome and to monitor the status of the remainder of the patient's dentition.

Commentary

Human clinical studies conservatively estimate that approximately 0.6 to 1.0 mm of recession of the labial marginal peri-implant soft tissues typically occurs in the first year following delivery of a definitive esthetic implant restoration.[86,87,90] These changes are thought to be the result of the biologic width phenomenon and represent apical migration of the peri-implant bone and soft tissues. In effect, *biologic width* is a clinical term used in dentistry that represents the immune system–mediated walling-off phenomenon commonly observed elsewhere in the body when microorganisms pose a threat to host tissue. An example of this phenomenon is the formation of granulomatous inflammation and tissue

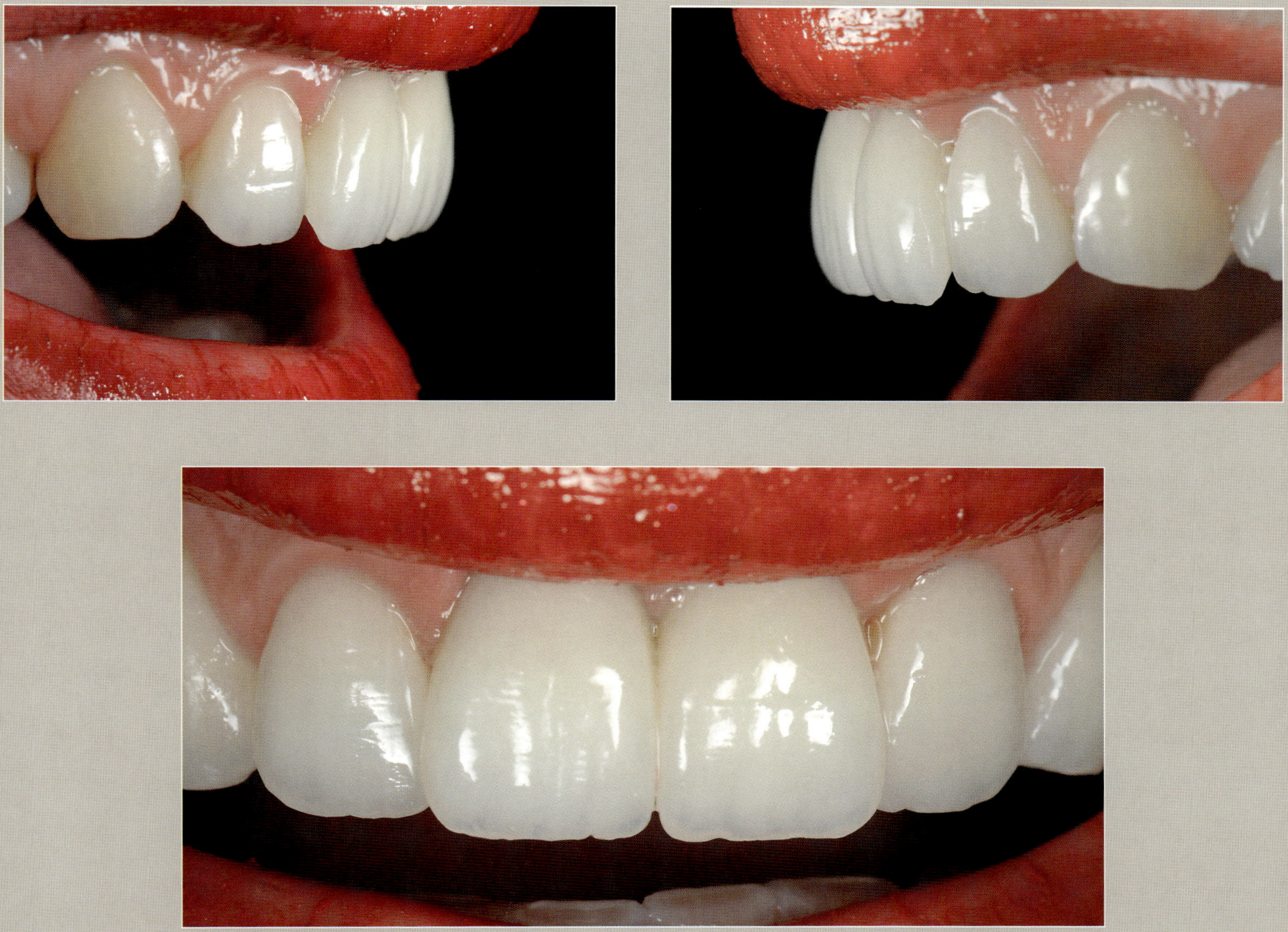

Lateral and frontal close-up views of smile.

fibrosis (Ghon focus) surrounding mycobacterium bacilli (tuberculosis) organisms in the lung.

In our clinical experience, when the labiopalatal dimensions of peri-implant soft tissues are 2.5 to 3.0 mm, long-term maintenance of pleasing esthetic outcomes can be expected. Conversely, when the labiopalatal dimensions are less than 2.5 mm, the risk of progressive deterioration of esthetic implant outcomes is greatly increased. Because few patients possess tissues of sufficient thickness to satisfy the vertical or lateral biologic width requirements that promote long-term esthetic stability, peri-implant soft tissue augmentation is almost always required for cases in which there is high esthetic concern.[12] In this case, significant loss of peri-implant hard and soft tissues had already occurred in the 5 years following the delivery of the initial esthetically compromised definitive prosthesis. While the loss of the interimplant bone height was not reparable, the papilla-sparing flap used for the site development procedures prevented further compromise of the interimplant and adjacent bone crests and allowed for soft tissue augmentation of the papillae and reconstruction of sufficient labiopalatal peri-implant soft tissue thickness to satisfy the horizontal biologic width requirement of the site.[44,45,51–56] In addition, this approach provided the necessary tissue bulk required for successful prosthetic tissue shaping.

You may now place the corresponding posttreatment overlay found in the separate folder over the pretreatment periodontal chart on page 395.

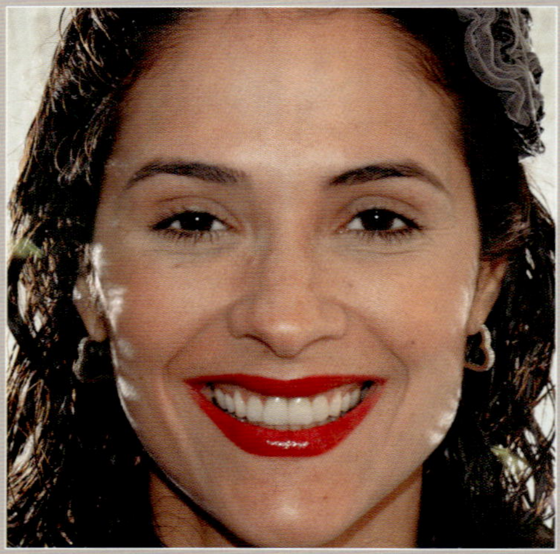

Facial view of smile at 1-year follow-up.

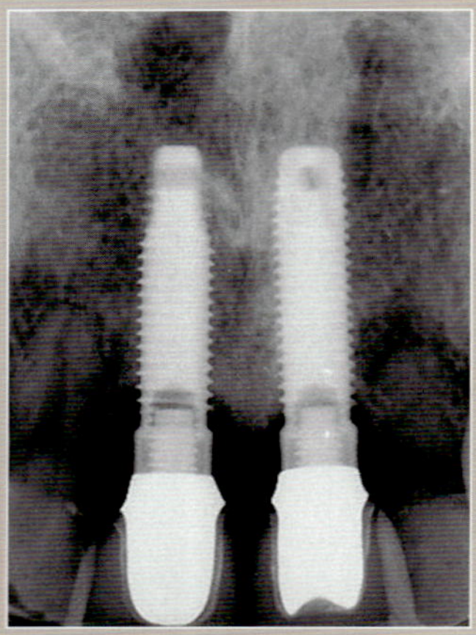

Radiograph at 1-year follow-up.

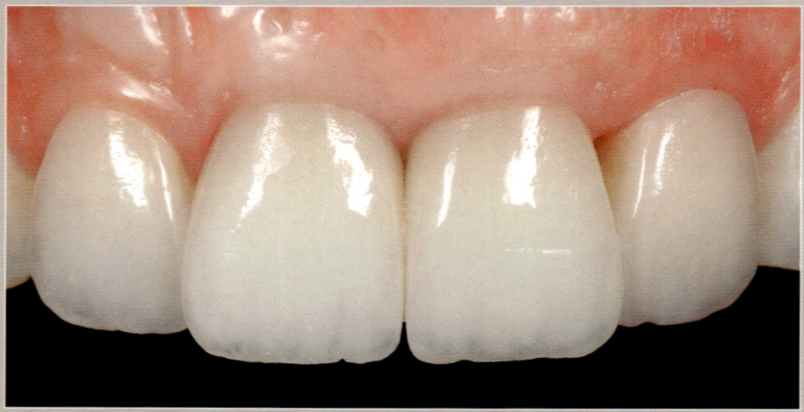

Intraoral view at 1-year follow-up.

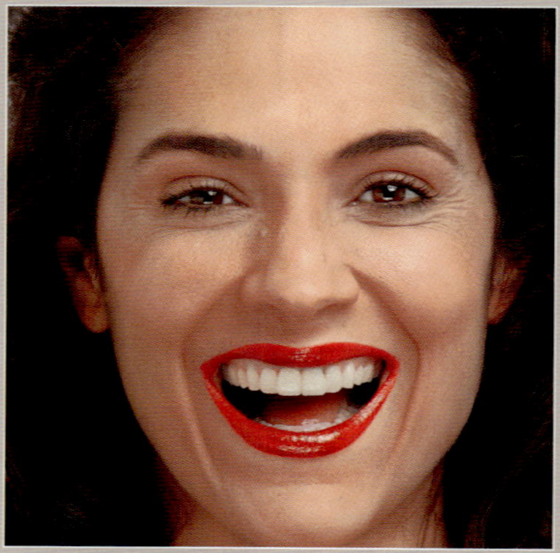

Facial view of smile at 2-year follow-up.

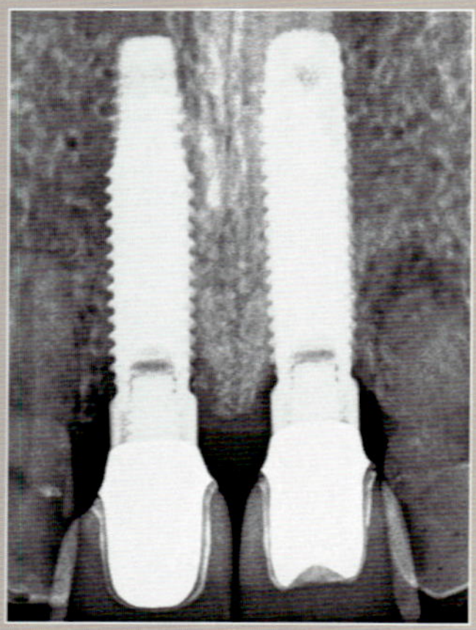

Radiograph at 2-year follow-up.

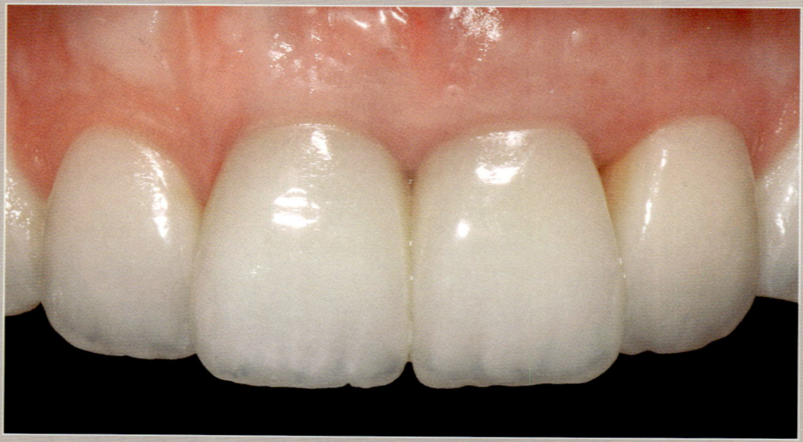

Intraoral view at 2-year follow-up.

Case Summary

The etiologic factors that contributed to this esthetic implant complication were as follows:

- Failure to initiate an interdisciplinary treatment-planning process prior to removal of the failing central incisors
- Failure to perform a systematic esthetic evaluation and identify risk factors associated with esthetic implant complications prior to initiating treatment
- Failure to perform ridge preservation procedures
- Failure to properly execute hard tissue ridge augmentation
- Inappropriate choice of biomaterials for hard tissue ridge augmentation
- Inappropriate (excessive) healing time allotted after hard tissue ridge augmentation
- Failure to perform peri-implant soft tissue augmentation
- Failure to execute ideal three-dimensional implant placement
- Failure to use implant provisional restorations to develop esthetic peri-implant soft tissue contours
- Failure to diagnose the existing clinical problems and refer to an experienced team

The management of this case exemplifies how interdisciplinary treatment planning and precise execution of biologically acceptable prosthetic and surgical protocols are essential to avoid and manage complications in esthetic implant therapy. Although one of the main issues in this case was the labial malposition and inclination of the implants, there were multiple errors and omissions in the diagnostic and treatment-planning phases of the patient's care that contributed to the complication. The damage was compounded by the several failures in the execution of the surgical and restorative procedures, resulting in this disfiguring esthetic implant complication.

The decision to perform reparative procedures while maintaining the fixed provisional restorations in place was based on an understanding of the underlying anatomical and biologic principles related to achieving success with the reparative implant site development procedures.

In addition to the requirement for the malposed implants to emerge 1.0 to 1.5 mm palatal to the emergence of the adjacent teeth at the gingival level (ie, within the alveolar housing), another key factor that influenced our decision to proceed with the reparative procedures was the fact that previous attempts at surgical repair were not performed and that evidence of fibrotic wound healing typically associated with diminished wound healing potential was not observed.

It is also very important to understand that if the emergence of the implants was labial to the emergence of the adjacent teeth (ie, outside of the alveolar housing), then we would have chosen to remove, permanently submerge, or possibly reposition the implants (using segmental osteotomy) because reparative site development procedures would likely fall short of fulfilling the treatment objectives for this patient.

Finally, temporary submergence of the implants in preparation for reparative procedures should always be considered because the recipient sites for implant site development procedures benefit from additional circulation and wound healing potential with this approach. Clear communication among the knowledgeable and skilled treatment team facilitated optimal sequencing and timing of the restorative and surgical procedures, which were precisely executed. As a result, a pleasing esthetic outcome was achieved for this patient.

ACKNOWLEDGMENT

Dr Nuria Otero and I would like to thank Stefano Inglese, RDT, for his contribution to the management of this difficult esthetic implant complication. We gratefully recognize the ingenuity, artistry, and precision that he brought to the laboratory phases of this case, without which a successful outcome would not have been possible.

REFERENCES

1. Sclar AG. Esthetic implant complications: Prevention and management. J Oral Maxillofac Surg 2006;64(9 suppl):4–5.
2. Martin WC, Morton D, Buser D. Preoperative analysis and prosthetic treatment planning. In: Buser D, Belser U, Wismeijer D (eds). ITI Treatment Guide, Vol 1: Implant Therapy in the Esthetic Zone for Single-Tooth Replacements. Berlin: Quintessence, 2007:9–24.
3. Wheeler S. Implant complications in the esthetic zone. J Oral Maxillofac Surg 2007;65(7 suppl):93–102.
4. Belser U, Bernard JP, Buser D. Implant-supported restorations in the anterior region: Prosthetic considerations. Pract Periodontics Aesthet Dent 1996;8:857–883.
5. Palacci P, Ericsson I. Esthetic Implant Dentistry: Soft and Hard Tissue Management. Chicago: Quintessence, 2001.
6. Sclar AG. Esthetic implant therapy: A comprehensive approach. In: Soft Tissue and Esthetic Considerations in Implant Therapy. Chicago: Quintessence, 2003:189–261.
7. Sclar AG. Treatment algorithms for esthetic implant therapy. In: Soft Tissue and Esthetic Considerations in Implant Therapy. Chicago: Quintessence, 2003:261–275.
8. Belser U, Buser D, Hess D, Schmid B, Bernard JP, Lang K. Aesthetic implant restorations in partially edentulous patients: A critical appraisal. Periodontol 2000 1998;17:132–150.
9. Belser U, Buser D, Higginbottom F. Consensus statements and recommended clinical procedures regarding esthetics in implant dentistry. Int J Oral Maxillofac Implants 2004;19(suppl):73–74.
10. Belser U, Buser D, Higginbottom F, Buser D. Outcome analysis of implant restorations located in the anterior maxilla: A review of the recent literature. Int J Oral Maxillofac Implants 2004;19(suppl):30–42.
11. Buser D, Belser U, Wismeijer D (eds). ITI Treatment Guide, Vol 1: Implant Therapy in the Esthetic Zone for Single-Tooth Replacements. Berlin: Quintessence, 2007.
12. Chiche GJ, Pinault A. Esthetics of Anterior Fixed Prosthodontics. Chicago: Quintessence, 1994.
13. Phillips K, Kois JC. Aesthetic peri-implant site development. The restorative connection. Dent Clin North Am 1998;42:57–70.
14. Sclar AG. Ridge preservation technique for optimal esthetics and function: The Bio-Col technique. Compend Contin Educ Dent 1999;6(suppl):3–11.
15. Sclar AG. Preserving alveolar ridge anatomy following tooth removal in conjunction with immediate implant placement: The Bio-Col technique. Atlas Oral Maxillofac Surg Clin North Am 1999;7(2):39–59.
16. Kois JC, Kan JY. Predictable peri-implant gingival aesthetics: Surgical and prosthodontic rationales. Pract Proced Aesthet Dent 2000;13:691–698.
17. Sclar AG. The Bio-Col technique. In: Soft Tissue and Esthetic Considerations in Implant Therapy. Chicago: Quintessence, 2003:75–112.

18. Kois JC. Predictable single-tooth peri-implant esthetics: Five diagnostic keys. Compend Contin Educ Dent 2004;25:895–896,898,900.
19. Evans CD, Chen ST. Esthetic outcomes of immediate implant placements. Clin Oral Implants Res 2008;19:73–80.
20. Chen S, Buser D. Recommendations for selecting the treatment approach. In: Buser D, Wismeijer D, Belser U (eds). ITI Treatment Guide, Vol 3: Implant Placement in Post-Extraction Sites: Treatment Options. Berlin: Quintessence, 2008.
21. Chen ST, Buser D. Clinical and esthetic outcomes of implants placed in postextraction sites. Int J Oral Maxillofac Implants 2009;24(suppl):186–217.
22. Kan JY, Rungcharassaeng K, Lozada JL. Bilaminar subepithelial connective tissue grafts for immediate implant placement and provisionalization in the esthetic zone. J Calif Dent Assoc 2005;33:865–871.
23. Chen ST, Darby IB, Reynolds EC, Clement JG. Immediate implant placement postextraction without flap elevation. J Periodontol 2009;80:163–172.
24. Higginbottom F, Belser U, Jones J, Keith S. Prosthetic management of implants in the esthetic zone. Int J Oral Maxillofac Implant 2004;19(suppl):62–72.
25. Garber DA, Belser UC. Restorative-driven implant placement with restoration-generated site development. Compend Contin Educ Dent 1995;16:796–804.
26. Lindhe J, Karring T, Lang NP. Clinical Periodontology and Implant Dentistry, ed 3. Copenhagen: Munksgaard, 1998.
27. Sclar AG. Beyond osseointegration. In: Soft tissue and Esthetic Considerations in Implant Therapy. Chicago: Quintessence, 2003:1–12.
28. Sclar AG. Soft tissue grafting in implant therapy. In: Soft Tissue and Esthetic Considerations in Implant Therapy. Chicago: Quintessence, 2003:113–162.
29. Chen LC, Lundgren T, Hallström H, Cherel F. Comparison of different methods of assessing alveolar ridge dimensions prior to dental implant placement. J Periodontol 2008;79:401–405.
30. Lekholm U. Surgical considerations and possible shortcomings of host sites. J Prosthet Dent 1998;79:43–48.
31. Fu JH, Yeh CY, Chan HL, Tatarakis N, Leong DJ, Wang HL. Tissue biotype and its relation to the underlying bone morphology. J Periodontol 2010;81:569–574.
32. Kan JY, Morimoto T, Rungcharassaeng K, Roe P, Smith DH. Gingival biotype assessment in the esthetic zone: Visual versus direct measurement. Int J Periodontics Restorative Dent 2010;30:237–243.
33. De Rouck T, Eghbali R, Collys K, De Bruyn H, Cosyn J. The gingival biotype revisited: Transparency of the periodontal probe through the gingival margin as a method to discriminate thin from thick gingiva. J Clin Periodontol 2009;36:428–433.
34. Kan JY, Rungcharassaeng K, Morimoto T, Lozada J. Facial gingival tissue stability after connective tissue graft with single immediate tooth replacement in the esthetic zone: Consecutive case report. J Oral Maxillofac Surg 2009;67(11 suppl):40–48.
35. Spray JR, Black CG, Morris HF, Ochi S. The influence of bone thickness on facial marginal bone response: Stage 1 placement through stage 2 uncovering. Ann Periodontol 2000;5:119–128.
36. Sullivan HC, Atkins JH. Free autogenous gingival grafts. I. Principles of successful grafting. Periodontics 1968;6:121–129.
37. Kan JY, Rungcharassaeng K, Sclar AG, Lozada JL. Effects of the facial osseous defect morphology on gingival dynamics after immediate tooth replacement and guided bone regeneration: 1-year results. J Oral Maxillofac Surg 2007;65(7 suppl 1):13–19.
38. Buser D, Dahlin C, Schenk RK (eds). Guided Bone Regeneration in Implant Dentistry. Chicago: Quintessence, 1994.
39. Buser D. 20 Years of Guided Bone Regeneration in Implant Dentistry. Chicago: Quintessence, 2009.
40. Miller PD. A classification of marginal tissue recession. Int J Periodontics Restorative Dent 1985;5:9–13.
41. Miller PD. Periodontal plastic surgical techniques for regeneration. In: Polson AM (ed). Periodontal Regeneration: Current Status and Directions. Chicago: Quintessence, 1994:53–70.
42. Kassolis JD, Baer ML, Reynolds MA. The segmental osteotomy in the management of malposed implants: A case report and literature review. J Periodontol 2003;74:529–536.
43. Sclar AG. Cosmetic soft-tissue enhancement for dental implants. Alpha Omegan 2000;93(3):38–46.
44. Sclar AG. Surgical techniques for management of peri-implant soft tissues. In: Soft Tissue and Esthetic Considerations in Implant Therapy. Chicago: Quintessence, 2003:70–74.
45. Romeo E, Lops D, Rossi A, Storelli S, Rozza R, Chiapasco M. Surgical and prosthetic management of interproximal region with single-implant restorations: 1-year prospective study. J Periodontol 2008;79:1048–1055.

46. Giannopoulou C, Bernard JP, Buser D, Carrel A, Belser UC. Effect of intracrevicular restoration margins on peri-implant health: Clinical, biochemical, and microbiologic findings around esthetic implants up to 9 years. Int J Oral Maxillofacial Implants 2003;18:173–181.
47. Lang NP, BerglundhT, Heits-Mayfield LJ, Pjetursson BE, Salvi GE, Sanz M. Consensus statements and recommended clinical procedures regarding implant survival and complications. Int J Oral Maxillofac Implants 2004;19(suppl):150–154.
48. Persson LG, Berglundh T, Lindhe J, Sennerby L. Re-osseointegration after treatment of peri-implantitis at different implant surfaces. An experimental study in the dog. Clin Oral Implants Res 2001;12:595–603.
49. Parlar A, Bosshardt DD, Çetiner D, et al. Effects of decontamination and implant surface characteristics on re-osseointegration following treatment of peri-implantitis. Clin Oral Implants Res 2009;20:391–399.
50. Renvert S, Polyzois I, Maguire R. Re-osseointegration on previously contaminated surfaces: A systematic review. Clin Oral Implants Res 2009;20(suppl 4):216–227.
51. Wilderman MN. Exposure of bone in periodontal surgery. Dent Clin North Am 1964;8:23–26.
52. Bernimoulin JP, Luscher B, Muhlemann HR. Coronally repositioned periodontal flap. Clinical evaluation after one year. J Clin Periodontol 1975;2:1–13.
53. Bahat O, Handelsman M, Gordon J. The transpositional flap in mucogingival surgery. Int J Periodontics Restorative Dent 1990;6:472–482.
54. Wood DL, Hoag PM, Donnenfeld OW, Rosenfeld LD. Alveolar crest reduction following full and partial thickness flaps. J Periodontol 1972;43:141–144.
55. Bragger U, Pasquali L, Kornman KS. Remodeling of interdental alveolar bone after periodontal flap procedures assessed by means of computer-assisted densitometric image analysis (CADIA). J Clin Periodontol 1988;15:558–564.
56. Azzi R, Takei HH, Etienne D, Carranza FA. Root coverage and papilla reconstruction using autogenous osseous and connective tissue grafts. Int J Periodontics Restorative Dent 2001;21:141–147.
57. Sclar AG. Strategies for management of single-tooth extraction sites in aesthetic implant therapy. J Oral Maxillofacial Surg 2004;62(9 suppl 2):90–105.
58. Sclar AG. Anterior aesthetics with single-staged implants and site development procedures. Implantol 2003: 29–36.
59. Artzi Z, Tal H, Dayan D. Porous bovine bone mineral in healing human extraction sockets. Part 1: Histomorphometric evaluations at 9 months. J Periodontol 2000;71:1015–1023.
60. Danan M, Degrange M, Vaïdeanu T, Brion M. Immediate replacement of a maxillary central incisor associated with severe facial bone loss: Use of Bio-Oss collagen—Case report. Int J Periodontics Restorative Dent 2003;23:491–497.
61. Meijndert L, Raghoebar GM, Schüpbach P, Meijer HJ, Vissink A. Bone quality at the implant site after reconstruction of a local defect of the maxillary anterior ridge with chin bone or deproteinized cancellous bovine bone. Int J Oral Maxillofac Surg 2005;34:877–884.
62. Meijndert L, Raghoebar GM, Meijer HJ, Vissink A. Clinical and radiographic characteristics of single-tooth replacements preceded by local ridge augmentation: A prospective randomized clinical trial. Clin Oral Implants Res 2008;19:1295–1303.
63. Marx RE, Carlson ER, Eichstaedt RM, Schimmele SR, Strauss JE, Georgeff KR. Platelet-rich plasma: Growth factor enhancement for bone grafts. Oral Surg Oral Med Oral Pathol Oral Radiol Endod 1998;85:638–646.
64. Yassibag-Berkman Z, Tuncer O, Subasioglu T, Kantarci A. Combined use of platelet-rich plasma and bone grafting with or without guided tissue regeneration in the treatment of anterior interproximal defects. J Periodontol 2007;78:801–809.
65. Thor A, Wannfors K, Sennerby L, Rasmusson L. Reconstruction of the severely resorbed maxilla with autogenous bone, platelet-rich plasma, and implants: 1-year results of a controlled prospective 5-year study. Clin Implant Dent Relat Res 2005;7:209–220.
66. Whitman DH, Berry RL, Green DM. Platelet gel: An autologous alternative to fibrin glue with applications in oral and maxillofacial surgery. J Oral Maxillofac Surg 1997;55:1294–1299.
67. Whitman DH, Berry RL. A technique for improving the handling of particulate cancellous bone and marrow grafts using platelet gel. J Oral Maxillofac Surg 1998;45:1217–1218.
68. Krupski WC, Reilly LM, Perez S, Moss KM, Crombleholme PA, Rapp JH. A prospective randomized trial of autologous platelet-derived wound healing factors for treatment of chronic nonhealing wounds: A preliminary report. J Vasc Surg 1991;14:526–532.

69. Knighton DR, Ciresi KF, Fiegel VD, Austin LL, Butler EL. Classification and treatment of chronic nonhealing wounds: Successful treatment with autologous platelet-derived wound healing factors (PDWHF). Ann Surg 1986;204:322–330.
70. Jung UW, Um YJ, Choi SH. Histologic observation of soft tissue acquired from maxillary tuberosity area for root coverage. J Periodontol 2008;79:934–940.
71. Azzi R, Takei HH, Etienne D, Carranza FA. Root coverage and papilla reconstruction using autogenous osseous and connective tissue grafts. Int J Periodontics Restorative Dent 2001;21:141–147.
72. Sorni-Bröker M, Peñarrocha-Diago M. Factors that influence the position of the peri-implant soft tissues: A review. Med Oral Patol Oral Cir Bucal 2009;14:e475–e479.
73. Abrahamsson I, Berglundh T, Lindhe J. The mucosal barrier following abutment dis/reconnection. An experimental study in dogs. J Clin Periodontol 1997;24:568–572.
74. Berglundh T, Lindhe J, Jonsson K, Ericsson I. The topography of the vascular systems in the periodontal and peri-implant tissues in the dog. J Clin Periodontol 1994;21:189–193.
75. Gargiulo AW, Wentz FM, Orban B. Dimensions and relations of the dento-gingival junction in humans. J Periodontol 1961;32:261–267.
76. Maynard JG, Wilson RD. Physiologic dimensions of the periodontium significant to the restorative dentist. J Periodontol 1979;50:170–174.
77. Abrahamsson I, Berglundh T, Glanzt PO, Lindhe J. The mucosal attachment at different abutments. An experimental study in dogs. J Clin Periodontol 1998;25:721–727.
78. Abrahamsson I, Berglundh T, Sekino S, Lindhe J. Tissue reactions to abutment shift: An experimental study in dogs. Clin Implant Dent Relat Res 2003;5:82–88.
79. Parma-Benfenati S, Fugazzotto PA, Ruben MP. The effect of restorative margins on the postsurgical development and nature of the periodontium. Part I. Int J Periodontics Restorative Dent 1985;5(6):30–51.
80. Parma-Benfenati SP, Fugazzotto PA, Ferreira PM, Ruben MP, Kramer GM. The effect of restorative margins on the postsurgical development and nature of the periodontium. Part II. Anatomical considerations. Int J Periodontics Restorative Dent 1986;6(1):64–75.
81. Hämmerle C, Jung R. Prosthetic management of implants in the esthetic zone: General principles and scientific documentation. In: Buser D, Belser U, Wismeijer D (eds). ITI Treatment Guide, Vol 1: Implant Therapy in the Esthetic Zone for Single-Tooth Replacements. Berlin: Quintessence, 2007:38–46.
82. Hinds KF. Custom impression coping for an exact registration of the healed tissue in the esthetic implant restoration. Int J Periodontics Restorative Dent 1997;17:584–591.
83. Jung R. Replacement of an upper right central incisor with a regular neck implant, restored with an all-ceramic crown, transocclusally screw-retained. In: Buser D, Belser U, Wismeijer D (eds). ITI Treatment Guide, Vol 1: Implant Therapy in the Esthetic Zone for Single-Tooth Replacements. Berlin: Quintessence, 2007:49–57.
84. Markus SJ. Interim esthetic restorations in conjunction with anterior implants. J Prosthet Dent 1999;82:233–236.
85. Pisis P. Emergence profile considerations of implant abutments. Pract Periodontics Aesthet Dent 1994:6(7):69–78.
86. Grunder U. Stability of the mucosal topography around single tooth implants and adjacent teeth: 1-year results. Int J Periodontics Restorative Dent 2003;20:11–17.
87. Mankoo T. Contemporary implant concepts in aesthetic dentistry—Part 1: Biologic width. Pract Proced Aesthet Dent 2003;15:609–616.
88. Hermann JS, Buser D, Schenk RK, Schoolfield JD, Cochran DL. Biologic width around one- and two-piece titanium implants. Clin Oral Implants Res 2001;12:559–571.
89. Hermann JS, Buser D, Schenk RK, Higginbottom FL, Cochran DL. Biologic width around titanium implants. A physiologically formed and stable dimension over time. Clin Oral Implants Res 2000;11:1–11.
90. Tarnow DP, Cho SC, Wallace SS. The effect of inter-implant distance on the height of inter-implant bone crest. J Periodontol 2000;71:546–549.

16

The Periodontal-Prosthodontic Interface Around Natural Teeth and Implants

Eric Van Dooren, DDS
Murilo Calgaro, CDT

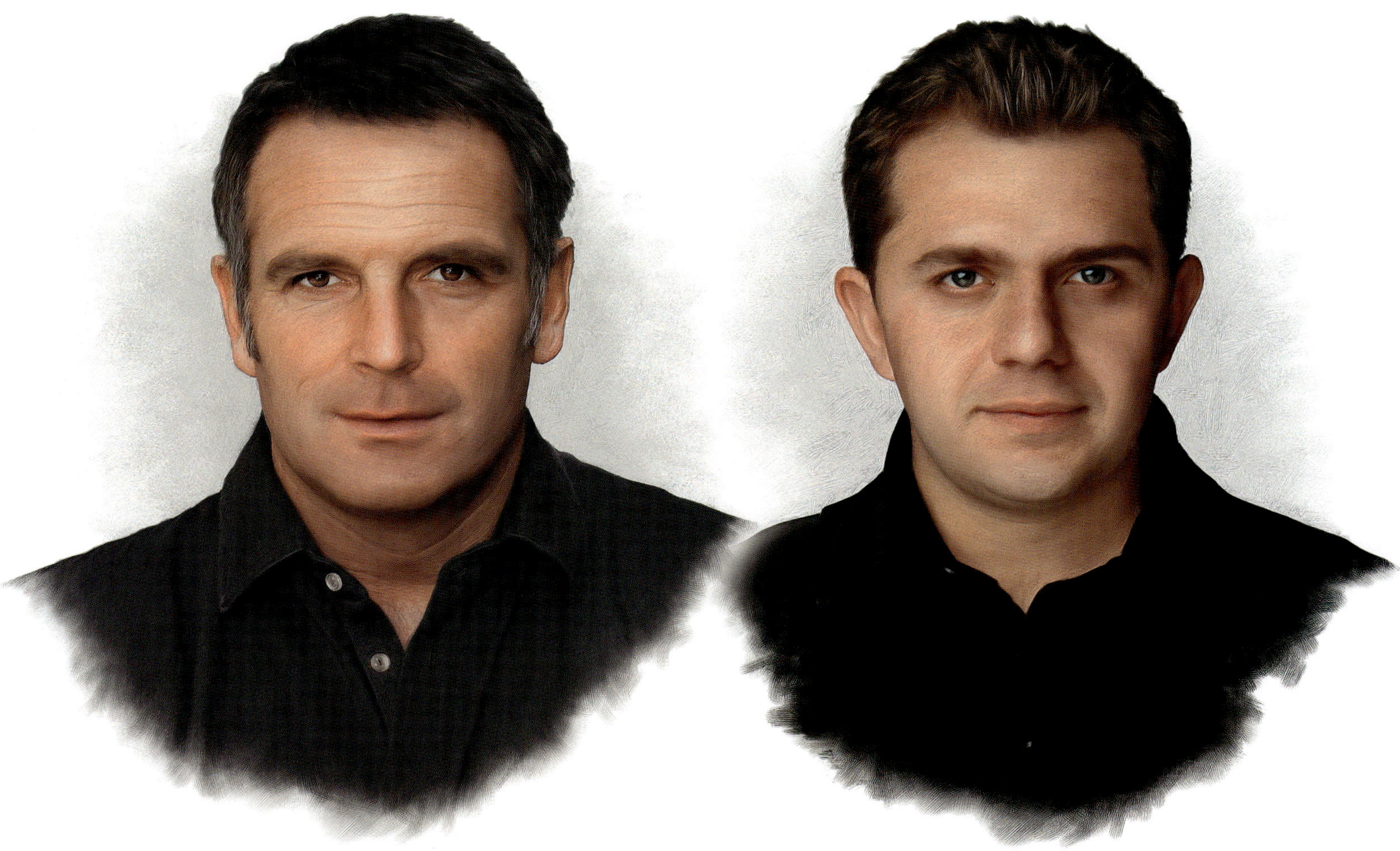

Often, the problem for most dentists is how to analyze and manage the vertical deficiencies that exist in the esthetic zone.

Philosophy and Background

During my 27 years in dental practice, I have encountered many treatment-planning challenges. In this chapter, I share some of the concepts and solutions I have employed to overcome esthetic and functional failures so that the reader may avoid the same disappointing experiences that many clinicians have faced in the past.

Dr Pat Allen, who has become a friend, mentor, and genuine inspiration, has helped me to acquire a greater understanding of esthetic dentistry and to become a more complete clinician. I have come to appreciate the importance of the interaction between prosthetics and periodontal plastic surgery (often combined with implant surgery) in achieving more successful and satisfying esthetic results.

One of the most important lessons I have learned and would like to impart is that in order to optimize tooth proportions and esthetic outcomes, the challenge is really not achieving "white esthetics." The difficulty is in addressing the prosthetic–soft tissue interface. Particularly in implant dentistry, it can become quite onerous to establish a balance between pink and white at this critical junction. By gaining a clear understanding of the very specific challenges of restoring implants in the esthetic zone, uncovering and analyzing different parameters, and synthesizing this information into a meaningful and effective treatment plan, we set the stage for long-term success.

Advances in dental technology have created avenues for treatment never before possible, especially in the field of dental implantology. As clinicians always striving for improvement, we are impressionable and sometimes susceptible to setting unrealistic expectations after seeing ideal cases presented in the literature and at national meetings. Unfortunately, clinical reality can be different. Without proper diagnosis and treatment planning, esthetic results can be very disappointing and unacceptable for both dentist and patient. In many situations, obtaining and creating ideal soft and hard tissue contours around implant restorations can be quite difficult.

In implant dentistry, minor errors can lead to major soft tissue discrepancies. A lack of knowledge of prosthetic components and restorative materials commonly can result in visual nightmares in the esthetic zone. For this reason, it is even more important to understand the limitations of the surgical and prosthetic protocols and techniques related to implant restorations.

There is a dearth of information in the literature (and among the most capable of clinicians) related to treating severe anterior esthetic failures with implant restorations. Often, the problem for most dentists is how to analyze and manage the vertical deficiencies that exist in the esthetic zone.

Treatment planning the case selected for this chapter should help the reader better appreciate the complexities faced and demands placed on the treatment team in resolving these challenging esthetic issues. The importance of the laboratory technician as an integral member of this team should also become clear. The laboratory technician can, in many cases, visualize less-than-desirable esthetic outcomes that may not be initially perceived by other team members. Having the technician involved in case planning has other advantages as well, including:

- More effective communication related to the desired function and appearance of the definitive restorations
- Improved planning for the interaction between the clinician and technician during treatment
- Better communication between the clinician and technician regarding the patient's goals and objectives

The reason for choosing this clinical case is that it clearly summarizes all the current thinking on:

- Analysis of anterior soft tissue defects and prosthetic problems
- The limitations of cosmetic periodontal and ridge augmentation surgery
- Communication with the lab technician
- Information transfer to casts
- Evaluation of wax-ups and mock-ups
- Innovations in noninvasive surgery
- New trends in abutment design and fabrication
- Definitive restoration

During the case presentation, I offer my thoughts on:

- Analyzing anterior soft tissue deficiencies
- Transferring intraoral information to the lab and translating it into a comprehensive wax-up
- Understanding soft tissue behavior related to prosthetic pressure, especially in thin phenotype cases
- Establishing a comprehensive treatment-planning protocol for anterior implant restorations

It can be very frustrating to be present at a lecture where the problems are recognizable but the solutions appear unattainable, at least in the hands of most in attendance. The goal of this chapter is to help the reader find practical solutions to the most challenging problems through a better understanding of esthetic diagnosis and treatment planning.

—Eric Van Dooren

Case Presentation

Treating clinicians
Periodontist, implant surgeon, and prosthodontist: Eric Van Dooren, DDS
Restorative dentist: Cláudio Pinho, DDS
Endodontist: Ralph Lemmens, DDS
Laboratory technician: Murilo Calgaro, CDT

Clinical Treatment Planning

Age at initial presentation: 45 years
Initial presentation: August 2008
Active treatment completed: January 2009

Introduction and background

A 45-year-old woman presented with a significant esthetic problem associated with failing anterior restorations on teeth nos. 9 and 10. The previous treatment was performed 3 years prior to the initial examination as a result of a bicycling accident. Endodontic therapy had been completed on both teeth. Subsequently, an apicoectomy was performed on tooth no. 10. These teeth had been restored with metal-ceramic crowns.

The patient was willing to undergo comprehensive treatment to achieve her esthetic goals but was reluctant to proceed with any surgery unless it would be minimally invasive in nature. She insisted that treatment be simple and limited to as few procedures as possible.

Medical history

- No significant findings

Diagnostic findings

Extraoral and facial findings

- Very high smile line

Intraoral findings

Dental

- Spacing of the mandibular anterior teeth
- Metal-ceramic crowns on teeth nos. 9 and 10 with unnatural tooth proportions
- Interproximal caries on tooth no. 7 and a deficient composite restoration on the mesial of tooth no. 8
- Light discoloration on the buccal aspect of tooth no. 8

Periodontal

- Thin gingival phenotype
- Generalized periodontal probing depths of 2 to 3 mm
- Generalized high scalloping of gingival margins
- Localized moderate gingival inflammation around teeth nos. 9 and 10
- Slight gingival recession on most of the mandibular anterior teeth
- Buccal fistula on tooth no. 10, probably due to failing surgical treatment (apicoectomy)
- Scar tissue and soft tissue discoloration apical to teeth nos. 9 and 10
- Good home care with minimal amounts of plaque present

Occlusal notes

- Angle Class I occlusion
- Slight centric relation–centric occlusion shift upon closure
- Horizontal overlap: 1 mm
- Vertical overlap: 1 mm
- Mandibular range of motion within normal limits

Pretreatment

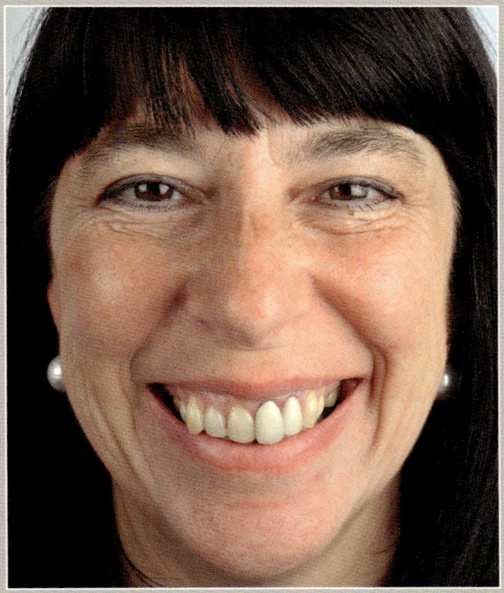

Facial view of smile.

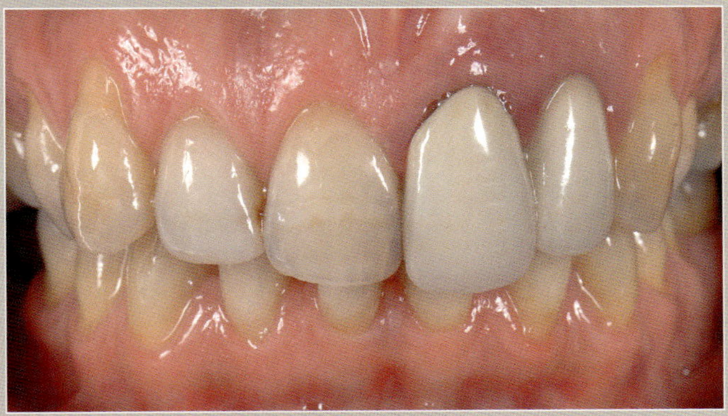

Frontal view of occlusion.

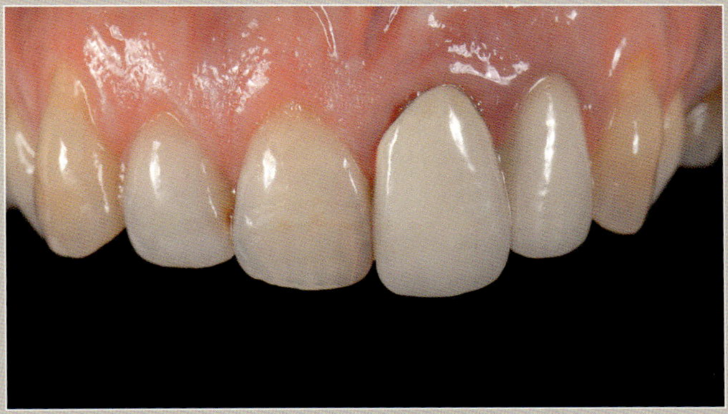

Frontal view of maxilla.

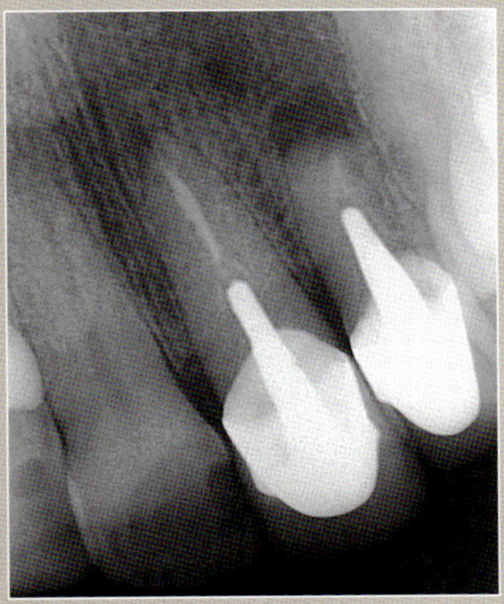

Radiograph of teeth nos. 9 and 10.

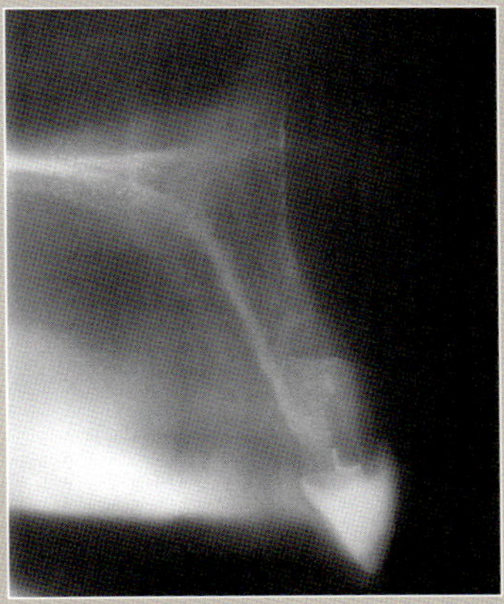

Tomography scan of tooth no. 10.

Radiographic findings

- Mild bone loss between teeth nos. 9 and 10
- Extensive periapical endodontic lesion on tooth no. 10
- Open margins and imprecise fit of full-crown restorations on teeth nos. 9 and 10

Diagnosis

- Localized gingivitis around teeth nos. 9 and 10
- Moderate bone and papilla height loss around and between teeth nos. 9 and 10

Prognosis

- Excellent general prognosis
- Good prognosis for tooth no. 9 and extremely poor for tooth no. 10

Summary of concerns

1. Even if the patient is willing to consent to surgical soft tissue grafting, how much can we realistically expect to gain and will we be able to meet or exceed this patient's expectations?
2. How do we communicate the treatment options, emphasizing the attendant risks, to the patient?
3. If a decision is made to replace the existing crowns and to try to restore harmony and balance in the face and smile, how can this be accomplished in a minimally invasive way?
4. Recognizing that we may be limited in the amount of vertical height that can be achieved, how will we be able to compensate for this restoratively to enhance the esthetic outcome?

Treatment-planning considerations

This patient expressed an interest in a noninvasive, nonsurgical approach to treatment. She qualified her wishes by stating that if surgery was unavoidable to achieve a successful result, she wanted it to be minimal and limited to one procedure.

This patient wanted treatment only on the esthetically failing teeth and on the replacement of tooth no. 10 with an implant restoration.

The patient expressed some concerns about her smile, especially about the incisal length of teeth nos. 9 and 10 and the subsequent disharmony between the right and left sides. She was also concerned about the lack of symmetry of her anterior teeth in length and form.

Although orthodontic forced eruption was considered as a treatment option to improve function and esthetics, the patient did not agree to proceed with this.

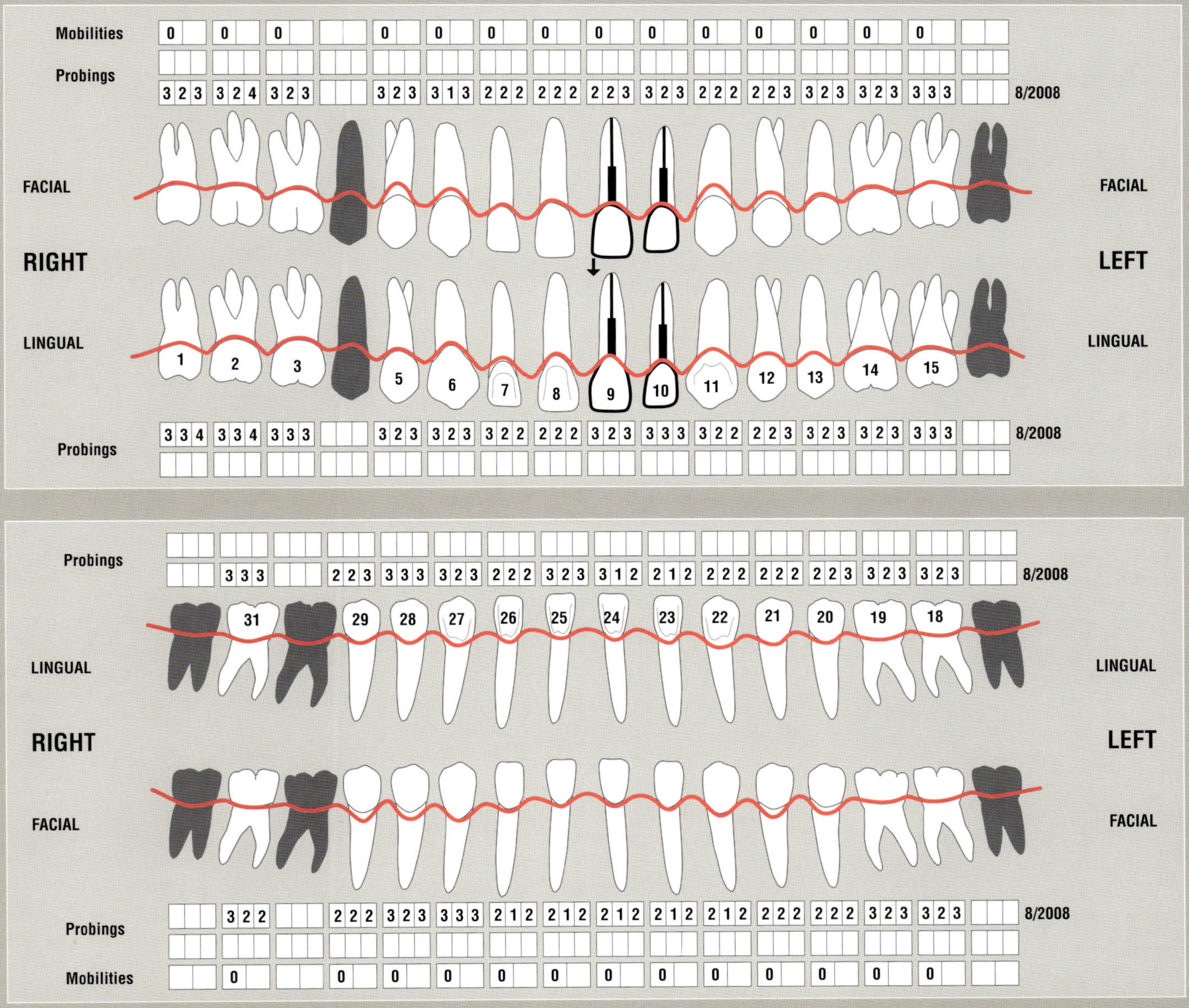

As a learning exercise, you may now outline goals/objectives of treatment and a treatment plan.

Proposed Treatment Plan

Goals/objectives of treatment

The goals and objectives of treatment for this patient were to accomplish a fixed method of rehabilitation without involving nonrestored teeth and to achieve optimal esthetics. The patient limited possible therapeutic options by requesting the fewest number of surgical and prosthetic procedures and a minimally invasive approach.

Phase I: Data gathering and digital planning

1. Intraoral and full-face digital photos in order to evaluate and establish:
   - Proper incisal edge position on teeth nos. 9 and 10
   - Ideal tooth proportions
   - Optimal gingival contour

Phase II: Transfer of data to the cast and fabrication of an ideal wax-up

2. Optimization of "white esthetics": Establish ideal incisal edge position, form, and gingival root emergence on a plaster cast
3. Optimization of "pink esthetics": Evaluate soft tissue deficiency and analyze the size of the defect

Phase III: Fabrication of a provisional fixed partial denture

4. Removal of old restorations; evaluation of tooth locations and form; fabrication of anterior provisional fixed partial denture with silicone index
5. Evaluation of design and implementation of minor changes in form, if necessary, by applying flowable composite
6. Finalization of surgical plan and protocol related to exact implant location and supporting soft tissue procedures to attenuate the influence of the anterior vertical bony defect, with the goal of obtaining an optimal gingiva-tooth interface with as "natural" an appearance as possible
7. Esthetic and functional evaluation to establish incisal edge position, soft tissue contours, lip support, and tooth form, which should provide an overall facial balance and harmony
8. Patient approval obtained

Phase IV: Establishing the final treatment plan

9. Final improvements in the plan based on the patient's preferences
10. Final adjustments to maximize soft tissue harmony, gain optimal soft tissue contours, and optimize selection of prosthetic materials

Phase V: Surgical treatment

11. Surgical therapy, including implant placement
12. Connective tissue grafting where indicated to improve soft tissue thickness both around the natural tooth and the implant restoration
13. Postoperative care and healing

Phase VI: Definitive restorations

14. Definitive tooth preparation
15. Impression taking and master cast fabrication
16. Fabrication of definitive restorations
17. Try-in of restorations

Active Clinical Treatment

Review of the goals/objectives of treatment

The goals and objectives of treatment for this patient were to accomplish a fixed method of rehabilitation without involving nonrestored teeth and to achieve optimal esthetics. The patient limited possible therapeutic options by requesting the fewest number of surgical and prosthetic procedures and a minimally invasive approach. This is not unlike the requests of many patients that we treat every day. Our concept of the "ideal treatment plan" is not necessarily for everyone. The patient declined minor orthodontic therapy and gingival plastic surgery on the nonrestored teeth, including the two canines. Despite these significant constraints, we were commissioned to meet or exceed her treatment expectations.

Phase I: Data gathering and digital planning

Photographic and dynamic video data were gathered on the patient. Intraoral and full-face smile images were taken. Today, in our office, the video images become increasingly important not only for data gathering but also for dynamic evaluation of the case during treatment and following case completion. This data was going to be important in establishing proper incisal edge position, tooth form, tooth preparation, and gingival contours. In our opinion, this is one of the most important steps in planning the case. Radiographs were taken.

Phase II: Transfer of data to the cast and fabrication of an ideal wax-up

A silicone impression material (Virtual light body and heavy body, Ivoclar Vivadent) was used to take mandibular and maxillary impressions. Care was taken to secure a very precise impression of both teeth and the surrounding gingiva. Two sets of casts were poured. This allowed us to maintain casts of the original situation for comparison and use as an ongoing reference.

In this particular case, a few important details became evident when we looked at the casts and the intraoral and facial photos and analyzed the existing esthetic deficiency:

- There were some potential ramifications of the existing incisal edge positions of teeth nos. 9 and 10, and this would influence our treatment approach.
- Most importantly, there were major concerns regarding the gingival contour of the crowns of teeth nos. 9 and 10 and the labioversion of the gingival portion of the root, especially of tooth no. 9. This became evident when the plaster cast was evaluated from an incisal angle. Understanding that this was the real issue in this case allowed us to finalize the surgical treatment plan and to focus on optimizing the natural root and transgingival abutment contours for ideal soft tissue support and long-term soft tissue stability.

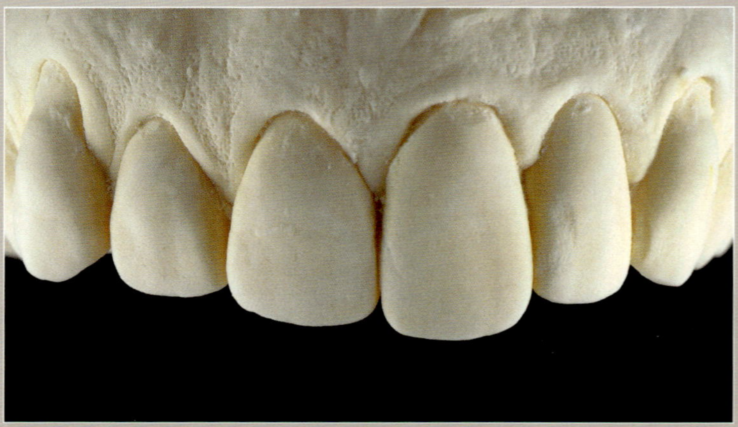

Frontal view of the maxillary cast.

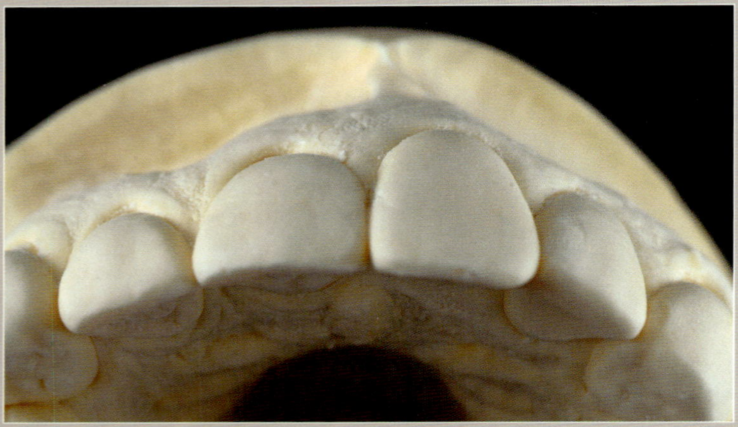

Incisal view of the maxillary cast.

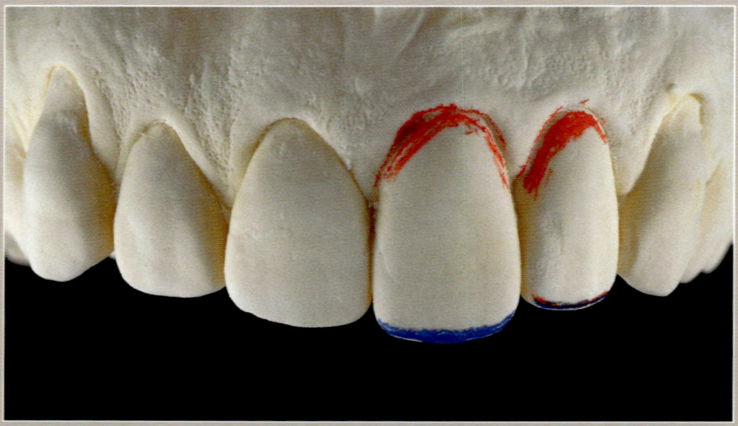

Frontal view of the maxillary cast marked for reshaping.

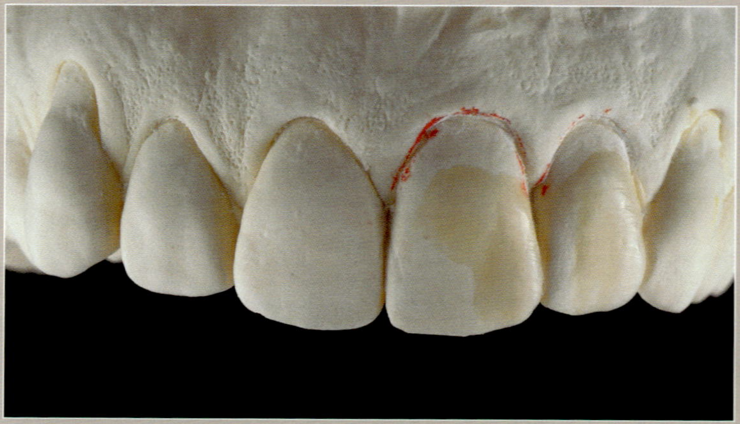

Frontal view of the maxillary cast after reshaping.

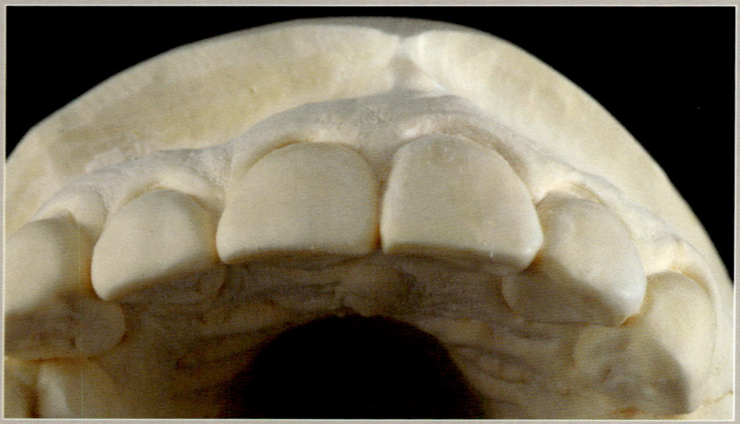

Incisal view of the maxillary cast after reshaping.

At this point, we needed to make a wax-up that would become a "project" and guide us through the whole surgical and prosthodontic treatment. The problem for the dental technician was not really to establish the ideal and symmetric incisal edge position and form but to understand the ideal three-dimensional (3D) gingival contour of the restorations that would allow ideal prosthetic soft tissue support. This is why the dental technician needed to understand the clinical impact of gingival tooth forms and emergence and submergence angles. Close cooperation and teamwork between dental technician and surgeon or prosthodontist were essential in optimizing long-term soft tissue stability.

First, the dental technician selectively removed plaster with a bur and reshaped areas such as the incisal edge and the gingival contour. Wax was then added to optimize tooth form and to mimic the tooth contralaterally. Paying attention to the details made all the difference in this case. When finalized, a silicone index was made from this wax-up. This allowed us, on the day of removal of the old restorations, to make a provisional fixed partial denture that we would also be able to use as a mock-up for esthetic evaluation.

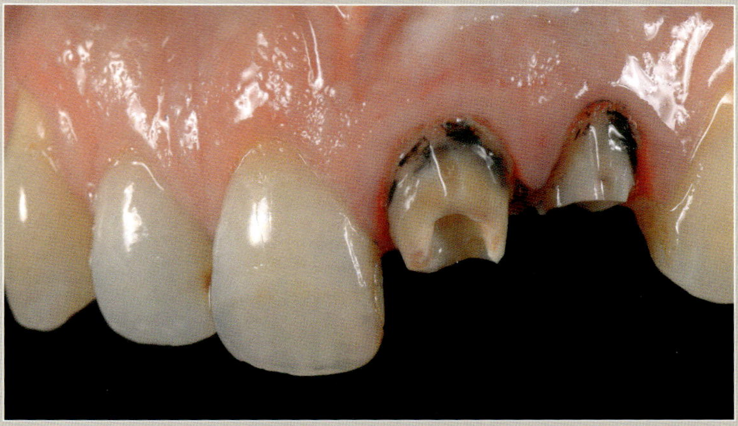

Existing preparations after removal of old restorations.

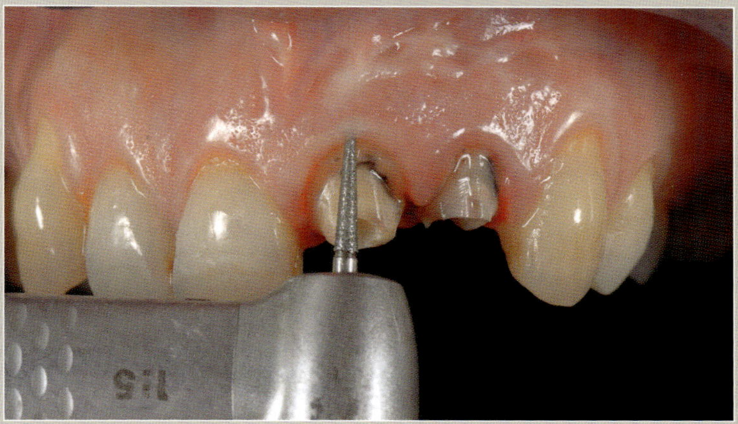

Modification of root profile of tooth no. 9 after placement of a more coronal chamfer preparation.

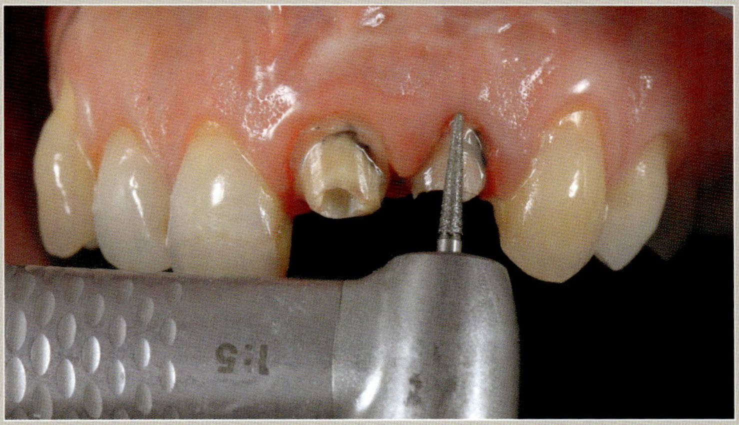

Modification of root profile of tooth no. 10.

Phase III: Fabrication of a provisional fixed partial denture

We evaluated the wax-up "project" intraorally. The old restorations were removed. At this point, a composite material (Luxatemp, DMG) was injected in the silicone index and applied intraorally.

The "project" was then evaluated. The old preparations exhibited severe staining, and gingival levels were very asymmetric compared with the contralateral side. A crack in the coronal part of the root was observed on tooth no. 10. During probing, no associated bone loss was apparent.

After showing the patient the mock-up, I decided to try to modify the gingival levels nonsurgically. The idea was to reduce the pressure on the marginal soft tissue by altering the root convexity or root profile in the transgingival zone (in the dental sulcus to the level of crestal bone).

On tooth no. 9, a new chamfer preparation was placed in a more coronal position, symmetric with the cementoenamel junction (CEJ) of the contralateral tooth no. 8. A sharp diamond bur was used to accomplish this. Although we planned to extract tooth no. 10, the root profile was also aggressively modified. In this way, I was able to move the tissue coronally in rapid fashion (1 week).

The most critical part of esthetic or cosmetic plastic surgery, especially in implant surgery or with gingival recession coverage, is to control the vertical component of the defect. This simple root-recontouring concept allowed us to alter the gingival levels nonsurgically, thus avoiding a more invasive procedure. The effect of the recontouring is almost immediate and easy to achieve. It is very predictable but should be reserved only for nonvital teeth. Two weeks after the provisional fixed partial denture was placed, we compared the soft tissue levels with the preoperative situation, and the advantage of this concept became quite evident.

Esthetic and functional evaluation occurred at this point. The objective was for the incisal edge position, soft tissue contours, lip support, and tooth form to create an overall balance and facial harmony. Once the projected esthetic outcome was approved by the patient, we were ready to establish a final treatment plan.

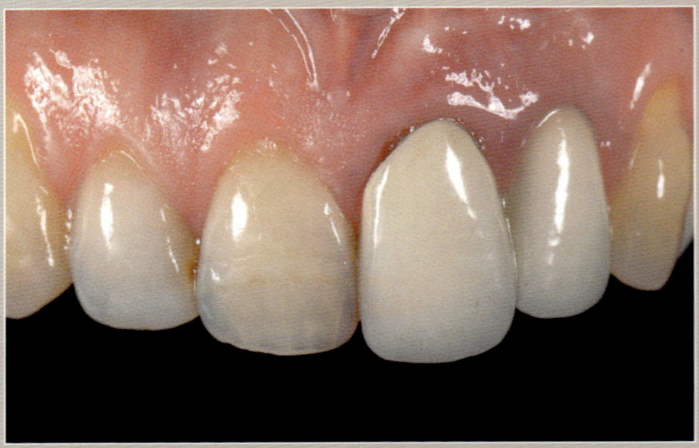

Preoperative clinical situation.

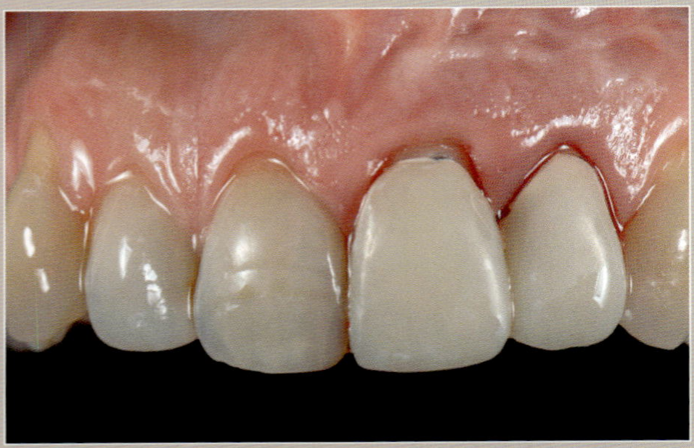

Placement of the provisional fixed partial denture and appearance of soft tissue levels on the day of root profile modification of teeth nos. 9 and 10.

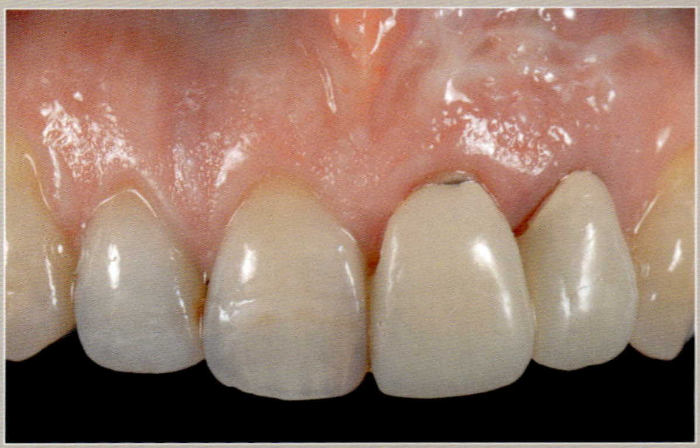

Improvement in soft tissue levels 2 weeks after placement of the provisional fixed partial denture.

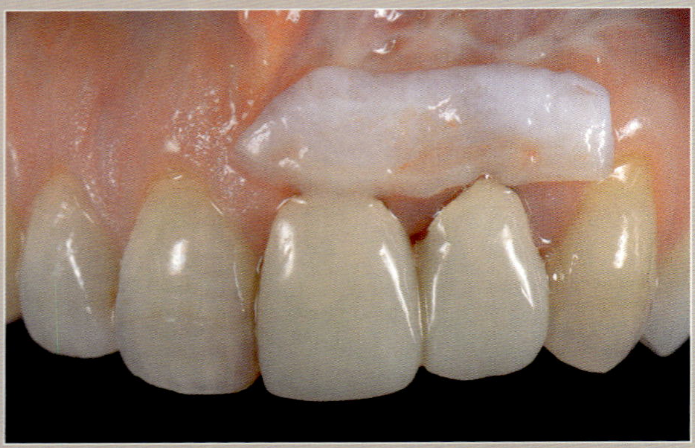

Soft tissue graft.

Phase IV: Establishing the final treatment plan

The wax-up "project" and the intraoral design were translated into a final treatment plan. At that time, we contemplated what we could do to maximally enhance the final esthetic and functional outcomes, considering that the patient wanted little or no surgery and that the existing ridge deficiency could not be restored surgically if we wanted any symmetry in soft tissue levels and papilla heights.

The following ideas were planned:

- We would improve soft tissue harmony and achieve a better balance in soft tissue levels by covering the remaining buccal recession on tooth no. 9 with a connective tissue graft.
- We would extract tooth no. 10 and replace it immediately with an implant.
- We would endeavour to optimize the prosthetic materials.

All-ceramic single crowns (e.max Press, Ivoclar Vivadent) were to be fabricated on teeth nos. 9 and 10. For the abutment, a lithium disilicate individualized pressed component would be bonded to a provisional titanium cylinder.

Phase V: Surgical treatment

A connective tissue graft was harvested from the maxillary tuberosity area and inserted in a split-thickness lateral pouch, starting from the distal aspect of tooth no. 9 and extending to the mesial aspect of tooth no. 11. Care was taken to maximize soft tissue thickness in the area where the implant would be placed. Seralene 6-0 sutures (American Dental Systems) were placed to secure the soft tissue graft into position.

Tooth no. 10 was extracted atraumatically, and aggressive curettage and debridement of the extraction socket was performed. Immediate implant placement (NobelActive NP, Nobel Biocare) was guided by a surgical stent designed and

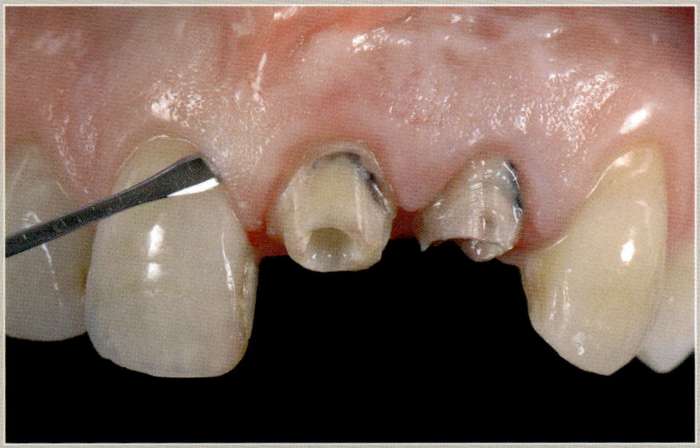

Incision for soft tissue graft placement.

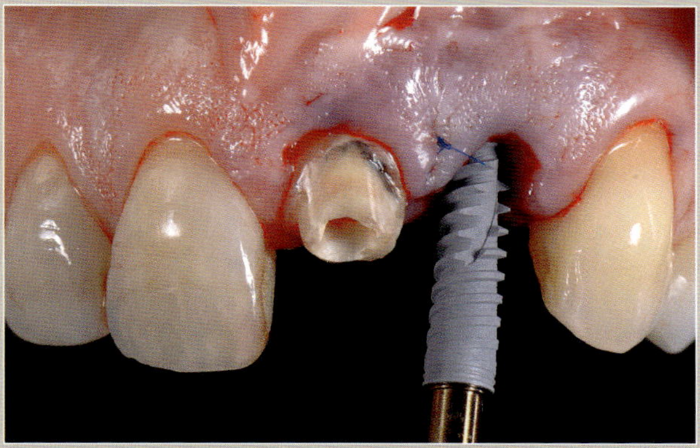

Implant placement.

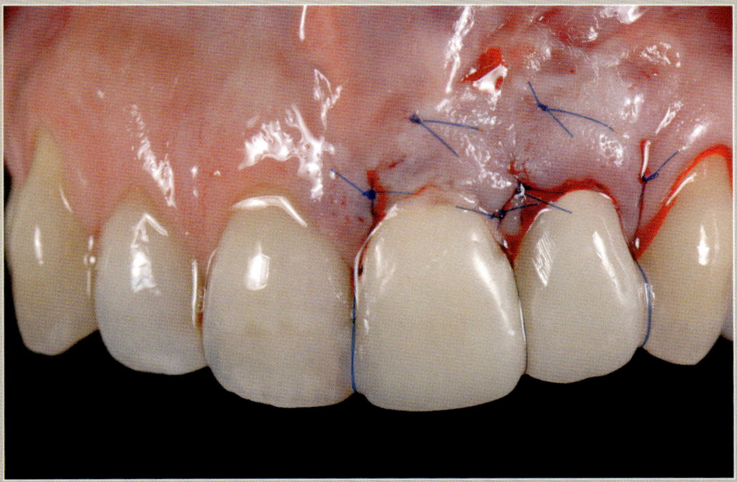

Frontal view of maxillary anterior teeth following soft tissue grafting and implant placement.

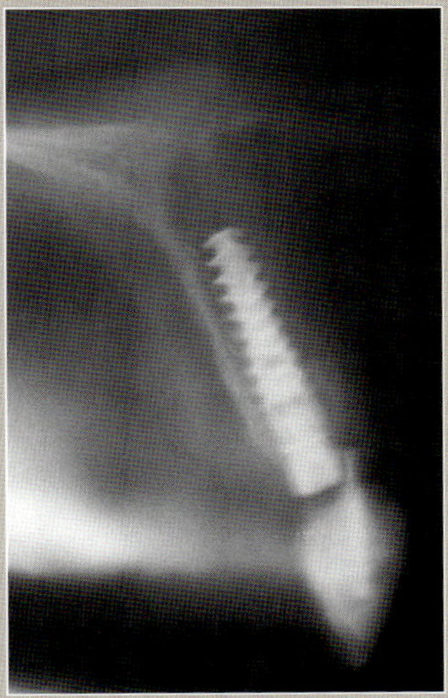

Tomography following implant placement.

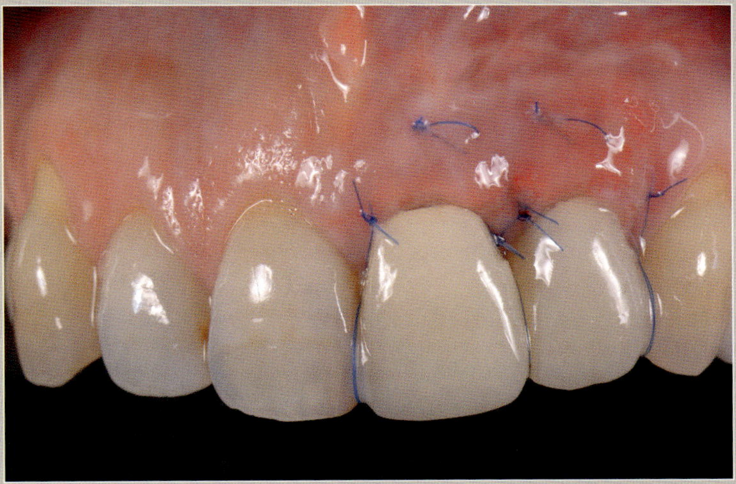

Frontal view of maxillary anterior teeth 1 week after soft tissue grafting and implant placement.

fabricated from the wax-up of the approved provisional restoration. Care was taken to leave a gap between the buccal bone and the implant. A narrow healing abutment was placed, and the gap was filled with a bovine filler material (Bio-Oss, Geistlich). The provisional restoration was cemented.

On the postoperative computed tomography (CT) scan, the ideal 3D implant position was evaluated. The fill of the gap and the buccal defect with bovine bone was clearly visible on the same CT scan. Healing was uneventful, and the sutures were removed after 1 week.

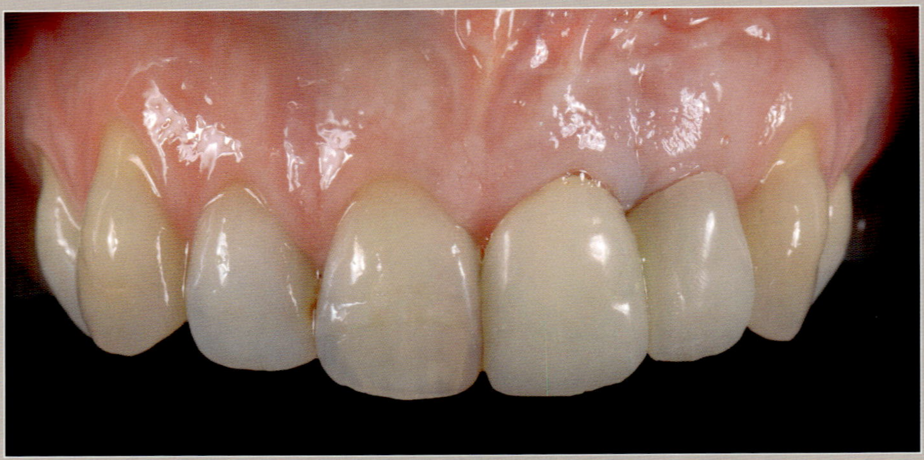

Three months after soft tissue grafting and implant placement.

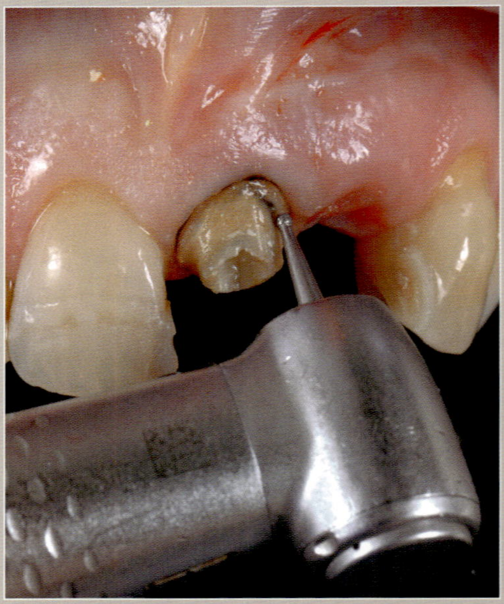

Removal of dentinal staining on tooth no. 9.

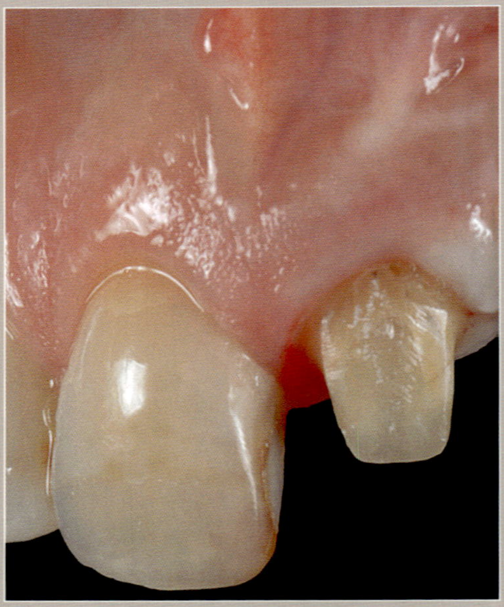

Final tooth preparation.

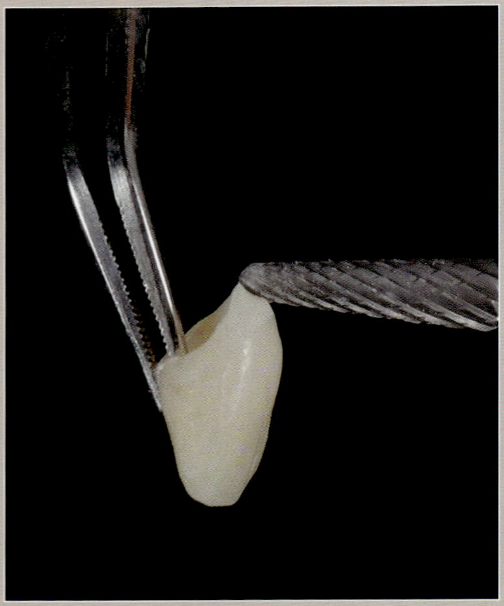

Optimizing the emergence profile of the provisional restoration.

Phase VI: Definitive restorations

Three months postoperatively, final tooth preparation was initiated. At that time, it was important to redo the endodontic treatment. The very dark stains in the dentin on tooth no. 9 were removed as much as possible, and an adhesive composite buildup, combined with placement and bonding of a fiber post (Paracore, Colténe Whaledent), was completed.

Care was taken to maintain a minimally invasive approach and to achieve biologically compatible preparations and impressions. Because tooth no. 9 was discolored, the preparation was placed subgingivally to minimize the effect of the root color and preparation on the gingival marginal color. The gingival color at the periodontal-prosthodontic interface is the critical zone for the esthetic outcome.

The disadvantage of a subgingival preparation in this case could be the combined effect of the preparation and convex contour of the crown on the vertical soft tissue level and soft tissue long-term stability. In situations in which a thin gingival phenotype is combined with discolored roots, we strongly prefer to make the preparation subgingival, but only if combined with a negative transsulcular profile.

In order for us to visualize this concept and evaluate the soft tissue behavior, the provisional fixed partial denture was relined and adapted to the new subgingival final tooth preparation after bonding. Care was taken to have a negative or

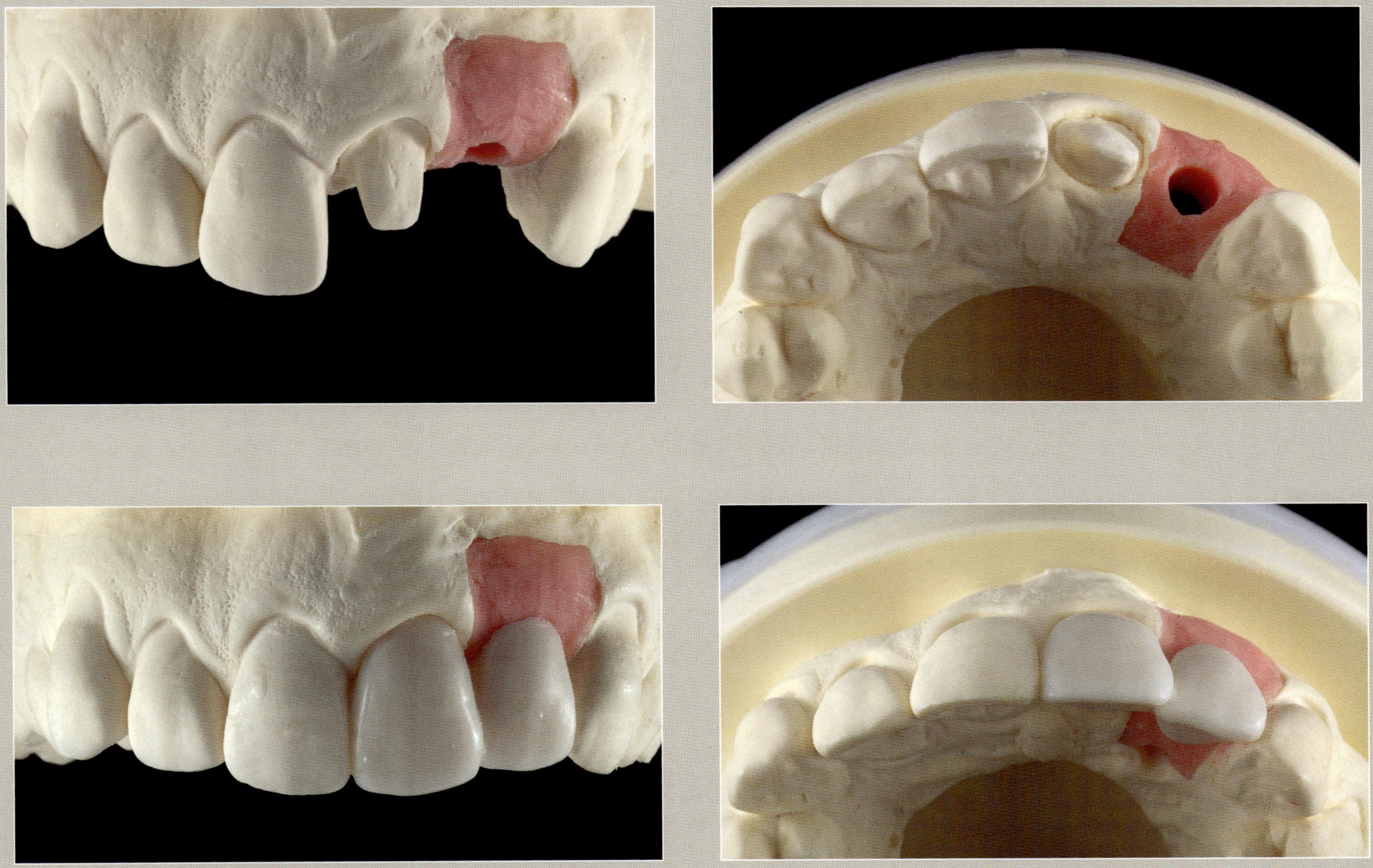

Wax-up incorporating the ideal form and 3D gingival tooth position.

concave transsulcular emergence profile on the gingival part of the provisional fixed partial denture. No attempt was made at this moment to optimize the gingival contours around the implant. The soft tissue contours could be optimized easily and very predictably on a cast in the laboratory.

The final impression was taken 2 weeks after the final preparation and evaluation of the final gingival contour around tooth no. 9. A narrow impression coping was deliberately used to take the implant impression. Final plaster casts were poured and mounted on an articulator.

The most critical factor in optimizing the soft tissue appearance around implant restorations is probably the concept of cast-based soft tissue recontouring. The dental technician needs to have a full understanding of ideal tooth diameters at the CEJ as well as the need to leave space (ie, transmucosal buccal concave forms) for soft tissue thickness (ie, connective tissue fibers) at the interface. The combination of these two parameters is essential. The images clearly demonstrate our ideas and concepts for abutment design in this particular case.

A high-quality, full-contour esthetic and functional wax-up was made. It was important at that time to incorporate the ideal form and 3D gingival tooth position in this wax-up. From the wax-up, a silicone index was fabricated. This allowed us to have an ideal reference, especially of the gingival position of both teeth, at any given moment.

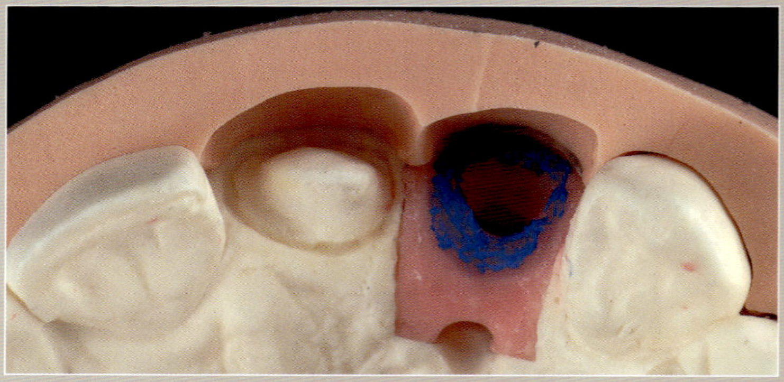

Silicone index fabricated from the wax-up. The blue line indicates the ideal buccogingival contour of the implant restoration.

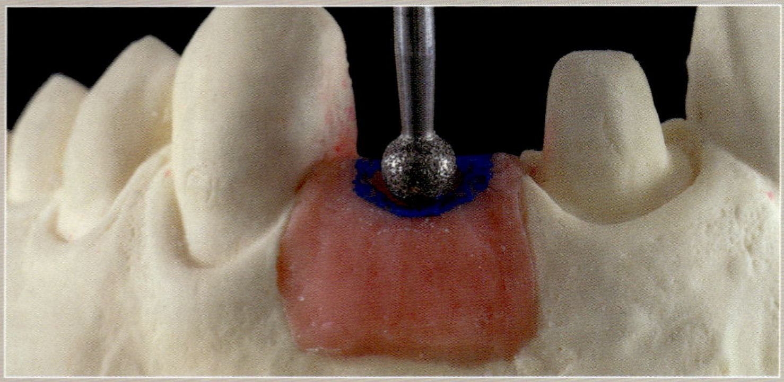

Adjustment of the transgingival space with a round diamond bur.

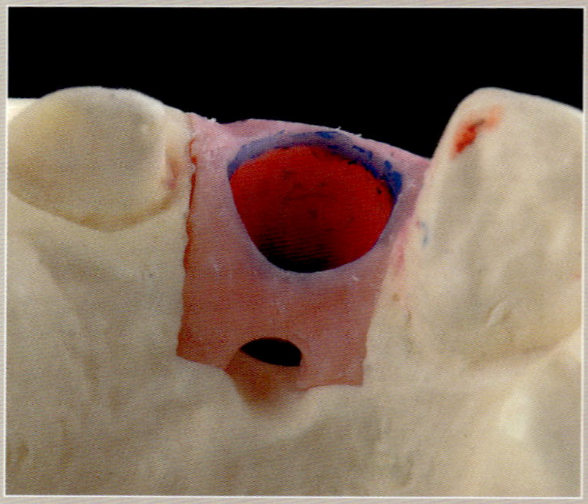

Palatal view of the final gingival contours around the implant.

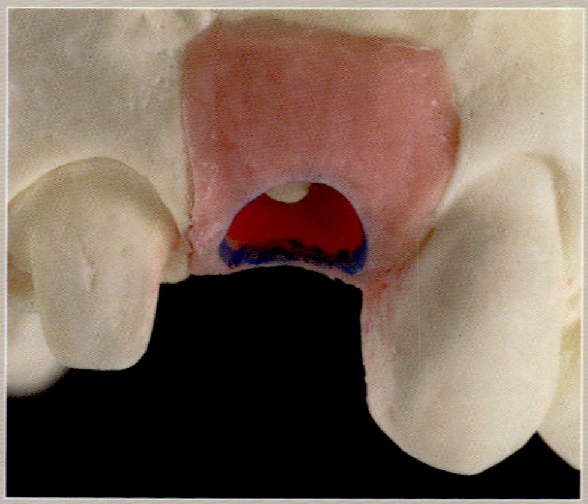

Anterior view of the final gingival contours around the implant.

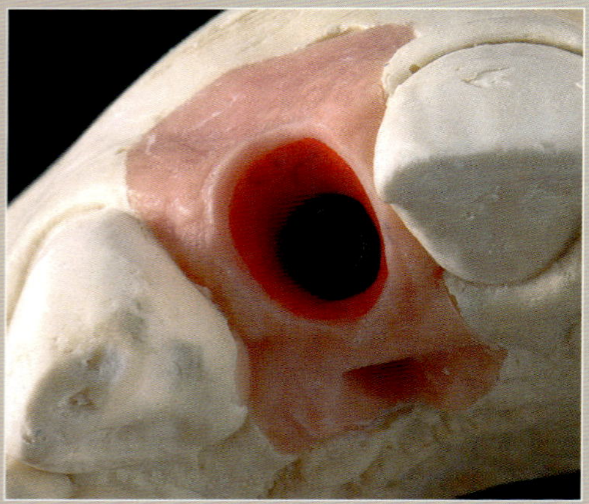

Occlusal view of the final gingival contours around the implant.

With a blue pencil we drew a line on the buccal aspect of the implant restoration, following the gingival contour in the silicone index (ie, a copy of the buccal contour of the wax). We could then transfer the ideal buccogingival contour of the implant restoration. However, the objective is not to meet this ideal line exactly but to stay 0.5 mm away from it. The most common error in implant restorations is trying to meet the ideal line or position and thereby creating excessive gingival pressure on the prosthetic components, which causes apical migration or recession of the marginal gingival tissue. As a result, the dental technician must create an optical illusion to compensate and optimize the final esthetic result. The full contour of the transgingival space was adjusted with a round diamond bur to best relate to the soft tissue mask, using this line as a reference.

The perfect implant restoration would be one in which the abutment occupies 90% of the transgingival space and the crown only emerges in the last 1 mm, or 10% of the transgingival space. From this point, the objective is to mimic the preparation of a natural tooth, with the abutment margin being positioned in the sulcus.

Zirconia computer-aided design/computer-assisted manufacture (CAD/CAM) abutments (Procera, Nobel Biocare) are the gold standard, especially for external hex connections. However, with internal connections, combining an internal hex with a morse taper design, we prefer a titanium connection. The best way for us to combine strength and esthetics is to bond a pressed part on a titanium provisional cylinder.

A provisional titanium cylinder (NobelActive) was adapted in length with the silicone index, and thus in relation to the definitive tooth form. Care was taken to leave sufficient space for the female pressed part of the abutment and the crown. The retention grooves were filled with wax, and a pattern resin project of the abutment was fabricated.

This resin abutment project was pressed (e.max Press) and bonded to the titanium cylinder in the lab with a cement (Multilink, Ivoclar Vivadent) after internal surface treatment of the pressed part (ie, etching for 20 seconds, silane application, and bonding). A high-opacity ingot (e.max Press HO, Ivoclar Vivadent) was selected to mask the underlying gray color of the titanium sleeve. The excess cement was then removed with a sharp blade after curing, and the surface was polished. Before intraoral use, the surface was cleaned with ethanol in an ultrasonic device for 10 minutes. This allowed for surface decontamination and eventual promotion of cellular adhesion on the titanium surface. All-ceramic single porcelain crowns (e.max Press MO/e.max Ceram, Ivoclar Vivadent) were fabricated.

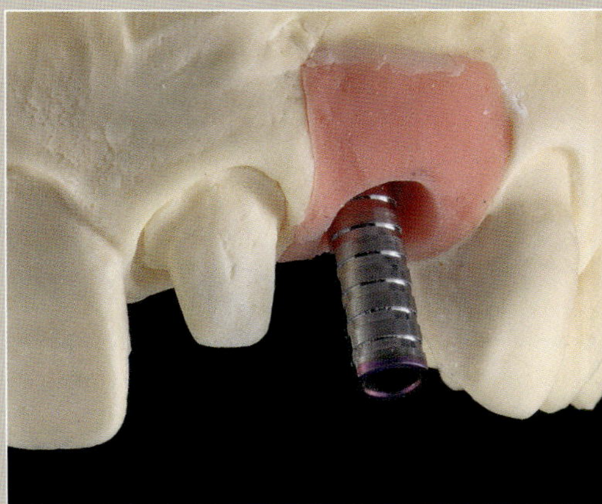

Provisional titanium cylinder prior to length reduction.

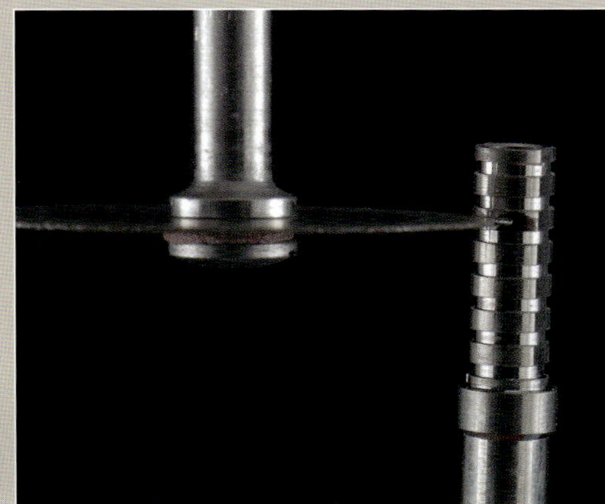

Diamond metal disc used to cut and adjust the length of the provisional titanium cylinder.

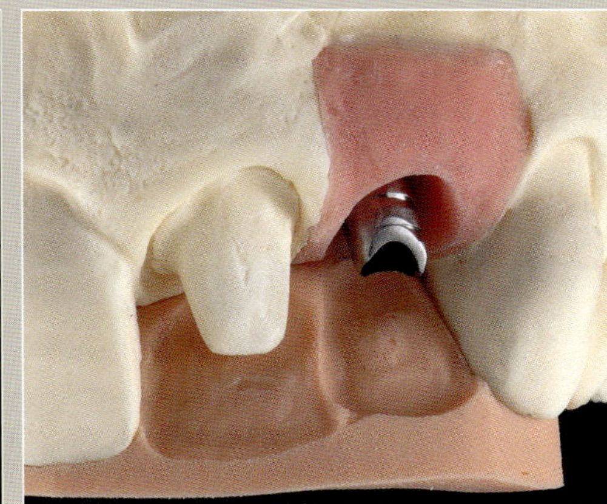

Provisional titanium cylinder adjusted in length to match the final tooth form.

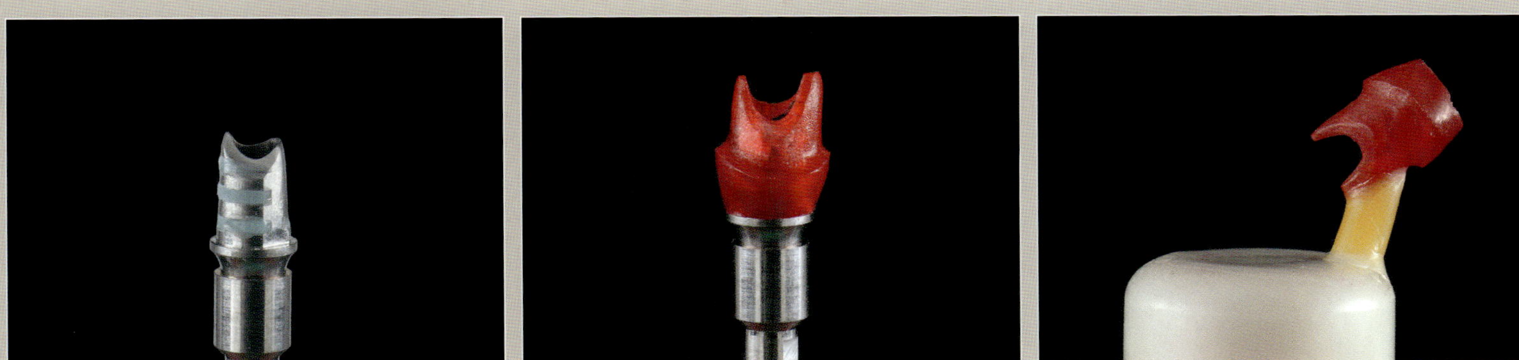

Filling the grooves of the provisional cylinder with wax, designing the proper abutment form (female part) in resin, and preparing for pressing.

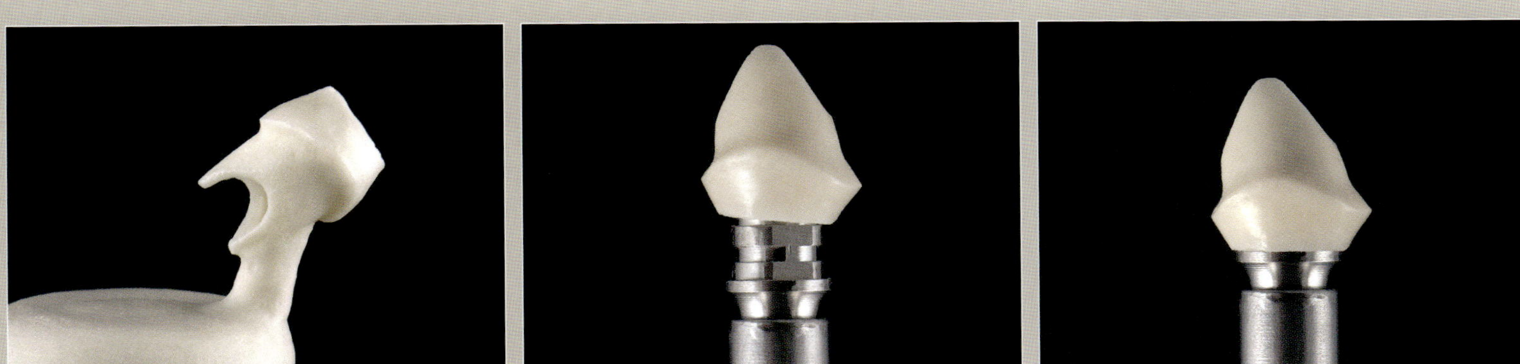

Abutment (female part) after pressing and refining fit and form.

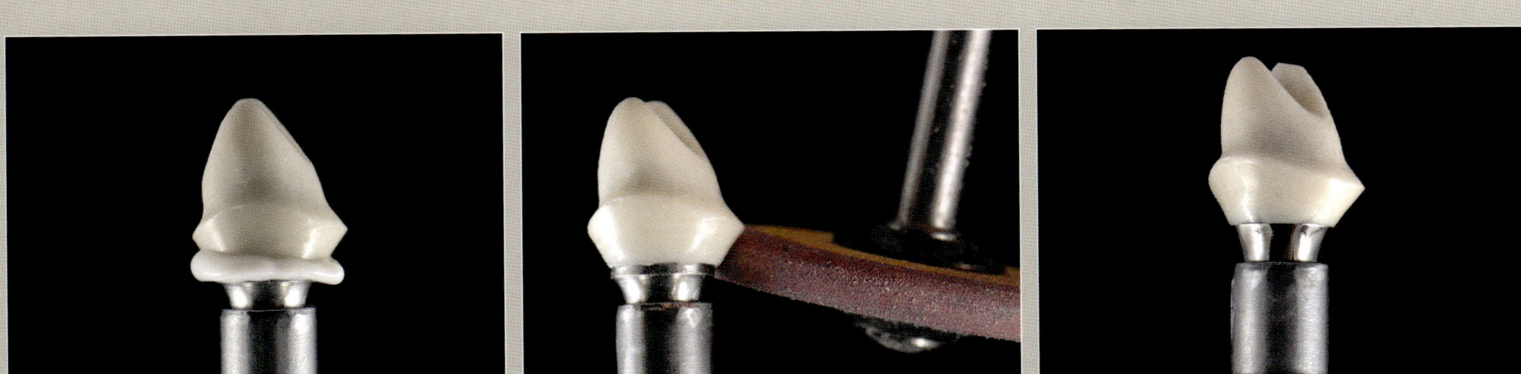

Bonding the pressed part to the titanium cylinder with Multilink cement and final polishing.

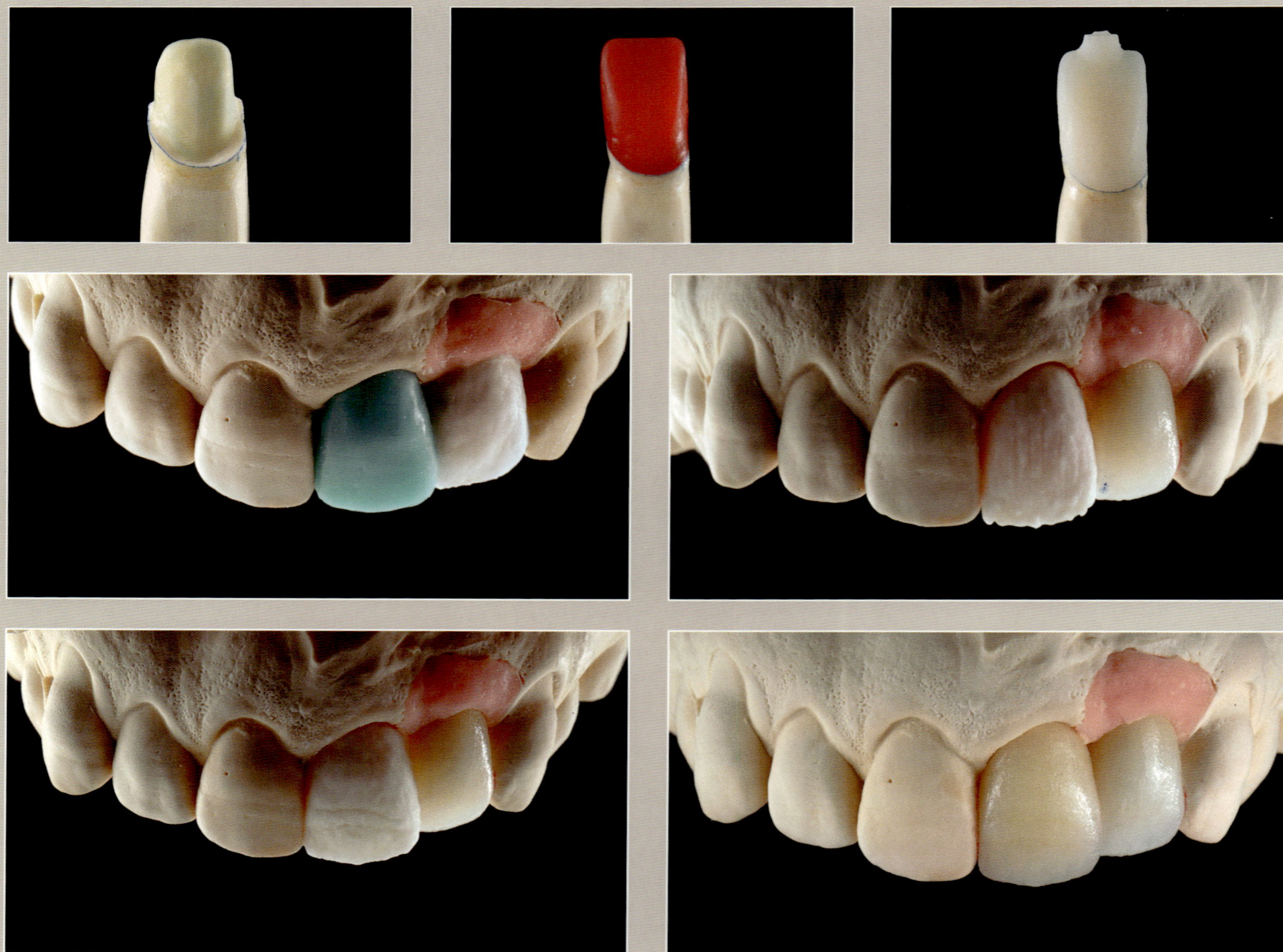

Fabrication of all-ceramic porcelain crowns.

At this stage, all prosthetic components and crowns were tried in and minor modifications made. This was necessary to evaluate color, form, and especially the prosthetic soft tissue support. We waited 30 minutes after inserting the abutment to evaluate the soft tissue contours to allow the blanching and compression of the marginal tissues to subside. The definitive soft tissue profile and position around the implant restoration are dependent upon the amount of prosthetic pressure and the prosthetic contour. In most cases, only very minor corrections are necessary.

A prefabricated gingival former was fabricated on a cast in the lab using a provisional titanium cylinder and composite. This former had the same profile as the final abutment and was used to keep the tissue in place and to prevent collapse while we made minor modifications in the lab to improve the profile of the abutment after the try-in.

Once the ideal contour had been obtained with the abutment, the contours of the crowns were finished intraorally. Line angle position was evaluated and modified to alter the visual perception of tooth width. The color details were finalized using a low-fusion glaze paste on both the natural tooth and crown and by applying stains intraorally. Photos were taken of these details. This gave the technician a clear idea of the colors and details needed to start the last bake and to finish the surface texture and luster.

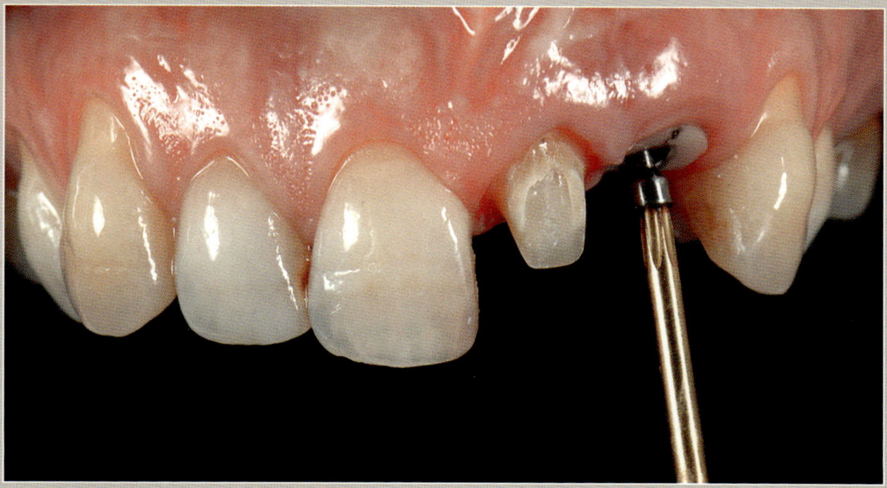
Placement of gingival former.

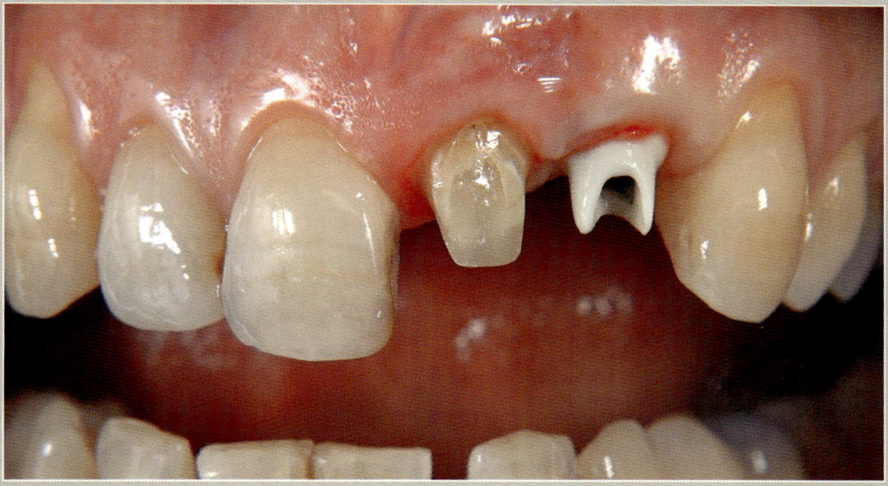
Final abutment in place.

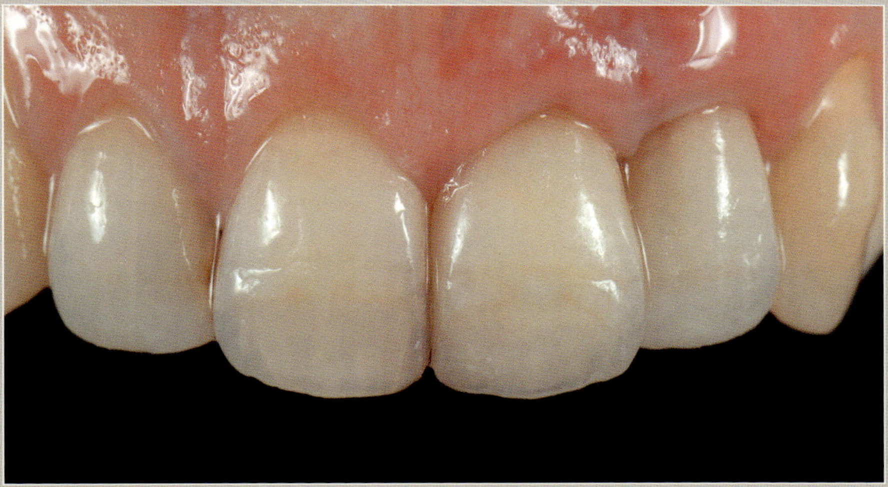
Finalizing the color details on the natural teeth and crowns.

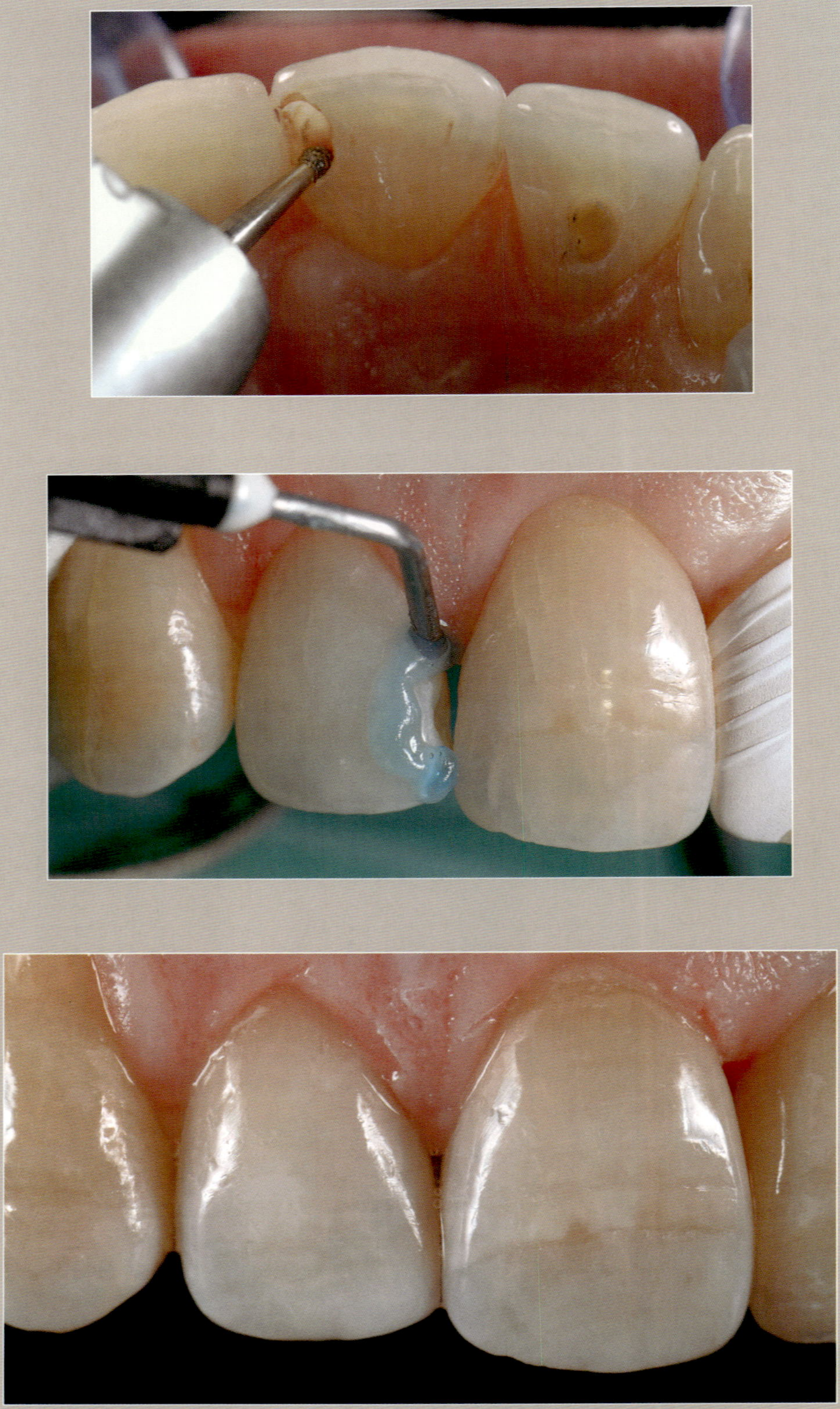

Replacement of existing composite restorations on teeth nos. 7 and 8
and treatment of caries on mesial aspect of tooth no. 7.

The abutment was torqued at 32 Ncm. The screw access hole was closed with polytetrafluoroethylene, and the crowns were adhesively cemented with a composite cement (Variolink II, Ivoclar Vivadent). Care was taken to follow the prescribed protocol for internal crown surface treatment before cementation.

Occlusion and hygiene were then checked, and the patient was placed on a 6-month periodontal and restorative maintenance program. After 6 months, the old mesial and palatal composite restorations on teeth nos. 7 and 8 were replaced. At the same time, the caries on the mesial aspect of tooth no. 7 was excavated and treated in a minimally invasive way.

Posttreatment

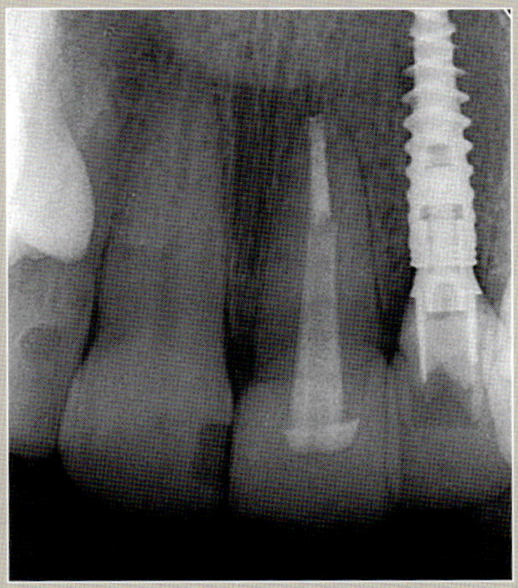

Radiograph of maxillary anterior teeth.

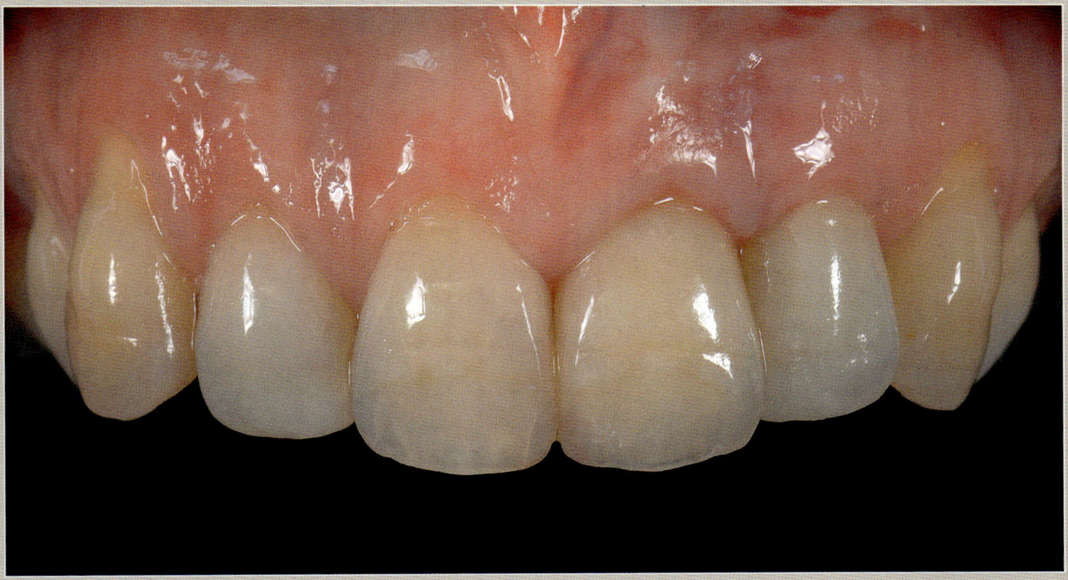

Intraoral view of maxillary anterior teeth.

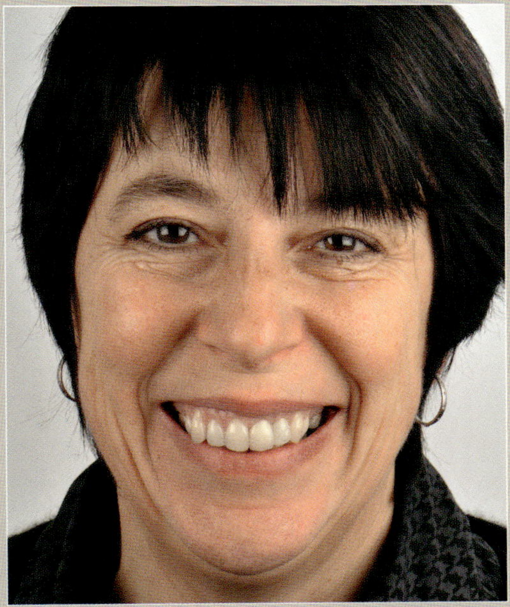

Facial view of smile.

You may now place the corresponding posttreatment overlay found in the separate folder over the pretreatment periodontal chart on page 421.

Commentary

This case presentation provides a snapshot of where we are with implant dentistry today. Treatment was not the most ideal, but this is the clinical reality. In most cases, reality dictates what our patients are willing to accept. Although from a technologic standpoint we are now able to provide restorations that are virtually indistinguishable from natural teeth, the state of the art in surgical reconstruction is not quite as predictable. In other words, in many cases we are faced with patients who are unwilling to take the steps necessary to achieve optimal esthetic results or we are not able to predictably achieve surgical results that provide the foundation for the most pleasing outcomes. This results in compromise; however, compromise does not have to be seen as one's enemy. In fact, compromise can be viewed as a friend because it provides the opportunity to make patients happy according to their own terms. This may result in more challenging treatment for the clinician but also provides the opportunity for great satisfaction when definitive outcomes ultimately meet or exceed patient expectations.

This case clearly had limiting factors from the start. A major obstacle was the papilla height between teeth nos. 9 and 10. This was not really clear at the start, especially because the papilla was swollen and irritated. It became more evident after initial periodontal therapy, with soft tissue healing taking place, and following provisionalization. This is one of the reasons we proposed orthodontic therapy to alter tooth position, which would positively impact soft tissue height. However, the patient was not willing to accept this approach.

The papilla height decreased slightly again after implant placement and connective tissue grafting. Although papilla height at 18 months had improved compared with that at 2 months postoperative, it would never be ideal compared with the contralateral side.

In retrospect, there may be some reasons why the papilla was not perceived as a problem at the onset of treatment. The fact that the papilla was larger (ie, inflamed) and more fully filled the interproximal space has already been mentioned. Another thought is that from an esthetic standpoint, the poor crown form and unattractive incisal length of the neighboring teeth may have distracted attention away from the papilla. Once the tooth form and incisal length issues were resolved and the teeth appeared more natural, the deficiency in papillary height was more obvious. This is something that is best diagnosed prior to treatment so that it can be addressed in collaboration with the laboratory and the necessary strategies can be considered. The laboratory technician is an integral part of the interdisciplinary treatment team and should be involved in all aspects of case planning from the very beginning. To date, the re-establishment of lost papillary height is still unpredictable at best, and the only solution is to try to mask these defects by creating optical illusions with the help of the laboratory technician.

When we approach difficult and challenging implant cases, it is often attention to the small prosthetic and surgical details that makes the greatest difference in the definitive treatment outcome. From the surgical side, improving the periodontal-prosthodontic interface with connective tissue grafting (especially in implant cases, but also around natural teeth with very thin gingival phenotypes) is one of the most effective treatment modalities for achieving long-term soft tissue stability. From the prosthetic side, using soft tissue–friendly materials and designs, understanding the effect of gingival prosthetic contours, and implementing abutment designs that improve tissue thickness and stability are of equal importance.

The last but probably most important remark is on the issue of precision. Most clinicians understand the importance of focusing on function, biology, and esthetics in achieving long-term treatment success, but few also recognize the value of precision as an equally significant determinant. Soft tissue health and ultimately esthetics cannot be achieved without prosthetic precision. This underscores the importance of the use of higher-magnification instruments such as loupes and microscopes by all treatment team members. In the laboratory, the entire cycle, from die preparation to finishing of the porcelain margins, should be accomplished under the microscope. Clinical observation has shown that the soft tissue condition and stability will be improved substantially by working with these immeasurably valuable tools.

What would I have done differently? It most likely would be preferable to bond the composites on the adjacent teeth before making the crowns. However, I planned to have these composite restorations fabricated by Dr Cláudio Pinho from Brazil, who is an expert in this area. Because he was only coming to Europe after the definitive placement of the crowns, this necessitated treatment in the reverse order. This certainly made the case more challenging for him.

To date, the patient has not been interested in covering exposed root surfaces on the facial of teeth nos. 7 and 11. It might have been better to propose to treat these areas at the same time that the implant was placed because I was already harvesting soft tissue from the palate to place around the implant. Instead, we suggested changes in the patient's brushing habits in order to avoid further apical migration of the tissue around these teeth.

The pressable ingots (e.max Press) do not really have the shades to match the adjacent root color. Also, the pressable material that we used in this case has very low fluorescence. This is certainly a concern. In the natural dentition, the greatest fluorescence is exhibited around the CEJ, in the gingival portion of the crown, and in the first part of the root surface. This fluorescence will affect the brightness and light reflection of the substrate and ultimately affect the appearance of the peri-implant soft tissue. In the future, many companies will need to improve the qualities of these materials in order to be able to mimic the natural dentition.

Acknowledgment

I am very fortunate and grateful to have a technician like Murilo Calgaro, who understands soft tissue contours and is a master at creating optical illusions. His assistance has been invaluable in overcoming many of the challenges in these complex and demanding cases.

17

A Comprehensive Approach to a Complex Case of Dysgnathia

Siegfried Marquardt, DDS

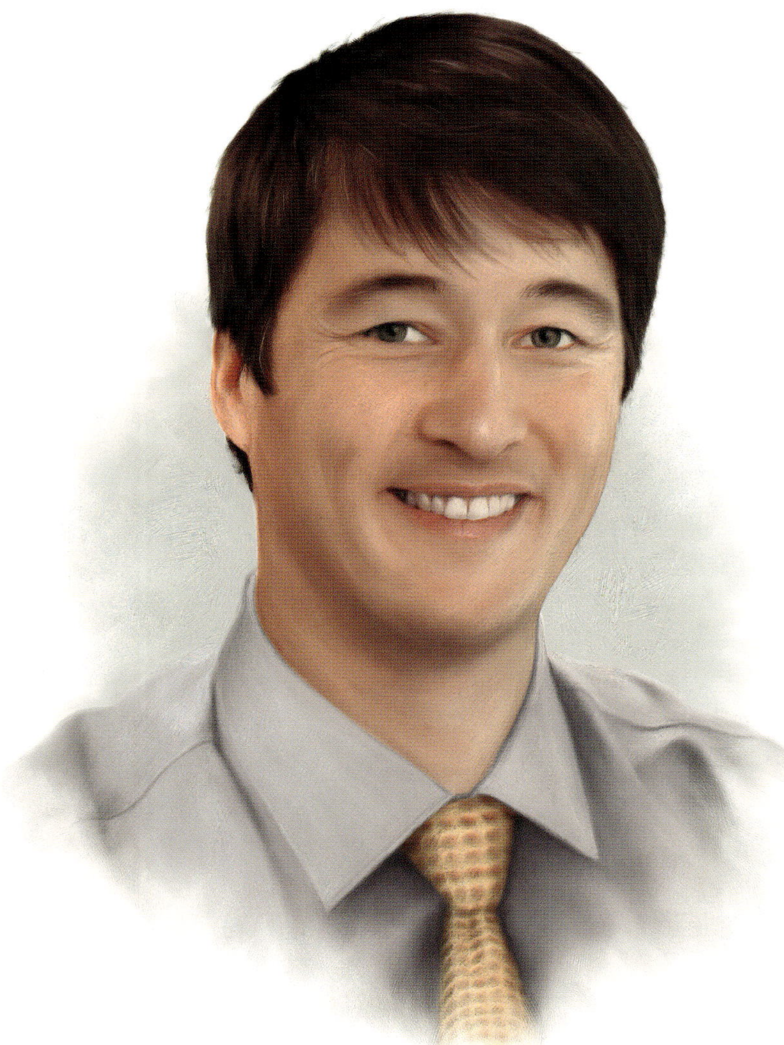

Today, we are not only dealing with evidence-based dentistry but also with an entirely different level of patient expectation arising from social trends and lifestyle-related concerns.

Philosophy and Background

One of the greatest challenges we face in our profession is how to develop and maintain a suitable interdisciplinary approach when dealing with complex cases. The treatment-planning philosophy and principles of the Seattle Study Club are some of the most helpful educational tools I have encountered in my professional life. Based on the concepts we have learned, my colleagues and I have incorporated a fixed series of theoretical steps, such as appropriate background questions, comprehensive data collection, analysis of this data, and synthesis of this information into a meaningful and effective treatment plan, into our daily practice. Consequently, the treatment-planning protocol that we have implemented now results in more optimal and predictable long-term outcomes.

Areas where differences and difficulties can arise are with the treatment solutions themselves, treatment implementation, and communication between treatment team members. Finding the right balance between several theoretical, treatment-based options and what the patient may see as the only right way can often be a dilemma. In addition to the purely technical and medical facts, we also must navigate patient expectations, psychologic and financial issues, and time management challenges. The key to successful treatment and to achieving a workable solution is optimal coordination and interaction of all the above factors. Without an interdisciplinary approach, this may become a hopeless undertaking.

The following three points illustrate my rationale for selecting this particular patient for the treatment-planning exercise that follows:

1. It illustrates a multidisciplinary approach at a complex level.
2. There is a discrepancy between patient expectations and the optimal treatment options, and it is interesting to see how these two gradually converge.
3. Some principles that may offer new treatment options for the reader are addressed.

This chapter will examine and demonstrate how to manage maxillary retrognathia or mandibular prognathism in adult patients. This is a common form of dysgnathia in which the maxilla has grown too slowly, resulting in a mandible that is positioned too far forward in relation to the opposing jaw,[1] or mandibular growth has been excessive in comparison with that of the maxilla. Determining the type of dysgnathia is usually accomplished by analyzing a lateral cephalogram and the patient's profile.

The term *dysgnathia* is defined as the summary of defective developments of the teeth, the jaws, and/or the masticatory apparatus. The anomalies may affect the position of the teeth, the form of the jaws, the position of the jaws in relation to each other, or the location of the jaws within the skull; such anomalies may lead to esthetic and functional impairments. When diagnosing dysgnathia, it is important to differentiate between the skeletal and dentoalveolar forms.

Skeletal dysgnathia refers to the abnormal position and dimension of the maxilla and mandible to the base of the skull. The classification is described in different ways. To identify a skeletal dysgnathia, it is necessary to analyze clinical signs, lateral cephalograms, and study casts.[2] Malpositions in the sagittal, vertical, and/or transverse directions are possible. Four basic forms of skeletal dysgnathia have been described:

- Class II dysgnathia
  1. Maxillary prognathia
  2. Mandibular retrognathia
- Class III dysgnathia
  3. Maxillary retrognathia
  4. Mandibular prognathia

Dentoalveolar dysgnathia refers to pure dentoalveolar malformations with a normal relationship of the jaws to the base of the skull. Edward Hartley Angle (1855–1930) defined three classes focused only on the occlusion in the posterior region[3]:

1. Class I: Normal occlusion
2. Class II: Disto-occlusion
3. Class III: Mesio-occlusion

Skeletal forms of dysgnathia are usually treated with surgical intervention, while in most cases dentoalveolar forms of dysgnathia can be treated with orthodontic treatment.

Orthodontic analysis must be used to determine whether there is dentoalveolar compensation related to a skeletal dysgnathia. The problems presented by such patients are complex and multifaceted. In addition to the esthetic problems, patients have difficulties chewing and biting because of the reverse vertical overlap of the anterior teeth. Furthermore, there can be additional complicating factors such as poor alignment of the teeth and temporomandibular joint (TMJ) dysfunction.[4,5] The most common characteristics of these patients are:

- Mandible too far forward in relation to the maxilla
- Concave facial profile
- Dominant nose and distinctive nasolabial sulcus
- Positive lip step (upper lip is behind the lower lip)
- Restricted nasal respiration
- Class III negative overjet

When approaching these complex situations, gathering an interdisciplinary team of specialists for case planning is invaluable. In most cases, the expertise of the dental technician, the orthodontist, the endodontist, and the oral and maxillofacial surgeon is required. By working together in a collaborative, interdisciplinary environment in which data analysis can be exchanged and individual knowledge shared, clinicians can create an optimal treatment plan.

The following case illustrates how we use a team approach with the goal of giving the patient a result that is as satisfying as possible. Both functional and esthetic needs led this patient to consider undergoing long-term treatment, although she had lived with her situation for more than 30 years without any problems. This is a point of great interest because we are seeing an increasing number of patients with similar conditions in our office. As they get older, patients become more aware of their dental health and the esthetic possibilities of dental treatment. Higher life expectancy also plays a role, as do high expectations with regard to the quality of life in middle and old age.

Today, we are not only dealing with evidence-based dentistry but also with an entirely different level of patient expectation arising from social trends and lifestyle-related concerns. This is what makes our profession so unique and interesting.

Case Presentation

Treating clinicians
Implant surgeon and restorative dentist: Siegfried Marquardt, DDS
Orthodontist: Haschem Abrischami, DDS
Maxillofacial and plastic surgeon: Kay Sauckel, DDS, MD
Endodontist: Franz Hagg, DDS
Ceramist: Andreas Reischl, CDT

Clinical Treatment Planning

Age at initial presentation: 54 years
Initial presentation: March 2007
Active treatment completed: December 2009

The focus of this case presentation is on the patient's goals and objectives and on how we were able to achieve a positive long-term prognosis with a high degree of predictability.

Introduction and background

This 54-year-old patient presented with a high degree of maxillary retrognathia, a potentially disfiguring disorder in which the mandible outgrows the maxilla, usually resulting in an extended chin. It most often has a genetic etiology. In this case, the maxillary retrognathia was pronounced by the congenitally missing maxillary lateral incisors.

The patient had not experienced problems with this condition in the past due to the dentoalveolar compensation for the underlying skeletal malformation. However, as a result of this compensation, the patient's dental restorations often fractured shortly after replacement, requiring her to frequently consult her dentist for re-treatment. Following the removal of amalgam fillings a few years previously by another dentist, she had been unhappy with her new crowns and other restorations, complaining of bad breath and slight sensitivity to pressure. In addition, she felt that she could not bite on both sides in comfort and could not chew properly. She felt that her "bite had become weaker" over time. Furthermore, she was unhappy with her prominent chin, rather flat face, and deep nasolabial folds. Additionally, she wished to achieve a more "appealing" smile and a "better and more stable bite."

It was clear that the psychologic strain felt by the patient was so high that she was willing to undergo whatever treatment was necessary to achieve an optimal result. Nevertheless, the initial challenge we faced was to deal sensitively with her wish to avoid surgical treatment and to use an approach to altering tooth structure that was as minimally invasive as possible.

Medical history

- Healthy 54-year-old woman
- Low blood pressure
- No current medications
- No known drug allergies
- Noncontributory medical history
- Slight hay fever
- Nonsmoker for more than 20 years

Diagnostic findings

Extraoral and facial findings

- Flat to slightly concave facial profile (midface hypoplasia)
- Acute (small) nasolabial angle (less than 90 degrees)
- Little to no incisor display at repose
- Incisor display while smiling (4 mm)
- Prominent chin on lateral profile
- Appearance suggestive of maxillary retrognathia
- Maxillary teeth almost invisible while smiling
- Maxillary midline in line with patient's facial midline
- Inverse smile line
- Low lip line; reduced maxillary and mandibular incisor display (3 to 4 mm) with broad smile
- Size and form of lips symmetric during smile and repose
- Mandibular dental midline is slightly deviated 1 to 2 mm to the patient's left compared with the maxillary dental midline

Pretreatment

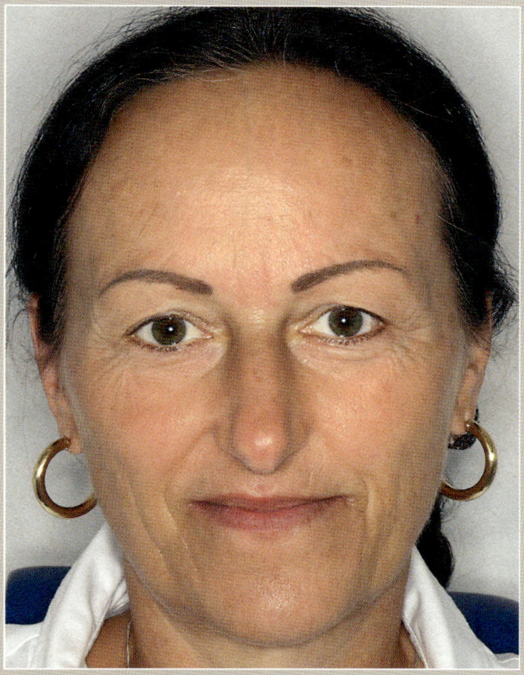

Frontal facial view.

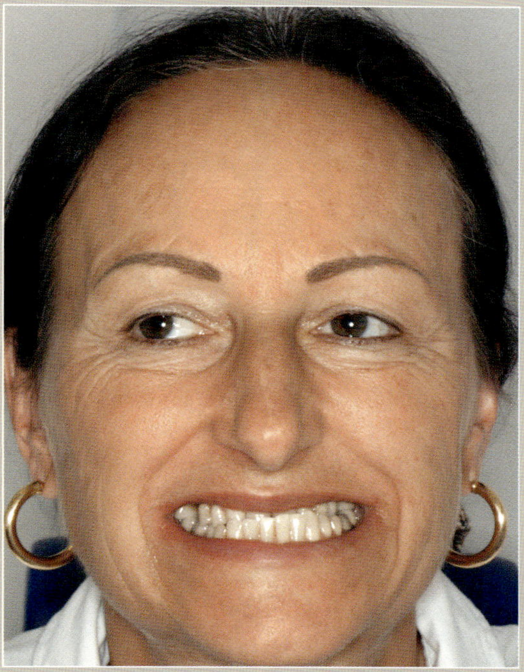

Frontal facial view of full smile.

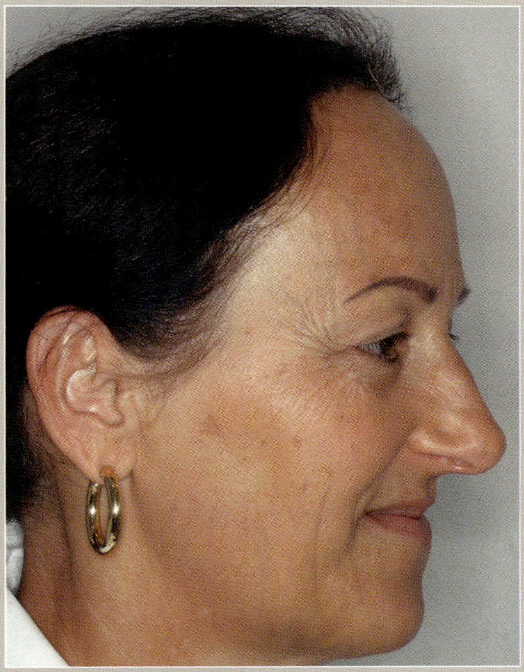

Lateral facial view.

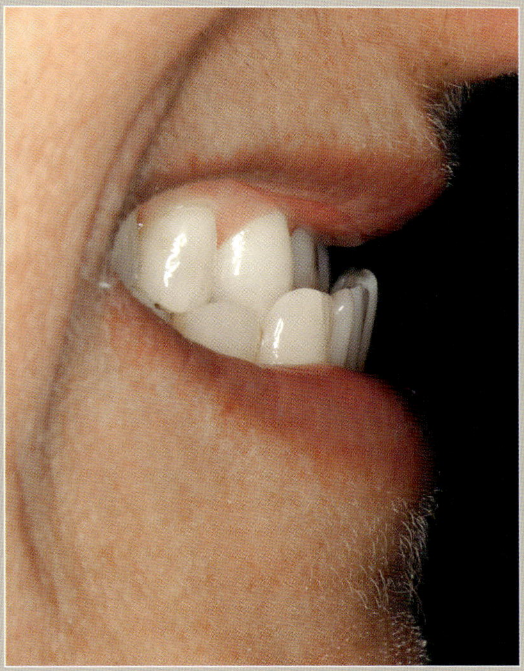

Lateral facial view of full smile.

TMJ and mandibular range of motion

- No joint clicking or popping
- Range of motion within normal limits; no deviation on opening
- Slight feeling of pressure in the right joint area during chewing movements
- Limited occlusal stability in maximal intercuspal position due to an inverse vertical overlap and reverse articulation (left)
- Slight discomfort upon opening and closing

Intraoral findings

Dental

- Missing teeth nos. 1, 7, 10, 14, 16, 17, 31, and 32
- Implant restoration at site no. 31
- Edentulous spaces of missing teeth nos. 7 and 10 have closed
- Poorly shaped mandibular and maxillary dental arches
- Crowding and supraeruption of the mandibular anterior teeth
- Extensive wear, fractured crowns, and erosion at teeth nos. 8, 9, 13, and 30
- Active caries not apparent
- Incomplete endodontic fill of teeth nos. 3 and 19

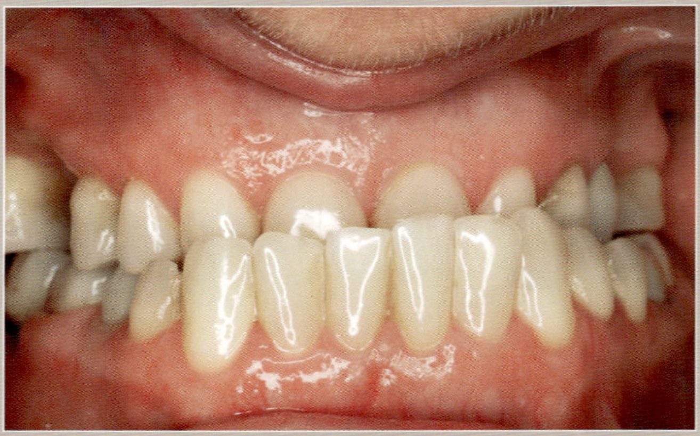

Intraoral anterior view.

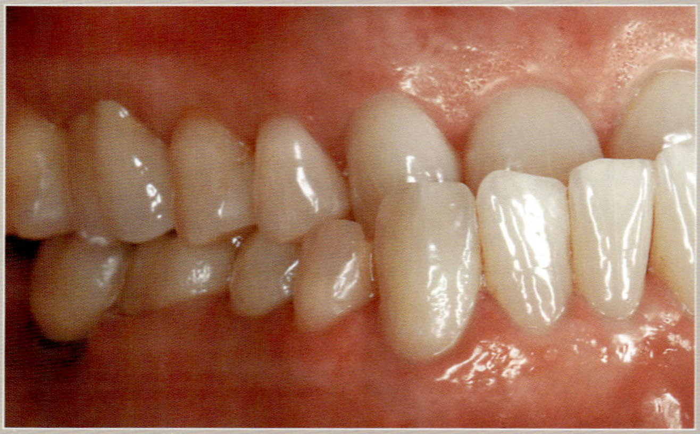

Intraoral right lateral view.

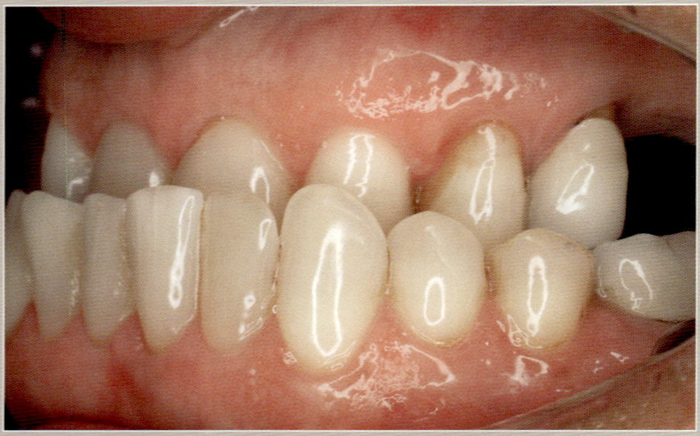

Intraoral left lateral view.

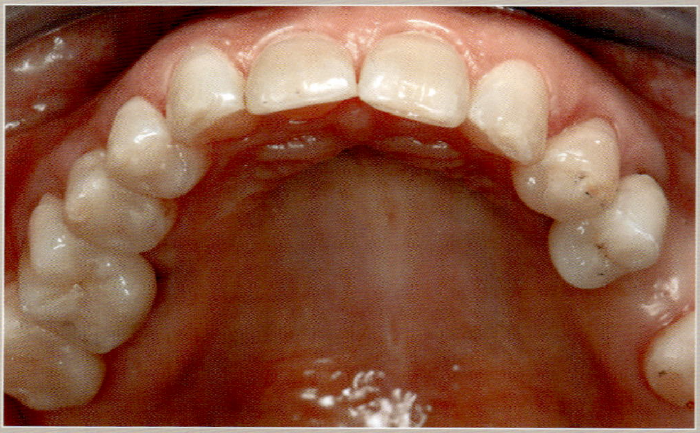

Occlusal maxillary view.

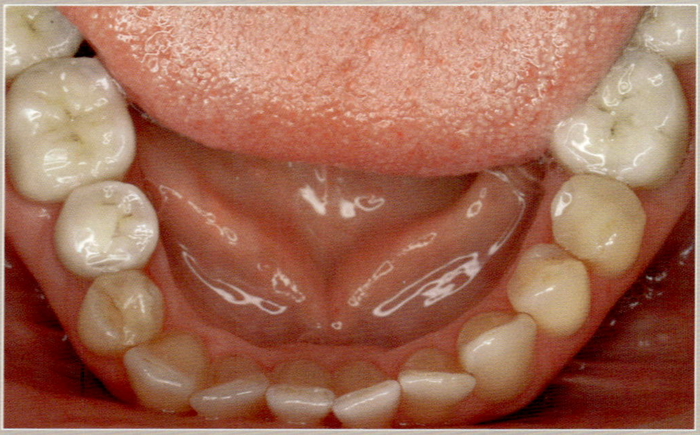

Occlusal mandibular view.

Periodontal

- Intraoral soft tissues appear normal
- Negative oral cancer examination
- Gingival line on facial of mandibular anterior teeth altered as a result of supraeruption of these teeth
- AAP Type II
- Generalized thin to normal gingival phenotype
- Generalized gingivitis
- Root perforation and localized periodontitis on tooth no. 3
- Bleeding on probing: 41%
- Plaque Index: 48%
- Probing depths generally less than 4 mm
- Probing depths in tooth no. 2 up to 5 mm and in tooth no. 3 up to 8 mm
- Generalized minimal bone loss with more significant bone loss around tooth no. 3

Occlusal notes

- Angle Class I occlusion
- Skeletal Class III dysgnathia
- Reverse overbite (vertical overlap): 2 mm
- Inverse overjet (horizontal overlap): 2 mm
- Mandible: anteroposterior stepped occlusal plane
- Reverse articulation (left)
- Habitual occlusion is not coincident with centric relation
- No contact between teeth nos. 13 to 15 and18 to 20

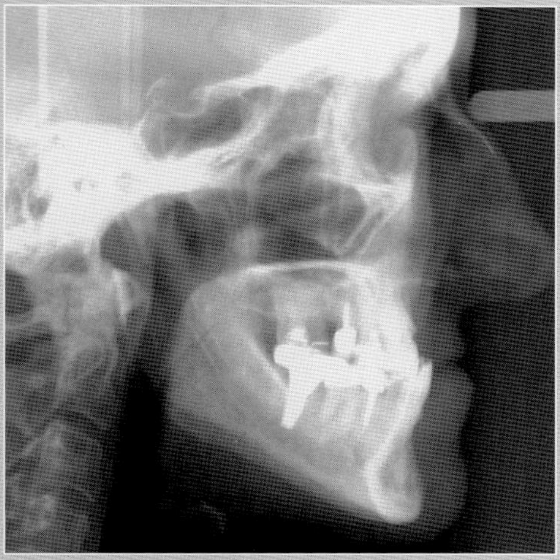

Pretreatment cephalometric radiograph, 2007.

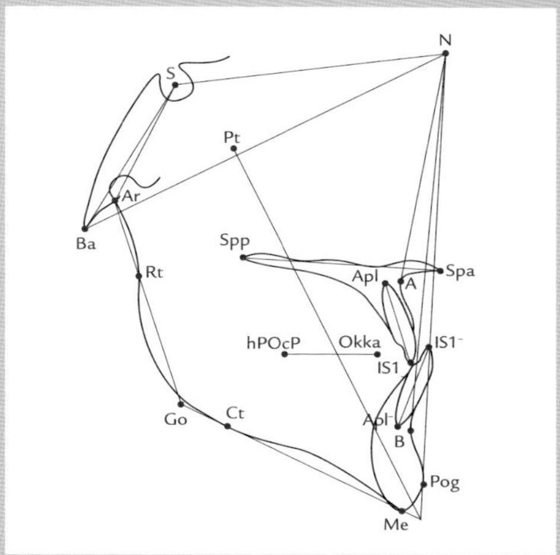

Pretreatment cephalometric tracing, 2007.

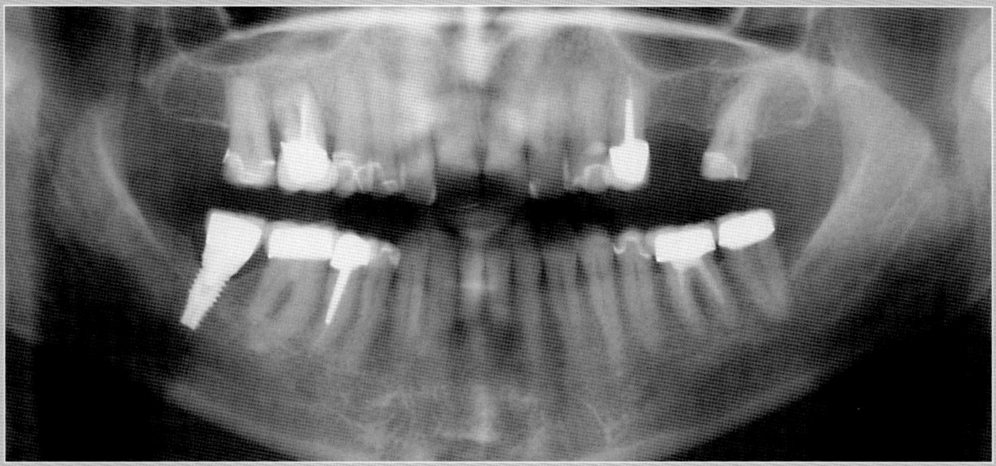

Pretreatment panoramic radiograph, 2007.

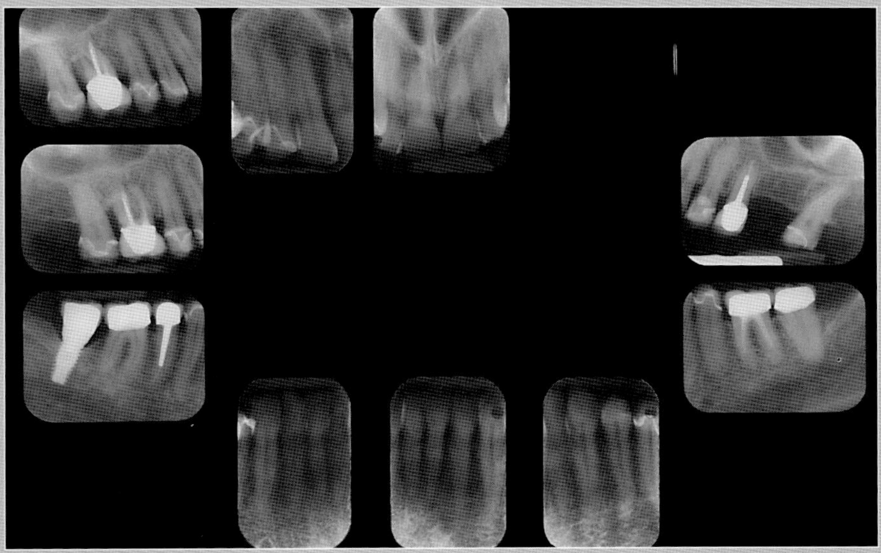

Pretreatment periapical radiographs, 2007.

Radiographic findings

- Endodontically treated teeth nos. 3, 13, 19, and 29
- Incomplete endodontic fill of teeth nos. 3 and 19
- Implant replacing tooth no. 31
- No apparent pathology in joint areas
- Generally minimal horizontal bone loss, with exception of tooth no. 3, where some vertical bone loss is noted

Cephalometric analysis

- Slightly steep position of the maxillary anterior teeth
- Mesiobasal jaw relation
- Midface hypoplasia
- Acute nasolabial angle

Diagnosis

- Skeletal Class III malocclusion with maxillary retrognathia
- AAP Type II
- TMJ within normal limits
- Reverse articulation and malocclusion on left side
- General moderate attrition in both arches except the mandibular anterior teeth
- Tooth erosion
- Partial edentulism
- Failing restorations

Etiology

Because of missing teeth nos. 7 and 10, the maxilla is smaller than the mandible. There is also an anterior forced bite—that is, the patient can only function by bringing the mandible completely forward of the maxillary anterior teeth. The patient had adjusted to this over the years.

Prognosis

- Periodontal: good overall with the exception of tooth no. 3, which is hopeless
- Biomechanical: generally good
- Functional: fair without surgery, good with surgery
- Esthetic: fair without surgery, good with surgery

The prognosis for the entire dentition becomes guarded if the orthognathic problems are not successfully addressed due to the potential for continued TMJ disease. The prognosis for the teeth will significantly improve if a mutually protected articulation can be established. The prognosis for the entire dentition would also improve from fair to excellent if orthodontic and surgical therapy could be implemented.

Summary of concerns

1. The patient feels her midface is too flat and her chin too prominent. Will the amount of maxillary advancement necessary to correct the malocclusion be sufficient for the patient to feel satisfied with the soft tissue changes?
2. Will the maxillary advancement worsen the nasolabial angle? If so, can the favorable anterior maxillary extrusion counteract this effect sufficiently?
3. If the patient declines orthognathic surgery, can she be adequately treated by orthodontic and prosthodontic treatment alone?
4. If the patient chooses an orthodontic and prosthodontic approach, what (if any) soft tissue treatment will be necessary to provide for a successful esthetic outcome?
5. How can we increase the vertical dimension to facilitate occlusal function before surgery?
6. What are the key functional and esthetic considerations in the achievement of a stable result with minimally invasive tooth treatment?
7. How can we stabilize the occlusion in the long term?

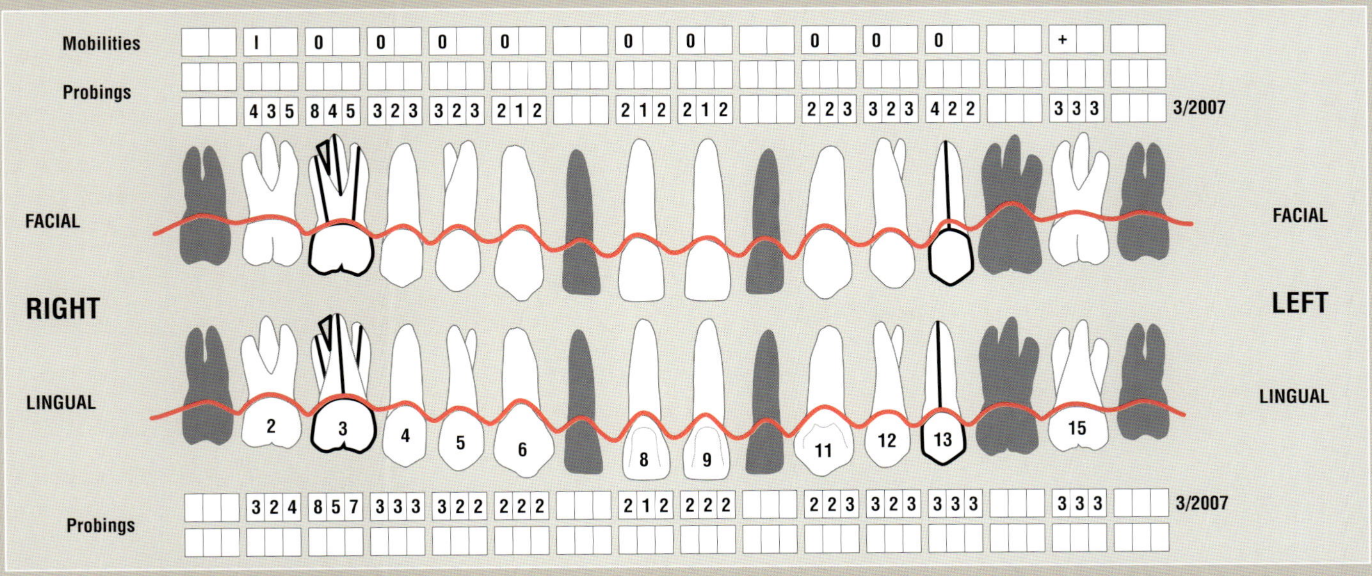

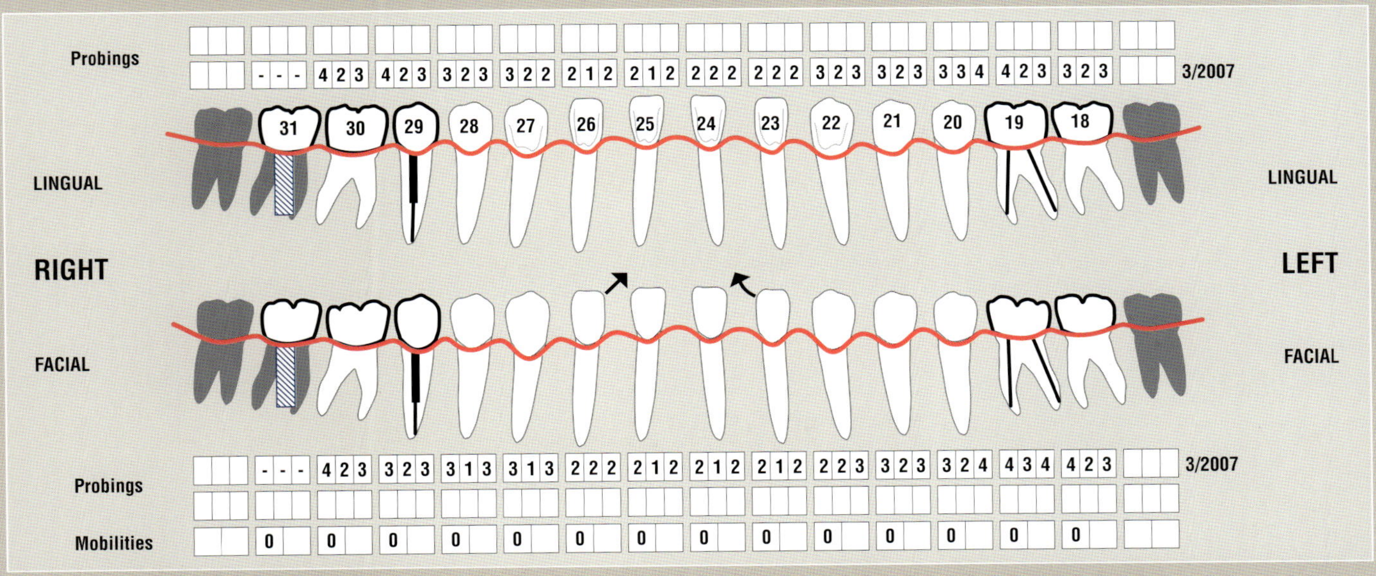

As a learning exercise, you may now outline goals/objectives of treatment and a treatment plan.

Proposed Treatment Plan

Goals/objectives of treatment

- Resolve the skeletal and dental abnormalities that have resulted in a poorly functioning dentition while establishing a more pleasing esthetic treatment outcome
- Achieve a stable occlusion with the aid of orthodontic therapy
- Replace poorly fitting restorations and increase the vertical dimension of occlusion
- Accomplish all of our goals and objectives without maxillofacial surgery

Phase I: Initial therapy

1. Initial records (including maxillary and mandibular casts, intraoral images, facebow transfer, centric relation record, radiographic examination)
2. Generalized root planing and scaling, prophylaxis, and oral hygiene instruction
3. Referral to orthodontist and oral and maxillofacial surgeon for orthodontic and orthognathic evaluation and consultation
4. Consultation with interdisciplinary team to develop and discuss possible treatment options

Phase II: Diagnostic wax-up and functional therapy with an occlusal guard

5. Data collection, including two sets of individual articulated casts—one set to produce an occlusal guard for evaluating the feasibility of changing the vertical dimension of occlusion and to relax the muscles and one set to fabricate a diagnostic wax-up and surgical guides

Phase III: Extraction of tooth no. 3 and preprosthodontic mock-up

6. Fabrication of "tabletops" (ie, unprepared onlays) for the posterior teeth to increase the vertical dimension of occlusion and to open the inverse anterior vertical overlap; this is important to enable the orthodontic forces to procline the maxillary anterior teeth and to retrude the mandibular anterior teeth

Phase IV: Orthodontics with or without orthognathic surgery

7. The following options were discussed using an interdisciplinary team approach, incorporating orthognathic and/or orthodontic therapy and prosthodontic treatment:

- Option 1
  - Orthodontic presurgical treatment: Correct the crowded mandibular anterior teeth. Resolve the space deficit by proclining the mandibular teeth, thereby enhancing the negative sagittal step. Shape and align the maxillary and mandibular teeth.
  - Orthognathic surgery: Perform maxillary correction with a Le Fort I osteotomy, clockwise rotation, advancement (3 mm), and anterior extrusion (2 mm) and mandibular correction with a bilateral sagittal split osteotomy and setback (3 mm).
  - Postoperative orthodontic completion: Finalize appropriate tooth alignment.
- Option 2
  - Orthodontic presurgical treatment: Resolve the space deficit in the mandible by removing tooth no. 24. Shape and align the maxillary and mandibular teeth.
  - Orthognathic surgery: Perform maxillary correction with a Le Fort I osteotomy, clockwise rotation, advancement (4 mm), and anterior extrusion (2 mm).
  - Postoperative orthodontic completion: Finalize appropriate tooth alignment.
- Option 3
  - Orthodontic therapy (nonsurgical treatment approach): Resolve the space deficit in the mandible by removing tooth no. 24. Procline the maxillary anterior segment and retrude the mandibular anterior segment to correct the negative sagittal overjet. Shape and align the maxillary and mandibular teeth.

Phase V: Endodontic re-treatment of tooth no. 19

Phase VI: Implant placement at sites nos. 3 and 14

Phase VII: Provisional restorative treatment

Phase VIII: Definitive restorative treatment

8. Individual abutments and implant-supported metal-ceramic crowns on implants in sites nos. 3, 14, and 31
9. Individual metal-ceramic crowns on teeth nos. 13, 18, 19, 29, and 30
10. Individual full-ceramic overlays on teeth nos. 2, 4, 5, 12, 15, 20, 21, and 28
11. Restoration of teeth with composite material on teeth nos. 7, 8, 9, and 10

Phase IX: Re-evaluation and maintenance

Active Clinical Treatment

Review of the goals/objectives of treatment

Overall goals

- Resolve the skeletal and dental abnormalities that have resulted in a poorly functioning dentition while establishing a more pleasing esthetic treatment outcome
- Achieve a stable occlusion with the aid of orthodontic therapy
- Replace poorly fitting restorations and increase the vertical dimension of occlusion
- Accomplish all of our goals and objectives without maxillofacial surgery

Specific objectives

- Reduce the flatness of the midface
- Correct the prominent chin or sagittal chin-midface relationship
- Establish a mutually protected articulation and stable occlusion
- Maintain periodontal health
- Create a natural-looking smile with normal incisor exposure in repose
- Protect the dentition from parafunctional habits, creating long-term stability

Phase I: Initial therapy

After completing a comprehensive examination, the patient participated in a thorough oral hygiene instruction program. We emphasized that this was of vital importance for the success of her treatment.

The consultation with the orthodontist and the maxillofacial surgeon generated several treatment options as outlined above. After much deliberation and weighing all of the potential risks and rewards, the patient opted for a nonsurgical approach to treatment.

Phase II: Diagnostic wax-up and splint therapy

After evaluation of the diagnostic wax-up, the interdisciplinary team decided to first implement splint therapy to increase the vertical dimension, relax the muscles, and observe whether the patient was subsequently more comfortable. The reversible occlusal therapy with the occlusal guard was also an important step in being able to demonstrate what could be accomplished related to her TMJ areas and muscles. Would we be able to eliminate the sense of pressure in her right joint area on chewing? Would she be able to tolerate her new vertical dimension of occlusion? Could we alter the joint areas to gain a relaxed centric relation position?

The patient wore the occlusal guard for about 3 months and then confirmed that she was quite comfortable. At this point, we were ready to consider instituting the "tabletop" treatment. The wax-ups on the casts allowed for constant comparison and evaluation during all phases of treatment.

Phase III: Extraction of teeth nos. 3 and 24, preprosthodontic mock-up, and preorthodontic treatment

As previously discussed, the treatment team complied with the patient's wishes and instituted a nonsurgical course of treatment. This included orthodontic therapy to attempt to retrude the mandibular anterior teeth. To address the mandibular anterior crowding, tooth no. 24 was extracted. This allowed for harmonization of the anterior segment independently of the decision for surgical treatment. Tooth no. 3 was also extracted due to its hopeless prognosis.

In addition, the orthodontist first corrected the reverse articulation on the left side using a quad-helix in the maxillary arch for 4 months; this also served to procline the anterior teeth. After the reverse articulation had been corrected, the laboratory fabricated "tabletops" with composite resin (Gradia Indirect, GC) for the posterior teeth to increase the vertical dimension of occlusion and to open the vertical overlap. These "tabletops" were fixed adhesively (Variolink, Ivoclar Vivadent). (Tabletop is an unprepared restoration in composite or ceramic fixed on the natural teeth or established restorations to optimize the occlusion.) In this case, these provisional restorations enabled the orthodontist to procline the maxillary anterior teeth and to retrude the mandibular anterior teeth.

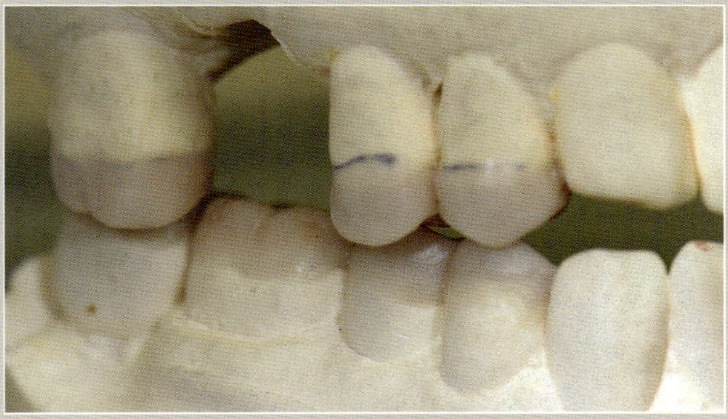

Right lateral view of diagnostic wax-up.

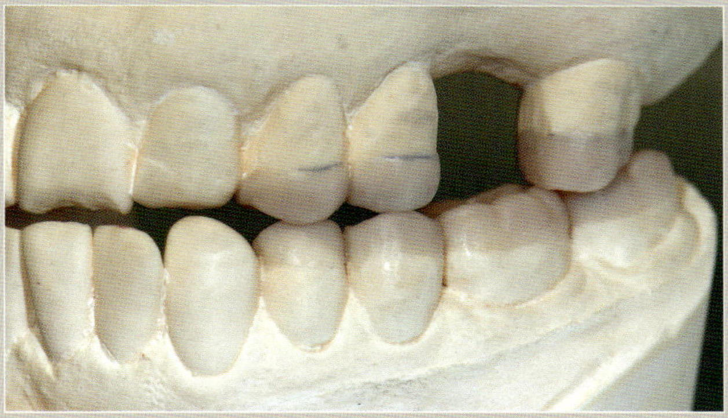

Left lateral view of diagnostic wax-up.

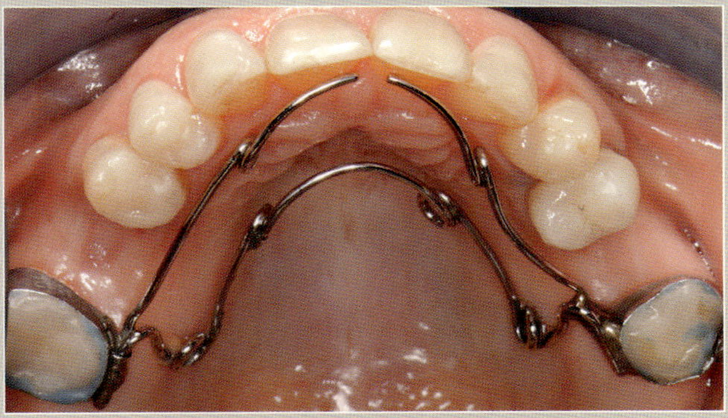

Maxillary occlusal view of quad-helix.

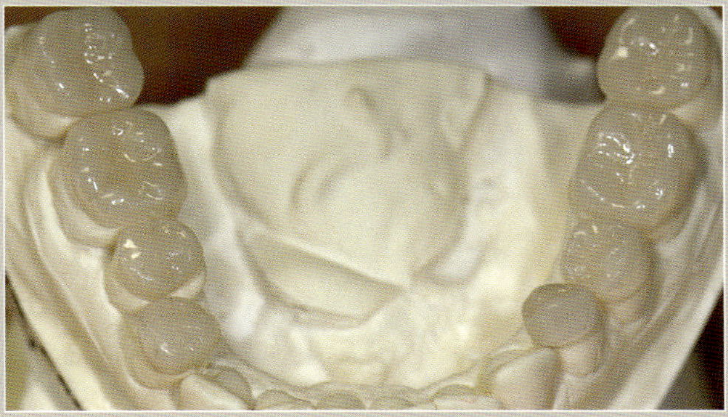

Composite resin "tabletops" on the mandibular cast.

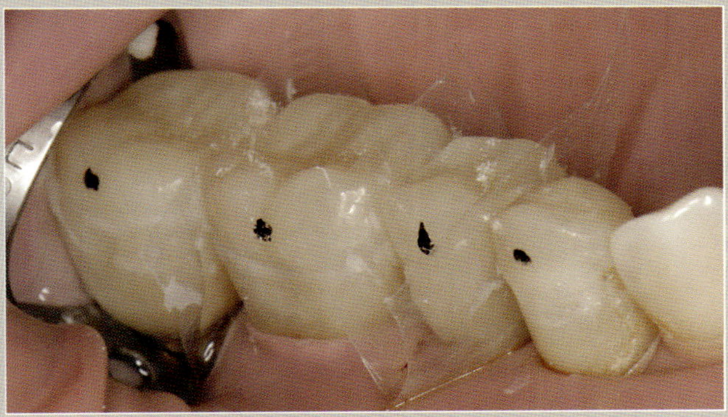

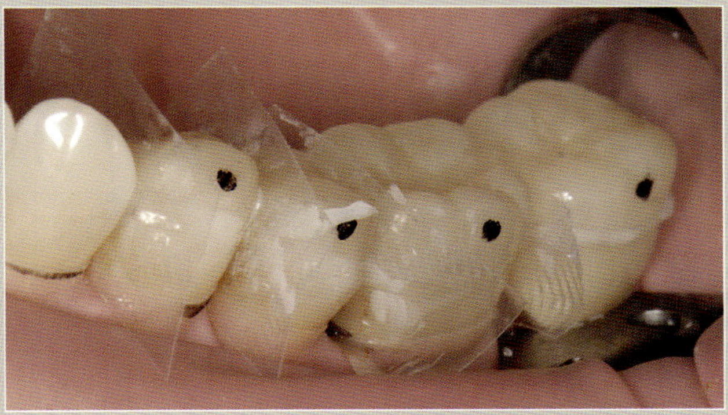

Mandibular posterior views of the composite resin "tabletops."

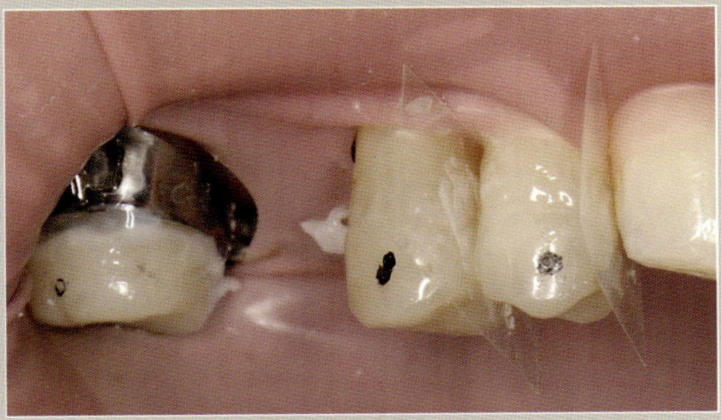

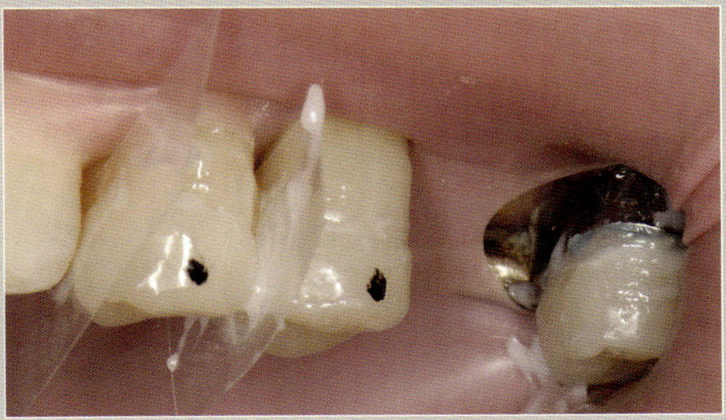

Maxillary posterior views of the composite resin "tabletops."

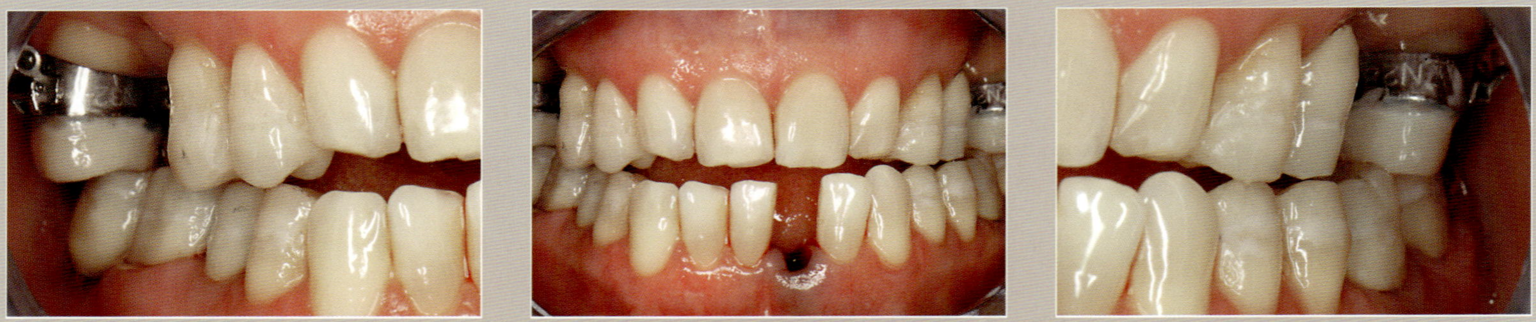

Intraoral views of occlusion following placement of composite resin “tabletops” and extraction of teeth nos. 3 and 24.

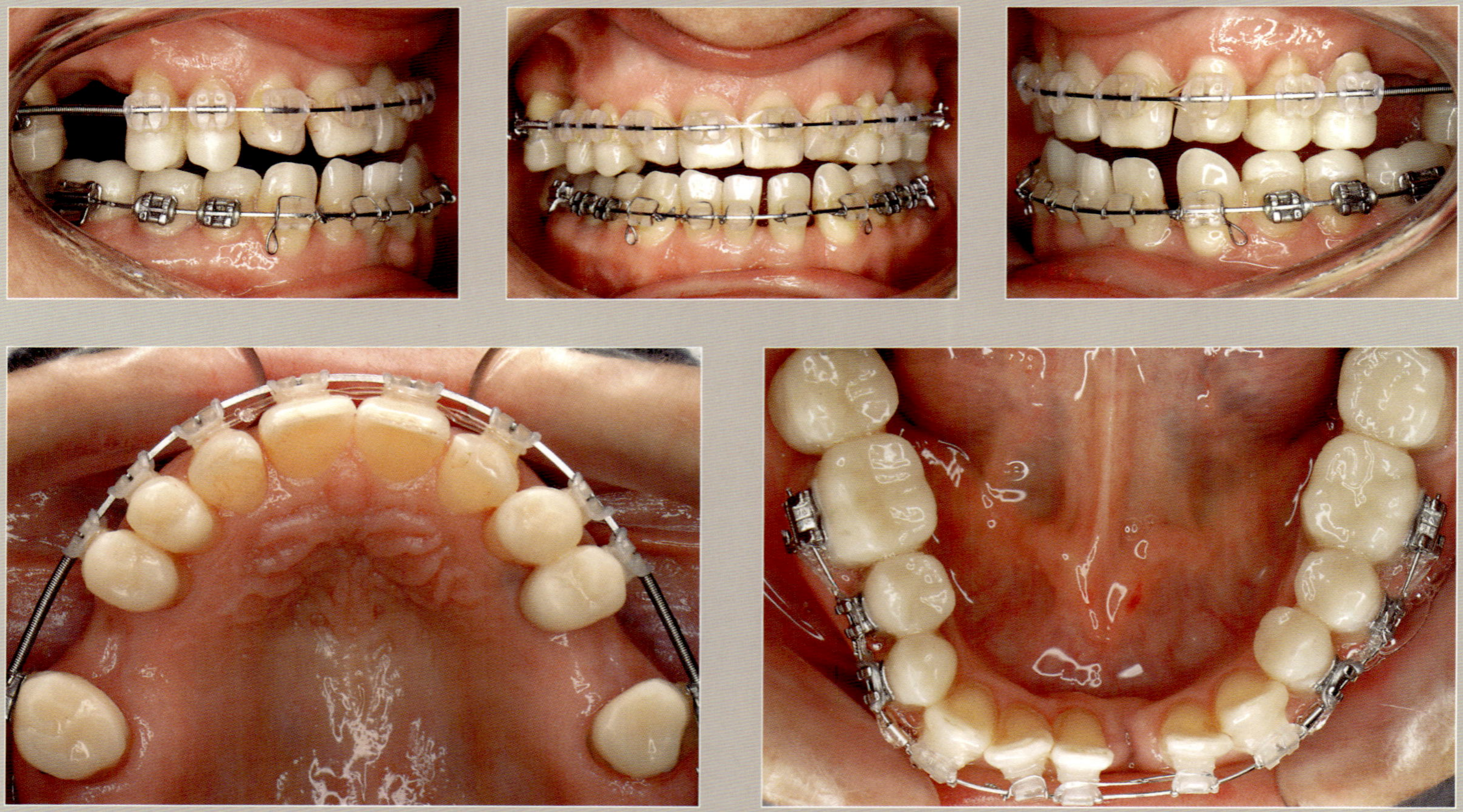

Intraoral views during orthodontic therapy to shape and align the maxillary and mandibular arches.

Phase IV: Orthodontic and surgical treatment

Orthodontic treatment was initiated. Once the brackets were fixed on all teeth, archwires were changed every 4 to 6 weeks. After 6 months of orthodontic treatment, it was evident that nonsurgical correction of the malocclusion would not be possible, and the patient agreed to proceed with option 2, which included orthognathic surgery.

The space increase in the mandible had been created by the removal of tooth no. 24, and the shaping and aligning of the maxillary and mandibular arches was almost complete, but the reverse vertical overlap and the occlusion were still inadequate. Furthermore, the profile was not satisfactory from an esthetic point of view.

Orthognathic surgery was the only viable option, and the surgeon started with a standard procedure that involved maxillary correction by means of Le Fort I osteotomy, clockwise rotation, advancement (4 mm), and anterior extrusion (2 mm). A 6-week period of postoperative retention was necessary.

Subsequently, the orthodontist completed treatment with up-down elastics to facilitate definitive positioning of the teeth and to allow the occlusion to settle in for approximately 3 months. The brackets and archwires were needed for space management to accommodate teeth nos. 3 and 19.

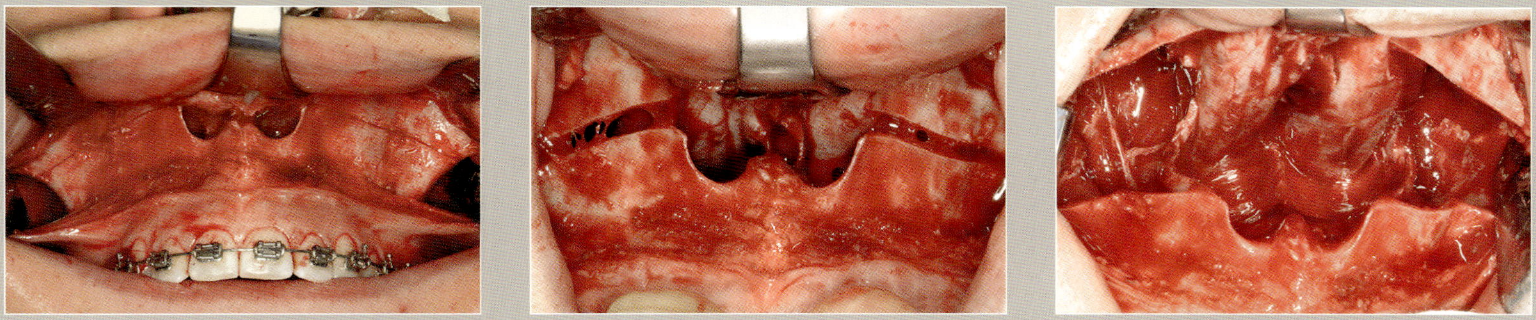

Le Fort I osteotomy, clockwise rotation, advancement, and anterior extrusion of the maxilla.

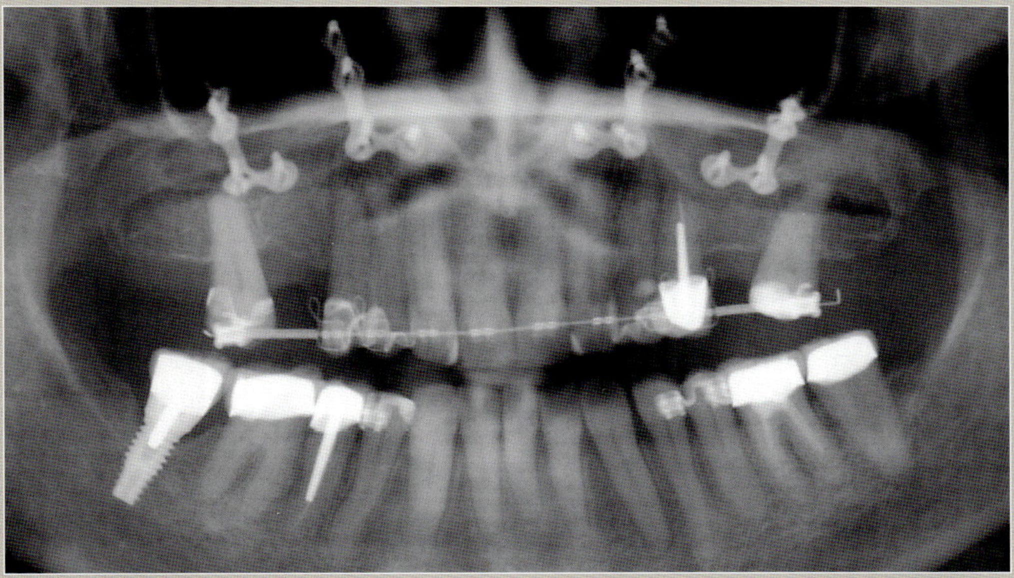

Panoramic radiograph after orthognathic surgery.

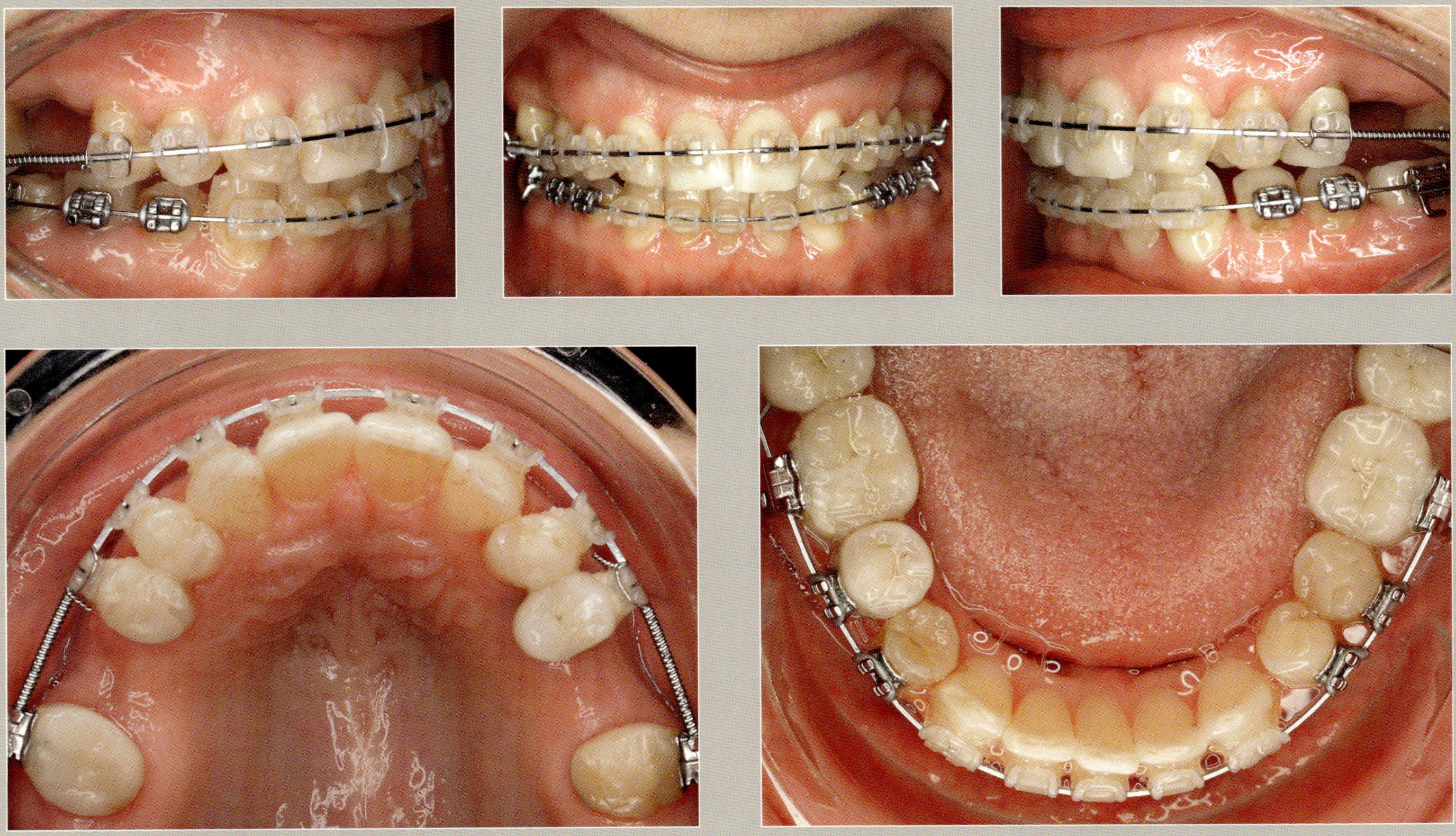

Intraoral views following orthognathic surgery.

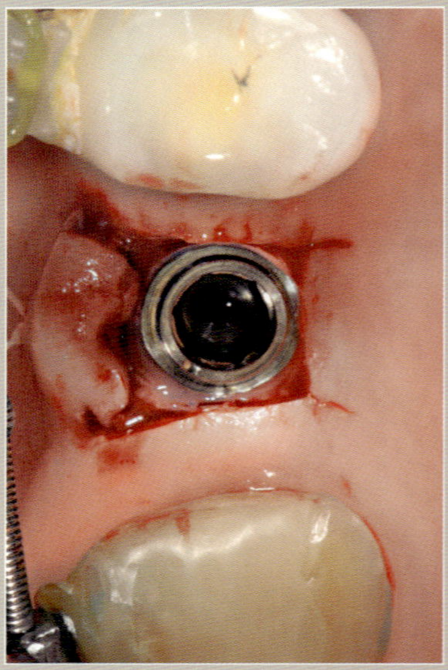

Flap elevation 4 months after placement of implant at site no. 3.

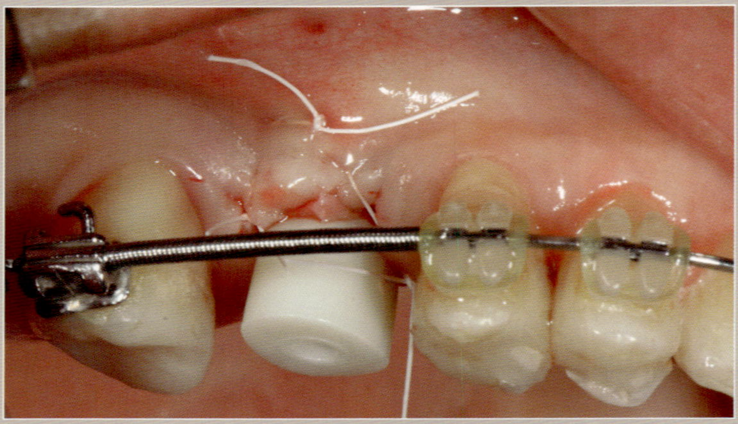

Healing abutment in place on implant at site no. 3.

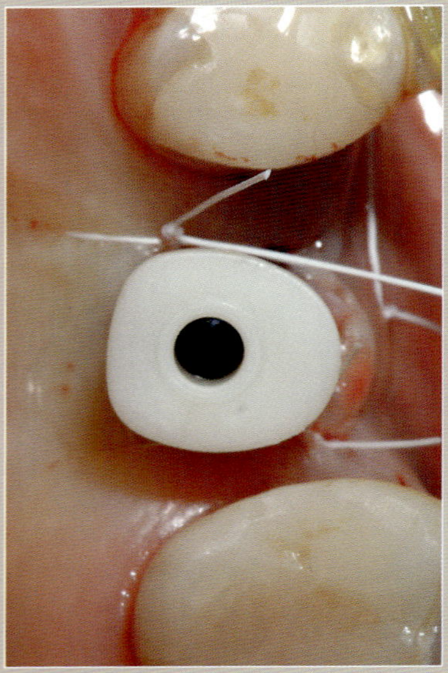

Healing abutment in place on implant at site no. 14.

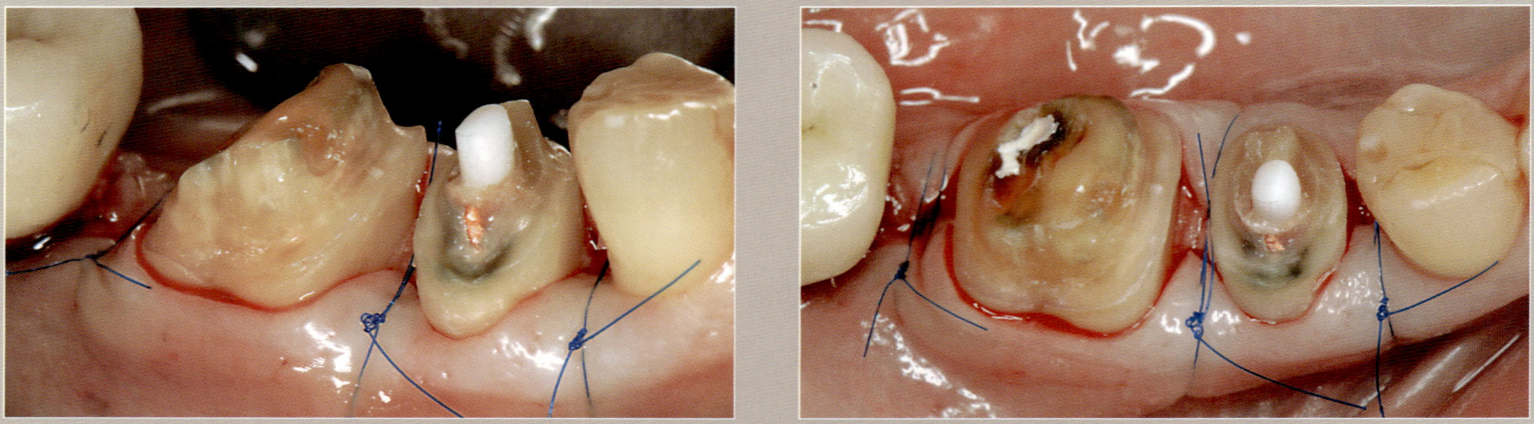

Crown lengthening procedure on teeth nos. 29 and 30.

Phase V: Endodontic treatment of teeth nos. 18 and 19

The existing endodontic fill on tooth no. 19 was incomplete and required re-treatment, which was successfully accomplished.[6-8] In addition, tooth no. 18 developed acute inflammation and was treated endodontically.

Phase VI: Implant placement and periodontal surgery

The implants in the areas of missing teeth nos. 3 and 14 were placed for four reasons:

1. To avoid the need for preparation of the adjacent teeth for crowns
2. To maintain the existing bone in those areas long term
3. To establish maximum biomechanical strength
4. To create a more maintainable hygienic environment

Both implants (SPI Element, Thommen Medical) were placed in conjunction with indirect sinus elevation procedures using the Summers technique.[9,10] This technique circumvents the need to enter the sinus laterally. It is also called the *osteotome technique* because the sinus membrane is raised through the base of the implant socket by osteotome instruments (indirectly). In addition, bone graft material is transported and placed through the implant bed using osteotomes.

In the case of teeth nos. 18, 19, 29, and 30, it became apparent after the removal of the crowns that the biologic width was inadequate to maintain periodontal health. Therefore, crown lengthening surgery was performed to establish stable, long-term soft tissue–crown relationships around these teeth.[11,12]

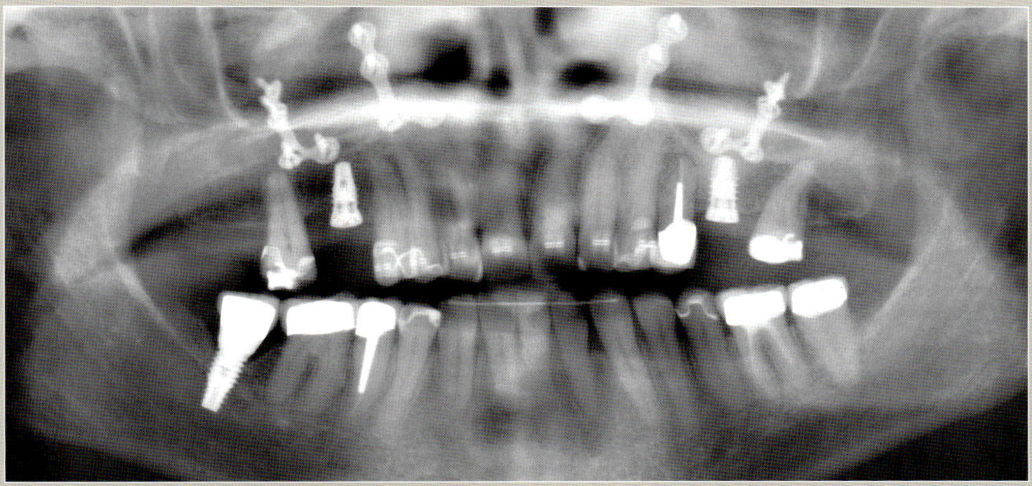

Panoramic radiograph after implant surgery.

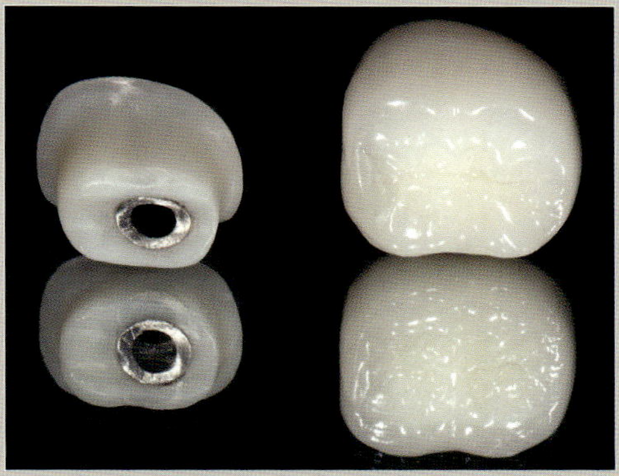

Definitive restorations with titanium base covered by a zirconia body.

Phase VII: Provisional restorative treatment

After a healing period of 4 weeks following the crown lengthening procedure and 4 months after implant placement in the maxilla, the preparations were made, and the patient was fitted with a provisional prosthesis for a period of about 2 months.

During that time, healing screws were placed on the implants at sites nos. 3 and 14 to create a proper emergence profile. These special healing screws (Thommen Medical) are titanium based and covered by acrylic resin to form the individual healing abutments.

After confirmation from the patient that she had no discomfort with function, laughing, or speaking and that centric relation was stable, final impressions were taken and sent to the laboratory for fabrication of the definitive restorations. A triple-check registration procedure with step-by-step comparison in each quadrant guaranteed the right translation to centric occlusion.

Phase VIII: Definitive restorative treatment

Individual abutments and implant-supported metal-ceramic crowns on the implants in sites nos. 3, 14, and 31 were then fabricated. Customizing the abutments and crowns presented some major advantages:

- More flexibility in restoration design
- Retrievability should a single implant or tooth fail in the future
- Improved access for effective oral hygiene

The abutments were titanium based and covered by an individualized computer-aided design/computer-assisted manufacture (CAD/CAM) zirconia body (luted with Multilink, Ivoclar Vivadent). The crowns were created at the crest of the gingival margin, which facilitated excess cement removal and provided for a more natural anatomical emergence profile. This also resulted in more esthetically pleasing restorations. With this procedure, we can solve three problems related to the emergence profile of implant restorations:

1. Biomechanics: Knowing that zirconia is very stiff, hard, and inelastic compared with titanium, it does not appear advisable to bring both materials together at the junction between the implant (titanium) and the abutment (zirconia), where the strongest forces will develop. Therefore, we always try to connect titanium with titanium to avoid distortion on the implant platform.
2. Biocompatibility: As we know from the literature, gold and aluminum oxide are not as biocompatible as zirconia and titanium.[13,14] That is the reason we only use titanium and zirconia for implant abutments.
3. Esthetics: If we fabricate the abutments as described, an individual emergence profile can be developed, and the outcome will be very anatomical. The natural form will improve the esthetic result, and the handling of the crown margin will be very predictable.

Individual metal-ceramic crowns on teeth nos. 13, 18, 19, 29, and 30 as well as individual full-ceramic overlays on teeth nos. 2, 4, 5, 12, 15, 20, 21, and 28 (e.max, Ivoclar Vivadent) were then delivered. To minimize the loss of tooth structure in preparation and still achieve a pleasant and harmonious esthetic outcome, teeth nos. 7 to 10 were restored with a direct composite resin material (Enamel Plus HFO, Micerium).

Posttreatment

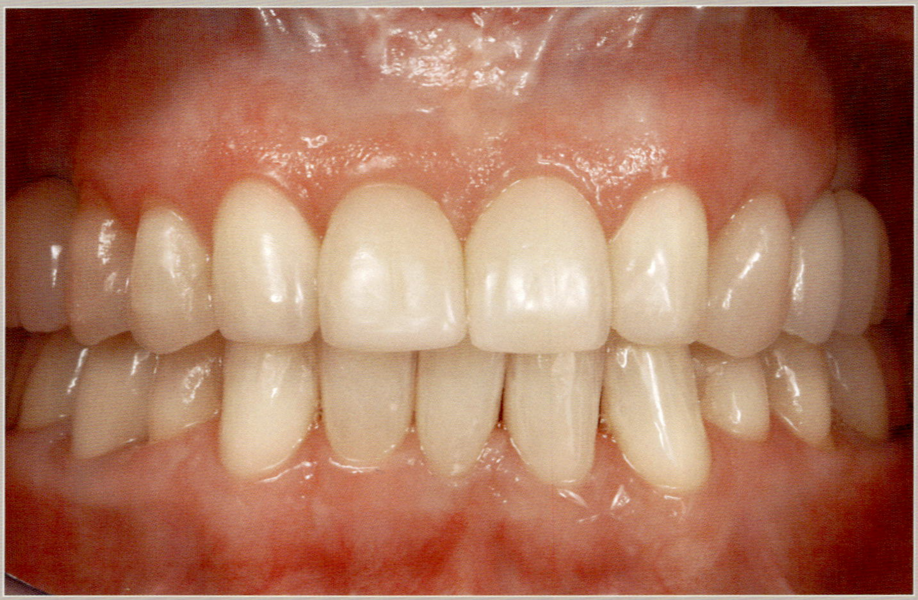

Intraoral anterior view.

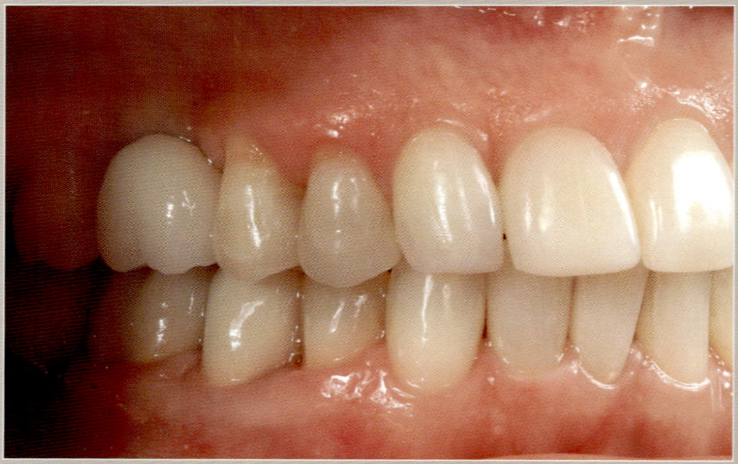

Intraoral right lateral view.

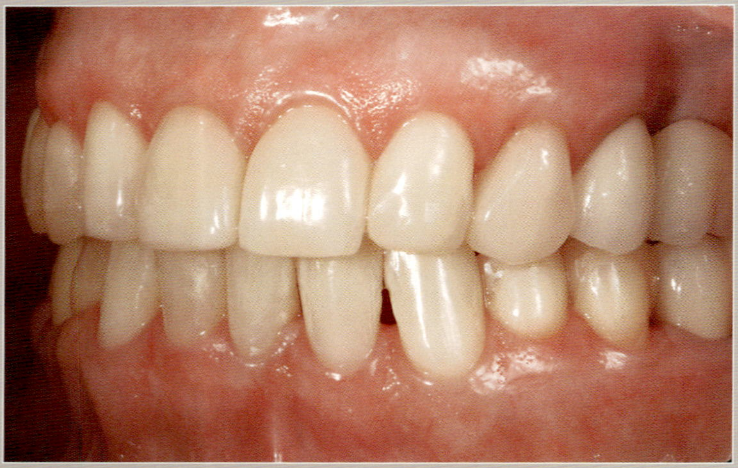

Intraoral left lateral view.

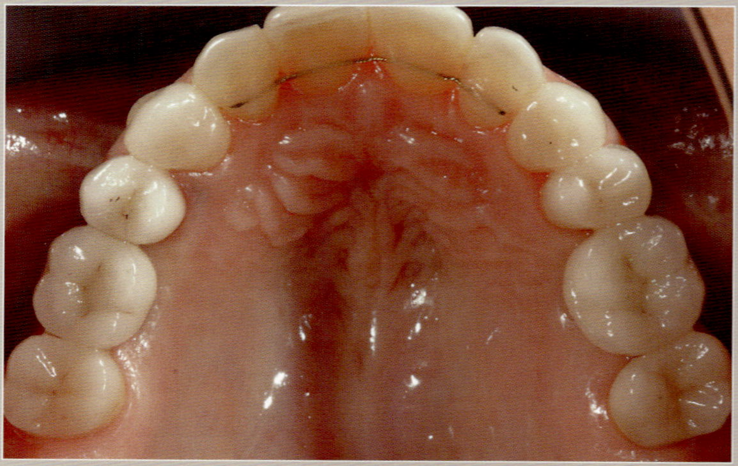

Occlusal maxillary view.

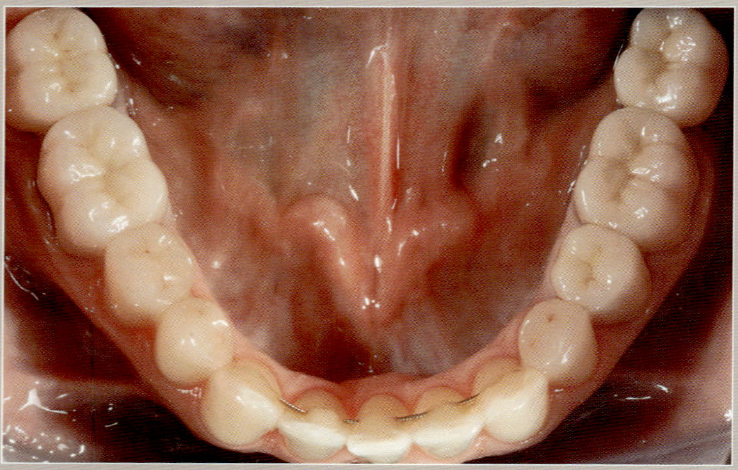

Occlusal mandibular view.

Phase IX: Re-evaluation and maintenance

At the 4-month recall, the patient complained of hot and cold sensitivity on tooth no. 2. Two months later, the same problem arose with tooth no. 15. Subsequently, endodontic therapy was performed on these teeth. Almost 1 year later, the occlusion is stable, the discomfort is gone, and the patient is thrilled with her bite and her smile.

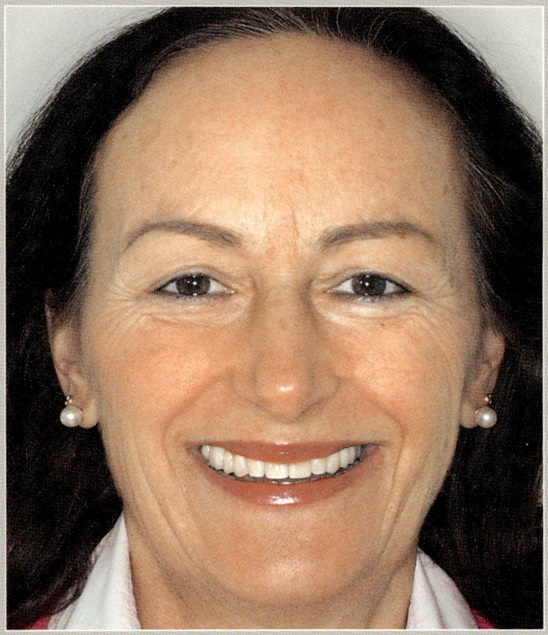

Facial view of smile.

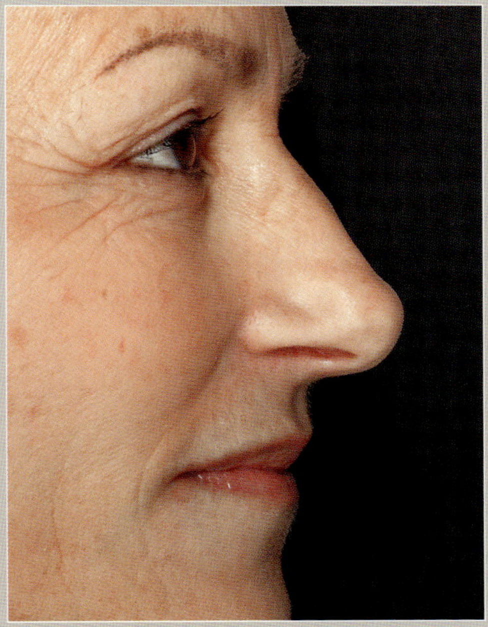

Lateral facial view.

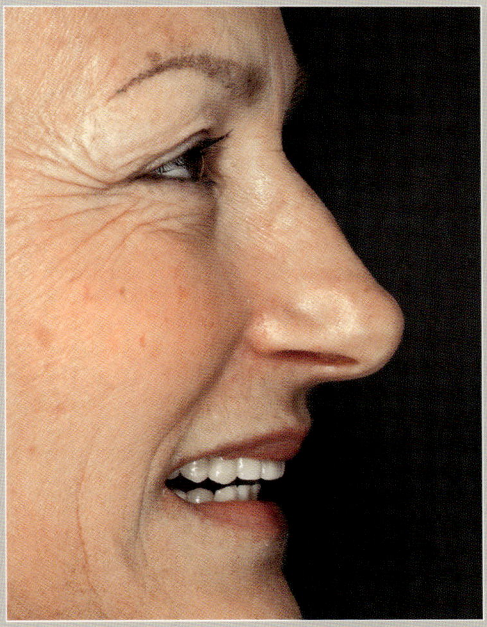

Lateral facial view of smile.

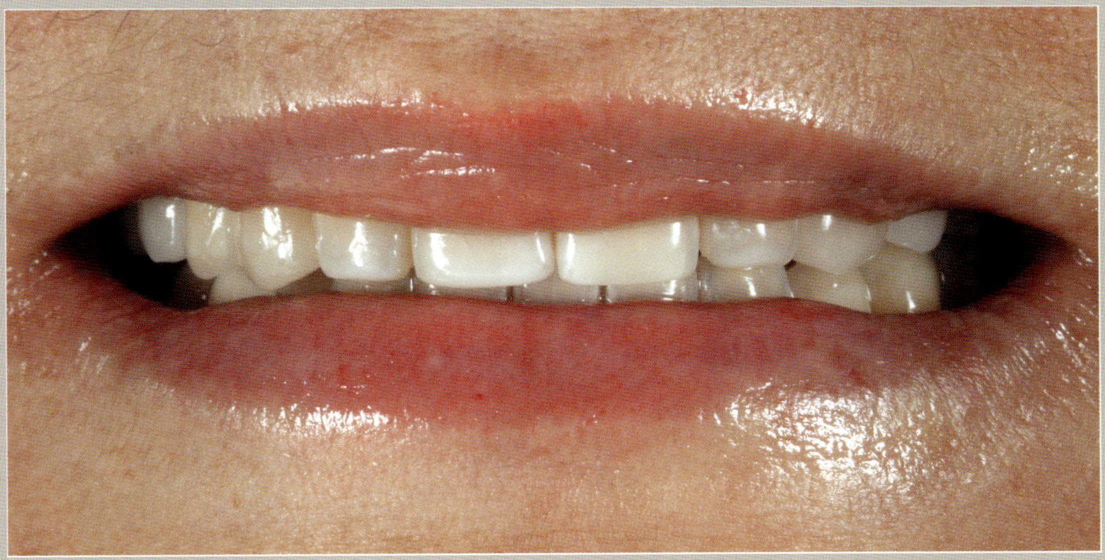

Close-up view of smile.

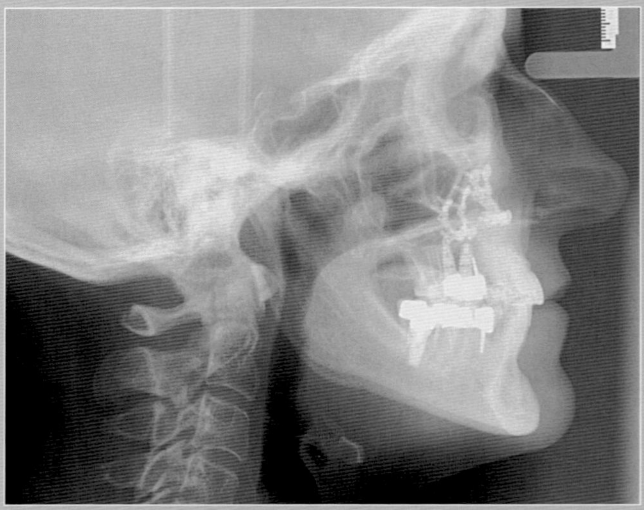

Three-year posttreatment cephalometric radiograph.

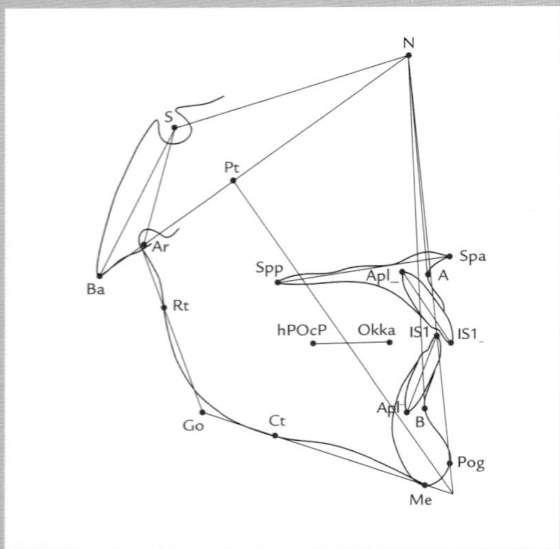

Three-year posttreatment cephalometric tracing.

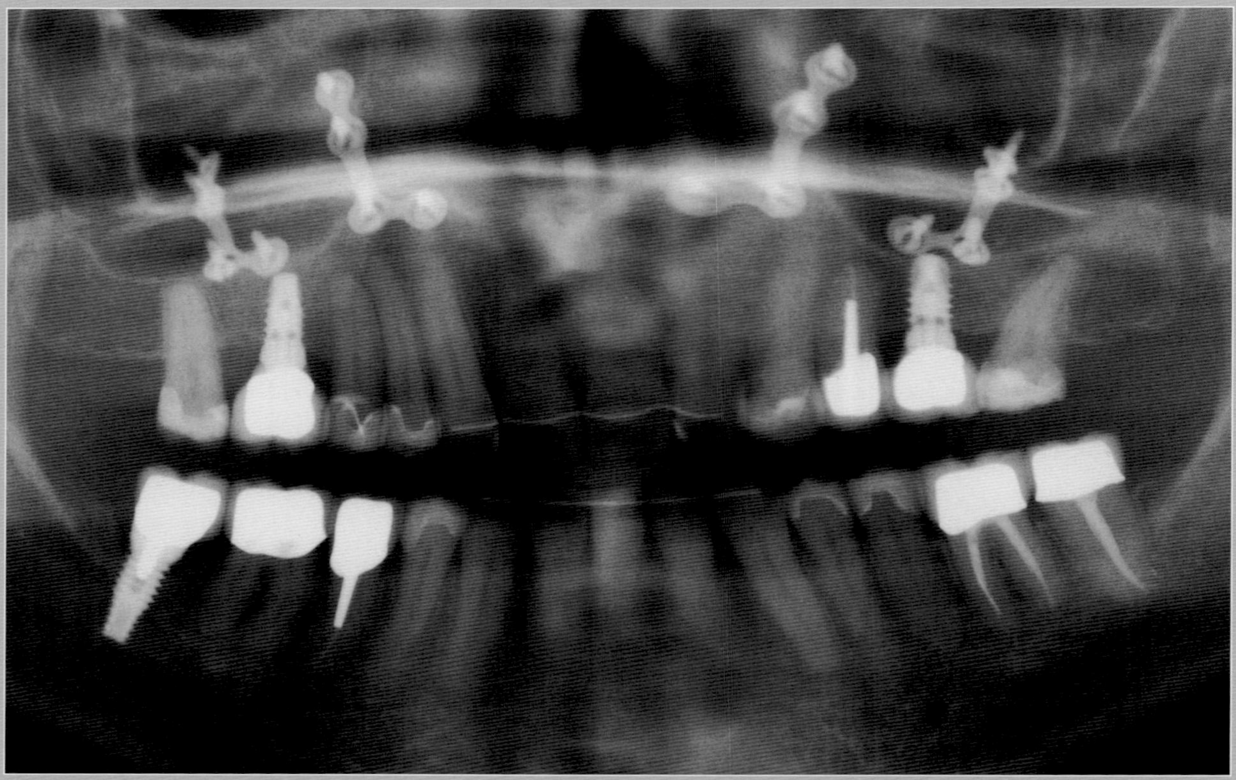

Three-year posttreatment panoramic radiograph.

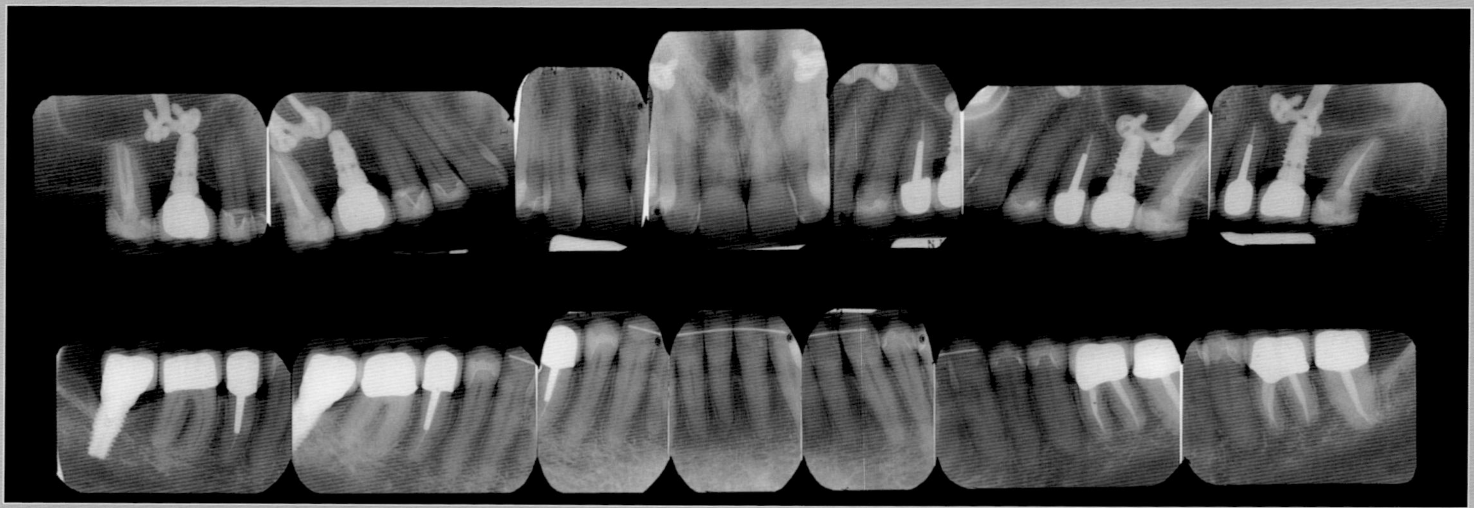

Three-year posttreatment complete-mouth series.

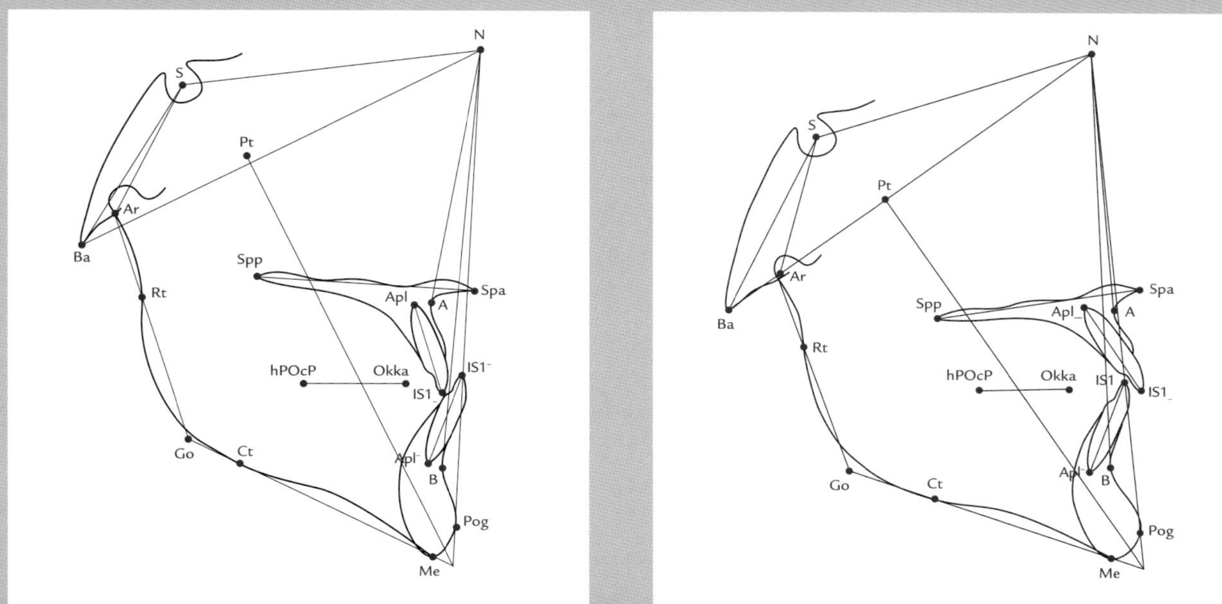

Comparison of pretreatment and posttreatment cephalometric tracings. For exact measurements, see Table 1 below.

TABLE 1 ANTEROPOSTERIOR POSITION OF THE MAXILLA AND MANDIBLE BEFORE AND AFTER TREATMENT

Angle	Before treatment (degrees)	After treatment (degrees)
SNA	72.3	77.3
SNB	77.8	75.0
ANB	-5.5	2.3

You may now place the corresponding posttreatment overlay found in the separate folder over the pretreatment periodontal chart on page 447.

Commentary

In hindsight, a number of core issues can be identified in treating this patient. First, the case is an impressive example of how the synthesis of data from multiple disciplines and comprehensive interdisciplinary collaboration is essential to achieve predictable treatment success. Important orthodontic, surgical, periodontal, and restorative decision making was born out of these valuable discussions.[15–17]

Option 1 was a nonextraction proposal. Retaining tooth no. 24 would result in enlargement of the negative sagittal step. This, in turn, would necessitate maxillomandibular surgery in order to create a stable result. Advantages to this approach include a reduction in chin prominence in the new mandibular positioning and a slight gain in midfacial fullness. However, the risks associated with such extensive surgery and the ability to resolve the reverse vertical overlap and significantly improve the facial profile were still uncertain enough to question the value of the procedure. In addition, the extent that the teeth would have to be moved to meet the esthetic goals would involve significant torque and could potentially result in gingival recession with this patient's thin gingival phenotype. There was also a risk of root and bone resorption.

Option 2 focused on maxillary advancement alone (Le Fort I osteotomy). This proposal would create greater midfacial fullness and ameliorate the chin-midface relationship as well. The alteration in the esthetic profile would be positive and pleasing with a more natural smile line. The surgical procedure is well described and the results are stable over years.[4,18–22]

An alternative surgical procedure not discussed in option 2 was a mandibular bilateral sagittal split osteotomy. This was never a viable alternative because of the negative influence of the smile line; also, the midface hypoplasia could not be altered. Moreover, although this approach might work from a functional point of view, the risk of damage to the mandibular nerve could not be underestimated.

The patient's preference was option 3. This was understandable because it had the lowest risk and was the least-invasive approach. However, at the same time, the treatment outcome would be the most questionable and least predictable. A benefit to this course of treatment (and the rationale used by the treatment team to proceed with this plan) was that with unsatisfactory results or failure, it would be possible to switch to treatment option 2. Although success with this approach was somewhat dubious, the team wanted to honor the patient's wishes and, at the same time, cater to her psychologic needs.

The treatment team also discussed the possibility of a nonorthodontic, nonsurgical plan. The patient's situation probably could have been improved with restorations alone, with some gain in occlusal stabilization. However, this would not have altered the reverse vertical overlap. Long-term predictability would have remained in question, with the prognosis significantly compromised. There would be no reason to think that any new restorations would not also fail, and the patient's esthetic goals would not have been met.

It could be argued that because the patient presented with a Class III skeletal dysgnathia, any nonsurgical alternative would fail. However, the treating clinicians felt that if the case had been diagnosed earlier and pretreated orthodontically during the growth phase with headgear, the dentoalveolar compensation could had been optimized and surgical intervention would had been much less invasive.

This case demonstrates that in adults whose function has been compromised by skeletal abnormalities, careful planning in an interdisciplinary team environment is not only valuable but essential in achieving long-term treatment success. In this case, comprehensive treatment should help provide this patient with a long-term stable occlusion, prevent future TMJ damage, and pave the way for a new dimension of quality of life.

REFERENCES

1. Schamsawary S. Dysgnathien [in German]. München: Urban & Fischer, 2007.
2. Hausamen JE, Becker FW, Neukam RA, Reichart PA, Schliephake H, Schmelzeisen R. Curriculum Chirurgie. Vol 3: Mund-, Kiefer- und Gesichtschirurgie [in German]. Berlin: Quintessenz, 2002.
3. Angle EH. Classification of malocclusion. Dental Cosmos 1899;41:248–264,350–357.
4. Bell WH. Le Fort I osteotomy for correction of maxillary deformities. J Oral Surg 1975;33:412–426.
5. Clark GT. Etiologic theory and the prevention of temporomandibular disorders. Adv Dent Res 1991;5:60–66.
6. de Chevigny C, Dao TT, Basrani BR, et al. Treatment outcome in endodontics: The Toronto study—Phases 3 and 4: Orthograde retreatment. J Endod 2008;34:131–137.
7. Farzaneh M, Abitbol S, Friedman S. Treatment outcome in endodontics: The Toronto study. Phases I and II: Orthograde retreatment. J Endod 2004;30:627–633.
8. Ng YL, Mann V, Gulabivala K. Outcome of secondary root canal treatment: A systematic review of the literature. Int Endod J 2008;41:1026–1046.
9. Summers RB. A new concept in maxillary implant surgery: The osteotome technique. Compendium 1994;15:152,154–156,158.
10. Summers RB. Sinus floor elevation with osteotomes. J Esthet Dent 1998;10:164–171.
11. Becker W, Ochsenbein C, Becker BE. Crown lengthening: The periodontal-restorative connection. Compend Contin Educ Dent 1998;19:239–240,242,244–246.
12. de Waal H, Castellucci G. The importance of restorative margin placement to the biologic width and periodontal health. Part II. Int J Periodontics Restorative Dent 1994;14:70–83.
13. Abrahamsson I, Berglundh T, Glantz PO, Lindhe J. The mucosal attachment at different abutments. An experimental study in dogs. J Clin Periodontol 1998;25:721–727.
14. Hisbergues M, Vendeville S, Vendeville P. Zirconia: Established facts and perspectives for a biomaterial in dental implantology. J Biomed Mater Res B Appl Biomater 2009;88:519–529.
15. Arnett GW, McLaughlin RP. Facial and Dental Planning for Orthodontists and Oral Surgeons. New York: Mosby, 2004.
16. Kokich VG, Kokich VO. Interrelationship of orthodontics with periodontics and restorative dentistry. In: Nanda R (ed). Biomechanics and Esthetic Strategies in Clinical Orthodontics. St Louis: Elsevier, 2005:348–373.
17. Andrews LF. The six keys to normal occlusion. Am J Orthod 1972;62:296–309.
18. Janson M, Janson G, Sant'Ana E, Nakamura A, de Freitas MR. Segmental LeFort I osteotomy for treatment of a Class III malocclusion with temporomandibular disorder. J Appl Oral Sci 2008;16:302–309.
19. Rosen HM. Miniplate fixation of the Le Fort I osteotomies. Plast Reconstr Surg 1986;78:748–754.
20. Welch TB. Stability in the correction of dentofacial deformities: A comprehensive review. J Oral Maxillofac Surg 1989;47:1142–1149.
21. Bell WH, Proffit WR, White RP. Surgical Correction of Dentofacial Deformities. Philadelphia: Saunders, 1980:271.
22. Obwegeser HL. Surgical correction of small or retrodisplaced maxillae. The "dish-face" deformity. Plast Reconstr Surg 1969;43:351–365.

18

A Path to Interdisciplinary Care for the Dental Team

George Duello, DDS, MS

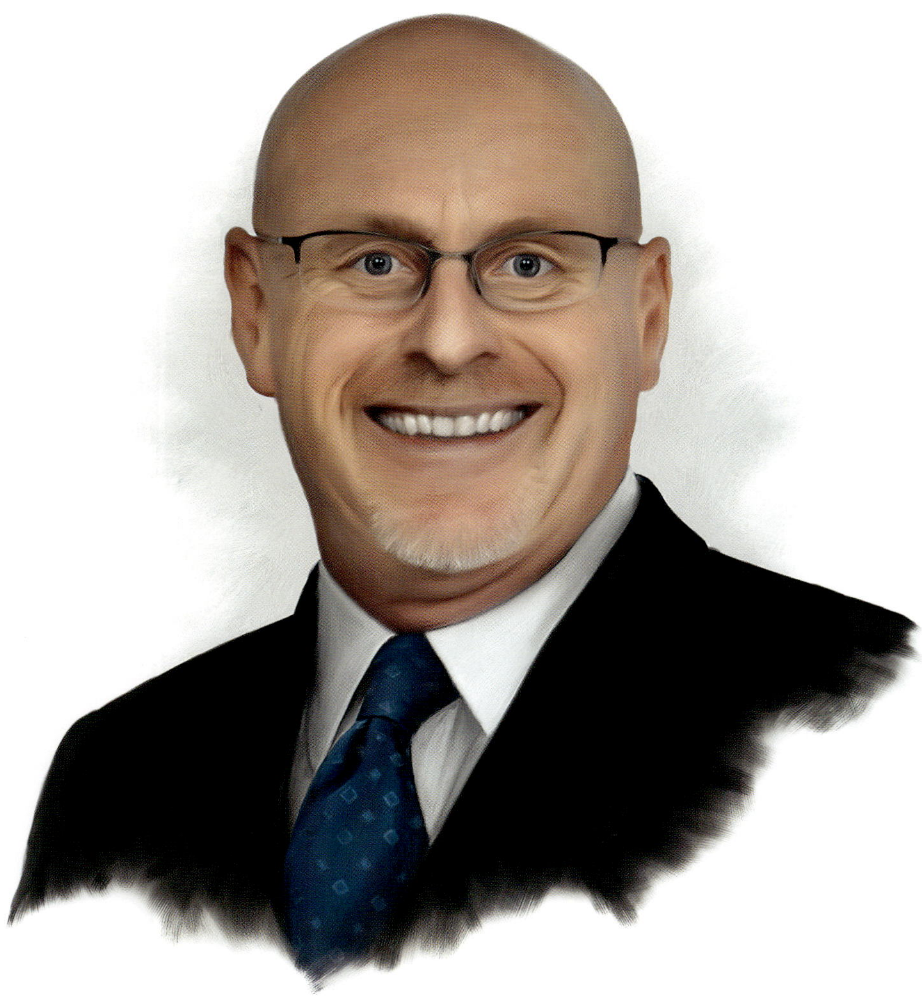

"Before enlightenment, chop wood and carry water.

After enlightenment, chop wood and carry water."

—Zen proverb

Philosophy and Background

My personal path to becoming a dentist started when I was very young. My grandfather was a general dentist who practiced in a small town in Missouri for 29 years. We both shared the same first name, a plan well orchestrated by my mother, which gave me an early bond with my first dental mentor. He would take me to the office and I would get to see and feel how a dentist of his era practiced and took care of patients in his two-room office. Fortunately, I chose the profession of dentistry based on this early exposure through my grandfather. When I graduated from dental school in 1979, I vividly remember asking him what makes a good dentist. He did not hesitate in his short but revealing answer: "A good dentist keeps the front teeth looking good and the back teeth from hurting and breaking."

The foundation for the Seattle Study Club is the use of interdisciplinary treatment to provide optimal dental care by a team of dentists using their collective knowledge and skills in a collaborative group setting. In order to provide comprehensive care, these clinicians need to start collecting the objective and subjective data on the present state of the patient prior to developing a presumptive diagnosis. The editor of this textbook has stated, "Treatment planning from a scientific standpoint can be perplexing and quite challenging. When human variables are added to the mix, case planning becomes even more demanding and difficult."[1]

Patients seek dental care to relieve pain and suffering from dental disease, to improve or relieve problems caused by poor function, and to enhance their personal appearance and self-esteem through cosmetic dental procedures. It is the veracity and integrity of the professional who respects the patient's autonomy to make decisions based on informed consent that can set the stage for quality dental care that meets the individual needs and wants of the patient.

In dentistry, there are so many approaches to therapy that it can sometimes be difficult to see the bigger picture that guides the selection of different modalities and how they interconnect in practice. In particular, there is a need to appreciate the concepts of complicated and complex problems in our patients. These intricate clinical situations are not always appreciated within the context of their presentation by clinicians who want to make everything simple. According to Sholom Glouberman and Brenda Zimmerman of the University of Toronto, systems can be understood as being simple, complicated, or complex.[2] Simple systems, such as following a recipe or protocol, may involve some basic issues of technique and terminology, but once these are mastered, following the protocol carries with it a very high assurance of success. The placement of an occlusal sealant on a recently erupted permanent molar would be an example of a simple dental technique.

Complicated problems, like sending a rocket to the moon, are different. Their complicated nature is often related not only to the scale of a problem (compared with simple systems) but also to issues of coordination or specialized expertise. However, rockets are similar to each other, and because of this, following one success, there can be a relatively high degree of certainty of outcome repetition. A dental analogy would be the use of a particular orthodontic system to treat a Class I dental malocclusion with mild crowding. In this situation, removable computer-aided design/computer-assisted manufacture (CAD/CAM) appliances or fixed orthodontics technologies could be used to achieve clinically acceptable intra- and interarch alignments.

In contrast, complex systems are based on relationships and their properties of self-organization, interconnectedness, and evolution. Research into complex systems demonstrates that they cannot be understood solely by simple or complicated approaches to evidence, policy, planning, and management. The metaphor that Glouberman and Zimmerman use for complex systems is raising a child. Formulae have limited application. Raising one child provides experience but no assurance of success with the next. Expertise can contribute but is neither necessary nor sufficient to assure success. Every child is unique and must be understood as an individual. A number of interventions can be expected to fail as a matter of course. Uncertainty of the outcome remains. The parts cannot be separated from the whole.

Treatment planning for patients exhibiting extensive dental pathology associated with significant medical and psychologic cofactors would be an illustration of a complex dental patient in need of an interdisciplinary approach. Complex dental care requires the expertise of a social network of clinicians that share a common philosophy in data gathering, diagnosis, treatment planning, and behavioral/anxiety analysis. Using many "eyes on the problem" may help distinguish between simple, complicated, and complex etiologies that will require the skill and judgment of a well-seasoned team approach.

The information obtained from the patient can be organized in a manner to meet the collective goals of the patient. Depending on the accuracy with which symptoms of disease were elicited, the acuity with which the signs were observed, and the diagnostician's prior knowledge of the disease manifestations, the initial assessment can provide the team with the causes of dental disease affecting the patient. Once the course of the disease has been determined, the team and the patient can set a path toward dental health using the scientific method with inductive and deductive reasoning. This journey is commonly referred as the *treatment plan*.

A treatment plan is a road map to address the etiologic factors that have led to the symptoms present. In some cases, the etiologic factors may be a collection of biologic, physical, mechanical, and/or psychologic issues. The sequence by which the team addresses the causative agents has been debated by clinicians in texts, periodicals, and lecture series. Patients, dentists, and dental laboratories can also formulate treatment sequencing to minimize risk factors identified in each patient. Any journey can lead to unexpected outcomes or difficulties, which are like detours on a long automobile trip. The key is to remain vigilant and flexible when challenges occur during the establishment of the presumptive diagnosis and then during the course of treatment.

In addition, contemporary treatment planning makes use of evidence-based literature, supported by the clinician's long-term experiential observations, and the patient's value system to achieve successful therapeutic outcomes in complex and complicated cases.[3] The purpose of this chapter is to highlight my collective experience over 31 years of clinical practice using the aforementioned information in a case requiring interdisciplinary care.

This case was selected based on the need to document the treatment of a patient experiencing a common midlife dental phenomenon—the absence of anterior guidance in an existing Class II skeletal malocclusion with physiologic wear of the anterior teeth that had resulted in fracture of several posterior teeth and unfavorable anterior esthetics. As an adolescent, this patient received orthodontic care that included dental compensation and growth management without definite treatment of the underlying Class II skeletal malocclusion. The reason for this specific orthodontic treatment is unavailable for discovery or historical speculation. Some of the posterior teeth have been periodontally compromised by genetic root length, previous endodontics, and prior surgical procedures, leaving them at risk for traumatic injury under normal or excessive occlusal loading.

Many textbooks have illustrated these types of patients in descriptive case reports using systematic checklists to document the patient's pathognomonic findings.[4] Depending on the individual and/or collective philosophy of the clinicians treating the patient, a treatment approach can be formulated that establishes the goals of therapy from various specialties involved in the interdisciplinary team. For the treating clinicians, it is important to establish agreed-upon criteria for success and goals of therapy based on the patient's motivation for treatment, extraoral and intraoral clinical examinations, and adequate informed consent regarding the consequences of treatment or nontreatment of clinical pathologies.

Numerous lectures and meetings have been organized for the sole purpose of solving these common dental puzzles. Semi-adjustable and fully adjustable instrumentation has been designed and developed for the purpose of accurately transferring clinical information from the operatory to the lab bench so that the deleterious effects of occlusion can be studied. A thorough cast analysis supported by additional photographic and radiographic data can allow the clinician to have greater insight in establishing the diagnosis and then formulating a treatment methodology.

Yet, despite all the available knowledge and technology, many patients still receive dental care one tooth at a time, as they fracture or become clinically symptomatic. Treatment may include single-tooth endodontics, crown lengthening, post-core buildups, and complete-coverage single-tooth prosthetics in centric occlusion. In some cases, the tooth is beyond repair, leading to extraction with various forms of irreversible dental therapy.

The purported reasons for providing care one tooth at a time are based on several unfounded theories. The various hypotheses for this treatment philosophy have been:

- Patients will not accept complete-mouth therapy even when they present the need for it.
- Patients will not invest the necessary time for a thorough examination and detailed treatment planning.
- Patients will not consent to complete-mouth therapy because of the financial commitment required.
- Individual patient demographics dictate that patients will not accept complete-mouth therapy.
- If the patient's insurance benefits are limited, then it is unlikely that the patient would be willing to pay out of pocket for more involved treatment.

It is noted that many of these opinions rarely include a statement regarding the wisdom and experience of the dental provider or team in handling the complexity of physical and mental challenges facing patients who require complete-mouth reconstructive dentistry. Dentists make many judgments regarding their patients' attitudes and beliefs based on their own personal beliefs and preferences. Most dental professionals agree that "do no harm" is a guiding principle for their clinical advice and care. In addition to this, it is the responsibility of clinicians to present all possible treatment options to patients and allow them to decide rather than making limited treatment recommendations based on what the clinician thinks the patient will or should accept.

The theory of cognitive dissonance proposes that people are motivated to reduce discord. Changing attitudes, altering beliefs, and ultimately modifying clinical examinations and treatment recommendations can decrease dissonance.[5] Unfortunately, clinicians may also reduce dissonance by providing clinical modalities that fail to meet the rigors of the scientific method despite contrary evidence-based protocols in the dental literature. By aspiring to less-than-ideal goals, treating over a shorter time interval, or adopting a "do our best" attitude, the course of therapy may lead to esthetic relapses, facial imbalances, periodontal decline, fractured teeth, inadequate airway space, and patient dissatisfaction.

Despite these observations, over many years of clinical practice and lecturing throughout the country, I have found that there are many practitioners who have mastered the science and the art of interdisciplinary complete-mouth care for patients in need of these services. Therefore, this chapter is dedicated to those who have helped me understand how to serve patients and challenge clinicians to discover how to unlock the mysteries surrounding comprehensive dental therapy. It is my hope that the presentation of the treatment of this patient will inspire the reader to embark on a path of self-discovery and personal and professional development similar to the one that I feel so lucky and honored to have traveled, guided by my mentors, over my professional career.

Case Presentation

Treating clinicians
Periodontist: George Duello, DDS, MS
Restorative dentist: Jack Marincel, DDS
Restorative dentist: Kevin Thorpe, DMD
Laboratory technician: Gerry Jacobi, CDT

Clinical Treatment Planning

Age at initial presentation: 53 years
Initial presentation: July 2004
Active treatment completed: January 2006

Introduction and background

The patient was referred to Dr Duello for implant consultation to support her general dentist's initial treatment plan. The patient was aware that she had some decayed and fractured teeth that were not restorable. During the codiscovery phase of the examination process, the patient became concerned about the wear and cosmetics of her maxillary anterior teeth. This patient also had financial concerns and understood that she would have to accept some compromise regarding the choice of restorations.

Medical history

- Good general health
- Gastroesophageal reflux disease (GERD), treated for 5 years with famotidine (Pepcid, Merck)
- Hysterectomy

Dental history

- Orthodontic therapy at St Louis University Graduate Orthodontics Clinic in 1963
- Admitted to clenching under stress
- Same general dentist for 23 years

Diagnostic findings

Extraoral and facial findings

- Within normal limits

TMJ and mandibular range of motion

- Within normal limits

Intraoral findings

Dental

- Dental caries
- Chemical erosion
- Enamel abfractions
- Tooth fractures
- Defective restorations on teeth nos. 4, 13, and 30

Periodontal

- Chronic plaque-induced gingivitis
- Chronic localized early to moderate periodontitis
- Chronic gingival recession
- Localized furcation involvement

Pretreatment

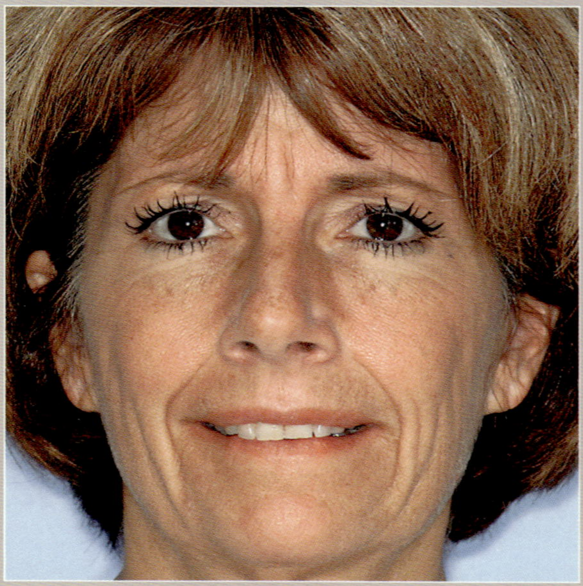

Facial view.

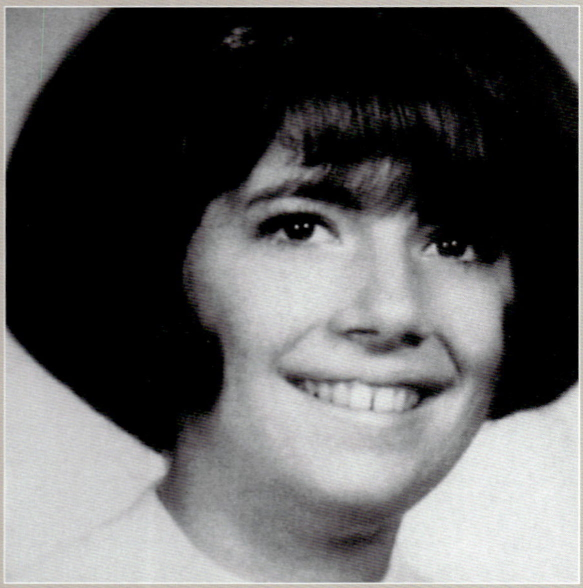

Patient at 17 years old.

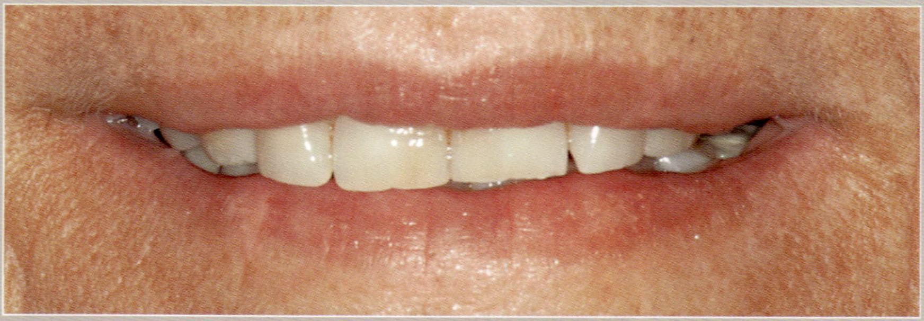

Close-up view of smile.

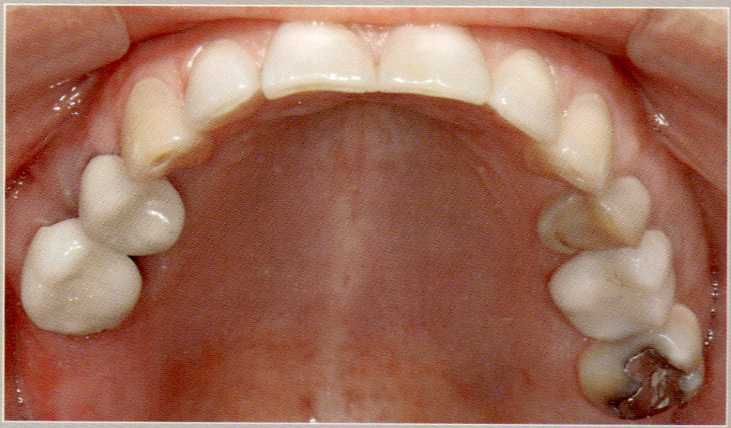

Maxillary occlusal view.

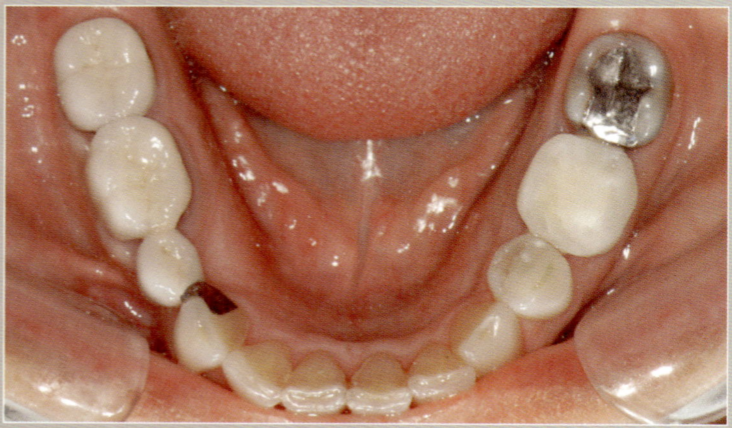

Mandibular occlusal view.

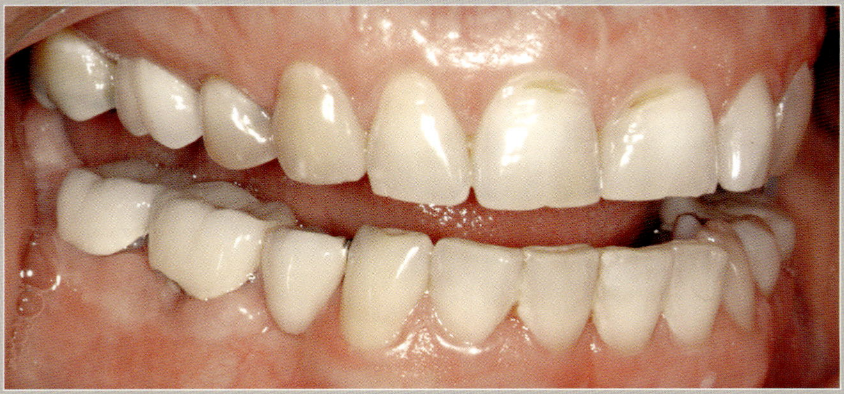

Intraoral right lateral view.

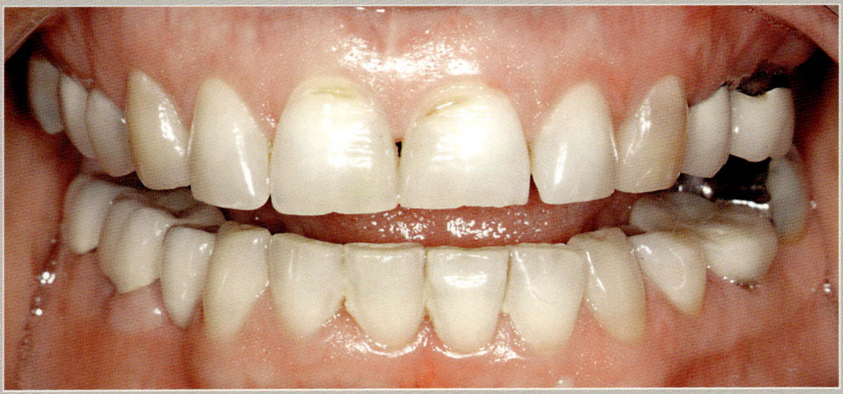

Intraoral anterior view.

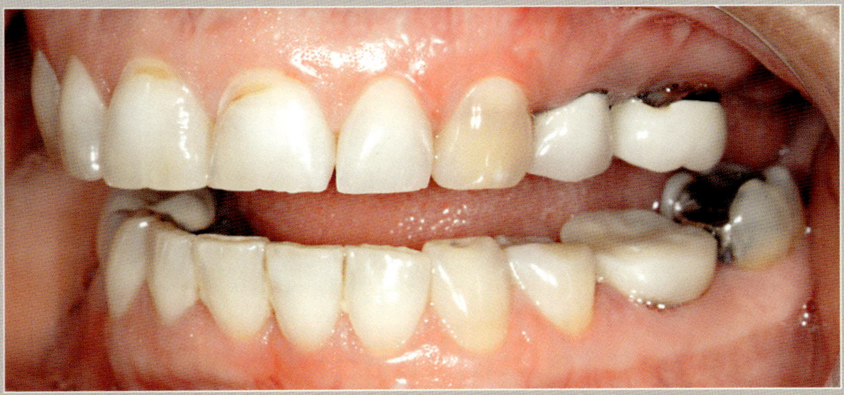

Intraoral left lateral view.

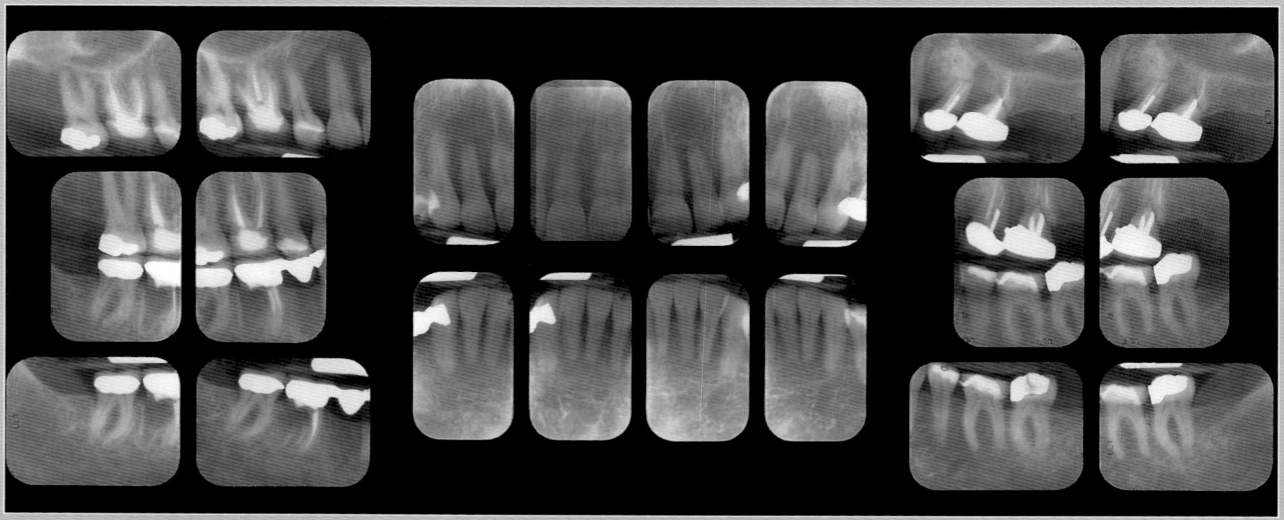

Complete-mouth radiographs.

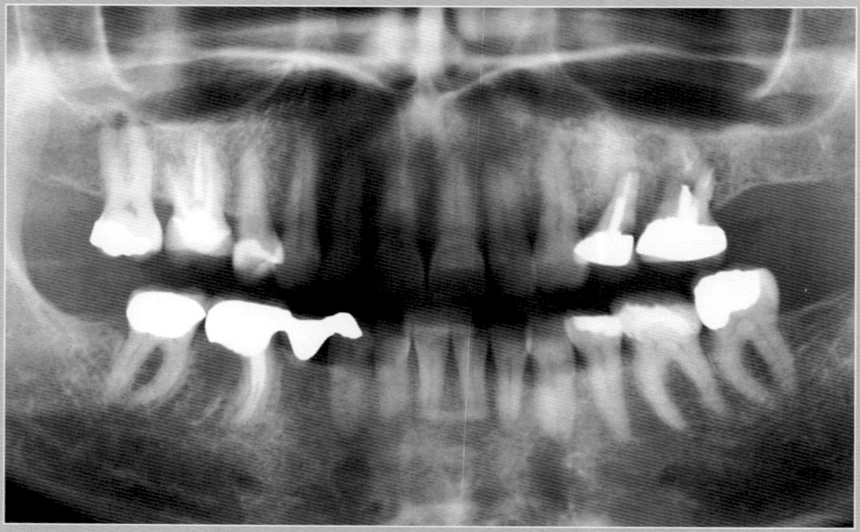

Panoramic radiograph.

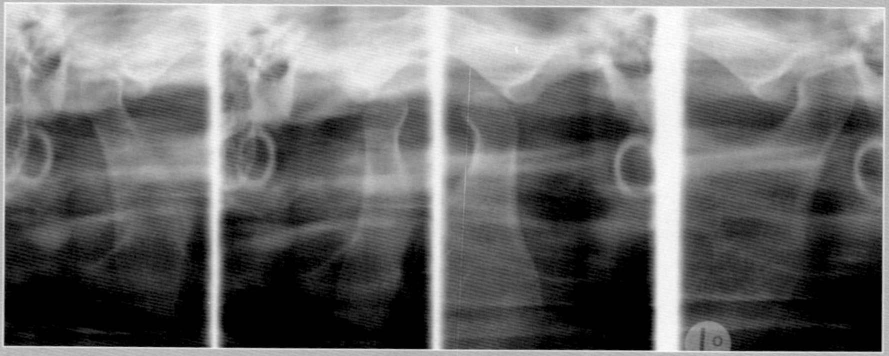

TMJ radiographs.

Radiographic findings

Complete-mouth series

- Short clinical roots
- Fractured tooth no. 14
- Provisional crown on tooth no. 19
- Previous root amputation in tooth no. 30
- Caries on tooth no. 13
- Pulpal sclerosis in tooth no. 11

Cephalometric

- Moderate to severe skeletal Class II
- Brachycephalic tendency
- Extremely upright/vertical maxillary incisors
- Compensation in mandibular incisors

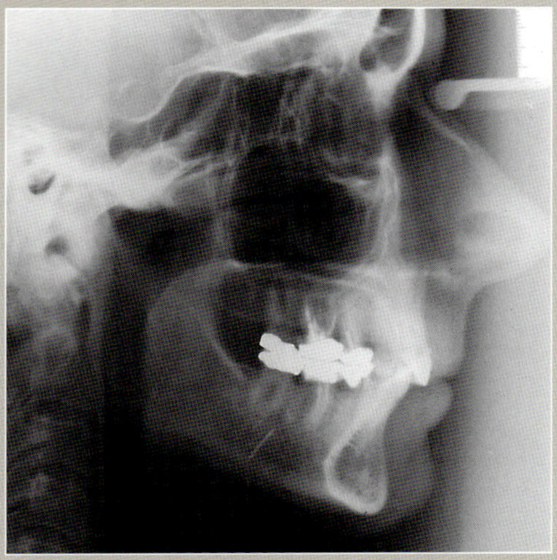

Cephalometric radiograph.

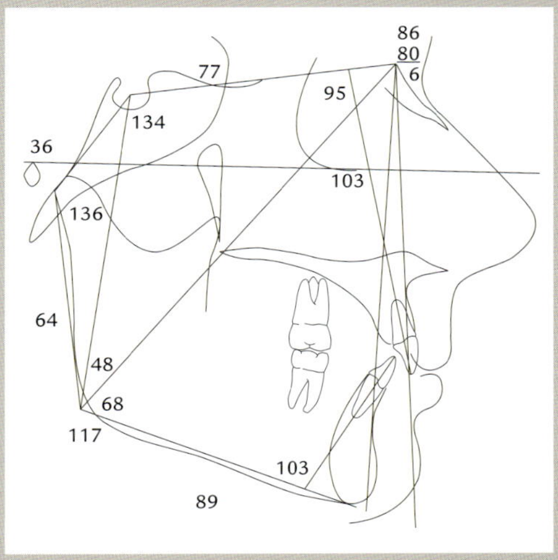

Roth cephalometric analysis.

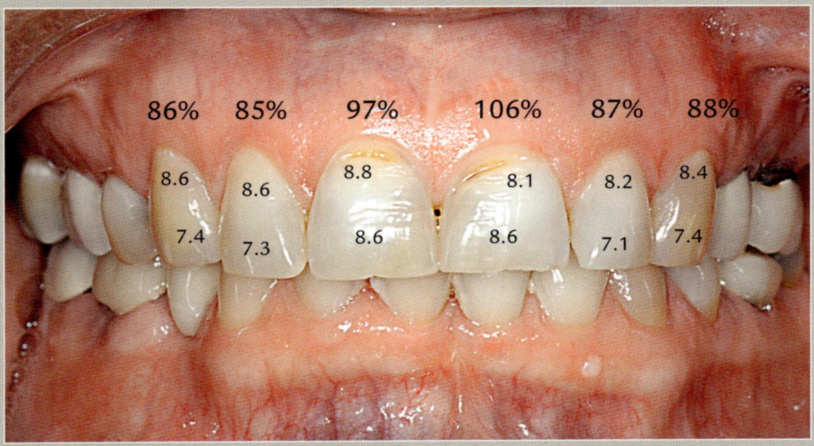

Width-to-length ratios according to the Chiche smile analysis.

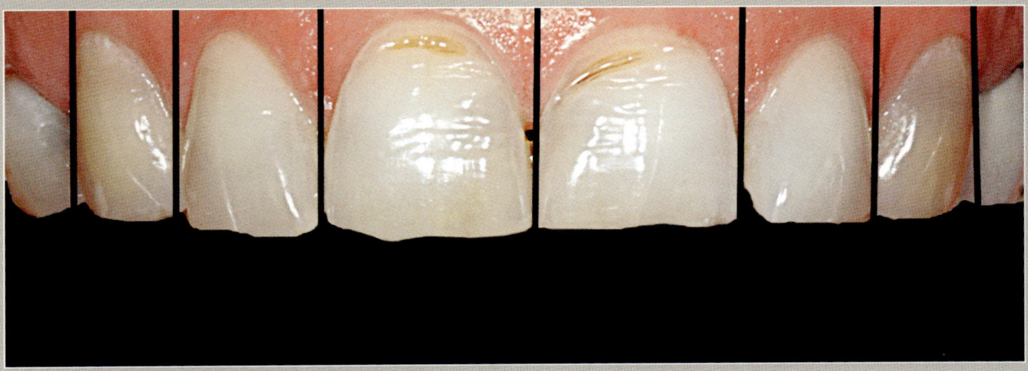

Application of golden proportions to maxillary anterior teeth.

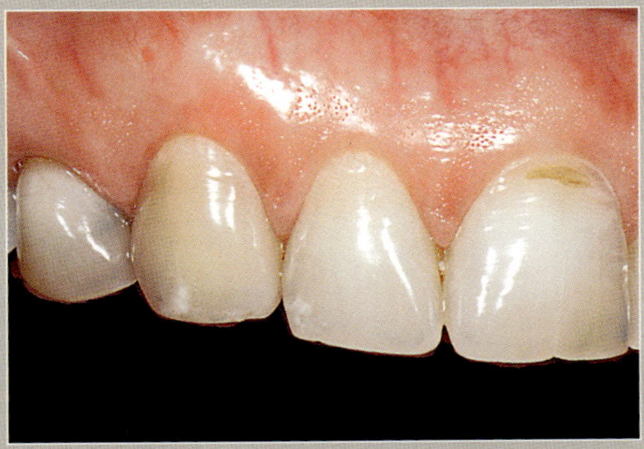

Maxillary right lateral view.

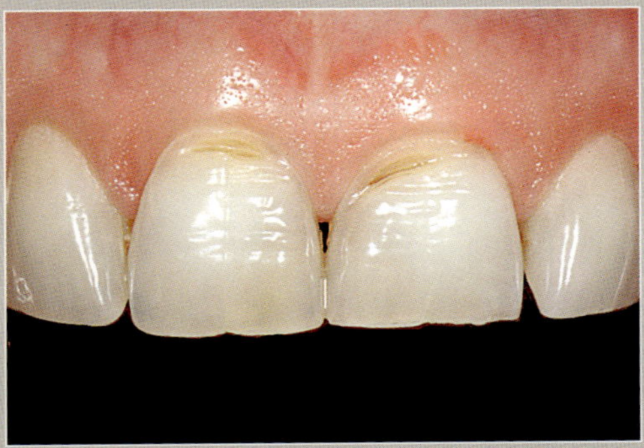

Maxillary anterior view.

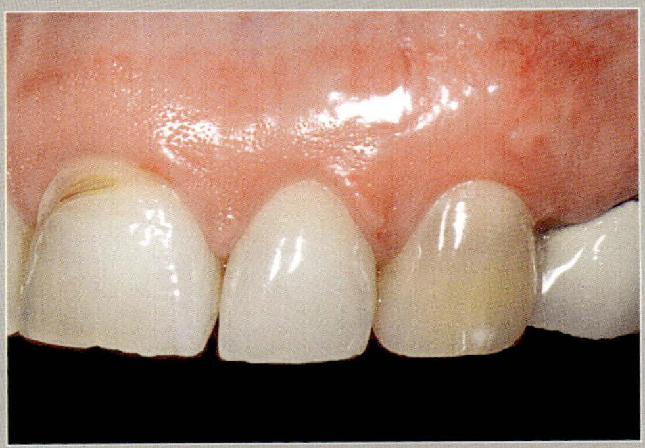

Maxillary left lateral view.

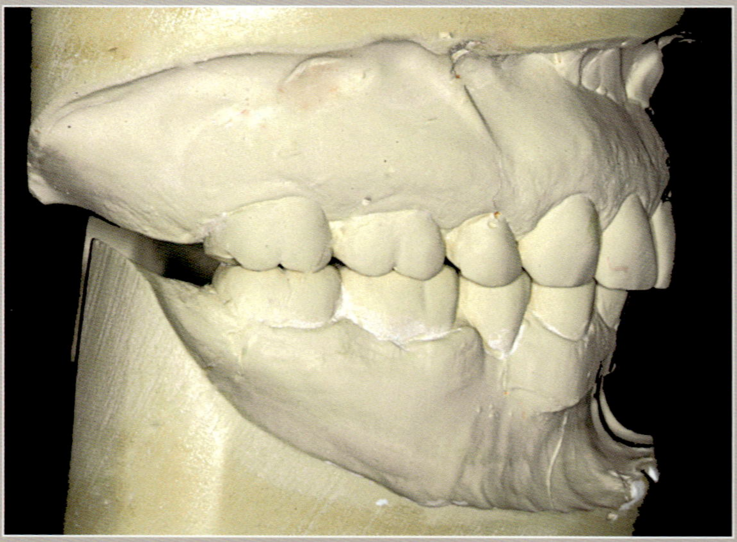

Right lateral view of study casts.

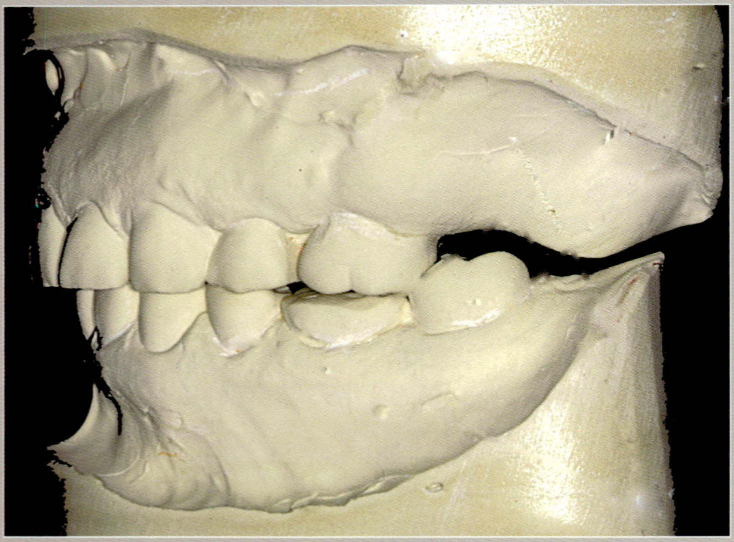

Left lateral view of study casts.

Diagnosis

- Moderate to severe skeletal Class II with orthodontic compensations
- Primary and secondary occlusal trauma
- Short clinical roots
- Fractured and carious teeth
- Defective restorations and prostheses
- Irregular tooth form and asymmetry of maxillary anterior teeth
- Medium lip dynamics, with thin upper lips
- Chronic plaque-induced gingivitis
- Chronic early to moderate periodontitis
- Chronic localized furcation involvement

Prognosis

- Overall: good
- Teeth nos. 13, 14, and 30: poor

Summary of concerns

1. Will definitive treatment for the correction of the skeletal Class II relationship be necessary, or can this patient be treated in her present state?
2. Is a phased approach possible given the extent of the problems in multiple segments?
3. Are the cosmetic concerns raised during the codiscovery phase a higher priority for the patient than the caries, defective restorations, and long-term prosthetic needs?
4. Does the patient have the time and financial resources for comprehensive treatment, or will alternative plans be more appropriate?

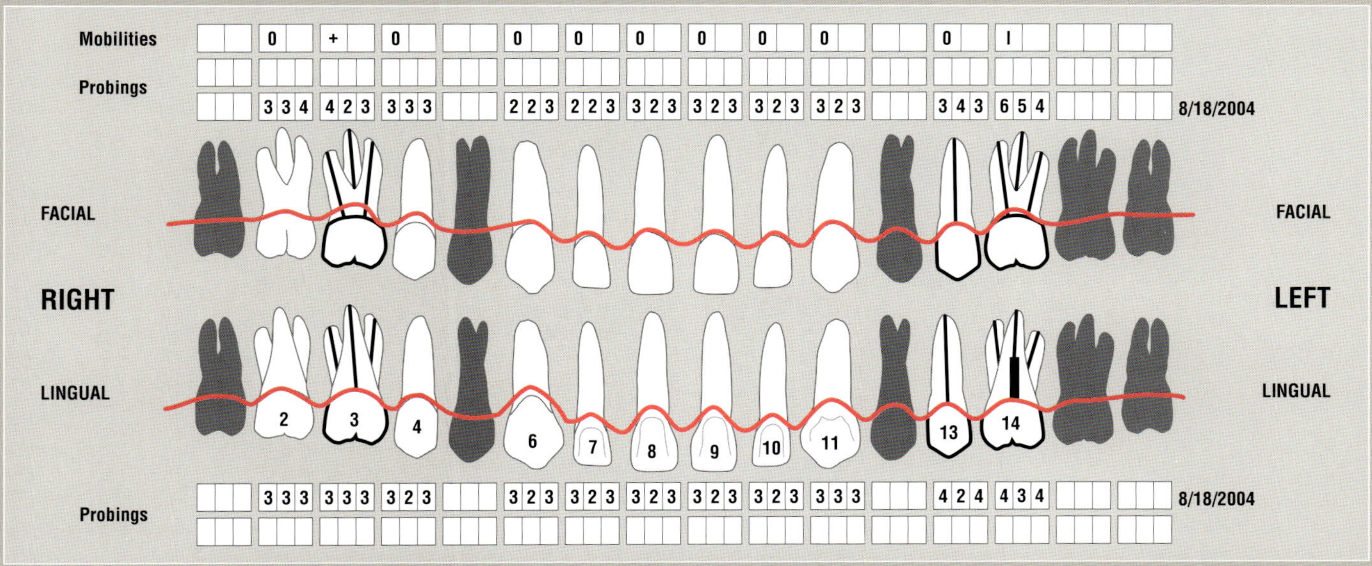

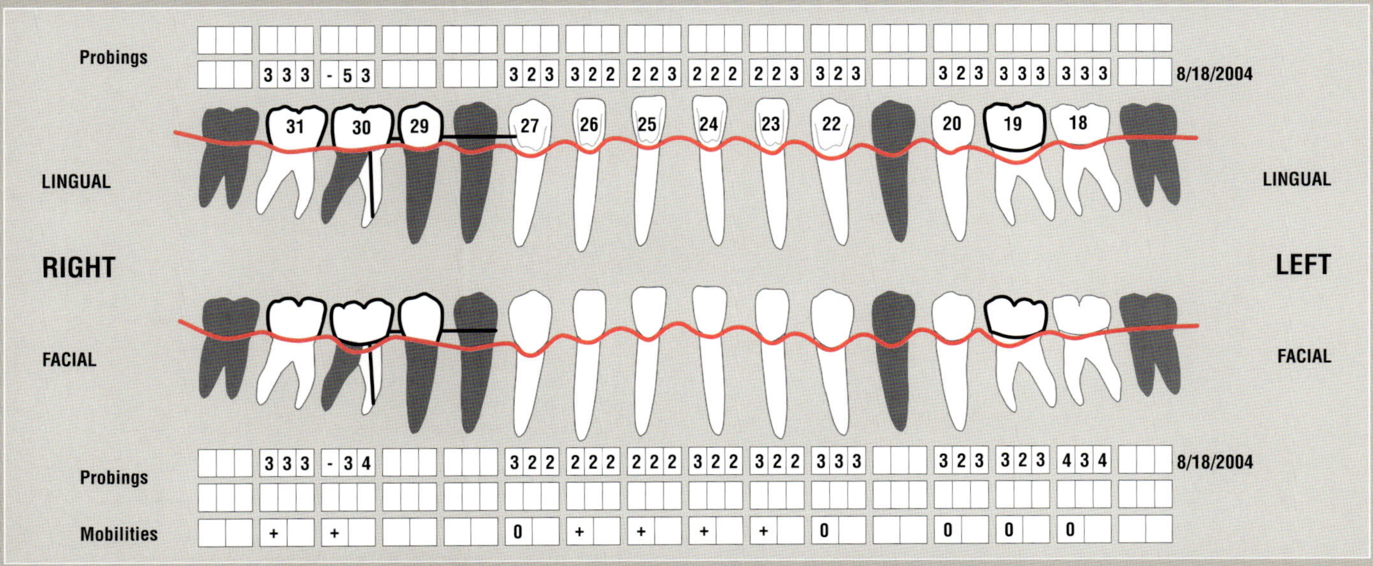

As a learning exercise, you may now outline goals/objectives of treatment and a treatment plan.

Proposed Treatment Plan

Goals/objectives of treatment

The patient was initially seen for implant therapy. However, during the consultation and codiscovery phase she expressed esthetic concerns, specifically the color and wear of her anterior teeth. This patient was presented at the Gateway Study Club in St Louis, Missouri, as part of a web-based treatment-planning session with Dr John Kois. During this session, the goals mutually established for this patient were:

- Elimination of oral pathology through strategic extractions
- Functional therapy to reduce or eliminate the occlusal dysfunction and replacement of strategically extracted teeth with implant prostheses
- Dentofacial treatment to improve the shape, surface texture, and color of the anterior teeth

Phase I: Diagnosis, case presentation/ discussion, and initial restorative treatment

1. Diagnostic wax-up to aid in finalizing the treatment plan, for the fabrication of provisional restorations, and to provide indices for the definitive treatment results
2. Consultation with treatment team members
3. Consultation and case presentation with patient
4. Mesio-occlusodistal direct composite resin restoration of tooth no. 4 to replace defective restoration
5. Complete full-crown restoration on tooth no. 19, which had previously been provisionalized
6. Caries control

Phase II: Occlusal and caries treatment

7. Fabrication of a mandibular Tanner bite splint for an occlusal evaluation for 3 months
8. During this period, extraction of teeth nos. 13, 14, and 30 with socket preservation and augmentation
9. After 3 months of occlusal treatment, evaluation and possible occlusal equilibration via selective grinding
10. Provisional direct bonding with composite on the maxillary anterior teeth to evaluate the patient's envelope of function, esthetics, and phonetics and to serve as a mock-up for future diagnostic casts, silicone index prep guides, and reduction templates

Phase III: Stage-one implant surgery

11. Implant placement in the maxilla and mandible in sites nos. 13, 14, 29, and 30 with immediate provisionalization and immediate loading
12. Sinus elevation employing the Summers osteotome technique may be required in the maxillary left segment

Phase IV: Limited/comprehensive orthodontics

13. Minor orthodontic treatment to procline the mandibular and maxillary teeth to facilitate improved function and esthetics associated with the definitive cosmetic procedures in the maxillary arch
14. Discussion with the patient regarding definitive facial and orthodontic procedures to correct the Class II skeletal malocclusion

Phase V: Prosthetic phase

15. Preparation of the maxillary anterior teeth for veneers based on the previous composite mock-up provided by the restorative dentist and laboratory
16. All-ceramic veneers on teeth nos. 6 to 11
17. Definitive metal-ceramic full-crown restorations on teeth nos. 13, 14, 29, and 30 on custom implant abutments
18. Occlusal device for nighttime wear

Active Clinical Treatment

Review of the goals/objectives of treatment

- Elimination of oral pathology through strategic extractions
- Functional therapy to reduce or eliminate the occlusal dysfunction and replacement of strategically extracted teeth with implant prostheses
- Dentofacial treatment to improve the shape, surface texture, and color of the anterior teeth

Phase I: Diagnosis, case presentation/ discussion, and initial restorative treatment

The patient was advised of the need for comprehensive occlusal and orthodontic evaluations. Cephalometric radiographs were taken, followed by tracings and analysis, in addition to a centric relation record and mounting on a Panadent articulator.

Doppler TMJ analysis was performed to evaluate the competency of the joints, and the findings were within normal limits.

Pretreatment diagnostic digital photographs were taken, and esthetic enhancements were performed in Adobe Photoshop CS using the methods of Dr Greg Lutke of Dallas Dental Solutions, Dallas, Texas. All diagnostic information was summarized using the Ten-Step Diagnostic Opinion Form developed by Dr John Kois at the Kois Center in Seattle, Washington. Based on the conclusions of the Seattle Study Club web-based program with Dr Kois, a definitive treatment plan for the patient was collectively formulated by the Gateway Study Club for the treating clinicians.

The patient accepted the plan and restated her desire to achieve a more beautiful smile. She also understood the necessity of all of the treatment being recommended.

Initially, the plan was to address a few teeth requiring immediate care. A mesio-occlusodistal direct composite resin restoration was placed on tooth no. 4 because the existing restoration was defective and bothering the patient. A metal-ceramic crown was fabricated for tooth no. 19 and cemented with a composite resin cement, replacing the existing provisional acrylic crown.

Following these procedures, irreversible hydrocolloid impressions were made for the fabrication of at-home bleaching trays for use with 15% carbamide peroxide gel. After successful home bleaching, the patient was seen for initial direct composite resin restorations on all of the maxillary anterior teeth. A silicone putty index was used along with a three-tier layering technique to lengthen the maxillary and mandibular incisal edges based on the esthetic imaging, occlusal analysis, and the diagnostic wax-up, emulating the methods of Dr Pascal Magne.[6]

Following completion of the maxillary anterior restorations, an acute periodontal abscess developed in the region of tooth no. 30 and was treated with systemic amoxicillin. The patient was immediately referred to the periodontist for more definitive treatment of that tooth and other necessary periodontal therapy that had been originally treatment planned.

To address the patient's interim esthetic and functional needs, Valplast acrylic interim removable partial dentures were made for the maxillary left and mandibular right sextants. The patient was experiencing constant discomfort while wearing the mandibular partial denture and consequently wore the appliance minimally after insertion. As soon as the implants were placed in the mandibular right sextant, the interim removable partial denture was converted to an immediately loaded provisional screw-retained prosthesis. In the maxillary left sextant, the patient had no discomfort and was compliant with the use of the Valplast interim removable partial denture. During the surgical phase, modification and finishing of the maxillary anterior restorations were accomplished to meet the esthetic goals of the patient. This precluded the use of the Tanner appliance planned in the proposed treatment.

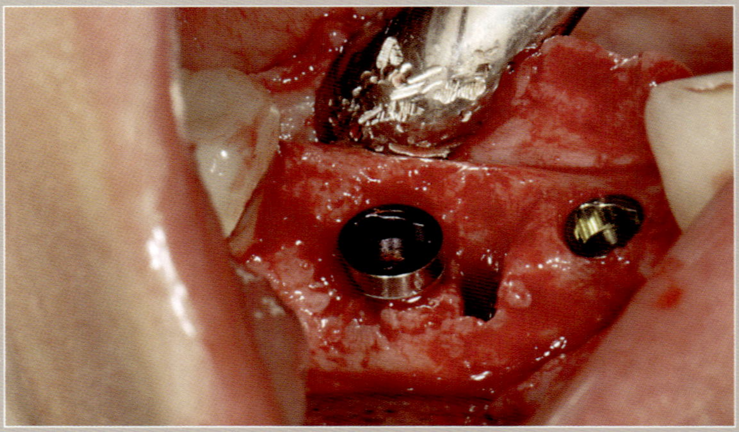

Implant placement in sites nos. 29 and 30.

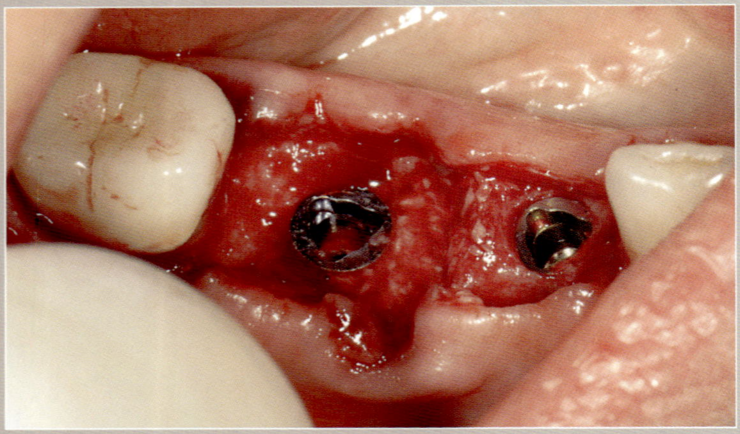

Placement of allograft in residual defects.

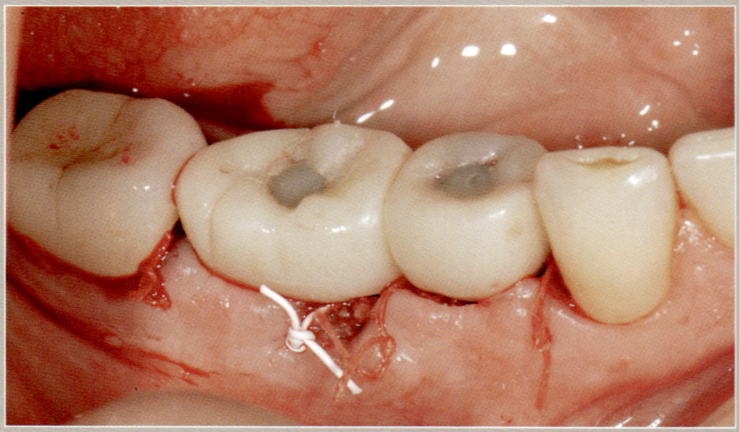

Immediate screw-retained provisional restorations.

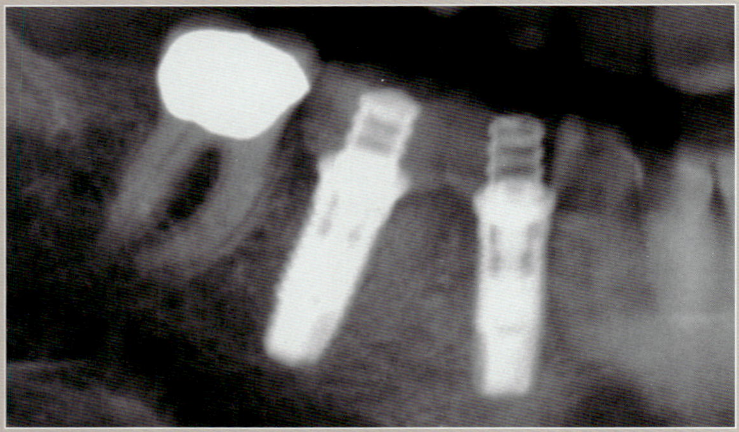

Periapical radiograph of provisional restorations.

Phase II: Mandibular surgical phase

The initial treatment plan sequence called for therapy to begin on the maxillary left posterior sextant with the mandibular right posterior sextant to follow. However, the patient traumatically fractured the distal abutment tooth, hemiresected tooth no. 30, in March 2005. Therefore, surgical therapy was initiated in the mandibular right sextant with the strategic extraction of the residual mesial root of tooth no. 30, after sectioning the connector on the mesial abutment retainer.

After extraction and site inspection, it was deemed feasible to perform immediate one-stage implant placement in sites nos. 29 and 30. Parallel-walled endosseous implants were placed in type 2 to 3 bone and were deemed stable at 45 Ncm. Screw-retained composite resin provisional restorations were fabricated for immediate provisional loading of the implants after allograft bone placement. The soft tissue was sutured and allowed to heal for 3 to 4 months with a screw-retained provisional restoration. The postoperative course for this treatment was uneventful.

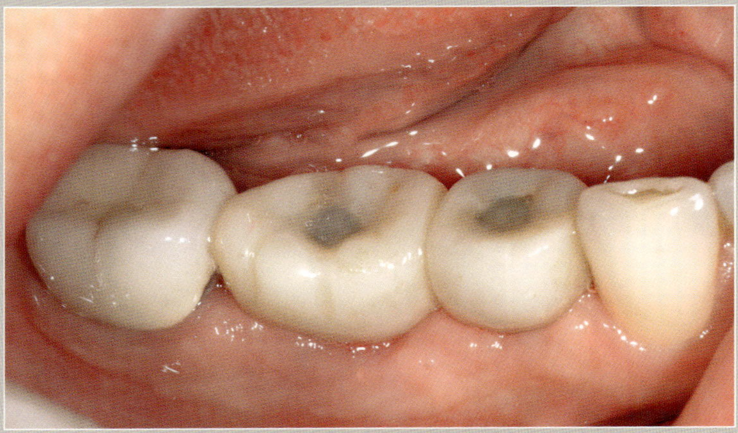

Healing of soft tissues around provisional restorations.

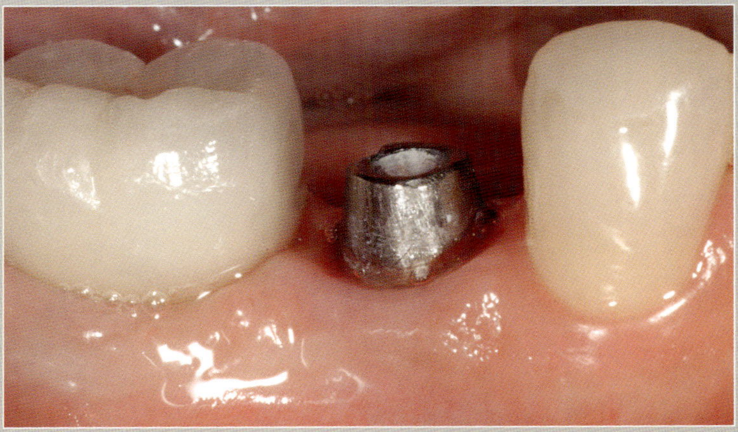

CAD/CAM titanium Procera abutment.

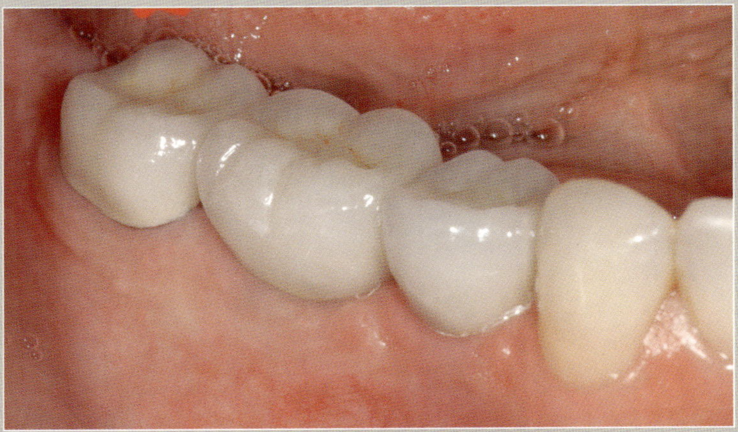

Definitive porcelain metal-ceramic crowns.

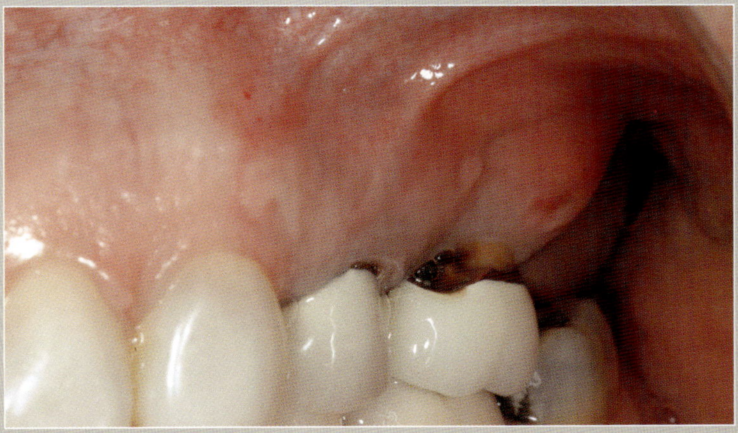

Root fracture of tooth no. 14 with periodontal abscess.

Phase III: Mandibular prosthetic phase

After surgical therapy and healing were completed, the patient was seen for definitive mandibular restorative therapy. She had declined orthodontic therapy. The healing abutments were removed and implant-level open-tray impressions were made. Stone casts with soft tissue indices were made by the laboratory technician for fabricating custom abutments. The abutment wax patterns were scanned with a Nobel Biocare Procero scanner for CAD/CAM custom titanium abutments for teeth nos. 29 and 30. These titanium abutments served as platforms for metal-ceramic crowns for teeth nos. 29 and 30.

Phase IV: Maxillary surgical phase

Following healing and definitive prosthetic rehabilitation of the mandibular right sextant, surgical therapy was performed in the maxillary left posterior sextant. The roots of teeth nos. 13 and 14 had remained asympto-matic until July 2005, when the root of tooth no. 14 experienced additional fractures. These fractures led to an acute periodontal abscess that was initially managed with the administration of systemic antibiotics, immediately followed by strategic extraction of teeth nos. 13 and 14.

After debridement of the sockets, it was deemed possible to place immediate implants in the sockets without sinus elevation. Two parallel-walled endosseous implants were

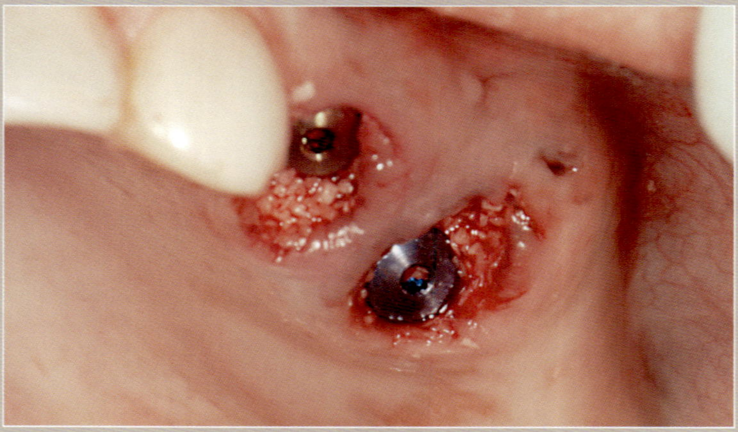

Immediate implant placement with allograft socket augmentation.

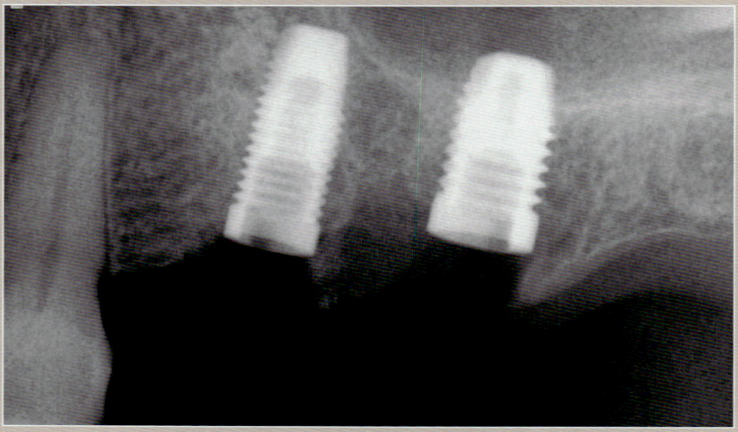

Radiograph of implants at placement.

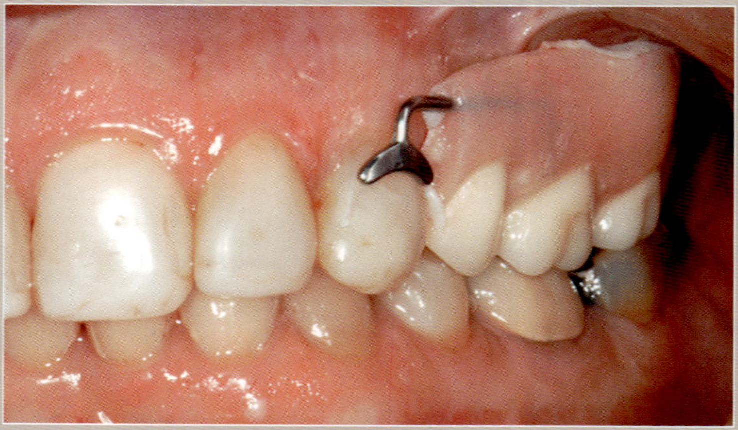

Maxillary provisional removable partial denture after implant placement.

placed in type 3 bone in the maxillary left sextant and were deemed stable. However, these implants did not meet either the mechanical or the biologic requirements for immediate loading. Mineralized allograft mixed with medical-grade calcium sulfate was placed to augment the peri-implant spaces in the socket, followed by the insertion of low-profile healing abutments. At the patient's request, a Valplast acrylic interim removable partial denture was fabricated by the general dentist during the healing phase in this sextant. The postsurgical course was uneventful, and osseointegration was confirmed by radiographic and standard clinical methods. The patient was referred back to the general dentist for the definitive restorative phase.

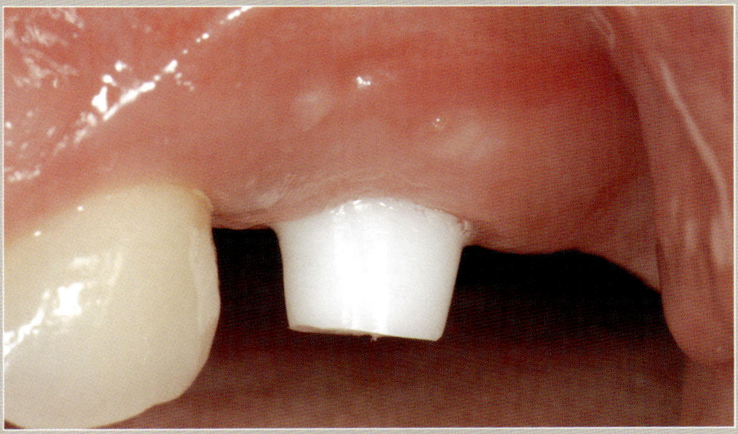

CAD/CAM Procera zirconia abutment.

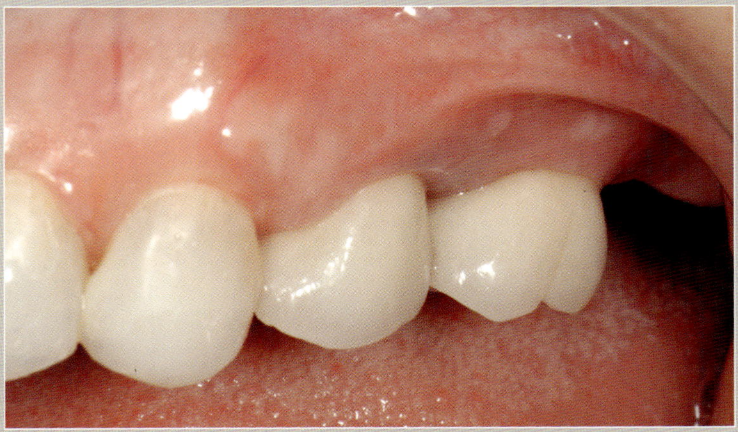

Definitive Procera AllZirkon crowns.

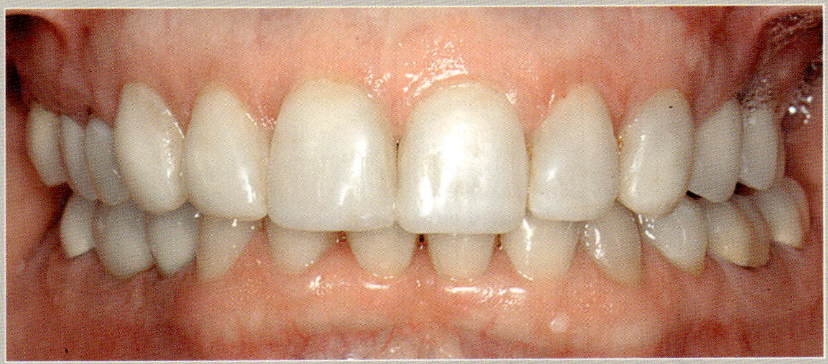

Intraoral view in centric occlusion after direct composite restoration of anterior teeth.

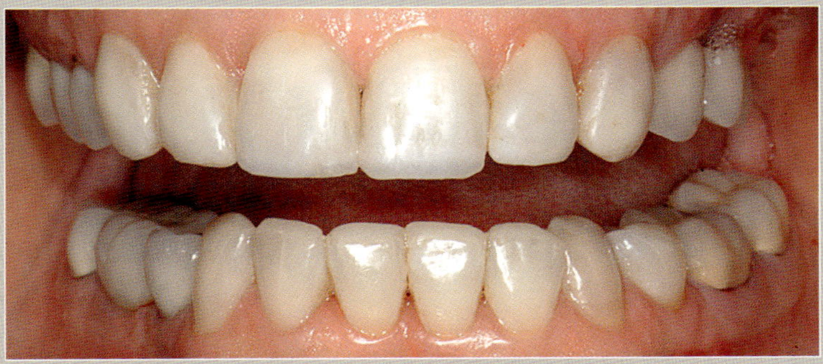

Intraoral view upon opening after direct composite restoration of anterior teeth.

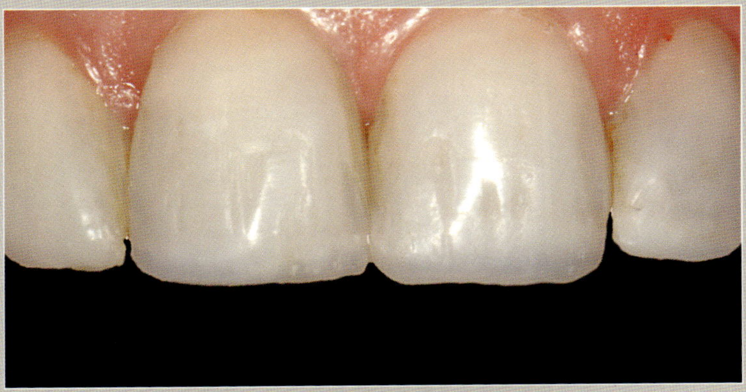

Maxillary incisal edges after cosmetic bonding.

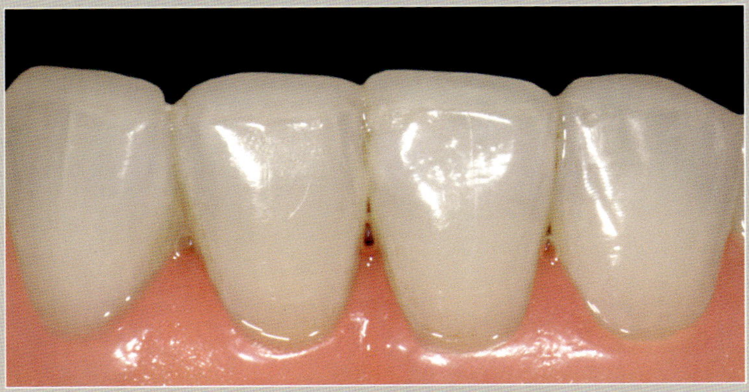

Mandibular incisal edges after cosmetic bonding.

Phase V: Definitive prosthetic phase

After surgical therapy was completed, the patient was seen for definitive restorative therapy. The healing abutments in the maxillary left were removed, and implant-level open-tray impressions were made. Stone casts with soft tissue indices were made by the laboratory technician for fabricating custom abutments. The abutment wax patterns were scanned with a Nobel Biocare Procera scanner for CAD/CAM custom zirconia abutments for teeth nos. 13 and 14.

Upon return and modification of the zirconia abutments, the maxillary zirconia abutments were scanned for zirconia copings to serve as an infrastructure for Procera AllZirkon crowns for teeth nos. 13 and 14. In conjunction with the

Posttreatment

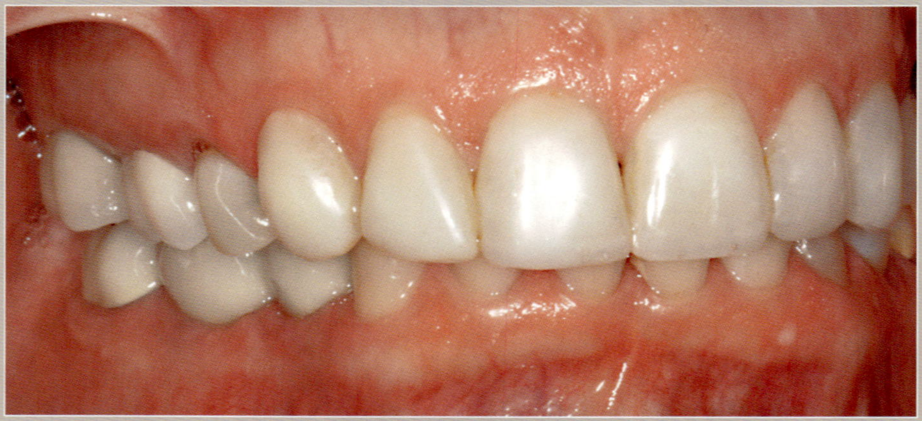

Right lateral view of definitive restorations.

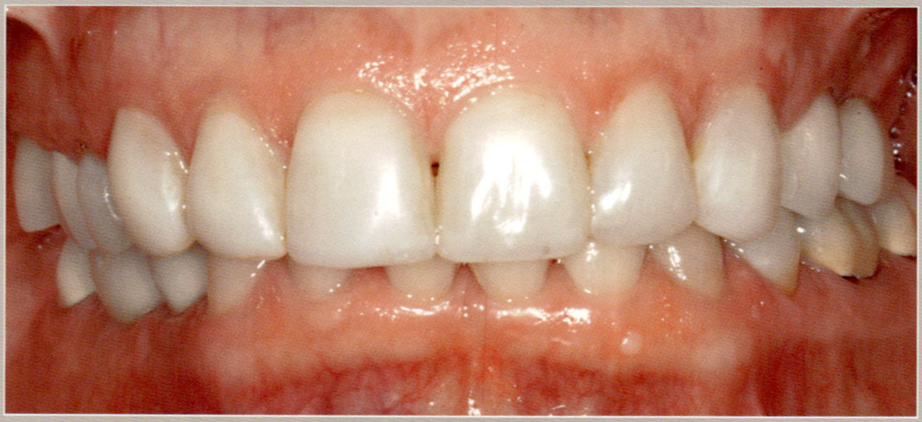

Anterior view of definitive restorations.

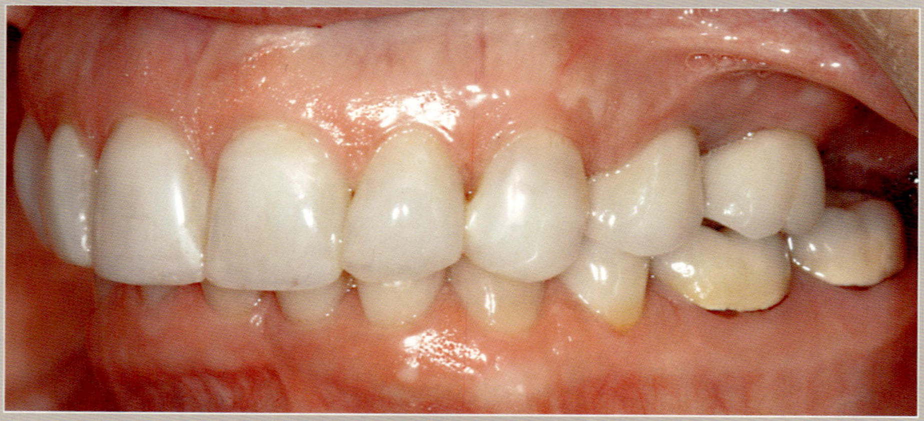

Left lateral view of definitive restorations.

overall occlusal reconstruction, teeth nos. 2, 18, 19, and 31 received new metal-ceramic crowns that were permanently cemented with resin-modified glass ionomer cement (RelyX Luting Cement, 3M ESPE). Tooth no. 2 became symptomatic with pulpalgia after cementation, and the patient was referred to an endodontist for therapy. After successful endodontic treatment and cessation of the patient's symptoms, placement of a new metal-ceramic crown was elected for tooth no. 2. Subsequently, a maxillary clear, hard acrylic occlusal nightguard was delivered to the patient.

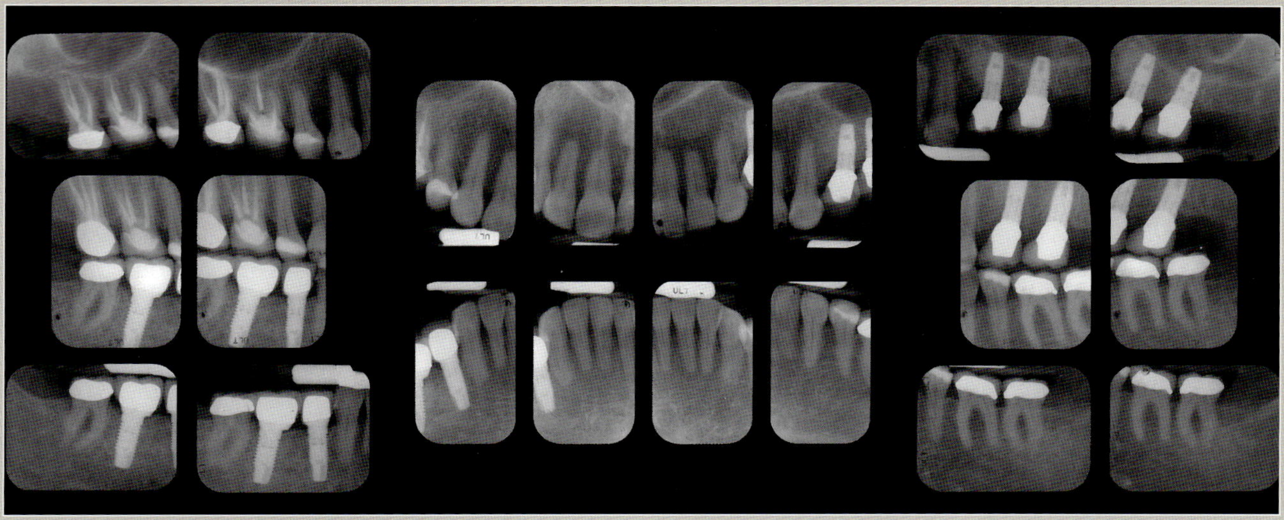

Complete-mouth radiographs.

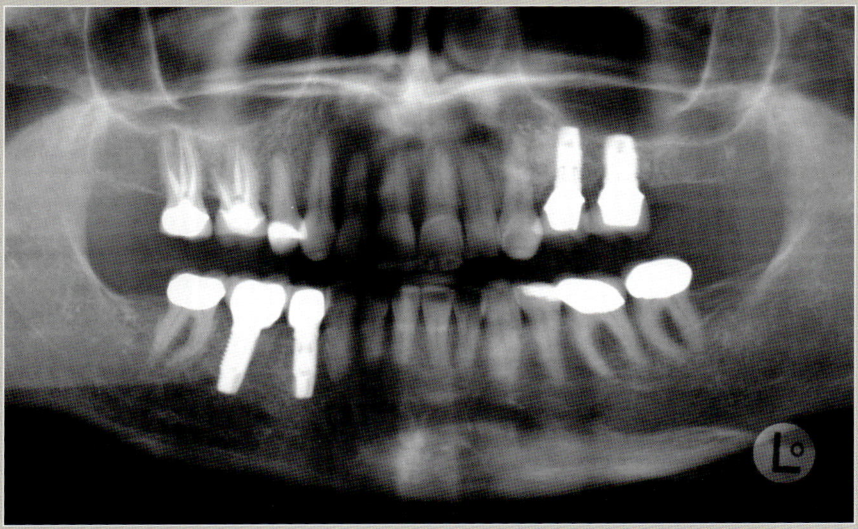

Panoramic radiograph.

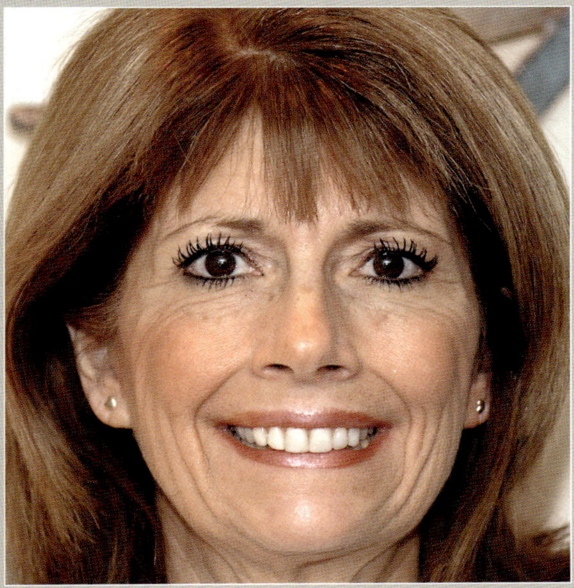

Facial view.

You may now place the corresponding posttreatment overlay found in the separate folder over the pretreatment periodontal chart on page 473.

Commentary

Given the extensive time devoted to the treatment planning and sequencing for this patient, it may be assumed that treatment would proceed as planned. However, the experienced clinician knows that treatment rarely follows the ascribed blueprints exactly, and we need to be ready to modify our therapeutic protocols appropriately, based on the many twists and turns that can occur related to the needs of the patient and unexpected treatment outcomes. Initial treatment planning for this patient emphasized the use of felspathic translucent porcelain laminate veneers for the maxillary anterior teeth. Even though financial constraints prevented us from proceeding in that direction, the patient was extremely pleased with the definitive result of the direct-bonded composite resin veneers on the maxillary and mandibular anterior teeth. At this time she has declined the recommended porcelain laminate bonded veneers. Although the clinicians are disappointed by this decision, the clinical option for esthetic porcelain laminate veneers in the maxillary anterior teeth to achieve the optimal luster and surface characteristics may be possible in the future.

The presentation of significant pre-existing conditions that are outside the control of interdisciplinary teams can be the greatest challenges facing the successful treatment outcome for the patient. These conditions include previous disease, physiologic and chronologic aging, traumatic injuries, and previous dental care. In some cases, these past events can present significant risks for current treatment.

When a team of dentists encounters a patient with this type of history, it may be difficult to determine where to begin the diagnostic process. The use of standardized procedures, forms, and checklists may aid the team in collection of necessary data. Once all the data is available, then a plan based on four general goals of dental treatment planning can be formulated:

1. Eliminate pain and suffering
2. Restore function
3. Achieve proper esthetics
4. Prevent future recurrence of disease by primary prevention

The order in which these goals are met is highly variable, and the sequence of treatment to achieve these goals can be individualized based on the acute and/or chronic nature of the symptoms presented by the patient.[7]

This patient presented with a worn anterior dentition that was not protecting the posterior teeth in function due to an existing Class II skeletal malocclusion. As a result of unabated skeletal development and previous orthodontic treatment, the posterior teeth were experiencing mechanical overload and structural wear with overt fractures. Initial interviewing supported by patient codiagnosis also revealed dissatisfaction with the esthetics of the anterior teeth. However, the patient had limited financial resources to commit to definitive long-term restoration of the anterior teeth with single-crown prosthetics or with bonded ceramic veneers.

It could be strongly debated that correction of the malocclusion would allow for an envelope of function that would be less harmful and more protective in nature and therefore limit future consequences of occlusal dysfunction.[8] This recommendation was discussed with the patient during codiscovery and during the extended course of clinical treatment. It also was a repeated topic of debate among the treating clinicians. However, despite the dental team's passionate occlusal philosophies, the patient declined the orthodontic/orthognathic approach.

The ethical and professional boundary for patients who defer definitive correction of malocclusions is a challenge for both clinicians and patients. These cases are complicated, and all the variables need to be considered. These variables include cultural difference, personal preferences, the orthodontist's view, surgical expertise, and financial considerations. In this case, one complicated problem led to more complex restorative problems that arose from continued primary and secondary occlusal trauma due to a lack of protective anterior guidance. Although photographic evidence presented in this case demonstrates improved esthetics and acceptable fixed prosthodontics on teeth and implants at the time of case completion, the veteran clinician knows this is not the end of the story. Even in the presence of occlusal protection offered by bite appliances of varying types, this patient is at risk for continued deterioration of the new reconstruction. Only time and continued observation by this team will confirm this suspicion.

In order to provide an upgradeable option, direct-bonded composite veneers were placed to enhance anterior esthetics, serve as a temporary guide for future prosthetics, and to provide some level of protection from continued wear. The posterior reconstruction of this patient was performed using single-tooth prosthetics on either natural teeth or endosseous root-form implants. By using the aforementioned dental technologies, the patient still has an opportunity in the future to consider the recommendations for comprehensive dentofacial therapy. It is assumed after the occlusal therapies the patient would have a more harmonious and protective stomatognathic system allowing for recommendations for either all-ceramic veneers or complete-coverage metal-ceramic or all-ceramic single-tooth prosthetics on the anterior teeth.

As the proposed treatment of this patient unfolded, new clinical findings required the team to reshape the working diagnosis and proposed treatments. These adjustments can cause additional financial considerations and anxiety for all concerned. Fortunately for the team and this patient, the unanticipated twists and turns experienced during treatment were overcome by a great collaborative effort on the part of the treatment team. In this case, some of the implants were immediately provisionalized while others required a conventional two-stage loading protocol. Treatment of the posterior teeth was performed in sextants to allow the patient and team to proceed in the most cost-effective manner, with a true sensitivity to the patient's budget.

It is important at the outset of complicated long-term treatment plans for the treating team to present the patient with realistic goals, risks, and potential complications that may be encountered. The definitive treatment solution for this patient differed greatly from the initial proposal but, in the clinicians' opinion, ultimately provided the patient with a result that dramatically improved her esthetic appearance with stabilization of the posterior dentition.

One of my mentors, Dr Henry Tanner, improved my understanding of treatment planning when he stated, "There is a right treatment plan for every patient—it is our responsibility to find the one inside the patient who is in front of us and have the patient take ownership for it" (personal communication, 1995). Sometimes the "right" treatment plan does not present itself at the outset of treatment but may surface somewhere along the path to completion. This patient's care required knowledge, flexibility, and perseverance on behalf of the patient and treating team.

The American College of Dentists has published several core values to act as a guide for ethical conduct and to serve as a foundation for providing exceptional care for patients.[9] Three of the core values played a pivotal role in this patient's treatment and represent important takeaway messages from this chapter. The first is the patient's right to personal autonomy in making treatment decisions on his or her own after weighing all of the benefits versus the attendant risks. However, this statement does not imply that a patient's right to self-determine treatment is absolute; rather, it should be supported by the counsel of capable and caring clinicians who make recommendations derived from evidence-based protocols.

The final two core values are, in my opinion, intimately tied together and are consistent with a philosophy taught to the author by clinical instructors in undergraduate and graduate dental school and later by a long list of professional mentors. These two values are competence and beneficence. Competence is a by-product of the relentless pursuit of knowledge. Competence, however, is only part of the equation in becoming a complete clinician. The other part is beneficence, which relates to never losing sight of human caring and kindness.

George Leonard, in his book *Mastery,* stated, "The human individual is equipped to learn and go on learning prodigiously from birth to death, and this is precisely what sets him or her apart from all other known forms of life."[9] Although many dental schools strive to provide their students with a basic foundation for clinical care, it is clear that most graduates are "safe beginners" at best and do not have the skills to handle more complex and advanced treatment. Unfortunately, these dentists who are starting out in practice are usually in survival mode and are faced with the dilemma of prioritization. They must decide whether continuing education can wait until when they can better afford it or if the need to acquire the knowledge that will fuel practice and personal growth overrides the strain on their resources.

However, continuing education is not only for beginners; regular participation also offers great benefit to the seasoned veteran. One of the most valuable assets one can acquire is the support of fellow clinicians in a study club environment. The collective wisdom of my dental elders led me to believe in the strength of using group expertise, putting multiple sets of eyes on problems, and building a team that shares responsibility for complex circumstances. I hope in some way I have honored those who have helped me on this path, including my grandfather, with this chapter. After all, someone needs to continue "chopping wood and carrying water."

Acknowledgments

I would like to thank the members of the Gateway Study Club, a Seattle Study Club, in St Louis for the memories, lessons, and experiences we have shared over the past 10 years. The case presented in this textbook was part of an ongoing educational process over the last 11 years. The individual team members in the Gateway Study Club who treated this patient were general dentists Drs Kevin Thorpe and Jack Marincel. I thank them for their patience and understanding in this project. Our laboratory partner was Mr Gerry Jacobi, Jacobi Dental Lab, who provided the outstanding definitive treatment result for this patient.

My staff also played a key role in the preparation of this manuscript. They helped prepare the patient, take photographs, and comfort the patient during multiple diagnostic and surgical treatments. I would especially like to thank my personal dental assistant, Ms Stephanie Barlow, for her great efforts with the patient and me.

Lastly, I would like to thank our patient for her understanding and patience throughout the duration of this treatment marathon. She endured the setbacks, the multiple therapies, and the disappointments with grace and dignity. It is only with her permission that we were able to share this experience of learning and demonstrate an interdisciplinary team striving to achieve the best outcomes.

References

1. Cohen M. Interdisciplinary Treatment Planning: Principles, Design, and Implementation. Chicago: Quintessence, 2008.
2. Gawande A. The Checklist Manifesto—How to Get Things Right. New York: Metropolitan, 2009.
3. Sackett D, Rosenberg W, Gray J, Haynes R, Richardson W. Evidence-based medicine: What it is and what it isn't. BMJ 1996;312:71–72.
4. Dawson PE. Functional Occlusion—From TMJ to Smile Design. St Louis: Mosby-Elsevier, 2007.
5. Travis C, Aronson E. Mistakes Were Made (But Not by Me): Why We Justify Foolish Beliefs, Bad Decisions, and Hurtful Acts. Orlando: Harcourt, 2007.
6. Magne P, Belser U. Bonded Porcelain Restorations in the Anterior Dentition: A Biomimetic Approach. Chicago: Quintessence, 2003.
7. Spear FM. Occlusal considerations for complex restorative therapy. In: McNeill C (ed). Science and Practice of Occlusion. Chicago: Quintessence, 1997:437–456.
8. Arnett GW, McLaughlin RP. Facial and Dental Planning for Orthodontists and Oral Surgeons. St Louis: Mosby, 2004.
9. Leonard G. Mastery: The Keys to Success and Long-Term Fulfillment. New York: Penguin, 1992:53.

19

The Difficult Deep Bite Dilemma

J. William Robbins, DDS, MA
Robert "Tito" Norris, DDS

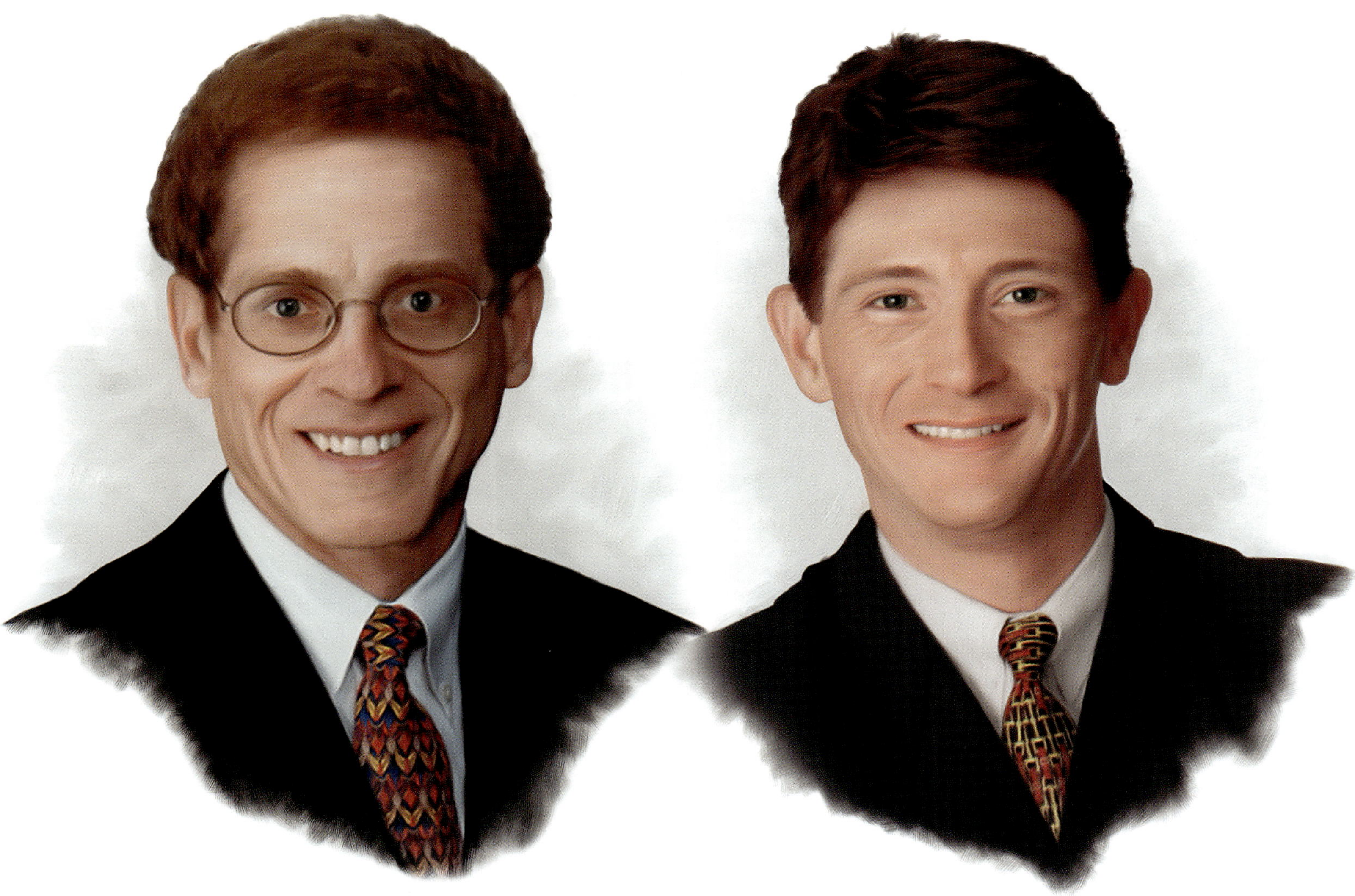

Patients with deep bite malocclusions and small teeth often believe that their esthetic issues can be resolved with restorative dentistry alone.

PHILOSOPHY AND BACKGROUND

Patients with a deep bite commonly present with excessive display of the maxillary anterior teeth in both repose and full smile. Additionally, the retroclination of the maxillary incisors appears unnatural and can be quite unsightly. Deep bite malocclusions also can lead to several long-term problems for the untreated patient.

The first problem is excessive wear of the anterior teeth. Due to the constricted envelope of function and/or parafunction, the incisolingual surfaces of the maxillary anterior teeth and the incisolabial surfaces of the mandibular anterior teeth are subject to damaging forces. The resultant wear can be progressive and ultimately make restoration of these teeth impossible.

Another issue is occlusal instability. Because the maxillary and mandibular teeth are not coupled at an acceptable angle (ie, 130 degrees), the teeth tend to supraerupt. This supraeruption may result in impingement of the mandibular incisors on the palatal tissue and can result in subsequent trauma to the alveolar support. The instability of the anterior incisal relationships and lack of proper guidance can result in instability of the posterior teeth as well.

The deep bite also can result in a constricted chewing pattern, which can significantly affect the patient's functional chewing cycle. This constricted envelope of function can result in muscle fatigue and myofascial pain.

Finally, smile presentation and esthetics are commonly compromised in deep bite patients. Patients with deep bite malocclusions and small teeth often believe that their esthetic issues can be resolved with restorative dentistry alone. However, it is impossible to adequately treat these individuals with only bonding, veneers, or full-crown restorations. These patients very likely require more comprehensive care, which often involves orthodontic therapy.

Helping a patient to make a decision to pursue interdisciplinary treatment, including orthodontics, requires excellent verbal and behavioral skills on the part of the restorative dentist and, ultimately, the treatment team. The patient is almost always surprised to hear that orthodontics is a necessary part of the treatment plan.

Once the patient understands the necessity of orthodontic treatment, the next challenge for the treatment team is the complexity of the treatment planning required with the deep bite patient. When the anterior teeth are moved into esthetically pleasing positions, there is inevitably a problem with excess interdental space. Additionally, it is usually very difficult to develop coupling of the maxillary and mandibular anterior teeth at an angle that will result in long-term occlusal stability.

Initially, it is the responsibility of the restorative dentist to lead the patient through the diagnostic discovery process. The predictability of case acceptance is much higher when the patient understands and takes ownership of all of the problems associated with his or her malocclusion.

We chose this case because of the generally difficult nature of treating a patient with a Class I deep bite malocclusion. In designing the treatment plan, it is important to focus on the consequences of changing tooth positions as it relates to coupling of the anterior teeth and the effect treatment will have on the management of interdental spacing.

We recognize that a case of this nature cannot be adequately managed by the restorative dentist alone. It requires a comprehensive approach to treatment planning. When designed from this perspective, the plan is more likely to be not only esthetically pleasing but also functionally sound in the long term.

Case Presentation

Treating clinicians
Restorative dentist: J. William Robbins, DDS, MA
Orthodontist: Robert "Tito" Norris, DDS
Oral and maxillofacial surgeon: B. D. Tiner, DDS, MD
Laboratory technician: Dene LeBeau, CDT

Clinical Treatment Planning

Age at initial presentation: 22 years
Initial presentation: December 2006
Active treatment completed: February 2010

Introduction and background

This 22-year-old man presented with concern about his appearance. He was a college graduate and had recently begun working as a pharmaceutical representative. He was concerned that his teeth and smile would have a negative impact on his career. Additionally, he complained of jaw pain after chewing and thought that this was related to his bite. He had only received routine restorative dentistry in the past. His primary goals were to look better, improve his bite, and to become pain free.

A CORE Global Diagnosis form was used in the dentofacial analysis of this patient (see Commentary section).

Medical history

- Reported seasonal allergies and carried an albuterol inhaler for use as needed
- Allergic to penicillin

Diagnostic findings

Extraoral and facial findings

- Relatively flat facial profile
- Good frontal symmetry
- Thin lips
- Lower third of the face slightly longer than middle third of the face
- Normal maxillary lip length (22 mm) and lip mobility (6 mm)
- Excessive amount of maxillary central incisor visible in repose (5 mm)
- Acceptable relationship of the incisal edges of the maxillary anterior teeth to the lower lip in full smile
- Excessive buccal corridors with negative spaces

TMJ and mandibular range of motion

- No joint sounds noted; however, the patient reported a past early opening click in the left joint area
- Range of motion: 12 mm on both sides
- Maximum opening: 51 mm
- Mild tenderness in the right masseter muscle
- No tenderness of either joint on loading
- Patient reported that he could not chew gum due to jaw fatigue

Dental cast analysis

- Significant generalized spacing secondary to proportionally small teeth
- Retroclined maxillary incisors

Pretreatment

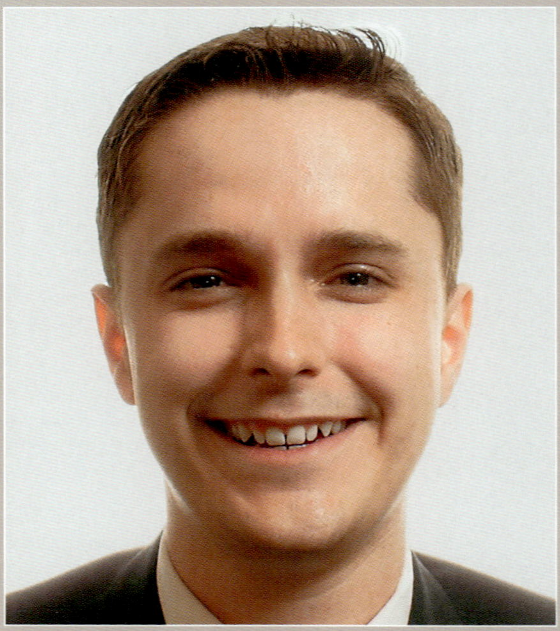

Facial view of smile.

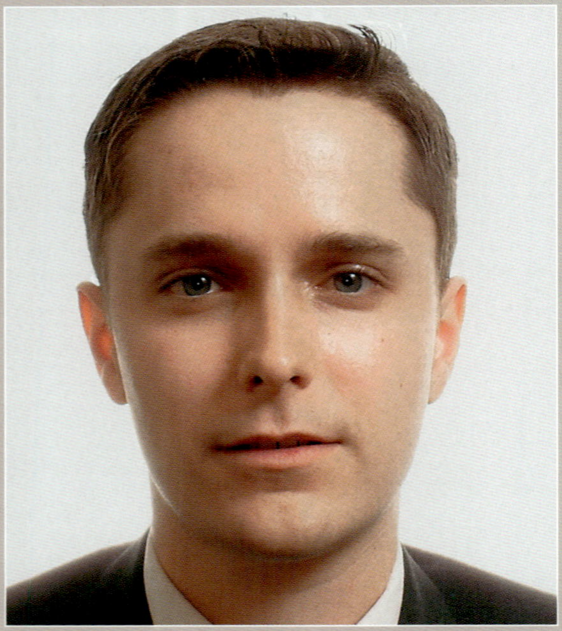

Facial view of lips in repose.

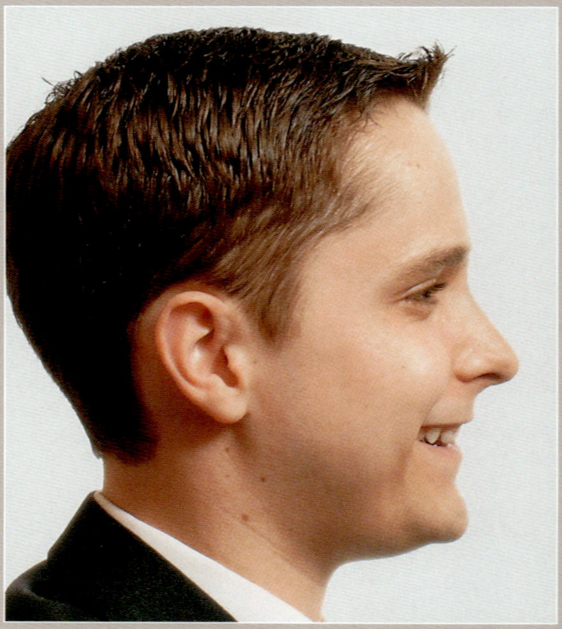

Profile view of smile.

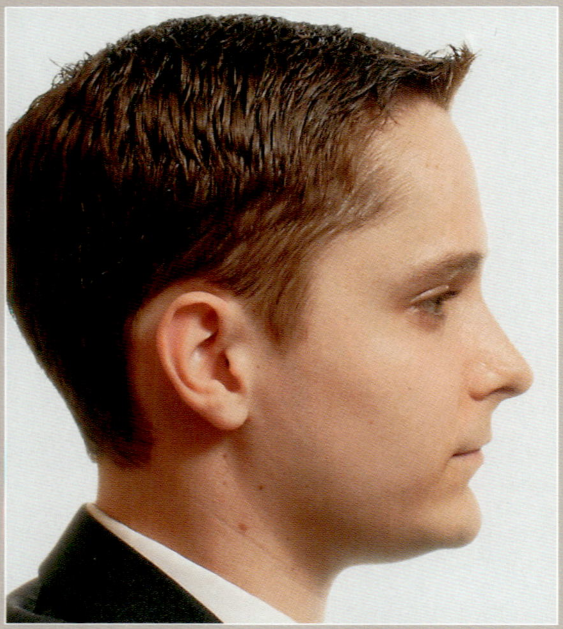

Profile view of lips in repose.

Intraoral findings

Dental

- Generalized spacing of the maxillary teeth
- Short maxillary anterior teeth
- Proportionally small maxillary lateral incisors
- Concave maxillary gingival line from canine to canine
- Cementoenamel junctions (CEJs) not palpable in the sulci
- Retroclined maxillary incisors
- Altered passive eruption of maxillary teeth
- Dentoalveolar extrusion of maxillary incisors
- Occlusal pit caries on teeth nos. 18 and 20
- Lingual pit caries on teeth nos. 7 and 10
- Existing restorations on teeth nos. 2, 3, 13, 14, 15, 18, 19, 30, and 31

Periodontal

- AAP Type I
- Healthy gingival tissues and excellent home care

Occlusal notes

- Angle Class I malocclusion with deep overbite
- No demonstrable centric relation–maximal intercuspal position discrepancy
- Angle Class I molar and canine relationships

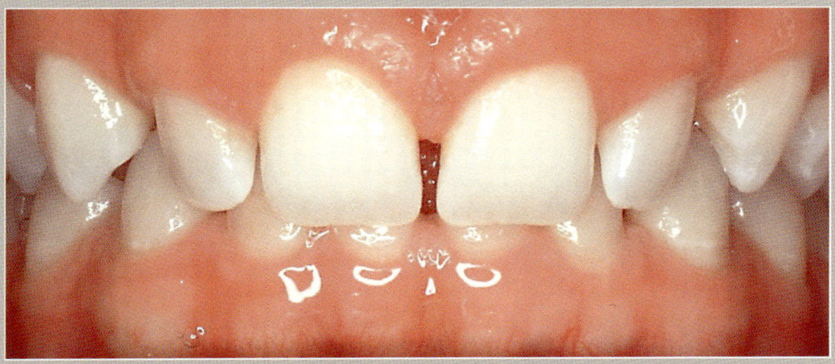

Intraoral anterior view.

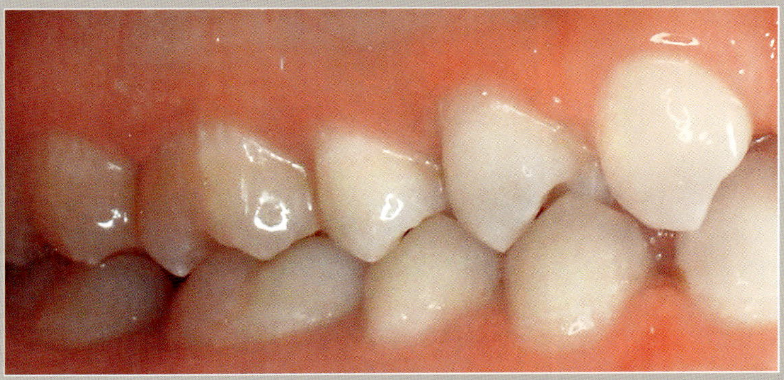

Intraoral right lateral view.

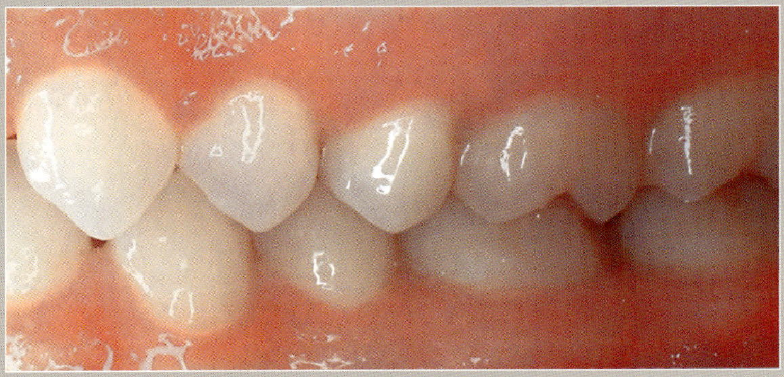

Intraoral left lateral view.

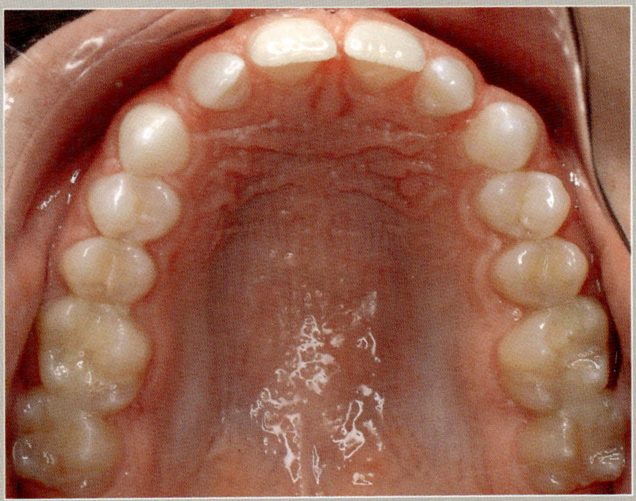

Maxillary occlusal view.

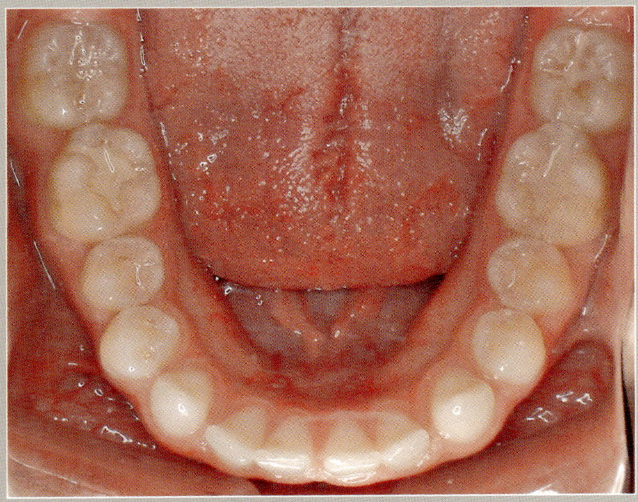

Mandibular occlusal view.

Radiographic findings

- Normal bone levels in anterior and posterior regions
- No evidence of caries

Cephalometric analysis

- Normocephalic skeletal pattern
- Normal facial proportions
- Retroclined maxillary incisors with excessive interincisal angle

Diagnosis and prognosis

- AAP Type I
- Angle Class I malocclusion
- Retroclined maxillary incisors
- Microdontia with spacing
- Dentoalveolar extrusion of the maxillary incisors
- Altered passive eruption of the maxillary teeth
- Excessive space in the buccal corridors
- Overall prognosis for the dentition: excellent

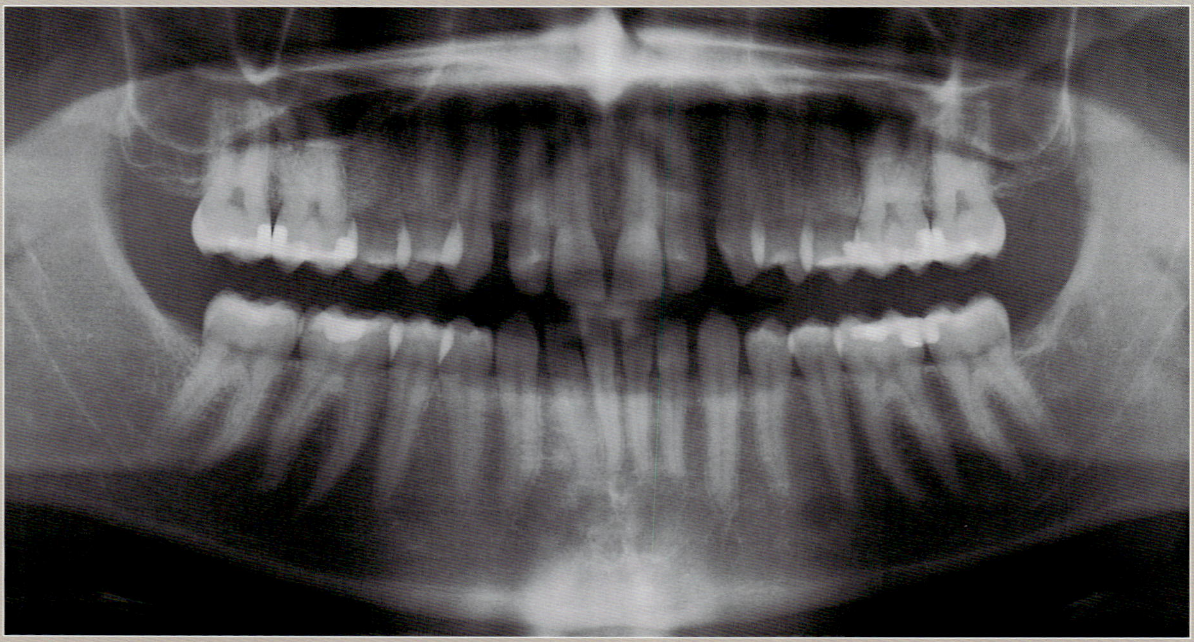

Panoramic radiograph.

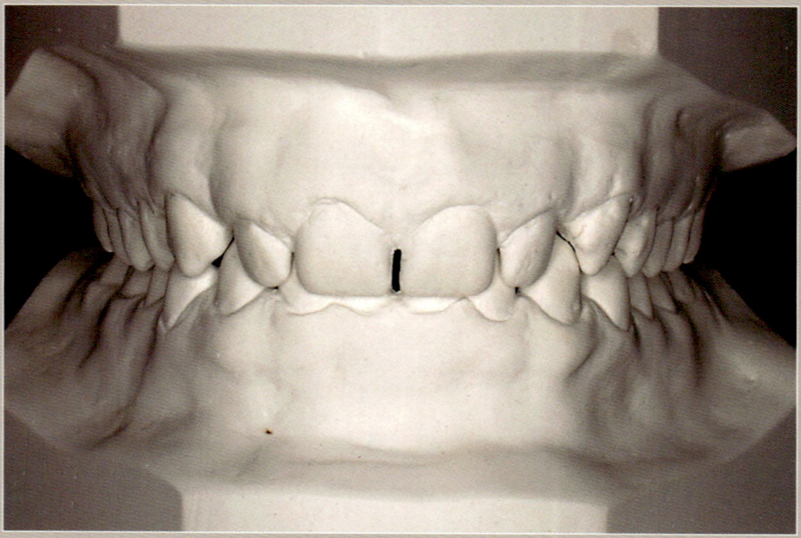

Anterior view of the study casts.

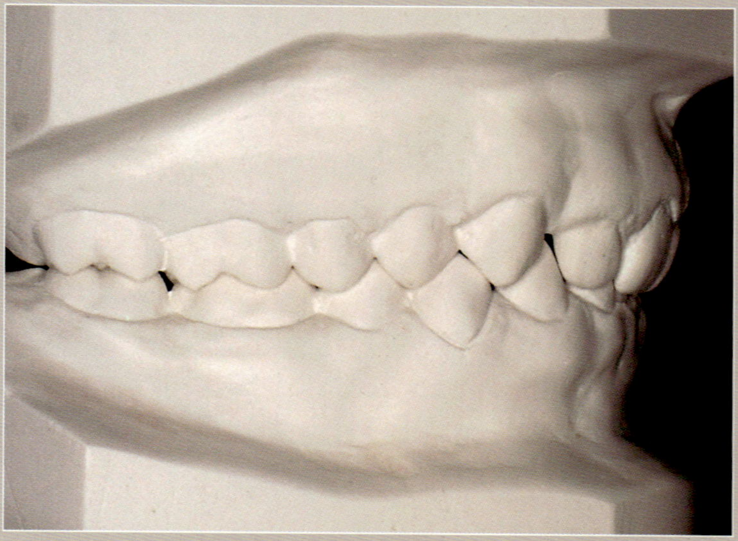

Right lateral view of the study casts.

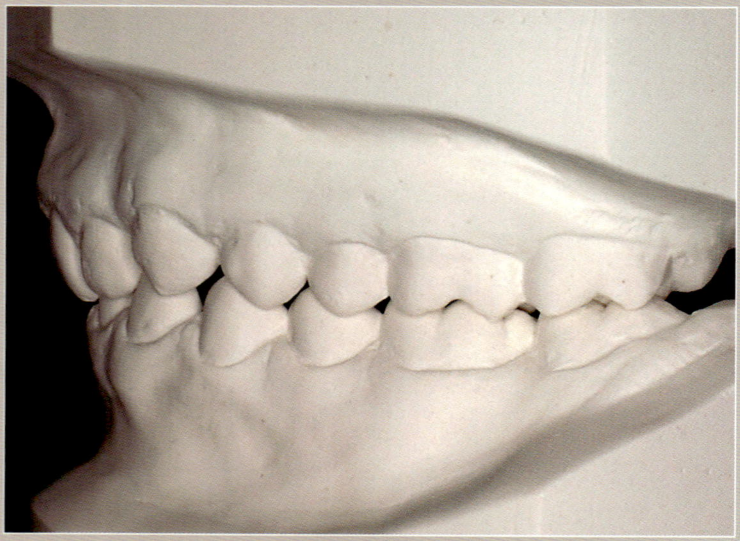

Left lateral view of the study casts.

CORE DENTISTRY "Global" Analysis Diagnosis

Face Height Mid 65 mm Lower 67 mm

Lip Length 22 mm mm Lip Mobility 6 mm mm

Dental / Facial Midline OK R/L

Central Exposed in Repose 5 mm mm

Gingival Line to Upper Lip in Full Smile Concave +1 mm +/- mm

Distal Extent of Smile (Tooth#) #3 R #13 L

Incisal Edges to Lower Lip (Follows Smile Line, Covered by Lip, Reverse, Irregular)

Follows Smile Line +3 mm at Central Incisors

Buccal Corridors — Negative Spaces Y/N Excessive on Right and Left

Length of Maxillary Anteriors — (Chart)

Tissue Levels — (Chart)

Angle of Incisal Plane — (Chart)

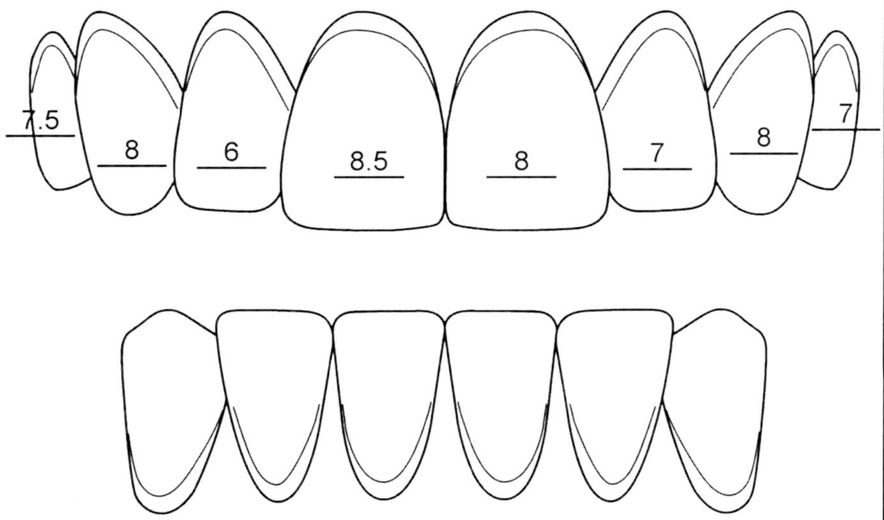

Pathologic Tooth Wear — Y/N Tooth #'s None

CEJ Located Y/N No on Maxillary Teeth

Posterior Occlusal Plane (OK, Step Up, or Step Down, Cant) OK

Tooth Color A-1

Tooth Alignment (Spacing, Overlap) Spacing in Maxillary Anterior Teeth

DR. NOTES

Deep Bite

Dentoalveolar Extrusion of Maxillary Anterior Teeth

Altered Passive Eruption of Maxillary Teeth

Microdontia of Maxillary Anterior Teeth With Spacing

Excessive Space in Buccal Corridors

CORE Global Diagnosis form.

Summary of concerns

1. The patient has significantly retroclined maxillary anterior teeth that are proportionally small, resulting in an unesthetic appearance. If we are to consider instituting orthodontic therapy, how will we be able to close the spaces, which will open (ie, increase in size) as a result of the tooth movement?
2. The patient has a constricted envelope of function related to the retroclined maxillary anterior teeth, resulting in muscle discomfort and fatigue. Will the orthodontic treatment improve the patient's function and eliminate the symptoms?
3. The patient has short teeth secondary to altered passive eruption. How and when in treatment can this best be resolved?
4. How will we be able to improve the maxillomandibular relationship, manage excess spacing, and maintain coupling in the anterior teeth?
5. What impact will space closure have on the lip support, buccal corridors, and facial profile in this patient, who has thin lips and a flat facial profile?

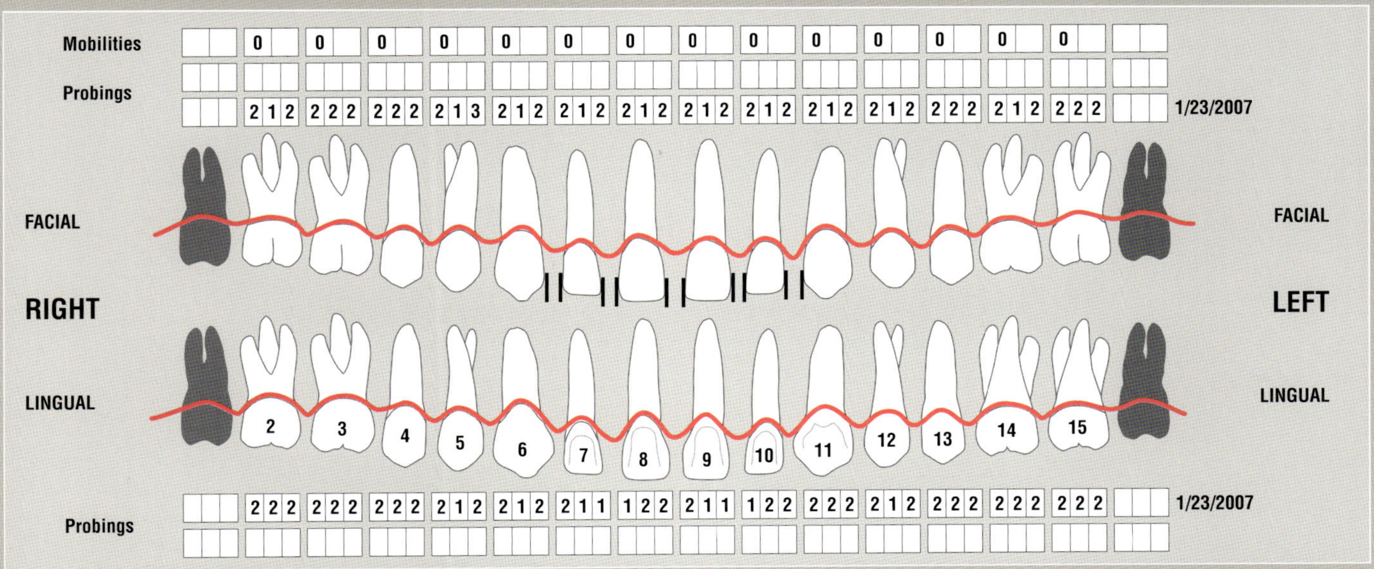

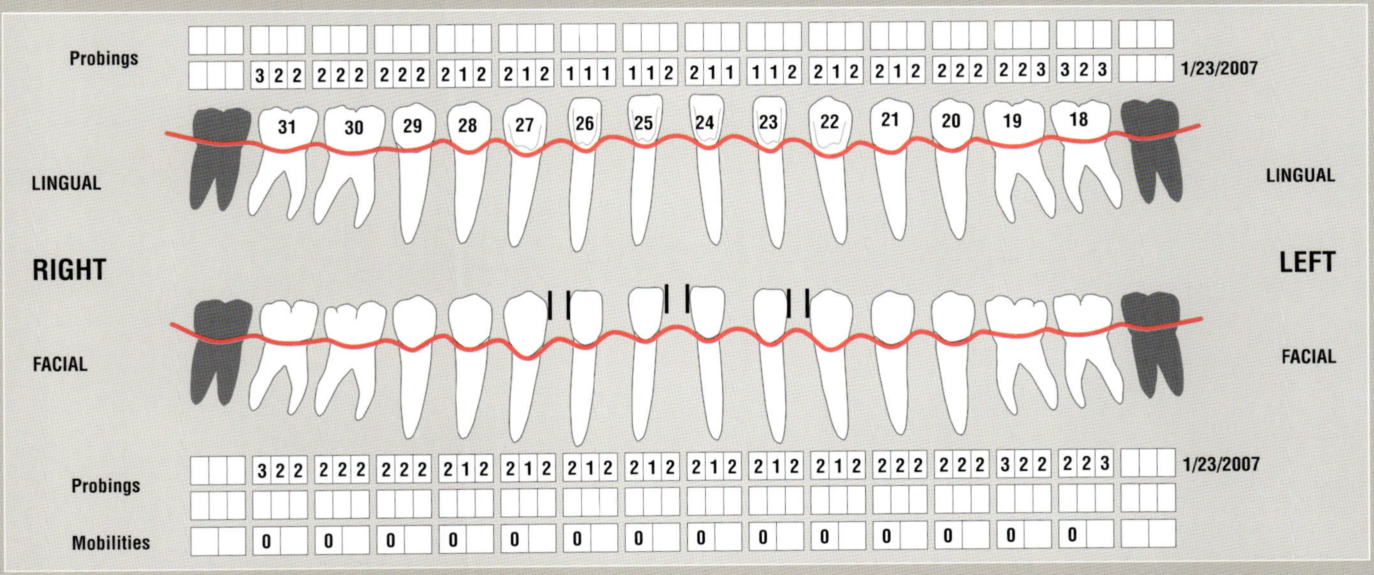

As a learning exercise, you may now outline goals/objectives of treatment and a treatment plan.

Proposed Treatment Plan

Goals/objectives of treatment

- Improve function, achieve a pleasing smile, and eliminate the existing pain and discomfort
- Restore the caries lesions
- Procline the maxillary anterior teeth
- Open the deep bite
- Broaden the dental arches
- Provide for long-term occlusal stability
- Create space for implant crown restorations mesial to teeth nos. 5, 12, 21, and 28
- Gain sufficient crown length in maxillary teeth
- Treat microdontia in the maxillary anterior segment to improve overall esthetics

Phase I: Initial case planning

1. Examinations followed by collaborative treatment planning between the restorative dentist and orthodontist
2. Diagnostic wax-up to determine possibility of placing implants
3. Consultation with the restorative dentist
4. Consultation with the orthodontist
5. Examination and consultation with the oral and maxillofacial surgeon
6. Interdisciplinary team meeting with all involved in treatment to review and finalize the treatment plan
7. Consultation and patient case presentation

Phase II: Initial restorative care

8. Dental prophylaxis and oral hygiene instruction
9. Restoration of pit caries

Phase III: Orthodontic therapy

10. Bracket placement on the maxillary and mandibular teeth
11. Consolidation of the anterior teeth and creation of space for four extra first premolars
12. Opening of the deep bite
13. Widening of the dental arches

Phase IV: Treatment of altered passive eruption

14. Esthetic crown lengthening surgery

Phase V: Surgical treatment

15. Placement of implants in sites mesial to teeth nos. 5, 12, 21, and 28

Phase VI: Definitive restorative therapy

16. Bleaching of teeth
17. Placement of porcelain veneer restorations on teeth nos. 7 to 10
18. Placement of porcelain crowns on implants
19. Delivery of maxillary occlusal appliance (nightguard)

Active Clinical Treatment

Review of the goals/objectives of treatment

Simply stated, the goals of treatment were to improve function, achieve a pleasing smile, and eliminate the patient's existing pain and discomfort.

Initially, the restorative dentist and the orthodontist met to begin the process of developing an interdisciplinary treatment plan for this patient. The oral surgeon would join the team discussions after examining the patient a short time later.

Given the patient's desire for a broader smile, the presence of multiple proximal spaces, negative spaces in the buccal corridors, and retroclined maxillary incisors, we felt that the patient would be best served by orthodontically broadening the patient's dental arches and proclining his maxillary incisors. Both of these orthodontic objectives would create more space in the dental arches. It was agreed that anterior proclination and space consolidation were necessary. This left three options for posterior space elimination following anterior space consolidation:

1. Protraction of all posterior teeth (a challenging and time-consuming procedure requiring multiple temporary anchorage devices)
2. Surgically protracting the buccal segments (an extremely invasive and technique-sensitive procedure)
3. Orthodontically opening spaces for an additional premolar in each quadrant

We chose the third option and decided to restore the first premolar spaces with dental implants rather than fixed partial dentures.

The orthodontist created a diagnostic wax-up to simulate the treatment results that could be achieved. Denture tooth pontics were placed in the setup, and anterior crown lengthening was also simulated.

Phase I: Initial therapy

Initial treatment included necessary dental prophylaxis and oral hygiene instruction.

At the same time, caries control was initiated with the restoration of the lingual pit caries on teeth nos. 7 and 10 and the occlusal pit caries on teeth nos. 18 and 20.

Phase II: Orthodontic therapy

The orthodontic treatment began with bracketing of the maxillary and mandibular teeth. Open coil springs were placed between the canines and premolars in each quadrant, and an elastic chain was placed from canine to canine in each arch. As the archwires were increased in size and rigidity and the dental arches were broadened, the open coil springs and elastic chains were reactivated. Following adequate space creation for an implant in each quadrant, a panoramic radiograph was taken to ensure root parallelism and adequate interradicular space. The denture pontic teeth were removed from the diagnostic wax-up, bracketed, and placed on the orthodontic archwire to preserve the spaces and improve esthetics. Concurrently, the other orthodontic objective was also addressed by proclining the maxillary anterior teeth.

When the anterior and posterior occlusions were appropriately coordinated from an orthodontic standpoint, the patient was seen by the restorative dentist for final approval before the appliances were removed. Following approval by the restorative dentist, impressions were made, and Hawley retainers were fabricated using the same denture pontic teeth that were used in the diagnostic wax-up and as space maintainers during the orthodontic finishing process. Note that these retainers should be fabricated quickly (same day if possible) to ensure the accuracy of their fit.

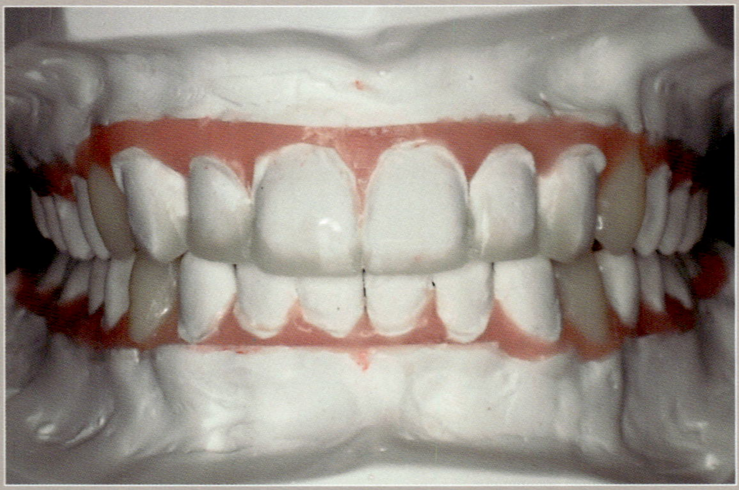

Anterior view of the diagnostic wax-up.

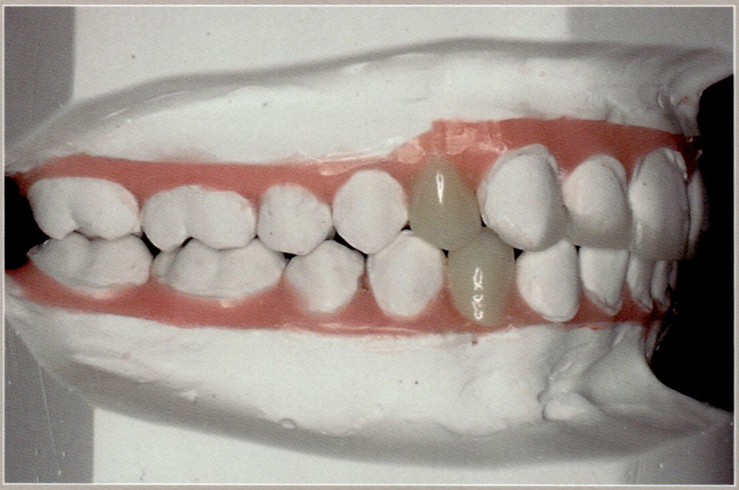

Right lateral view of the diagnostic wax-up.

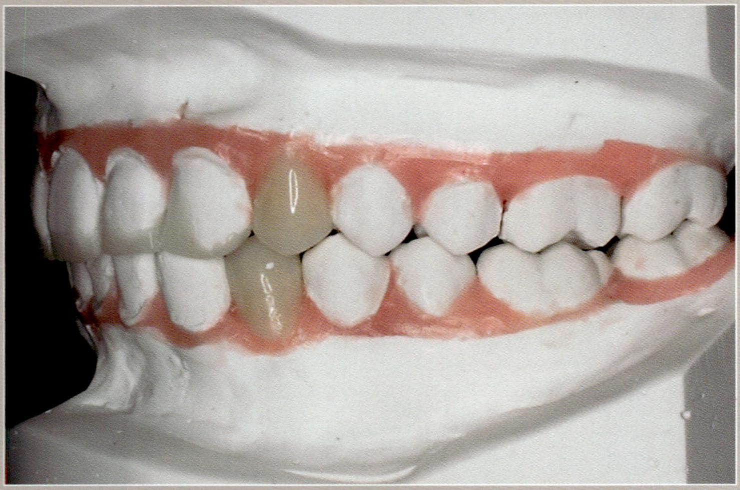

Left lateral view of the diagnostic wax-up.

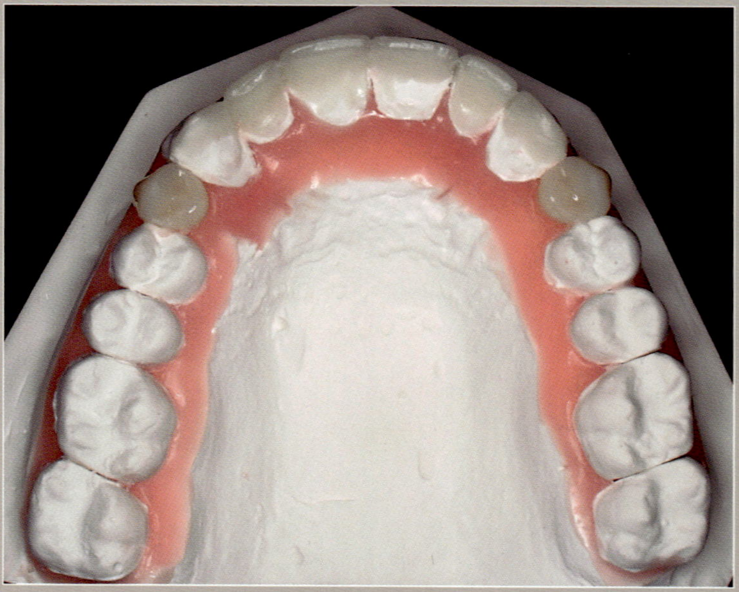

Occlusal view of the maxillary diagnostic wax-up.

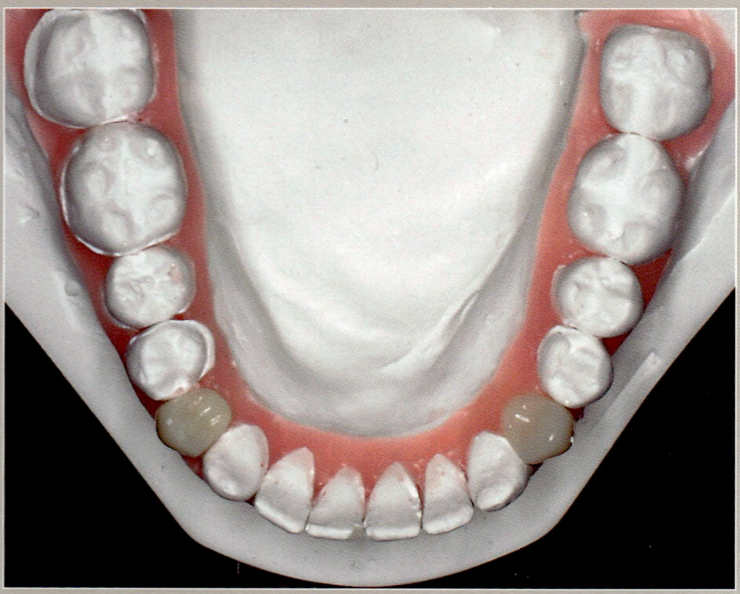

Occlusal view of the mandibular diagnostic wax-up.

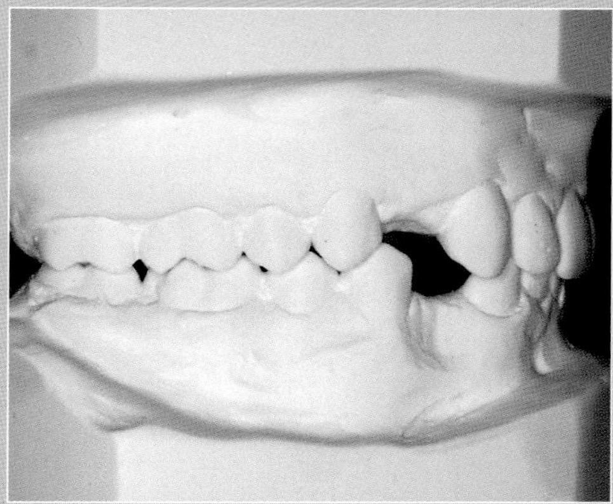

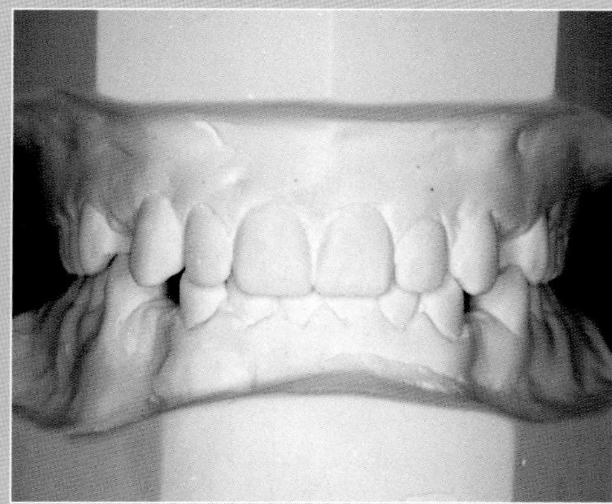

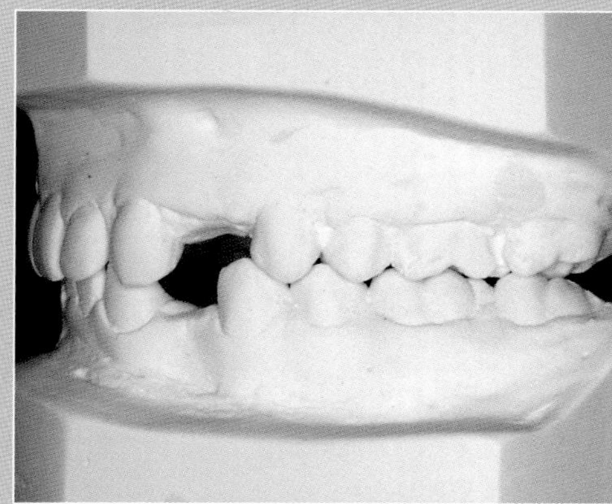

Postorthodontic treatment casts.

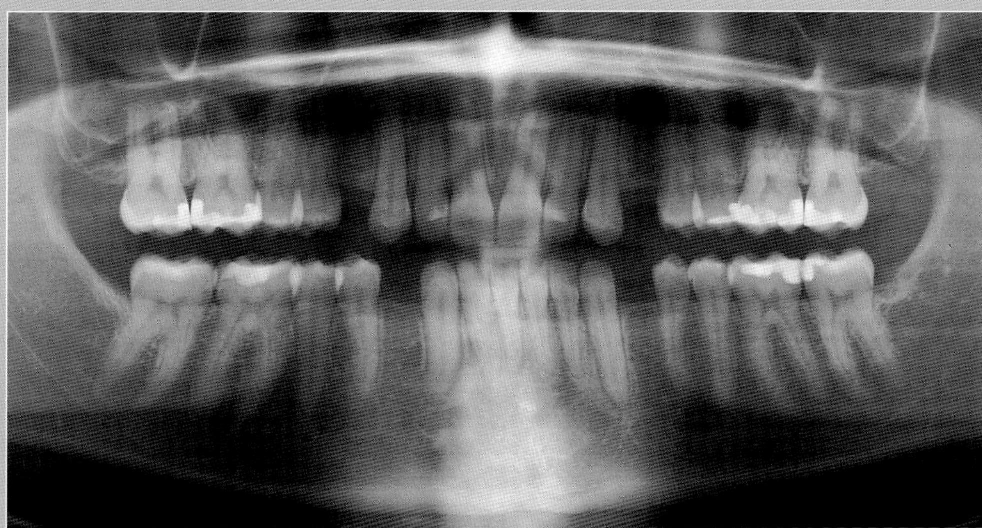

Panoramic radiograph prior to implant placement.

Phase III: Treatment of altered passive eruption

With approximately 6 months remaining in active orthodontic treatment, the restorative dentist consulted with the patient, who was very pleased with the progression of treatment and the esthetic improvement in his smile presentation. At this time, he decided against porcelain veneer restorations. Therefore, there was no reason to perform the esthetic crown lengthening surgery during active orthodontic therapy because the incisal edge positions of the maxillary anterior teeth would not be lengthened restoratively.

Upon completion of orthodontic treatment, appliances were removed and the patient received a comprehensive dental prophylaxis. Approximately 1 month after removal of orthodontic appliances, esthetic crown lengthening surgery was completed on teeth nos. 3 to 14. It was important to do the crown lengthening surgery prior to the placement of the implants in order for the surgeon to determine the correct position for implant platform placement.

Phase IV: Surgical treatment

Approximately 2 months after the esthetic crown lengthening surgery, the implants were placed in the four prepared sites. These sites were mesial to teeth nos. 5, 12, 21, and 28. The implants were allowed to integrate for 3 months. Postoperative healing was uneventful.

Posttreatment

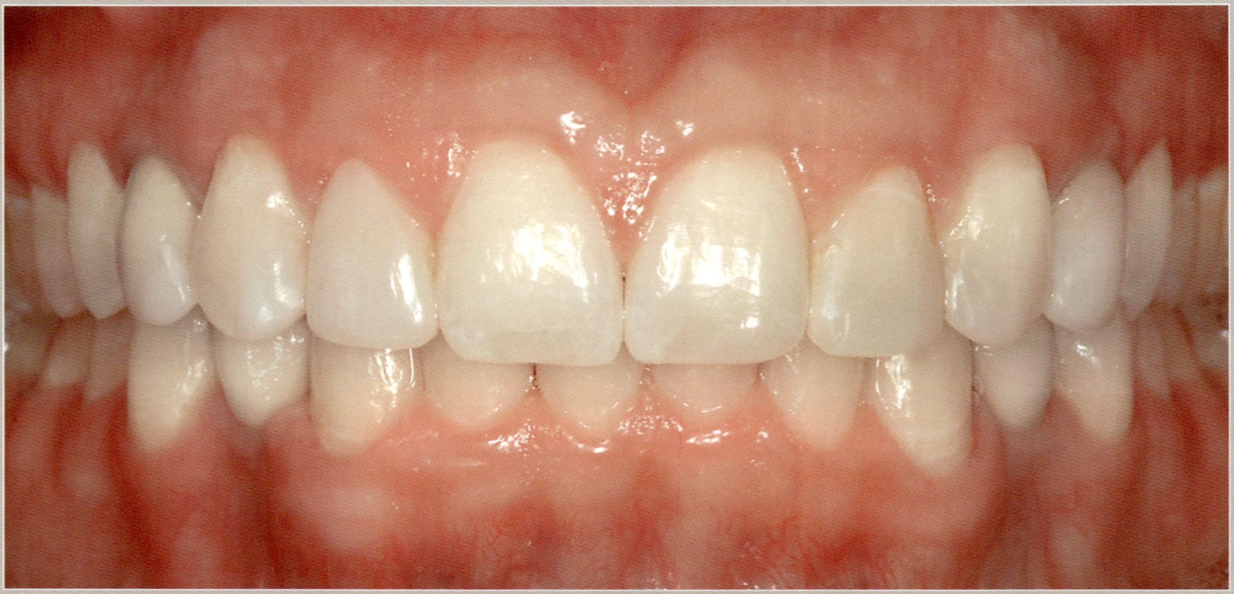

Postoperative intraoral anterior view.

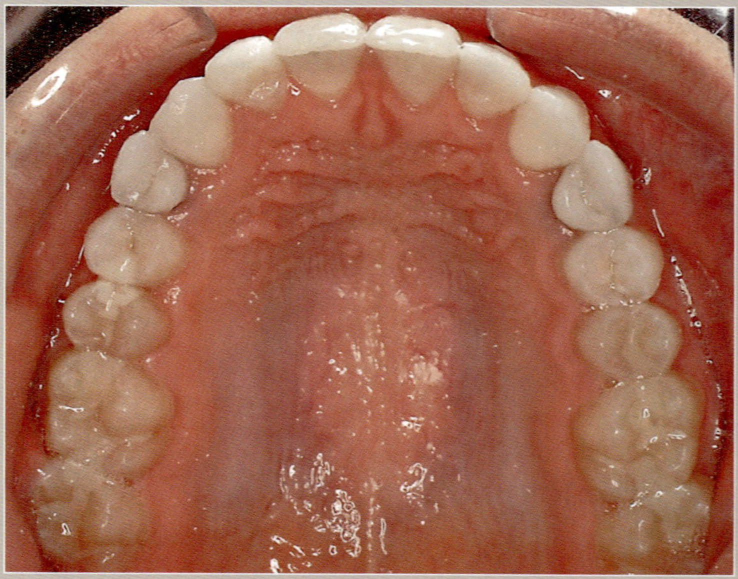

Postoperative maxillary occlusal view.

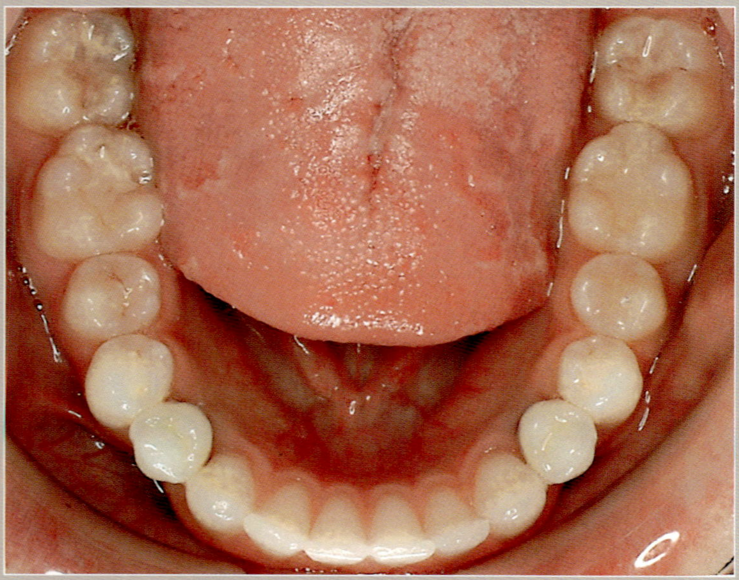

Postoperative mandibular occlusal view.

Phase V: Definitive restorative therapy

Upon completion of healing after the surgical phase, the patient was ready for definitive restorative treatment. He desired lighter-colored teeth and was given a home tray bleaching system for this purpose. Once the desired tooth color was obtained, impressions were made to restore the four implants. Following insertion of the implant crowns, direct composite bonding was used to improve the contours of the six maxillary anterior teeth. The composite bonding was placed on the mesial surface of tooth no. 6, mesial and distal surfaces of tooth no. 7, distal and incisal surfaces of teeth nos. 8 and 9, mesial and distal surfaces of tooth no. 10, and the mesial surface of tooth no. 11. Finally, a maxillary nightguard appliance was fabricated and inserted. This also served as a maxillary orthodontic retainer.

The patient's treatment goals were all met at the completion of treatment. He was very pleased with his appearance. Additionally, his bite was very comfortable. He no longer experienced fatigue after prolonged chewing and had no muscle discomfort.

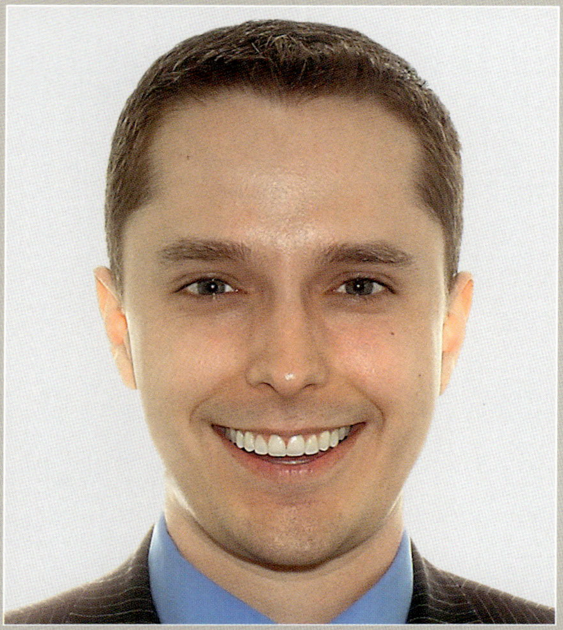

Facial view of smile.

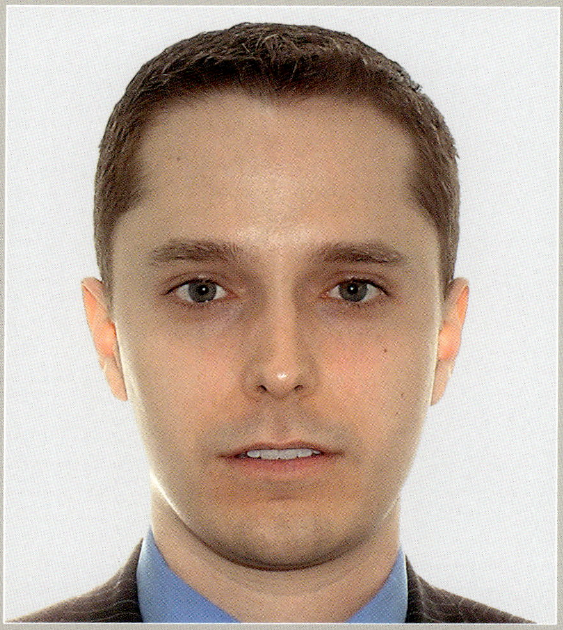

Facial view of lips in repose.

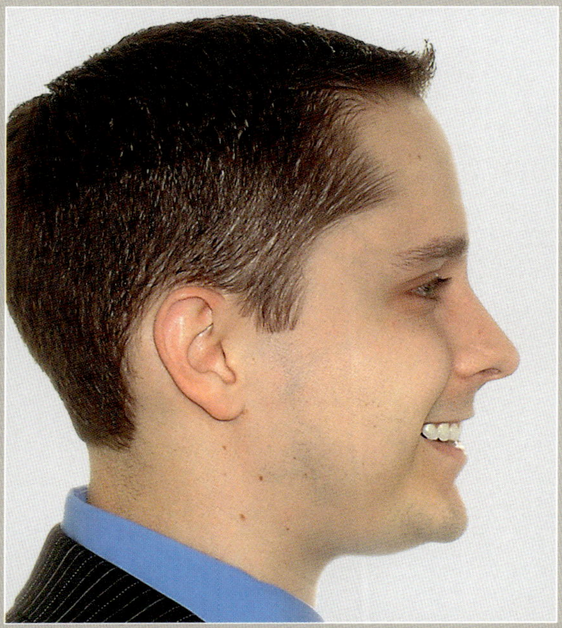

Profile view of smile.

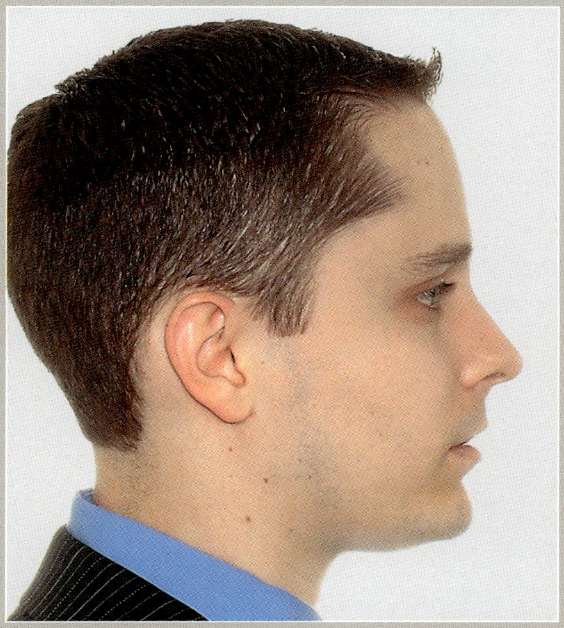

Profile view of lips in repose.

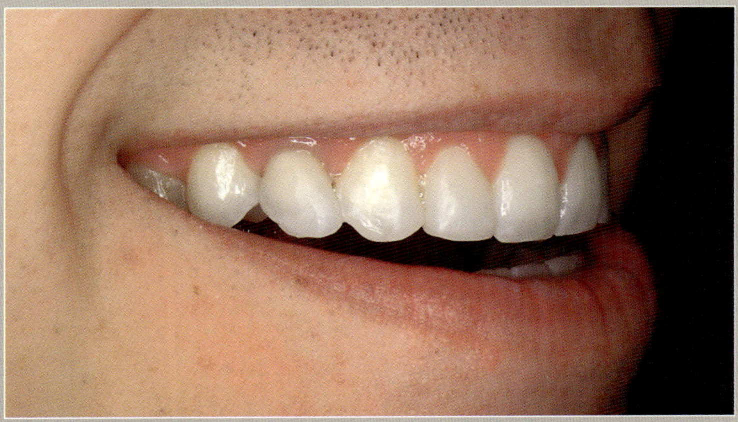

Right oblique close-up view of smile.

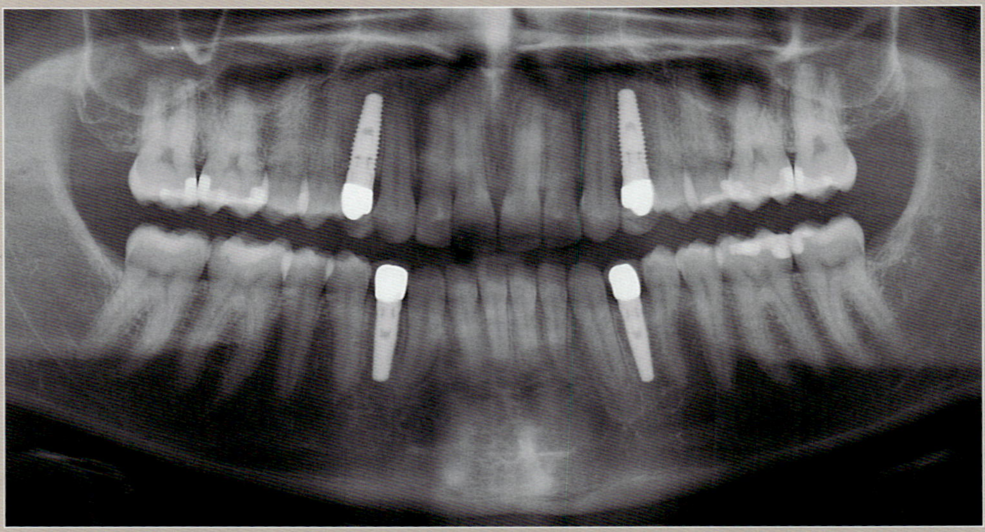

Panoramic radiograph after implant placement and restoration.

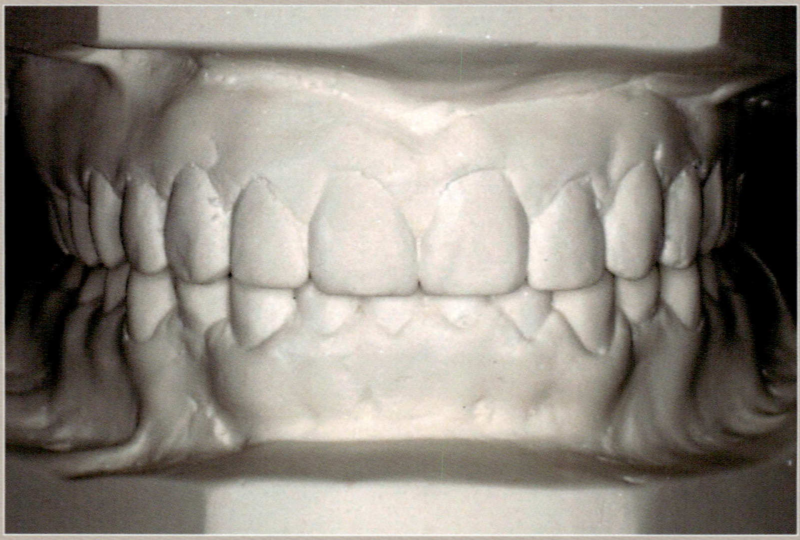

Anterior view of the definitive casts.

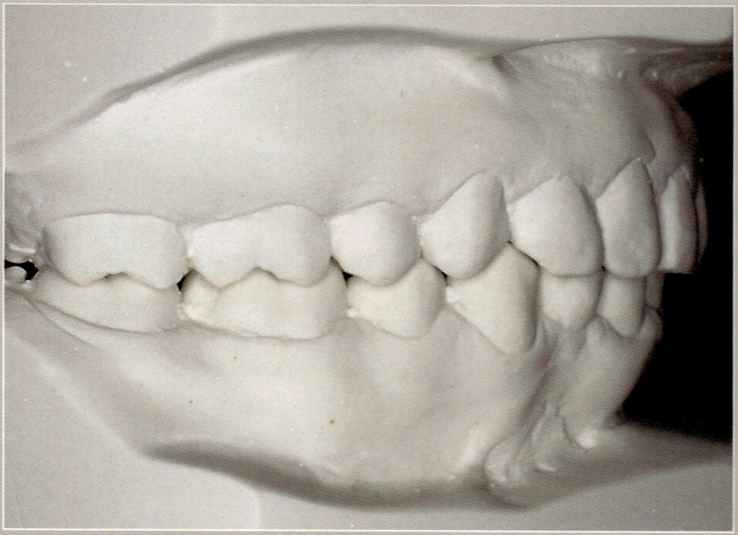

Right lateral view of the definitive casts.

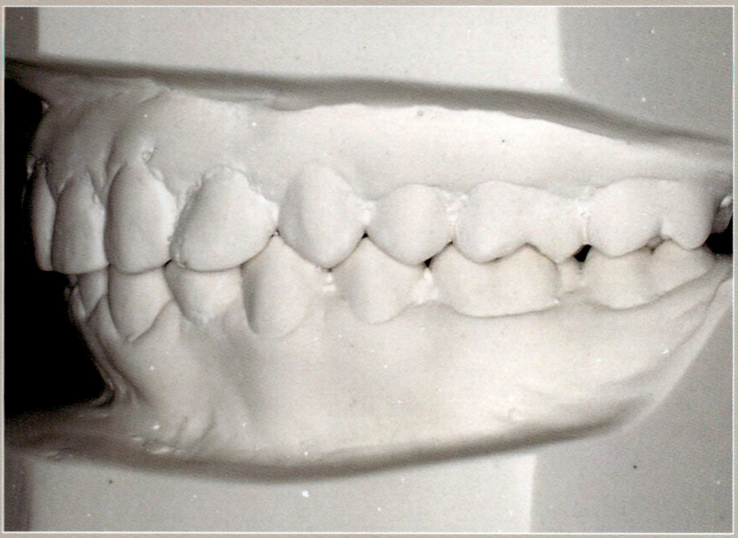

Left lateral view of the definitive casts.

You may now place the corresponding posttreatment overlay found in the separate folder over the pretreatment periodontal chart on page 493.

Commentary

Dental diagnosis and treatment planning continue to become more complex with the increased emphasis on multi-specialty treatment. Traditional data collection involves gathering a vast amount of information and then synthesizing it into a meaningful comprehensive treatment plan. This can present real challenges in terms of data organization.

Once all of the patient records are collected and evaluated, conventional protocol is to make a series of "regional" diagnoses (eg, periodontal, pulpal, skeletal, occlusal, and caries status). Although these are important in designing and sequencing a treatment plan, one important guiding element is often missing: the placement of the teeth in the correct position in the face. Without considering this factor, it is very difficult to know where to begin treatment.

In treating this case, we arrived at what we have termed a "global" diagnosis, which helped determine the overall position of the teeth in the face. This provided excellent guidance in visualizing the proposed definitive restorative outcome and aided in incorporating all of the regional issues into a comprehensive interdisciplinary team treatment approach.

We call our approach to diagnosis and treatment planning the CORE Global Diagnosis System.

CORE Global Diagnosis System parameters

When using the CORE Global Diagnosis System, the dentist must first collect a set of data that is not commonly gathered in a traditional dental examination and then interpret the information based on normative data.

Face height

In the proportional face, the length of the middle third of the face and the length of the lower third of the face should be equal. The middle third is measured from the mid-brow point (glabella) to under the base of the nose (subnasale). The lower third of the face is measured from subnasale to under the chin (menton). These measurements are made with the patient in a repose position. The repose position is with the lips and teeth slightly apart in a relaxed posture. Additionally, the proportions in the lower third of the face must be evaluated. With the patient in the repose position, a horizontal line is drawn through the center of the labial commissure. Above the line is the maxilla and below the line is the mandible. The normal proportion is one-third maxilla and two-thirds mandible.

Lip parameters

The average length of the upper lip is 20 to 22 mm in the young (ie, age 25 to 30 years) woman and 22 to 24 mm in the young man. Age is important because, as the patient ages, the upper lip tends to increase in length. A second parameter that must be evaluated is lip mobility. The mobility of the upper lip is measured from the repose position to the most superior position in full smile. The average translation of the upper lip from repose to full smile is 6 to 8 mm.

Gingival line in relation to the horizon

In the anterior maxilla, a line may be drawn from canine to canine at the most apical point of the gingival margin. This line is termed the *gingival line*. When viewed from the front, the gingival margins of both central incisors should fall on this line. The lateral incisors may either be on the line or up to 1.5 mm below the line. Additionally, this line should be parallel to the horizon. Similarly, the bilateral posterior gingival lines should reveal a smooth transition from canine to first molar. The mandibular gingival line may also be evaluated in relation to horizon.

Tooth length and width

The average length of the maxillary central incisor is 10 to 11 mm. The average height-width ratio in the maxillary central incisor is 1.2:1, ie, the width of the central incisor is approximately 75% to 80% of its height. This same ratio (1.2:1) holds in the comparison of the measured width of the maxillary central incisor to that of the maxillary lateral incisor, with the width of the lateral incisor being 75% to 80% of the width of the central incisor.

Palpability of the CEJ in the gingival sulcus

A dental explorer is used to palpate the CEJ. It is placed on the enamel surface just coronal to the gingival crest. It is kept in contact with the tooth surface and gently moved into the sulcus. In a normal periodontal-restorative interface, as the explorer moves into the sulcus, first the roughness of CEJ and perhaps a small amount of rougher root surface is felt before the tissue blanches as the explorer reaches the base of the sulcus.

The five CORE questions

Upon completion of the data collection, the clinician must answer five questions, which will lead to a global diagnosis or diagnoses.

1. What are the facial proportions?

If the lower third of the face is long in comparison to the middle third of the face, this defines a global diagnosis of vertical maxillary excess. This patient commonly presents with excess gingival display in both the anterior and posterior maxilla. If the lower third of the face is shorter than the middle third, this is commonly due to an underdeveloped maxilla. Both of these conditions may be treated with orthognathic surgery.

2. What is the length and mobility of the upper lip?

If the upper lip is shorter than normal or hyperactive, this may result in excess gingival display during full smile. There is much anecdotal information regarding an upper lip plication procedure that removes vestibular mucosa and sutures the mucosal surface of the lip to the attached gingiva. However, there is no long-term prospective data that defines the morbidity of this procedure. Therefore, the primary treatment for the short or hyperactive upper lip is onabotulinumtoxinA (Botox, Allergan). It is injected into the facial muscles responsible for upper lip mobility and temporarily paralyzes these muscles. This is a very effective short-term (3- to 6-month) solution for the reduction of lip mobility.

3. What is the relationship between the gingival line and the horizon?

When teeth overerupt, they bring bone and gingiva with them, resulting in a concave rather than a straight gingival line. This is termed *dentoavleolar extrusion* and may occur with or without incisal attrition. It is most common in the anterior region but may occur anywhere in the mouth and on any number of teeth. There are several treatment options for the patient with dentoavleolar extrusion, but the two primary treatment options are *(1)* orthodontic intrusion followed by restoration when required and *(2)* functional crown lengthening surgery followed by restoration.

4. What are the lengths of the maxillary central incisors?

When a maxillary central incisor is short compared with normative measurements, there are three possible etiologies:

1. Microdontia
2. Loss of incisal length due to attrition
3. Altered passive eruption

If the etiology is microdontia, the maxillary anterior teeth will not be proportionally correct. If the etiology is due to incisal attrition, the normal incisal edge anatomy will be altered. Otherwise, the etiology is altered passive eruption, subject to confirmation by the answer to the following question.

5. Is the CEJ palpable in the gingival sulcus?

If the tooth is short by measurement and the CEJ is not palpable in the sulcus, the etiology of the short tooth is altered passive eruption. The gingival tissue has not migrated to its correct position to within approximately 1 mm of the CEJ, resulting in excessive coverage of enamel. Altered passive eruption is treated with esthetic crown lengthening surgery.

Applying the CORE Global Diagnosis System

The CORE Global Diagnosis System is a diagnostic approach that leads the dentist through a systematic process of developing a problem list that then leads to a therapeutic answer for each diagnosed problem. Once the global diagnosis is made, an interdisciplinary treatment strategy can be developed for placing the teeth and gingival complex in the correct positions. This information can then be combined with the regional diagnoses (eg, periodontal, pulpal, and occlusal status), and the definitive comprehensive treatment plan can be finalized and implemented.

In the patient presented in this chapter, the CORE Global Diagnosis System was used in creating the definitive treatment plan. The five CORE questions revealed that the patient's lower third of the face was slightly longer than the middle third. However, his facial presentation was not consistent with vertical maxillary excess, so that condition was ruled out.

The lip length and lip mobility were within normative values. The gingival line from maxillary canine to canine was concave, which is consistent with dentoalveolar extrusion. The maxillary teeth were short by measurement. Incisal edge wear was ruled out. The height-width ratios of the maxillary lateral incisors were outside the normative numbers and consistent with microdontia. However, the CEJs could not be detected with an explorer in the sulci of the maxillary teeth, which confirmed the diagnosis of altered passive eruption.

The five CORE questions revealed the following global diagnoses:

- Dentoalveolar extrusion without wear, which required orthodontic intrusion and flaring
- Microdontia, which required restorative therapy
- Altered passive eruption, which required esthetic crown lengthening surgery

These global diagnoses dictated the treatment approach in this case.

The CORE Global Diagnosis System presents an organized and methodical way to gather and evaluate diagnostic data. The results then can be easily and logically incorporated into a comprehensive case plan that will best meet the patient's and clinician's treatment expectations.

Acknowledgments

The authors wish to thank their families for their unending support and understanding. We also want to thank Dr B. D. Tiner for his expertise in the surgical placement of the implants. Finally, we want to thank Dene LeBeau, CDT, and his wonderful team of dental laboratory technicians for the creation of the porcelain crown restorations.

Seattle Study Club Chapters Worldwide

If you are interested in becoming more involved in interdisciplinary treatment planning, please contact a Seattle Study Club in your area.

AUSTRALIA

Adelaide Seattle Study Club
Rick Sawers
Adelaide, SA
+61 8 8232 1366

The Cutting Edge
David Bachmayer
Baulkham Hills, NSW
+61 2 8850 6733

DMF Study Club of Western Australia
Chris Wholley
Perth, WA
+61 8 9300 9975

Melbourne Seattle Study Club
Ray Stabey
Melbourne, VIC
+61 3 9848 7490

CANADA

Comprehensive Dentistry Study Club of Hamilton
Daniel Zeiter
Tamara Jackson
Hamilton, ON
(905) 318-4330

Hands On Training Institute
Ken Hebel
Reena Gajjar
London, ON
(519) 439-4111

Island Pursuit of Dental Excellence
Stephen Crowley
Robert Sorochan
Claudio Sansalone
Nanaimo, BC
(250) 753-6671

Limestone City Study Club
Paul D'Aoust
Kingston, ON
(613) 634-6221

North Fraser Seminars for Dental Excellence
Tobin Bellamy
Mike Henry
Coquitlam, BC
(604) 941-2312

Northwest Dental Study Club
Paul Jang
Langley, BC
(604) 546-1133

PA Study Club
Len Diamond
Michael Gangbar
Leo Gerzcuk
Mississauga, ON
(905) 279-3364

Vancouver Implant Study Club
Tassos Irinakis
Vancouver, BC
(604) 876-9777

VIP Study Club
Sonia Leziy
Brahm Miller
North Vancouver, BC
(604) 983-9836

Winnipeg Progressive Dental Study Club
Paresh Shah
Tim Dumore
Winnipeg, MB
(204) 837-4517

GERMANY

SSC, Study Club Hamburg
Oender Solakoglu
22359 Hamburg
+49 4 047 2638

SSC Tegernsee
Siggi Marquardt
83684 Tegernsee
+49 8 022 1505

GREAT BRITAIN

British Dental Forum
Nat Tiebrewal
Leeds, UK
+44 11 3248 0589

SPAIN

Campus Stellae Study Club
Julio Tojo
Santiago de Compostela
+34 981 57 0607

TAIWAN ROC

Taiwan Seattle Study Club
Paul Lin
Taipei 100
+886 2 2393 6772

USA

ALABAMA
Wiregrass Study Club
Dan Pittman
Dothan, AL
(334) 793-7232

ARIZONA
Comprehensive Care Continuum
Greg Kammeyer
Sun City West, AZ
(623) 556-5442

Saguaro Study Club
Dale Lentz
Tempe, AZ
(480) 838-5675

Smile Synergy Study Club
Mark Waring
Mesa, AZ
(480) 775-2656

ARKANSAS
Hot Springs Study Club
Daron Praetzel
Hot Springs, AR
(501) 623-4485

NWA Study Club
Boyd Whitlock
Springdale, AR
(479) 751-1103

CALIFORNIA
Advanced Dental Seminar
Tim Shahbazian
Dale Minkin
Fremont, CA
(510) 797-9100

Bay Area Study Club
Anthony Rega
San Ramon, CA
(925) 830-0800

Central Valley Dental Forum
Tony Jonker
Ron Northrop
Reed Van Wagenen
Fresno, CA
(559) 432-4911

Delta Study Club
Sloan McDonald
Bob Deloso
Antioch, CA
(925) 778-2100

Diablo Study Club
Nestor Karas
Walnut Creek, CA
(925) 933-6190

East Bay Study Club
Keith Gronbach
Lafayette, CA
(925) 283-4050

Modesto Study Club
Stan Baker
Modesto, CA
(209) 527-5050

Monterey Bay–Salinas Study Club
Jochen Pechak
Monterey, CA
(831) 648-8800

Mt Baldy Study Club
David Gilbert
Upland, CA
(909) 982-8888

Mt Palomar Study Club
Allen Pulsipher
Murrieta, CA
(951) 600-7457

North Coast Dental Institute
James Hargas
Jaime Quejada
Oceanside, CA
(760) 433-0393

Northern California Dental Forum
Mark Zablotsky
Sacramento, CA
(916) 641-1200

PRIME Study Club
Stephen Smith
Monterey, CA
(408) 779-8686

Palo Alto Study Club
Mark Beckstead
Los Altos, CA
(650) 941-7300

Peninsula Study Club
Bryan Pope
Stephen Pickering
Brenda Lewis
San Mateo, CA
(650) 348-4030

Redding Advanced Dental Studies Forum
Russ Holpuch
Redding, CA
(530) 241-3302

San Diego Advanced Study Group
Fred Hammond
Tim Smith
Larry Addleson
San Diego, CA
(619) 298-2200

San Francisco Study Club
Steve Lim
San Francisco, CA
(415) 776-4040

San Joaquin Study Club
Randy Gordon
Lodi, CA
(209) 367-1484

San Jose Study Club
Louis Poulos
San Jose, CA
(408) 356-9736

Santa Barbara Dental Study Group
Ray Kubisch
Dennis Shanelec
Santa Barbara, CA
(805) 687-7417

Santa Monica Interdisciplinary Dental Study Group
Howard Park
Santa Monica, CA
(310) 315-1034

Silicon Valley Study Club
Rik Vanooteghem
Sunnyvale, CA
(408) 738-3424

Sonora Study Club
Slim Bouchoucha
Sonora, CA
(209) 532-5578

South Bay Study Club
Mark Oseas
Torrance, CA
(310) 373-7773

Wine Country Study Club
Paul Steigerwald
Santa Rosa, CA
(707) 525-1228

COLORADO
5280 Study Club
Mike Burnham
Thornton, CO
(303) 451-6767

Colorado Academy of Excellence in Dentistry
Erik Mathys
Greenwood Village, CO
(303) 741-3300

Mile High Dental Study Club
Cherie Brown
Tony Kardelis
Lakewood, CO
(303) 986-2212

Rimrock Seminars
Greg Hunter
Grand Junction, CO
(970) 424-5014

Seattle Study Club of Southern Colorado
Jeff Dombrowski
Colorado Springs, CO
(719) 264-6070

Study Club of the Rockies
Todd Singiser
Loveland, CO
(303) 772-8551

CONNECTICUT
Connecticut Study Club for Excellence in Dentistry
Joel Rosenlicht
Manchester, CT
(860) 649-2272

Greenwich Study Club
Eman Traynor
Greenwich, CT
(203) 661-5885

River Valley Study Club
Jim McAraw
Lee Cantner
Matt Cantner
Old Saybrook, CT
(860) 388-4439

Smooth Sailing Study Club
Marianne Urbanski
Meriden, CT
(203) 630-1312

FLORIDA
Central Florida Occlusal Study Club
Michael Langan
Orlando, FL
(407) 843-2261

DEAL Study Club
Stephen Rimer
Boca Raton, FL
(561) 368-3170

Greater Pensacola Study Club
David Williams
Pensacola, FL
(850) 433-1543

Intracoastal Dental Study Club
Barry Kligerman
Ft Lauderdale, FL
(954) 776-9090

Manatee Study Club
Lindsay Eastman
Bradenton, FL
(941) 792-3899

Miami Comprehensive Team Approach
Pepe Mellado
Ed del Amo
Hialeah, FL
(305) 558-2200

Perio-Prosthetic Study Club of St Petersburg
Greg Langston
St Petersburg, FL
(727) 579-8487

Pinnacle Study Club of Tampa Bay
Michael Pikos
Palm Harbor, FL
(727) 786-1631

Rolling Hills Study Club
Dennis Davis
Lady Lake, FL
(352) 259-6799

Sailfish Study Club
Ed Lippisch
Shawn Engebretsen
Jeff Brown
Stuart, FL
(772) 223-0600

Seaside Study Club
Wael Garine
Jupiter, FL
(561) 747-4272

Seattle Study Club, Tampa
Rick Rasmussen
Patrick Abbey
Barry Levine
Tampa, FL
(813) 977-2928

Shark Tooth Study Club
Cara Overbeck
Venice, FL
(941) 488-8788

South Florida Dentists in Pursuit of Excellence
Jorge Ramirez
South Miami, FL
(305) 665-6575

Speed Coast Study Club
Joh Akers
Richard Gaines
Curt Schalit
Daytona Beach, FL
(386) 252-6438

Triple-Win Study Club
Andy Alpert
N Miami Beach, FL
(305) 935-0122

GEORGIA
Accelerated Dental Studies
Phil Parham
Dalton, GA
(706) 278-5344

Atlanta Seattle Study Club
Tom Osborne
Tucker, GA
(770) 723-9965

Cherokee Study Club
John Carey
Canton, GA
(770) 345-8118

Institute for Excellence in Dentistry
Lyle Zuck
Lawrenceville, GA
(770) 995-7960

Rivertown Study Club
Rob Vazquez
Columbus, GA
(706) 596-8850

Seattle Study Club of Atlanta
Colin Richman
Roswell, GA
(770) 442-1011

Southern Crescent Study Club
Bruce Anderson
Vince Perciaccante
Jeff Schultz
David Timmis
Peachtree City, GA
(770) 692-0453

HAWAII
Hawaii Dental Forum
Clyde Umaki
Honolulu, HI
(808) 955-2275

Hawaii Interactive Peer Practicum
David Hiranaka
Kailua-Kona, HI
(808) 236-2040

Maui Postgraduate Dental Forum
Peter Fay
Mike Clarke
Kahului, HI
(808) 242-0077

IDAHO
High Desert Sage Study Club
Michael Florence
Jack Lincks
Boise, ID
(208) 385-9228

Intermountain Odontology Study Club
Brad Morlock
Lewiston, ID
(208) 743-1114

ILLINOIS
Contemporary Dental Forum
Ian Elliott
Naperville, IL
(630) 862-3600

Elite Dental Group
Scott Frank
Buffalo Grove, IL
(847) 520-1300

Illinois River Valley Study Club
Chris Couri
Peoria, IL
(309) 674-4148

Northwest Suburban Chicago Study Club
Mike Jones
Crystal Lake, IL
(815) 356-3977

PDL Seminars
Rich Marinello
Skokie, IL
(312) 641-2572

Windy City Seminars
Rick Munaretto
Richard Munaretto
Raymond Munaretto
Keith Sommers
Elmwood Park, IL
(708) 456-7787

INDIANA
Dental Study Club of Northwest Indiana
Gene Ranieri
Highland, IN
(219) 838-6500

The Fort Study Club
Mike Stronczek
Fort Wayne, IN
(260) 423-2340

The Greater Lafayette Study Club
David Alexander
Lafayette, IN
(765) 447-9319

Hoosiers for Dental Excellence
Mark Sutor
Bloomington, IN
(812) 333-4550

Select Study Club
Jim Woodyard
Newburgh, IN
(812) 473-4833

Sonar Downtown Study Club
Stephen Towns
Indianapolis, IN
(317) 269-0402

IOWA
North Iowa Dental Seminars
Lyell Hogg
Todd Juhlin
Mason City, IA
(641) 424-1656

KANSAS
CREATE Dentistry Study Club
Jason Wagle
Mark Moxley
Wichita, KS
(316) 208-6481

Great Plains Study Club
Rich Oakley
Mission, KS
(913) 722-3253

KENTUCKY
Premier Dental Study Club of Lexington
Greg Vance
Lexington, KY
(859) 264-1854

LOUISIANA
Crescent City Study Club
Paul Walters
Marc Smith
Gretna, LA
(504) 378-3005

Lake Pontchartrain Study Club
Tom Mabry
Slidell, LA
(985) 646-1421

River Cities Study Group
Steve Guier
Shreveport, LA
(318) 798-1201

MAINE
Casco Bay Study Club
Peter Then
South Portland, ME
(207) 774-5527

MARYLAND
Comprehensive Care Study Sessions
Tony Rose
Chevy Chase, MD
(301) 652-3355

Greater Chesapeake Study Club
Leo Trail
Bel Air, MD
(410) 569-8567

Maryland Dental Forum
Tom Daley
Jim Kassolis
Kathy Mutzig
Towson, MD
(443) 219-0805

Triple Crown Study Club
David Mugford
Crofton, MD
(410) 721-7801

MASSACHUSETTS
Boston Dental Alliance
Sharona Dayan
Weston, MA
(781) 894-3223

Shamrock Study Club
Bill Lane
Plymouth, MA
(508) 746-8700

SSC of Central New England
Gene Mariani
Worcester, MA
(508) 754-1122

MICHIGAN
Grand Traverse Study Club
Jeff Link
Traverse City, MI
(231) 933-1220

Port Huron Study Club
Dale Sweeney
Port Huron, MI
(810) 985-6600

MINNESOTA
City of Lakes Study Club
Mark Wilson
Minneapolis, MN
(612) 332-0869

Great Lakes Study Club
Duncan Puffer
Marty Espe
Duluth, MN
(218) 722-8377

Great River Study Club
Don Primley
St Cloud, MN
(320) 252-3611

Northern Lights Dental Forum
Larry Palmersheim
Mark Roszkowski
Burnsville, MN
(952) 435-0310

Southside Comprehensive Study Club
Jim Jensen
Russ Dylla
Edina, MN
(952) 922-6949

True North Professional Studies
Marty Wade
Woodbury, MN
(651) 578-7000

West Suburban Study Club
Neil Covin
Teri Bretz
St Louis Park, MN
(952) 920-9209

MISSISSIPPI
Golden Triangle Study Club
John Griffin
Columbus, MS
(662) 327-2100

MidSouth Dental Study Club
Michael Perry
Oxford, MS
(662) 513-4619

MISSOURI
Gateway Study Club
George Duello
St Louis, MO
(314) 965-3271

MONTANA
Blue Ribbon Seminars
Brian Chisdak
Bozeman, MT
(406) 587-0767

NORTH CAROLINA
Carolina Mountain Dental Education
Ty Hornsby
Hendersonville, NC
(828) 693-4163

Central Carolina Dental Continuum
Gary Jones
Fayetteville, NC
(910) 483-9216

Foothills Dental Continuum
David Darab
Paul Richardson
Hickory, NC
(828) 322-1667

Greater Charlotte Study Club
Ray Haigney
Huntersville, NC
(704) 987-3132

Greater Forsyth Study Club
Todd Smith
Winston-Salem, NC
(336) 765-9550

High Point Dental Study Club
Karen Lanier
High Point, NC
(336) 889-5466

Nu-Image Advanced Dental Seminars
Kevin Neshat
Raleigh, NC
(919) 841-1720

Outer Loop Education of Charlotte
Priveer Sharma
Charlotte, NC
(704) 541-6070

Port City Study Club
Phyllis Cook
Wilmington, NC
(910) 256-8486

Sandhills Symposium
Steven Van Scoyoc
Southern Pines, NC
(910) 692-6270

Southern Wake Dental Institute
Paul Kazmer
Cary, NC
(919) 468-6410

The W Group FIX
Jeff Thomas
New Bern, NC
(252) 633-1631

NORTH DAKOTA

Heartland Study Club
Michael Noffze
Fargo, ND
(701) 232-9565

Red River Valley Study Club
Marcus Tanabe
Grand Forks, ND
(701) 772-7379

NEVADA

Las Vegas Study Club
David Trylovich
Gary Goaslind
Ryan Gifford
Las Vegas, NV
(702) 877-0022

Sierra Society for Dental Excellence
Steve Robinson
Reno, NV
(775) 827-3302

Southern Nevada Premier Study Club
Ed De Andrade
Henderson, NV
(702) 270-4600

NEW JERSEY

3rd Millennium Dental Study Club
Ed Galkin
Michael Kleiman
Woodbridge, NJ
(732) 634-3300

Advanced Dental Seminars
Barry Elbaum
Freehold, NJ
(732) 431-3400

Apex Seminars
Harout Barsemian
Morristown, NJ
(973) 538-5660

Jersey Coast Dental Forum
Tony DiCesare
Buck DiCesare
Red Bank, NJ
(732) 747-2888

Journey for Excellence
Jeff Zissu
Cheryl Robins
Millburn, NJ
(973) 467-5567

The Mountain Lakes Study Club
Scott Cohen
Denville, NJ
(973) 627-6006

Pinnacle Dental Study Club
Ben Calem
Medford, NJ
(609) 953-3700

Princeton Group for Dental Excellence
Richard Staller
Princeton, NJ
(609) 921-6610

Seminars for Advancement of Dental Excellence
Michael Singer
Ed Rosenbaum
Bernard Barrish
Randolph, NJ
(973) 328-1555

Somerset Study Club
Marty Cornick
Peter Cornick
Somerville, NJ
(908) 526-0545

NEW MEXICO

High Desert Dental Colloquium
Brian Dennis
Albuquerque, NM
(505) 292-1051

NEW YORK

Capital District Continuum for Advanced Dental Education
Fred Marra
Cohoes, NY
(518) 237-0019

Empire State Academy of Continuing Dental Education
Gary Wadhwa
Clifton Park, NY
(518) 348-0634

Greater New York Study Club
Martin Prager
Jeffrey Shapiro
New York, NY
(212) 393-1113

Long Island Dental Forum
Alan Farber
Hauppauge, NY
(631) 265-4442

The Seattle Study Club of Manhattan
Harrison Chen
Andrew Kim
New York, NY
(212) 755-5570

SSC of Rochester
Suresh Goel
Pittsford, NY
(585) 385-4867

OHIO

Central Ohio Study Club
Fred Sakamoto
Mark Klabunde
Columbus, OH
(614) 575-0070

Cleveland Comprehensive Care Study Group
Paul Ricchetti
Mayfield Heights, OH
(440) 461-6008

Comprehensive Dental Excellence Forum
Constantin Farah
Canton, OH
(330) 494-7004

The Great Black Swamp Dental Study Club
Brian O'Neill
Toledo, OH
(419) 385-5743

K2 Peak Performance Study Group
Mark Silvers
Cincinnati, OH
(513) 271-1101

Seattle Study Club of Akron
Don Raabe
Akron, OH
(330) 836-9341

Sfumato
Jason Stoner
Dublin, OH
(614) 889-8222

Southwest Ohio Study Club
Larry Martin
Mason, OH
(513) 829-8999

Western Ohio Dental Study Club
Ed Rugh
Ryan Harris
Beaver Creek, OH
(937) 426-5411

OKLAHOMA

Red Earth Study Club
Vince Montgomery
Norman, OK
(405) 292-8900

Tulsa Study Club
E.J. Vaught
Brent Burchard
Tulsa, OK
(918) 748-8868

OREGON

Alpha Omega Study Club
Marv Johnson
McMinnville, OR
(503) 472-1468

Capitol Study Club for Excellence in Dentistry
Ronald Levine
Salem, OR
(541) 686-2443

Exploring Excellence Study Club
Tim Welch
Eugene, OR
(541) 465-3939

Mind Dental Studies
Rob Henshaw
Portland, OR
(503) 531-3550

Mt Bachelor Dental Seminars
Nick Misischia
Bend, OR
(541) 317-0255

Two Rivers Study Club
Erik Richmond
Brian Humble
Gresham, OR
(503) 667-1431

PENNSYLVANIA

Allegheny Restorative Study Club
Barry Stein
Stephen Engroff
State College, PA
(800) 446-5680

Dentists for Comprehensive Care
Veasey Cullen
York, PA
(717) 755-1200

Discovery Study Club
Mark Silberg
Robinson Twp, PA
(412) 787-8590

Extra Mile Study Club of Delaware County
Joe Havrilla
Springfield, PA
(610) 328-9608

Pittsburgh Dental Network
Mark Weingarden
Allison Park, PA
(412) 487-8288

Pittsburgh East Suburban Study Club
Jim Tauberg
Pittsburgh, PA
(412) 244-9044

Quakertown Dental Study Club
Sid Lyons
Quakertown, PA
(215) 538-9505

Susquehanna Valley Dental Study Club
Steven Sudbrink
Lititz, PA
(717) 733-8645

RHODE ISLAND

Providence Plantations Dental Study Club
Ed Katz
Greg Theberge
Johnston, RI
(401) 233-9800

SOUTH CAROLINA

Carolina Dental Forum
Ken Barrack
Mayur Patel
Mt Pleasant, SC
(843) 849-9044

Upstate Study Club
Rip Owings
Greenville, SC
(864) 232-7348

TENNESSEE

Middle Tennessee Society for Advanced Dentistry
Mark Hardison
Murfreesboro, TN
(615) 893-7736

Oral Design and Implant Study Club
Lee Ann Hovious
John Sterrett
Knoxville, TN
(865) 539-1113

Pinnacle Study Club of Nashville
Michael Skinner
Brentwood, TN
(615) 370-9486

Summit Institute
Gary Cohen
Hendersonville, TN
(615) 824-8929

TEXAS

Central Texas Study Club
Lyn Machen
Austin, TX
(512) 912-9750

Dallas Study Club
John Wallace
Steve Sherry
Dallas, TX
(214) 363-9946

The DDS Study Club
Donald Steinberg
Steven Alspach
Ed Tanur
Bedford, TX
(817) 267-1851

El Paso del Norte Study Club
Stephen Caldwell
John Purdy
El Paso, TX
(915) 598-6702

Excellence in Restorative Dental Education
Eric Rindler
San Antonio, TX
(210) 497-6677

IMPACT Austin
Mike Williamson
Austin, TX
(512) 346-2782

Knowledge Bank, SSC
Southeast Houston
Frank Frishkey
Houston, TX
(281) 484-9400

Lone Star Dental Seminars
Rob Naples
Round Rock, TX
(512) 388-4412

Nautilus Educational Group
James Gossett
New Braunfels, TX
(830) 625-6914

North Houston Seattle Study Club
Robert Stanton
Victor Manon
Humble, TX
(281) 358-2997

Odyssey Study Group
John Schmitz
Shavano Park, TX
(210) 444-9312

Permian Basin Dental Continuum
Marshall Morgan
Odessa, TX
(432) 367-0401

Seattle Study Club of South Texas
Gary Schwarz
McAllen, TX
(956) 687-7141

Seattle Study Club of The Woodlands
Colby Ferguson
The Woodlands, TX
(281) 298-3244

South Texas Advanced Restorative Seminars
Amir Hosseini
San Antonio, TX
(210) 614-4700

Southwest Academy of Comprehensive Dentistry
Kent Stobaugh
Paul Metz
Houston, TX
(713) 464-2833

Southwest Restorative Esthetic Forum
Barry Bartee
Lubbock, TX
(806) 792-0030

Texas Advanced Dental Seminars
Larry Pritchard
Waco, TX
(254) 751-1171

Thunderbird Study Club
Cinco Feuille
El Paso, TX
(915) 845-7979

University Dental Study Club of Houston
David Dennison
Houston, TX
(713) 523-9040

VIRGINIA

Big Lick Study Club
Barry Wolfe
Roanoke, VA
(540) 772-2913

Colleagues in Comprehensive Care Seminar
Bruce Barr
Virginia Beach, VA
(757) 422-0005

Commonwealth Study Club
Bob McGrail
Fredericksburg, VA
(540) 373-3066

Greater Loudoun Study Club
Steve Dorsch
Andy Bluhm
Jay Vandervort
Leesburg, VA
(703) 771-1771

NOVA Institute for Advanced Dental Education
Brian Feeney
Pete Passero
McLean, VA
(703) 821-4040

Southwest Virginia Advanced Seminars
Rick Boyle
Blacksburg, VA
(540) 951-8777

WASHINGTON

Great Blue Heron Seminars
Michael Cohen
Bob Gottlieb
Coury Staadecker
Kenmore, WA
(425) 489-2002

Great Blue Heron Seminars, East
Bob Gottlieb
Michael Cohen
Richland, WA
(509) 946-9313

Greater Pierce County Seminars
Minou Karbakhsch
Silvia La Rosa
Tacoma, WA
(253) 752-6336

Insight Study Club
Jack Neal
Craig Neal
Galia Leonard
Seattle, WA
(206) 363-3010

Meridian Dental Study Group
Lauralee Nygaard
Spokane, WA
(509) 927-3272

Mt Baker Study Club
Kathleen Stambaugh
Roger Stambaugh
Burlington, WA
(360) 757-7667

Olympic Peninsula Study Club
Stig Osterberg
Port Townsend, WA
(360) 385-5121

Rainy Day Dental Study Club
Peter Agnos
Everett, WA
(425) 252-1136

Renaissance Study Club
Lloyd Tucker
Seattle, WA
(206) 937-8253

SouthShore Study Club
Allen Chen
Dick Quinn
Renton, WA
(425) 271-5812

Spokane Study Club
David Engen
Spokane, WA
(509) 326-4445

St Helen's Shadow Study Club
Greg Boice
Vancouver, WA
(360) 260-3290

WISCONSIN

Central Wisconsin Dental Forum
John Stilp
Wausau, WI
(715) 845-4511

Greater Green Bay Study Club
Doug Pierre
Marty Williams
Green Bay, WI
(920) 499-2991

Milwaukee Study Club
Constantine Stamatelakys
Brookfield, WI
(414) 282-2642

Seattle Study Club of Madison
Scott Hoyer
Madison, WI
(608) 274-0770

Third Coast Study Group
Phil Hawkins
Tim Hart
Milwaukee, WI
(414) 257-1161

West Central Wisconsin Study Club
Slavko Ivankovic
Eau Claire, WI
(715) 834-8414

Winnebagoland Dental Study Club
Chris McFarlane
Oshkosh, WI
(920) 231-4600

INDEX

Page numbers followed by "f" denote figures; those followed by "t" denote tables

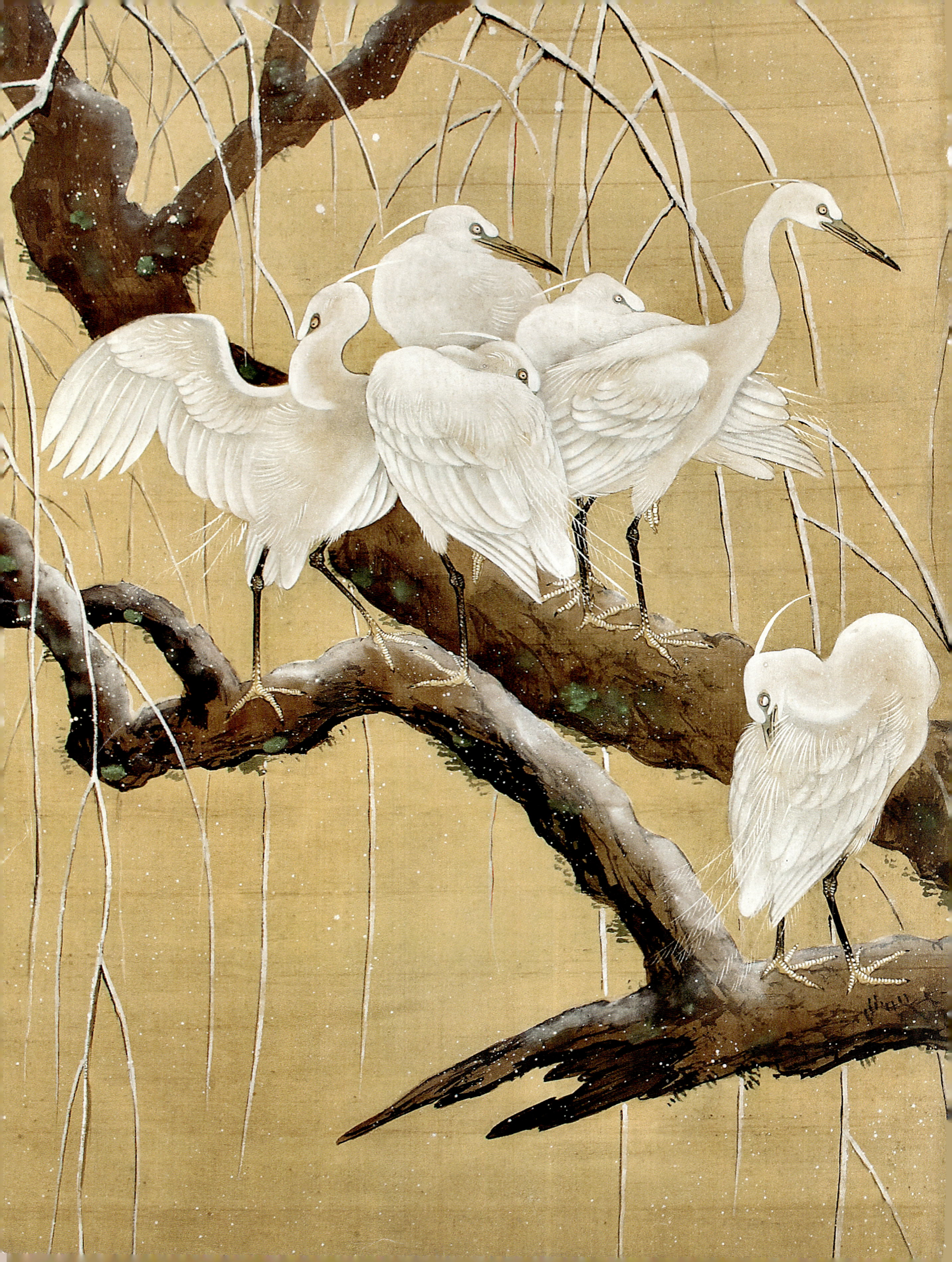